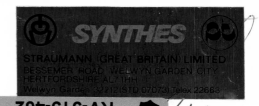

Materials and Orthopaedic Surgery

Materials and Orthopaedic Surgery

By DANA C. MEARS,
B.M., B.Ch., Ph.D., M.R.C.P., F.R.C.S.(C)

Associate Professor of Orthopaedic Surgery and
Director of Orthopaedic Research, University of Pittsburgh.

Staff, Presbyterian-University Hospital,
Children's Hospital, Pittsburgh, Pennsylvania.

Consultant, Veteran's Administration Hospital, Pittsburgh, Pennsylvania.

Fellow, American Academy of Orthopaedic Surgeons.

Member, British Standards Committee for Surgical Implants.

American Society for Metals.

Fellow, Nuffield Orthopaedic Research, North American Orthopaedic Travelling,
Orthopaedic Audio-Synopsis Travelling.

With 900 Illustrations

THE WILLIAMS & WILKINS COMPANY
Baltimore

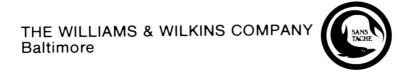

Library of Congress Cataloging in Publication Data

Mears, Dana C
    Materials in orthopaedic surgery.

    Bibliography: p.
    Includes index.
    1. Orthopedic implants.   2. Orthopedic surgery.
I.   Title. [DNLM: 1. Orthopedics. 2. Prosthesis. WEl68 M483m]
RD755.5.M4   617′.3′028   78-690
ISBN 0-683-05901-7

Composed and printed at the
Waverly Press, Inc.
Mt. Royal and Guilford Aves.
Baltimore, Md 21202, U.S.A.

Foreword

When *Metals and Engineering in Bone and Joint Surgery* was originally published in 1959, it sold to a small group who had become interested in the possibilities for improvement in internal fixation and prosthetic replacement devices. It was described then as being ahead of its time because widespread interest had not yet occurred. Instrument companies bought the book for their personnel, but the fact that treatment failures could be ascribed to materials and the design of those materials was certainly not generally apparent. In addition, the widespread use of prosthetic replacement devices had not as yet occurred. It took the dawning of a new era perhaps symbolized by the widespread use of prosthetic replacement, particularly the total hip replacement and the novel engineering redesign exemplified by the AO group with its laboratory in Davos, Switzerland, to awaken an interest which had to lead to the event symbolized by the publication of *Materials and Orthopaedic Surgery* whose father, or perhaps grandparent, was authored by Patrick Laing, Charles Bechtol and myself.

The growth of the audience created a demand for information in this field which would be readily and completely available. Now there had to be an author who demonstrated a command of the engineering, materials composition and properties and who, in addition, was an outstanding orthopaedic surgeon. Just as the growth of the times created the audience it also created the man.

It began years ago when a summer student worked in the Orthopaedic Laboratory at the University of Pittsburgh. This boy's father had made many important contributions in the field of metallurgy—one which intrigued me the most was the explanation of the development of "whiskers" on metal surfaces.

The young student found his way through college at Cornell and then was off to his Ph.D. work in engineering at Cambridge University. This research was productive and academically alarming since it was evident that a most unusual individual was developing. Research contributions confirmed this. Medical school at Oxford followed with prizes for outstanding work readily achieved. It was apparent that an intellect that could retain and use information to a degree that was remarkable was growing by leaps and bounds.

He was tenderly nurtured through his surgical and orthopaedic training at Pittsburgh while he maintained his laboratory interest. For a year he returned to the Oxford Infirmary for further training in trauma and since has been on the staff at the University of Pittsburgh. Here he has a busy orthopaedic practice and in addition works in and directs what may well be the best equipped and active biomaterials-engineering laboratory now existing.

It's hard to explain how deep and sophisticated research can be combined with a heavy involvement in the clinical practice of orthopaedic surgery without coming to the conclusion that a most unusual talent, intellect and drive has been combined in one individual. Those who have met him as he has traveled around the world on speaking and traveling fellowships are aware of the nature of the author of this new book which grew out of the old and is now entitled *Materials and Orthopaedic Surgery*.

The unique combination of surgeon and Ph.D. scientist in one individual makes this book possible. The audience now interested in this field has grown in depth and numbers and will appreciate the opportunity to aid their patients through the availability of the information brought concisely into this volume.

ALBERT B. FERGUSON, JR., M.D.

Preface

In 1959 a new volume entitled *Metals and Engineering in Bone and Joint Surgery,* by Bechtol, Ferguson and Laing, appeared on the orthopaedic bookshelf. At that time there was no single work which could illuminate the bioengineer and the orthopaedic surgeon on the complex biological and engineering principles that are the foundation for modern orthopaedic implantation. That volume stimulated great interest among orthopaedists and bioengineers alike and was partially responsible for developments beyond the wildest dreams of the previous authors. In particular, the design and implantation of devices, which are meant to perform for the duration of a patient's lifetime, have proliferated into both a major science and a vast industry. Total joint replacement of the hip and knee lead the field although work is progressing on arthroplasties of many other diarthrosial joints, implants for replacement of bone, tendon and ligaments, devices for internal and external fixation of fractures and for stabilization of the spine.

With the great increase in knowledge and in the clinical implantation of orthopaedic implants, it seemed timely that Bechtol, Ferguson and Laing's volume should be revised. The title has been changed to indicate the significance of a variety of nonmetallic materials in orthopaedic practice, notably: high density polyethylene, methylmethacrylate cement and silicon elastomers, and to reflect the new methods for their clinical application.

The volume is enlarged to provide new knowledge on the behavior of foreign materials in the human body and its response to surgical implants. The subject matter is organized into three categories. Chapters 2 and 3 describe the physical and mechanical behavior of the materials that are being used or considered for orthopaedic implants. Chapters 4 to 7 present the biological responses of human tissues to the presence of orthopaedic implants. Chapters 8 to 15 relate the clinical applications of orthopaedic implants and the problems associated with their use. Every attempt has been made to use terminology that will be understood by the diverse audience who might read the present volume.

Lastly, I should like to express my gratitude to my teachers who have prepared me to write this book: Professor Sir Allan Cottrell and the late Dr. T. P. Hoar in metallurgy; Dame Honour Fell, Professor Leonard Weiss and Dr. Stephan Perren in pathophysiology of bone; and Professors Robert Duthie, Albert Ferguson, Jr., Martin Allgöwer and Hans Willenegger in orthopaedic surgery.

DANA C. MEARS

Contributors

Daniel H. Brooks, M.D., *Head, Division of General Surgery, Allegheny General Hospital, Pittsburgh, Pennsylvania.*

M. A. R. Freeman, M.D., F.R.C.S., *Consultant Orthopaedic Surgeon, London Hospital, London, England, Director, Biomechanics Unit, Imperial College, London, England.*

Robert Hamas, M.D., *Resident in Plastic Surgery, University of Pittsburgh, Pittsburgh, Pennsylvania.*

Joseph E. Imbriglia, M.D., *Assistant Professor of Orthopaedic Surgery, University of Pittsburgh, Pittsburgh, Pennsylvania.*

G. P. Rothwell, M.A., Ph.D., C.Chem., M.R.I.C., M.I.M., F.I.Corr. T., *Head, National Corrosion Service, National Physical Laboratory, Teddington, Middlesex, England.*

Michael F. Schafer, M.D., *Assistant Professor of Orthopaedic Surgery, Northwestern University, Chicago, Illinois.*

Alfred B. Swanson, M.D., F.A.C.S., *Chief, Orthopaedic Surgery and Orthopaedic Research, Blodgett Memorial Hospital, Grand Rapids, Clinical Professor of Surgery, Michigan State University, Lansing, Michigan.*

Acknowledgments

While writing this book, I have received considerable assistance from many of my friends whose contributions I am happy to mention. For many years, Albert Ferguson has provided vigorous encouragement and a highly productive environment in the Department of Orthopaedic Surgery at Pittsburgh. With his critical eye and pen Peter Rothwell revised the chapters on the physical and chemical properties of implantable materials. Michael Schafer kindly offered to prepare the chapter on spinal instrumentation. Michael Freeman, Alfred Swanson and Joseph Imbriglia provided detailed surgical descriptions of their clinical experience with total knee, wrist and finger joint replacements respectively. Robert Hamas organized his recent studies on the biomechanics of the wrist. Daniel Brooks described his observations on the general surgical complications of total hip joint replacement.

In addition, I have received technical support from several others. My wife, Yvonne, typed much of the original draft and cheerfully tolerated my long hours at work. Nan Wholey prepared many excellent drawings of the surgical procedures. Annette Alberth provided a few thousand photographs with her characteristic high standard of work. Drew Steis undertook editorial assistance with his usual aplomb. Carol Crawford, Sally Greenwood, and Colleen Dunwoody spent many long evenings and weekends of assistance with typing and proofreading. In addition to her hectic schedule of handling harassing telephone calls, bills and records, my secretary, Jan Westwood, gave freely of her time to type and review the manuscript and to encourage the boss. In addition to his patient and skillful proofreading Robert Bruce Mears provided sagacious paternal support throughout my prolonged period of training and during the preparation of this manuscript.

The publishers have made every effort to trace the copyright holders for borrowed material. If they have inadvertently overlooked any, they will be pleased to make the necessary arrangements at the first opportunity.

DANA C. MEARS

Contents

7. The Biological Response to Implanted Materials *196*

8. The Design, Use and Care of Implants   *258*

9. Fractures and Methods of Internal Fixation   *279*

10. Clinical Methods of Fracture Treatment

11. Percutaneous Pin Fixation

12. Instrumentation in Spinal Surgery

13. Reconstruction of Articular Joints

14. Clinical Methods of Total Joint Replacements

15. Supplementary Implants in Musculoskeletal Surgery 690

16. Future Developments 720

Index 737

Manufacturers' Index of Currently Available Surgical Implants and Tools 757

1

Introduction

While the use of metals can be traced for thousands of years, their widespread application as surgical implants is limited to the past century. Prior to the development of aseptic surgery with anesthesia and the availability of X-ray control most of the sporadic attempts to employ implants were painful, ineffective and exceptionally hazardous in view of the likelihood of wound infection. The present chapter records the principal milestones in materials science and the advancement of orthopaedic implants. During the period from 1860 to 1900, while metallurgy was transforming rapidly from an empirical art into a highly complex technology that would revolutionize most aspects of Western life, orthopaedic surgery was in its infancy. After 1940, when the Age of Plastics began to compete with steel, the use of orthopaedic implants first began to receive the close scrutiny which has evolved into an exacting technology that now rests firmly on the biomechanics and pathophysiology of musculoskeletal organs, the structural attributes of inert materials and sound clinical acumen.

One of the great stages in man's development was the discovery that he could change the nature of materials such as the thermal conversion of clay to stone.[1] The nearly unlimited formability of clay is replaced by high stabi..ty in stone because of changes in the complex relationship between the microcrystals of the clay and water and the chemical change and complete recrystallization that occurs on firing above a red heat. The use of ceramics exemplified the diversity of structure and related physical properties in several ways. Shaping involved moisture dependent plasticity and thixotropy. Decorative textures were derived from vitrification and devitrification, a nucleation of various gases in crystalline phases and local variations of the expansivity, viscosity and surface tension. Colors depended upon various states of oxidation, abnormal ionic states and structural imperfections in crystals. All these phenomena were discovered for aesthetic pleasure rather than utility. The earliest use of metal followed closely after the widespread use of fire-hardened clay. Metals owe their main utility to their rigidity below a certain stress but plasticity above other stress which can be surpassed locally by the concentrated action of a tool. Above another tempera-ture they become liquid to facilitate alteration of shape by casting.

Several thousand years ago man discovered and collected native metals such as copper, gold, silver and meteoric iron. Initially, the specimens were used in their natural shape although gradually man learned to fashion them for his own needs. Brightly colored ornamental stones were accidentally heated and observed to yield molten metal. From *circa* 3000 B.C., copper was smelted with lead, silver and antimony to form bronze. The Age of Bronze spread from Egypt to Mesopotamia and persisted until 1000 B.C. The metal was wrought and cast in various alloys to provide functional and ornamental objects. Subsequently, the Age of Iron evolved wherein different techniques for smelting were necessary. Where smelted iron yielded slag and droplets of iron a reheating process was necessary after which the material was hammered into a compact mass of wrought iron.

In the 16th Century, practical metallurgists such as Georgius Agricola began to record their empirical knowledge (Fig. 1-1) and to instruct others.[2] This transition reflects the technology of printing and also a change of direction for technologists who became interested in the documentation of applications of metals in mining, ore dressing and smelting. Slow progress occurred in the working and joining of metals and in their fabrication. Between 1600 and 1750, the main advances represented practical adaptation of the older processes on a larger scale. From 1750 to 1830, the use of iron increased substantially in the sophistication of its applications. As shown in the next subsection, however, it was the period from about 1860 to 1880 when man's basic material changed with extraordinary rapidity from wood to iron and subsequently to steel, to create the modern industrial civilization.

Once steel could be reproducibly heat treated it represented a notable improvement in technology. Prior to the 19th Century pure iron was unmeltable in any available furnace. If iron is heated in a fire long enough to absorb carbon from the charcoal fuel, it changes its properties greatly, becoming first steel and then cast iron. The latter is relatively brittle but it is not much more difficult to melt than copper. Shaping was undertaken by skillful use of the hammer but

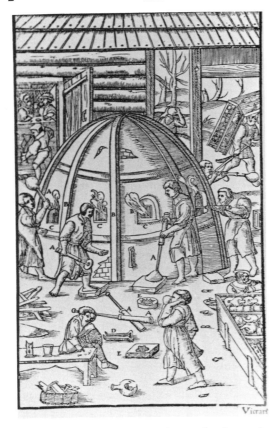

Figure 1-1. A beehive-shaped furnace for glass making and a man blowing glass with blow pipes is seen in this print from the work of Georgius Agricola, *De Re Metallica* (1556).

such wrought iron always contained residual inclusions of the slag and rocky matter that greatly weakened it. The subsequent stages in the development of steel have been well documented by Smith.[1, 2] This striking transformation was an indication of man's technical ingenuity in fashioning the raw materials of nature for human application.

Materials in Orthopaedic Surgery

Prior to 1860 when Lister introduced the aseptic surgical techniques, any surgical procedure was exceptionally hazardous in view of the likelihood of postoperative wound infection, particularly if the procedure involved the insertion of a foreign material into the wound. There were many isolated attempts by bold surgeons who employed various metallic devices to assist in the repair of broken bones (Fig. 1-2). Most of the devices consisted of wires or pins made of iron, silver, gold or platinum. A few signs of rational progress, however, were made. In 1804, Bell[3] observed galvanic corrosion of steel-tipped silver pins used to close wounds. Levert[4] made the first study of the suitability of implant materials in experimental animals. In 1829 he implanted gold, silver, lead and platinum specimens in dogs. Of the buried wire sutures, platinum was the least irritating. In 1849, Malgaigne[5] postulated that metallic implants were a source of hospital gangrene. In an effort to immobilize unstable fracture fragments he devised a series of adjustable metal hooks that pierced the skin to provide stability. Once early osseous repair had occurred the hooks were withdrawn. The introduction of two volatile anesthetic agents, ether and chloroform, by Morton and Simpson respectively, between the years 1846 and 1850 was crucial to the evolution of modern surgery.[6]

MATERIALS AND IMPLANT SURGERY AFTER 1860

Materials

During the 17th Century numerous great advances were made in physics and chemistry. These studies had no immediate effect on the metallurgical industries which had reached a stage of empirical development far beyond the theoretical understanding of the day.[1, 2] During the 1800's, however, the situation changed rapidly. Great advances in the methods of chemical analysis, largely by Swedish chemists, led to the discovery of many new metals and provided assays for revealing minor amounts of impurities.[7] Previously impurities had not been recognized as the responsible agent for vastly different qualities of iron from individual ores and for the differing results from various methods of processing. After 1800 the nature of various alloys could be determined with increasing sophistication. For example, carbon was identified as the substance in iron responsible for its transformation into hardenable steel and then into fusible cast iron. In 1786, several independent workers including Morveau, Vandermonde Berthollet and Mange confirmed the modern concept that steel is an alloy of iron containing carbon. Aristotle's concept that steel was a more refined form of iron had been proved. Over the following century the modern theory of the nature of steel alloys eventually evolved.

In 1863, Henry Sorby in Sheffield, England, undertook the first microscopic study of metals

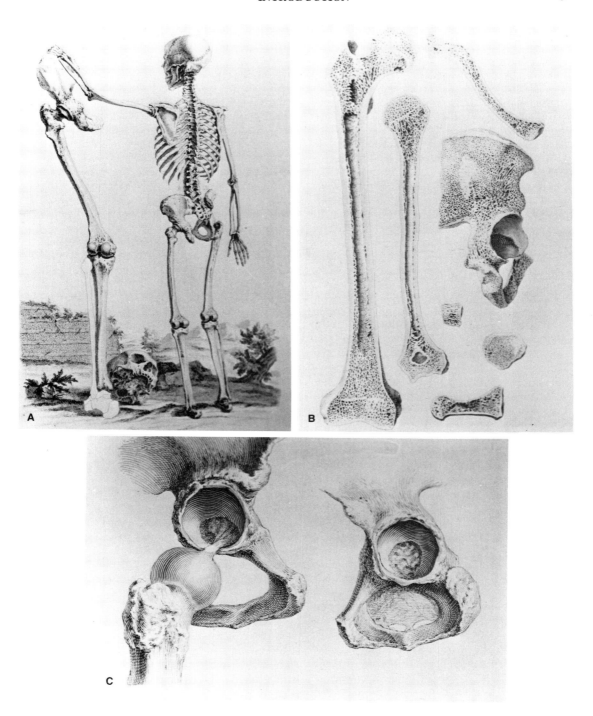

Figure 1-2. Prior to the time of Lister most of the critical investigations relevant to surgery comprised anatomical dissections of the musculoskeletal system. The first great illustrated work by Andreas Vesalius, *De Humani Corporis Fabrica* (1543), was followed by other contributions. In addition to their elegant anatomical detail to show the entire skeleton (*A*), sections of bones (*B*) or joints (*C*), the volumes represent exceptional artistic achievements with their format, typography and illustrations.

and identified different chemical phases in iron.[7] Sorby showed how the minute crystals in iron were packed together, how they could be deformed by working and how they could recrystallize on heating. Steel was observed to undergo a complete change in structure when it was hardened. In 1887, Floris Osmond in France combined microscopic observations and thermal analyses to show the temperatures at which structural changes occurred in iron and steel. In 1889 the American, Willard Gibbs, applied the concept of "phase rule" and formulated diagrams to depict the dependence of microstructural constitution on temperature and composition. By the early 20th Century metallurgists had systematically collected data on the constitution of alloys, related microstructural details to service failures and learned to use structure as the key to the control of reproducible quality in production operations.

Meanwhile mineralogists had been studying the symmetries of the external shapes of crystals and developing the mathematics of the crystal lattice without recognition of the nature of these units. The previous observations of Johannes Kepler and Robert Hooke on the stacking of spheres in contact to give rise to crystalline polyhedrons was forgotten. The basic conceptual unit of matter had become prismatic boxes in which molecules were situated. Molecular composition rather than crystal structure was the basis of almost all 19th Century physical and chemical discussions of solids. In 1912, X-ray defraction was discovered and soon applied to the structural solids by Lawrence Bragg and his followers. Immediately it provided immeasurable physical meaning to structure on an atomic scale and it rapidly superseded the larger-scale structures that had been revealed by Sorby's microscopic methods. At first X-ray defraction patterns were interpreted in an excessively idealized picture of highly regular, indeed, perfect crystal lattices. Subsequently the role of imperfections in crystals was discovered to explain the deformability of metals as well as the nature of the interface between crystal grains. Foremost in the new understanding of materials was the realization that the properties of all types of materials arise from their structure, from the manner in which their constituent atoms aggregate into hierarchies of molecular crystalline order or into disordered amorphous structures. Moreover the properties of all matter depend largely upon the structure of imperfections, either purely architectural or chemical, in their main array. Most of the properties observed and exploited in materials are cooperative properties of the aggregate rather than of the constituent atoms and simple molecules that were previously overemphasized.

Mechanical properties have been the main criteria for the selection of materials from ancient times to the present. Previously the principal aim of a scientific metallurgist was to comprehend the structural basis of strength and ductility. The development of heat-treatable alloy steels that provide high strength in large cross section coincided with their need in the first automobile. It excited an initial wave of metallurgical research that has persisted to the present time.

The unraveling of the microstructures of metals was paralleled by the development by the mathematical theory of elasticity and strength in materials. Laboratory tests for mechanical strength, ductility, hardness and fatigue resistance provided a quantitative assessment on the effectiveness of the compositional and structural changes created by metallurgists. Also it gave a numerical basis for engineering design. During the 1800's a variety of steel alloys was developed for particular applications and in the 1820's Berthier introduced the chrome steels. In the 1850's, the tungsten-tool steels emerged in Austria and England. The highly corrosion resistant alloys of steel and other ferrous materials, however, would not appear until the 1920's.

Corrosion Resistance

Without chemical stability in the environment no other property of a material can be utilized. Until fairly recent times man had no useful way to alter the inherent corrosion resistance of a particular metal or alloy in a particular environment. Certain noble metals such as gold were observed to be more inert than others, such as iron. In 1779, Luigi Galvani of Bologna documented the first useful electrochemical experiment.[8] While investigating the susceptibility of nerve to irritation he showed that nervous action could be induced by electrical phenomena. Galvani studied a frog nerve-muscle preparation in which a series of dissimilar alloys was employed (Fig. 1-3). In the upper drawing a brass rod contacts the frog's foot while a silver rod touches the spinal cord. When the free ends of the rods are brought together contraction of the leg muscles ensues. In the lower drawing the spinal cord and legs rest respectively on brass and copper foil. When the rod touches the pieces of foil

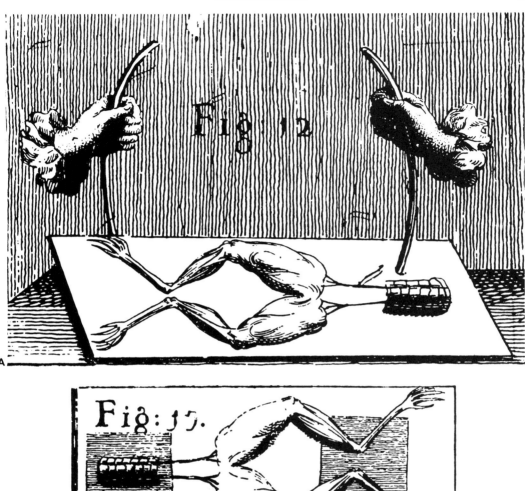

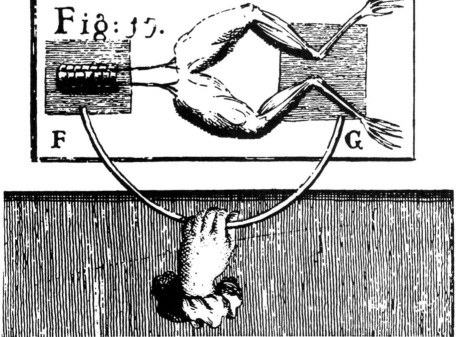

Figure 1-3. *A* and *B*. Galvani's experiments on animal electricity (Galvani, *De viribus electricitatis,* Modena, 1792). (Reproduced with permission of C. Singer and E. A. Underwood.[8])

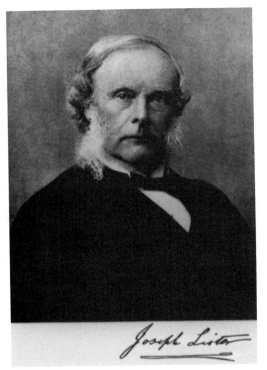

Figure 1-4. Joseph Lister originated aseptic surgery and successfully used silver wire sutures for internal fixation of fractures. (Reproduced with permission of *Surgery, Gynecology and Obstetrics, 1912.*)

simultaneously the leg contracts. At that time many observers attributed these events to a novel type of "animal electricity" they called "galvanism." In 1800, Alexandra Volta of Pavia showed that galvanism is devoid of inherent animal relationship and that muscle is induced to contract by electrical stimulation.[8] The practical application of the galvanic effect was elucidated by Sir Humphrey Davey[9] of London. He was invited by the Royal Navy to undertake an investigation of the nature of corrosion observed on the copper sheathing used to encase the wooden hulls of vessels to prevent encrustation with barnacles. Certain copper sheets immersed in sea water were observed to undergo rapid corrosion. It was widely believed that impurities in the copper provoked the rapid dissolution. Davey was able to show that copper deliberately contaminated with a small amount of zinc was rendered immune from corrosion. Instead the zinc underwent rapid anodic dissolution.

In the 1860's Michael Faraday at Cambridge undertook a series of experimental observations on the corrosion of iron from which would evolve the concept of corrosion as an electrochemical phenomenon.[10] The concept was rigorously confirmed in the 1930's by U. R. Evans and his school,[11, 12] also in Cambridge.

Implants in Orthopaedic Surgery

Between 1860 and 1870 Joseph Lister (Fig. 1-4) introduced the aseptic surgical techniques and thereby initiated enormous strides in all aspects of surgery especially in orthopaedics.[13] The techniques of internal fixation of fractures emerged in various parts of the world. One of the first workers to report the use of plates for internal fixation was Hansmann[14] in 1886. He applied metallic strips, preferably of unhardened nickel-plated sheet steel, with numerous screw holes. Nickel-plated screws were used to secure the plate to the bone. One end of the plate showed a 90 degree bend which permitted it to protrude through the skin for easy removal 4 to 8 weeks after implantation. Widespread application of onlay plates and screws for the treatment of fresh uncomplicated fractures was rare until after 1900. At that time the clinical application of X-rays revealed to surgeons the poor reductions of fractures that previously had been considered to be acceptable.

As early as 1862, Gurlt[15] published a book in which a number of patients with fresh broken bones underwent open reduction of intra-articular fractures as well as nailing, screwing and wiring. This documentation was exceptional because at that time open reduction of fractures was indicated only in cases where prolonged conservative treatment had failed. Exceptions were made only for fractures that occurred in subcutaneous bones such as the patella and the olecranon process. For example, wiring of a fractured patella was one of the earliest forms of internal fixation. Toward the end of the 19th Century with the development of aseptic surgical technique, operative fracture treatment emerged from a position as a supplementary form of treatment to a primary role for certain fractures. Among the pioneers of the technique were the German surgeon, Fritz Koenig, Elie and Albin Lambotte of Belgium, Lane of England and Cudder of the United States.

Perhaps the first workers to appreciate the full significance of internal fixation were Fritz Koenig[16] of Altona-on-the-Elbe and the two Lambotte brothers.[17] Koenig attempted to define the indications for the conservative and the operative methods of management and to use internal fixation for the realization of early postoperative mobilization without the need for plaster cast fixation. Koenig, however, was well

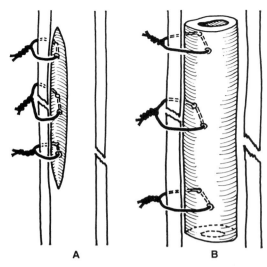

Figure 1-5. Stabilization of bone sutures with ivory pegs (*A*) or bone inserts (*B*) after Fritz Koenig. (Reproduced with permission of M. E. Müller, M. Allgöwer, H. Willenegger.[18])

aware of the inadequacy of materials then available for internal fixation. This ingenious worker recommended the use of hemi-cerclage wiring to preserve the nutrition of bone. He attempted to improve stabilization by the use of ivory pegs and bone inserts (Fig. 1-5). In Belgium, Elie Lambotte systematically treated oblique fractures of the lower leg by open reduction and fixation with wire sutures or screws. His method was described in the *Presse Medicale Belge* of 1890. Despite the good results of his method Lambotte met with overwhelming criticism, became discouraged and withdrew from the controversy. His brother, Albin, pursued the study of internal fixation at the Stuivenberg Hospital where he advocated the use of internal fixation with a plate and external clamps (Fig. 1-6*A* and *B*). For periarticular fractures he created curved and Y-shaped plates with an improved application of screw fixation (Fig. 1-6*C*). In 1907, his first monograph entitled *Open Reduction of Recent and Old Fractures,* was published. In 1913, a second revision entitled *The Operative Treatment of Fractures,* elucidated the functional principles of internal fixation. Early mobilization of joints in the absence of weight bearing was the principal goal. He was especially concerned about the rigid fixation of interarticular fractures (Fig. 1-7). He developed a thin nail for use in small interarticular fragments such as internal fixation of the scaphoid and the radial styloid (Fig. 1-8).

Lambotte also assessed the use of a variety of alloys in the body. In 1909, he reported the use of brass plates as well as aluminum, silver and copper.[19] All of these materials were discarded for their excessive malleability. When he combined magnesium plates with steel screws he observed rapid dissolution of the plate which vanished prior to repair of the fracture. He recommended the use of a soft steel plated with gold or nickel. Numerous applications of the plate have been well illustrated by Müller, Allgöwer and Willenegger.[17]

A closer scrutiny of the cellular reaction to metallic implants buried in tissues for prolonged periods was reported by von Baeyer[20] in 1908. After copper and zinc were implanted close together he observed axial alignment of the adjacent reparative connective tissue cells along the anticipated pathway of the corrosion current. The current also appeared to provoke rhythmic muscular contractions. Von Baeyer confirmed the selective dissolution of zinc in the bimetallic couple. He first raised the possible application of bimetallic couples to provide selective immunity from corrosion of the principal implant alloy. In 1913, Hey-Groves[21] reported on tissue tolerance for a variety of implant alloys applied

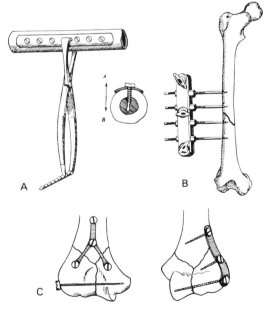

Figure 1-6. *A.* Forceps and bone plates after Lambotte. *B.* External fixation clamps with transfixing pins after Lambotte. *C.* Internal fixation of the distal humerus after Lambotte. (*A, B,* and *C* Reproduced with permission of M. E. Müller, M. Allgöwer, and H. Willenegger.[18])

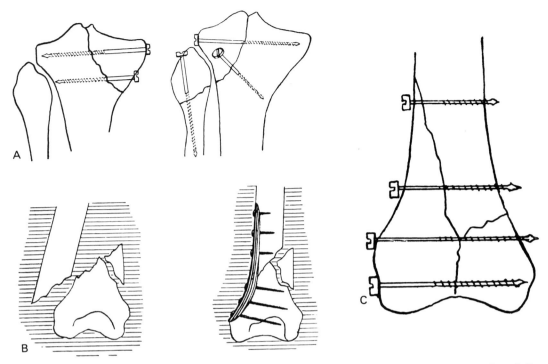

Figure 1-7. Internal fixation of intra-articular fractures of the proximal tibia (A) and the femur (B and C), after Lambotte. (Reproduced with permission of M. E. Müller, M. Allgöwer, and H. Willenegger.[18])

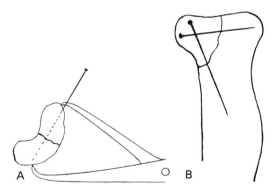

Figure 1-8. Method of immobilizing a scaphoid fracture (A), and a fracture of the radial styloid (B), after Lambotte. (Reproduced with permission of M. E. Müller, M. Allgöwer, and H. Willenegger.[18])

in the form of plates, screws and intramedullary pegs. He confirmed the rapid dissolution of magnesium, the relative inertness of nickel-plated steel, and the relative tolerance of tissues to the presence of fairly inert and aseptic alloys. In these and other experiments Hey-Groves observed the influence of motion between the implant and the adjacent bone. He deduced that continuous movement, even of small amplitude,

between a plate and the bone initiates a mechanical irritation with resorption of bone, inflammation with drainage and sinus formation and finally sepsis. The clinical significance of this striking observation would remain obscure until the studies undertaken by Willenegger and others in the 1970's.

In the early 1900's Lane[22] of England, considered methods for the introduction of implants into the body without bacterial contamination. He developed a "no-touch" technique by which his plates (Fig. 1-9A) were implanted with minimal direct handling. With the low rate of postoperative wound infections in his patients, he was able to distinguish the failures provoked by rapid corrosion of metallic implants. Subsequently, Sherman,[23] of Pittsburgh, applied the Lane plate in 55 midshaft femoral fractures of which three plates underwent mechanical failure. As shown in Figure 1-9A, the fractures in the Lane plate all occurred at the junction of the central metal bar and the first screw hole. Sherman studied the optimal mechanical properties and the ideal design of the bone plate. He reasoned that the previously employed high-strength, brittle, high carbon tool steels possessed great elastic limits but poor ductility.

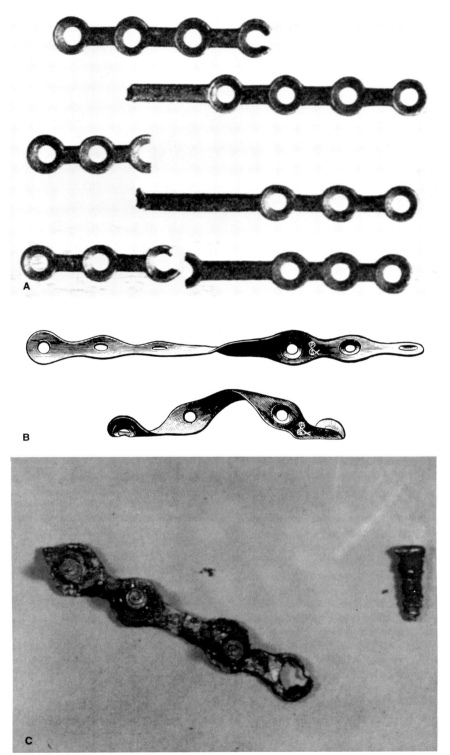

Figure 1-9. *A.* Three examples of a Lane plate used by Sherman which underwent fracture at the junction of the first screw hole and the center bar. *B.* A Sherman plate, which can be deformed without breakage, was made of a vanadium steel. *C.* A vanadium steel plate and screw implanted for 30 years is shown after removal when it has lost its mechanical integrity and consists primarily of rust. (*A,* Reproduced with permission of *Surgery, Gynecology and Obstetrics,* 1912; *B* and *C,* reproduced with permission of C. O. Bechtol, A. B. Ferguson, Jr., and P. G. Laing.[24])

Sherman assumed that the ideal steel for a bone plate should possess a sufficient elastic limit and great ductility so that, under load, it would deform progressively rather than undergo abrupt fracture. Sherman introduced the use of high carbon steel alloyed with vanadium to increase toughness. He also altered the design of bone plates by reduction in the number of screw holes with diminution in the amount of necking of the plate between the screw hole (Fig. 1-9B). When he removed a series of vanadium alloy plates 6 weeks after implantation he noted that the surrounding tissues were stained with iron. He denied that the corrosion of the plate influenced its performance. Other surgeons, however, noted the staining of adjacent tissues with loosening of the plates and related clinical failures. One corroded vanadium steel implant is shown in Figure 1-9C.

In summary, during the first half century after Lister's advancement of aseptic surgery a few surgeons were stimulated to initiate studies on, and the clinical applications of, devices for internal fixation. They showed the potential for the satisfactory application of implants to facilitate the union of fractures. Many of the general principles that govern the modern applications of internal fixation were noted by a few astute but isolated, traumatic surgeons whose observations were generally discredited or ignored. The surgical alloys then available possessed inadequate inertness and unsuitable mechanical properties. While Sherman and others had shown the need for sound metallurgical and engineering consideration for the improvement of techniques in internal fixation, such a rational approach would not be witnessed again for another 20 years.

MATERIALS AND ORTHOPAEDIC SURGERY 1920-1950

Materials

After 1920 an extraordinary burst of scientific energy was invested in a scrutiny of numerous ferrous alloys and in the chemical constitution of matter, including metals. One example is the development of dislocation theory in metals. Dislocations were first introduced into physical theory as part of a study of a so-called mechanical "aether". In 1892, Burton[25] postulated that any given portion of matter consists of modifications in the regular structure of the material, which were called "aether." When the matter is altered in shape it is merely the modifications of

structure which are transferred from one region to another.

The theory of dislocations in an elastic continuum was developed by the Italian school and by Timpe from 1900 to 1920 but it did not influence the then current ideas of crystal plasticity. In 1928, Prandtl[26] explained the mechanical hysteresis observed during the deformation of material in terms of the translational periodicity of the crystal lattice. He visualized sheets of atoms jumping irreversibly from one position of equilibrium to another. His model, however, did not contain the idea essential to the development of the modern theory of crystal dislocations, namely of a boundary between a region which has jumped and a region which has not. The foundations of the modern dislocation theory were laid by Orowan,[27] Polanyi[28] and Taylor[29] in 1934. The first major survey of the practical application of dislocation theory to crystal physics was made by Seitz and Read[30] and was soon followed by those of Mott[31] and Cottrell.[32] The relationships between the theory of plastic deformation and the geometrical and elastic properties of dislocation in crystal lattices were summarized by Cottrell in about 1950.[33] By this time an elaborate theory of the microstructure of metals and the predictable changes in microstructure with mechanical deformation or alloying had evolved. After 1950 elegant microstructural analysis with electron microscopy, electron probe microanalysis, field ion and field emission microscopy would confirm these findings down to the atomic level.[34]

In the early 1900's plastics were introduced with the preparation of cellulose acetate by alteration of cellulose from wood. This, the first plastic, was widely employed for the manufacture of films and lacquers.[35] The next available plastics evolved from the ready availability of formaldehyde which was combined with phenol or urea-form compounds. For example, Leo Baekeland developed his Bakelite, the first marked success in the history of plastics. Even in 1929 celluloid remained the dominant plastic. After 1930, however, the Age of Plastics began whereby materials were produced synthetically from organic compounds especially from the gases, acetylene and ethylene. Under selected and controlled conditions of temperature, pressure and special catalysts, up to several hundred thousand of the small units were linked together by chemical bonds. During and after World War II nylons, in which amino residues served to link long chains of carbon atoms, were developed. In 1954 two new methods to manufacture polymers were introduced. One, the Zeigler process, is used to produce the polyethylene employed in total joint replacements. The technique occurs at low temperatures and low pressures with the use of oxide catalysts. Silicones, in which the connecting link is silicone, and the urethanes, derived from isocyanates, emerged during this period. Numerous ancillary materials such as plasticizers, stabilizers and mould-release agents were developed.

In recent years an increasing diversity of materials has evolved to compete with steel in terms of mechanical criteria and economic factors. The new research workers have been willing to examine a wide variety of materials for their potential applications rather than focusing excessive attention on ways to alter one material. This concept has only recently been recognized by many of the surgeons with particular interest in implantable materials. Until the present decade these workers have attempted to adapt the few available implantable materials to serve various mechanical applications for which their properties often were greatly over-extended. At present bioengineers are studying an extraordinary range of implantable materials which will become evident in subsequent chapters.

Corrosion

In the early 19th Century, Michael Faraday reduced electrolysis to quantitative terms by elaboration of what are now known as Faraday's laws. He introduced the term electrode, anode and cathode and described a variety of corrosion reactions of which one was anodic protection. From about 1920 several workers renewed studies on the nature of metallic corrosion. In 1916, Aston[36] had described electric or corrosion currents established by differences in the oxygen concentration within the solution around the metallic specimen. From about 1930, U. R. Evans and his school[11, 12] in Cambridge undertook quantitative studies on the rates of corrosion of iron and aluminum immersed in sodium chloride solutions. These workers confirmed that corrosion is one of the several types of electrochemical events that obey Faraday's law. Evans[37] and Mears and Brown[38] undertook further quantitative assessment of corrosion by the application of statistical techniques. Numerous laboratory tests[39] were developed after 1930 for rapid and accurate estimation of the anticipated corrosion behavior for metals exposed to various environments. The first quantitative assessment was a record of weight loss of specimens after periods of exposure to an accurately simulated environment. After 1940 Edeleanu[40] and others attempted to develop quantitative electrochemical analyses such as potentiostatic and potentiodynamic evaluation. The Belgium school of Pourbaix[41] introduced the concept of potential pH diagrams as an indication of the thermodynamic conditions under which metals could be expected to be inert or to corrode rapidly. While this thermodynamic approach provided great stimulation for experimentalists it ignored certain kinetic attributes of electrochemical phenomena which often dictated the rates of corrosion that are observed under service conditions.

From 1940, a variety of mechanisms of mechanochemical dissolution were studied intensively. Mears, Brown, and Dix[42] and Hines and Hoar[43] described stress corrosion cracking of aluminum and austenitic stainless steels in chloride containing solutions. Other workers focused their attention on fretting and fatigue corrosion which remains poorly understood to the present time.[44]

Implants in Orthopaedic Surgery

The great wars of the last century have provided much of the impetus for improvement in the care of trauma. In 1870 during the Franco-Prussian War, the French orthopaedic surgeon Louis Ollier[45] introduced a technique of complete immobilization of a limb in a plaster of Paris cast. Ollier devised his treatment as a method to isolate the wound from infective germs and to afford the region complete rest. In 1898, Friedrich,[46] a German surgeon, published experimental findings which showed conclusively that the excision of dead tissue in open wounds was crucial. His study provided a scientific basis for techniques of debridement that Botallo, Desault and Larrey had applied empirically over the previous century or more.[47]

In the early part of World War I surgeons with British, German and French armies independently recognized the importance of primary debridement of open wounds with secondary closure when possible. Robert Jones (Fig. 1-10) of England reintroduced the use of the Thomas splint when he recognized the importance of rest for the treatment of open wounds. Between 1918 and 1920 Winett Orr, the American surgeon, documented that soldiers admitted to his hospital showed better conditions of their open and infected fractures when the wounds were enclosed in a plaster cast to facilitate transport to America.[47] In spite of the presence of bacterial infection the granulation process proceeded undisturbed and the patients showed no clinical

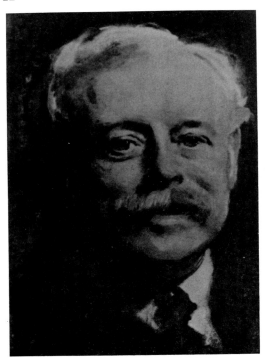

Figure 1-10. Sir Robert Jones, 1857–1933. (Reproduced with permission of Williams & Wilkins Co., Baltimore.)

evidence of sepsis. This notable observation was documented in his book, *Osteomyelitis and Compound Fractures* (1929). Orr applied his methods of treatment primarily to patients with chronic osteomyelitis rather than to those with recent open and contaminated fractures. By 1929 Joseph Trueta[47] in Barcelona had applied the method of Orr to over 40 cases of osteomyelitis and was highly impressed with its success. He questioned whether the technique could be extended to the management of acute contaminated fractures. At the time of initial treatment Trueta lengthened the open wound to facilitate excision of the devitalized tissues. Then he resutured each end of the initial incision to leave open the length of the initial wound. The open area was packed with fine mesh gauze and, in certain cases, suction irrigation drainage was applied. At the time of the outbreak of the Spanish Civil War in 1936, Trueta was chief surgeon at the General Hospital in Catalonia. During the war he had ample opportunity to confirm the highly favorable results of his method. Subsequently, he had to flee to England where he continued his techniques at the Nuffield Orthopaedic Centre in Oxford. In his book

entitled, *Principles and Practices of War Surgery* (1943), Trueta divided the treatment of open fractures into two stages. The first was the removal of various noxious factors such as foreign bodies, bacteria and devitalized tissue. The second was the treatment of the general condition of the patient and an attempt to stimulate rapid healing at the fracture site. In his research laboratories, Trueta studied the healing mechanisms of bone and other tissues. Trueta confirmed that the application of a plaster of Paris cast to an open fracture enhanced the rates of epithelialization and collagen regeneration as well as the tensile strength of the wound. No further improvement in the care of open fractures would be widely observed until the 1960's.

After 1920, attempts to employ surgical implants were still hampered by the limitations of available materials. In 1924, Zierold[48] published a study on the reactions of tissues, including skulls, tibiae and ribs of dogs, to a variety of metals. Iron and steel, the most widely employed materials at the time, were noted to dissolve rapidly and to provoke erosion of adjacent bone. Substantial discoloration of tissues was observed around specimens of copper, nickel, zinc, magnesium and an aluminum alloy embedded in bones. No deleterious tissue reaction was observed around gold, silver, lead or pure aluminum but these materials were too soft or weak for most applications other than sutures, wires or thin platings on other metals. Stellite, a cobalt-based alloy, was observed to have satisfactory tissue tolerance but surprisingly, in view of its high strength, further studies on the material were not undertaken at that time. In 1926, 18% chromium-8% nickel (18-8) stainless steel was introduced into surgical applications. This material was observed to be more corrosion resistant in body fluids than vanadium steel, although in certain instances it, too, underwent rapid dissolution. It was, however, the precursor of the molybdenum-bearing austenitic stainless steels which show much greater resistance to corrosion in saline solutions. Large[48a] reported the favorable inertness observed *in vivo* for a molybdenum-bearing stainless steel in 1926 but its general application was delayed for many years.

In 1929 another cobalt-based alloy, Vitallium was developed and shortly thereafter was introduced as a dental alloy. In 1936, Venable and Stuck[5] initiated an extensive search for more inert implant alloys. These workers observed that Vitallium was completely inert in the body and provoked minimal destruction of bone around implanted specimens. At about the same time Burch, Carney and others[5] observed a similar inertness for specimens of tantalum *in vivo*. In view of limitations in techniques of purification and manufacture, tantalum showed poor mechanical attributes which rendered the material unacceptable to the orthopaedic surgeon. It was employed by neurosurgeons and plastic surgeons for applications that required lower strength. The next alloy to be introduced into orthopaedic practice was titanium and its alloys. About 1947 Joseph Cotton, a metallurgist in Birmingham, England, discussed its possible applications for surgical implants with a few local surgeons and businessmen.* The pure metal had shown excellent inertness in an environment of sea water so that corrosion resistance seemed likely to be good in the human environment. A few surgical implants were made and inserted in human subjects. Upon their removal excellent corrosion resistance was confirmed. Subsequently Maurice Down introduced a variety of titanium orthopaedic fracture devices such as plates and screws. By 1947 the United States Committee on the Treatment of Fractures of the American College of Surgeons had accrued enough evidence so that material specifications for bone plates and screws were established.[49] The recommended materials were Vitallium, a 19% chromium-9% nickel stainless steel, the 18% chromium-8% nickel-2-4% molybdenum stainless steel, or pure tantalum.

Of the multitudinous fracture problems confronting the traumatic surgeon, fractures in the region of the neck of the femur were the most widely encountered complex problem. Most fractures of the shaft of the femur, tibia, or more distal bones could be treated satisfactorily by conventional means. In the geriatric population who sustain most femoral neck fractures the healing potential of the bone is poor and non-operative methods of treatment were generally unsatisfactory. The intense pain associated with motion at the fracture causes a self-imposed immobilization by the patient which frequently culminates in associated pulmonary or urinary tract infections of high mortality. Various unsuccessful attempts were made to drive nails or screws into the neck of the femur to secure the detached fragment. Prior to radiological visualization of the fragment, success was unlikely. In 1922, Martin and King[49] achieved better results by the application of X-rays to position nails through the greater trochanter into the femoral

head and neck. Alternatively, Hey-Groves[21] advised the application of bone or ivory pegs to immobilize the fracture with subsequent biodegradation of the implant. The most significant advances, however, were made by Smith-Petersen, Cave and Vangorder[50] in 1931. Smith-Petersen (Fig. 1-11) devised a nail with three radial flanges which possessed good rigidity in bending to resist the shear forces of the fracture interface and satisfactory resistance to rotational forces. The nail had a sharpened point to facilitate introduction through the neck of the femur. While the first Smith-Petersen nails were manufactured of stainless steel they were soon made available in Vitallium. Johannsen modified the "trifin" nail with a central hole so that a small wire could be driven into the bone across the fracture site for radiological confirmation of satisfactory position and alignment. Subsequently the nail could be introduced over the guide wire. Other workers undertook numerous modifications of the original hip nails, many of which are still in use.

One of the principal problems of the Smith-Petersen nail was migration of the implant after

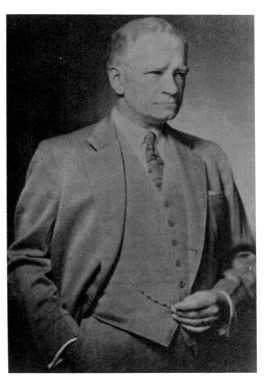

Figure 1-11. Marius N. Smith-Petersen, 1886–1953. (Reproduced with permission of *J. Bone Jt. Surg.,* 35A: 1043, 1953.)

---

* M. Down, personal communication, 1974.

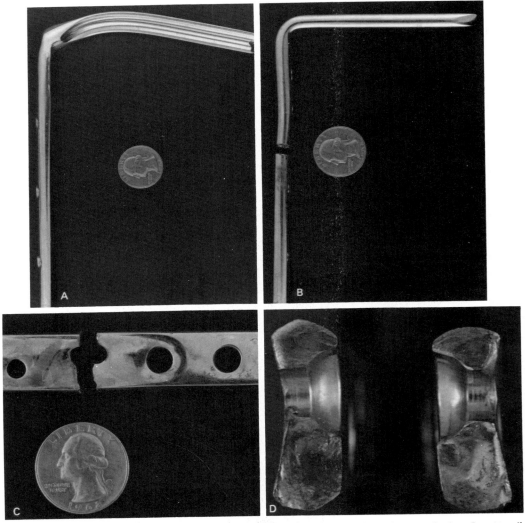

Figure 1-12. Photographs reveal two types of failure of hip nails that continue to occur. In A, a Jewett nail-plate device shows deformation of the three flanged cannulated nail. Figures B–D show three views of a fatigue fracture through the site of a screw hole in a blade-plate device employed in the proximal femur. The clinical and biomechanical factors associated with such failures are reviewed in Chapters 9 and 10.

its initial insertion. The nail tended to withdraw with loss of fixation of the fracture. In 1937 Thornton and McLaughlin attached a plate to the distal end of the Smith-Petersen nail and secured the plate to the shaft of the femur by the use of screws.[51] Since then numerous other refinements and modifications of these devices have been made which are described in Chapters 9 and 10. Despite the alterations in design, mechanical failures continued to be a problem of which two examples are shown in Figure 1-12.

In 1940, Küntscher,[52] in Germany, presented a major advancement in internal fixation with the V-shaped medullary nail. During the next year he modified his device to elaborate the rigid slotted medullary nail with a clover-leaf cross section for use in the femur. In 1950, Herzog[17] modified the nail with an anterior curve to introduce the era of rigid medullary nailing for fractures of the tibia. The concept of reaming the intramedullary cavity was provided by Maatz in 1942, who sought a perfect fit between the metal and the bone. By 1951 Küntscher had employed reaming and the use of much thicker nails to increase stability both for pseudoarthroses and for fresh fractures. Alternatively,

Hackethal[17] in Europe, and Rush[53] in the United States introduced the use of multiple intramedullary wires or pins.

From the early studies reported by Lambotte in 1907, numerous isolated workers had employed external fixation clamps with transfixing pins for certain difficult fracture problems. In the presence of open contaminated fractures, or infected nonunions external fixation possesses several attractions. Internal fixation is generally undesirable in these situations because the implant may serve as a foreign body to increase the likelihood of a clinical infection and to accelerate the rate of progression of an established infection. If a plaster cast is used to immobilize the fracture, the inspection and care of the open wound with daily dressing changes, is rendered more difficult. External fixation may provide adequate immobilization without impingement of the device on the fracture site or obliteration of the wound. Technical problems with the external devices including difficulties in assembly, loss of stability and pin track infections had thwarted their general application. In 1938 Raoul Hoffmann[54] introduced another external fixation device which permitted three-plane corrections in alignment after its application. While this device was otherwise not notably superior to its competitors in the 1960's it would be modified by Vidal et al.[55] and Adrey[56] to provide an extraordinarily rigid and versatile external fixation device.

From 1920 to 1950, most of the progress made in internal fixation focused on improvements in the alloys themselves or in the surgical implants. Few workers, however, considered the theoretical principles governing the influence of internal fixation on fracture healing. The Belgian orthopaedic surgeon, Danis,[57] contributed substantially to internal fixation in his monograph entitled, *Theory and Practice of Internal Fixation* (1947). To provide stability and compression of a fracture site he designed a special compression plate which provided rigid stabilization especially in a midshaft forearm fracture. His foremost contribution was a biological concept of primary bone healing. With rigid compression and fixation of fractures of the shaft of the radius and ulna, Danis observed that healing transpired without radiological signs of callus formation. He assumed that under the influence of axial compression, the cortex was capable of primary bone union. He believed that the healing process under the influence of rigid fixation followed a different course from that which occurs with conservative treatment where the biological basis for union is visible external callus formation. The recognition of these distinct mechanisms of fracture healing gave internal fixation a scientific background and stimulated much further research in the 1960's which will be presented shortly.

The treatment of joint stiffness or ankylosis had aroused the curiosity of surgeons for centuries. After 1800, many ingenious but isolated attempts were made by several surgeons to surgically correct stiff joints. In his monograph entitled: *Arthroplasty* (1955), Buxton[58] has documented a multitude of extraordinary procedures. Prior to aseptic, anesthetic surgery little real progress was made. In 1913 William Baer of Baltimore, outlined six methods of treatment for ankylosis: manipulation; injection of fluid into the joint cavity to separate the opposing surfaces; surgical creation of a pseudoarthrosis, or false joint, in the neighborhood of the ankylosis; resection of the adjacent bone ends at a joint such as the elbow; transplantation of a joint such as the knee, which was performed on two occasions by Lexer in 1908; and arthroplasty. The last refers to the restoration of an anatomic-like joint with or without the use of man-made materials. Interpositional materials to be employed in arthroplastic procedures were classified as to their organic, inorganic and biodegradable constituents. Baer was aware of experiments performed by Chulmsky in which tin, zinc, silver, rubber and other materials were employed for interposition in animal joints. At that time, fascia, as a free graft or a flap, was the most popular interpositional agent. Prior to 1930, most interpositional arthroplasties were performed as the late reconstructive treatment for previously infected joints. In view of the great limitations of the then available implant alloys, and of the indication for surgery, it is not surprising that most interpositional arthroplasties performed with foreign bodies were unsuccessful.

In summary, prior to about 1930, most surgeons feared that surgical measures would aggravate joints afflicted by various arthritides. Most orthopaedic procedures were directed toward the treatment of malunited or ununited fractures or to joint infections.

In the 1930's, McMurray and Whitman,[59] rekindled interest in reconstructive joint procedures with their osteotomies of the proximal femur. It was observed that many patients with early degenerative arthritis of the hip joint prior to the onset of profound stiffness, showed reversal of their disease when the femoral neck was divided and allowed to heal. McMurray applied

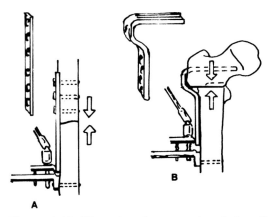

Figure 1-13. The external compression device of Müller is shown schematically as applied to a shaft of a long bone (*A*) and to a proximal femoral osteotomy (*B*). In both cases the fracture surfaces are compressed to provide rigid stabilization.

a hip spica cast for immobilization. In 1943 Blount and in 1944 A. T. Moore described a blade plate for the fixation of a high subtrochanteric osteotomy. After 1950 Müller in Switzerland, and Ferguson and Laing in Pittsburgh popularized the application of internal fixation with nail or nail-plate devices to facilitate the immobilization. The blade plate designed by Müller employed a tension device (Fig. 1-13) to provide rigid stabilization of the osteotomy site. While the procedure has fairly narrow indications, many highly satisfactory results were documented both by elimination of joint pain and stiffness and by radiological evidence of restitution of the articular surfaces.

The crucial studies on the potential for arthroplasty of joints were made by Smith-Petersen of Boston.[60] He undertook carefully documented experimental studies in which a solid material or "mould" was positioned between the head of the femur and the acetabulum (Fig. 1-14). Chronologically he used glass in 1923, viscalloid in 1925, Pyrex in 1933, Bakelite in 1937 and Vitallium in 1938. The last material provoked the least tissue reactions and in perhaps 30 to 40% of the patients, a mobile, pain-free reconstructed joint was encountered. The operation, postoperative treatment and convalescence required a highly ordered program tailored to the precise specifications established by Smith-Petersen. An accurate fit of the implant to the bone was essential. Prolonged physical therapy, which has now become virtually cost prohibitive, also was necessary. While this procedure has ceased to have very widespread ap-

plication, nevertheless, it is Smith-Petersen who enlightened orthopaedic surgeons with the potential for reconstruction of joints if initially a sound experimental program was undertaken.

The principal surgical alternative to mould arthroplasty is joint replacement of one or both surfaces of the joint. In retrospect it seems surprising that probably the first application of total joint replacement was performed in 1938 by Wiles[61] of England, who inserted six such appliances. The prosthetic acetabulum was stabilized in rotation by two pelvic screws. The femoral head component was situated on the end of a bolt inserted through the femoral neck. The bolt was stabilized by a plate with screws into the proximal femoral shaft. X-rays taken 10 years after implantation, reveal osseous change around both components highly suggestive of loosening. In 1940, several designs of total hip joint replacement, such as the one seen in Figure 1-15, were considered although the problems of satisfactory anchorage to bone and the provision for satisfactory articular surfaces were unsolved.

Perhaps the first serious and systematic attempt to design a prosthetic femoral head was initiated by the Judet brothers and co-workers[63] with their prosthesis introduced in 1946 (Fig. 1-14). They attempted to employ biomechanical principles although, as subsequently emerged, their parameters for design were ill-conceived. For the principal articular component of the device, they employed a thermoplastic, polymethylmethacrylate or acrylic. In the 1930's the material was first used as a dental implant. In 1943, Harmon reported a few trials with arthroplastic cups made of acrylic in which the results were better than with the standard Vitallium cups. Frequently the Judet brothers had observed settling of the cup on the femoral head. With degenerative arthritis, the femoral head may be seriously weakened so that the bone readily impacts and the implant migrates. In the Judet prosthesis the articular surface, therefore, was supported by a metallic cylinder in the femoral neck. In the hands of the originators good results were reported although other surgeons described numerous failures. The reasons for the discrepancy include the vast experience of the Judet brothers with their prosthesis, probably their careful selection of patients, and rigid adherence to their operative technique. Nevertheless, several justifiable criticisms were leveled against the Judet prosthesis. As Scales and Zarek[64] have reported, the biomechanical analysis of the hip joint by Judet underestimated the mechanical forces to which the hip joint is ex-

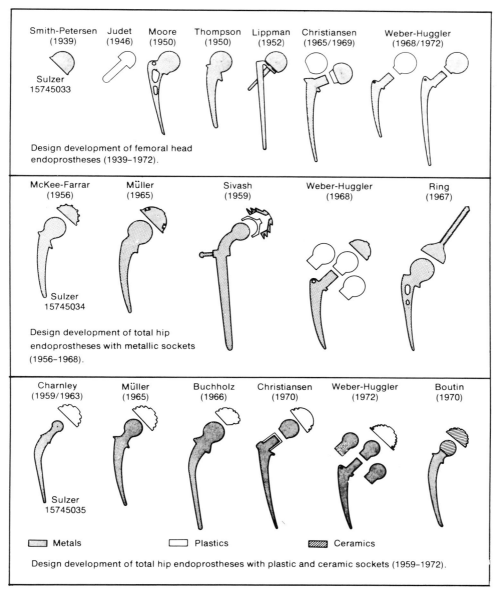

Figure 1-14. The stages in the development of arthroplastic devices for the hip joint are shown schematically. (Reproduced with permission of Sulzer Bros., Ltd. Winterthur, Switzerland).

posed. Furthermore, the accelerated laboratory tests on the wear resistance and mechanical properties of polymethylmethacrylate were unduly optimistic. Fractures of the prosthetic stems and rapid erosion of the articular surfaces were encountered. When conventional sterilization with rapid cooling was employed, the mechanical properties of the acrylic were compromised. Alternatively, after sterilization of the implant by exposure to formalin, a noxious dis-

charge from the patient's wound was observed. Crevice corrosion of the stainless steel rod at the interface with the acrylic articular component was encountered while surface "crazing" of the acrylic was noted. Nevertheless, as Scales[65] emphasized, despite the widespread failures encountered with the Judet procedure, it, like the Smith-Petersen cup, ranks as a milestone in orthopaedic surgery. It stimulated enormous efforts toward the improvement of arthroplasty

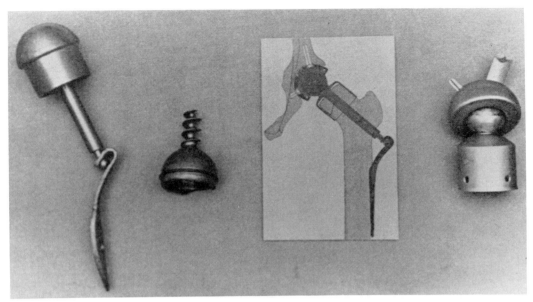

Figure 1-15. Photographs of a total hip joint prosthesis considered for use in 1940. (Reproduced with permission of G. K. McKee.[62])

and in elucidation of the biomechanics of the hip joint as well as the careful laboratory assessment of the mechanical, chemical and mechanochemical properties of implantable materials.

THE RECENT PERIOD

Materials

In the past 20 years material science has been characterized by its extraordinary diversification to study almost a continuous spectrum of materials ranging from metal, glasses, ceramics, polymers to composites.[66] Numerous organizations have created laboratory facilities wherein novel materials can be developed to satisfy peculiar applications. While materials of an incredible breadth of mechanical attributes can be tailor-made, the cost of the novel material frequently is in excess of what the market is willing to support. The cost analysis has become ever more influential in the selection of untried implant materials. The facilities necessary to devise superior materials require complex accelerated testing apparatus that permit accurate simulated tests of the particular environment. Before the test can be undertaken the precise nature of the service conditions must be defined. For improvement in surgical implants, understanding of the human environment has been one of the foremost obstacles. In the early part of this century, little interest was expressed in

the biomechanics of the musculoskeletal system. A few workers such as Koch[67] had reported a mathematical analysis of the trabecular pattern in bone to show how the configuration of trabeculae and the shape of the whole bone was best suited to resist the principal weight bearing forces (Fig. 1-16). Among the early workers Wolff[68] is credited with defining the relationships between structure and function of tissues. Nevertheless, the first detailed account of a mechanical analysis of bones and their microstructure and indeed of numerous other tissues was provided by D'Arcy Thompson[69] in his book *On Growth and Form,* which first appeared in 1917. Thompson was particularly interested to understand how the form of living organisms could be explained in terms of physical considerations and mathematical formulae. After 1950, a number of other workers became interested in the biomechanics of the musculoskeletal system. Workers such as Evans,[70] Hirsch,[71] Frankel,[72] Frankel and Burstein,[73] Yamada[74] and others provided analyses of the forces acting upon bones and joints at microscopic and macroscopic levels. In one example, shown in Figure 1-17, the anisotropic nature of bone and cartilage is documented. Concurrently much new knowledge on the gross and microanatomy of bone, as indicated in Figure 1-18 and the pathophysiology of bone was accrued. These studies provide the necessary background in which the striking ad-

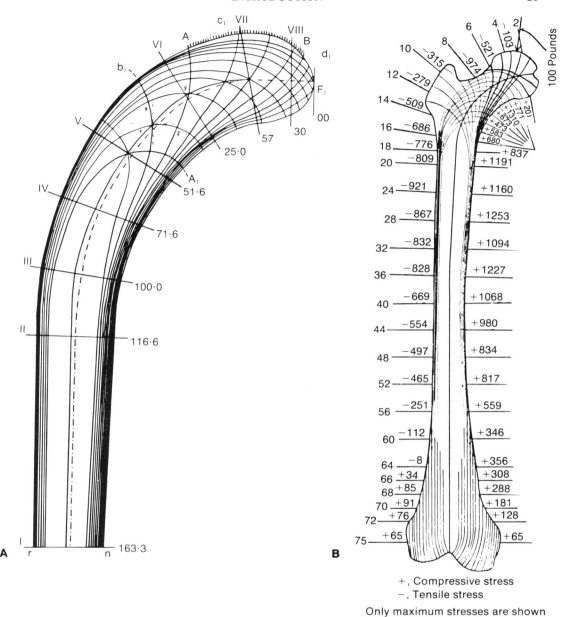

+, Compressive stress
−, Tensile stress

Only maximum stresses are shown
(in pounds per sq. in)

Note: Stresses due to other
loads may be found by
multiplying the stresses in
the figure by the ratio between
the load and 100 pounds.

Figure 1-16. Culmann's trajectory diagram of a Fairbairn crane, *A* reveals the biomechanical concept of the proximal femur as appreciated in 1870. *B*. The stresses determined mathematically by Koch in a femur under the imposition of a vertical load are shown schematically. (*A*, Reproduced with permission of *Virchow's Archiv. Path. Anat., 50,* 1870; *B*, reproduced with permission of *Am. J. Anat., 21*; 243, 1917).

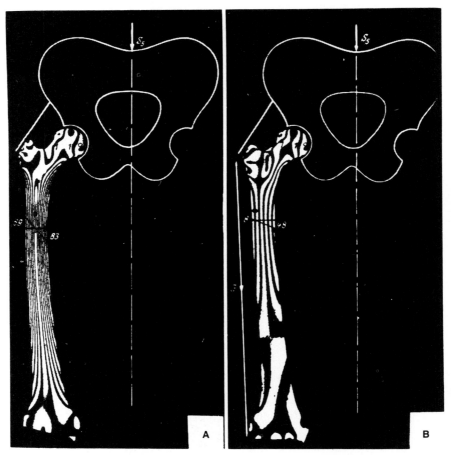

Figure 1-17. Photoelastic patterns in models of a femur reveal local variations and the profiles of stress distribution in the bone. (Reproduced with permission of F. G. Evans.[75])

vances in the use of surgical implants could arise in the 1960's.

Corrosion

After 1950 systematic attempts to elucidate corrosion resistant ferrous alloys and those based on nickel, cobalt, titanium, zirconium and tantalum were undertaken.[44] By adaptation of the thermodynamic data of Pourbaix, theoretically attractive materials were readily prepared. Numerous electrochemical methods were developed which provided rapid accelerated tests to eliminate from consideration all but the most likely candidates and to limit the costly experimental studies in animals. Certain electrochemical tests as described in Chapter 4 were developed which permitted an assessment of the corrosion resistance of implants in humans and other animals.

Recent Developments in Orthopaedic Implants

The past 25 years have witnessed extraordinary advances in the application of implants to orthopaedic surgery. Perhaps the single most influential reason for the rapid progress has been the close co-operation between surgeons, biologists, and bioengineers. The application of implantable materials in the human body rests heavily upon sound knowledge of the biomechanical properties of musculoskeletal tissues and the kinematics of articular joints. Unless a bioengineer possesses a precise tabulation of the mechanical properties of a tissue which he is requested to replace, he is hard pressed to provide a suitable manmade alternative. Similarly for the development of total joint replacements an engineer requires a rigorous description of the planes of motion of an articular joint, the

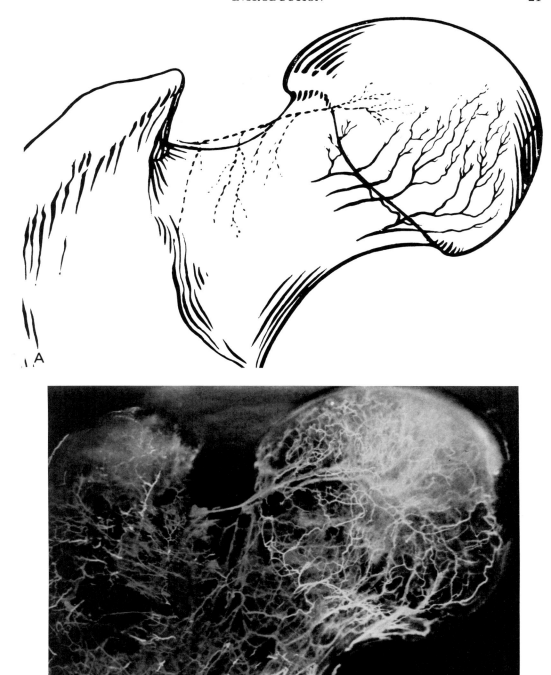

Figure 1-18. *A.* The schematic drawing reveals the terminations of the posterior ascending cervical arteries and their epiphyseal branches in the proximal femur as determined by injection of the arteries with red latex rubber. In *B*, the terminal portions of posterior ascending cervical branches of the arterial ring of the femoral neck are highlighted in this cross section of the bone. (*A*, Reproduced with permission of H. Crock[76]; *B*, reproduced with permission of H. Crock.[77])

Implant material	Used for				
	Cup	Socket	Sphere	Shaft	Anchoring to surrounding tissue
CoCrMo casting alloy (HS-21/PROTASUL-2)	+ +	+ +	+ +	+ +	+
FeNiCrMo forging steel (AISI-316)	+ +	−	+ +	+ +	−
CoNiCrMoTi forging alloy (MP-35N/PROTASUL-10)	−	−	−	+ +	+
TiAlV-forging alloy (IMI-318A)	−	−	+	+	+
Polymethyl methacrylate (Plexiglas)	+ −	− −	− −	− −	+ +
Polytetrafluoroethylene (Teflon/Fluorosint)	− −	+ −	− −	− −	+
High-density polyethylene (RCH-1000)	−	+ +	+	−	+
Polyethylene terephthalate (Polyester KVP-4022/AP4)	− −	+ −	+ −	−	−
Polyoxymethylene polyacetal (Ertacetal[1], Delrin-AF[2], Hostaform-C[3])	− −	+[2,3]	+ −[1]	+[3]	+[3]
Aluminum oxide ceramic	+	+	+	+	+

+ +   Clinically tested for many years
+   Undergoing clinical testing
+ −   Unsuitable following clinical testing
−   Not yet tested
− −   Unsuitable from standpoint of materials experience
[1] Polyacetal homopolymer, [2,3] polyacetal copolymer

Figure 1-19. A list of the principal implantable materials for artificial hip joints employed since 1939 is shown. (Reproduced with permission of Sulzer Bros., Ltd., Winterthur, Switzerland).

magnitude, direction and frequency of application of weight-bearing forces, and the mechanisms of lubrication. The mechanical failures currently witnessed in presently available total joint replacements can be explained in large part by faulty or limited knowledge of complex human joints such as the knee or the elbow. Another strong impetus for improvement was the accelerating cost of prolonged hospital admission. Previous methods of treatment such as prolonged skeletal traction or the extended period of physical therapy needed after cup arthroplasty stimulated surgeons to develop techniques of internal fixation suitable for early weight bearing and discharge from hospital in the former case and total joint replacement for the latter. Concurrent improvements in industrial facilities provided novel materials for potential use as surgical implants which are listed in Figure 1-19. Superior methods were developed to characterize the mechanical environment of the body and testing procedures were devised to determine both suitabilities of materials in the laboratory and *in vivo*. Most of these recent developments are discussed in more detail in subsequent chapters.

In recent years perhaps the outstanding improvements in techniques of internal fixation have been made by the AO* group in Switzerland. In the early 1950's Müller, Allgöwer and Willenegger, three Swiss surgeons, questioned how they might undertake to improve the available surgical implants. They were fortunate to collaborate with Straumann of Waldenburg. As a result of their discussions, a large part of the Straumann Institute was converted from the study of improvements in alloys for use as main springs in watches to the improvement of surgical implants. In 1958, 15 Swiss general and orthopaedic surgeons joined together to further this study on the operative treatment of fractures. In 1965, they published their first manual on fracture treatment entitled, *Technique of Internal Fixation of Fractures.*[17] Meanwhile they had documented open fracture treatment on over 4000 cases. Their primary goal was to improve the clinical methods of open fracture care where well established principles of fracture treatment dictated an operative approach. As a result of their collaboration, however, numerous other improvements in fracture treatment were to evolve. The different surgeons provided various improvements in the design of individual surgical implants. In turn the implants were organized into compact units, the sum total of which could be applied to treat most types of fractures. A set of tools powered by compressed air was devised to complement the implants. The contributions by the AO group, however, have extended far beyond the simple development of surgical tools and implants. They encouraged documentation of novel techniques undertaken in large series so that the relative merits of different methods of treatments could be established. They undertook further research in a series of Swiss research laboratories to understand the nature of primary bone healing, bone biochemistry and histology and the relevant physical and chemical metallurgy necessary to improve implantable materials. Their investigations raised the crucial question of the optimal mechanical properties needed for various surgical implants. Whereas previous workers had attempted to employ the strongest and most rigid

material, the Swiss workers clarified the superiority of softer, ductile materials which could be shaped to closely coadapt to the surfaces of irregular bones and which provided less relief of strain from a plated bone. They studied the influence of motion on infected fractures to determine the nature of healing in infected nonunions. As will be shown subsequently, Rittmann and Perren[78] undertook a series of animal experiments with the application of compression to infected osteotomies which confirmed the superiority of primary bone healing with rigid stabilization in the presence of bony infection. The proliferative infective bone, or callus formation seen in Figure 1-20, that would otherwise ensue does not tend to occur. This and allied observations provided a marked alteration in the optimal form of management for these difficult fracture problems. Previous workers recommended the removal of all foreign bodies from infected fractures, whereas Rittmann and Perren emphasized the need for rigid stabilization. The irony of internal fixation of infected nonunions is that the implant facilitates healing provided that an adequate degree of stability is realized. If, however, the bone is excessively soft or friable, or, if an inadequate selection of implants is available so that rigid stabilization is not realized, internal fixation of the infected fracture may be deleterious. The implant may serve as an additional stimulus for further spread of the infection.

Another area where extraordinary advances were made in stabilization was in the treatment of spinal deformity.[79] The principal deformity, scoliosis refers to a lateral displacement with rotation seen in Figure 1-21. Less frequently other deformities and instability secondary to fractures or fracture dislocations provide indications for internal stabilization. For centuries treatment of scoliosis by the application of external splinting with braces and casts has been undertaken with limited success. In certain patients with rapid progression of their deformity, posterior fusion of the deformity was performed after which the patient was immobilized in bed for 4 to 6 months with a body cast to provide adequate immobilization for the fusion to unite. During the 1950's Harrington[80] in Texas, attempted to apply internal fixation to scoliotic spines, particularly in children afflicted with polio. The instrumentation consisted of a metallic rod and fixation hooks which could provide distraction to the relevant spinal segment. In 1962, he reported the results of his 13-year survey which provoked immediate interest and widespread application of his methods. More re-

---

* AO, Arbeitsgemeinschaft fur Osteosynthesefragen (Association for the study of the problems of internal fixation).

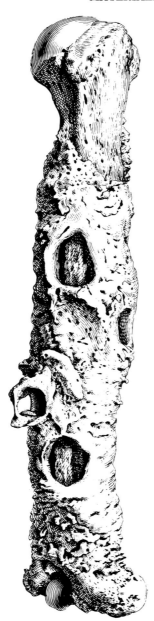

Figure 1-20. A schematic diagram of a humerus with osteomyelitis reveals the proliferative callus or involucrum that is encountered also in an infected nonunion.

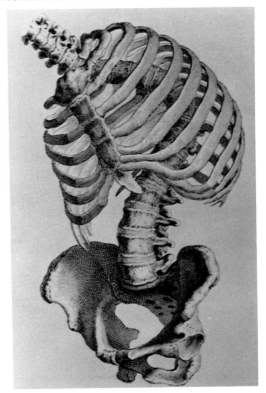

Figure 1-21. The drawing from the 18th Century reveals a deformed spine with idiopathic scoliosis. The lateral and rotational deviations are evident.

cently, Dwyer[81] in Australia, has devised supplementary techniques of anterior spinal instrumentation with the use of a cable and vertebral stabilizing elements. These and other diverse applications of spinal instrumentation are described in Chapter 12.

Perhaps the single development since 1950 which has excited the most widespread interest, not only among orthopaedic surgeons but within the whole medical community has been the evolution of arthroplastic procedures for treatment of the arthritic hip. As mentioned in the previous section, the attempts by the Judet brothers for hemiarthroplasty of the hip had culminated in numerous clinical failures. Nevertheless, many other workers were stimulated to undertake comparable studies. In 1950, Moore and Thompson, in the United States, independently produced their straight and curved stemmed metallic femoral head replacements.[59] Initially the devices were employed for treatment of degenerative arthritis where they encountered limited success. They were also used, however, for treatment of grossly displaced subcapital femoral fractures in the geriatric population where the incidence of nonunion and death of the proximal fragment is exceptionally high. In this application they encountered considerable success so that the method has gained an established position. In the 1950's, Charnley of the Wrightington Hospital in England (Fig. 1-22), initiated his attempt to develop a successful arthroplasty for

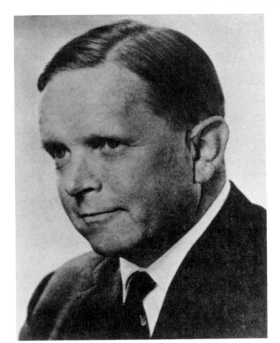

Figure 1-22. Sir John Charnley 1911–Present. (Reproduced with permission of *Clin. Orthop., 95:* 5, 1973.)

the hip.[65] The two principal problems were a method to anchor the implantable devices to bone and suitable materials for the articulating surfaces. On a trip to California, Charnley learned about the use of self-curing polymethylmethacrylate in dental surgery. Charnley questioned whether the material could be used to anchor orthopaedic implants. Subsequent experiments showed that a mixture of polymethylmethacrylate monomer and prepolymerized polymethylmethacrylate could be inserted into the intramedullary cavity between the prosthetic stem of an implant and the adjacent cortical bone of the femoral shaft where polymerization provided a solid "cement" fully occupying the space. The reaction was exothermic in nature with the evolution of considerable heat. Certain volatile moieties were generated during polymerization which in some instances initiated transient toxic reactions. Nevertheless, these problems were overcome and a suitable technique for attachment of an orthopaedic implant was devised. Charnley questioned whether a stainless steel alloy could articulate satisfactorily against a suitable polymer. His initial attempt to employ polytetrafluoroethylene in a series of more than 100 patients proved to be disastrous with rapid erosion of the "Teflon" and the production of toxic wear particles. Charnley had the

resolution to continue his research and shortly he was rewarded by the discovery of a second highly satisfactory polymer, high density polyethylene. Between 1959 and 1963 his techniques evolved to provide the most satisfactory arthroplastic procedure ever devised.[82] As shown in Figure 1-14, numerous other workers have continued these studies to provide subtle improvements in the design of implants. Various articulations in surfaces of different geometries and compositions have been employed. Whereas the high density polyethylene showed excellent wear resistance when employed in total hip joint replacements, it underwent much more rapid deterioration in the form of abrasive wear and creep (Fig. 1-23) when used to fabricate total knee joints and other arthroplasties. Most recently workers have attempted to replace the plastic articular component with a ceramic although it seems unlikely that these highly brittle materials will prove to be superior. Many workers also have attempted to devise comparable arthroplastic devices for other articulating joints. None of the other devices has proved to be as satisfactory as total hip joint replacement. They are fully discussed in Chapters 13 and 14.

The attempts to devise finger joint prostheses have required the consideration of other materials with different mechanical properties. Perhaps the most satisfactory of these has been silicone rubber, polydimethylsiloxane. As employed by Swanson[83] and other workers this material can undergo repeated deformation to serve as a hinge without showing evidence of fatigue failure. To date comparable attempts to develop articulating metallic hinges for finger joint replacement as undertaken by Brannon, Klein and Flatt[84] have not shown comparable satisfactory results.

Perhaps the greatest problem that faces arthroplastic reconstruction with total joint replacements and internal fixation of fractures is the risk of infection. Most wound infections arise from intraoperative contamination, or in the case of open fractures, of contamination at the time of the injury. It is now evident that total joint replacements have a life-long predilection for infection that may arise from organisms that enter the blood from another site such as a pulmonary, urinary tract or cutaneous infection. It will be recalled that the landmark in surgery which permitted the initiation of internal fixation of fractures or arthroplastic procedures was aseptic surgery. In 1932, Domagk and his collaborators devised the sulfa drugs, such as Prontosil, from derivatives of azo dyestuffs.[85] These

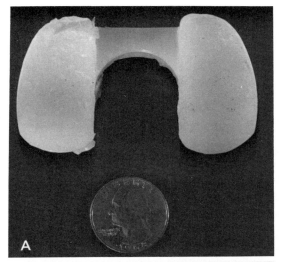

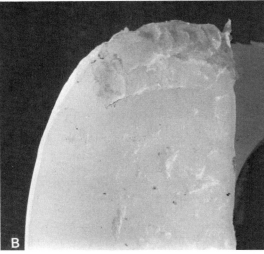

Figure 1-23. *A.* The polyethylene component of a geometric total knee joint replacement removed 3 years after insertion is shown. The implant was removed after an initial good result when the patient began to complain of knee pain associated with activity. As revealed in *B*, the implant has undergone substantial erosion with fracture and creep of the anterior rim. The whitish discoloration seen in the close-up, *B*, represents particulate polymethylmethacrylate cement which serves as an abrasive agent to enhance the rate of wear of the polyethylene.

were the first generally available chemotherapeutic agents which showed selective toxicity to bacteria without harmful side effects to most living tissues. Soon afterwards Fourneau in Paris, showed the lethal effect of para-amino-benzene sulfonamide against streptococci. A widespread search was initiated to discover other antimetabolites which were ingested by bacteria because of their chemical similarity to metabolically required materials. The antimetabolites were lethal to the cells from one of several effects. Soon an entire family of sulfa drugs emerged. In 1928, Alexander Fleming of London made the accidental discovery of a mold, *Penicillium notatum,* which showed a selective toxicity for various infective organisms. In 1943, under the direction of Howard Florey in Oxford, production of the antibiotic penicillin was introduced. The application of these and other antibiotics spread rapidly throughout the spectrum of clinical practice. Certain deleterious side-effects of the use or abuse of antibiotics soon appeared. Highly resistant organisms evolved which were not influenced by the presence of the previously lethal antibiotic. In certain cases the antibiotic appeared to become a favored nutrient of the organisms! In other instances patients treated with a single broad-spectrum antibiotic or several antibiotics developed "super infections" with organisms of low grade pathogenicity, such as a variety of yeasts, which were extremely difficult to eradicate. Nevertheless, a variety of attempts were made to incorporate antibiotic therapy into the use of surgical implants. The precise role of antibiotics remains controversial to the present time.[86] For the treatment of open fractures, especially where internal fixation is employed, prophylactic antibiotics are widely recommended although certain workers disagree vigorously with this application. In the United States most centers undertaking total joint replacements employ a short course of intravenous antibiotics from about the time of surgery to a few days later as discussed in Chapters 9, 10, 13 and 14. The relationships between total joint replacements and postoperative wound infections of great morbidity has caused numerous workers to study methods to limit the incidence of infection. Perhaps the most significant of these was that undertaken by Charnley whose studies re-emphasized the need for rigorous aseptic technique as originally defined by Lister. As Charnley[87] reasoned, since most of the infections arose from intraoperative contamination they should be eliminated by rigorous exclusion of organisms from the intraoperative field. A whole discipline of "clean air" surgery evolved in which a high rate of sterile air flow was directed across the patient and the operative wound site. The surgical team and indeed the patient himself were shielded in garments much like the space suits used by astronauts so that their own airborne waste products could be withdrawn without an opportunity to circulate around the open wound. By the application of these and other methods postoperative wound infection rates were diminished to exceptionally low values, well below 1%. While further studies are underway the exceptionally good results have rendered further improvements difficult to document because it is hard to accumulate adequate numbers of procedures undertaken in identical fashion to provide useful statistical confirmation of the efficacy of new techniques.[88] In Chapter 8, this field is reviewed.

Most recently numerous workers have attempted to develop surgical implants that incorporate the unique attributes of living tissues with implantable materials.[89] The ingrowth of bone into a porous implant provides a method of skeletal attachment in which at least part of the interface is living and able to undergo continuous repair and to show inherent resistance to infection. As discussed in Chapter 16 other attempts are underway to stimulate the regeneration of numerous musculoskeletal tissues in porous implants. The implant serves as a method of attachment and as a means to direct the growth of healing tissues along the optimal anatomical configuration. It seems likely that further studies in the use of implants will focus much of their attention on methods to influence the regeneration of tissues.

In these and other ways the progress of the next 20 years is likely to be as dramatic as that observed in the past.

REFERENCES

1. Smith, C. S. *Sci. Am.*, *217*:69, 1967.
2. Smith, C. S. Metallurgy in the 17th and 18th centuries. In *Technology in Western Civilization* edited by M. Kranzberg and C. W. Pursell, Jr., p. 142, Oxford University Press, London, 1967.
3. Bell, B. A. *A System of Surgery*, p. 22, Penniman, Troy, NY, 1804.
4. Levert, H. S. *Am. J. Med. Sci.*, *4*:17, 1829.
5. Venable, C. S., and Stuck, W. G. *The Internal Fixation of Fractures*, p. 5, Charles C Thomas, Springfield, Ill., 1947.
6. Singer, C., and Underwood, E. A. *A Short History of Medicine*, p. 341, Clarendon Press, Oxford, 1962.
7. Smith, C. S. Metallurgy: Science and practice before 1900. In *Technology in Western Civilization* edited by M. Kranzberg and C. W. Pursell, Jr., p. 592, Oxford University Press, London, 1967.
8. Singer, C., and Underwood, E. A. *A Short History of Medicine*, p. 159, Clarendon Press, Oxford, 1962.
9. Davy, H. *Phil. Trans. Roy. Soc.*, *114*:151, 1824–1825.
10. Singer, C., Holmyard, E. J., and Hall, A. R. (editors) *A History of Technology*, p. 375, Oxford University Press, London, 1954.
11. Evans, U. R., Bannister, L. C., and Britton, S. C. *Proc. Roy. Soc.*, *131*:355, 1931.
12. Evans, U. R., and Hoar, T. P. *Proc. Roy. Soc.*, *137*:343, 1932.
13. Singer, C., and Underwood, E. A. *A Short History of Medicine*, p. 352, Clarendon Press, Oxford, 1962.
14. Hansmann, H. *Verein Deutsches Gesellschaft fur Chir.*, *15*:134, 1886.
1ᵇ. Gurlt, E. *Handbuch der Lehre von den Knochenbruchen*, p. 119, Berlin, 1862.
16. Koenig, F. *Langenbechs. Arch. Klin. Chir.*, *76*:23, 1905.
17. Müller, M. E., Allgöwer, M., and Willenegger, H. *Techniques of Internal Fixation of Fractures*, p. 1, Springer-Verlag, Berlin, 1965.
18. Müller, M. E., Allgöwer, M., and Willenegger, H. *Techniques of Internal Fixation of Fractures*, Springer-Verlag, Berlin, 1965.
19. Lambotte, A. *Presse Med. Belge*, *17*:321, 1909.
20. von Baeyer, H. *Munchen. med. Wchnschr.*, *56*:2416, *1909; Beitr. Klin. Chir.*, *58*:1, 1908.
21. Hey-Groves, E. W. *Br. J. Surg.*, *438*:501, 1913.
22. Lane, W. A. *The Operative Treatment of Fractures*, p. 71, Medical Publishing Co., London, 1914.
23. Sherman, W. D. *Surg. Gyne. & Obst.*, *14*:629, 1912.
24. Bechtol, C. O., Ferguson, A. B., Jr., and Laing, P. G. *Metals and Engineering in Bone and Joint Surgery*, p. 6, Williams & Wilkins Co., Baltimore, 1959.
25. Nabarro, F. R. N. *Theory of Crystal Dislocations*, p. 1, Clarendon Press, Oxford, 1967.
26. Prandtl, L. *Z. angew Math. Mech.*, *8*:85, 1928.
27. Orowan, E. *Z. Phys.*, *89*:634, 1934.
28. Polanyi, M. *Z. Phys.*, *89*:660, 1934.
29. Taylor, G. I. *Proc. Roy. Soc.*, *45A*:362, 1934.
30. Seitz, F., and Read, T. A. *J. appl. Phys.*, *12*:100, 1941.
31. Mott, N. F. Research, *2*:162, 1949.
32. Cottrell, A. H. *Prog. Met. Phys.*, *1*:77, 1949 and *4*:205, 1953.
33. Cottrell, A. H. *Theory of Crystal Dislocations*, p. 80, Blackie & Son, London, 1964.
34. Cottrell, A. H. *Sci. Am.*, *217*:90, 1967.
35. Farber, E. Man Makes His Materials. In *Technology in Western Civilization*, edited by M. Kranzberg and C. W. Pursell, Jr., p. 183, Oxford University Press, London, 1967.
36. Aston, J. *Trans Am. Electrochem. Soc.*, *29*:449, 1916.
37. Evans, U. R. *The Corrosion and Passivation of Metals*, p. 911, E. Arnold, London, 1960.
38. Mears, R. B., and Brown, R. H. *Industr. Eng. Chem.*, *29*:1087, 1937.
39. Mears, R. B., and Brown, R. H. *Industr. Eng. Chem.*, *33*:1001, 1941.
40. Evans, U. R. *The Corrosion and Oxidation of Metals*, p. 219, Edward Arnold, London, 1960.
41. Pourbaix, M. *Z. Elektrochem.*, *62*:670, 1958.
42. Mears, R. B., Brown, R. H., and Dix, E. H. *Symposium on Stress-Corrosion Cracking*, Am. Soc. Test. Mater./Am. Inst. Min. Met. Eng., p. 323, 1944.
43. Hines, J. G., and Hoar, T. P. *J. Appl. Chem.*, *8*:764, 1958.
44. Mears, D. C. *Int. Met. Rev.*, *Rev. 218*:119, 1977.

45. Ollier, L. *Bull Acad. de med Paris, 2:*1, R 413, 1872.
46. Friedrich, P. L. *Arch. f. Klin. Chir., 57:*288, 1898.
47. Trueta, J. *Principles and Practice of War Surgery,* p. 30, C. V. Mosby, St. Louis, 1943.
48. Zierold, A. A. *Arch. Surg., 9:*365, 1924.
48a. Large, M. *Z. Orthop. Chir., 47:*520, 1926.
49. Williams, D. F., and Roaf, R. *Implants in Surgery,* p. 10, W. B. Saunders Co., London, 1973.
50. Smith-Petersen, M. N., Cave, E., and Vangorder, G. W. *Arch. Surg., 23:*715, 1931.
51. Thornton, L. *Piedmont Hosp. Bull., 10:*21, 1937.
52. Küntscher, G. *The Practice of Intra-medullary Nailing,* p. 21, Charles C Thomas, Springfield, Ill., 1967.
53. Rush, L. V. *Atlas of Rush Pin Techniques,* p. 5, Berivan Co., Meridian, Miss., 1955.
54. Hoffmann, R. *Acta. Chir. Scand., 107:*72, 1954.
55. Vidal, J., Rabischong, P., Bonnel, F., and Adrey, J. *Montpellier Chir., 16:*53, 1970.
56. Adrey, J. *Le Fixateur Externe d'Hoffmann,* p. 25, Paris Ed. Gead, Paris, 1970.
57. Danis, R. *Theorie et pratique de l'osteosynthese,* p. 9, Masson & Cie, Paris, 1947.
58. Buxton, St. J. D. *Arthroplasty,* p. 5, J. B. Lippincott Co., Philadelphia, 1955.
59. Tronzo, R. G. *Surgery of the Hip Joint,* p. 6, Lea & Febiger, Philadelphia, 1973.
60. Aufranc, O. E. *J. Bone Jt. Surg., 37A:*237, 1957.
61. Wiles, P. *Br. J. Surg., 45:*488, 1957.
62. McKee, G. K. *Clin. Orthop., 72:*85, 1970.
63. Judet, J., Judet, R., Legrange, L., and Dunoyer, J. *Resection Reconstruction of the Hip. Arthroplasty with Acrylic Prosthesis,* p. 45, E. & S. Livingstone, Edinburgh, 1954.
64. Scales, J. T., and Zarek, J. M. *Br. Med. J., 1:*1907, 1954.
65. Scales, J. T. Arthroplasty of the hip using foreign materials; a history. In *Lubrication and Wear in Living and Artificial Human Joints,* paper 13, Inst. Mech. Eng., London, 1967.
66. Mott, N. *Sci. Am., 217:*80, 1967.
67. Koch, J. C. *Am. J. Anat., 21:*177, 1917.
68. Wolff, J. *Das Gesetz der Transformation der Knochen,* Berlin, 1892.
69. Thompson, D. W. *On Growth and Form,* p. 997, University Press, Cambridge, 1959.
70. Evans, F. G. *Stress and Strain in Bones,* p. 16, Charles C Thomas, Springfield, Ill., 1957.
71. Hirsch, C. Harrington rods in scoliosis. In *Proceedings of Symposium on Operative Treatment of Scoliosis,* Nijmegen, Amsterdam, 1971.
72. Frankel, V. H. *The Femoral Neck,* p. 15, Almqvist & Wiksells, Uppsala, 1960.
73. Frankel, V. H., and Burstein, A. H. *Orthopaedic Biomechanics,* p. 119, Lea and Febiger, Philadelphia, 1970.
74. Yamada, H. *Strength of Biological Materials,* p. 19, Williams & Wilkins Co., Baltimore, 1970.
75. Evans, F. G. *Stress and Strain in Bones,* p. 30, Charles C Thomas, Springfield, Ill., 1957.
76. Crock, H. *The Blood Supply of the Lower Limb Bones in Man,* p. 14, Williams & Wilkins Co., Baltimore, 1967.
77. Crock, H. *J. Anat. Lond., 99:*77, 1965.
78. Rittmann, W. W., and Perren, S. M. *Cortical Bone Healing after Internal Fixation and Infection,* p. 14, Springer-Verlag, Berlin, 1974.
79. Bradford, D. S., Moe, J. H., and Winter, R. B. Scoliosis. In *The Spine,* edited by R. H. Rothman and F. A. Simeone, p. 271, W. B. Saunders Co., Philadelphia, 1975.
80. Harrington, P. R. *J. Bone Jt. Surg., 44A:*591, 1962.
81. Dwyer, A. F. *Clin. Orthop., 93:*191, 1973.
82. Charnley, J. *J Bone Jt. Surg., 54B:*61, 1972.
83. Swanson, A. B. *Flexible Implant Resection Arthroplasty in the Hand and Extremities,* p. 235, C. V. Mosby, St. Louis, 1973.
84. Flatt, A. E. *The Care of the Rheumatoid Hand,* p. 206, C. V. Mosby, St. Louis, 1974.
85. Singer, C., and Underwood, E. A. A Short History of Medicine, p. 693, Oxford University Press, London, 1962.
86. Bowers, W. H. *Instruct. Course Lect. A.A.O.S., 26:*30, 1977.
87. Charnley, J. *Clin. Orthop., 87:*167, 1972.
88. Dixon, R. E. *Cleveland Clin. Quart., 40:*115, 1973.
89. Klawitter, J. J., Weinstein, A. M., Hulbert, S. F., and Sauer, B. W. Tissue ingrowth and mechanical locking for anchorage of prostheses in the locomotor system. In *Artificial Hip and Knee Joint Technology,* edited by M. Schaldach and D. Hohmann, p. 422, Springer-Verlag, Berlin, 1976.

2

The Structure and Properties of Materials

D. C. MEARS AND G.P. ROTHWELL

Throughout the ages human cultures have utilized a variety of materials for constructional purposes, for weapons and in art forms. In earliest times the materials available were governed by the technology available for mining and fabrication, and many of the cultures were identified by the principal materials they employed (*e.g.,* the Ages of Gold, Bronze and Iron). As the range of materials available increased, materials could be selected to match the needs of a particular technology, but it was not until very recently that man had the need to make significant modifications to the properties of available materials to meet particular technological requirements. Indeed it is only during the past 50 years that knowledge of the structure of materials on an atomic scale and of the relationship between the structure and the bulk properties has been developed, knowledge which makes it possible to make such modifications to the properties of materials on a rational basis. Armed with this knowledge, we are currently in a position to *design* the properties of a material for a specific end use, rather than simply to *select* from a limited range of materials. Few areas should benefit more from this ability than that of surgical implants, where a range of extremely inert materials is required with particular mechanical and physical properties. It should be stated, however, that the market in materials for implantation is too small to warrant the vast expenditure of large scale materials development, save in extremely special cases, and most benefits may be expected to be gained from the application of developments in related fields. The fact remains, however, that the proper understanding of current materials and the development of potentially superior ones are based on the detailed knowledge of the structure of the materials and the relation between structure and properties.

STRUCTURE OF MATERIALS

While the study of the structure of matter on a scale finer than the atomic can perhaps be safely left to the endeavors of the physicist, the manner in which individual atoms aggregate into more ordered hierarchies is of the greatest importance in determining the mechanical and physical properties of solid materials.[1] Most of the observed properties are cooperative properties of the aggregate rather than those of the individual atoms, and in fact the properties of real materials depend strongly on the presence of either purely architectural or chemical imperfections in such arrays.

Figure 2-1 shows a periodic table in which the 92 naturally occurring elements are tabulated in seven horizontal *periods* of increasing atomic number and in vertical groups of elements with similar chemical properties. This type of classification was proposed by Mendeleev (1869), based on observed similarities between the then known elements, but it has long been clear that the similarities in properties arise broadly because the elements in each group have the same number of electrons in the outermost shell of the atom. It is these *valence* electrons which determine the types of bond which an element can form, and thus the structures of the element itself and of its compounds with other elements. Figure 2-2 illustrates the arrangement of the valence electrons of a variety of atoms, and Figure 2-3 shows schematically the five types of bonding which determine the structure of all solid materials. In the ionic bond and the covalent bond, stable structures are developed by the atoms either transferring electrons or sharing electrons in order to produce complete octets in the outer shell. Thus the sodium atom and the chlorine atom have 1 and 7 valence electrons respectively. If a sodium atom loses its valence

Figure 2–1. The periodic table of the elements. Key: H, chemical symbol; 1, atomic number; 1.008, atomic weight.

H 1 1·008																	He 2 4·003
Li 3 6·939	Be 4 9·012											B 5 10·81	C 6 12·01	N 7 14·01	O 8 16·00	F 9 19·00	Ne 10 20·18
Na 11 22·99	Mg 12 24·31											Al 13 26·98	Si 14 28·09	P 15 30·97	S 16 32·06	Cl 17 35·45	A 18 39·95
K 19 39·10	Ca 20 40·08	Sc 21 44·96	Ti 22 47·90	V 23 50·94	Cr 24 52·00	Mn 25 54·94	Fe 26 55·85	Co 27 58·93	Ni 28 58·71	Cu 29 63·54	Zn 30 65·37	Ga 31 69·72	Ge 32 72·59	As 33 74·92	Se 34 78·96	Br 35 79·91	Kr 36 83·80
Rb 37 85·47	Sr 38 87·62	Y 39 88·90	Zr 40 91·22	Nb(Cb) 41 92·91	Mo 42 95·94	Tc 43 (97)	Ru 44 101·1	Rh 45 102·9	Pd 46 106·4	Ag 47 107·9	Cd 48 112·4	In 49 114·8	Sn 50 118·7	Sb 51 121·8	Te 52 127·6	I 53 126·9	Xe 54 131·3
Cs 55 132·9	Ba 56 137·3	La* 57 138·9	Hf 72 178·5	Ta 73 180·9	W 74 183·9	Re 75 186·2	Os 76 190·2	Ir 77 192·2	Pt 78 195·1	Au 79 197·0	Hg 80 200·6	Tl 81 204·4	Pb 82 207·2	Bi 83 209·0	Po 84 (210)	At 85 (210)	Rn 86 (222)
Fr 87 (223)	Ra 88 226·0	Ac 89 (227)	Th 90 232·0	Pa 91 (231)	U 92 238·0	†											

* The *rare earths* occur here (La(57), Ce(58), Pr(59), Nd(60), Pm(61), Sm(62), Eu(63), Gd(64), Tb(65), Dy(66), Ho(67), Er(68), Tm(69), Yb(70), Lu(71)).

† The *transuranic* elements follow here: *e.g.,* Np(93), Pu(94), Am(95), Cm(96), Bk(97), Cf(98), Es(99), Fm(100), Md(101), No(102).

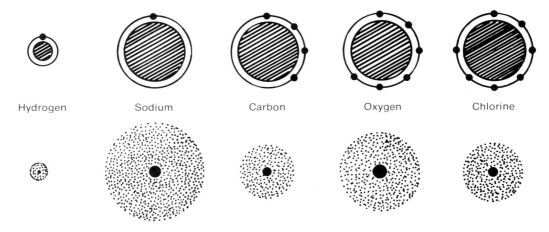

| Hydrogen | Sodium | Carbon | Oxygen | Chlorine |

Figure 2-2. Atoms are represented schematically (*top*) and more realistically (*bottom*). In the schematic representation the *dots* indicate valence, or outer, electrons. The *gray area* is the inner electron "core." In the more realistic representation the electrons are shown as a cloud around a black nucleus. The atoms at the *bottom* are drawn to scale according to their size when they are electrically neutral.

electron the new outer shell of the sodium *ion* is stable with 8 electrons, and if a chlorine atom gains this electron the chloride *ion* is stable with an outer shell of 8 electrons. The sodium and chloride ions are thus bound together by the electrostatic attraction resulting from the charge transfer, and the lattice geometry is determined by the relative ionic sizes. In the covalent bond, on the other hand, stable outer shells are produced by sharing electrons. Thus, for example, 2 chlorine atoms with 7 valence electrons can combine to form a linear Cl_2 molecule by sharing with each other 1 of the 7 electrons; the shared electrons orbit around both nuclei. Similarly, a

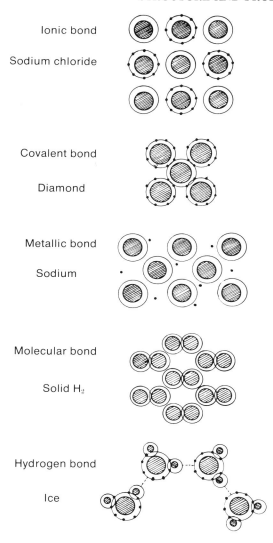

Ionic bond

Sodium chloride

Covalent bond

Diamond

Metallic bond

Sodium

Molecular bond

Solid H_2

Hydrogen bond

Ice

Figure 2-3. Five types of bond that hold all materials together are shown schematically. In the ionic bond the atoms have either lost an electron or gained one so that their outer electron shell is complete. While they cannot share electrons they are electrically charged by the presence of the additional or the lost electron so that they are attracted to atoms of the opposite charge. In the covalent bond pairs of atoms share their outer electrons in filling their outer shells. In the metallic bond all the atoms share all the valence electrons. The molecular, or van der Waals, bond arises from the displacement of charge within electrically neutral atoms or molecules, which produces a weak attraction between them as they approach each other. The hydrogen bond is mediated by the hydrogen atom. This weak bond depends upon the small size of the atoms and the ease with which the charge can be displaced. All of these bonds are idealized and most materials involve some combination of them.

carbon atom with 4 valence electrons can form a stable configuration by sharing an electron with each of *4* other carbon atoms. The only way this can be accommodated spatially is in the tetrahedral structure of diamond, which owes its extreme hardness to the strength and rigidity of its bonding.

Metallic bonding is in fact akin to ionic bonding, and the valence electrons of the metal atoms can be thought of as donated to an electron "gas." The structures are then based on close-packed arrays of metal *ions* held together by their electrostatic attraction to the electron gas. This is by no means a rigorous model of metallic structure, but it is one which enables many of the structure/property relationships of metallic phases to be interpreted.

Secondary or van der Waals bonds are weaker forces resulting from the internal electrical dipoles arising either in asymmetrical molecules or as a result of the statistical variations in electron density which occur in symmetrical atoms or molecules. Thus, for example, it is van der Waals bonding which binds together the H_2 molecules in solid hydrogen. The hydrogen bond is a particular type of van der Waals bond, in which a covalently bound hydrogen atom in a molecule is weakly attracted also to the electron clouds around atoms in an adjacent molecule. For example, the hydrogen nuclei in water molecules are attracted to the electrons around the oxygen of adjacent water molecules, and the resultant binding force significantly modifies the physical properties of water and ice. In fact, the bonding in most real compounds tends to be hybrid (*i.e.,* individual bonds have a partly ionic, partly covalent character) or mixed (bonds of different types exist within the same molecule). Nevertheless, the atomic and molecular architecture of the solid state may be considered to be determined by the properties attributable to the five simple bond types discussed above.

In 1911 William and Lawrence Bragg developed the technique of X-ray crystallography, which enabled the arrangement of atoms in many solids to be determined. Solids were thus categorized as crystalline or "amorphous," although the latter designation strictly indicates those solids in which no substantial order can be measured by a particular type of technique rather than signifying a genuine and total lack of form or structure. The crystalline group includes the metals and most minerals, in which the atoms are demonstrably packed in a geometrically regular manner.[2] In many metals, such as copper and nickel, the atoms are packed

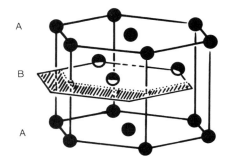

A

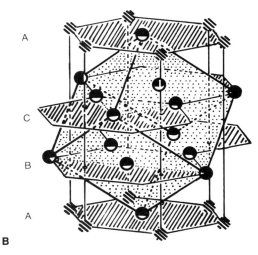

B

Figure 2-4. *A*. Hexagonal-packed structure, a lattice arrangement common to many metals, is erected of tightly nested layers of atoms. Three layers of hexagons provide the 17 atoms that comprise a crystal unit. Atoms in the layers labeled *A* fall directly over one another. Three atoms in layer *B* are situated inside the hexagonal lattice arrangement. *B*. An alternative close-packed structure can be erected from layers of hexagons stacked in the sequence *ABCA*. In this configuration 12 atoms can be selected that form a face-centered cube with the same packing density at the hexagonal close-packed structure. Metals often crystallize in either the hexagonal or the face-centered configuration. A less common form of metal crystal is the body-centered cubic one.

together just as one would pack balls into a box in order to house the maximal number (Fig. 2-4). In other metals, such as iron at room temperature, the structure is body-centered cubic; that is, the 8 atoms at the corners of the cube are in contact with a 5th at the center. The arrangements of atoms in all crystalline solids fall into 14 crystallographic categories, shown in Figure 2-5. In the structure of crystalline compounds points of the *space lattices* in Figure 2-

5 may represent the position of a definite group of atoms rather than an individual atom. The same element or compound may also exist in more than one structure. Two forms of carbon with markedly different properties are illustrated in Figure 2-6. The hardness of diamond with its strong, spatially rigid bonding has already been mentioned. Graphite, on the other hand, although rigidly bonded in planar layers, exhibits much weaker bonding between the layers, which are thus able to slide relatively freely over one another.

The most common compounds in the amorphous group are the glasses. The atoms in a glass are arranged in a much less ordered way than in a crystalline solid, although there is still some short range order, and the structure is much more difficult to determine. A comparison of the structure of silica as a crystal and as a possible glass is shown in Figure 2-7.

METALLIC MATERIALS

The nondirectional nature of the metallic bond has been introduced above. Since all atoms share the valence electron "gas," the binding is equally strong in all directions, and the primary requirement of the atomic arrangement is to achieve the closest possible packing of the atoms. This is achieved in face-centered cubic (FCC) and hexagonal close-packed structures (HCP). The body-centered cubic (BCC) structure adopted by some metals is not quite close-packed, but it gives about 90% of maximum packing efficiency. The closeness of packing and the nondirectional bonding lie behind the density, the resistance to tensile forces and the comparative ductility of metallic materials.

Two defects in the regular pattern of bonding must be introduced in order to be able to predict the mechanical behavior of real materials. In the 1930's Taylor reasoned that the regular atomic structure alone could not account for the ease of deformation of metallic materials. He suggested that deformation must occur by the movement of an extra plane of atoms through the regular array of rows of atoms; one such arrangement is shown in Figure 2-8. The application of transmission electron microscopy to thin films of metals in the last 30 years has both proved the existence of dislocations and enabled very complex determinations of their interaction within the structure and their effects on material properties. The second type of defect is the point defect, either a vacant lattice site or an interstitial or substitutional atom, which is important

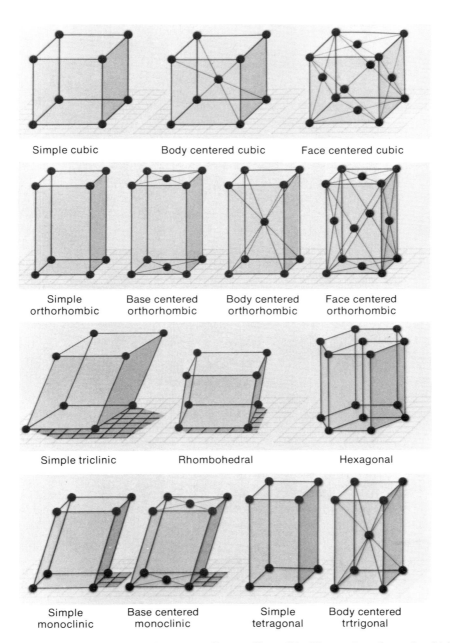

Simple cubic   Body centered cubic   Face centered cubic

Simple orthorhombic   Base centered orthorhombic   Body centered orthorhombic   Face centered orthorhombic

Simple triclinic   Rhombohedral   Hexagonal

Simple monoclinic   Base centered monoclinic   Simple tetragonal   Body centered trtrigonal

Figure 2-5. Fourteen crystal configurations cover all crystalline solids. The number of ways in which atomic arrangements can be repeated to form a solid is limited to 14 by the geometries of the space division. A crystalline material consists of one of the lattice structures repeated in space. (Reproduced with permission of Sir Neville Mott.[3])

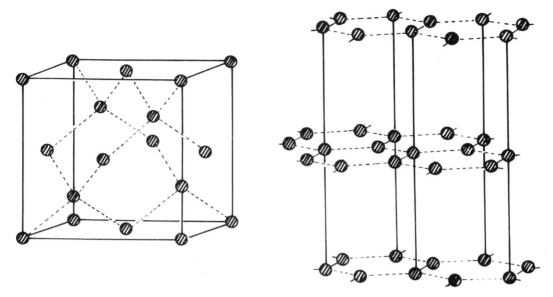

Figure 2-6. Two forms of carbon exhibit markedly different properties because of their different crystal structure. Diamond (*left*) consists of pairs of carbon atoms and a face-centered cubic array. Each carbon atom is tightly bound to 4 others in the lattice and contributes to the hardness of diamonds. Graphite (*right*), a soft material, possesses carbon atoms arranged in layers that are bound by weaker forces. (Reproduced with permission of Sir Neville Mott.[3])

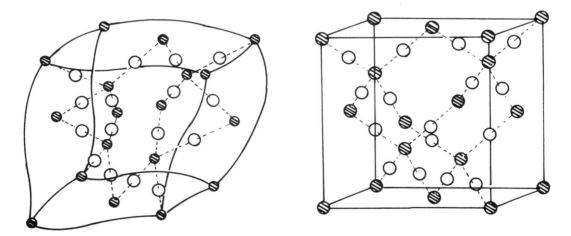

Figure 2-7. Two forms of silica show how molecules of the same composition can exist either as a crystal or as a glass. Crystobalite (*left*), a high temperature form of quartz (SiO₂), possesses a face-centered cubic structure similar to diamond. Silicon atoms (*gray*) occupy the sites filled by carbon atoms in the diamond lattice. An oxygen atom, also, sits between adjacent silicon atoms. A schematic diagram of a glass structure (*right*) resembles a crystobalite structure that has been distorted. The three rings, each with 6 silicon atoms, found in the crystobalite cell have been reconnected to form two rings with 4 silicons and one with 8. (Reproduced with permission of Sir Neville Mott.[4])

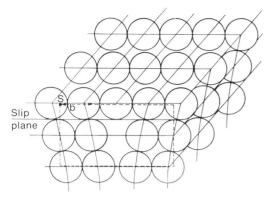

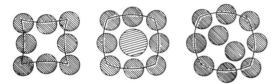

Figure 2-8. An edge dislocation indicating that the dislocation is similar to a tunnel forcing through the crystal. The lattice around the line of the dislocation is distorted. (Reproduced with permission of J. B. Moss.[5])

Figure 2-9. The three types of point-defects or imperfections in a crystal are shown. On the *left* a vacancy is present, in which an atom is missing. In the *center* a substitutional atom is shown in which a different atom is present. On the *right* an interstitial is seen in which an extra atom is present. Each type distorts a cubic crystal lattice in a characteristic way (*black line*). Point defects often interact with linear defects called dislocations.

to the surface of the metal. Each grain, however irregular in shape, is a single crystal, and a piece of metal thus consists of a multitude of differently oriented crystals joined along common boundaries. These observations, which originally derived from the work of Henry Sorby in 1864, have been confirmed by direct observation of the grain structure and grain boundaries at the atomic level by the recent application of field ion microscopy (Fig. 2-11). Optical microscopy also gives information on the *phase structure* of a specimen, that is, the distribution of different alloy phases in complex materials.

Thus it is possible to determine the microstructure, the atomic structure and the defect structure of a metallic specimen, and with this information a significant insight can be gained into the properties of the material under consideration.

Plastic Deformation

If a polished metallographic specimen is lightly deformed, it is frequently possible to observe an array of fine lines on the surface. The lines run straight and parallel in well defined

in predicting diffusion behavior and some strengthening processes (Fig. 2-9).

If a suitable metallic specimen is polished plane and scratch-free and examined under an incident light optical microscope, a uniformly bright image is observed. If the surface is lightly etched by an appropriate chemical reagent, it is possible to reveal the irregular honeycomb of boundaries which divide the metal into small polyhedral grains, typically 0.01 inch across (Fig. 2-10). Some etching reagents attack the grain boundaries to produce deep grooves. Others reveal the microstructure by their attack on the grains themselves, giving a distribution of light and shade among the grains which varies as the angle of incidence of the illumination is changed. Each grain surface consists of an array of narrow, reflecting terraces all set at the same inclination

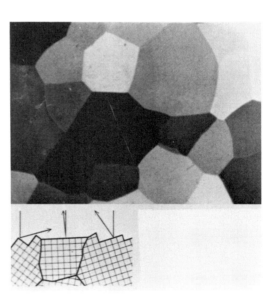

Figure 2-10. Grains in aluminum seen by reflected light in a photomicrograph. The sample was electrolytically etched and oxidized as seen schematically (*below*). Some grains have crystal orientation that reflect most of the incident light and therefore appear to be bright. Others reflect less light and appear darker. ×39 diameters. (Reproduced with permission of A. H. Cottrell.[6])

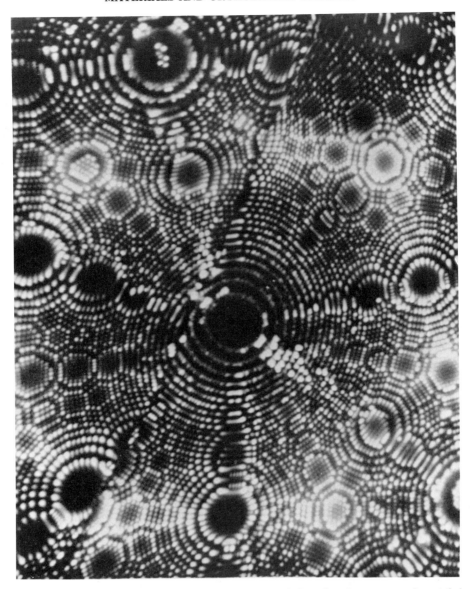

Figure 2-11. A field ion micrograph reveals the presence of a grain boundary between metal crystals but only a few atoms in width. Here the tip of a tungsten needle is enlarged about 5 million diameters. Each *bright spot* represents a tungsten atom. The pattern depends upon the way that the curve surface of the tip intersects successive crystal planes. The pattern changes abruptly at the grain boundary (*bottom left* to *top right*). (Reproduced with permission of A. H. Cottrell.[6])

directions within each grain (Fig. 2-12). They are in fact the traces of steps formed where neighboring thin sections of the crystal have slid past one another, like sliding cards in a deck. Study of the deformation of single crystal specimens shows that the sliding occurs on particular planes of atoms and along particular directions within these planes. The mechanism of deformation is thus very different from the flow of liquids or gases, and depends upon the perfectly regular structure of the crystal which allows atom planes to slide over one another in an organized manner and yet at each step to restore the original properties and internal order of the crystal. The question still arises, however, why most metals exhibit a high degree of ductility while the majority of nonmetallic crystals such as diamond or sapphire are brittle.

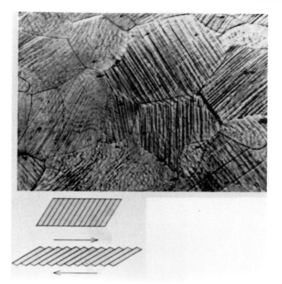

Figure 2-12. Plastic deformation reveals the slip planes in the crystals of a metal. The photomicrograph shows deformation of aluminum. The *parallel lines* within each grain are steps formed when the metal is stressed and slip occurs on certain crystal planes in each crystal. ×37 diameters. (Reproduced with permission of A. H. Cottrell.[7])

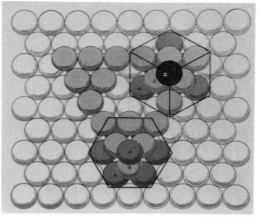

Figure 2-13. The two close-packed atomic structures, characteristic of most metals, are shown. They are modeled by layers of close-packed spheres. On a first layer of spheres at site *A* a second layer is placed at site *B*. There are two sets of sites for a third layer. They may be positioned at *A*, above the first layer, or at *C*. If the layers are stacked *ABCABC*, face-centered cubes are formed as seen in the *top right*. If the layers are stacked *ABABAB*, as seen in the *bottom*, hexagonal close-packed structures are formed. (Reproduced with permission of A. H. Cottrell.[8])

The close-packed structure of metals has been introduced earlier. As Figure 2-13 illustrates, each trio of spheres in a close-packed layer provides one hollow in which a sphere from the next layer can rest.[9] For the complete *A* layer, there are two complete sets of hollows providing the sites for further close-packed layers. If these sets are labeled *B* and *C* respectively, the face-centered cubic structure is obtained when layers are stacked in the sequence *ABCABC,* and the hexagonal close-packed structure when the sequence is *ABABAB*. In metals, slip occurs along the close-packed directions. With their high symmetry, cubic crystal structures are close-packed in several directions, and deformation is thus made easier. Again, if the crystal can slip in several directions simultaneously, it can assume any shape while maintaining the same volume. Thus a metal specimen can be deformed and the grains can change their shape as required while still preserving grain boundary cohesion, without cracks or disintegration. The hexagonal structure has lower symmetry and hexagonal metals are correspondingly less easy to work mechanically and more brittle.

Examination of Figure 2-14 reveals the nature of close-packed rows in more detail. The close-

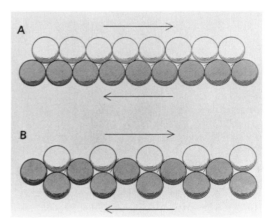

Figure 2-14. Plastic flow of metal occurs when planes of atoms slip passed one another. Close-packed planes do this more easily (*A*) than planes aligned in another direction (*B*). The atoms in a row are closer and the rows are further apart in *A* then they are in *B*, so that less force is required for a given horizontal displacement, as suggested by the pitch of the oblique lines placed between adjacent atoms. Less displacement, also, is required to move atoms into unstable positions from which they will be advanced into stable ones when the stable positions are closer together (*A*). (Reproduced with permission of A. H. Cottrell.[8])

packed rows in (*A*) are clearly further apart than the less closely packed rows in (*B*). There is thus less obstruction to sliding in configuration *A* than in *B*. More precisely, a *smaller force* is required to deform the close-packed configuration, since the atoms have to climb less to produce a given deformation, and also *less deformation* is required to induce flow, since the horizontal distance a close-packed atom has to move to reach the unstable position directly above the atom of the layer below is minimized. Both factors contribute to the ease of deformation along close-packed rows within close-packed planes of atoms, which in turn suggests why, under most conditions, only the close-packed metallic structures among the crystalline materials display such remarkable ductility.

While this argument explains the ductility of cubic metals such as aluminum and copper, it fails by orders of magnitude to predict the shear strength of metals. Early calculations of the ideal shear strength suggested that a metal should deform elastically by 3 to 10% before the onset of plastic flow. In fact, however, single crystals of pure metals usually flow at deformations as low as 0.01%. The 1000-fold disparity between ideal and real shear strength arises because of the invariable occurrence of dislocations in the crystal structure of useful metals.[10] In fact, the strength of thin single crystal "whiskers" may approach the ideal, but, in larger specimens, the presence of dislocations provides an easier mode of deformation. It is analogous to moving a large heavy rug across a floor. There is great resistance to sliding the entire rug in one piece, but it is relatively easy to introduce a wrinkle at one end of the rug and advance this across the floor, enlarging the slipped region behind it at the expense of the unslipped region ahead of it.

Similarly, in a metal crystal, the dislocation (Fig. 2-15) represents the boundary in the slip plane between the slipped and unslipped regions. The detailed geometry of real dislocations is complex and not relevant to the present discussion; it is the principle which is important. If a single dislocation in an otherwise perfect crystal were stressed, it would run out of the crystal and leave a step of one atomic spacing. In reality, crystals contain complex networks of dislocations, which are both interconnected and bound to other defects in the lattice. When the dislocations begin to move under stress, therefore, their ends remain bound, and they cannot run out of the operating slip planes. Indeed, the dislocations multiply during deformation.

The magnitude of the stress required to move

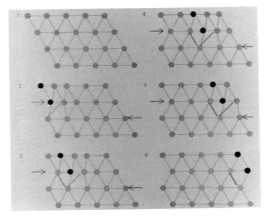

Figure 2-15.. Dislocations enable metals to flow more easily than the mechanism outlined in Figure 2-14 would suggest. Dislocations advance through a metal crystal by one line of atoms at a time. The diagrams show plastic flow in a close-packed crystal (*1*). In the presence of a shearing force (*2*) a plane of atoms (like spheres) moves (*2*) and a bond is broken (*broken line*). The extra plane (*solid black circle*) continues to move. Bonds break and subsequently reform (*solid black lines*) as the dislocation passes (*3 to 5*). When the dislocation (region of broken bond to edge of extra plane) has traversed the crystal, the crystal is deformed by one atomic spacing (*6*). (Reproduced with permission of A. H. Cottrell.[11])

a dislocation in a slip plane depends both on the resistance of the ideal crystal to the passage of dislocations and on the presence of obstacles which may impede their progress. As the dislocation moves through the crystal, the atoms immediately ahead of it resist its approach, because the dislocation forces them out of their stable crystal sites. On the other hand, the atoms immediately behind it push the dislocation forward, for the further it moves the more completely they can assume their new stable sites. When the dislocation region is wide, so that the transition from slipped to unslipped regions is gradual, the forward and backward forces on the dislocation are approximately balanced and the resistance of the crystal to the passage of the dislocation is virtually zero. This is the situation which one obtains in pure close-packed cubic metals, as illustrated by the extreme softness of pure gold, copper and aluminum. However, when the dislocation is very narrow, there are too few displaced atoms to maintain symmetrical forces and a finite stress is required to move the dislocation. As the dislocation width falls to a single atomic spacing, the stress required to move the dislocation approaches the ideal shear strength. Thus although it is possible to describe dislocations in structures such as diamond or corundum, the structure and rigid bonding demand that such dislocations are extremely narrow, and under normal conditions they offer no easy shear mechanism.

Useful engineering materials are generally required to have significantly greater strength than the pure metals which we have been describing, and there are a number of techniques which can be used in a controlled manner to produce the required resistance to deformation. Foreign atoms dissolved in the metal lattice produce local distortion of the crystal structure, by reason of their dissimilar size, and suitable alloying additions are thus extremely valuable in increasing strength. In some alloys, for example, the aluminum-copper alloy, Duralumin, suitable heat treatment can produce a structure in which the foreign atoms are organized into "clumps," increasing their strengthening effect. Again, dislocations are arrested, or at worst slowed down, by grain boundaries, and so metals can be hardened somewhat by reducing the grain size and so increasing the grain boundary area. In fact, many practical alloys consist of several different phases, and the dislocation movement can be impeded by the presence of second phase regions of different crystal structure. Finally, it is well known that the hardness of a metal can be increased by deformation by hammering, rolling or the like. The deformation generates progressively more dislocations, which ultimately obstruct one another as they move along intersecting slip planes. Paradoxically the dislocations, the source of easy plastic deformation, become in turn the obstacles to deformation.

THE ULTIMATE MECHANICAL PROPERTIES OF SOLIDS

During the past 25 years, the development of dislocation theory has given insight into methods for the design of stronger and tougher materials. Moreover, it has provided an understanding of the ultimate mechanical properties of solids and led to techniques for the development of these properties both in the laboratory and in industry. While the subject is fully reviewed by Cottrell,[12] the following brief resumé is helpful.

Ideal Strength

Consideration of a range of different materials reveals that materials with different types of atomic bonding display widely different strengths. Nevertheless, although they may fail at widely different values of stress, the bonds in these materials all fail at approximately the same elongation, that is, when the atoms are distracted to a strain of 0.2 to 0.4. Thus the basic property of the material appears to be ideal strain rather than ideal strength, and apart from polymeric materials, which deform by a unique mechanism, other solids show a remarkably consistent geometry of deformation and failure.

The ideal tensile strength, σ_m, may be represented by

$$\sigma_m = \alpha E$$

where E is Young's modulus and α has the dimensions of strain. Usually α is between 0.05 and 0.2, and it is smaller than the ideal strain because the stress falls below that predicted by Hooke's law at large elastic strains (Fig. 2-16). For a strong material we require high values of α and E. A high E provides elastic stiffness, which is an essential feature for most strong engineering structures, and, since it is an intrinsic property of the particular solid, correct selection of the material is necessary at the outset. For a selected material there are then numerous methods of improving α. Of the materials currently available, graphite shows the highest value of E at 144×10^6 psi. Many refractory oxides, carbides and borides exhibit values in excess of 60×10^6 psi, while common metallic materials shows values around 30×10^6 psi. Because of the low density of the refractory

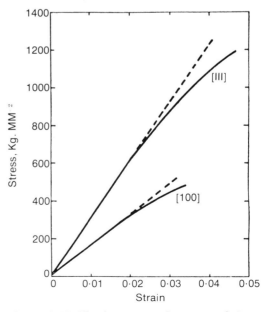

Figure 2-16. Elastic stress-strain curves of strong iron "whiskers" are shown. (Reproduced with permission of A. H. Cottrell.[12])

oxides, their strength-to-weight ratio is very attractive compared with common metals. As a practical target for future strong materials, an E value of 50×10^6 psi coupled with a working elastic strain of 0.02 would enable a working stress of 10^6 psi to be attained, which is an order of magnitude better than materials available at present.

Observed Strength

Ordinary commercial materials usually fail at stresses where $\alpha \simeq 0.001$. If the materials are ductile, they are weakened by the propagation of dislocations; if brittle they fail by the propagation of sharp cracks. This is the dilemma in the design of strong materials: resistance to yield and resistance to brittle fracture are usually contradictory properties. Mobile dislocations provide resistance to cracking by allowing plastic deformation. Nevertheless, remarkably high strengths have been attained in practice, particularly in whiskers and fibers (Table 2-1). Not only do the strengths of these materials confirm the order of magnitude of ideal strengths, but with the development of fiber-reinforced materials, in which large numbers of strong fibers are bonded together by a relatively ductile matrix, the technological exploitation of such high strengths has become commercially feasible.

In fiber-reinforced materials, the problem of fracture is overcome not by mobility of disloca-

tions but by the geometry of the system. The fibers constrain cracks to be either very short if transverse or harmlessly oriented along the fiber if lengthy. Since dislocations are no longer needed to provide resistance to cracking, they may be eliminated by using brittle, noncrystalline materials. Brittle behavior ceases to be synonymous with low crack resistance. In fact, the use of strong ductile materials in fiber-reinforced composites is a distinct disadvantage. In 1952 Herring and Galt[13] prepared single crystal tin "whiskers" 1 μm in diameter which had extremely high strengths, and strengths in the range $0.01 < \alpha < 0.1$ have subsequently been measured for whiskers of many materials. The whiskers contain no dislocations, at least none which would facilitate slip. To prepare such dislocation-free whiskers on an industrial scale would be prohibitively difficult and expensive, and furthermore the whiskers are continuously liable to generate dislocations if handled or exposed inappropriately. Thus the use of noncrystalline materials, in which dislocations cannot form, or brittle materials, in which they are not mobile, is favored for fiber reinforcement, and hard, brittle and elastically rigid nonmetals such as alumina, silica, boron and boron nitride are of particular interest.

Bulk Strength

Large pieces of brittle solids are weak if they contain deep, sharp cracks or other features which can act as stress concentrators. These defects are often mechanical scratches or sites of chemical attack on the surface, and the elimination of surface blemishes by chemical polishing or other means may significantly enhance bulk strength. Nevertheless, such finishing methods cannot make possible the use of monolithic brittle materials in engineering applications because of the catastrophic loss of strength which might follow accidental surface damage.

Let the bulk strength of a solid (failure load per unit area) be σ, and the local strength at the root of a notch be σ_y, as in Figure 2-17A. When the notch depth $c = 0$, $\sigma = \sigma_y$, and the brittle solid shows enormous strength, $\sigma \simeq E/10$. However, the bulk strength falls rapidly with increasing depth of the notch as described by Griffiths' formula (curve a of Figure 2-17A). For practical purposes, a material with much less notch sensitivity is required (curve b). To determine the shape of such curves, consider the behavior of a small element of material at the root of the notch. If the material has strength σ_y and elongates by an amount U_f before fracture, then the

Table 2-1
Observed Tensile Strengths (10^6 psi)

Graphite whiskers	Up to 3.5
Alumina whiskers	Up to 2.2
Iron whiskers	Up to 1.9
Silica glass fibers	Up to 0.8
Asbestos fibers	Up to 0.8
Drawn high-C steel wire	0.6
Piano high-C steel wire	0.35
Heat-treated steel (bulk)	0.35
Fiberglas rod (bulk)	0.2
Flax (cellulose)	0.16
Low alloy steel (bulk)	0.1
Hard copper	0.08
Nylon thread	0.08
Cotton thread	0.06
Hard aluminum	0.06
Catgut	0.06
Cast iron	0.045
Polyester fiber	0.035
Spider thread	0.03
Tendon	0.015
Hardwood	0.015
Glass	0.015

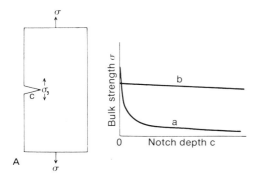

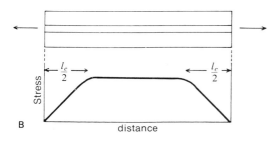

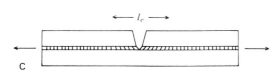

Figure 2-17. *A.* Effect of notch depth (*c*) on strength σ of notch-sensitive (*a*) and insensitive (*b*) solids. (Reproduced with permission of A. H. Cottrell.[14]) *B.* The enhancement of stress toward the center of a strong elastic fiber along the axis of a plastically yielding tensile rod is shown. (Reproduced with permission of A. H. Cottrell.[15]) *C.* The dispersion of stress at the end of a crack by shear along a weak interface is seen. (Reproduced with permission of A. H. Cottrell.[16])

work done per unit area of the element on fracture is given by

$$2\gamma \simeq \sigma_y U_f.$$

For an ideally brittle material α is equal to the specific surface energy. It can be shown that the bulk strength, σ, of a specimen with a crack of depth, *c,* is given by

$$\sigma \simeq \sqrt{\frac{E\gamma}{c}}$$

For simple brittle solids, γ is very low; for example, a crack 0.001 inch in depth can reduce

the strength of glass to approximately 15×10^3 psi, a fraction of its ideal strength. In contrast, for a ductile metal, dislocation glide occurs at stresses which are well below the fracture strength, and failure occurs by plastic elongation at the root of the notch. Thus U_f is greatly increased, and γ is increased to values far exceeding the surface energy. In such circumstances, the σ *vs. c* curve hardly falls unless extremely deep notches are considered.

Ductile Metals

Ductile metals show a very high intrinsic resistance to crack propagation, but the mobility of dislocations stands in the way of achieving high strengths. Traditional metallurgical methods of hindering plastic flow include alloying, cold working and heat treatment to provide obstacles to the motion of the dislocations. On the other hand, if the dislocations are totally immobilized, the problem of brittle fracture returns. A method of overcoming this problem is provided in the structure of the precipitation-hardened or dispersion-hardened alloys, in which fine, hard particles are dispersed in the ductile matrix. The particles obstruct the movement of long dislocation lines, and so the material is hard. On the other hand, dislocation movement between the particles keeps the local stress below the ideal fracture strength, and so the alloy has good crack resistance.

$$\sigma \simeq \mu b/l$$

where μ is the shear modulus, *b* is the atomic spacing in the direction of motion of the dislocation line and *l* is the separation of the particles. If *l* is too small, the dislocations cut through the particles rather than passing between them. The optimum spacing is about 100 Å, which corresponds to observed strengths of $E/100$ in Nimonic (nickel-chromium) alloys, aluminum alloys and quenched and tempered steels. The problem with such fine dispersions is thermodynamic instability, and increased stability is obtained in alloys with coarser dispersions. While such alloys are initially softer in view of the larger value of *l,* they work-harden rapidly. The particles disturb the regular flow of metal around them and produce a more "turbulent" flow pattern which produces many dislocations with intersecting planes; rapid work hardening thus ensues. Again, since the matrix slips and the particles do not, much of the applied load is borne by the particles. They may be viewed as pegs which immobilize the slip planes of the alloy, a concept discussed fully by Kelly.[17] The most satisfactory materials for the particles are insoluble refractory oxides.

Two problems remain however. The soft matrix can deform plastically around the particles, and ultimately ductile rupture occurs near each particle. Again, unless the work-hardening curve can be made steeper so that the maximum strain is reduced to an elastic order of magnitude, the precipitation-hardened alloys still show appreciable deformation at fracture. Both of these problems are reduced if the particles are replaced by long fibers. Figure 2-17B shows the simple situation where tensile stress is applied axially along a single fiber and its metal matrix. As the stress is increased, the metal yields and starts to flow along the fiber. Because of the adhesion at the interface, the stress is transferred to the fiber, and the stress and elastic strain in the fiber increase from the ends of the fiber toward the middle. At a distance $l_{c/2}$ from the end of the fiber, the elastic strain in the fiber is equal to the overall strain of the composite. Further toward the middle of the fiber, the stress no longer rises since the fiber is now deforming as much as the metal. The weakness of the soft matrix is overcome provided the fiber is long compared with l_c, and the metal then serves merely to transfer the stress smoothly to the fiber. The problem of excessive deformation is also overcome, for the overall elongation cannot exceed the elastic elongation of the fibers. Thus the composite stress/strain curve rises elastically up to the breaking stress of the fibers even though the metal becomes plastic at a much lower stress. The composite deforms in an elastic manner up to its fracture stress.

Crack Resistance

In most ductile metals crack resistance is provided at mobile dislocations. Since the dislocations produce plastic weakness of the metal, an alternative obstacle is required to prevent crack propagation in strong materials. The best obstacle to propagation of a crack is a weak interface, perpendicular to the crack. Several stress relaxation effects are provided thereby, as shown schematically in Figure 2-17C. With an interface weak in shear, propagation of the crack provides motion of the opposing surface and dispersion of the stress at the end of the crack over a transfer length l_c, in a manner similar to that shown in Figure 2-17B. Maximum fracture toughness will be achieved with a composite structure in which the tensile members of the load-bearing constituent are separated from each other by thin layers of a second constituent which is soft and

shears easily. Thus the fiber composite model shows optimum performance not only on strength considerations but on grounds of toughness. Toughness ensues from the deliberate use of weak interfaces, provided that the fibers are long enough in relation to the transfer length. Again the model allows the selection of brittle materials to obtain toughness. From this point of view, the traditional microstructure of metals and alloys with continuous paths through the grains or along the grain boundaries is inherently unsatisfactory for crack resistance. Once a crack starts in such a homogeneous microstructure it can propagate across the whole specimen by the same process. Less ductile metals are thus plagued by brittle fracture and more ductile ones by fatigue fracture. Interruption of cracks requires a heterogeneous microstructure interrupted by weak interfaces. These interfaces should not be in sheets; otherwise, when these are inclined to the tensile axis the shear stress can be relaxed and strong stress concentrations are produced at their edges. This problem does not arise with long thin fibers. A parallel bundle of fibers provides the best one-dimensional strength along the axis of the bundle. Two-dimensional strength is achieved by arrangements of the fibers randomly in mats, and three-dimensional strength is possible with randomly interpenetrated fibers. As indicated below, recent advances in technology have made it feasible to consider such novel materials for use as surgical implants.

FIBER-STRENGTHENED METALS

From three independent considerations of the engineering properties of materials the common conclusion has been reached that the fiber-reinforced composite provides the best microstructure for utilizing ultimate mechanical properties of solids on a practical scale. These are (1) the study of the crack resistance conferred by the shape of glass fibers and brittle whisker crystals, (2) consideration of the further development of dispersion-strengthened metals and alloys and (3) consideration of the best microstructure for toughness of the bulk material.

It seems likely that composite materials will be developed for strong, wear-resistant implants of the future. Brittle, elastically strong fibers, perhaps of refractory oxides, will be bound in an inert elastically rigid metal such as titanium. It is useful to consider more closely such a composite with aligned fibers. As tensile force is applied, the strains in the fibers and in the matrix are virtually equal. The stress within the fibers, however, is enormously greater than that in the matrix. The difference is so marked that an estimate of the breaking strength of the composite shows a negligible contribution by the matrix. When the fibers are highly stressed, some which have cracks will break. The unique attribute of the composite is that such a crack is insignificant, since propagation is hindered by the softness of the matrix, and if the adhesion of the matrix to the fiber is poor, a crack propagating across a fiber will be deflected along the weak fiber/matrix interface and rendered harmless for tensile failure of the composite. For the crack to propagate across the specimen, either all the fibers would have to fail in the same plane or the fibers would have to be pulled out of the matrix as they broke. The first possibility is extremely unlikely and, while composites do fail in tension by pulling out of the fibers, this requires considerable work and contributes significantly to the work of fracture in fiber-reinforced materials.

So far the discussion has centered on the strength and failure of a composite under tension in a direction parallel to the fibers. When the material is subjected to compression parallel to the fibers, it fails by buckling and shear. For compressive loading the stiffness of the fibers should be high to resist buckling, and the fiber/matrix interface should show great adhesion to resist splitting. However, for the material to resist cracking under tension, a weak interface is required. Thus, for resistance to both tension and compression some compromise must be adopted.

Compromise is also required when a composite is to resist shearing forces at an angle to the fibers. The composite is significantly less able to resist shear than tension, and the strength of a composite tends to be highly directional just as wood is strong parallel to the grain and weak at right angles to it. Composites can be laminated, like plywood, to counteract weakness under compression and shear. The laminated material, however, is weaker in any particular direction than it would be if all the fibers were oriented in that direction. The human femoral neck is an outstanding example of a composite in which the fibers are oriented in several directions to resist a complex stress geometry, and it has recently become technically possible to produce commercial materials which reproduce this multiaxial strength. These are under intense scrutiny to assess their possible use for surgical implants.

When fibers of an extremely brittle material such as glass are used in a composite, they will always be marred by some flaws. The application of stress to such a composite causes failure at some of the fibers before others. Obviously the parts of a broken fiber close to the break will not support any load. A short distance from the break, however, the unbroken parts of that same fiber will carry as much load as the surrounding unbroken fibers. When the fiber breaks, the two ends attempt to pull away from each other but are prevented from doing so by the adhesion of the matrix to the fiber, and the flow of the matrix parallel to the stress counteracts the tendency of the fiber to relax. Shear forces come into play and build stress back into the broken fiber. Thus the principle of combined action would be realized even if all the fibers were broken. The same effect is also achieved with large numbers of small fibers. Composites can thus be made with a short length of fiber, none of which traverses the entire specimen. The use of numerous small fibers allows multidirectional orientation and strength to be achieved. Furthermore, short single crystal whiskers, the strongest materials known, may be used for reinforcement. Whisker-reinforced composites have shown remarkable properties in the laboratory, although commercial techniques are not yet available for their application in the surgical implant field.

Fibers of graphite and boron now in production are more than twice as stiff as steel. With a density less than one-third that of steel, they may lead to composite materials which show a stiffness per unit weight very much higher than that of steel. The fibers are also extremely strong; such a composite would also show much greater strength per unit weight than steel.

A further approach to fiber-reinforced materials is to prepare the matrix and the fiber in a single operation by controlled solidification of certain eutectic alloys, so that one phase of the alloy grows into parallel whiskers and the other becomes a matrix for the whiskers. The result is a whisker-reinforced composite of great strength. One such alloy consists of niobium carbide whiskers in a niobium matrix. It provides a new approach to the development of strong, wear-resistant alloys for use in many fields, including orthopaedic surgery.

Creep

From the discussion above, it might seem that a given stress always produces the same strain, for no matter how long it is applied. This is never strictly true and not even approximately true at high temperatures. Plastic glide is a form of flow, like fluid flow, except that the atomic movements are crystallographically organized, and it can occur, as *creep,* at constant stress. Closely related to creep is *stress relaxation,* the slow replacement of elastic strain by plastic strain at constant total strain, which, for example, may cause high temperature bolts to lose their grip with time. The low strain rates associated with creep, compared with the high rates resulting from the movement of dislocations under stress, indicate that creep is a thermally activated process. The creep strain produced depends on the experimental temperature, and creep rates at a given stress usually double or treble for each 10°C rise in temperature. For implant alloys exposed to body temperature or the temperature required for heat sterilization, creep does not present a significant problem, since appreciable creep rates only occur in most metals at temperatures approaching one-half of the absolute melting point. As might be anticipated, creep is more important in polymers, since at room temperature they are much nearer to their melting points. Furthermore, many plastics readily undergo creep in the elastic region, under the application of very low stresses. In many such cases, the strain is largely recoverable, given sufficient time after removal of the load; this phenomenon is called *viscoelasticity.*

METALS AVAILABLE FOR IMPLANTATION

Despite the great number of metals and alloys known to man, remarkably few warrant even preliminary consideration for use as implantable materials. The highly corrosive environment combined with the poor tolerance of the body to even minute concentrations of most metallic dissolution products eliminates from discussion all except certain materials based on iron, cobalt, nickel, titanium, tantalum, zirconium, silver, gold and the noble metals. Of this group, tantalum and the noble metals do not have suitable mechanical properties for the construction of most orthopaedic tools and implants, while zirconium is in general too expensive. The following discussion is limited to potentially useful alloys.

All of the implantable metallic materials are used as alloys, either wholly of metallic compo-

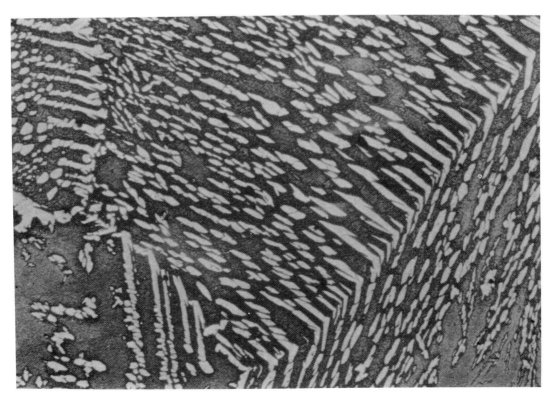

Figure 2-18. Photomicrograph of a 60:40 brass alloy is shown, etched in alcoholic ferric chloride. ×50. (Reproduced with permission of D. F. Williams and R. O. Roaf.[18])

nents or containing some minor amounts of non-metallic elements such as carbon, sulfur or oxygen. The precise composition of an alloy has a profound effect on its phase structure and hence on its properties. For example, copper and nickel are very similar elements, with face-centered cubic structures and roughly the same atomic radius. Each is continuously soluble in the other by lattice substitution over the whole range of composition, giving a single phase FCC solid solution. In other cases, if the metals involved are of less similar size and structure, the range of solubility is limited, and a number of intermediate phases may be formed. The phase structures are usually readily distinguished by optical microscopy of polished and etched surfaces. For example, Figure 2-18 shows the duplex structure of a brass containing 60% copper and 40% zinc.

Some of the nonmetals (*e.g.,* carbon, nitrogen) have atomic radii significantly smaller than most metals and, instead of combining to form alloys by substitution, they form interstitial alloys by fitting into the spaces between the close-packed atoms of the parent metal. Even so, solubility is usually limited to a few per cent, and is strictly controlled by size considerations. Again, if the solubility limit is exceeded, a second phase usually separates with a nonmetallic structure.

Steels

The most common example of interstitial alloying is the case of carbon in iron, where the solubility limit is less than 0.02% at ambient temperature. Beyond this limit the stable phase is *cementite,* iron carbide (Fe_3C) which contains 6.7% carbon. This is the basic alloy system of the steels.[2] The carbon steels usually used contain between 0.15 and 1.5% carbon and may consist of just two phases, ferrite, the saturated solution of carbon in BCC α-iron, and cementite. On the other hand, iron is polymorphic, and different phase structures are stable at different temperatures (Fig. 2-19A). Above 910°C, iron exists as the FCC γ-phase called austenite. Austenite can contain more carbon in solid solution than ferrite, the maximum solubility being 2.06% at 1147°C. If the austenite is cooled slowly, the atoms rearrange themselves to reform ferrite and cementite. If, however, the austenite is cooled rapidly, the atoms may have insufficient time to rearrange before the temperature falls so low that they do not have sufficient energy to move. In this event, the metastable phase *martensite* is formed, a strained body-centered tetragonal structure in which all of the carbon is

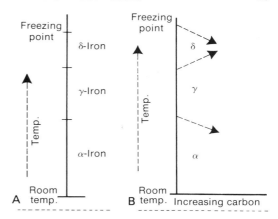

Figure 2-19. *A.* The constitutional diagram for iron is shown. As molten iron cools, initially, it freezes or solidifies as δ-iron or ferrite, with a body-centered cubic (BCC) structure. On further cooling it converts first to γ-iron, or austenite, with a face-centered cubic (FCC) structure; then it converts back to BCC, known as α-iron. (Reproduced with permission of C. O. Bechtol, A. B. Ferguson, Jr., and P. G. Laing.[19]) *B.* The effect of carbon on the constitution of iron is shown. The addition of small quantities of carbon depresses the freezing point of molten iron, elevates the temperature at which BCC converts to FCC and depresses the temperature at which the alloy reverts to the BCC structure. It thereby widens the austenitic range. (Reproduced with permission of C. O. Bechtol, A. B. Ferguson, Jr., and P. G. Laing.[19])

retained in solution. Martensite is thus much harder than either austenite or ferrite, and is widely used to provide a hardened steel to take a cutting edge.

Much more complex phase structures can be produced by different heat treatment cycles, all of which have their place in the engineering use of steels. Further alloying additions may considerably alter the relationships between ferrite, austenite and martensite and the other phases, and may also have an important effect on the mechanical properties and the corrosion behavior exhibited by ferrous alloys. The only ferrous alloys which are of practical importance in orthopaedic surgery are the stainless steels, and the effects of each of the principal alloying elements which are combined in the stainless steels are considered in turn.

Carbon

The addition of carbon to iron lowers the melting point, raises the temperature at which austenite is formed on cooling and lowers the temperature at which ferrite is formed on cool-

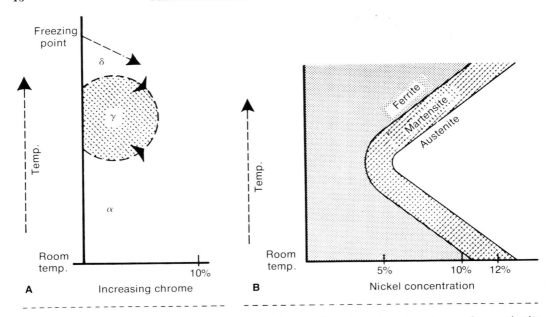

Figure 2-20. *A*. In the closed loop of austenite, the influence of supplementary chromium on the constitution of low carbon steel is shown. With elevation of chromium concentration the temperature at which BCC transforms to FCC is elevated and then lowered. Conversely with a diminishing concentration of chromium conversion back to BCC occurs initially at a lower temperature but subsequently at an elevated temperature. In this way the austenite range forms a closed loop. (Reproduced with permission of C. O. Bechtol, A. B. Ferguson, Jr., and P. G. Laing.[19]) *B*. The effect of supplementary nickel to a chrome steel with concentrations of chromium exceeding the range at which the closed austenitic loop prevails is shown. With higher concentrations of nickel, the austenitic structure FCC reverts to a stable phase at room temperature. There is an intermediate range, however, when cooling the austenitic structure partially transforms it into ferrite and forms the hard martensitic steels. (Reproduced with permission of C. O. Bechtol, A. B. Ferguson, Jr., and P. G. Laing.[19])

ing. Thus increasing carbon content has the effect of increasing the temperature range over which the austenite phase is stable. These effects are shown schematically in Figure 2-19*B*. In addition, particularly in the ferrite region, the carbon may exist in discrete carbides. In the simple binary system the phase formed is cementite as described above, but in many alloy steels the carbon has a greater affinity for some of the other alloying elements and may preferentially form carbides of chromium, for example. The carbide-forming tendencies in this latter case may be so great under certain circumstances that the matrix becomes depleted in chromium, and the corrosion resistance of steels in which this occurs is seriously jeopardized.

Chromium

Chromium itself has a remarkable resistance to corrosion because of the formation of a compact, resistant film of chromium oxide. It is also freely soluble in iron, to which it is able to confer a similar resistance to corrosion because above quite low concentrations of chromium the same resistant film is formed on the surface of the alloy. Addition of chromium alone to iron first expands the range of austenite stability, but then contracts it markedly. Above 13% chromium, ferrite is the stable phase at all temperatures (Fig. 2-20*A*), although more chromium is required to give an α-phase at all temperatures if carbon is present. These alloys are the ferritic stainless steels. If, for example, 3% of nickel is added to a 13% chromium steel, the stable structure is austenitic at high temperatures and ferritic at low temperatures. If these alloys are quenched rather than slowly cooled, or if they are mechanically worked under appropriate conditions, a martensitic phase is formed. The martensitic stainless steels are strong, and can take and retain a cutting edge, but they are less corrosion-resistant than the austenitic steels. For orthopaedic bone screws, partial conversion of austenite to martensite by mechanical working during manufacture appreciably augments the thread strength.

Table 2-2

Composition and Mechanical Properties of Metal Alloys for Surgical Implants

	Stainless Steel ASTM F55 or F56 316 or 316 L: Wrought	CO-CR ASTM F75 ASTM F75 (Vitallium, Zimalloy Vinertium, Allivum, Protasul-2): Cast	CO-CR ASTM F90 (Protasul-10:) Wrought
Composition (weight %)			
Carbon	0.08 max. (0.03 max.)	0.35 max.	0.05–0.15
Manganese	2.00 max.	1.0 max.	2.0 max.
Phosphorus	0.03 max	—	—
Sulfur	0.03 max.	—	—
Silicon	0.75 max.	1.00 max.	1.00 max.
Tungsten	—	—	14–16
Cobalt	—	Bal. (57.4–65)	Bal. (46–53)
Chromium	17–20	27–30	19–21
Nickel	10–14	2.5 max.	9–11
Molybdenum	2–4	5–7	—
Iron	Bal. (59–70)	0.75 max.	3.0 max.
Properties			
Hardness	R_B85–95	R_C25–34	R_B98–100
Hardness (CW)[a]	R_C30	—	R_C65
UTS	80,000 psi	95–105,000	130,000
UTS (CW)	140,000	—	250,000
0.2% YS	35,000	65,000	55,000
0.2% YS (CW)	115,000	—	190,000
Max. strain	55%	8%	50%
Max. strain (CW)	22%	—	10%
Modulus (0.2%)	17.5–57.5×10^6 psi	32.5×10^6	27.5–95×10^6

	MP35N AMS 5758 Vacuum Remelt: Cast-Wrought	Titanium (pure) ASTM F67 Cast-Wrought	Titanium 6Al-4V Alloy ASTM F136 Cast-Wrought
Composition (weight %)			
Carbon	0.25 max.	0.10 max.	0.08 max.
Manganese	0.15 max.	—	—
Phosphorus	0.015 max.	—	—
Sulfur	0.01 max.	—	—
Silicon	0.15 max.	—	—
Oxygen	—	0.45 max.	0.13 max.
Cobalt	Bal. (30.25–38)	—	—
Chromium	19–21	—	—
Nickel	33–37	—	—
Molybdenum	9–10.5	—	—
Iron	1.0 max.	0.5 max.	0.25 max.
Aluminum	—	—	5.5–6.5
Vanadium	—	—	3.5–4.5
Titanium	—	Bal. (99+)	Bal. (88.5–92)
Properties			
Hardness	R_C50 (R_C8)	R_B100	Depends on surface finish
UTS	125,000 (325,000) psi	90,000	125,000–130,000
0.2% YS	60,000 (235,000)	80,000	115,000–120,000
Max. strain	70% (10%)	18%	10%
Modulus (0.2%)	30–117.5×10^6 psi	40×10^6	60×10^6

[a] CW indicates the value obtained for maximal cold reduction. Modulus (0.2%) is the apparent Young modulus at 0.2% strain.

Table 2-3
Mechanical Properties of Various Materials

	Tensile Strength (N/m^2)	Yield Strength (N/m^2)	Elongation at Fracture (%)	Hardness (V.P.N.)	Young's Modulus (n/m^2)	Shear Modulus (N/m^2)	Fatigue Limit (N/m^2)
Metals							
316 Stainless steel, annealed	$6.5 \cdot 10^8$	$2.8 \cdot 10^8$	45	190	$21 \cdot 10^{10}$	$8.4 \cdot 10^{10}$	$2.8 \cdot 10^8$
316 Stainless steel, cold-worked	$10.0 \cdot 10^8$	$7.5 \cdot 10^8$	9	325	$23 \cdot 10^{10}$	—	$3.0 \cdot 10^8$
Wrought cobalt-chromium alloy, cold worked	$15.4 \cdot 10^8$	$10.5 \cdot 10^8$	9	450	$24 \cdot 10^{10}$	—	$4.9 \cdot 10^8$
Cast cobalt-chromium alloy	$6.9 \cdot 10^8$	$4.0 \cdot 10^8$	8	300	$24 \cdot 10^{10}$	—	$3.0 \cdot 10^8$
MP35N	$16.7 \cdot 10^8$	$7.8 \cdot 10^8$	13	—	$24 \cdot 10^{10}$	—	—
Titanium 160, annealed	$7.1 \cdot 10^8$	$4.7 \cdot 10^8$	30	—	$12 \cdot 10^{10}$	$4.6 \cdot 10^{10}$	$3.0 \cdot 10^8$
Ti-6Al-4 V alloy	$10.0 \cdot 10^8$	$9.7 \cdot 10^8$	12	—	$12 \cdot 10^{10}$	—	—
Plastics							
Nylon 66	$8.5 \cdot 10^7$		90		$2.8 \cdot 10^9$	$1.0 \cdot 10^9$	
Polymethyl methacrylate	$7.0 \cdot 10^7$		5		$3.0 \cdot 10^8$	$1.1 \cdot 10^9$	
Polypropylene	$3.5 \cdot 10^7$		500		—	—	
Polyethylene (H.D.)	$3.0 \cdot 10^7$		800		$0.4.10^9$	$0.14.10^9$	
Polytetrafluoroethylene (PTFE)	$2.3 \cdot 10^7$		600		$0.5 \cdot 10^9$	$0.18 \cdot 10^9$	
Silicone rubber	$0.5 \cdot 10^7$		600		—	—	

Nickel

Addition of nickel to chromium steels widens the austenite range again (Fig. 2-20B), and also tends to lower the tensile strength and hardness and decrease the rate of work hardening. If the combined addition of nickel and chromium is at least 24% and neither component is less than 8%, the steel is austenitic at all temperatures. The austenitic stainless steels are the most corrosion-resistant of the stainless steels. Since the nickel expands the austenite range, it permits the addition of larger amounts of chromium and also of molybdenum, both of which impart greater strength and corrosion resistance, especially for exposure in acid- and chloride-containing solutions.

For use in surgical implants the only alloys recommended are the molybdenum-bearing austenitic steels with 18 to 20% chromium and 10 to 14% nickel. Recommended alloys are AISI (American Iron and Steel Institute) type 316, or 316L, with up to 2.5% molybdenum, and type 317, with up to 3.5% molybdenum. These are fully characterized in Tables 2-2 and 2-3 within the specifications compiled by ASTM,[20] the British Standards Institution[21] and standardization organizations in many other countries. Published documents from such organizations clearly specify the recommended compositions, mechanical properties and the accepted manufacturing practices, testing and labeling procedures for all orthopaedic implants made in these materials.

Within the range of acceptable surgical grades of austenitic stainless steel, considerable variation in grain structure is encountered. Figure 2-21A is a photomicrograph of a recrystallized type 316L stainless steel from a surgical implant. The fine grain structure with minimal inclusions is evident. In contrast, Figure 2-21B is a photomicrograph of a Spanish surgical grade stainless steel alloy which is not of remelted quality. Numerous inclusions are seen. The inclusions may affect both the mechanical properties and the corrosion resistance. Figure 2-21C is a photomicrograph of a cold-worked implant made of vacuum-remelted type 316L stainless steel. Comparison of Figure 2-21A with Figure 2-21C

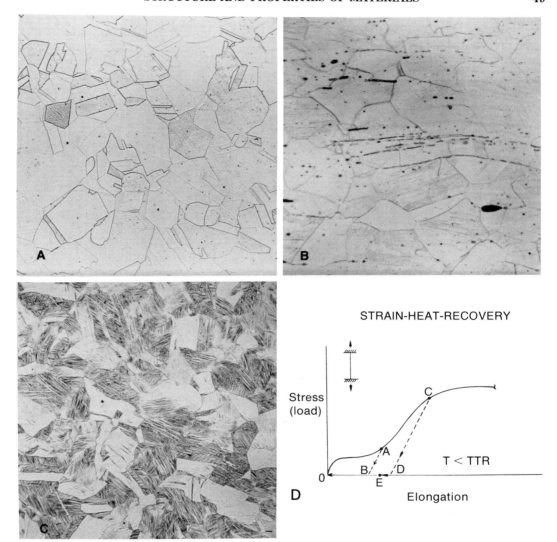

STRAIN-HEAT-RECOVERY

Figure 2-21. *A.* Photomicrograph of the grain structure of American Iron and Steel Institute (AISI) 316L stainless steel of recrystallized quality that was prepared from a surgical implant. ×100. (Reproduced with permission of Miss O. Pöhler.) *B.* Photomicrograph showing the grain structure of a surgical grade stainless steel of a Spanish implant that was not a remelted quality. ×360. (Reproduced with permission of Miss O. Pöhler.) *C.* Photomicrograph of the grain structure of a cold-worked implant as shown which is constructed of stainless steel type 316L of remelted quality. ×160. (Reproduced with permission of Miss O. Pöhler.) *D.* Changes in dimensions for a Nitinol alloy after plastic deformation, when heated above its transition temperature. (Reproduced with permission of Dr. James Hughes.)

readily reveals the changes in microstructure engendered by cold working.

Nickel-based Alloys

While nickel-based alloys are not currently used for orthopaedic implants, both their mechanical properties and their corrosion resistance suggest that they would be satisfactory for the manufacture of implants which are at pres-

ent made from the less expensive, but otherwise comparable, stainless steel. Pure nickel is a FCC metal with good corrosion resistance and moderate strength.[22] There are many types of nickel alloy available, but two have been considered for orthopaedic purposes. The first group are the Inconels, nickel-chromium alloys containing about 76% nickel, which have high resistance to both corrosion and wear. The second group are the Nimonic alloys, based on nickel, chromium and iron. These are rather complex alloys and were designed as creep-resistant materials. Not only are these alloys inert, they are also, or may be, precipitation-strengthened. Typical of this group of alloys is Nimonic 75 which contains roughly 20% chromium and 5% iron, with small additions of other elements and the balance nickel.

Travis and Johnson[23] have described the equiatomic nickel-gold alloy, which has excellent strength and inertness and is biologically acceptable. The alloy would appear to be prohibitively expensive for normal use. Another remarkable nickel alloy, the nickel-titanium "memory" alloy Nitinol, has recently been the subject of detailed study for its applications in orthopaedics. This alloy has the ability to return precisely to its original dimensions after plastic deformation, if heated above its transition temperature, as shown in Figure 2-21D. The alloy has been studied by Castleman et al.[24] for its potential as a compression plate for internal fixation of fractures. Hughes and Perren* have studied its potential as a fixation device for femoral neck fractures in osteoporotic bone. Another possible application is the fixation of the spine in scoliosis, or spinal deformity. In all of these situations, the "memory" effect can be used to reduce the length of all or part of the device to provide firm anchorage or to correct deformity. The transition temperature can be varied widely by small adjustments in composition, and it can be adjusted to approximately body temperature so that tissue is not damaged by excessive heat. Only a brief application of heat is required for transformation. Both of the authors cited above report that the alloy has excellent corrosion resistance and compatibility with tissues both in experimental animals and in cell and tissue cultures *in vitro*.

Cobalt-based Alloys

Cobalt is also polymorphic with a HCP α-form stable at room temperature and a FCC β-structure at high temperature. Chromium is readily soluble in cobalt, so that a large range of cobalt-chromium alloys is available. Carbon has an effect on cobalt rather similar to that on iron. In general, surgical alloys consist of a matrix of cobalt-rich solid solution containing chromium-rich carbides. The other principal alloying elements are molybdenum and tungsten which, like

chromium, raise the α- to β-transition temperature, and iron and nickel which depress this temperature. Two main types of cobalt-based alloys are used in surgery. Stellite 21 consists typically of 61 to 62% cobalt, 28 to 29% chromium, with 5 to 7% molybdenum, 1.5 to 2% nickel and less than 0.6% iron. As cast it has a duplex α-β-structure seen in Figure 2-22. When annealed it is entirely β-phase. Despite recent improvements,[25] this alloy has a high rate of work hardening and is therefore difficult to machine and must be cast. Expensive tests for casting defects must therefore be carried out on every implant. The relative cost of cobalt-chromium-molybdenum is slightly higher than that of austenitic stainless steel, although this is not a major factor. A somewhat similar alloy, Stellite 25, is a machinable alloy containing typically 20% chromium, 10% nickel, 15% tungsten and the balance, cobalt. As shown below, this alloy has superior mechanical properties to cast cobalt-chromium-molybdenum, although it is somewhat less resistant to crevice corrosion. A detailed survey of the compositions of cobalt-based alloys is shown in Tables 2-2 and 2-3.

Another new alloy, MP35N, is a nickel-cobalt-based alloy characterized by a high tensile strength combined with good ductility, toughness and corrosion resistance.[26, 27] For several years it has been used satisfactorily in Europe under the trade name Protasul-10. Its nominal composition is 35% nickel, 35% cobalt, 20% chromium and 10% molybdenum. Like other multiphase materials it is easily fabricated when annealed. However, it work-hardens rapidly when machined, and this hampers certain techniques of fabrication. It is considerably more expensive than austenitic steel, but in view of its superior strength and inertness it is likely to increase in popularity. Its microstructure is shown in Figure 2-22E.

Titanium-based Alloys

In pure form titanium has a HCP α-structure at room temperature which transforms into a BCC β-structure at 880°C. In fact, commercially pure forms of titanium contain small amounts of other elements, mainly oxygen and iron, which markedly affect the grain structure and the mechanical properties (Tables 2-2 and 2-3). The microstructures of two commercially pure titanium implants are shown in Figure 2-23, A to C.

The addition of elements such as chromium, molybdenum, vanadium, niobium and tantalum affects the α-β-transition temperature (Fig. 2-24), and by substantial addition of these ele-

---

* J. L. Hughes and S. M. Perren, private communication, 1975.

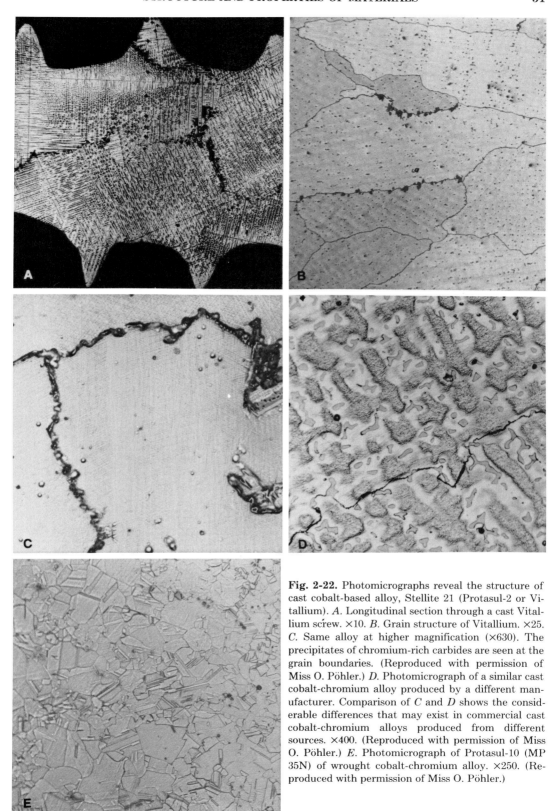

Fig. 2-22. Photomicrographs reveal the structure of cast cobalt-based alloy, Stellite 21 (Protasul-2 or Vitallium). *A.* Longitudinal section through a cast Vitallium screw. ×10. *B.* Grain structure of Vitallium. ×25. *C.* Same alloy at higher magnification (×630). The precipitates of chromium-rich carbides are seen at the grain boundaries. (Reproduced with permission of Miss O. Pöhler.) *D.* Photomicrograph of a similar cast cobalt-chromium alloy produced by a different manufacturer. Comparison of *C* and *D* shows the considerable differences that may exist in commercial cast cobalt-chromium alloys produced from different sources. ×400. (Reproduced with permission of Miss O. Pöhler.) *E.* Photomicrograph of Protasul-10 (MP 35N) of wrought cobalt-chromium alloy. ×250. (Reproduced with permission of Miss O. Pöhler.)

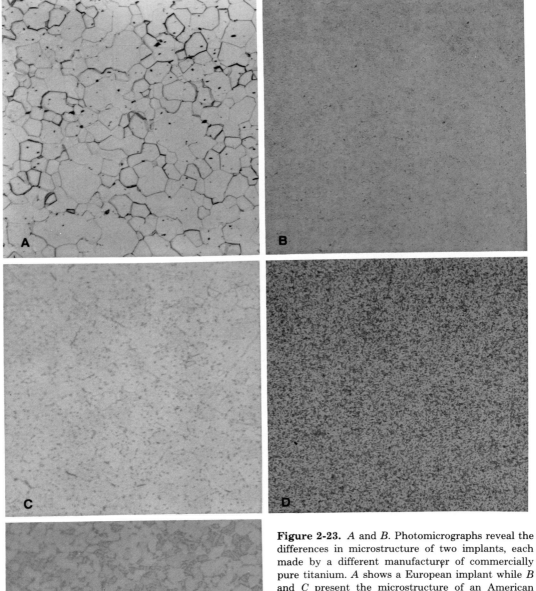

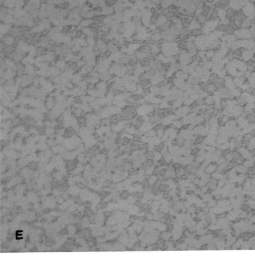

Figure 2-23. *A* and *B*. Photomicrographs reveal the differences in microstructure of two implants, each made by a different manufacturer of commercially pure titanium. *A* shows a European implant while *B* and *C* present the microstructure of an American titanium bone screw at two different magnifications. While the pure titanium is comprised primarily of a HCP α-structure, the alloys seen in *B* and *C* contain a fine dispersion of another phase. Figure 2-23*A*, ×100. Figure 2-23*B*, ×100. Figure 2-23*C*, ×500. (Figure 2-23*A* reproduced with permission of Miss O. Pöhler; Figure 2-23, *B* and *C*, reproduced with permission of Zimmer-USA.) *D* and *E*. Microstructure of an H-Beam nail manufactured from Ti-6A1-4V alloy. Figure 2-23*D* (×100) shows the fine dispersion of the α- and β-structures while Figure 2-23*E* (×500) reveals the microstructures of the individual phases. (Reproduced with permission of Zimmer-USA.)

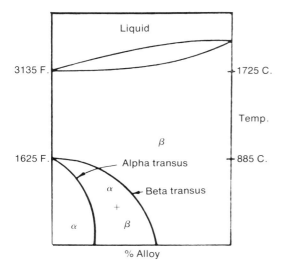

Figure 2-24. A schematic phase diagram for a representative titanium alloy is shown. α refers to the small HCP α-structure while the β refers to the BCC structure. Under certain conditions duplex alloys of α- and β-combinations are stable. (Reproduced with permission of C. O. Bechtol, A. B. Ferguson, Jr., and P. G. Laing.[19])

ments the β-structure can be made stable at room temperature.[28] With intermediate amounts of alloying elements, both phases may be stable, as seen in Figure 2-23, D and E which show the microstructure of Ti-6A1-4V alloy. The phase diagram for a representative titanium alloy is shown in Figure 2-24. The duplex alloys are substantially stronger than pure titanium, and they have been used with advantage in implant surgery primarily in the form of Ti-6A1-4V alloy. In addition they are easily weldable, machinable and extraordinarily inert in body fluids. Their principal drawback is poor resistance to erosion, which makes them unsatisfactory for the bearing surfaces of total joint replacements. Some examples are shown in Tables 2-2 and 2-3.

Zirconium-based Alloys

Zirconium is very similar to titanium. Like the latter it shows a HCP α-structure at room temperature and undergoes allotropic transformation to β-zirconium, a BCC phase, at elevated temperature.[29] Its strength rivals that of titanium and it can be cold-worked. It can be machined almost as easily as stainless steel. On the other hand, it is considerably more costly than titanium and thus appears unlikely to be employed widely for the construction of surgical implants.

Tantalum-based Alloys

Tantalum is an inert metal, closely related to niobium, with which it is usually found.[30] It has excellent fabricability, even under conditions of the operating room. In the past, it has gained a reputation for rapid corrosion *in vivo*. With substantial modern improvements in the techniques of manufacture, however, its corrosion resistance is no longer suspect. It is satisfactory for use as surgical wire or staples and as pliable sheets. It is not sufficiently rigid for many other orthopaedic applications.

The Noble Metals

Apart from silver, the noble metals—platinum, palladium, iridium, rhodium and gold—show excellent resistance to corrosion in chloride-containing solutions.[31] Silver dissolves slowly with the formation of innocuous corrosion products. As pure metals the noble metals show unsatisfactory strength for applications in orthopaedic surgery. Alloys of the noble metals, however, such as platinum—10% iridium, show adequate strength and other mechanical properties but they are prohibitively expensive.

NONMETALLIC MATERIALS

The nonmetallic materials include a wide and varied array of substances, but for present purposes they may usefully be organized into the amorphous glasses, the crystalline ceramics and carbon and the polymeric materials. To these are added consideration of the potentially useful composite materials and of plaster of Paris. While the latter is not an implantable material, it is so widely used in orthopaedic surgery, often in conjunction with implanted materials, that some consideration of its properties seems appropriate.

Glasses

Glasses have not been widely used as implantable materials for orthopaedic surgery, and it may seem irrelevant to devote much space to this group of materials. In the past decade, however, there has been perhaps more research into the possible uses of glasses in this field than into any single similar group of materials. The explanation of this intense interest is the similarity between the elements which constitute certain glasses and ceramics and those of which bone matrix is comprised. Some glasses exhibit slow dissolution of the free surface which favors the development of adhesive bonds with adjacent

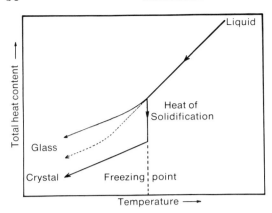

Figure 2-25. The solidification of liquid can produce either a crystal or a glass. When a liquid solidifies into a crystal, it releases a burst of heat at some particular temperature which identifies its freezing point. This burst, or heat of solidification, coincides with the final ordering of atoms or molecules into a crystalline array. Liquids that cool to the rigid state without crystallizing are called glasses. Glasses that are cooled slowly (*broken grain curve*) more closely approach the crystalline state than glasses that are cooled rapidly (*solid gray curve*). (Reproduced with permission of R. J. Charles.[32])

bone. With other compositions not only does it seem to be possible to prepare a synthetic bone mineral, but even a biodegradable form of material for bone replacement which will be dissolved by conventional mechanisms of bone degradation. Furthermore, it is probable that the degradation products could be converted by the bone cells into live bone matrix so that the implant is wholly converted into a biological supportive structure. This is perhaps the most exciting concept of the century in biomaterials. It is described in detail in Chapter 16. The glasses and ceramics are therefore given emphasis not because of the extent of their present application but because of their great potential for the future.

The Structure of Glass

The classification of solids is largely determined by the geometrical arrangement of their atoms or molecules. Glasses are distinguished from other solids by their lack of crystallinity in the solid state. It is useful to contrast the crystallization of a solidifying metal with solidification of a glass which maintains its amorphous structure even when solid.

If a pure liquid metal such as titanium, is slowly cooled, a sudden release of heat to the surroundings occurs at the freezing temperature

(Fig. 2-25). At the same time the atoms which were in a substantially disordered state in the liquid solidify to form ordered crystalline arrays. The release of latent heat is in fact the work done by the attractive forces between the atoms when the atoms move from random to ordered sites in the system. In fact, the specific volume of the liquid decreases continuously during the initial cooling, indicating that gradual ordering proceeds in the cooling liquid phase as the solidification temperature is approached.

Before a liquid can crystallize, it must contain "seeds" or minute crystal nuclei. These seeds often consist of groups of atoms attached to foreign particles in the melt or to irregularities on the surface of the container. Under certain circumstances, however, small random groups of atoms will aggregate spontaneously to form a crystal nucleus on which other atoms can deposit. With extremely small aggregates, the relatively large contribution from the surface energy may swamp the decrease in energy due to ordering of the atoms and the total energy per unit weight may be too high for the aggregates to be stable. If a critical size can be reached, there is a net decrease in energy and the seed is able to continue to grow, with a reduction of the overall energy of the system. The critical nucleus size is temperature-dependent and, in order for the probability of such an occurrence to be significant, the melt must be supercooled somewhat below the thermodynamic freezing temperature.

To change their configuration, the atoms or molecules of a liquid must be able to move past one another. For many common liquids, the individual atoms or molecules approximate to spheres, and sliding proceeds with ease. The attractive forces between the atoms or molecules are sufficient to move them into place at normal rates of cooling, and in such liquids crystal nuclei form and grow with only a few degrees of supercooling. Certain liquids, however, become particularly viscous near the freezing point and formation and growth of nuclei are prevented even when the cooling rate is low. Unable to crystallize, these liquids follow the supercooled route to the solid state (Fig. 2-25). As the viscosity increases with the fall in temperature, their molecular structure lags further behind as the temperature continues to fall. The structure at any instant, therefore, corresponds to the equilibrium structure at a temperature much higher than the actual temperature.

If cooling is continued until the glass becomes rigid, random structures characteristic of the liquid at much higher temperatures will be frozen in. As the cooling rate is increased, the glass structure corresponds to the equilibrium liquid structure at progressively higher temperatures. Thus the structure and properties of glasses depend both on their composition and on their thermal history, and the commercial manufacture of glasses requires precise schedules of quenching and annealing if predictable products are to be obtained.[33, 34]

Mechanical considerations suggest that a structure consisting of flexible chains or of chains cross-linked into three-dimensional networks should be particularly conducive to high liquid viscosities and inhibited crystallization. Thus the elements sulfur, selenium and tellurium, which form many membered ring structures and long chain molecules, form glasses readily. Similarly the oxides of silicon, boron, germanium, arsenic and phosphorus, which form network structures, and the silicates, borates and phosphates are ready glass formers. Many organic compounds behave similarly, and some alcohols, glycerol and glucose can be supercooled to form glasses, as can many polymeric materials.

The unit of structure of the glass-forming oxides is a small, highly charged positive ion, for example, silicon or boron, surrounded by a polyhedron of oxygen ions. In the solid or liquid, sharing of the oxygen ions at their corners bonds large numbers of the polyhedra together. Thus in silica, each silicon is surrounded by a tetrahedron of oxygen ions, and tetrahedra are bound together by sharing the oxygen at their corners. The solid may be crystalline, if the tetrahedra are arranged appropriately, as in crystobalite, or glassy if the ordering is prevented. Similar criteria apply to the triangular array of oxygen ions which surround boron in B_2O_3 (Fig. 2-26A, B). Zachariasen's rules for ready glass formation by oxides suggest that each oxygen should be linked to no more than 2 positive ions, not more than 3 or 4 oxygen ions should surround each positive ion, the oxygen polyhedra should share corners rather than edges (i.e., 2 positive ions should not share more than 1 oxygen ion between them) and enough of the polyhedra should share corners to make a three-dimensional network of bonds. The oxides which obey these rules have virtually the same energy in the crystalline and glassy phases, so the glassy phase is as stable as the crystalline form.

Such pure oxide glasses, like their crystalline

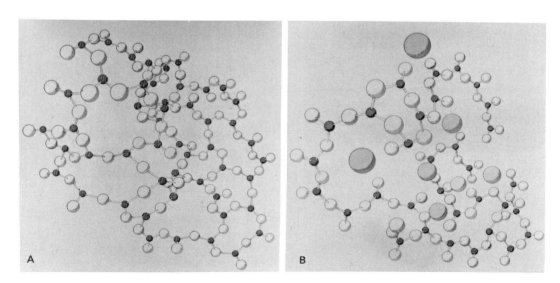

Figure 2-26. *A.* The schematic diagram shows the structure of a pure oxide glass with a random three-dimensional network in which each oxygen atom (*white*) is bonded to 2 atoms of a metal such as boron. Here each metal atom is bonded to 3 oxygen atoms. Other kinds of glass, such as silica glass, produce more complex networks in which each metal atom is bonded to 4 oxygen atoms. (Reproduced with permission of R. J. Charles.[35]) *B.* The schematic diagram shows a flux containing glass with a random three-dimensional network except that flux atoms such as sodium (*unattached gray spheres*) have reduced the amount of cross-linking. Some oxygen atoms therefore are strongly bonded to a single atom and have weaker ties with 1 or more flux atoms which are not shown. Such glasses have a reduced melting point. (Reproduced with permission of R. J. Charles.[35])

counterparts, have high softening temperatures. The extent of cross-linkage can be reduced and the softening temperature lowered by introducing into the melt readily ionizable atoms such as sodium or potassium, which form weak ionic bonds with the oxygen ions and terminate the chains (Fig. 2-26B). These fluxing ions are used extensively in glass technology to lower the melting point, inhibit crystallization and control the viscosity of the glass.

The addition of fluxing and other foreign ions into oxide glasses produces profound changes in structure, and on cooling the melt may separate into phases of markedly different composition. The distribution of such phases after solidification may greatly alter properties such as mechanical strength, chemical inertness, electrical conductivity or optical clarity. By careful manipulation of such phase separation phenomena, it is possible to produce technical glasses with a range of industrially valuable properties. Two examples of crystalline structures in glass-forming substances are shown in Figure 2-27.

A wide variety of two-phase structures are present in many commercial glasses. More recently multiphase "crystallizable" glasses have also become available. After producing the required shape of article, such glasses are subjected to an appropriate heat treatment which converts them into strong and durable structures with a uniform dispersion of fine crystals strengthening the glass matrix. Such materials include Pyroceram, CERVIT and Re-X.[37] They show high strength, great impact resistance and low chemical reactivity.

Most elements can be dissolved in glasses to a considerable degree, and in doing so they ionize to a greater or lesser extent and become involved with the ionic equilibria of the glass. It is no surprise, therefore, that chemical reactions such as precipitation, dissolution, decomposition, ion exchange, oxidation and reduction can be carried out in molten glasses. Moreover, these reactions can be halted at any desired stage. This control enables glasses to be produced which exhibit semiconductivity, photoconductivity, fluorescence, selective ionic transport and many other properties. A detailed description of this aspect of the subject is available elsewhere.[38]

Crystallization of Glass

Glass is metastable with respect to crystalline phases at temperatures below its equilibrium liquidus temperature, which for alkaline silicate

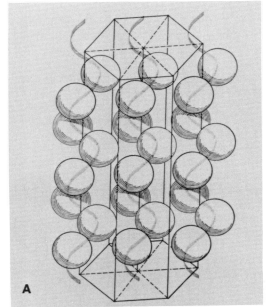

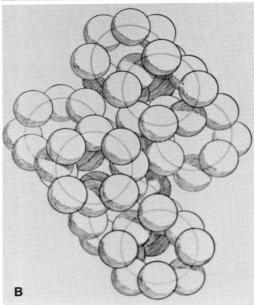

Figure 2-27. Glass-forming substances may crystallize to take the form of spiral chains in a hexagonal array (A) or nests of eight-numbered rings (B). Selenium and tellurium exhibit the spiral structure. Selenium also crystallizes in the ring structure, as does sulfur. When such ring structures are heated in a melt, the rings tend to open and link up into extended chains. If the melt is quickly cooled, the rings do not have time to reform and a glass results. Glasses are also readily produced from spiral chain arrays. (Reproduced with permission of R. J. Charles.[36])

glasses is usually higher than 700°C. Surface crystallization of glass may produce deterioration of the mechanical properties, since nonuniform contraction on cooling may cause high surface stresses to be developed. Glass technologists have evolved empirical criteria for the avoidance of surface crystallization. Recent experimental and theoretical studies on glass crystallization now allow crystallization rates for new compositions to be predicted and the limiting times and temperatures for treatment of the glasses to be defined.

In the discussion of the crystallization of glasses it is useful to consider separately nucleation behavior and crystal growth.

Nucleation. A variety of methods has been used to nucleate uniform crystallization in glass. Fine metal particles formed in the glass can act as centers of crystallization, and thereby enhance the nucleation rate. "Nucleating agents" such as the platinum metals in concentrations of 0.001 to 0.1% catalyze crystallization in lithium silicate glass.* The metal is added to the melt as a compound, after which it decomposes to form a fine dispersion of metal particles about 50 Å in diameter. Other metals such as gold, silver and copper may function similarly.[39] The most commonly used nucleating agent, however, is titanium dioxide, TiO_2, while others include phosphorus pentoxide, P_2O_5[40] and a number of transition metal oxides.[41] Fluorides have a similar application in alumino-silicate glasses[42] and soda-lime glasses.[43] Crystallization may require a two-stage heat treatment, a nucleation treatment just above the annealing temperature, to form the required number and size of nuclei, followed by a higher temperature treatment to permit rapid growth of the crystals.

Chance impurity particles can also nucleate crystals in glasses,[44] and in surface crystallization such impurities are the main source of nucleation. As the melt cools, dust particles can adhere to the surface and provide nucleation sites, and other impurities such as alkalis can attack the surface and provide regions of reduced surface energy, at which nucleation is favored. It is important, therefore, to protect the glass surface from dust and other impurities until it is well below temperatures at which these effects can take place.

Crystal growth. The rate of growth of a crystal from a melt is controlled both by considerations of heat flow and of atomic rearrangement at the growing interface. As the temperature is reduced below the freezing point, the heat transfer from the growing crystal is improved, and the rate of crystallization initially increases. On the other hand, the ease of atomic rearrangement is decreased as the temperature falls, and this has the effect of reducing the rate of crystallization. The observed growth rate therefore passes through a maximum at a critical temperature determined by the balance of the two competing effects.

Theories of varied complexity have been put forward to explain the kinetics of crystallization from the melt. The validity of the various theories remains a matter of considerable controversy, and the reader is referred to a more detailed account elsewhere.[38]

Chemical and Surface Properties

The nature of physical and chemical adsorption onto glass is strongly dependent upon the structure of the surface.[45] In oxide glasses such as silicates the surface provides a high concentration of "dangling" (*i.e.,* unsatisfied) oxide bonds, such as —Si—O—. These react readily with atmospheric water to form —Si—OH groupings or comparable hydroxides of other metals. The thickness and structure of the hydrated layer depend on the composition and thermal history of the glass, its surface treatment after cooling and the humidity of the environment. The surface hydroxyl groups provide the most important sites for the surface chemical reaction of glasses and in particular for adsorption processes. The hydroxyl groups can also be replaced by halogen atoms to give substantially altered surface properties. Consideration of the adsorption processes involves many factors, including *inter alia* the surface change of the silinol groups, the nature and amounts of trace elements in the glass and the pH and chemical constitution of the solution. It is known that the surface chemistry of some glasses enables them to act as catalysts for biochemical reactions, for example, the clotting of blood. On the other hand, there are few observations available which allow this information to be applied to the use of glass implants in a biological environment.

The Strength and Fracture of Glass

Modeling of the bonding forces between atoms has been widely used to estimate the strength of materials.[46] With the strong bonding in glasses,

---

* British Patent No. 863, 569, 1961.

a mathematical determination would suggest an ultimate tensile strength for silica glass of about 2×10^6 psi (1.8×10^{10} N/m^2); the values measured in practice are 5 to 15×10^3 psi (3×10^7 to 10^8 N/m^2). On the other hand, the elastic modulus and compressive strength are high, and reflect the calculated bond strength. The very low tensile strength is typical of most brittle materials, and, as has been suggested earlier, it arises because inherent faults and microcracks at the surface can concentrate the applied stress so that the theoretical strength is exceeded locally at the tip of the crack and failure ensues. Griffith calculated the stress at the tip of the crack, σ_c, as

$$\sigma_c \simeq \sqrt[2]{\frac{L}{R} \cdot \sigma_A}$$

where L is the length of the flaw, R is its root radius and σ_A is the applied tensile stress normal to the plane of fracture.

The inherent flaws in a brittle material, arising by normal handling abrasion, are minute, with root radii of atomic dimensions (approximately 2×10^{-10} m). These produce a dramatic concentration of stress which in brittle materials cannot be dissipated by plastic blunting of the crack. Indeed L/R, and therefore σ_c, increases as the crack grows. The same considerations make thermally induced nonuniform dimensional changes very much more significant in glasses than in metals. In compression, however, inherent defects tend to be closed so that the material may show exceptional strength. Similar principles apply to the mechanical behavior of crystalline ceramics.

The great strength of very fine filaments of glass, which can be produced essentially free from surface flaws, has already been discussed, and provides practical validation of the Griffith approach for the analysis of the strength of glasses.

Strengthening of Glass

Since the marked difference between the theoretical and practical strengths of glasses has been related to the presence of surface defects, a variety of surface treatments has been used to overcome the problem.[47]

Defects may be removed from the glass surface by fire polishing[48] or chemical etching or polishing.[49, 50] The glass is then protected from further damage by the application of a protective coating. These latter, however, are far from perfect, and tend to be too soft and themselves

Table 2-4
Strengthening of Glasses

Methods	Maximum Strengthening Factor
Quench hardening	×6
Ion exchange	×10
Surface crystallization	×17
Ion exchange and surface crystallization	×22
Etching	×30
Fire polishing	×200
Second phase particles	×2
Factor required for theoretical strength	×2000

easily damaged or too hard and induce stresses and surface damage in the glass.

A second type of treatment involves the introduction of compressive stresses into the glass surface to enhance the breaking strength. Compressive stresses may be introduced by rapid cooling,[47] ion exchange with metal ions larger than those in the glass matrix[51-53] and surface crystallization.[54] All of these processes are used commercially. Again, combinations of treatments may provide improved strength and abrasion resistance.[49, 55] None of these steps, however, allows glasses to approach their theoretical strength, as shown in Table 2-4.

An entirely different approach to strengthening of glasses is the introduction of fine crystalline second phase particles.[56] Composites of glass and alumina have been prepared by hot pressing a mixture of 5 μm of borosilicate glass powder with 35 to 44 μm of alumina, and the strength of the glass was thereby doubled. Lange[57] explains the increase in strength in terms of pinning of the propagating crack by the particles, which thus increases the energy required for fracture.

Mechanochemical Failure of Glass

The strength of glass deteriorates when it is held under stress in the atmosphere. The extent of deterioration depends on the amount of water in the air.[58] It occurs by reaction of water with the glass surface, leading to stress-induced dissolution at the tips of surface cracks. Hillig and Charles[59, 60] have explained this "static fatigue" of glass by assuming that the rate of reaction of water with glass controls the rate of change of the crack tip profile. The reaction of water with the silica network allows the load-bearing —Si—O—Si— bonds to be broken to form —Si—OH linkages, with change in shape at the crack tip. Under stress the reaction is accelerated:

$$V = V_0 \exp B_0,$$

where V is the velocity of reaction under stress, V_0 is the velocity of reaction in the absence of stress and B_0 is the measure of the stress susceptibility of the reaction.[61] Fracture is assumed to occur when the stress at the crack tip reaches the theoretical fracture stress of the glass.

On the other hand, in the absence of stress, reaction with the environment tends to blunt the cracks rather than sharpen them. There is thus some small stress at which the crack tip profile is preserved as attack proceeds. At this stress the strength of the glass is independent of time; the stress is called the static fatigue limit. It can be seen then that in a given environment the strength of a glass and the rate of crack growth leading to mechanical failure are closely related to the chemical durability of the glass, a concept quite similar to some types of environment-sensitive failure of metallic materials. The mathematical formulation of engineering design criteria for the use of glasses is thus rendered substantially more complex.[62, 63]

Glasses of Orthopaedic Interest

Of the many types of glasses being studied as possible implantable materials, the calcium phosphate glasses have shown the most promise. In the biological environment, all glasses undergo slow but finite degradation by hydrolysis, and in many cases this may lead to deterioration of mechanical properties or toxic tissue response. This is particularly likely with porous coated structures which show a large surface area but limited ionic diffusion in the interstices. Nevertheless, some workers such as Hensch and Paschall[64, 65] have attempted to exploit this dissolution. Their results are discussed in detail in Chapter 16. In brief, they have observed that the rate of dissolution of glasses can be controlled by modification of their composition. With slow dissolution a firm adhesive bond may develop between the bioglass implant and the bone that is stronger than the cohesive strength of the bone itself. With more rapid dissolution of a porous bioglass, "creeping substitution" may be realized, so that the entire implant is ultimately replaced by live bone.

In addition, intramedullary implants have been coated with porous calcium phosphate glasses to improve fixation by bony ingrowth.[66] Early clinical success has been reported for fem-

oral head replacements. Similar attempts are in progress to obtain superior fixation of soft tissues such as tendons and ligaments to implants[67] (see Chapter 16).

Ceramics and Carbon

The Nature of Ceramics

The term ceramic is applied to two related groups of materials. The first consists of strong, crystalline, high melting pure metallic oxides, carbides, nitrides and borides, in which the large, usually closely packed, anions form the skeleton of the structure, with the smaller metallic ions lodged in the interspaces. Examples appear schematically in Figures 2-28 and 2-29. The second group contains compounds which are mixtures of these materials and which, although not so pure, so strong or so temperature-resistant, provide the basic materials for many areas of commercial high temperature technology. The strength, hardness and thermal resistance of the ceramics arise from their strong directional bonding, which may be ionic or covalent, or mixed, depending on the compound in question. Most ceramic materials are crystalline in nature, although the structures involved are necessarily more complex than those in metallic crystals since atoms of widely different sizes must be accommodated. However, the distinction between those ceramics which are amorphous or

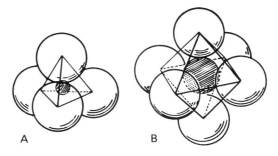

A   B

Figure 2-28. The schematic diagrams show two simple ceramics. Oxygen and metal atoms (or semimetals such as silicon) are the basis of most ceramics. In the simplest ceramics equal numbers of oxygen (*white*) and metal (*gray* or *black*) atoms are packed together in an arrangement that depends largely on the relative sizes of the ionized atoms. In beryllium oxide (*A*) the "coordination number" is 4; each beryllium atom is surrounded by 4 oxygens (and each oxygen atom by 4 beryllium atoms, although only 1 is shown). In magnesium oxide (*B*) each atom has 6 nearest neighbors. The ceramic bond is primarily ionic. Each metal atom surrenders 2 electrons to each oxygen. (Reproduced with permission of J. J. Gilman.[69])

glassy and some of the glasses which have high melting points is somewhat difficult to draw.

Two types of crystalline ceramics, silica and alumina, have received close examination for

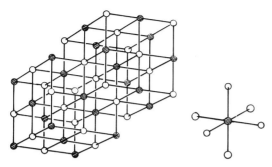

Figure 2-29. The schematic diagrams show the structure of magnesium oxide, or periclase. The ball and stick model (*left*) shows the relative locations of the atoms in the magnesium oxide crystal lattice which is face-centered cubic. The lattice consists of interpenetrating face-centered cubic structures, one of magnesium and one of oxygen (*right*). (Reproduced with permission of J. J. Gilman.[69])

their suitability in orthopaedics. They are considered briefly here; more extensive reviews are available elsewhere.[46, 48]

Silica, SiO_2, is an allotropic compound which, as well as its glassy form, can exist in three crystalline modifications at various temperatures: quartz, crystobalite and tridymite. All the structures contain Si^{4+} ions tetrahedrally surrounded by 4 $O^=$ ions as shown in Figure 2.30A. Polymerization of the $[SiO_4]$ tetrahedra to form a network in three dimensions leads to the crystal structures of the various crystalline modifications (see Fig. 2-30B). In contrast, when the arrangement of the tetrahedra ceases to show appreciable long range order, amorphous silica, or silica glass, results. The pure silica structures are wholly covalently bonded. On the other hand, the $[SiO_4]$ group may form ionic bonds with a number of metal ions, reacting as the silicate ion, SiO_4^{4-}, as seen in Figure 2-30C. For example, magnesium silicate, Mg_2SiO_4, is the important refractory forstenite. If there are insufficient metal cations available to form the stoichiometric compound, some of the $[SiO_4]$

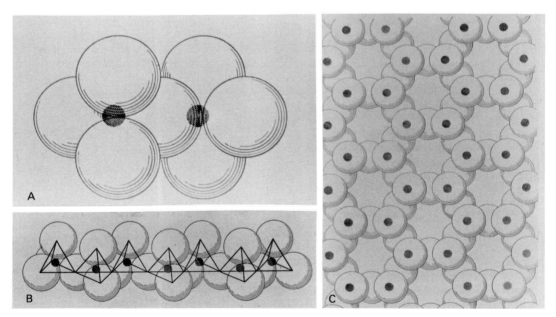

Figure 2-30. *A.* The schematic diagram shows a silicate unit, a primary building block of many ceramics. It consists of a silicon atom surrounded by 4 oxygen atoms in a tetrahedronal arrangement as in beryllium oxide as shown in Figure 2-28A. (Reproduced with permission of J. J. Gilman.[70]) *B.* A chain of silicate groups is shown. Each of the silicon atoms has 4 valence electrons to surrender to each 1 of the 4 surrounding oxygen atoms. Each oxygen atom remains deficient of 1 electron in its outer shell. It can obtain that electron from another silicon atom by linking two groups. (Reproduced with permission of J. J. Gilman.[70]) *C.* Silicate sheet formed by linked chains. Each silicon atom (*gray*) is surrounded by 4 oxygen atoms (*white*). Each tetrahedron shares 3 of its oxygen atoms with 3 other tetrahedrons. A hexagonal pattern of "holes" appears in the sheet. (Reproduced with permission of J. J. Gilman.[70])

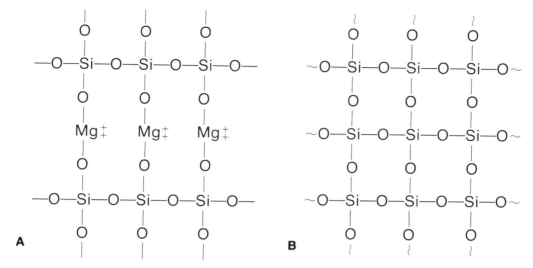

Figure 2-31. *A.* Polymerization of the SiO_4^{-4} tetrahedron has long chains. This chemical diagram should be compared with the same material shown in Figure 2-30C. The ionic bonds across the chains are not as strong as the covalent bonds along the chains. Such structures tend to cleave easily parallel to the chains. The fibrous nature of asbestos is representative of such internal structure. *B.* Extension of the polymerization of the silicate group in two dimensions produces feet-like structures typical of clay minerals, mica and talc. The figure shows a plan view of such a sheet. (Reproduced with permission of J. B. Moss.[5])

groupings undergo partial or complete polymerization to form long chains and network structures, and multivalent metal cations may provide the bridges to cross-link between the chains or network structures. An example of a typical silicate structure is shown in Figures 2-30C and 2-31. The ionic bonds between the chains are not quite as strong as the covalent bonds within the chains, and such structures may cleave easily parallel to the chains, as in asbestos for example. If sheet structures are continued indefinitely, it is possible for all the oxygen atoms to have saturated bonds within the plane, and adjacent sheets are then only held together by weak van der Waals forces. Thus the sheets can readily slide over one another, as occurs, for example, in kaolinite, china clay, which is a hydrated aluminosilicate.

When aluminum hydroxide is heated to a sufficiently high temperature it loses water and forms alumina, Al_2O_3. This is a remarkably inert material, which melts above 2000°C, and is used as a refractory material for industrial applications. Pure alumina is colorless, but it can be colored by traces of transition metal oxides such as Fe_2O_3 or Cr_2O_3. Synthetic rubies are made by mixing Al_2O_3 and Cr_2O_3 powders and dropping them through the flame of an oxyhydrogen torch. Such synthetic jewels are remarkably hard, and have been considered for resurfacing articular joints, although a resilient subarticular surface would have to be interposed between the ruby and the underlying bone to provide a more gradual transition in elastic modulus. An aluminate sheet appears in Figure 2-32A.

As indicated above, most commerical ceramics consist of two or more constituents. These may occur together in nature, or they may be mixed together in manufacture, and they are formed and fired at a high temperature before use. One example, kaolinite, a "laminate" of silicate and aluminate sheets is shown in Figure 2-32B. During firing and cooling, partial fusion and phase changes occur, and the final structure may be predicted from phase diagrams prepared for the system. Figure 2-33 shows the phase diagram for the Al_2O_3—SiO_2 system. At high temperatures a number of phases exist which are not relevant to ambient temperature application. At room temperature three phases are stable, and these give rise to phase compositions of trydimite plus mullite, pure mullite and mullite plus corundum (Al_2O_3) depending on the proportions of SiO_2 and Al_2O_3 in the material. Mullite is a distinct compound with a composition close to $2SiO_2 \cdot 3Al_2O_3$. Each of these phases and phase

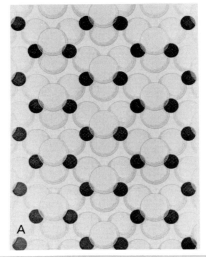

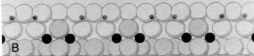

Figure 2-32. *A.* An aluminate sheet consists of aluminum ions (*black*) and hydroxyl (OH) ions (*white*). The *top layer* of hydroxyls has a hexagonal pattern. If the two sheets are superimposed they mesh to form kaolinite. (Reproduced with permission of J. J. Gilman.[70]) *B.* A kaolinite sheet is shown schematically. From such a side view it appears as a "laminate" of the silicate and aluminate sheets shown in Figures 2-30*C* and 2-32*A.* In kaolinite each of the aluminum ions is surrounded by neighboring oxygen or hydroxyl ions. (Reproduced with permission of J. J. Gilman.[70])

mixtures has characteristic mechanical and physicochemical attributes and finds appropriate uses.

The Response of Ceramic Materials to Stress

The crystalline ceramics contain dislocations, as metal crystals. Unlike metals, however, they show almost no capacity to undergo plastic deformation except at very high temperatures, and in consequence are usually extremely brittle materials. The reason for this difference is 2-fold. In the first place the ceramics contain ions of different sizes, all of which must be moved to equivalent positions if a dislocation is to move through the lattice. This "cooperative" slip is extremely difficult except at high temperatures, where diffusion can assist the process, or at extremely high stresses. Second, the slip process would require ions of the same charge to pass close to one another, so there is a considerable electrostatic opposition to this type of movement. Thus, while these materials display the

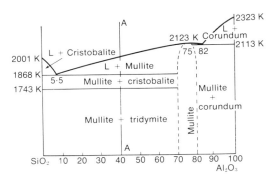

Figure 2-33. A phase diagram for the SiO_2—Al_2O_3 system is shown. (Reproduced with permission of J. B. Moss.[5])

high elastic moduli and compressive strengths which the extremely strong bonding would predict, they generally fail at tensile stresses much lower than those which might produce slip, since the tensile strength is severely compromised by the Griffith's crack mechanism discussed for glasses.

Available Ceramics

Of the large number of different ceramics, three types have been considered for surgical implantation. Calcium phosphate ceramics, crystalline variants of the bioglasses described previously, have been studied.[71] Their properties do not differ markedly from those of their amorphous counterparts, although recent reports indicate a marked reduction in fatigue strength in aqueous environments, a further example of mechanochemical interaction which is discussed in Chapter 4. A second group of materials includes the calcium aluminates, titanates and zirconates and alumina and titania. Hulbert and his colleagues[72, 73] have reported extensively on studies of porous ceramics for segmental bone replacements. In summary, they observe that a variety of these ceramics provokes no evidence of toxicity in experimental animals. When porous implants are inserted adjacent to bone, ingrowth of unmineralized, or even fully mineralized, bone may follow, provided that the pore diameter is sufficiently large. These workers and others have subsequently developed a variety of possible clinical applications of ceramics. While early results are encouraging, especially in the area of bone replacement, two problems remain: the marked difference in elastic modulus between bone and most ceramics, and the low resistance to infection of implants or implant/tissue interfaces compared with living tissue. Further studies by Griss *et al.*[74] have shown that aluminate wear particles are well tolerated by a variety of experimental animals. Finally, there have been recent reports on the compatibility of a ceramic coating on the femoral component of a total hip replacement in humans.[75] These observations are discussed in Chapters 13 and 16.

Carbon

Not surprisingly, carbon is one of the most compatible materials for implantation.[76] The great dissimilarity between the two allotropic forms of carbon is a function of the different types of bonding, as has been discussed. In diamond, each carbon atom has four nearest neighbors, and the atoms form a three-dimensional network of interlocking tetrahedra. In graphite, on the other hand, each carbon atom has only three nearest neighbors and the structure consists of giant sheets of atoms, strongly bonded within the sheet, but relying on much weaker van der Waals forces for bonding between adjacent sheets. Figure 2-34 shows a schematic diagram of the graphite structure. Thus massive graphite is a soft, gray high melting solid with a dull metallic luster. The softness is a result of the weak intersheet bonding which allows adjacent sheets to slide over one another with ease. Graphite is thus a good lubricant, and has been studied as a possible articular component for total joint replacement. Porous forms of graphite are available, somewhat akin to coke or charcoal,

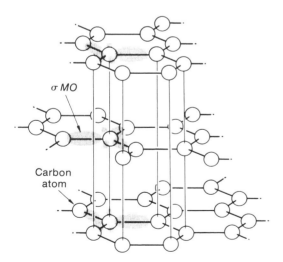

Figure 2-34. Schematic illustration showing the structure of graphite. The molecular orbital (*OM*) indicates hybridization directional bonding consistent with covalent bonding. In graphite each carbon atom bonds primarily with 3 other carbon atoms to produce a sheet type structure. Separate sheets are held together by weak van der Waals bonding. (Reproduced with permission of A. G. Guy.[77])

and their great surface area lends itself to tissue ingrowth for anchorage of osseous implants. Several types of graphite have been studied[78] and, as discussed below, they have been considered for femoral head replacement. Isotropic pyrolytic carbon has been produced by hydrocarbon pyrolysis.[79] The isotropic material has mechanical properties superior to other synthetic graphites or glassy carbons. More recently, graphite composites formed by pyrolysis of a hydrocarbon gas to deposit carbon onto carbon fibers have provided materials of superior strength which can be produced in intricate shapes.[80] Other two-phase graphite composites are available. For example, by pyrolysis of a mixture of hydrocarbon gas and silanes, silicon carbide whiskers may be formed within a pyrolytic graphite matrix. This material shows good strength, a fairly low elastic modulus and can be machined readily. All of these materials show good biological compatibility.

Apart from massive graphite, carbon fibers may also be used to reinforce organic polymers or metals, as is discussed below.

POLYMERIC MATERIALS

A polymer is composed of giant molecules produced by repetition of a simple unit called a mer.[81, 82] The number of mers per molecule may range from hundreds to tens of thousands. Carbon is the principal element which has the ability to form polymers, but silicon also possesses this capacity to a degree, and silicone fluids and silicone rubbers are examples of silicon polymers. The organic (carbon-based) polymers are discussed first.

The process of polymerization involves either addition or condensation reactions. Addition polymerization involves breaking a double bond in the monomer and saturating the broken bonds by combining the monomers into a chain structure. Usually the presence of a catalyst is required, but application of heat or pressure may also be used. The process can occur without any byproducts. The simplest example of addition polymerization is the formation of polyethylene. The ethylene monomer

$$\begin{array}{c} H \quad H \\ | \quad | \\ C = C \\ | \quad | \\ H \quad H \end{array}$$

polymerizes to yield a structure

$$\cdots \begin{array}{cccc} H & H & H & H \\ | & | & | & | \\ C - C - C - C \\ | & | & | & | \\ H & H & H & H \end{array} \cdots$$

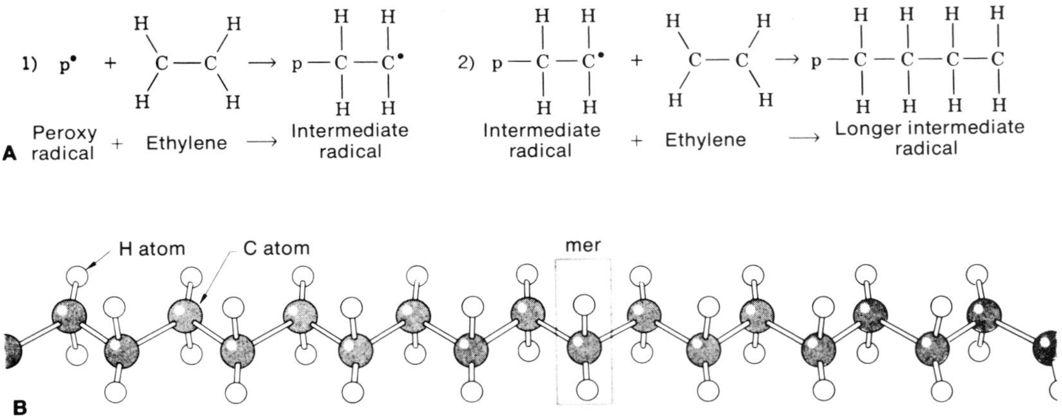

Figure 2-35. The polarization of ethylene molecules to form polyethylene is shown. The stages of the reaction are indicated in *A*. The *black dot* indicates the role of free radicals in the initial steps of polarization of ethylene. In *B* a straight portion of a typical chain of polyethylene is shown. Each unit of the chain is called a mer. The entire chain may contain 50,000 monomer units. (Reproduced with permission of A. G. Guy.[77])

Figure 2-35 is a graphic portrayal of the polymerization of polyethylene. If a polymer is constructed from a single monomer it is called a homopolymer. If different monomers are combined, the product is termed a co-polymer. Co-polymers are the organic analogue of metallic alloys, and offer similar opportunities to tailor the properties of the material to suit a particular application. For example, polystyrene is a stiff rigid compound, but if styrene is co-polymerized with butadiene, a rubber-forming monomer, a styrene-butadiene rubber is obtained with superior properties to the straight polybutadienes.

Condensation polymerization depends on reaction at active sites on the monomers, and double bonds are not required. A byproduct is always produced. The product of the condensation need not be a linear molecule. For example, condensation between phenol, C_6H_5OH and formaldehyde, HCHO, produces a phenol-formaldehyde resin (Bakelite):

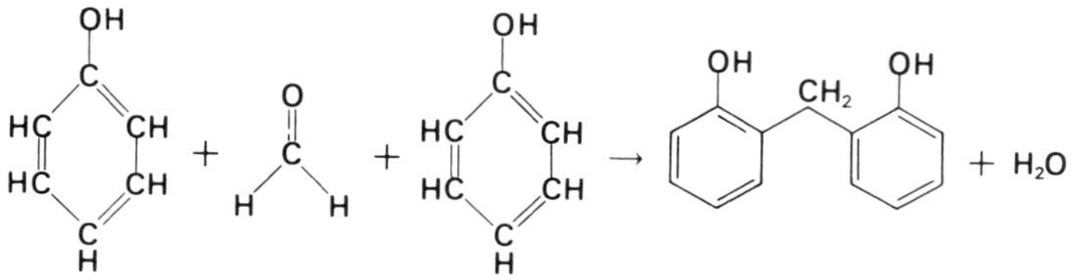

Thermoplastics and Thermosets

Those polymers like polyethylene, polyamides and polyacetals, which show a linear configuration of molecules, rely solely on van der Waals bonds to bind adjacent chains together. Under stress the chains can slide past one another, and this mobility is enhanced by temperature. These *thermoplastics* are characterized by their ability to form viscous fluids at elevated temperatures, and reverse the change on cooling. In contrast, the other major class of polymers, the *thermosets,* show no viscid state prior to thermal decomposition of the resin. In the main, the thermoplastics tend to be tough and resilient, whereas the thermosets are hard, rigid materials. Table 2-5 shows the structures of some thermoplastics with medical applications, while the structure of phenol-formaldehyde is typical of a thermosetting resin in which covalent bonds may link the separated molecules. With heating,

A network molecule is produced and 1 molecule of water is rejected per reaction event. During polymerization any of the hydrogens on the benzene ring, except the hydroxyl hydrogen, may react in this way and a complicated cross-linked polymer results.

further cross-linking occurs to transform the material into a hard rigid mass.

Structure of Polymers

As well as their composition, polymers may be classified in terms of the long range arrange-

Table 2-5

Structures of Thermoplastics with Medical Applications

Polymer	Repetitive Structure	$T_g{}^a$
		$°K$
Polyethylene	H H H H | | | | —C—C—C—C— | | | | H H H H	153
Polypropylene	H CH_3H H | | | | —C—C—C—C— | | | | H H H CH_3	260
Polytetrafluoroethylene (PTFE)	F F F F | | | | —C—C—C—C— | | | | F F F F	399

Polymethylmethacrylate (acrylic)	H CH_3 H CH_3
	| | | |
	—C——C——C——C—
	| | | |
	H C H C
	    ⫽ | ⫽ |
	  O OCH_3 O OCH_3	

Polyamide (nylon 66)	H H O H O H ┌ | ┐ | ‖ ┌ | ┐ ‖ | C —N—C— C —C— —N— | | H ┘$_6$ H ┘$_4$	
Polyethylene terephathalate (Dacron, Terylene)	H H O O | | ‖ C—C ‖ O—C—C—O—C—|C_2 C—C— | | C＝C H H | | H H	

^{a} T_g (°K), glass transition temperature in degrees kelvin.

ment of their molecules. Three types may be considered, the amorphous and crystalline thermoplastics and the cross-linked thermosets.

Amorphous thermoplastics show random distribution of the long chain molecules without crystallinity or cross-linkage, much like a mass of cooked spaghetti. Many of these, for example, polymethylmethacrylate, tend to be glass-like and transparent. With the random mode of polymerization, the chain lengths vary considerably and a particular sample of polymer may be characterized by its average molecular weight. The molecular weight of a polymer controls properties such as viscosity and response to temperature changes. Such a material shows a num-

ber of different physical states which depend on the temperature and the molecular weight, as illustrated in Figure 2-36. At low molecular weight a definite melting point exists, whereas in high molecular weight commercial polymers there is a diffuse transition from solid to liquid. Over a narrow range of temperature, the glass transition temperature, these rigid polymers transform into a rubbery condition with marked change in mechanical properties. At higher temperatures, the rubbery state gradually transforms into a liquid.

The glass transition temperature (T_g) may be defined as the temperature at which, on cooling, molecular rotation about the carbon-carbon

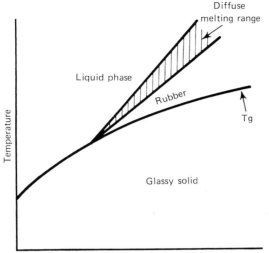

Figure 2-36. A phase diagram for amorphous polymer (a thermoplastic), such as polymethylmethacrylate, is shown. T_g refers to the glass transition temperature, a narrow range of temperature where the polymer passes from a rigid to a rubber-like condition. The glass transition temperature, T_g, is often defined as the temperature at which, on cooling, molecular rotation above the —C—C— backbone bonds becomes restricted. (Reproduced with permission of J. B. Moss.[5])

bond becomes restricted. Above T_g, in the rubbery state, the molecules prefer to assume a coiled configuration. With the application of stress the molecules may uncoil by rotation about C—C bonds. Removal of stress allows the molecules to coil again. However, hysteresis determines that the deformation lags behind the application and removal of stress. The deformation characteristics of a polymer in its rubbery state above T_g, therefore, depend upon the rate of application of stress. A material which behaves like a rubber when stress is applied slowly may appear to be quite rigid and brittle if loaded suddenly.

If an amorphous polymer in its rubbery state is stressed, its molecules align themselves in the direction of the stress. If the polymer is subsequently cooled below T_g while the stress is still applied, the new orientation is retained, and the anisotropic material shows higher strength parallel to the preferred direction. This strengthening by stress-induced orientation is common practice in the production of filament and film.

To use a thermoplastic, a knowledge of the difference between the glass transition temperature and the ambient temperature is essential. Considerably below T_g the material is rigid and

able to bear stress whereas above T_g the material is rubbery. The value of T_g can be altered by several factors including the type of carbon backbone, cross-linkage between adjacent polymer chains, the presence of large side chains and the presence of plasticizers. Cross-linkage or bulky side chains tend to stiffen the polymer and elevate T_g. Plasticizers, high molecular weight solvents for the polymer, enhance chain mobility to lower T_g. Co-polymers usually have a value of T_g intermediate between those of the respective homopolymers.

Crystalline thermoplastics also show a glass transition temperature. T_g for a crystalline polymer may be appreciably below room temperature even though the material is not rubbery. In contrast to an amorphous polymer where the properties are a function, T_g, in relation to ambient temperature, the behavior of crystalline polymers is determined primarily by the degree of crystallinity. While no polymer is wholly crystalline, most display zones of crystallinity separated by amorphous regions. A degree of crystallinity over 80% is rare and most crystalline polymers contain about 50% crystalline and 50% amorphous material. The crystalline regions confer rigidity while the amorphous zones give toughness.

Crystallinity denotes the presence of long range ordering of the atoms. The ordering of polymers arises by three main mechanisms (Fig. 2-37). The simplest model of ordering entails the matching of parts of neighboring chains. A major source of crystallinity is derived from recurrent folding of the chains at intervals of about 10^{-10} cm along their lengths, to yield close-packed lamellae. A third source arises by matching of coils along helical chain molecules. The crystalline zones, called spherulites, confer mechanical strength and raise the softening temperature. Maximum rigidity is therefore attained when the spherulites are closely spaced. Crystallinity may be enhanced by stretching the chains, which untangles and orients them to provide greater symmetry among chain segments. This technique is widely used in the commerical production of nylon and Dacron filaments.

The ability of a polymer to crystallize is a function of the regularity of its molecular structure. Irregular or random structures favor the production of amorphous polymers. Regularity of molecular structure is reduced by irregular substitution of foreign atoms or branching side chains of polymers, and co-polymerization or lack of stereoregularity. The bonds to carbon atoms are oriented tetrahedrally, and a chain molecule is therefore not planar but in the form

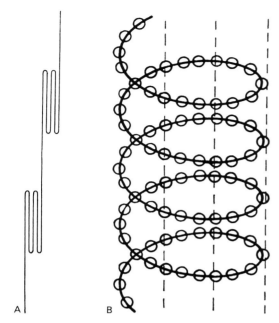

Figure 2-37. Schematic diagram indicating two types of long range ordering in polymeric molecules that contribute to the crystalline state. *A.* Recurrent folds in chains, at intervals of about 100×10^{-10} m along their length. The folds produce matched close-packed lamella, a major source of crystallinity. *B.* A helical chain molecule that occurs by the matching of adjacent coils. The crystalline zones are referred to as spherulites. (Reproduced with permission of J. B. Moss.[5])

of a zigzag or helix, so that different forms or isomers of the same molecule may exist. *Isotactic polymers* are highly crystalline because all the substituent groups are regularly arranged and matching across chains is highly probable.

Syndiotactic polymers exhibit regular alternation of the substituent groups, with only a limited ability to crystallize.

If the arrangement of substituted groups is completely random, the polymer will be amorphous; this is the *atactic* condition.

Three of the polymers with medical applications show varying degrees of crystallinity. Polytetrafluoroethylene (PTFE) has a very regular chain and can exist in a highly crystalline form. While polyethylene possesses a simple structure, many of the chains are branched and this produces great variation in crystallinity (Fig. 2-38). With a greater degree of crystallinity, the chains are packed more closely, with a resultant increase in density. Low density polyethylene, therefore, contains many branched chains. By the use of particular catalysts during manufacture, more linear chains may be produced to yield high density polyethylene. For polypropylene, stereoregularity is extremely important, since a high degree of molecular orientation is required to provide adequate strength for use in certain joint replacements.

In *cross-linked thermosetting polymers,* covalent bonds occur between adjacent chains instead of the usual van der Waals bonds. Such cross-linkage may encourage the formation of recurrent folds or helical coils as seen in Figure 2-38. Regulation of the amount of cross-linking allows the production of a range of products from viscous liquids to hard, rigid solids.

A typical lightly cross-linked material is the highly elastic natural latex rubber, polyisoprene. It exhibits a large hysteresis in deformation in response to stress and is useful only at normal temperatures. By vulcanizing with sulfur, further covalent bonds are formed which increase rigidity, the rate of response to applied load and the range of operating temperature. On the other hand, for applications as implants the vulcanized rubbers display considerable toxicity while the pure natural rubber is tolerated far better.

Inorganic Polymers

Silicon, like carbon, is a tetravalent element capable of covalent bonding, and polymers are available with a backbone of silicon atoms. Compounds of the type

do exist but they become unstable with more than 6 silicon atoms. Such short chains hardly qualify to be called polymers. The siloxane grouping, however, is much more stable:

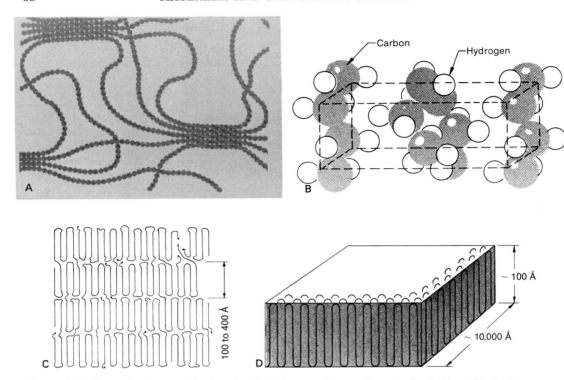

Figure 2-38. Stages in the crystallization of polyethylene are shown schematically. *A.* Crystallization between adjacent chains or of a single chain on itself, characteristic of lower temperatures. *B.* The orthorhombic unit cell in crystalline polyethylene. *C.* The interweaving of polyethylene molecules through a folded chain lamellae. *D.* The close-packed structure of adjacent lamellae formed by a folding polyethylene chain. Each of the *gray dots* indicates an individual

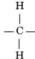

mer. (*A, B* and *D* reproduced with permission of A. G. Guy.[77] *C* reproduced with permission of R. D. Deaning.[83])

This is the basis of the silicones or silicon polymers. With short polymeric chains of low molecular weight, the polymers may be fluid, but with longer chains and cross-linking various grades of silicone elastomers are formed.[84, 85] In silicone rubber, used for surgical applications, the radical —R is the methyl group, CH_3, forming polydimethylsiloxane.

Biodegradable Polymers

For the orthopaedic surgeon, degradable polymers which do not induce an excessive toxic or inflammatory response are of limited application. While the ideal resorbable suture remains to be developed, polyglycolic and polylactic acids have been suggested as biodegradable su-

ture materials.[86, 87] Control of the degradation rate has been a difficult problem, and is critically dependent upon the polymeric structure.[88]

Plastics

The vast majority of polymers are used in a modified form. After the admixture of one or more of a great variety of additives the end product usually is called a plastic. Typical additives include plasticizers, fillers, pigments, heat stabilizers, ultraviolet light stabilizers and lubricants. The main additives for biomedical plastics are introduced to improve mechanical properties or inertness, and examples are given in subsequent sections.

Fibers

In orthopaedic surgery, the application of polymers in fiber form is limited to suture materials such as nylon (polyamide), Dacron or Terylene (polyethylene terephthalate) and PTFE (polytetrafluorethylene). The sutures may be monofilaments or multistranded. As mentioned above, the molecular chains in a fiber are aligned primarily with axial orientation to give maximum strength in the direction of the fiber. During fabrication, multistranded fibers can be woven with a variety of geometries.

Bone Cement and Grouting Agents

Twenty years ago unsuccessful attempts were made to prepare polymeric adhesive agents for immobilization of fractures from polyurethane[89-91] and polystyrene.[92] Subsequently, little work has been reported on true adhesive agents for use in bone surgery. Recent studies by Hench and Paschall[64, 65] on the nature of chemical bond between bone and bioglasses provide the sort of groundwork which will be necessary to make progress in this field. About 15 years ago Charnley introduced polymethylmethacrylate[93, 94] into orthopaedic surgery as a grouting agent. While the term bone cement or glue is frequently applied in the literature it should be clearly understood that this polymer is a poor adhesive agent and does not function in that capacity. In fact, the cement is used to secure implants, usually total joint replacements, to bone by the extrusion of dough-like polymer into interstices in the bone and corresponding recesses or slots in the implant. The implant is forced into close proximity with the bone and, within 10 min after application, the cement solidifies to provide a mortice fit between the implant and bone.

The cement consists of a liquid and a powder; the liquid contains mainly methylmethacrylate monomer, with hydroquinone to prevent premature polymerization which might occur under certain conditions such as exposure to light or to elevated temperature, and N,N-dimethyl-p-toluidine to promote cold curing of the mixture. The liquid is sterilized by membrane filtration. The powder is a fine granular mixture of methylmethacrylate-styrene copolymer with 15 to 16% polymethylmethacrylate. Up to 10% of barium sulfate may be added to make the cement radiopaque for postoperative identification of the cement by X-rays. In addition, small amounts of benzyl peroxide, another activator, may be present. The powder component is ster-ilized by γ-irradiation. The powder and liquid are mixed at the time of use and within 3 to 5 min polymerization yields a soft pliable dough-like mass, at which time the cement is applied. Within 8 to 12 min after mixture, a hard, cement-like compound is formed. During solidification the exothermic reaction is accompanied by a considerable rise in temperature of the mass of cement. The temperature usually rises to between 40°C and 80°C, although it may rise to 100°C, and precautions may be necessary to prevent thermal damage to adjacent tissues. The mechanical properties, techniques of application and deleterious side effects of methylmethacrylate are described in later sections (Chapters 3, 7, 13 and 14).

COMPOSITES

A composite material was originally considered simply as a combination of two materials. Two classic examples are two phase metallic alloys and the lamination of sheets of wood, as plywood. In these cases the objective is to provide a material with somewhat better strength or thermal resistance than would be exhibited by the individual constituents. While such combinations are of course composites, the combinations provided by modern technology are unique in that they may possess properties which are not exhibited by either material.

An elementary example of the newer concept of composites is the bimetal strip. This might consist of a flat piece of brass and a similar piece of iron bonded together. If the two pieces were heated separately the brass would expand more than the iron. If the composite is heated, the expansion of the brass forces the iron to bend, and the bending of the iron forces the brass to bend. The bending can be used to indicate temperature or to activate an on-off switch. Neither metal alone could achieve this effect.

Like synthetic polymers, modern composites imitate nature. Bone, for example, is a composite of the strong but soft protein collagen and the hard but brittle mineral hydroxyapatite. Wood is a composite of strong flexible cellulose fibers and a cement-like substance, lignin, which binds the fibers to stiffen the material. Modern composites achieve similar results even more effectively by the combination of strong fibers of a material such as carbon in a soft matrix such as epoxy resin. A familiar example is Fiberglas (fiber glass reinforced plastic) which consists of glass fibers in resin. The new materials provide strength, stiffness and lightness and are also

Table 2-6
Observed Tensile Strengths (10^6 psi)

Graphite whiskers	Up to 3.5
Alumina whiskers	Up to 2.2
Silica glass fibers	Up to 0.8
High carbon steel wire	0.6
Fiberglas rod (bulk)	0.2
Nylon thread	0.08
Catgut	0.06
Polyester	0.035
Spider thread	0.030
Glass	0.015
Bone	0.015
Tendon	0.015

inert. In view of the current interest in the application of composite materials for orthopaedic implants, it is useful to consider briefly how composite materials derive their outstanding attributes. More detailed accounts are recommended for the interested readers.[12, 17, 95]

Table 2-6 illustrates some of the remarkably high strengths which have been achieved in whiskers and fibers. The commercially available materials have much lower strengths. The reason for this marked discrepancy in strengths is of course that the high strength of whiskers and fibers is realized only when the specimens have a surface without cracks, notches or steps and have no internal cracks. The significance of cracks and other superficial blemishes has already been discussed, but an example is of interest. At a stress of 100,000 psi a steel specimen would tolerate a notch up to 1 inch deep while in aluminum the crack can be no deeper than 0.016 inch. Glass, on the other hand, fails if the crack is deeper than 10^{-4} inch.

The measure of the ability of a material to retain its strength in the presence of cracks is given by the work of fracture or the energy required to break the material. Glass has a very low work of fracture, while that for a strong steel is very high. The inherently strong materials such as graphite, alumina, boron and silicon carbide all behave somewhat like glass. Their work of fracture is small and they are vulnerable to the presence of small cracks. Metal and polymeric materials, with their high resistance to cracks, are widely used as engineering materials.

While an unscratched ceramic can be very strong, flaws enable it to be easily broken. If the ceramic is divided into minute pieces, as in a powder, any crack present cannot find a continuous path through the material. For the particles, or more usually fibers, to form a useful structural material, however, they must be bound together in a matrix. The properties of the matrix are of great importance. It must not scratch the fibers and introduce cracks, it must transmit stress to the fibers, it must be plastic and adhesive to immobilize the fibers securely and, finally, it must deflect and control cracks within the composite.

Metals such as aluminum or titanium or polymers provide all the required mechanical attributes for a matrix. They are soft or weak in shear so that they do not scratch the fibers. Under tensile load, virtually all the stress is carried by the fibers, so that the matrix makes a negligible contribution to the breaking strength of the composite. Under stress, the fibers with cracks may break, but the soft matrix hinders propagation of the crack. The fibers do not fail at one plane, so that progression of the crack completely across the material occurs only if the fibers are withdrawn from the matrix. Considerable work must be expended to pull out the fibers, and the pull-out work represents a large portion of the work of fracture of composites. If the adhesion is low, a crack that initially runs at right angles to the fibers will be deflected along the weak interface and rendered harmless as far as tensile strength of the composite is concerned. As discussed earlier, for resistance to tension, shear stress and compression, a compromise is required, and multiple orientations of fibers provide moderate strength in many directions of stress although the absolute strength in any one axis will be compromised.

For most industrial applications the immense stiffness and great strength of composites with ceramic fibers in a metallic matrix, which have already been outlined, provide the optimal mechanical properties. For internal reconstruction of the skeleton, however, the stiffness of such composites would be a disadvantage because it is so different from that shown by bone. To use the rigid implant materials some method of providing a gradual transition in stiffness across the bone implant interface would be necessary. At present, composites are under consideration which may provide both superior metals and polymers for implantation.[96] Fiber-reinforced metals, with graphite and boron fibers, are being studied as possible total joint replacements, and carbon fiber-reinforced polyethylene shown in Figure 2-39A-C, is undergoing clinical trial for use in total hip joint replacements. Reinforcement of methylmethacrylate cement with particles of carbon and cobalt-chromium alloy is

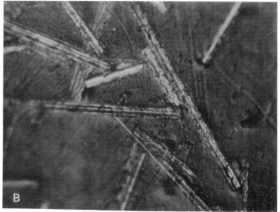

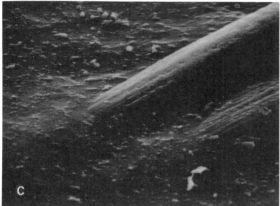

Figure 2-39. *A* and *B*. Photomicrographs of a carbon fiber-reinforced ultra high molecular weight polyethylene matrix. *A,* ×32. *B,* ×260. (Reproduced with permission of Zimmer-USA.) *C*. A scanning electronmicrograph reveals the carbon fiber-ultra high molecular weight polyethylene matrix interface of the same material that is seen in *A* and *B*. ×1600. (Reproduced with permission of Zimmer-USA.)

also under investigation. The results are discussed in Chapters 3 and 13.

PLASTER OF PARIS

For over a century, plaster of Paris has been the most widely used material for external immobilization. It has a unique combination of physical and mechanical properties which makes it an almost ideal material for the construction of most casts.

Plaster of Paris is manufactured from gypsum, calcium sulfate dihydrate.[97] Gypsum, a solid crystalline material, is pulverized and then ignited at 120°C, at which temperature it loses 75% of its water of crystallization. The fine white powder which remains is plaster of Paris.

$$2 \, [CaSO_4 \cdot 2H_2O] \xrightarrow{heat} \quad 2CaSO_4 \cdot H_2O + 3H_2O$$
$$\text{Gypsum} \qquad\qquad \text{Plaster of Paris}$$

When water is added to the plaster, the reaction is reversed and the plaster recrystallizes or "sets" back into solid gypsum. It expands slightly and

evolves heat. Long, thin closely interlocking crystals form rapidly and give the plaster much of its ultimate strength. During the period of recrystallization, however, if the plaster is disturbed by excessive molding or bending, short stubby crystals are formed which are loosely interlocked, and a weak cast ensues.

The Setting Process

Plaster requires more water to bring it to a fluid, workable state than is needed to satisfy the chemical requirements. The crystals that form during the setting process contain about 20% water of crystallization, although several times this amount of water may be present in the fresh cast. After the cast has set, the excess water evaporates from the surface before the cast can attain its maximum strength, and air voids replace the water to produce a highly porous cast which permits air to pass through it to the skin. Naturally, the cast also becomes highly absorbent of blood or purulent drainage from wounds. The absorbancy of the plaster is one of its outstanding attributes in immobilization of open or infected wounds.

Thermal Effects

The chemical reaction which occurs when plaster recombines with water is exothermic. The evolution of heat is not appreciable with thin casts, but with excessively thick casts the rise in temperature may be sufficient to make a patient apprehensive. In extreme conditions, thermal damage to the skin may occur. The conditions can be regulated to a considerable extent by the person who applies the cast. While the quantity of heat produced by a given amount of plaster is constant, the maximum temperature will vary with the technique of application and the conditions surrounding the cast. A thicker cast will reach a higher maximum temperature, bandages with faster setting time reach a higher temperature than bandages with a slower setting time and raising the dipping water temperature, the room temperature and the humidity will cause an increase in the maximum temperature of the cast. During the drying period, increased circulation of air around the cast will reduce the maximum drying temperature, since evaporation of excess water is increased. The maximum temperature of the cast is usually achieved within 5 to 15 min, after which it cools rapidly.

Setting Time

Most plaster bandages and splints can be classified either as fast setting (5 to 8 min) or as extra fast setting (2 to 4 min). The time is measured from complete wetting of the plaster until the cast has become firm. The setting time is a function of several variables. Soaking the bandage in warm water hastens setting while soaking it in cool water retards setting. Application of a very wet bandage delays setting while the use of a bandage that is wrung dry hastens solidification. Accelerators such as potassium sulfate or sodium chloride or retarders such as sodium citrate or borax may be added to the saturation water to adjust the rate of setting. The addition of such agents, however, may limit the strength of the cast. Saturation water must be changed frequently, for the plaster residue in the pail also acts as an accelerator.

Cast Strength

It is important that a cast has adequate "green" strength. It is probable that most cases of premature mechanical failure of a cast are initiated while the cast is in the green state, before its maximum strength is attained. Each additional layer of plaster bandage should be rubbed into the previous layer to avoid delamination. If less water is carried into the cast in each bandage, the cast will dry and achieve maximum strength more rapidly. The addition of extraneous ingredients to the plaster usually weakens the cast. For example, the addition of a small quantity of a smoothing agent to increase the creaminess of a bandage may decrease cast strength by up to 25%. One exception to this rule is the resin-plaster bandage where the addition of a synthetic plastic resin substantially increases cast strength, as well as resistance to deterioration on exposure to water.

In the same way as described above for other brittle materials, plaster fractures by propagation of a crack from a notch or other blemish in the surface. The susceptibility of plaster to brittle fracture is greatly reduced if the surface is rubbed to an extremely smooth finish during the application of the cast. Smoothing is improved if the surgeon wears rubber gloves that are wetted immediately before starting to rub the cast.

The Optimum Thickness of Casts

Plaster casts should be made as thin as the required strength, rigidity and degree of immobilization permit. Usually a thickness of ¼ inch gives adequate strength and yet is sufficiently light in weight that it does not retard activity or exercise by the patient. Excessive thickness of the cast may be associated with thermal damage to the skin, delay in drying out and difficulty in removal of the cast. Also, X-rays are clearer when taken through a thin cast. When a cast shows repetitive premature breakage, two courses should be considered. Selective reinforcement with plaster splints may greatly increase the strength of the cast without excessive bulk. Since plaster is much stronger in compression than in tension, the splints should be applied to the concave side of joints. In addition, immobilization of successively more proximal joints may considerably limit the trauma to which the cast is subjected. The latter course is particularly helpful with children. Finally, the resin-plaster bandage is preferred where greatest strength is needed.

Recently a Fiberglas cast, Lightcast II (Merck Sharp & Dohme), has become generally available. The material is a Fiberglas tape coated with a photo-sensitive resin supplied in various widths. The cotton orthopaedic sockinet is replaced by polypropylene material which resists water, and a web strap, also of polypropylene, is available to pad bony prominences. The cast is applied in a manner similar to plaster casts. To harden the material, it is exposed to a special ultraviolet lamp which provides a wave length of 3500 to 3900 Å. Polymerization requires between 5 and 30 min, depending on the thickness of the cast. After the cast is fully hardened, it may be soaked in water without deleterious side effects. The Fiberglas cast is considerably stronger and lighter in weight than a comparable plaster cast. However, there are disadvantages, including prolonged time for application, greatly increased cost, sharp irregular edges of the cast, occasionally hypersensitivity to the cast and the need for a diamond-edged blade for removal of the cast. The results of a large clinical trial with the material have recently been published[98]; a generally favorable impression was obtained. With its light weight, strength and water tolerance it is of particular value for athletes. In addition, it allows hydrotherapy or treatment of soft tissues with medical solutions. In view of its prolonged application time, sharp edges and cost, however, it is not generally favored for routine use.

REFERENCES

1. Mott, N. *Sci. Am., 217:*80, 1967.
2. Cottrell, A. H. *An Introduction to Metallurgy,* p. 150. Edward Arnold, London, 1968.
3. Mott, N. *Sci. Am., 217:*85, 1967.
4. Mott, N. *Sci. Am., 217:*84, 1967.
5. Moss, J. B. *Properties of Engineering Materials,* Butterworths, London, 1971.
6. Cottrell, A. H. *Sci. Am., 217:*92, 1967.
7. Cottrell, A. H. *Sci. Am., 217:*93, 1967.
8. Cottrell, A. H. *Sci. Am., 217:*94, 1967.
9. Cottrell, A. H. *The Mechanical Properties of Matter,* p. 64. John Wiley & Sons, New York, 1964.
10. Cottrell, A. H. *Theory of Crystal Dislocations,* p. 1. Blackie & Son, London, 1964.
11. Cottrell, A. H. *Sci. Am., 217:*95, 1967.
12. Cottrell, A. H. The ultimate mechanical properties of solids. In *Metallurgical Achievements,* p. 259. Oxford Pergamon Press, Oxford, 1965.
13. Herring, C., and Galt, J. K. *Phys. Rev., 85:*1060, 1952.
14. Cottrell, A. H. The ultimate mechanical properties of solids. In *Metallurgical Achievements,* p. 264, Pergamon Press, Oxford, 1965.
15. Cottrell, A. H. The ultimate mechanical properties of solids. In *Metallurgical Achievements,* p. 268, Pergamon Press, Oxford, 1965.
16. Cottrell, A. H. The ultimate mechanical properties of solids. In *Metallurgical Achievements,* p. 270, Pergamon Press, Oxford, 1965.
17. Kelly, A. *Strong Solids,* p. 35. Oxford University Press, Oxford, 1966.
18. Williams, D. F., and Roaf, R. O. *Implants in Surgery,* p. 46, W. B. Saunders Co. Ltd., London, 1973.
19. Bechtol, C. O., Ferguson, A. B., Jr., and Laing, P. G. *Metals and Engineering in Bone and Joint Surgery,* Williams & Wilkins Co., Baltimore, 1959.
20. *Annual Book of ASTM Standards,* Part 46. American Society for Testing Materials, Philadelphia, 1974.
21. British Standard 3531: 1962 and 1968. *Specification for Metal Implants and Tools used for Bone Surgery,* p. 2, British Standards Institution, London, 1968.
22. Moss, J. B. *Properties of Engineering Materials,* p. 118. Butterworths, London, 1971.
23. Travis, W. C., and Johnson, A. A. The behavior of a wrought equiatomic gold-nickel alloy as an implant material in living rats. In *Biomaterials,* edited by L. Stark and G. Agarwal, p. 44. Plenum Press, New York, 1969.
24. Castleman, L. S., *et al. Nickel-Titanium "Memory" Alloy,* p. 1. J. A. Hartford Foundation Inc., New York, 1974.
25. Devine, T. M., Kummer, F. J., and Wulff, J. *J. Mater. Sci., 7:*126, 1972.
26. Semlitsch, M. *Sulzer Tech. Rev., 2:*1, 1973.
27. Escalos, F., Galante, J., Rostoker, W., and Coogan, P. S. *J. Biomed. Mater. Res., 9:*303, 1975.
28. Taylor, L., editor. *Metals Handbook,* p. 524. American Society of Metals, Metals Park, OH, 1971.
29. Taylor, L., editor. *Metals Handbook,* p. 1228. American Society of Metals, Metals Park, OH, 1971.
30. Taylor, L., editor. *Metals Handbook,* p. 1222. American Society of Metals, Metals Park, OH, 1971.
31. Taylor, L., editor. *Metals Handbook,* p. 1181. American Society of Metals, Metals Park, OH, 1971.
32. Charles, R. J. *Sci. Am., 217:*129, 1967.
33. Moss, J. B. *Properties of Engineering Materials,* p. 221. Butterworths, London, 1971.
34. Charles, R. J. *Sci. Am., 217:*126, 1967.
35. Charles, R. J. *Sci. Am., 217:*132, 1967.
36. Charles, R. J. *Sci. Am., 217:*134, 1967.
37. McMillen, P. W. *Glass-Ceramics,* p. 7. Academic Press, London, 1964.
38. Doremus, R. H. *Glass Science,* p. 15. John Wiley & Sons, New York, 1973.
39. Stookey, S. D., and Mauter, R. D. *Progress in Ceramic Science,* edited by J. E. Burke, p. 77. Pergamon Press, Oxford, 1962.
40. Sarvoir, I. *Glass Tech., 2:*243, 1961.
41. Rogers, P. S., and Williamson, J. *Glass Tech., 10:*128, 1969.
42. Lyng, S., Markali, J., Krogh-Mae, J., and Lundberg, N. H. *Phys. Chem. Glasses, 11:*6, 1970.
43. Mukherjee, S. P., and Rogers, P. S. *Phys. Chem. Glasses, 8:*81, 1967.
44. Doremus, R. H., and Turkalo, A. M. *Phys. Chem. Glasses, 13:*14, 1972.
45. Doremus, R. H. *Glass Science,* p. 93. John Wiley & Sons, New York, 1973.
46. Moss, J. B. *Properties of Engineering Materials,* p. 234. Butterworths, London, 1971.

47. Schroder, N., and Gliemeroth, G. *Naturwiss.*, 57:533, 1970.
48. Mould, R. E. *Fundamental Phenomena in the Materials Science,* edited by J. Boris, J. J. Duga and J. J. Gilman, vol. 4, p. 119. Plenum Press, New York, 1967.
49. Roy, N. H., and Stacy, M. H. *J. Mater. Sci., 4:*78, 1969.
50. Proctor, B. A. *Phys. Chem. Glasses, 3:*7, 1967.
51. Kistler, S. S. *J. Am. Ceram. Soc., 45:*59, 1962.
52. Nordberg, M. E., Machel, E. L., Garfunkel, H. M., and Oloott, J. J. *J. Am. Ceram Soc., 47:*215, 1964.
53. Krohn, O. A. *Glass Tech., 12:*36, 1971.
54. Olcott, J. S., and Stookey, S. D. *Advances in Glass Technology,* p. 400. Plenum Press, New York, 1962.
55. Faile, S. P., and Roy, R. *J. Am. Ceram. Soc., 54:*532, 1971.
56. Hasselman, D. P. H., and Fulrath, R. M. *J. Am. Ceram. Soc., 49:*68, 1966.
57. Lange, F. F. *J. Am. Ceram. Soc., 54:*614, 1971.
58. Baker, T. C., and Preston, F. W. *J. Appl. Phys., 17:*179, 1946.
59. Charles, R. J., and Hillig, W. B. *Symposium on Mechanical Strength of Glass,* p. 511. Union Scientifique Continentale du Verre, Charleroi, Belge, 1962.
60. Hillig, W. B., and Charles, R. J. *High Strength Materials,* edited by V. F. Jookey, p. 682. John Wiley & Sons, New York, 1965.
61. Stuart, D. A., and Anderson, O. L. *J. Am. Ceram. Soc., 36:*416, 1959.
62. Charles, R. J. *J. Appl. Phys., 29:*1549, 1958.
63. Mould, R. W., and Southwick, R. D. *J. Am. Ceram. Soc., 42:*582, 1959.
64. Hench, L. L., and Paschall, H. A. *J. Biomed. Mater. Res., 4:*25, 1973.
65. Hench, L. L., and Paschall, H. A. *J. Biomed. Mater. Res., 8:*219, 1974.
66. Homsy, C. A., Cain, T. E., Kessler, F. B., Anderson, M. S., and King, J. W. *Clin. Ortho. Rel. Res., 89:*220, 1972.
67. Gibbons, D. F. *Ann. Rev. Biophys. Bioeng., 4:*367, 1975.
68. Gilman, J. J. *Sci. Am., 217:*113, 1967.
69. Gilman, J. J. *Sci. Am., 217:*114, 1967.
70. Gilman, J. J. *Sci. Am., 217:*116, 1967.
71. McGee, T. D., and Wood, J. L. *J. Biomed. Mater. Res., 8:*137, 1974.
72. Hulbert, S. F., Klawitter, J. J., and Leonard, R. B. Use of porous ceramics as surgical implants. In *Medical Engineering,* edited by C. D. Roy, p. 1139. Year Book Medical Publishers, Chicago, 1974.
73. Hulbert, S. F., Matthews, J. R., Klawitter, J. J., Sauer, B. W., and Leonard, R. B. *J. Biomed. Mater. Res., 8:*85, 1974.
74. Griss, P., Krempien, B., von Andrian-Werburg, H., Heimke, G., Fleiner, R., and Diehn, T. *J. Biomed. Mater. Res., 8:*39, 1974.
75. Bouton, P. *Rev. Chir. Orthop., 58:*229, 1972.
76. Kadefors, R., Reswick, J. B., and Martin, R. L. *Med. Bio. Eng., 8:*129, 1970.
77. Guy, A. G. *Introduction to Materials Science,* McGraw-Hill Book Co., New York, 1971.
78. Funck-Bentano, J. L., *Biomat. Med. Dev. Artif. Org., 3:*339, 1974.
79. Bokios, J., *et al. Chemistry and Physics of Carbon,* edited by P. L. Walker, vol. 9, p. 103. Marcel Dekker, New York, 1972.
80. Olcott, E. L. *J. Biomed. Mater. Res., 8:*209, 1974.
81. Mark, H. F. *Sci. Am., 217:*148, 1967.
82. Moss, J. B. *Properties of Engineering Materials,* p. 172. Butterworths, London, 1971.
83. Deaning, R. D. *Polymer Structure, Properties and Applications,* Cahners Publishing Co., Boston, 1972.
84. Braley, S. A. *J. Macromol. Sci.-Chem., A4:*529, 1970.
85. Bloch, B., and Hastings, G. W. *Plastics in Surgery,* 2nd ed., p. 22. Charles C Thomas, Springfield, IL, 1972.
86. Kulkarni, R. K., Moore, E. G., Hegyeli, A. F., and Leonard, F. *J. Biomed. Mater. Res., 5:*169, 1971.
87. Frazzu, E. J., and Schmitt, E. *J. Biomed. Mater. Res. Symp., 1:*43, 1971.
88. Anderson, J. M., and Gibbons, D. F. *Biomat. Med. Dev. Artif. Org., 3:*235, 1974.
89. Macoomb, R. K., Hollenberg, C., and Zingg, W. *Surg. Forum., 11:*454, 1960.
90. Salvatore, J. E., and Mandarino, M. P. *Ann. Surg., 149:*107, 1959.
91. Bloch, B. *J. Bone Jt. Surg., 40B:*804, 1958.
92. Hudec, M. *Folia Morphol., 13:*57, 1965.
93. Charnley, J. *J. Bone Jt. Surg., 42B:*28, 1960.
94. Charnley, J. *Acrylic Cement in Bone Surgery,* p. 2. E. & S. Livingstone, London, 1970.
95. Kelly, A. *Sci. Am., 217:*161, 1967.
96. Clauser, H. R. *Sci. Am., 289:*36, 1973.
97. Salib, P. I. *Plaster Casting,* p. 9. Appleton-Century-Crofts, New York, 1975.
98. Leach, R. E., *et al. Clin. Ortho. Rel. Res., 103:*109, 1974.

3

The Mechanical Behavior of Real Materials

D. C. Mears and G. P. Rothwell

In the previous chapter, the inter-relation between the structure of a material and some of its fundamental strength properties was discussed in somewhat elementary terms. In the application of real materials in specific situations, however, rather more practical considerations must be made. The strength of the materials must be assessed in mechanical or engineering terms. For some applications, such as cardiac pacemakers or implantable power sources, the physical behavior of materials, their thermal, optical, electrical properties *etc.*, may be particularly relevant. In orthopaedic applications, however, purely physical properties are of less importance. The chemical performance of materials when exposed to body fluids is also a matter for careful consideration. Finally, the financial implications of all of these technical decisions must be carefully analyzed, for the material and manufacturing costs may completely over-rule other considerations which indicate a particular solution to be desirable. For example, the nickel-gold alloy mentioned in Chapter 2 shows excellent chemical and mechanical properties but its prohibitive cost rules out any practical use at present. This chapter deals with some mechanical and engineering properties of materials, including friction and wear, and makes brief comment on the physical properties relevant to orthopaedic applications.

The selection of a material for a given application is an extremely complex problem. Inevitably a compromise must be made between ideal and acceptable properties. For any particular implant, the component must support the loads which it will encounter in service when exposed to the corrosive environment of body fluids. In addition, the material must be able to be fabricated economically by available techniques and selection of a suitable material must include such considerations as shaping, joining and hardening. Few of these attributes can be defined as the direct consequences of one or two mechanical properties. They are rather the net result of many inter-related properties, and the selection process frequently rests more strongly on past experience than on short term laboratory measurements. Where short experimental study is the only available source of information, unexpected drawbacks of the material are likely to be encountered on exposure to novel environments.

Faced with a new material, an engineer designs a product against failure under particular conditions of service for a specific period of time. There are four principal modes of failure:

1. Excessive deformation. Perhaps the most frequently encountered failures of implants are the introduction of large, irrecoverable strains following static or dynamic overloading.

2. Fracture. After a material shows irrecoverable deformation it may fracture. In cases of ductile fracture, the component is usually deemed to have failed by excessive deformation, long before physical separation occurs. In contrast materials may fracture without appreciable plastic deformation under a variety of loading conditions such as high rates of deformation or fatigue conditions.

3. Abrasion or erosion. The material may undergo a process of gradual attrition or wear when two surfaces rub repeatedly.

4. Chemical attack. As described in Chapter 4 corrosion may lead to a mode of surface attack analogous to abrasion; alternatively it may initiate sudden failure by stress-corrosion cracking or corrosion fatigue analogous to brittle failure.

To design with an untested material so that it will function satisfactorily in a particular environment, it is clear that the characteristics of the environment must be rigorously defined. Regrettably, until recently the mechanical and chemical environment of the human body has been poorly characterized. Thus, even when a new material could be defined precisely by conventional mechanical testing methods, its suitability for a particular implant design could not be stated with confidence. A body of information is now slowly growing which should rectify this shortcoming.

MECHANICAL PROPERTIES

Elasticity

Elasticity can be studied by the use of a helical spring as indicated in Figure 3-1. When a load w, of 1 kg, is attached, the wire increases in length. The wire is said to be elastic for loads from 0 to 1 kg if the wire returns to its original length on removal of the weight. The extension, e, of the wire may be plotted as w is increased,

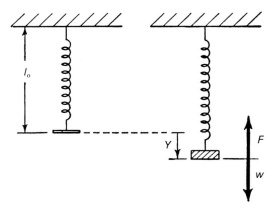

Figure 3-1. An experiment to demonstrate Hooke's law is shown. The force of the weight on the spring is w. The equal and opposite reaction of the spring on the weight is the elastic force, F. (Reproduced with permission from G. Shortley and D. Williams[1].)

as in Figure 3-2A. Initially a straight line OA is observed, followed by a curve, ABY. Until the point A is reached, the wire returns to its original length if the load is removed. Beyond A, however, the extension increases rapidly with increase in load, and the wire no longer returns to its original length when unloaded; it is thus permanently strained. A is called the *elastic limit* of the material.

Along the straight line OA, the extension is proportional to the load or tension in the wire until the elastic limit is exceeded. This is Hooke's law, after Robert Hooke who discovered the relation in 1676. The curve indicates that the use of such a wire as a surgical implant in the regime beyond A would be hazardous.

When the load exceeds the elastic limit, as indicated by the slight "kink" at B in Figure 3-2A, the material becomes plastic. The change from an elastic to a plastic stage is shown by a sudden increase in the extension. As the load is increased further the extension increases rapidly along the curve YN and the wire fails. The *breaking stress* of the wire is the force at failure per unit area of the wire. Substances such as lead, copper and soft iron which undergo considerable plastic deformation before failure are *ductile* materials. Other substances such as glass and high carbon steels, which fail immediately after the elastic limit is reached are known as *brittle* materials.

At the atomic or molecular level, the contrast between elastic and plastic deformation has been outlined in Chapter 2. During elastic deformation the atoms are distracted in such a way that they readily return to their original equilibrium

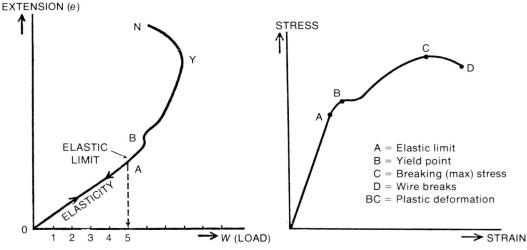

Figure 3-2. Graph A plots extension *vs.* load; graph B plots stress *vs.* strain.

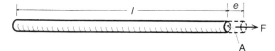

Figure 3-3. Tensile stress and strain in an elastic wire of original length, *l*, and area, *A*, shown when the wire is subjected to tensile stress, *F*.

positions when the material is unloaded. With the application of greater load, the available energy may exceed that necessary to break the bonds between the atoms, and create two new interfaces, and so the specimen fails. Alternatively, the atoms may find it energetically favorable to migrate into new, stable positions giving the same engineering strain while minimizing the interatomic distances. On removal of load, the atoms now have no driving force to revert to their original positions since the atoms are in identical positions with respect to their neighbors as if they were unstressed material. The dislocation mechanism by which the atomic rearrangement can most easily take place has already been outlined.[2]

Many materials, however, do not conform to the foregoing description of elasticity. The prime examples are rubbers and some other noncrystalline materials which possess a more flexible lattice arrangement. The force required to displace their atoms from equilibrium positions may vary considerably; indeed, it is not clear what should be these equilibrium positions. Such materials display "high elasticity," an attribute that is associated with long range rather than short range forces between the atoms.

It is useful to consider the technical terms used to describe deformation of materials.[3] When a force or tension *F* is applied to the end of a wire of cross-sectional area *A*, as in Figure 3-3,

tensile stress

$$= \text{force per unit area} = F/A.$$

If the extension of the wire is *e* and its original length is *l*,

tensile stress

$$= \text{extension per unit length} = e/l.$$

Stress has units such as dynes/cm^2, Newtons/m^2, kilograms/m^2 or pounds/inch^2 (psi). In contrast, strain, has no units because it is the ratio of two lengths. The actual value may be expressed as a fraction or it may be described as a percentage.

A modulus of elasticity of the wire, called

Young's modulus (*E*), is defined by the ratio

$$E = \frac{\text{tensile stress}}{\text{elastic strain}} = \frac{F/A}{e/l}.$$

Figure 3-2*b* shows the general stress/strain diagram for a ductile material; the slope of line *OA* is Young's modulus. The steeper the slope the higher the value of the modulus and the stiffer the material. Values of Young's modulus for a variety of materials are shown in Table 3-1, which shows that the ceramics tend to show the highest values. Metals may exhibit a wide variation of modulus. While values for polymers are included, these may not be strictly accurate; as will be shown below, polymers exhibit time-dependent elastic effects.

Materials also may be subjected to compressive forces (Fig. 3-4A). Compressive stress and strain are measured in an identical manner to tensile stress and strain. Materials may be subjected to shearing forces as illustrated in Figure 3-4B. If a specimen is subjected to a tangential force *F* on its top surface, the shape is altered by lateral displacement, although the volume remains unchanged. The *shear stress* acting on the material is equal to the applied tangential force per unit area of the top surface. The strain is a function of the angle θ through which the mass is sheared:

$$\text{shear strain} = \frac{\text{displacement of top surface}}{\text{thickness of specimen}}$$
$$= \tan \theta.$$

On an atomic scale, shear strain can be represented schematically as shown in Figure 3-4C. The bonds between atoms are deformed by a force at right angles to their original alignment. A geometrically complex system of shear is encountered in the torsion of a wire or rod, Figure 3-4D. In this case the applied torsional force, or torque, necessary to produce the twist about the longitudinal axis is directly related to the shear stress on the material. The angle of twist is proportional to the shear strain.

A material shows a different modulus in shear than in tension or compression since, on the atomic scale, shear forces operate in a different mode. The modulus is called either the shear modulus or the modulus of rigidity:

$$\text{shear modulus} = \frac{\text{shear stress}}{\text{shear strain}}$$

Again, shear modulus is measured in units of stress (dyne/cm^2 or Newton/m^2) and its value tends to be between 0.35 and 0.4 times the

Table 3-1
Young's Modulus, Shear Modulus and Poisson's Ratio for Some Materials

	Young's modulus (N/m^2)	Shear modulus (N/m^2)	Poisson's ratio
Metals			
Aluminum	7.0×10^{10}	2.6×10^{10}	0.345
Chromium	28.0×10^{10}	11.5×10^{10}	0.210
Copper	13.0×10^{10}	4.8×10^{10}	0.343
Pure iron	21.0×10^{10}	8.2×10^{10}	0.293
Stainless steel	21.0×10^{10}	8.4×10^{10}	0.283
Tantalum	18.0×10^{10}	6.9×10^{10}	0.342
Titanium	12.0×10^{10}	4.6×10^{10}	0.361
Ceramics			
Polycrystalline glass	9.0×10^{10}	3.6×10^{10}	0.25
Tungsten carbide	69.0×10^{10}	28.0×10^{10}	0.24
Graphite	0.7×10^{10}	0.3×10^{10}	0.14
Alumina	35.0×10^{10}	13.5×10^{10}	0.24
Silicon carbide	48.0×10^{10}	19.0×10^{10}	0.23
Polymers			
Epoxy resin	4.5×10^9	1.6×10^9	0.4
Polyethylene (medium-density)	0.4×10^9	0.14×10^9	0.45
Nylon 66	2.8×10^9	1.0×10^9	0.4
Polytetrafluoroethylene (PTFE)	0.5×10^9	0.18×10^9	0.4
Cast acrylic	3.0×10^9	1.1×10^9	0.4

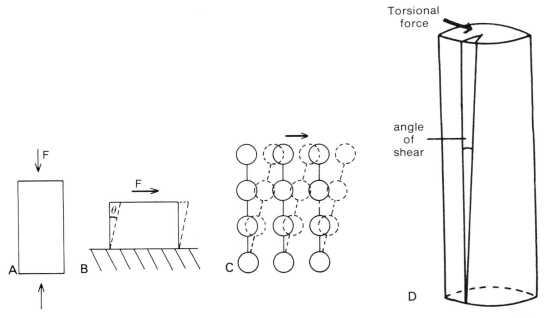

Figure 3-4. *A.* Definition of a compressive stress; *B.* Definition of a shear stress; *C.* Atomic movements in *D.* Shear stresses established by torsion of a rod. (Reproduced with permission from D. F. Williams and R. Roaf.[4])

Young's modulus. The shear modulus represents a measure of the resistance of a material to change in shape, and important practical applications in implants would include the torsion of screws or intramedullary rods or the elastic distortion of bone plates. Values of shear modulus also appear in Table 3-1.

While the strength, ductility, toughness or hardness of many materials may be readily altered by slight modifications in composition or heat treatment, the elastic moduli are intrinsic properties and are not easily changed. The measured elastic properties represent the average behavior of the bonds between adjacent atoms, and so sparsely intermingled foreign atoms in a lattice of pure metal provide no significant alteration in bulk elasticity. Table 3-1 confirms this observation for various pure metals and alloys. Apart from some exceptional polymeric materials, most structural materials show little alteration in stiffness or rigidity when subtle alloying adjustments are made.

When a metal is subjected to tensile stress, the longitudinal elongation is accompanied by a lateral contraction (*i.e.,* the material becomes thinner). For any material the ratio

$$\frac{\text{lateral contraction/original width}}{\text{longitudinal extension/original length}}$$

is a constant. The ratio is known as Poisson's ratio and is more properly written as

$$\frac{\text{transverse strain produced by axial stress}}{\text{axial strain produced by the same axial stress}}$$

Thus for any material, the transverse strain is proportional to the axial strain. If a material had a Poisson's ratio of 0, it would indicate an absence of reduction in thickness with elongation. On the other hand, at the maximum value of 0.5, the volume of the material is unchanged by deformation. In practice rubbery materials may show values approaching 0.5 and soft metals such as gold or lead, values of about 0.4 to 0.45. The majority of useful structural metals have values of about 0.28 to 0.35 while extremely hard materials show lower values of about 0.2. Some examples are shown in Table 3-1.

A second aspect of the deformation of materials is concerned with the geometry of the deformation. Some materials show physical properties which are independent of the direction in which the properties are measured; these are called *isotropic* materials. In contrast, *anisotropic* materials exhibit physical properties which vary with the direction of measurement. Wood is a familiar example of an anisotropic material. It has a grain and a structure which makes its physical properties quite different in the three principal directions. Bone is a similar example. A specimen of bone shows different compressive properties if the compressive stress is applied in different directions. These properties should be expressed by three separate Young's moduli in the principal directions rather than by a single value. Clearly single-valued moduli apply only to isotropic materials.

With certain exceptions, single crystals are anisotropic. They show different mechanical, optical and electrical properties in different directions. Metals are composed of large numbers of individual crystals, and while each crystal may be anisotropic, the crystals in bulk material are usually randomly orientated so that the metal as a whole behaves isotropically. It is possible, however, to fabricate polycrystalline metallic specimens in which most grains show a particular orientation; then, the material would be anisotropic. In polymers, the effect of anisotropy tends to be more pronounced because there are both interatomic and intermolecular forces of vastly different strengths. Fibrous polymeric materials derive particular benefit from such anisotropy, since the higher elastic moduli associated with the axial interatomic bonds dominate the bulk properties.

Plastic Deformation

When a material reaches the limit of elastic deformation, it may deform plastically when irrecoverable transposition of atoms or molecules occurs. The macroscopic features of plastic deformation may be observed when a specimen of material is subjected to a conventional tensile test. Figure 3-5 illustrates two examples of stress/strain curves resulting from this type of test. After the onset of plastic deformation, the curves have a lower slope than in the elastic region. With curves of type *B,* the change of slope is abrupt, although there may be subtle deviation from linearity immediately prior to the yield point. Most ferrous alloys show a characteristic yield point. At the atomic level, prior to deformation, there are strong forces resisting atomic movement of atoms to alternative sites. Once these forces are overcome, however, a certain amount of further deformation can continue

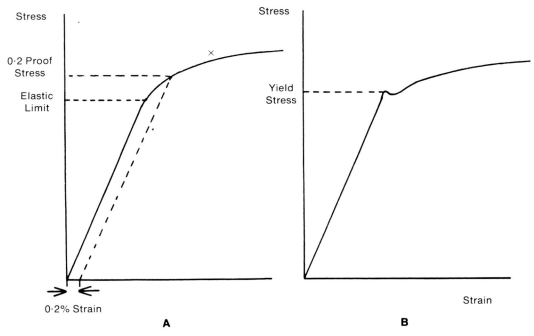

Figure 3-5. Stress-strain curves for materials deforming plastically are illustrated. In *A,* A gradual transition from elastic to plastic deformation appears; in *B,* a yield point is shown. (Reproduced with permission from D. F. Williams and R. Roaf.[4])

without increase of stress. Most plastics also exhibit a yield point although the subsequent change in stress is less abrupt.

On the other hand, many nonferrous alloys show curves such as that in Figure 3-5*A.* Here, the transition is sufficiently indistinct that it becomes difficult to define a precise elastic limit. In practice the curve may cease to be linear long before the elastic limit is reached. To overcome this difficulty engineers have adopted the quantity, 0.2% proof stress, the stress at which 0.2% plastic strain is reached, for design purposes.

The slope of the curve in the plastic region is less steep than in the elastic region. As the amount of plastic deformation increases, however, a continuous increase in stress is required to continue the deformation. The resistance of metal to additional plastic deformation is called work hardening or strain hardening. An explanation for this phenomenon has already been suggested in terms of the interaction or entanglement of mobile dislocations to inhibit further motion.

The plasticity of a material under tensile forces is called *ductility.* Ductility can be measured in several different ways. A specimen may be broken in tension and the reduction in cross-sectional area or the amount of plastic strain measured. The ductility may then be expressed as

$$ductility = \frac{change\ in\ length}{original\ length} \times 100\%,$$

or

$$ductility = \frac{change\ in\ cross\text{-}sectional\ area\ at\ fracture\ site}{original\ cross\text{-}sectional\ area} \times 100\%.$$

Useful ductile materials show values of ductility of as high as 60 to 90%. In contrast, plasticity in compression is called malleability. Most pure metals are highly ductile, since each atom in the bulk material is surrounded by identical atoms, and there are no directional bonds. Ductility is thus limited only by the interaction of dislocations. Fabrication often involves substantial deformation of a material, and such cold working imparts considerable strength. If the work-hardened material is heated above its "recrystallization" temperature, the atoms rearrange themselves into an entirely new array of strain-free grains. The process is shown schematically in Figure 3-6, in which the new grains grow from nuclei, generally at the grain boundaries of the

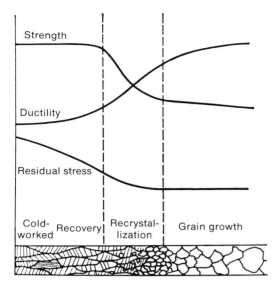

Strength

Ductility

Residual stress

| Cold-worked | Recovery | Recrystal-lization | Grain growth |

Figure 3-6. The effect of annealing on cold-worked metal is revealed. (Reproduced with permission from W. D. Biggs.[5])

deformed structure, until they impinge on each other. The driving force for recrystallization is the lowering of the overall energy of the system as the deformed grains are replaced by strain-free grains. For a given degree of strain hardening, the rate of crystallization is a function of temperature; the minimum recrystallization temperature is approximately $0.4\ T_m$ where T_m is the melting point of the material in degrees Kelvin. The recrystallized material is again capable of further deformation, and if extensive working of a sample is required, several intermediate annealings may be necessary.

Fracture

When the atoms in any part of a material are sufficiently stressed but unable to slip into new positions, fracture will ensue. Fracture may occur in brittle solids with virtually no prior plastic deformation. Alternatively, in ductile solids it may occur when the limit of plasticity has been reached. Either brittle or ductile solids may undergo fatigue fracture as a result of the repeated application of a stress which is lower than that required to cause failure in a single application. *Brittle fracture* occurs when the material fractures while it is still elastic. It occurs suddenly and the faceted fracture surfaces are geometrically similar and can be fitted together to form the original shape (Fig. 3-7). Brittle solids usually break at about $\frac{1}{1000}$ of Young's modulus. Calculations based on known bond strengths

predict theoretical fracture stresses much greater than the experimental values. As mentioned previously, the discrepancy arises from defects particularly at the surface of the material, which provide sites for stress concentration, and Griffith's analysis of this effect has been discussed. Even in the most brittle metals, however, there is some evidence of slight plastic deformation before brittle fracture.

Other materials under tensile stress extend until they narrow down to a point or edge and cohesion is lost. This type of *ductile fracture* is characteristic of hot glass and single crystals of metals such as zinc and cadmium. With most ductile materials, however, the "necked" region is highly localized so that deformation occurs in two distinct phases, uniform extension followed by localized extension at the neck (Fig. 3-8). It seems that more plastic strain is always needed to spread a crack once it has formed in ductile material so that the crack is perhaps best perceived as an internal cavity which grows outward as the narrowed region or neck continues to decrease in diameter. Such cavities are usually nucleated at foreign particles such as nonmetallic inclusions, so that a very pure metal would be expected to fail wholly by progressive reduction in area at the neck. Final separation occurs by shear along planes at 45° to the axis of the specimen.

A third mode of failure occurs as the result of many applications of a stress lower than that required to cause failure in a single application. Such *fatigue failure* occurs at significantly lower life times as the applied stress increases, although there may be a marked scatter in any one series of tests. For some metals and alloys such as steels, a stress level is observed below which failure does not occur; this "fatigue limit" is empirically observed to be about 0.4 times the ultimate tensile strength. As in other failure mechanisms, fatigue can be divided into stages of nucleation and propagation. The mechanisms are somewhat better understood in metals than in nonmetals. In metals, the crack usually initiates at the surface and grows slowly during the functional life of the specimen. Initiation seems to represent about 5 to 15% of the total functional life. Deformation tends to be localized within a few grains and develops into persistent slip bands, which cannot be removed by polishing and etching. At some stage of growth, cracks form in the slip bands, which may intersect a number of grains. This stage can be considered as a zig-zag crack which develops approximately at right angles to the direction of principal ten-

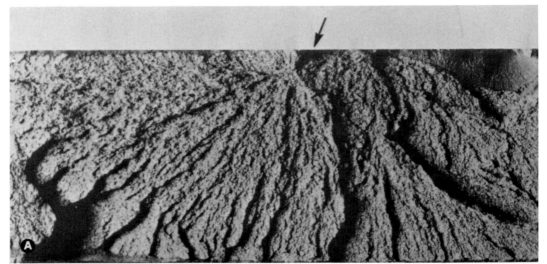

Figure 3-7. *A.* The "chevron" pattern points to the origin of a brittle fracture (*arrow*) in this specimen. A fracture surface is also apparent in the upper right hand corner. (Reproduced with permission from B. J. Wulpi.[6]) *B* and *C.* Brittle, cleavage fracture surface of a failed cast cobalt-chromium alloy is shown in the two scanning electron micrographs. *B,* ×120. *C,* ×1000 (Reproduced with permission from Miss O. Pöhler).

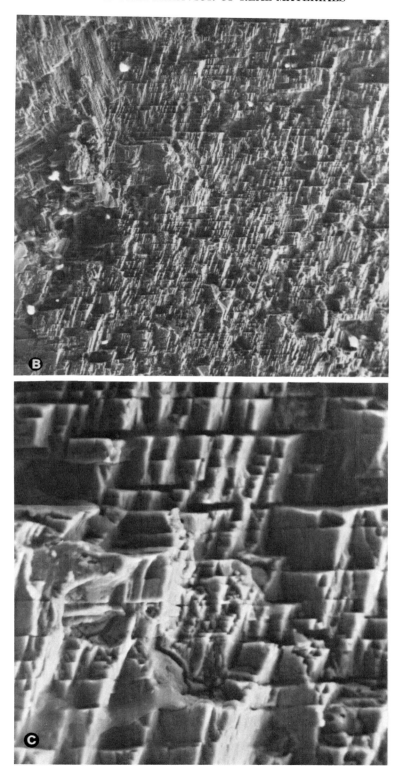

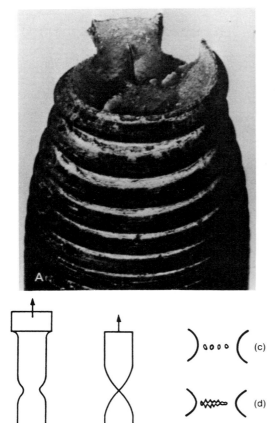

Figure 3-8. *A.* A photograph reveals an example of ductile failure. *B.* A schematic diagram illustrates the principal features of ductile failure. In (*a*) the formation of a tensile neck is seen. In (*b*) point rupture or chisel-edge rupture occurs, as seen in many soft metals that approximate ideal ductility. Alternatively, as seen in most metals, however, small holes usually form at weak or weakly adherent foreign inclusions. Rupture occurs by the growth and coalescence of holes in the neck (*c* and *d*) which ultimately lead to (*e*) fibrous cup-and-cone rupture.

sile stress. The stress concentration at the crack tip promotes further growth at each positive stress cycle, giving rise to the typical striated appearance of the fracture surface (Fig. 3-9). Finally, when the residual section is sufficiently small and highly stressed it fails by conventional overload mechanisms.

A number of factors affect fatigue life. Surface notches or holes severely reduce fatigue strength. Surface conditions are therefore exceptionally important in fatigue behavior, and a surface roughened by scratches or by corrosion may show a reduction in fatigue strength of up to 20%. Improvement in surface finish of specimens raises the fatigue strength and also reduces the scatter in results of fatigue tests. In general fine-grained materials show superior fatigue life. Localized precipitation of second phases within the grains has a similar effect. The shape and distribution of internal inhomogeneity such as oxides and inclusions is also an influential factor. One method for improving fatigue strength is to introduce residual compressive stresses into the surface of the specimen, for example by shot peening or surface rolling. In contrast residual tensile stresses are invariably deleterious.

Hardness

The term hardness is used in practice to describe two somewhat different, though related, mechanical properties. It is a measure of the resistance to abrasion, the ability of one material to scratch or be scratched by another. In Mohs' scale of hardness a series of standard materials is arranged in order, with talc at number 1, rising to diamond at 10. Each material will scratch any material lower in the table. Materials under test can be assigned a position in the series by similar scratch tests. Metals may show hardness values

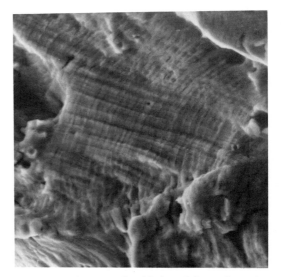

Figure 3-9. An example of fatigue failure of a stainless steel implant with scanning electron microscopy. ×1460. Reproduced with permission from Miss O. Pöhler).

on this scale ranging from <2 to >8, while plastics are normally in the range of 2 to 3.

More frequently hardness indicates resistance to indentation. In the usual form of test, a material is indented by a ball (Brinell test) or by a pyramidal diamond (Vickers test) or by a conical diamond (Rockwell test). The hardness is defined as some convenient function of the area of the indentation and the load and is usually expressed in kg/mm^2. High values indicate hard materials and low values, soft materials. Under some circumstances, the hardness assessed in this way may show a linear relationship with the yield stress in tension. Usually, however, indentation is accompanied by local work hardening so that hardness becomes a function of both yield strength and work hardening rate.

Time-dependent Deformation of Materials

Many materials are not perfectly elastic in their response to stress. Their deformation may be partly elastic but also have some of the characteristic flow of viscous liquids. Such phenomena can be divided into viscoelasticity and creep.

Linear polymers consist of long-chain molecules with only weak van der Waals bonds between chains. There is thus the possibility for these chains to slide past each other under stress to provide a viscous component to deformation under stress. In addition, the stretching of chains by rotation and extension of molecular bonds provides an elastic component. Viscoelasticity is also displayed by musculoskeletal tissues such as muscle, tendon or bone. This sort of behavior raises problems in design and in mechanical testing since the mechanical properties will be sensitive to the time over which the stress is applied and the temperature of testing.

In a somewhat comparable way, material may show progressive deformation with time under constant stress. This process of creep is markedly dependent on temperature. Noncrystalline materials are much more temperature-sensitive than metals and deform rapidly on exposure to quite low stresses. Creep tests are usually performed at constant temperature under constant load so that both of these quantities can be varied independently. A characteristic form of creep curve is shown in Figure 3-10. Three zones of behavior are evident, transient creep AB which may include an elastic component, steady state creep BC and tertiary creep CD. The transient stage is particularly evident in metals. It is associated with work hardening processes in

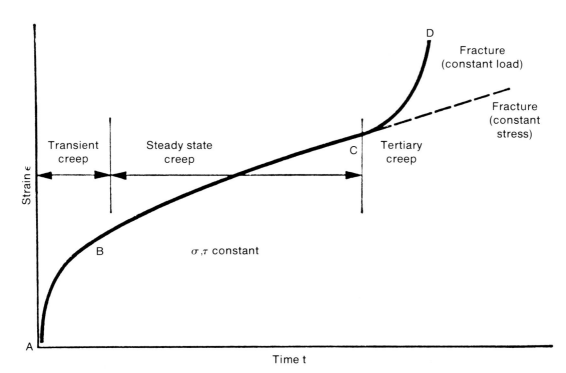

Figure 3-10. The general form of a curve relating strain and time under conditions where creep can occur is revealed. (Reproduced with permission from W. D. Biggs.[5])

which dislocations become entangled with each other and locked at grain boundaries. This process ceases when equilibrium is achieved under the particular conditions of stress and temperature. Steady-state creep denotes the equilibrium rate of deformation and may be either viscous or plastic in character depending on the magnitude of stress and temperature. It is a continuous thermally-activated process in which diffusion is the controlling mechanism. In tertiary creep, deformation occurs at an accelerating rate and the progressive damage culminates in fracture.

While the theories of creep are inadequate to allow accurate predictions of creep resistance of specific materials, certain guidelines are available. Favorable attributes of creep resistant alloys include a high melting point, face-centered cubic structure in which dislocations experience greater resistance to motion and the presence of stable precipitates which restrict dislocation movement. The creep resistance of plastics varies widely from one material to another, but resistance to creep deformation can be increased by the addition of fillers or other reinforcing materials which raise the viscosity. On the other hand, the creep resistance of plastics is seriously compromised by the presence of moisture which penetrates the material and functions as a plasticizer.

DESIRABLE PROPERTIES OF IMPLANTABLE MATERIALS

The discussion of materials has so far attempted to assess different mechanical properties.[7] The more difficult task is to determine the particular features of a material which are useful in a specific situation. Most favorable attributes of materials comprise a number of properties, the sum of which may be difficult to define precisely.

Strength has been previously defined as the resistance of a material to an applied stress. Tensile strength alone has remarkably little significance or descriptive value. For example, the tensile strengths of mild steel, Duralumin, natural silk, cotton and nylon all lie within the same range of 50,000 to 80,000 psi, but these materials are dissimilar in practically every other respect. Again, the tensile strength of a brittle solid is determined by the number, size and location of pre-existing flaws so that a particular value of tensile strength is of significance only if the scatter of the population of values is considered. Since the maximum and minimum values may differ by two orders of magnitude, it is essential to know which value is relevant before a design

figure is adopted. Clearly the strength of a material must be adequate for a particular application. Surprisingly low values of strength may suffice however, if other mechanical and physical properties are satisfactory. A similar rationale applies to considerations of stiffness or specific moduli of materials.

Toughness

Toughness may be the single most important attribute of structural materials. It is a measure of the energy necessary to produce fracture. The energy to produce tensile failure is determined as the area under the stress/strain curve (Fig. 3-11). A brittle material of high tensile strength may show a small area (curve A). Alternatively, as in curve B, a material may be highly ductile, but weak and again show only a small area. The area under curve C, and therefore the energy to fracture, is high, so that a material displaying this type of curve is tough. In general, it is easier to increase this area by increasing the breaking strain than by raising the ultimate tensile stress. High toughness and high ductility in terms of breaking strain have therefore come to be regarded as synonymous. Toughness and ductility may be considered to be the designer's insurance policy against accidental overload or localized strain.

Unfortunately the conventional impact tests to measure toughness do not yield particularly helpful results for design purposes. The susceptibility of a material to the effects of local concentrations of stress is assessed by means of a notched specimen which is broken in bending as

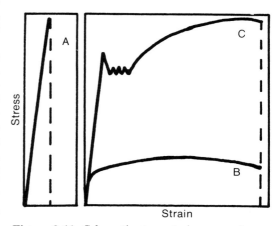

Figure 3-11. Schematic stress-strain curves show a low energy requirement to fracture A strong brittle and B weak ductile material and a high energy requirement to fracture C strong ductile material.

a beam (Charpy test) or as a cantilever (Izod test) under impact loading conditions. The test does not distinguish clearly between a material having a high rate of work hardening with low total deformation and one having a low rate of work hardening with a large deformation to fracture. In practice the impact test is most useful to exclude materials that show brittle behavior under some conditions of temperature or heat treatment. Problems with brittle materials are more apparent when they are subjected to impact loading conditions than with static or slow loading. With slow application of load a minute amount of plastic deformation may occur which will be adequate to inhibit the propagation of small cracks. Under high speed loading conditions there may be insufficient time for plastic deformation to precede the crack and the brittle failure is observed.

While for virtually all orthopaedic implants toughness is especially important, some appliances also require particularly high strength or rigidity, ductility or other attributes. The materials engineer must be able to select the most suitable material and modify it to match mechanical properties to the design criteria. The need for prior accurate assessment of the mechanical forces that will be imposed by the body on the implant and of the precise mechanical requirements for any particular application cannot be overemphasized.

MODIFICATION OF MECHANICAL PROPERTIES OF METALS AND ALLOYS

Certain applications of metallic implants require toughness combined with especially high strength. The three general mechanisms for strengthening metals are work hardening, solute hardening and fiber strengthening.

For implant alloys, perhaps the most widely used means of strengthening is work hardening. The simplest example of work hardening is the drawing of a wire. Various degrees of hardness and strength can be obtained, depending on the amount of work hardening. While this method reduces ductility, this can be restored in part by annealing the work-hardened material, accompanied by some reduction in ultimate strength. Annealing also may alter the structure of the metal to further modify the mechanical properties, and the combination of work hardening and annealing can be extremely useful.

The second mechanism of strengthening of metals is solute hardening. As described previously, the dispersion of foreign atoms of slightly different size into a lattice may inhibit the movement of dislocations and postpone the onset of plastic deformation. Rather than such substitutional alloying, interstitial atoms may be introduced which profoundly distort the crystal lattice. The foreign atoms may be metallic or nonmetallic atoms. Table 3-2 indicates the strength of titanium alloys containing different amounts of oxygen; variation of oxygen content of 0.25% results in nearly a 3-fold increase in 0.2% proof stress. Again as mentioned earlier, modification of phases in alloys may considerably alter their strengths. The introduction of body-tetragonal martensite into austenitic stainless steel by appropriate heat treatment increases the tensile strength significantly. Another example is the recently introduced multiphase cobalt-nickel-chromium alloy, MP35N, in which a similar method is applied to achieve great strength. The strength of titanium may also be greatly increased by the introduction of a second phase. The addition of molybdenum, tantalum, niobium or aluminum, vanadium and tin to alloys of titanium promotes the development of stable two-phase structures on heat treatment, with a corresponding increase in strength (Fig. 3-12).

Finally, the combination of different metals or metals with nonmetals to produce composites may provide materials of greatly improved strength and stiffness. The commercial techniques for achieving this are now becoming available at realistic cost. A further practical problem has been the construction of fiber-reinforced materials of adequate ductility so that the composites can be fabricated by conventional methods.

In the past complex implants with multiple components have been fabricated from a single alloy to avoid the risk of accelerated attack by galvanic corrosion. The corrosion of dissimilar metals is fully discussed in Chapter 4. It seems, however, that the corrosion of combinations of dissimilar passive or inert alloys has been greatly overemphasized, and a wide variety of inert alloys can probably be used in combination without deleterious side-effects. If the absence of undue risk is accepted from the corrosion standpoint, then combinations of dissimilar alloys for the construction of complex implants become extremely attractive. Previously, alloys such as austenitic stainless steel, which could be made with a range of mechanical properties, were used for the construction of complex implants, even if the range of mechanical properties was not as wide as would be ideal. Austenitic stainless steel may be treated to give values of yield strength

Table 3-2
Mechanical Properties of Various Materials

	Tensile Strength (N/m²)	Yield Strength (N/m²)	Elongation at Fracture (%)	Hardness (V.P.N.)	Young's Modulus (n/m²)	Shear Modulus (N/m²)	Fatigue Limit (N/m²)
Metals							
316 Stainless steel, annealed	$6.5 \cdot 10^8$	$2.8 \cdot 10^8$	45	190	$21.0 \cdot 10^{10}$	$8.4 \cdot 10^{10}$	$2.8 \cdot 10^8$
316 Stainless steel, cold-worked	$10.0 \cdot 10^8$	$7.5 \cdot 10^8$	9	325	$23.0 \cdot 10^{10}$	—	$3.0 \cdot 10^8$
Wrought cobalt-chromium alloy, cold-worked	$15.4 \cdot 10^8$	$10.5 \cdot 10^8$	9	450	$24.0 \cdot 10^{10}$	—	$4.9 \cdot 10^8$
Cast cobalt-chromium alloy	$6.9 \cdot 10^8$	$4.0 \cdot 10^8$	8	300	$24.0 \cdot 10^{10}$	—	$3.0 \cdot 10^8$
MP35N	$16.7 \cdot 10^8$	$7.8 \cdot 10^8$	13	—	$24.0 \cdot 10^{10}$	—	—
Titanium 160, annealed	$7.1 \cdot 10^8$	$4.7 \cdot 10^8$	30	—	$12.0 \cdot 10^{10}$	$4.6 \cdot 10^{10}$	$3.0 \cdot 10^8$
Ti-6Al-4V alloy	$10.0 \cdot 10^8$	$9.7 \cdot 10^8$	12	—	$12.0 \cdot 10^{10}$	—	—
Plastics							
Nylon 66	$8.5 \cdot 10^7$		90		$2.8 \cdot 10^9$	$1.0 \cdot 10^9$	
Polymethylmethacrylate	$7.0 \cdot 10^7$		5		$3.0 \cdot 10^8$	$1.1 \cdot 10^9$	
Polypropylene	$3.5 \cdot 10^7$		500		—	—	
Polyethylene (H.D.)	$3.0 \cdot 10^7$		800		$0.4 \cdot 10^9$	$0.14 \cdot 10^9$	
Polytetrafluoroethylene (PTFE)	$2.3 \cdot 10^7$		600		$0.5 \cdot 10^9$	$0.18 \cdot 10^9$	
Silicone rubber	$0.5 \cdot 10^7$		600		—		

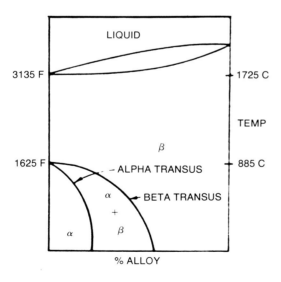

Figure 3-12. The constitutional diagram for some titanium alloys reveals the solidification of β-titanium with a body-centered cubic structure and transformation to the α-structure with a close-packed hexagonal form on further cooling.

between 250 and 770 MN/m², of tensile strength between 610 and 1000 MN/m² and of ductility between 36 and 8%. While this is certainly a wide range for a single material of this type, a much wider range is possible by the use of dissimilar alloys in combination.

For many orthopaedic implants the ideal modulus of elasticity or rigidity remains a controversial issue. In a few situations such as thin, small bone plates for application in the hand, or in Kirschner wires, a rigid material is clearly preferred. For application in most bone plates, in intramedullary rods or for total joint replacements the use of an implantable material more rigid than the bone may be detrimental. In such a situation, normal fatigue forces associated with weight bearing and physical activities will not be borne by the bone, and such "stress protection" may provoke osteoporosis or limitation in the normal rate of healing of bone at fractures.[8] Certainly where bony ingrowth into a porous coated implant unites the bone to a more rigid material, fatigue forces will lead to fatigue fracture of the bone at the interface. Unfortunately, most materials with low moduli also have low tensile strengths, and when such materials are used with bone, either their use must be limited to nonweight-bearing situations or they must be applied after the bone has been reconstructed so that it is inherently stable. In such cases minimal tensile forces or bending moments may be imposed on the implant. One example is the recent report of the application of polyethylene and polycarbonate plates to fractures in osteoporotic bone.*

Ductility of metals is highly desirable to facilitate fabrication of surgical implants. A few implants such as the titanium sheet for reinforcement of methylmethacrylate, require considerable fabrication by the surgeon at the time of implantation. Other implants such as bone plates may require modest shaping by the surgeon to contour the plate to match the bony surface. In such cases, titanium alloys or austenitic stainless steel are superior to the cobalt-chromium alloys. Most implants however are used without deliberate alteration of shape, so that ductility is an asset only for fabrication. While brittleness should be avoided, excessive ductility may lead to deformation during the period of implantation. For many implants such as intramedullary rods, bending of the implant, even after its functional life-time is completed, can impede removal.

Fatigue failure of surgical alloys has gradually become the principal cause of implant failure.[9] The reason for this is 2-fold. With the introduction of total joint replacements over the past decade, the prolonged implantation of metals has greatly increased. Since approximately 3 million flexions of the hip or spine per year is typical for a sedentary individual, the serious fatigue considerations for a total hip joint replacement or a Harrington rod for spinal immobilization may readily be appreciated. Unfortunately little information is available on the fatigue behavior of the currently available implantable alloys. The fatigue limits given by the British Standards Institution[10] and by others[11] are listed in Table 3-1. The highest values are obtained for wrought cobalt-chromium alloy while the purest grade of commercially pure titanium (Ti 115) shows the lowest value. The surgical grade of titanium (Ti 160), cold-worked or annealed stainless steel and cast cobalt-chromium alloy have similar values. In rotational-bending tests on machined specimens of 316 stainless steel Laing and O'Donnell[12] reported that for a variety of cross-sectional shapes of hip nails, the fatigue limits were as low as 10% of the yield point in bending. Clearly stress concentrations associated with implant design can have a critical effect on fatigue life.

Several authors[13-15],† have documented clinical examples of fatigue failure in orthopaedic implants, and a number of workers [16-18] have recently reported fatigue failures of the stems of total hip joint replacements of a wide variety of designs and materials. The incidence of such failures is extremely difficult to determine. Retrieval of implants has not been the subject of statistically valid surveys. After fracture, the opposing surfaces may fret and obliterate the telltale signs of a particular mode of failure. Similarly the surgeon may damage the fracture surfaces at the time of removal. Nevertheless, it is clear that there are more fatigue fractures of orthopaedic implants than is desirable. As in the case of structural failure in aircraft, bridges or buildings, the penalties associated with abrupt mechanical failure of many implants are unacceptably great.

The irony is that fatigue failure might appear to be more easily eliminated than other types of mechanical failure. Fatigue failure is usually associated with poor design, workmanship or handling. By the elimination of sites of stress concentration such as crevices, corners or other irregularities, the nucleation of fatigue cracks should be inhibited. In practice, however, even if great care is taken during fabrication, scratches will *inevitably* arise during surgical implantation. With the limitations imposed by the obvious need for outstanding corrosion resistance, the range of materials is severely reduced and many alloys with excellent fatigue resistance are excluded from consideration. Furthermore anatomical considerations frequently restrict the designer's freedom to exclude sites of stress concentration on many implants. As a result of such practical considerations, fatigue failure of metal implants is likely to remain a problem. The best hope for improvement rests on the possible introduction of a variety of fiber-reinforced composite materials that show remarkable resistance to fatigue.

The previous discussion has rested upon the assumption that the surgeon employs a particular implant to a particular role and in the

---

* R. Pilliar, personal communication, 1977.

† M. Allgöwer and T. Ruedi, personal communication, 1975.

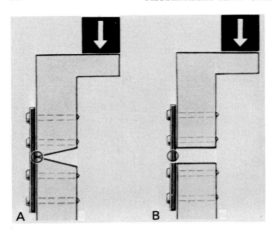

Figure 3-13. Two examples of the incorrect application of a bone plate to a fracture, without reconstruction of a solid column of bone at the fracture site are shown. If these situations are observed in a postoperative X-ray, fatigue failure of the implant can be predicted unless alteration of the postoperative management is initiated.

precise conditions of load for which the implant was designed. Until recent years, the operating conditions for particular implants were not well defined. For example bone plates frequently were applied to a fracture without accurate reconstruction of the adjacent bone with resumption of activity by the patient. The plate transmitted virtually all of the load imposed upon the limb. As described in Chapter 9, plates were not designed for this type of application which is shown in Figure 3-13. During the past decade, many workers have studied implant failures and have defined the conditions under which the implant is likely to function satisfactorily without fatigue failure. With the availability of this knowledge, it has become feasible to examine postoperative X-rays in internal fixation devices and decide whether the implant was used in a way that is likely to culminate in fatigue failure. Furthermore, the precise site on the implant where the implant will fail can be predicted accurately. With this knowledge, the surgeon can alter the anticipated postoperative course, by limiting the patient's activities, applying an external cast or support or undertaking surgical revision, so that failure of the implant does not occur. In the author's experience most of the fatigue failures of fixation devices are of this type. With superior education, surgeons of the future should be able to recognize unsatisfactory mechanical conditions for internal fixations and prevent most fatigue failures.

One further question which has rarely been considered is the optimum fatigue life for devices used in the internal fixation of fractures. The duration of normal fracture repair varies considerably, from about 3 weeks for small chip fractures of phalanges, to 3 to 6 months for fractures of the femoral neck or shaft. In some instances, for example with poor mechanical stabilization of avascular fragments of bone, or with malignancy or certain inflammatory conditions, the duration of fracture repair may extend indefinitely. In such circumstances fatigue fracture of the implant becomes highly likely. On the other hand, experience suggests that most fatigue fractures occur when the surgeon fails technically to achieve rigid stabilization with abutting bony fragments. In such cases, the probability of fatigue fracture could be predicted from the intraoperative X-ray in which the gap between bone fragments is apparent.[19] Clearly the plate then becomes subjected to large bending moments. If the surgeon recognizes the problem, he may prevent it by postoperative limitation of weight-bearing, external immobilization or by intraoperative alteration of the surgical procedure. In other situations fatigue fracture could not be eliminated simply by educating surgeons. For example, after intramedullary rod fixation of long bones, nonunion of the fracture is uncommon. However, when it does occur, the patient may have no symptoms because the rod provides adequate immobilization. Within 18 to 24 months after internal fixation, fatigue fracture of currently available rods is extremely likely to accompany a nonunion. Admittedly, radiography of the extremity prior to the fatigue failure might show evidence of the nonunion of bone, but with the mobility of modern life, many cases will arise where patients are lost at least temporarily to follow-up so that the X-rays are not taken.

Admittedly there are a few implants, in particular those with multiple components, that show designs which favor fatigue failure. The nail-plate assemblies for fixation of fractures of the femoral neck as shown in Chapter 9, and bone screws (Fig. 3-14) are prime examples. High concentrations of stress arise at small areas of contact. In addition, a small amplitude of movement frequently occurs between the components so that fretting and fatigue conditions prevail. As shown in Chapter 9, some recent designs appear to have overcome these problems.

In summary, apart from a few poorly designed implants most orthopaedic implants are subject to rigorous fatigue conditions, they may also

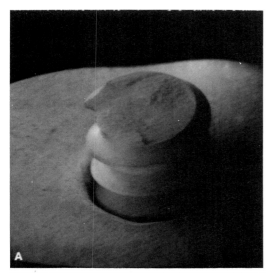

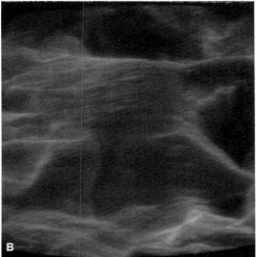

Figure 3-14. Scanning electron micrographs reveal the fracture surface of a titanium bone screw that underwent fatigue fracture. ×8. *B,* ×4000. (Reproduced with permission from Zimmer U.S.A.).

require design features that predispose to stress concentration. Implantation may aggravate the situation by damage to the surface of the implant. Elimination of fatigue failure is unlikely to be achieved by drastic changes in the designs of implants, the methods of fabrication or of implantation. An alternative route, the use of inert alloys of improved intrinsic resistance to fatigue failure appears to be the only mechanical solution. The optimal method of improvement is better education of surgeons to recognize satisfactory mechanical and radiological conditions which largely preclude fatigue failures.

MODIFICATION OF THE MECHANICAL PROPERTIES OF POLYMERS AND CERAMICS

The mechanical properties of polymeric materials may be modified by regulation of crystallinity, molecular weight and molecular linearity.[20] As suggested previously, crystallization is associated with an increase in strength. Elongation of material at constant load causes stress-induced ordering or crystallization, which leads to greater tensile strength. Crystallization also alters the viscoelastic behavior, widening the distribution of relaxation times and extending the relaxation of stress to much longer times. With increase in molecular weight polyethylene may show improvement of strength, with an increase of ultimate tensile stress from about $15.2 \, MN/m^2$ to about $27.6 \, MN/m^2$. At the same time the elongation to fracture is reduced from 620 to 500%. Similarly for polytetrafluoroethylene (PTFE), increased orientation of molecular chains by cold drawing may raise the ultimate tensile stress from about $17.2 \, MN/m^2$ to about $27.6 \, MN/m^2$. For linear crystalline polymers such as the polyamides (nylons), bonding between adjacent chains alters the mechanical properties. Nylon 66 has a high degree of hydrogen bonding between adjacent chains while nylon 610 has considerably less. In Table 3-3 the mechanical properties of these nylons and of a nylon co-polymer are shown. Nylon 66 shows the highest strength and elastic modulus. The co-polymer has a more random arrangement of amide groups and the least hydrogen bonding, and thus it shows the lowest strength and elastic modulus.

In other instances co-polymerization may be used to improve strength. For example the co-polymerization of propylene with ethylene may improve the impact strength as much as 10-fold. Many engineering thermoplastics rely on this principle, in which ordering of molecules is increased by the polymerization. Commercial techniques are available for regulation of the sites of the different units in co- or ter-polymers to produce block co-polymers and graft co-polymers. Thus, instead of random dispersion of monomeric units, the monomers may be arranged in blocks of the same type, or side chains formed from one monomer may be "grafted" on to a backbone formed from another. In this way the individual components may contribute more effectively to the provision of the required mechanical properties than if they were randomly dispersed.

Table 3-3
Mechanical Properties of Some Polyamides

Property	Nylon 66	Nylon 610	66/610/6 Co-polymer 40%/30%/30%
Yield stress MN/m^2	79.3	58.6	31.0
Elongation %	90	120	300
Elastic modulus MN/m^2	2965	2069	1379
Density kg/m^3	1140	1090	1080

Viscoelastic failure of polymeric components has become an urgent problem in recent years. Previously the major application of solid polymers was in total hip joint replacements. While high loads were transmitted, the hemispherical geometry of the articular surfaces limited the force per unit area, and Charnley et al.[21] discounted the possibility of such deformation contributing to polymeric failure. In total knee replacements and total ankle joint replacements, however, failure of high density polyethylene by creep has become a major mode of failure. In designs where complex radii of curvature are adopted in an attempt to mimic the geometry of human joints, failure by creep may occur within 2 to 5 years after implantation. While the addition of graphite fibers has improved wear or erosion resistance and toughness it has not improved creep resistance in these materials. Other commercial additives or fillers, which are frequently added to polymers to reduce the quantity of expensive polymer in the plastic, do not improve creep resistance either. Other polymers under examination, such as the polyesters, have failed to show significant superiority over polyethylene in respect to creep resistance. Further research is clearly essential.

While ceramics have high strengths, they are excessively brittle for most present surgical applications. Their attributes appear to limit their application to massive replacement of bone, and other roles for which metals are inherently unsuitable. However, the reinforcement of metals with ceramics is provoking particular interest. For example, at 8% carbon the tantalum-carbon system forms a eutectic which contains about 30 vol.% of the extremely strong intermetallic compound Ta$_2$C. During solidification, the Ta$_2$C can be grown in a rod-like form in the metal matrix so that the strength of alloy can be elevated from 45 MN/m^2 to over 1000 MN/m^2. Such research curiosities provide an insight into the possibilities of potential inert materials of superior strength, stiffness, and wear- and creep-resistance for surgical applications.

At present metal-ceramic mixtures, or cermets, such as bonded tungsten carbide, provide the best cutting edges for many orthopaedic tools; they can be fabricated by standard powder-sintering methods. While such materials possess excellent strength and creep resistance their inherent brittleness limits their use to cutting edges of surgical scissors or osteotomes, and the surfaces of jaws for holding instruments such as needle holders or hemostats.

FRICTION AND WEAR

With the rapid increase in the use of partial or total joint replacements in orthopaedic surgery, the friction and wear of materials for construction and the lubrication of joints has become a major field of concern. The characteristics of human joints and of possible joint replacements have been studied closely; the former are described in Chapter 5. One further feature of rubbing surfaces, transfer of material from one surface to the other, is discussed after a description of friction, wear and lubrication.

Coefficient of Friction

If two flat surfaces are moved one over the other, a frictional force is encountered which resists their relative motion. The limiting value of the tangential force for a given pair of surfaces is a constant fraction of the normal force pressing the two surfaces together. This fraction is the *coefficient of friction* for that pair of surfaces. The total frictional force to be overcome thus depends only on the normal force and not on the area over which it is distributed. When unidirectional sliding of flat surfaces is considered, therefore, experiments on any size of specimen should give the same value for the coefficient of friction.

When curved surfaces are considered the picture is more complex. For example, a spherical ball may be pressed into a matching hemispherical socket by means of a vertical force. A certain minimum turning moment is then required to make the ball rotate in any direction relative to the socket. The vertical force is transmitted from the ball to the socket as the sum of forces acting on small elements of the contact surface and therefore inclined at various angles to the vertical. Each of these small elements will contribute to the frictional force when movement is attempted or initiated and the turning moment which must be applied is that which balances the sum of the moments of all of these elemental frictional forces. Thus the relationship between the applied vertical force and the limiting frictional moment depends upon the distribution of pressure over the contact area and the extent of this area, as well as upon the coefficient of friction for the two materials. Conversely, if a coefficient of friction is sought from experiments on bearings with curved surfaces, the value cannot be determined without some knowledge of or assumptions about the distribution of pressure. The degree of congruity of the surfaces becomes a critical factor. If, for example, the socket of a ball-and-socket joint is slightly larger in diameter than the ball, most of the force will be transmitted through a small area of contact close to the load axis, and the frictional situation is similar to that when two flat surfaces are pressed together. If, however, the ball has the larger diameter, most of the force will be transmitted through the "equatorial" region. Large pressures will be exerted at the equator with correspondingly higher frictional forces. For a given vertical force acting on the whole joint an appreciably higher frictional moment will be developed than in a joint where the socket has the larger radius.

Lubrication

If a fluid film is present between adjacent surfaces the frictional forces are usually lower and may have considerably different characteristics from the forces exerted between dry surfaces. Under high magnification the dry surfaces are observed to be highly irregular. When the surfaces are opposed the actual contact area may be a small fraction of the total surface area. At very low velocities of relative motion, contacting surfaces develop points of attachment, or cold welds, which must be disrupted. In contrast, when the surfaces are lubricated they do not rub against each other. Rather, there is relative motion between minute volumes of fluid. Unlike the forces of solid friction, fluid frictional forces are extremely sensitive to velocity. If the velocity of the fluid "particles" inside a laminar stream is examined, a velocity gradient is observed from the center to the outside of the

moving stream, with particles in the center of the flow showing maximum velocity. The change in velocity of the fluid particles causes a frictional shearing force proportional to the change in fluid velocity per unit distance normal to the direction of flow. All fluids show a definite resistance to relative motion between adjacent fluid particles, a sort of internal friction, termed the viscosity. Viscosity, therefore, is a material property which helps to determine the suitability of a liquid as a lubricant. It is expressed in dyne-seconds per cm^2 or Poises. Some lubricants, such as synovial fluid in human articular joints, show large changes in viscosity with velocity gradient. Such a *thixotropic* fluid is in marked contrast to *Newtonian* fluids, such as water, in which viscosity is independent of velocity gradient.

The Nature of the Frictional Forces

Table 3-4 shows the wide variation of values of coefficient of friction for a range of systems.

A number of types of lubrication have been identified, which are associated with different orders of magnitude of coefficient of friction. The simple system of a dry block on a flat surface would show frictional characteristics depending on the nature of the surfaces in contact. Surface roughness is obviously relevant as is the cleanliness or degree of contamination of the surfaces. Ordinary metallic surfaces in air, for example, are always partially oxidized and usually have some water or other substances present. Such impurities restrict the frictional forces; with thoroughly clean surfaces, higher coefficients of friction are found, as shown in Table 3-4. In contrast, if the surfaces are deliberately contaminated with a substance able to remain adsorbed on the surfaces at a range of loads and rubbing speeds and with a molecular structure

Table 3-4
Typical Values of Coefficient of Friction[22]

System	Coefficient of friction
Clean, smooth metal surfaces	100
Rubber tire on dry road	1
Nylon on steel	0.2
Steel shaft on bronze bush, oiled	0.3
PTFE[a] on PTFE	0.07
Bearing hydrodynamically lubricated with oil	0.05
Ball bearing	0.001
Hydrostatic air bearing	0.0005

[a] PTFE, polytetrafluoroethylene.

Table 3-5

Coefficients of Friction of Present or Potential Combinations of Materials for the Construction of Total Joint Replacements

Materials	Lubricant	Coefficient of friction
Co-Cr alloy/Co-Cr alloy	Distilled water	0.377
Co-Cr alloy/HDPE[a]	Distilled water	0.044
Stainless steel/HDPE	Distilled water	0.043
Co-Cr alloy/polyester	Distilled water	0.041
Co-Cr alloy/vitreous carbon	Distilled water	0.12
Stainless steel/PTFE[a]	Distilled water	0.034
PTFE/PTFE	Distilled water	0.04
Human hip joint[22]	Distilled water	0.009

[a] HDPE, high density polyethylene; PTFE, polytetrafluoroethylene.

that offers little resistance to relative motion, boundary lubrication is said to exist. Both dry and boundary-lubricated surfaces exhibit frictional forces which approximately obey empirical laws of friction.

If the solid surfaces are completely separated by an unbroken film of fluid, the frictional forces depend on the properties of the fluid. If the film is thick enough to prevent contact between asperities on the surfaces, but not so thick as to permit turbulent motion within the film, the frictional force results from shearing of the fluid and depends on its viscosity. For Newtonian fluids the frictional force is directly proportional to the relative speed of the two surfaces and to the wetted area, and inversely proportional to the film thickness. For thixotropic fluids, such as synovial fluid, the frictional force does not increase as rapidly with increasing velocity. A thixotropic fluid, therefore, allows hydrodynamic lubrication at lower relative velocities and lower coefficients of friction at higher relative velocities.

The application of these principles to the study of human articular joints is complicated by the material properties of the articulating surfaces. Cartilage is a porous viscoelastic material. While the mechanisms of lubrication of human joints are considered in more detail in Chapter 5, the results of frictional measurements in entire joints indicate that boundary lubrication predominates, perhaps combined with fluid film lubrication, while the contribution to lubrication by the viscoelastic and spongy nature of cartilage appears to be small.

The coefficients of friction for a variety of materials used for the construction of present, and possibly superior, total hip joints have been recorded by many workers.[23-27] Typical values for a variety of materials are shown in Table 3-5. The results depend somewhat on the experimental conditions of lubricant, surface roughness, geometry of articular surfaces, sliding velocity and surface pressure. Specific variables which affect the design of total joint replacements are considered in Chapter 13. The results indicate that metal-on-plastic joints show coefficients of friction about $\frac{1}{10}$ the value of metal-on-metal articulations. The metal-on-plastic joints, however, show about 5 times greater coefficients of friction than a human hip joint given the same lubricant.

In practice the frictional force depends on the real area of contact. Where two dissimilar metals are in contact, the frictional behavior is controlled by the softer material, which yields plastically to give a larger contact area; it also undergoes shear during sliding. The harder material shows a smaller amount of deformation.

In ideal unlubricated conditions, the coefficient of friction would be independent of load, sliding speed, surface geometry and roughness. In practice this is never true because of the influence of surface contaminants and other factors. Another consideration arises because coefficient of friction is a function of the shear strength and the hardness of a material. The ratio of these two parameters, and thus the coefficient of friction, is surprisingly constant for a range of different materials. For clean metal surfaces the coefficient of friction is usually in the range 0.3 to 1.5, while clean plastic surfaces have coefficients of friction in the range of 0.4 to 0.6. In practice the observed frictional forces will show much greater variation because of contamination than because of changes of materials. An exception is the case of PTFE which is remarkably inert and has little affinity for any material which it contacts. A further group of low-friction materials possesses crystalline structures with layers of atoms strongly bound within the layers but with weak binding forces between layers. Shear between adjacent layers occurs readily, while compression normal to the layers is difficult. Examples are of course graphite and molybdenum disulfide.

A low coefficient of friction in a total joint replacement is important because the frictional force is transmitted to the implant/bone interface as a force which may potentially loosen the implant. While the frictional force has to be overcome by the patient, who actively initiates movement of a total joint replacement, no clinical evidence has ever been recorded to show that patients are aware of the additional work required to overcome the larger coefficients of friction of implanted joints compared with normal human joints. For the selection of implantable joint replacements another criterion, wear resistance, is far more significant than the coefficient of friction.

Wear Resistance

Wear represents the removal and relocation of material arising from the contact of two solids. Wear may occur as the result of one or more mechanisms[28]: abrasive wear, adhesion wear, corrosion and surface-fatigue wear. Abrasive wear occurs when a hard surface rubs across a softer surface or when hard particles slide or roll under pressure across a soft surface. Projections in the harder surface tend to scratch or gouge the softer material. The material from the scratches is displaced in the form of wear particles, which are often of a highly characteristic shape. Abrasive wear particles of metal look like minute chips from a lathe and take the form of spirals, loops and bent wires. The complexity of abrasive wear often hinders modification of materials, because of the risk of introducing other types of damage. For example increasing hardness may reduce abrasive wear but increase the likelihood of fracture or chipping.

Adhesive wear, or galling, scoring or seizing, occurs when microscopic asperities at the sliding interface weld together under high local pressure and temperature. After welding, sliding forces tear the metal from one surface, leaving a depression. The transferred metal provides a projection which may initiate further damage. Adhesive wear is the principal form of wear in total joint replacements. Metals which tend to be mutually soluble gall more readily than insoluble metals. When the metals are dissimilar, the majority of the wear particles are of the softer material, although some particles of the harder

material are also formed. For example, soft polymers such as PTFE will remove particles from very much harder metals. Recent observation of the highly characteristic morphology of metallic wear particles has revealed that the classic theory of adhesive wear is substantially in error for metal-on-metal articulations.[29-31] The wear particles appear as thin flakes of metal with extraordinarily smooth, highly polished surfaces. The rubbing of opposing surfaces polishes the surface and creates a layer that is different from underlying metal. This layer is similar to the layer first noted on polished metal surfaces by Sir George Beilby some 70 year ago, and named after him. The Beilby, or shear-mix, layer does not require direct metal-to-metal contact for its formation, although it is usually formed in that way. Polishing metal with a chamois leather or stropping a razor also produces a Beilby layer. The layer has the same composition as the parent metal but the long-range order is missing (Fig. 3-15). The material of the layer is almost superductile and spreads over cracks and other irregularities in the underlying metal. Repeated rubbing provokes fatigue failure of the Beilby layer so that particles flake from the surface.

The amount of adhesive wear is directly proportional to the applied load and to the distance of sliding and is inversely proportional to the hardness of the eroding surface:

Volume of transferred fragments
$$= \frac{\text{constant} \times \text{load} \times \text{distance of travel}}{3 \times \text{hardness}}.$$

The constant in the equation is called the *coefficient of wear*. Larger values of the constant

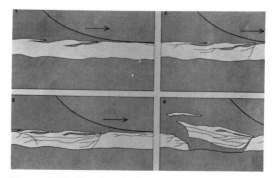

Figure 3-15. A series of schematic diagrams illustrate the mechanism of adhesive wear. The metal surface is covered with a shear-mix or Beilby layer. With rubbing this super ductile material spreads over the surface and subsequently flakes particulate matter of unique morphology. (Reproduced with permission from D. Scott, W. W. Seifert, and V. C. Westcott.[29])

Table 3-6
Wear Coefficient (k) of Various Sliding Combinations[32]

	k
Zinc on zinc	0.160
Mild steel on mild steel	0.045
Copper on copper	0.032
Stainless steel on stainless steel	0.021
Copper on mild steel	0.0015
Bakelite on Bakelite	0.00002

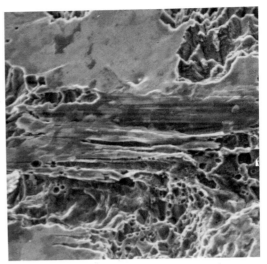

Figure 3-16. A scanning electron micrograph of the surface of a stainless steel plate that has undergone corrosive wear or fretting corrosion is shown. Linear striations indicate the mechanical erosion while the numerous hemispherical depressions, or pits, illustrate the corrosive process. ×335. (Reproduced with permission of Miss O. Pöhler).

indicate a greater susceptibility to wear. Some typical values for wear coefficients are shown in Table 3-6.

While adhesive wear is usually important in articulating joints, it also merits consideration when materials rub in other situations, such as the contact between surgical tools and implants. Such "metallic transfer" is discussed below.

Corrosive wear, or fretting corrosion, involves the removal of superficial oxide films that otherwise would provide resistance to corrosion. It is considered in Chapter 4. Corrosive wear frequently complicates the analysis of other types of wear, although unless the corrosion products are conspicuous it may be difficult to detect. A scanning electron micrograph of a surface with corrosive wear is seen in Figure 3-16.

Under conditions of repetitive loading and sliding, surface cracks may form which lead ultimately to the removal of particles. For metals, the particles which arise from contact stress fatigue have a highly characteristic "chunky" morphology in which the three perpendicular dimensions are roughly similar.[30] In steels, where the process has been most carefully studied, the cracks initiate primarily at the sliding surface and propagate into the material at a small angle to the surface. They later turn parallel to the surface, and eventually the cracks link so that rectangular chunks spall from the surface.

The highly distinctive morphologies of particles formed by abrasive, adhesive and surface-fatigue wear are emphasized because the pathological response varies enormously with the size and shape of foreign particles, as well as with the nature of the material.[33, 34] Current knowledge on the toxicity of foreign particles is described in Chapter 7.

Since the recent development of wear particle analysis by ferrography in 1971, the knowledge of mechanisms of wear and prognostication of future anticipated wear in a particular machine has increased greatly. Scott, Seifert and Westcott[29-31] have revealed that the particles contained in lubricating oils relay information about the condition of the machine in the form of particle shape, composition, size, distribution, and quantitative levels. The particle characteristics are sufficiently specific to the operating wear modes to enable a diagnosis of the machine to be made. If abnormal wear modes are detected, a prognosis of the imminent behavior of the machine can be estimated. More recently, Mears, Westcott, and Hanley[35] have confirmed that ferrographic analysis can be applied to total joint replacements in vivo and even to human degenerative joints.

With the Ferrograph analyzer 2 ml of the lubricant are pumped across a glass microscope slide subjected to a magnetic field (Fig. 3-17). Small, weakly paramagnetic particles in the fluid, often a fraction of a micrometer in size, are precipitated according to their volume and magnetic susceptibility. Larger particles are deposited near the entry end of the substrate. Further along the flow path progressively smaller particles are differentially deposited. Nonmagnetic particles such as polymers or articular cartilage or bone can be made susceptible to the magnetic field by the application of proprietary reagents of minute magnetic particles which are absorbed onto the surface of the relevant wear particles.

After preparation of the Ferrogram, the deposited particles are examined by various micro-

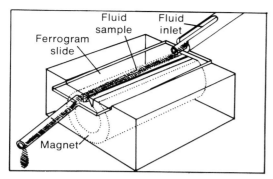

Figure 3-17. A ferrograph analyzer separates wear particles from a lubricant such as synovial fluid by precipitation in a strong magnetic field. Larger particles are deposited near the fluid inlet and smaller particles are deposited further along the slide. About 2 ml of fluid are pumped across the slide. Afterward, washing and fixing solutions can be pumped over the substrate on the slide to remove residual lubricant and to bond the particles to the surface. For biological wear particles such as fragments of articular cartilage or subchondral bone, proprietary reagents of minute, highly magnetic particles are absorbed onto the surfaces of the fragments prior to ferrographic analysis. Subsequently the biological particles possess sufficient magnetic susceptibility to permit routine separation.

scopic techniques. The bichromatic microscope employs simultaneously transmitted green light and direct red light and thereby permits easy identification of the metallic particles (Fig. 3-18). Metallic particles appear red due to the attenuation of the green transmitted light and reflection of the red direct light. Nonmetallic compounds vary in color from green to yellow to pink, depending upon their density and thickness. The metallic particles do not have to be highly reflective in order to be visible, and particles with different surface conditions are distinguished by the intensity of the light that they reflect. Polarized light microscopy permits characterization of nonmetallic compounds such as polyethylene and polymethylmethacrylate (Fig 3-19). Ancillary observations with transmission and scanning electron microscopy, combined with energy dispersion X-ray analysis, permit higher resolution of the particles and a chemical analysis of particulate constitution. For the analysis of wear particles in synovial fluid, 2 ml of fluid from a joint after total joint replacement or of a degenerative joint are aspirated by routine sterile technique. Alternatively, saline washings from arthroscopy can be used. Also the wear particles in synovial biopsies, or even in-

gested by individual cells, such as polymorphonuclear leukocytes, in synovial fluid samples can be identified.

Ferrographic analyses of total joint replacements *in vivo* and of human degenerative joints are discussed in Chapters 7, 13, and 16.

Seifert and Westcott[30] have differentiated five main mechanisms of wear. Rubbing or adhesive wear is the usual benign wear of sliding surfaces. After a normal break-in of a wear surface, a unique "shear-mix" layer is formed at the sur-

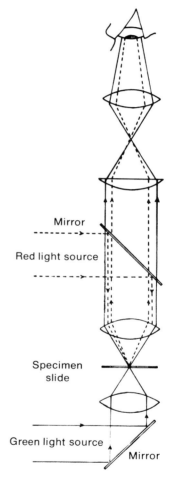

Figure 3-18. A bichromatic microscope has two light sources, one green and the other red. The green light is transmitted through the specimen and the red light is reflected from its surface. This arrangement permits distinction between free metal particles and oxides or other compounds. Free metal particles as small as 1 μm visibly reflect red light and appear red in color. Compound particles transmit green and, depending upon thickness, appear green, yellow, or pink. Polarized light can be used to distinguish polyethylene from methylmethacrylate particles.

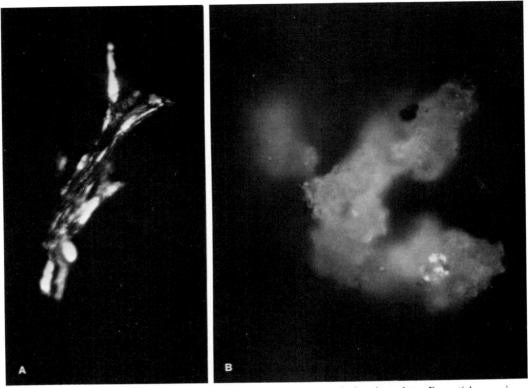

Figure 3-19. Photomicrographs reveal polyethylene, *A*, and polymethylmethacrylate, *B*, particles as viewed under polarized light. The difference in their appearance is clearly evident. The greater degree of crystallographic orientation of polyethylene is manifest as a large refraction of polarized light. The particles are about 10 μm in length.

face in which an amorphous metallic layer, about 1 μm thick, flows over the surface to cover scratches and irregularities. Rubbing wear particles (Fig. 3-20*A*) represent platelets of about 0.5 to 15 μm in major dimension that are exfoliated from the surface.

Excessive contaminants such as particulate polymethylmethacrylate, in a lubricating system with the softer high density polyethylene, can increase the rubbing wear generation rate by more than an order of magnitude without completely removing the shear-mixed layer. Impending trouble can be forecast by the dramatically increased quantity of particles.

Cutting wear particles (Fig. 3-20*B*) are generated as a result of one surface penetrating another. The effect is to generate particles much as a lathe tool creates machining swarf although at a microscopic level. Cutting wear may occur when a relatively hard component slides and penetrates a softer surface or when hard abrasive particles in the lubricating system become embedded in a soft wear surface. The abrasive particles protrude from the soft surface and penetrate the opposing wear surface. Particles generated in this way generally are coarse and large, averaging 2 to 5 μm wide and 25 to 100 μm long, although smaller particles may be encountered. Not only is the presence of cutting wear particles undesirable but a serial increase in the numbers of large (50 μm long) cutting wear particles within a lubricant indicates that a component failure is potentially imminent.

Rolling contact bearings such as total joint replacements may generate three additional distinct particle types: fatigue spall particles, spherical particles, and laminar particles (Fig. 3-20*A*). All three of the peculiar types of particles are indicative of abnormal, accelerated patterns of wear. The fatigue spall particles are flat platelets, up to 100 μm in maximal dimension with a major dimension to thickness ratio of about 10:1. Spherical particles have diameters between 1 and 5 μm. Laminar particles are thin free metal particles between 20 and 50 μm in major dimension with a thickness ratio of about 30:1.

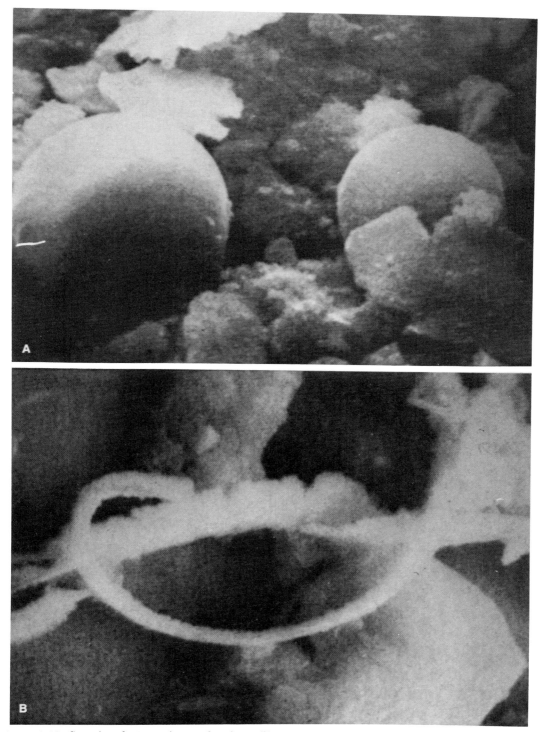

Figure 3-20. Scanning electron micrographs of metallic wear particles separated by ferrography. (*A*) A the micrograph reveals flat platelets of adhesive, or rubbing, wear particles and of spherical spall or surface fatigue particles. (*B*) An abrasive or cutting wear particle is present. The particles are about 2 μm across their major axes.

Combinations of wear mechanisms frequently occur. If wear surface stresses become excessive due to load and/or speed, the shear-mixed layer becomes unstable and large particles exfoliate with an accelerated wear rate. Ultimately complete surface breakdown may ensue with an associated catastrophic wear rate. Such severe sliding wear particles are larger than 20 μm in major dimension with a thickness ratio of about 10:1. Sliding of the particles may produce surface striations.

Wear In Total Joint Replacements

The rates of wear in previous assessments of total joint replacements can be of practical importance either because of mechanical deterioration of the implant or toxicity of the wear products. The rates of wear for a variety of designs of joint replacement and the mechanisms of toxicity caused by wear products are discussed in Chapters 13 and 7 respectively. Two different lines of approach have been pursued for the development of good bearing materials, the metal-on-metal system and the metal-on-plastic system.

In engineering practice metal bearings conventionally consist of a soft metal, a hard metal and a satisfactory lubricant. As described above, dissimilar metals tend to show low adhesive forces. Dissimilar alloys have not been used for joint replacements for two reasons. Of the three alloys available for the construction of most orthopaedic implants, austenitic stainless steel and titanium show a great tendency to gall or seize when they are rubbed against themselves or against other implant alloys. In addition, there has been great concern that the combination of dissimilar alloys in an implant could provoke rapid galvanic corrosion of the less noble alloy. In the context of currently available or of future implant alloys, it is felt that this fear has been exaggerated. A full description of galvanic corrosion follows in Chapter 4. By exclusion, the cobalt-chromium alloy/cobalt-chromium alloy system remains the sole metal-on-metal implant under consideration. Past clinical experience suggested that this combination was satisfactory for total replacement of the hip, knee and elbow. The wear process for McKee-Farrar total hip prosthesis has been described in detail by Walker *et al.*[36] The volumetric rate of wear is about 5 mm^3 per year, which is about $\frac{1}{10}$ of the rate observed for metal-on-plastic total hip replacements. Microscopy of the cobalt-chromium articular surfaces after implantation periods of about 4 years reveals three types of wear phenomena. There are scratches provoked by abrasive and adhesive wear and by contact stress fatigue. Susceptibility to the last mechanism arises from the stresses produced in the articular surface by polishing and grinding during fabrication. Apparently the original stressed surface is not strongly adherent to the mass of metal and hence not resistant to wear. Once this is eroded however, a new smooth surface is formed with great wear resistance. More recently, observations on the biological fate of cobalt-chromium wear particles have raised new doubts about prolonged application of metal-on-metal joints *in vivo*. The toxicological evidence is reviewed in Chapter 7.

The pattern of wear on the articular surface is asymmetrical, with maximum wear at the center of the articular surface and the least wear at the equator (Fig. 3-21). Deviations from roundness of both the femoral and articular components of at least several microns are observed. Metallographic analysis reveals the presence of several phases in the microstructure as well as the presence of numerous small voids resulting from the casting process. A network of carbide particles is evident along the grain boundaries. This observation suggests that the wear process is stimulated by motion of the extremely hard carbide particles against the moderately hard cobalt-chromium matrix. The pores may provide sites for adsorption of molecules from synovial fluid to provide boundary lubrication.

It can be concluded that the metal-on-metal bearing surfaces in total hip or other joint replacements show extremely high wear resistance. Nevertheless, as indicated in Chapters 7 and 13, biological observations have begun to reveal the unfavorable response of tissues to the minute concentrations of metallic wear products. If further histological evidence of toxicity accumulates, the biological disadvantages of cobalt-chromium/cobalt-chromium joint replacements may outweigh the mechanical advantages.

Metal-on-plastic joint replacements represent a logical application of the concept of a hard articular surface mated with a softer material. The modulus of elasticity of the plastic approaches that of bone or cartilage and provides better damping of shock forces than would a comparable metal component. While the strength of most thermoplastic polymers is much less than that of surgical alloys, and insufficient for the construction of supportive or an-

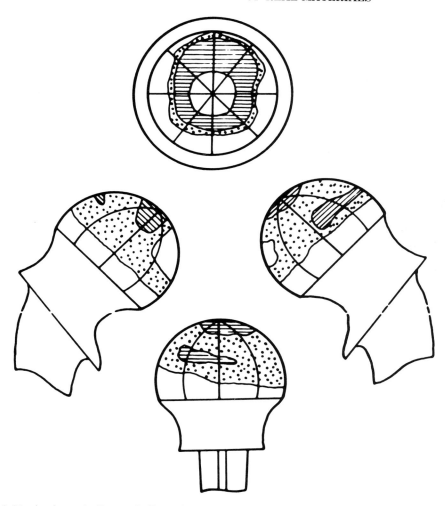

Figure 3-21. A schematic diagram indicates local variations in wear on the articular surface of a femoral head component of a cobalt-chromium total hip joint prosthesis. The wear pattern on the McKee femoral head component is shown schematically. *White* indicates unworn area; *dotted,* heavier wear with initial scratching and abrasive wear; and *cross-hatching,* lighter wear where initial scratching and abrasive wear was supplanted by smoothing and adhesive wear. (Reproduced with permission from P. S. Walker, E. Salvati, and R. K. Hotzler.[36])

choring portions of joint replacements, it is adequate for the articular portions of total joint replacements. Initially Charnley[38] favored the use of PTFE because of its remarkably low coefficient of friction. In simulated wear tests in the laboratory it showed negligible rates of adhesive wear when rubbed against austenitic stainless steel. Implantation of PTFE in humans as the acetabular socket of total hip joint replacements, however, was followed by a catastrophic wear accompanied by marked toxic response to the wear products, including fluoride ion. Subsequent studies have confirmed the difficulty in carrying out wear tests that accurately simulate conditions *in vivo,* especially for plastics and other nonmetallic materials. The premature erosion of PTFE has never been satisfactorily explained. One possibility would be corrosive wear of the polymer. Recent observations on other polymeric materials have shown that sorption of small amounts of lipids or plasma proteins may initiate serious mechanical deterioration of the materials.[37] The mechanism of such mechanochemical failure of nonmetallic materials is poorly understood. Another possible explanation of failure is adhesive wear of PTFE which occurs under high load conditions such as are encountered in the human hip joint. In any event, Charnley and Halley[38] replaced the PTFE sockets with high density polyethylene (HDPE), which has functioned satisfactorily. The rates of wear for the HDPE have been studied for over 10 years of implantation. While there is a wide scatter of individual wear rates, a linear wear of about 0.18 mm is usually observed for the first year *in vivo*, after which the rate of erosion declines to about 0.10 mm per year, so that the rate of wear for the first decade averages about 0.15 mm per year. A study of prematurely removed implants provides an explanation for the fall in the rate of wear of polymers.[24] In the early running-in period, virtually all of the erosion occurs on the polymeric surface. While much of the debris accumulates in the joint space, the articulating metal surface is gradually coated with a smooth layer of finely compressed polymeric particles. Ultimately both articular surfaces are equally covered by HDPE, and the rate of wear is correspondingly lower.

The surface finishes of present total hip joints are extremely good.[34] The typical center line average (CLA) of metal on metal joints is $\frac{1}{40}$ μm (1 μinch) for the femoral head prosthesis with $\frac{1}{5}$ to $\frac{1}{3}$ μm (8 to 12 μinch) for the acetabular component while for a Stanmore total hip prosthesis, the CLA is less than 0.025 μm with out of roundness less than 5 μm root mean square (RMS). CLA represents the average deviation of a surface profile from a line which makes the sum of the areas contained between itself and those parts of the profile which lie on either side of it. CLA represents sphericity at the equator of a sphere, whereas total indicator reading (TIR) represents the sphericity of sagittal sections through the sphere as well as the sphericity of the equators. The typical TIR of the best femoral head prosthesis is about 2.5 μm. RMS is an index of out of roundness that indicates both the width and the depth of surface irregularities. The friction in total joint replacements is proportional to the mode of lubrication, the nature of the materials, the geometry of the joint, and the load imposed upon the joint (0 to 4 times body weight for the hip joint).

On theoretical grounds it has been suggested that the surface finish on the metal and plastic surfaces should be of as high a quality as possible. Recent clinical observations fail to confirm improved wear characteristics associated with optimal surface finish of the metallic component.

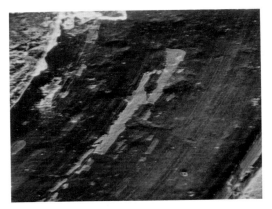

Figure 3-22. A photomicrograph reveals the articulating surface of an acetabular component manufactured of a composite material, polyethylene reinforced with graphite. Irregular, linear wear tracks are visible. ×50. (Reproduced with permission Zimmer U.S.A.).

In fact, since the metallic component is coated by HDPE during the running-in period, superior surface finish of the metal would be unlikely to diminish the rate of polymeric wear for more than the first few months after implantation.

The results recently published by Charnley and Halley[38] for the wear rates of HDPE hip sockets after 10 years of implantation provide the first useful check on the accuracy of long-term predictions based on accelerated laboratory wear tests. The best laboratory tests have predicted overly optimistic rates of wear that are about one-half of the rates observed for implants *in vivo*. The wide variation of rates of wear observed in individual total hip joint replacements remains a mystery. In the past, marked obesity of the patient, with excessive forces on the implant, or excessive physical activity have been implicated. In the prolonged study by Charnley,[38] neither obesity nor physical activity correlates with the observed rate of wear of the polymeric socket.

A variety of other polymers including PTFE, polyesters, polyterephthalate, polyamide, polyimide, polycarbonates, polysulfone and polyacetals have been tested for possible use in total joint replacements.[39–41] Apart from polyimides, all of the polymers show wear characteristics inferior to that of HDPE. The most wear-resistant polymeric material has proved to be HDPE with graphite fiber reinforcement. This material shows wear resistance 50 to 200% better than has been obtained with conventional HDPE. Unfortunately its resistance to creep is not improved. Clinical trials with this composite ma-

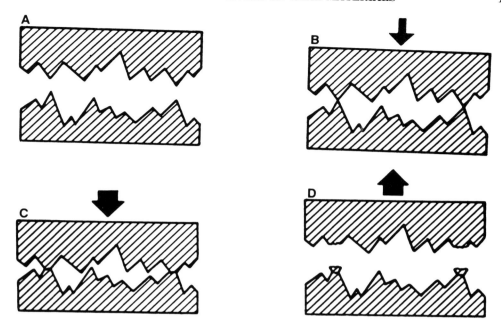

Figure 3-23. A schematic representation of metal transfer is shown. In *A*, two metal surfaces approach each other. The roughness is exaggerated. In *B*, contact has occurred between the "mountain peaks" in two places. In *C*, force is applied and the projection is flattened until their area of contact can resist the force. The asperities undergo cold welding, and in *D*, the two metal surfaces are separated. Two small pieces of the upper one remain cold-welded to the lower one. Metallic transfer has occurred. (Reproduced with permission from C. O. Bechtol, A. B. Ferguson, Jr., and P. G. Laing.[44])

terial for hip sockets are in progress. A photomicrograph of a composite acetabular wear surface is shown in Figure 3-22.

METALLIC TRANSFER

It is common observation that the application of a pencil point to paper produces a thin trace of graphite transferred from the pencil to the paper. For many years it has been known that rubbing one metal across another could produce a similar transfer of metal.[42, 43] The significance of metallic transfer between surgical tools and implants has been debated. While there is no doubt that such transfer does occur, the critical question is whether it is of clinical significance.

As mentioned above, even polished metallic surfaces show micro-roughness, with asperities and depressions. When two such surfaces are brought together (Fig. 3-23), a few opposing asperities make actual contact. At these sites the contact pressure may be so great that they cold weld together. When the two metals are slid or distracted apart, fracture occurs through the bases of peaks of the two metals, since metal

adjacent to the welds has undergone work hardening by the deformation of the initial contact. When dissimilar metals are brought into contact and separated, transfer of the soft metal to the harder one is favored.

Many years ago Bowden, Williamson and Laing[45] documented metallic transfer between a variety of surgical tools and implants (Fig. 3-24). The tips of screwdrivers and other tools were made radioactive and after insertion of surgical screws, the amount of metal transferred was determined by radiographic analysis. The results confirmed that the transfer is greater between similar alloys than between dissimilar alloys, provided that the alloys are of comparable hardness. Again, transfer was greater from softer alloys to harder ones than *vice versa*, and lubrication diminished the amount of transfer. When greater force was used during insertion of a screw, the amount of metallic transfer increased. Similar observations were made for a variety of orthopaedic tools and implants including nuts and bolts, osteotomes and mallets, and nails and mallets. When a hole is drilled in bone by insertion of the drill through a hole in a metal plate,

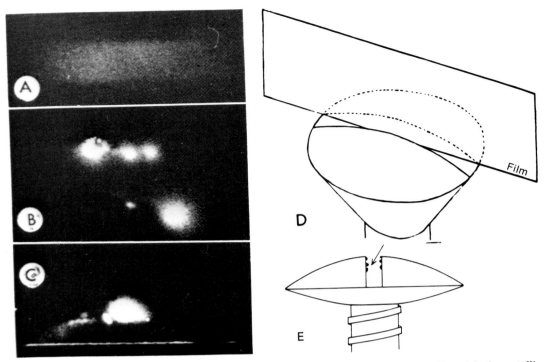

Figure 3-24. Radiographs of screw slots handled with radioactive screwdrivers acquire radioactivity by metallic transfer. *A.* Handled lightly with little slip, 22 mg of transferred metal. *B.* Slightly greater slip, 47 mg of transfer. *C.* Distribution of transferred metal within the screw slot. *D.* Position of film to obtain view shown in *C. E.* A diagram showing a screw head where adherent metal is detected. (Reproduced with permission from C. O. Bechtol, A. B. Ferguson, Jr., and P. G. Laing.[44])

accidental contact between the drill and the plate may cause transfer of several milligrams of metal. Numerous free fragments are also formed and contaminate local tissues, and histological studies readily identify the fragments in surrounding tissues (see Chapter 7).[46]

Bowden *et al.*[45] were of the opinion that metallic transfer and tool flaking are serious complications in implantation. There is no doubt that severe flaking of a screw head can damage the slot so that the screw driver cannot engage for complete insertion of the screw or for subsequent removal. Indeed this is one factor which strongly favors a hexagonal-recess screw head since a hexagon driver rarely slips within the head. The crucial question of metallic transfer, however, is the biological significance of the metal flakes and the possibility of enhanced rates of galvanic corrosion at sites of metallic transfer. The author believes that the biological significance of metallic transfer has been greatly overestimated, and is aware of no clinical evidence that metallic transfer has stimulated toxic response. The amount of corrosion observed on

screw heads is negligible compared with the crevice between a screw head and a bone plate. Constant microscopic motion also abrades the protective oxide film at the latter site, as described in Chapter 4. The combination of abrasion and crevice corrosion promotes increased removal of metal throughout implantation. Again, Bowden *et al.*[45] failed to consider that the tips or gripping surfaces of most surgical tools are harder than surgical implants. For example, many tools have tungsten carbide tips. Most metallic transfer thus occurs from the implant to the tool and the principal area of dissimilar metals is not implanted. Finally, as described in Chapter 4, dissimilar combinations of *currently available* surgical alloys do not show any significant galvanic effect nor would this be anticipated on theoretical or practical grounds.

In summary, severe flaking of metal at sites of contact between surgical tools and implants is obviously undesirable and may provoke mechanical failure of either component. With careful design however, such gross examples of metallic transfer are avoided. The less severe forms of transfer occur during the insertion or removal of surgical implants whenever there is direct contact with tools. At present there is not sufficient evidence to show that this transfer is of clinical significance.

PHYSICAL PROPERTIES OF IMPLANTABLE MATERIALS

In contrast with many other types of implants, orthopaedic implants make virtually no demands on properties such as electrical, magnetic or optical behavior. The reader is referred elsewhere for such information.[47-51] The only physical criteria of orthopaedic interest are those which relate to methods of sterilization, such as heat and irradiation, and the degree of radiotransparency of implantable materials. Sterilization of surgical tools and implants is described in Chapter 8.

Radiotransparency

Most orthopaedic implants should be sufficiently opaque to X-rays that they can be located and examined during and after implantation. X-rays are absorbed to varying degrees by all kinds of matter. When a beam of X-rays strikes a material, part of the energy is transmitted directly while the remainder of the beam is modified by the material.[52] The amount of energy that a particular material will absorb depends on the nature of the atoms, the thickness of the material and the wave length of the X-rays. The absorption of X-rays obeys an exponential law; I, the intensity after passage through a homogenous material of thickness x is given by

$$I = I_0 \, e^{-\mu x},$$

where I_0 is the initial intensity, and μ is the absorption coefficient. The absorption coefficient is characteristic of the material and the wave length. The principal property of a material which influences the absorption of X-rays is density, and there is a logarithmic increase in absorption with increase in density.

With standard implant alloys, most radiographs display shadows which readily differentiate even minute wires from soft tissue or bone. When polymers such as polymethylmethacrylate or HDPE are used, radiography of the implant may be difficult because the polymers absorb X-rays to a similar degree to the surrounding tissues. Where visualization of such a component is essential, a small metallic marker, usually a stainless steel or titanium wire, is secured to the implant. Alternatively a heavy metal may be incorporated into the formulation of the plastic. For example, 5 to 10% barium sulfate is frequently added to methylmethacrylate, although there is abundant evidence that such additions considerably alter the mechanical properties of polymers and may also affect their physical properties and biocompatibility.

REFERENCES

1. Shortley, G., and Williams, D. *Elements in Physics*, Prentice-Hall, Englewood Cliffs, N. J., 1955.
2. Cottrell, A. H. *The Mechanical Properties of Matter*, p. 32, John Wiley & Sons, New York, 1964.
3. Nelkon, M. *Mechanics and Properties of Matter*, p. 136, W. Heinemann Ltd., London, 1956.
4. Williams, D. F., and Roaf, R. *Implants in Surgery*, W. B. Saunders Co., London, 1973.
5. Biggs, W. D. *The Mechanical Behaviour of Engineering Materials*, Pergamon Press, Oxford, 1965.
6. Wulpi, B. J. *How Components Fail*, American Society for Metals, Metals Park, Ohio, 1966.
7. Cottrell, A. H. *An Introduction to Metallurgy*, p. 386, Edward Arnold, London, 1975.
8. Kiehl, K., and Mittelmeier, H. *Z. Ortho.*, 112:235, 1974.
9. Black, J. *Ortho. Clin. N. Am.*, 5:(4) 833, 1974.
10. British Standards Institution, *Specification for Metal Implants and Tools Used in Bone Surgery*, Part I, B.S. 351, London, 1968.
11. Grover, H. J. *J. Mater.*, 1:413, 1966.
12 Laing, P. G., and O'Donnell, J. M. *Surg. Gyne. Obst.*, 112:567, 1961.
13. Cohen, J. *J. Mater.*, 1:354, 1966.
14. Colangelo, V. J., and Greene, N. D. *J. Biomed. Mater. Res.*, 3:247, 1969.
15. Cahoon, J. R., and Paxton, H. W. *J. Biomed. Mater. Res.*, 2:1, 1968.
16. Galante, J. O., Rostoker, W., and Doyle, J. M. *J. Bone Jt. Surg.*, 57A: 230, 1975.
17. Markoff, K. L., and Amstutz, H. C. *J. Biomechanics*, in press.
18. Weightman, B. The stress in total hip prosthesis femoral stems. In *Advances in Artificial Hip and Knee Joint Technology*, p. 138, edited by M. Schaldach and D. Hohmann, Springer-Verlag, Berlin, 1976.
19. Muller, M. E., Allgöwer, M., and Willenegger, H. *Manual of Internal Fixation*, p. 162, Springer-Verlag, Berlin, 1970.
20. Deanin, R. D. *Polymer Structure, Properties and Applications*, p. 53, Cahners Books, Boston, 1972.
21. Charnley, J., Kamangar, A., and Longfield, M. D. *Med. Biol. Engng.*, 7:31, 1969.
22. Bowen, F. P., and Tabor, D. *The Friction and Lubrication of Solids*, p. 135, University Press, Oxford, 1954.
23. Ungethüm M. Requirements of operational tests and test result in total hip and knee arthroplasty. In *Advances in Artificial Hip and Knee Joint Technology*, p. 493, edited by M. Schaldach and D. Hohmann, Springer-Verlag, Berlin, 1976.

24. Walker, P. S., and Bullough, P. G. *Ortho. Clin. N. Am.*, *4*:275, 1973.

25. Wilson, J. N., and Scales, J. T. *Clin. Ortho. Rel. Res.*, *72*:145, 1970.

26. Swanson, S. A. V., Freeman, M. A. R., and Heath, J. C. *J. Bone Jt. Surg.*, *55B*:759, 1973.

27. Little, T., Freeman, M. A. R., and Swanson, S. A. V. Experiments on Friction in the human hip Joint. In *Lubrication and Wear in Joints*, p. 110, edited by V. Wright, Sector, London, 1969.

28. Wulpi, D. J. *How Components Fail*, p. 28, American Society of Metals, Metals Park, Ohio, 1966.

29. Scott, D., Seifert, W. W., and Westcott, V. C. *Sci. Am.*, *230*:88, 1974.

30. Seifert, W. W., and Westcott, V. C. *Wear, 21*:22, 1972.

31. Scott, D., and Westcott, V. C. *Wear, 44*:173, 1977.

32. Shortley, G., and Williams, D. *Elements of Physics*, p. 41, Prentice-Hall, Englewood Cliffs, N.J., 1955.

33. Winter, G. D. *J. Biomed. Mater. Res.*, *8*:11, 1974.

34. Mears, D. C., *Ortho. Survey*, *1*:65, 1977.

35. Mears, D. C., Hanley, E., Westcott, V. C., and Rutkowski, R. *Wear, 50*:115, 1978.

36. Walker, P., Salvati, E., and Hotzler, R. K. *J. Bone Jt. Surg.*, *56A*:92, 1974.

37. Swanson, A. B., Meester, W. D., Gide, G. Swanson, L. Rangaswamy and G. E. D. Schut, *Ortho. Clin. N. Am.*, *4*:(4) 1097, 1973.

38. Charnley, J., and Halley, D. K. *Clin. Ortho. Rel. Res.*, *112*:170, 1975.

39. Walker, P. S., and Erkman, M. J. *Adv. in Polymer Friction and Wear*, *5B*:553, 1973.

40. Walker, P. S., and Salvati, E. *J. Biomed. Mater. Res.*, *4*:327, 1973.

41. Amstutz, H. C. *J. Biomed. Mater. Res.*, *3*:547, 1968.

42. Bowden, F. P., and Tabor, D. *The Friction and Lubrication of Solids*, p. 199, Oxford University Press, London, 1954.

43. Bowden, F. P., and Williamson J. B. P. *Eng.*, *182*:619, 1956.

44. Bechtol, C. O., Ferguson, A. B., Jr., and Laing, P. G. *Metals in Engineering in Bone and Joint Surgery*, Williams & Wilkins Co., Baltimore, 1959.

45. Bowden, F. P., Williamson, J. B. P., and Laing, P. G. *Nature, 174*:834, 1954.

46. Bechtol, C. O., Ferguson, A. B., Jr., and Laing, P. G. *Metals and Engineering in Bone and Joint Surgery*, p. 77, Williams & Wilkins Co., Baltimore, 1959.

47. Williams, D. F., and Roaf, R. *Implants in Surgery*, p. 119, W. B. Saunders Co., Philadelphia, 1973.

48. Weymueller, C. R. *Met. Prog.*, *1*:77, 1968.

49. Zimon, J. *Sci. Am.*, *217*:180, 1967.

50. Ehrenreich, H. *Sci. Am.*, *217*:194, 1967.

51. Gibbons, D. F. Biomedical materials, In *Ann. Rev. Bio. Phys. BioEng.*, *4*:367, 1975.

52. Hall, E. J. Radiobiology for the radiologist, p. 12, Harper & Row Publishers Inc., Hagerstown, Md., 1973.

4

The Dissolution of Implantable Materials

For centuries attempts have been made to use metals for the repair or replacement of damaged human organs. The vast majority of the attempts failed, principally because of wound sepsis, but also for want of inert metals with appropriate mechanical properties. By 1930, surgeons with greatly improved technical skills were making frequent reference in the literature to the search for the "perfect implant alloy" with suitable inertness and mechanical properties for all implants. Subsequently, three alloys which largely fulfilled this need were introduced into general surgical practice, 316 stainless steel, cast cobalt-chromium, and pure titanium and surgeons were able to greatly increase the use of implants, principally in the stabilization of fractures. At the same time, implants of increased complexity, such as joint replacements, were being designed. Frequently the various parts of one implant were in marked contrast to each other with respect to mechanical criteria. The need arose to use combinations of dissimilar materials in the fabrication of implants. There was great reluctance to use dissimilar metals for fear of accelerated or galvanic corrosion of one of the pair of metals. For this and other reasons, a wide variety of nonmetallic substances including polymers, ceramics and silicones have been introduced, both singly and in combination with metals. While there was an introductory period of overoptimism about the degree of inertness of the nonmetallic substances, clinical experience gradually has revealed the universal liability of nonmetallic implants both to slow but finite rates of general dissolution and to rapid, highly localized forms of dissolution which may provoke mechanical failure of the implant. There has therefore been a resurgence of interest in laboratory studies of the behavior of materials exposed to body fluids. Early qualitative assessments[1] confirmed the universal nature of the corrosion of metals in body fluids. Subsequent studies have been undertaken to measure the absolute rate of corrosion of metal implants,

with estimates of the rates of corrosion of metal into soluble dissolution products.

In this chapter we examine the mechanisms by which materials dissolve when placed in body fluids. The liability of some materials to undergo a change from one mode of dissolution to another, often with greatly accelerated rates of dissolution, is discussed. Accelerated laboratory tests for the measurement of rates of dissolution of previously untried materials are presented. Finally, the behavior of combinations of dissimilar metals and of metals with nonmetallic substances is described.

ELECTROCHEMICAL PRINCIPLES OF CORROSION AND PASSIVATION OF METALS

Corrosion refers to a kind of deterioration in which metal leaves the metallic state to form aqueous cations in solution or is converted into solid compound. This is accompanied by the equivalent cathodic reduction of some constituent in the aqueous electrolyte. On corroding metals, these sites of the oxidation and reduction reactions may be a few atoms or a few centimeters apart. The basic reaction in corrosion is the removal of positive metal ions from their positions in the metal crystal lattice, where they are stabilized electrically by the electrons of the metal to positions in the environment where they are stabilized by negative anions. This is an anodic reaction and must be accompanied by a corresponding cathodic reaction in which the electrons thus freed from the metal remove cations from the environment, or create anions. Thus, for iron corroding in neutral aerated saline solution, the anodic reaction is:

$$Fe_{metal} \rightarrow 2e^-_{metal} + Fe^{2+}_{aqueous}$$

and the cathodic reaction is:

$$^1/_2 \, O_2 + H_2O + 2e^-_{metal} \rightarrow 2OH^-_{aqueous}$$

The latter reaction represents reduction of

dissolved oxygen in solution and electric current flows equivalent to the amount of metal that dissolves at the anode. Thus, corrosion is an electrochemical deterioration of metals which obeys Faraday's laws. This was confirmed by early workers [2, 3] who studied the corrosion of iron specimens partly immersed in stagnant saline solutions. The corrosion distribution found is shown in Figure 4-1*A*. Attack began at the edges, spread inwards, and then ceased to spread, while alkali was formed at and near the waterline where oxygen for the cathodic reaction was most readily replenished. Next, the plates were cut along the zone of demarcation, as shown in Figure 4-1*B*, and the pieces were joined through a milliammeter to measure current flow between corrosion sites and unattacked metal. In more complex experiments, the electrode potential at the anodic and cathodic zones on corroding metal was measured by means of capillaries leading to a standard electrode. The current corresponding to any particular potential was measured by applying a variable external electromotive force between separated anodes and cathodes. The resulting polarization curve (Fig.4-2*A*) allowed potential measurements to be used to estimate corrosion currents on metals carrying both anodic and cathodic reactions and thereby to deduce the corrosion rate.

Anodic Reactions of Metals in Passivity and Corrosion

When the currently used implant alloys are immersed in an aqueous buffered solution of pH 7 they become passivated immediately through the formation of a compact solid film of hydrox-

ide, or oxide. Usually, however, before exposure to the solution, the metal is covered with an air-formed oxide film, and exposure to the solution serves to provide a thickened film and better barrier to the egress of metal into solution.

In strongly acid solutions, the same metals may show different behavior.[4] The air-formed oxide film dissolves, and subsequently the bare metal dissolves with the formation of metallic cations in solution. If the anode potential is made more positive (Fig. 4-2*B*) by application of the potentiostatic technique, then the anodic current and rate of metallic dissolution increase. With further polarization and increase of potential beyond point *B*, the anodic formation of, say, $M(OH)_2$ or MO becomes thermodynamically possible and may well be kinetically easier than the formation of dissolved M^{2+} ions. The anode current density falls (*BC*, Fig. 4-2*B*) to a very small value, and the metal is *passive*. Further rise of anode potential leads to an increase (*CD*, Fig. 4-2*B*) of the very small anode current density or rate of conversion of solid metal to film substance although this falls with passage of time since the thickening solid film presents an improved barrier. Still further rise of anode potential may lead to one of several phenomena: (a) the film may be oxidized to a soluble product, whereupon the metal undergoes dissolution (*DE*, Fig. 4-2*B*) in the transpassive state; (b) a substance in the solution, such as hydroxyl ion, may become oxidized and oxygen gas is evolved (*FG*, Fig. 4-2*B*), the metal remaining passive; (c) in the presence of chloride-containing solutions, passive metals are liable to a third mode of behavior,[5] film breakdown. Passivation is nor-

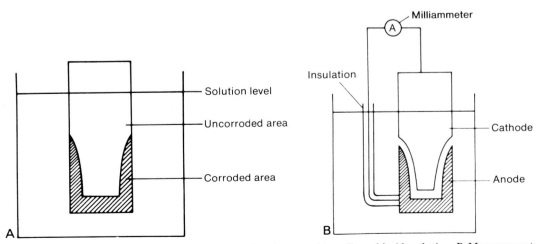

Figure 4-1. *A*. Distribution of corrosion on an iron plate immersed in sodium chloride solution. *B*. Measurement of the current flowing between anodic and cathodic areas on iron partly immersed in sodium chloride solution.

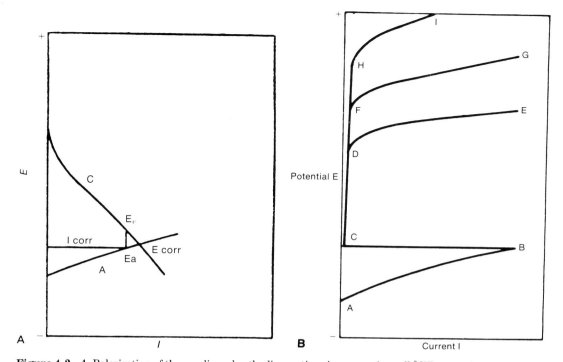

Figure 4-2. *A.* Polarization of the anodic and cathodic reactions in a corrosion cell.[3] When anodic and cathodic reactions occur on the same piece of corroding metal they mutually polarize one another, the potential of the more positive cathode tending to fall and that of the anode tending to rise. Polarization thus occurs to the values E_c and E_a where $E_c - E_a = IR$ the working electromotive force needed to drive the current I through the circuit of resistance R. For low-resistance metallic and electrolytic paths (anode and cathode are near together), R is sometimes small enough for E_c to approximate E_a to within 1 mV and each may be identified with E_{corr}, the corrosion potential. *B.* Schematic diagram of an anodic polarization curve for a passive metal. *AB*, active dissolution; this is the portion of the anodic curve shown in Figure 4-2 *A* where the classic "bare" metal dissolution is described. *BC*, passivating; rapid decrease in *rate* of metallic dissolution. *CD*, passive; slow rate of metallic dissolution through a protective "passive" film. *DE*, transpassive; oxidation of the passive film to a soluble form so that rapid metallic dissolution ensues. Pure chromium exhibits this behavior in sulfuric acid solution. *FG*, oxygen gas evolution; the metal remains passive. *HI*, chloride breakdown; resumption of rapid metallic dissolution occurs with the formation of brightened hemispherical pits. The anodic polarization curve shows the relationship between current flow and the potential of a metal. Other observations are required to determine the *nature* of the electrochemical reaction and the rate of metallic dissolution. Two or more anodic reactions may occur simultaneously on a metal surface. If the potential of the metal is lowered to point A, the corrosion rate is 0. This can be accomplished by cathodic protection. Alternatively by combination of the metal with an appropriate cathodic material, the potential of the metal can be regulated between *CD* so that the metal is passive (anodic protection). For satisfactory application of anodic protection to surgical alloys, conditions for *repassivation* are required in addition to *maintenance* of passivity. For fulfillment of this criterion, either an efficient cathode is needed which can provide adequate current to raise the potential past point B, or the "active loop", *ABC*, must be small enough so that the magnitude of current B for repassivation approximates the current of passive dissolution, *CD*.

mally greatly delayed or entirely prevented by the presence of chloride ions in solution. Often the chloride may be strongly adsorbed on the metal surface and prevent contact with water or oxygen-bearing anions, which is essential for the easy formation of adherent compact oxide or hydroxide layers. Furthermore, chloride ions tend to break down passive or air-formed oxide films where these have been formed. Above a critical potential (*HI*, Fig. 4-2B), chloride anion enters the passive films at singular points where the film is less regular than usual. The "contaminated" oxide so formed has a greatly increased ion conductivity which allows rapid egress of metal into solution. Hemispherical pits form at these sites on the metal surface. Present electrochemical techniques[6] allow accurate prediction of the behavior that will occur if a previously untried alloy is exposed to simulated body fluids for an indefinite length of time. As will be described shortly, these methods also allow prediction of the behavior of combinations of metals with respect to corrosion or passivation *in vivo*.

Cathodic Reactions in Corrosion

As was previously emphasized, whenever a metal dissolves as an anode, an equivalent cathodic reaction must occur. If all cathodic reactants could be removed from the environment, then a metal could not dissolve electrochemically. The principal cathodic reaction in the corrosion of surgical implants is the reduction of dissolved oxygen to hydroxyl ion.

$$\tfrac{1}{2}\,O_2 + H_2O + 2e^-_{metal} \rightarrow 2OH^-_{aqueous}$$

At a site of low oxygen concentration, however, such as a crevice between two components of an implant or between cement and an implant, water reduction may supercede the oxygen reduction cathode.

$$2H_2O + 2e^-_{metal} \rightarrow H_2 + 2OH^-_{aqueous}$$

It is possible that organic constituents of body fluids participate to a minor degree as cathodic reactants although, at present, little is known about their nature or significance.

Assessment of Liability to Corrosion and Rates of Passive Dissolution

With the proliferation of alloys available for a discipline where research expenditure is hampered by the small potential market, rapid, inexpensive methods are essential for the selection of materials which merit expensive and time-consuming biological tests. Previously the most widely used guide has been past industrial experience with materials upon exposure to sea water or in a desalinization plant. Also potential/pH, or Pourbaix, diagrams[7] (Fig. 4-3) may indicate the likelihood of passive behavior on exposure of an alloy to a solution of known pH such as pH 7.35 to 7.45 for extracellular fluid. The potential pH diagrams, however, do not indicate liability to breakdown of passivity in a chloride-containing environment, nor do they reveal the kinetic aspects of a particular mode of behavior (*e.g.*, rate of metallic dissolution).

Ultimately laboratory tests are required which allow accelerated prediction of the long-term behavior of materials when exposed to an environment that accurately simulates the human

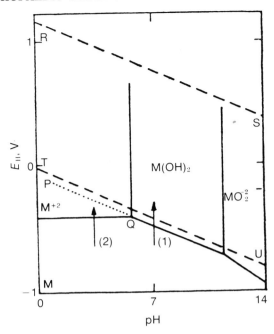

Figure 4-3. Schematic potential pH or Pourbaix diagram for a representative passive metal. Each line represents the conditions of some equilibrium. A *horizontal line* represents equilibrium for a reaction involving electrons (*e.g.*, $M \rightarrow M^{++} + 2e^-$). A *vertical line* represents an equilibrium involving H^+ or OH^- ions (*e.g.*, $M^{+3} + H_2O \rightarrow M\,(OH)_2^{++} + H^+$). A *sloping line* represents an equilibrium involving H^+ or OH^- ions and *also* involving electrons (*e.g.*, $2M^{+2} + 3H_2O \rightarrow M_2O_3 + 6H^+ + 2e^-$). The diagram can be divided into areas which represent immunity, passivation or corrosion. Immunity refers to an area where the metal (M) is thermodynamically stable or resistant to corrosion even though its exposed surface shows bare metal. Passivation refers to an area where a solid film ($M(OH)_2$) is formed. Provided that the film substance has appropriate physical characteristics as a compact solid and adherent layer, then the metal will exhibit passive behavior. Corrosion refers to regions where soluble species (*e.g.*, M^{+2}) are formed. It should be emphasized that the diagram makes no attempt to predict the kinetics of any corrosion reactions, nor does it account for the behavior when other anions such as chloride-ion are present.

environment. From a few weeks of study, one must predict how a material will perform *in vivo* if implanted for 50 years, or more. The traditional corrosion test is the measurement of weight change in a specimen during exposure to a corrosive environment. The specimen is weighed before and after exposure, and the decrease in weight represents the amount of metal that has been converted to soluble corrosion products. By use of numerous identical specimens in the same environment a graphic portrayal of change in corrosion rate with time is obtained (Fig. 4-4). For the assessment of passive alloys with low corrosion rates, the measurement of weight-loss is often obscured by weight *gain* in the specimen due to uptake of oxide or hydroxide as a compact solid passive film. Furthermore, the test gives no indication of whether corrosion has occurred uniformly over the exposed surface or whether it has been localized to a few sites which show enhanced susceptibility. However, the principal limitation of weight-loss measurements is the inability of the method to provide an accurate prediction of corrosion rate if exposure of the alloy to the corrosive environment is prolonged significantly longer than the period of experimental exposure (Fig. 4-4). Thus empirical observation shows that the measurement of weight loss is not a satisfactory form of accelerated test.

Some workers have recorded the uptake of metallic dissolution products in tissues around implants by the use of optical microscopy,[8] X-ray spectrography,[9] spectrochemical analysis[10] and electron probe microanalysis.[11] While these methods may provide useful information about the location of corrosion products, they are vitiated as measures of corrosion rates by the transport of corrosion products to more widespread tissues of the body and by excretion of corrosion products in urine, feces and sweat.

During the past two decades, electrochemical methods have been widely used for estimation of corrosion in surgical alloys. The first extensive electrochemical tests performed on alloys for implantation were described by Clarke and Hickman.[12] They reported the "anodic back EMF" (electromotive force) obtained by measurement of the potential difference across an electrochemical cell with a calomel electrode as cathode and a rotating rod of the test metal as anode in a bath of equine serum at 37°C, when known currents were passed. The technique required a complex bridge circuit for its operation but deserves considerable scrutiny. The method has never gained widespread use. In the author's opinion, its principal drawback is the provision of a single electrochemical index of inertness which attempts to combine the *liability* of a metal to dissolve with the actual *rate* of dissolution and thereby provides an unsatisfactory rating on both counts. Nevertheless, these workers did stimulate a resurgence of interest in the use of electrochemical methods for the study of metals for use in implantation.

In 1966, Hoar and Mears[6] published results of a variety of electrochemical tests performed on currently used, implant alloys and on many potentially superior ones. Their methods are now described in detail. First the potential time test (Fig. 4-5) is used to assess alloys immersed in such physiological solutions as Hanks' solution which, from the corrosion point of view, closely simulates the human environment. The potential of the metal with respect to a standard half cell, such as a silver/silver chloride or calomel electrode, is recorded serially for a few days or weeks. The results allow rapid classification of alloys into three categories: (a) alloys which show a decrease in potential with concomitant general dissolution; (b) alloys which show an initial rise in potential followed by a cyclic rise and fall which indicates sequential formation of pits, repassivation, and recurrent local break-

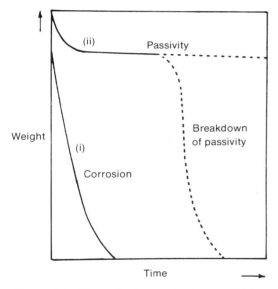

Figure 4-4. Schematic diagram to show weight-loss curves for metals that corrode or undergo passivity. The *solid lines* refer to the changes in weight that are observed during the longest tests that are feasible. Either the metal may dissolve rapidly (line *i*) with rapid change in weight or it may undergo passivity (line *ii*) to show stabilization in weight. The *dotted lines* show alternative forms of behavior that might be observed if the passive alloys were studied for a significantly longer period. Either passivity might be maintained, with insignificant change in weight of the specimen or, alternatively, breakdown of passivity might ensue with a markedly enhanced rate of corrosion and change in weight. Hence the curves confirm that weight-loss studies are not a satisfactory form of accelerated test to predict the breakdown of passivity.

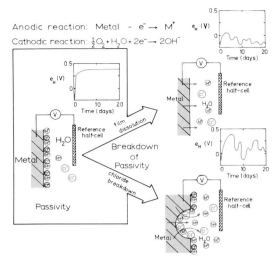

Anodic reaction: Metal $-$ e^- $\rightarrow$ M^+

Cathodic reaction: $\frac{1}{2}O_2 + H_2O + 2e^- \rightarrow 2OH^-$

Figure 4-5. Schematic diagram to show the mechanism of passivity with an appropriate potential/time curve and the mechanisms for breakdown of passivity and appropriate potential/time curves for active dissolution of metal and for chloride breakdown. Passivity occurs by formation of a compact, solid film of metallic oxide on the surface of the metal. Measurement of the change in potential of the specimen with reference to a standard half cell such as a silver-silver chloride reference electrode shows initial increase in potential followed by stabilization of the potential at above 350 mV. Alternatively, after exposure to solution, the metal may undergo generalized dissolution of the air-formed passive film with rapid dissolution. A potential/time curve shows rapid fall to a negative value which continues indefinitely. Another mode of rapid dissolution of metal with the formation of discrete pits may occur. Chloride anion enters the oxide film to provide a film that permits rapid conduction of metal ions across the film into solution. The potential/time curve shows an initial rise as passivation ensues. Subsequently it shows cyclic decline and elevation as pits form, heal with repassivation and new pits develop.

Red, anodic reactions with dissolution or passivation of metal. *Black*, cathodic reactions such as reduction of dissolved oxygen. *Green*, a combination of simultaneous anodic and cathodic reactions. Where a *red* anodic curve is superimposed on a *black* cathodic curve, the point of intersection(s) is shown as a *green dot*. Concurrent anodic and cathodic reactions polarize one another to about the same potentials. These corrosion potentials or passivation potentials are those recorded for potential/time experiments in natural environments.

down of passivity; and (c) alloys which show an initial increase of potential followed by maintenance of a constant potential within the passive region for an indefinite period of exposure. Only alloys showing the third type of behavior war-

rant further electrochemical study. It should be emphasized, however, that alloys which show satisfactory potential time behavior do not necessarily have adequate corrosion resistance. If exposed to body fluids for a period of time substantially longer than that used for such investigation, they may be liable to breakdown of passivity. Before costly and time-consuming animal tests or clinical trials are considered, it must be demonstrated that the alloys will remain passive for an extended period of exposure to the human environment. Furthermore, measurements of the actual rate of dissolution during passivity must be obtained.

Next, alloys which show satisfactory potential time behavior are studied with potentiostatic polarization[13] in order to observe whether they would be likely to undergo breakdown of passivity with the onset of rapid dissolution if exposed to body fluids for an extended period of time (*e.g.*, 50 years or more). Using the potentiostat a specimen is made anodic under conditions of slowly increasing polarization with an externally applied EMF. For example, if a specimen of 18% chromium 8% nickel stainless steel is immersed in Hanks' solution under potentiostatic conditions, the polarization curve (Fig. 4-2B) is obtained. The part of the curve *AB* represents increasing anodic dissolution in the active "bare metal" condition. *BC* represents the onset of anodic passivity caused by the growth of a passive film on the anodic surface. The potential *B* at which this reaction occurs is called the Flade potential. Curve *CD* represents passive behavior; it is caused by the formation of an oxide film on the metal surface. At point *D* a new anodic reaction supervenes. In neutral chloride-containing solutions, stainless steel alloys show either chloride breakdown (curve *HI*), with the formation of brightened hemispherical pits, or the evolution of oxygen gas (curve *FG*). Alternatively, other passive alloys such as titanium or tantalum may show marked thickening of the oxide film, so-called anodization. The particular reaction observed depends on the properties of the anodic film. Where the film is a compact solid layer and a good ionic conductor, pitting or even generalized brightening can be observed. Where the film is a poor ionic conductor but a good electronic conductor, evolution of oxygen gas or occasionally, in chloride solutions, chlorine gas is observed. Where the film is a poor ionic and electronic conductor then anodization will be found. The reader is referred to Hoar[14] and Young[15] for a more detailed account.

The situation becomes much clearer if the anodic and cathodic reactions are studied sepa-

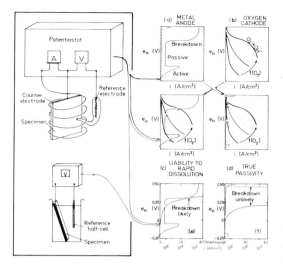

Figure 4-6. Schematic diagram of polarization curves. Measurements are performed by immersion of a flat plate of sample alloy in a physiological solution. The electropotential of the specimen is controlled by the potentiostat. The potential (V) is measured with reference to a standard reference electrode that is enclosed in a Luggin capillary. The dissolution rate is estimated by the corrosion current (A) that flows between the specimen and a concentric helical platinum counter electrode. (*a*) shows the anodic polarization of a sample metal which shows passive behavior (*dotted lines*) across most of the controlled potential. At the lowest potential applied to it, a minor elevation in corrosion rate with active dissolution is observed. The solid line portrays a metal which undergoes loss of passivity with active dissolution and chloride breakdown. (*b*) shows three cathodic polarization curves for solutions of different oxygen concentration. The lowest curve refers to the smallest oxygen concentration. In the next two figures, (*c*) and (*d*), the anodic polarization curves for the sample metal that is subject to loss of passivity and for the sample metal that is not liable to breakdown of passivity are superimposed on the cathodic polarization curves for solutions of different oxygen concentration. Since anodic and cathodic reactions polarize one another to the same potential in any given environment, the potentials that would occur *in vivo* are revealed by dots where the cathodic and anodic lines intersect. In (*c*) the three intersections correspond to active dissolution, passivity and chloride breakdown respectively. This observation confirms that this alloy could show great variation in corrosion rate, with change in oxygen content of the solution. In (*d*), the metal shows unchanged corrosion rate in the three solutions; its behavior is clearly preferred for use in the human body. (*e*) and (*f*) correlate the results of potential time measurements with polarization curves for two types of passive alloys. In (*e*) the magnitude of the chloride breakdown potential, as determined potentiostatically, is similar in magnitude to that of the long term rest potential of the same alloy when it is implanted in human subjects or experimental animals.

rately. This can be done for the anodic reaction if the solution is rigorously de-aerated so that no cathodic reduction of oxygen can occur. Then, a slow "potential sweep" leads to the curve shown in Figure 4-6*a*. At passivation the measured current (now equal to the anodic current) falls to a very low value, in favorable cases around 10^{-9}amps/cm^2. This corresponds to a dissolution rate of the anode of 0.1 ng/cm^2/hr. In the same solution but with oxygen present, a downward potential sweep of an inert electrode leads to cathodic curves such as are shown in Figure 4-6*b* for three different concentrations of oxygen. In Figure 4-6*c* and *d* the cathode current (*heavy lines*) is plotted on the same side of the diagram as the anode current. This emphasizes that quite a small variation of cathodic oxygen-reduction rate can lead to the establishment of either rapid dissolution conditions or *passive* conditions or of rapid dissolution with chloride breakdown. When anodic and cathodic reactions occur simultaneously on the same piece of metal they polarize each other to nearly the same potential, that of the intersection of the two potential/current polarization curves. While a relatively small cathodic reduction rate can maintain passivity, in the event of mechanical damage to the passivating film, the cathodic reaction cannot provide enough current to repassivate the specimen by repairing the film; whereas in the middle curve, the cathode can do so. Thus, quite small fluctuations in the degree of aeration of a solution, as may occur in crevices on implants, (Fig. 4-7), may provide conditions under which 18-8 stainless steel is rapidly attacked. The susceptibility of an alloy to crevice corrosion can be determined by scratch tests.[6] The alloy is im-

---

This indicates that chloride breakdown with formation of pits would be likely if the metal underwent prolonged exposure *in vivo*. In *f* the chloride breakdown potential, as determined potentiostatically, is considerably higher than the magnitude of the long term rest potential of the same metal studied *in vivo* although the breakdown potential is lower than the oxygen reversible potential. Here after prolonged exposure of the metal *in vivo* chloride breakdown is theoretically possible although exceedingly unlikely.

Red, anodic reactions with dissolution or passivation of metal. *Black*, cathodic reactions such as reduction of dissolved oxygen. *Green*, a combination of simultaneous anodic and cathodic reactions. Where a *red* anodic curve is superimposed on a *black* cathodic curve, the point of intersection(s) is shown as a *green dot*. Concurrent anodic and cathodic reactions polarize one another to about the same potentials. These corrosion potentials or passivation potentials are those recorded for potential/time experiments in natural environments.

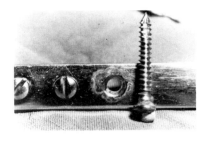

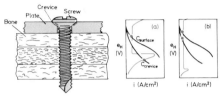

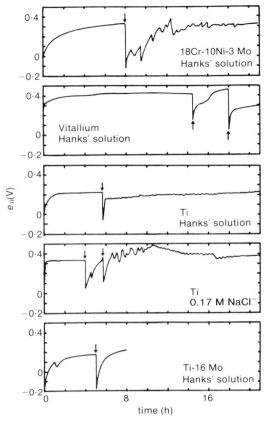

Figure 4-7. The photograph shows crevice corrosion of a stainless steel plate and screw at the areas of contact. The schematic diagram reveals the geometry of the crevice as a long narrow juncture. The polarization curve (*a*) shows a red anodic curve of a susceptible metal with the black cathodic curves for the oxygen cathodes on the metal surface and in the crevice respectively. The dots of intersection of the anodic and cathodic curves show increased rate of corrosion in the crevice. With motion of the screw head against the plate, the air-formed oxide film is abraded from the opposing surfaces. Film repair occurs by utilization of dissolved oxygen within the crevice. Continuous motion of the surfaces may create a need for constant replenishment of the dissolved oxygen within the crevice. Diffusion of oxygen from the bulk solution is greatly impeded, however, by the geometry of the crevice. Hence depletion of oxygen in the crevice may follow, whereupon conditions for active dissolution of metal ensue. Polarization curve (*b*) shows an alloy such as titanium which can rely on a water reduction cathode and remains passive despite total exhaustion of dissolved oxygen from the solution in the crevice.

Red, anodic reactions with dissolution or passivation of metal. *Black*, cathodic reactions such as reduction of dissolved oxygen. *Green*, a combination of simultaneous anodic and cathodic reactions. Where a *red* anodic curve is superimposed on a *black* cathodic curve, the point of intersection(s) is shown as a *green dot*. Concurrent anodic and cathodic reactions polarize one another to about the same potentials. These corrosion potentials or passivation potentials are those recorded for potential/time experiments in natural environments.

Figure 4-8. Schematic diagram to show potential/time curves of scratch tests of implant alloys in Hanks' solution and 0.17 M sodium chloride solution. 22°C: ↓ specimen scratched.

mersed in a physiological solution which is thoroughly deoxygenated. After deoxygenation, the metal must rely on the water-reduction cathode, the only cathodic reactant which is available in a crevice. Next the alloy is scratched with a diamond stylus, and the potential time curve is plotted (Fig. 4-8). For a metal such as titanium, which is resistant to crevice attack, repassivation occurs within a few seconds. The potential time transient shows an initial drop in potential at the time of scratch with a rapid rise in potential to the prescratch "passive" value. For alloys such as 18Cr-10Ni austenitic stainless steels, which require an oxygen cathode, a different potential time curve is recorded. At the time of the scratch, the potential drops to a value consistent with active dissolution of the scratch. It never returns to its prescratched value, since repassivation cannot occur.

From these considerations Hoar and Mears[6] were able to formulate the polarization diagram (Fig. 4-9) for the ideal implant alloy, which will behave solely in the passive mode. On mechanical destruction or removal of the passive film,

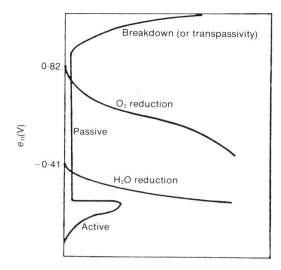

Figure 4-9. Schematic polarization curves for alloys that show optimal behavior in body fluids (pH 7). Such alloys show only passive dissolution *in vivo*. Combination of these alloys will not provoke more rapid dissolution of any constituent.

even in a poorly oxygenated crevice, rapid re-passivation is assured. Such alloys rely on a water reduction cathode for hydroxide or oxide film formation, which may occur in the complete absence of dissolved oxygen. The ability to re-form or repair a passive film in the absence of oxygen is a prerequisite for resistance to crevice corrosion. Alloys which show this behavior include titanium, zirconium, niobium, hafnium and tantalum. Furthermore, as will be shown subsequently, all of the ideal alloys of this type may be used in combination with one another without increased liability to passive breakdown with accelerated dissolution rate. To meet this criterion, the "ideal" alloy must behave in a passive manner across the range of potential between the water reduction cathode (−0.41V) and the oxygen reduction cathode (0.82V). These two cathodic reactions regulate the range of electrodepotential found *in vivo*, so that mixed potentials greater or less than this range will not occur for implants *in vivo*.

The question has been raised as to whether an alloy which shows a breakdown potential of 20V is more inert *in vivo* than an alloy which shows a breakdown potential of 2V. From the point of view of chloride breakdown *in vivo*, they are *equally* inert, since neither alloy may undergo chloride breakdown *in vivo* where the maximum potential that will be found with the

oxygen reduction cathode is 0.82V. However this test does not measure the absolute rate of passive dissolution. The alloy with the lower chloride breakdown potential may actually dissolve more slowly *in vivo* than the alloy with the higher chloride breakdown potential.

Another practical situation that gives rise to confusion is the relationship of the implant rest potential, as determined by potential time studies, to the chloride breakdown potential (Fig. 4-6 *E* and *F*). If the rest potential recorded for an alloy after 2 weeks' exposure to Hanks' solution or to implantation is higher than the breakdown potential, determined potentiostatically, then breakdown of passivity is inevitable. If the rest potential is similar to the breakdown potential, then with prolonged exposure to body fluids, loss of passivity is likely. If, as in the case of the cobalt-chromium surgical alloys, the breakdown potential is significantly higher than the rest potential, although lower than the oxygen reversible potential, then the liability to chloride breakdown becomes a remote possibility.

Other potentiodynamic techniques notably the polarization resistance technique,[16, 17] have been used to estimate the corrosion rates of implant alloys. The attractiveness of this method is its ability for establishing the instantaneous velocity of corrosion by measurement of the gradient of the polarization curve in the vicinity of the corrosion potential. As Prázak and Barton have shown,[18] a polarization curve (Fig. 4-10*A*) represents the relationship between the boundary between a dissolving electrode and the electrolyte. The gradient (dE/di) has the dimensions of an electrical resistance. As the rate of corrosion K on unit area of metal surface is proportional to the current i_{corr}, there exists a simple relationship according to Faraday's laws:

where

$$K = C/R_p$$
$$R_p = (d\,E/d_i)_{E_{corr}} \tag{1}$$

The constant c comprises a number of electrochemical constants that are characteristic of the metal and solution. Stern and Geary[19] derived (1) on the assumption that both anode and cathode E/i relationships are of Tafel form with linear slope as shown in Figure 4-10*A*. Whence

$$E = b_a \log i_a + A_{a'} \tag{2}$$

$$E = b_c \log i_c + A_{c'} \tag{3}$$

At a potential greater than the corrosion poten-

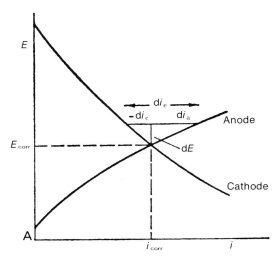

$$i_{\text{corr}} = \frac{b_a b_c}{2.303(b_c - b_a)}/(dE/di_e)\,E_{\text{corr}},$$

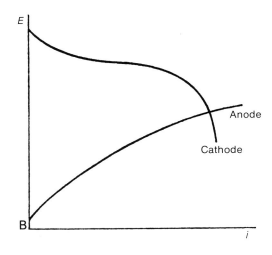

$$i_{\text{corr}} = \frac{b_a}{2.303}/(dE/di_e)E_{\text{corr}}.$$

Figure 4-10. *A.* Polarization curve idealized by Prázak and Barton for verification of their technique to use estimation of polarization resistance for the estimation of corrosion rates. *B.* Polarization curve for the system silver-acid-ferric-sulfate. Far from having a Tafel form as shown in *A*, the cathodic polarization curve may approach i_c constant.

tial E by an amount dE (Fig. 4-10), the external current $ie = i_a - i_c$,

and

$$\frac{di_e}{dE} = \frac{di_a}{dE} - \frac{di_c}{dE} \qquad (4)$$

Thus, with (2) and (3),

$$\left(\frac{di_e}{dE}\right)_{E_{\text{corr}}} = 2.303\, i_{\text{corr}}\left(\frac{1}{b_a} - \frac{1}{b_c}\right), \qquad (5)$$

whence

$$i_{\text{corr}} = \frac{b_a b_c}{2.303\,(b_c - b_a)}/(dE/di_e)_{E_{\text{corr}}} \qquad (6)$$

This is equivalent to (1) as used by Prázak and Barton.

As Hoar pointed out,[20] the anodic and cathodic polarization curves for metals in most natural corrosion environments fail to show these idealized linear slopes. In some systems, far from having a Tafel form, the form of the cathodic polarization curve may well approach i_c equals constant (Fig. 4-10*B*). Here, approximate experimental verification of (1) may still follow if the slope of the cathodic E/i curve is large compared with that of the anodic E/i curve, because then

$$b_c \gg b_a$$

and (5) reduces to

$$i_{\text{corr}} = \frac{b_a}{2.303}/(dE/di_e)E_{\text{corr}} \qquad (7)$$

Thus, as Hoar argues, there are two highly specific situations in which the polarization resistance technique might be useful for measurement of corrosion rate. In practice, neither of these is likely to be encountered in corrosion measurements *in vivo*; hence the results of linear polarization measurements will be subject to considerable experimental error.

The method has a second liability. It requires contact between an external probe and the implant for a few seconds or minutes. The probe is likely to scratch the implant and thereby alter the recorded corrosion rate greatly. Thirdly, as has been shown elsewhere, the rate of dissolution of imperfectly passive alloys is apt to vary by orders of magnitude from one moment to the next. The polarization resistance technique does not reveal the liability of an alloy to change from a minute rate of passive dissolution recorded in one experiment to a much greater rate of dissolution at some time in the future.

The potentiostatic technique can be used to estimate the minute rate of production of dissolution products of passive alloys *in vivo*. First, measurements of the resting potential of the alloy *in vivo* are undertaken over a protracted period. Initially such measurements were made on specimens exposed to physiological solutions, while more recently they have been made on animals and ultimately in human subjects.[6] The measurements can be undertaken in several ways. A probe electrode may be used which contains a central reference electrode carefully insulated electrically from an outer concentric probe (Fig. 4-11). The probe is inserted, preferably under X-ray control until it just touches the metal implant. Then the potential difference between the implant and the reference electrode is recorded on a millivoltmeter (Fig. 4-12). Alternatively, a conventional reference electrode may be placed in the animal's mouth beneath the tongue, and the potential reading can be recorded on a high resistance electronic millivoltmeter. The tissues and extracellular fluid between the reference electrode and the implant form a "salt bridge". The implant is contacted by a metal probe which is insulated apart from the pointed tip. A few implants such as many Kirschner wires or Steinmann pins protrude from patients. In such cases the exposed end may be secured with an alligator clip while the reference electrode is placed in the mouth. In all cases, potential measurements are recorded sequentially on each implant, over a period of time.

Next, specimens of the same alloy are exposed to physiological fluids in which all possible cathodic reactants, such as oxygen, have been completely removed. The potential of the metal is controlled by the potentiostat to the natural potential previously measured *in vivo*. The very small anode current flowing is a measure of the minute corrosion rate under natural conditions.

When the changes in corrosion rates with time are plotted graphically for a variety of alloys, four shapes of curves are observed (Fig. 4-13). Certain stainless steels show continuous cyclic variation of corrosion rate, which indicates imperfect passivity. In contrast, some cobalt-chromium alloys show a curve which after an initial period of equilibration, reaches a constant value. Afterward, the oxide film seems to dissolve, albeit slowly, as fast as it forms. Still other alloys show an initial drop in corrosion current followed by an increase, and subsequently a constant rate. This phenomenon may be similar to the micropore formation for the oxide film on

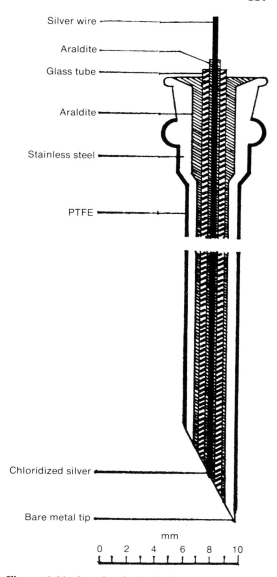

Figure 4-11. A probe electrode for measurement of the potential of an implant *in vivo*. PTFE, polytetrafluoroethylene.

Silver wire
Araldite
Glass tube
Araldite
Stainless steel
PTFE
Chloridized silver
Bare metal tip

mm
0   2   4   6   8   10

aluminum alloys described by Hoar and Yahalom.[21] Certain titanium alloys show continuous diminution of corrosion rate over a period of several weeks, the longest period of observation. This is the optimum situation, where the passive film continues to thicken over the entire period of study, the metal thereby dissolving ever more slowly. Ultimately, minute dissolution rates equivalent to 0.1 to 1.0 $ng/cm^2/hr$ have been recorded for several titanium alloys. Table 4-1 shows that these values represent dissolution

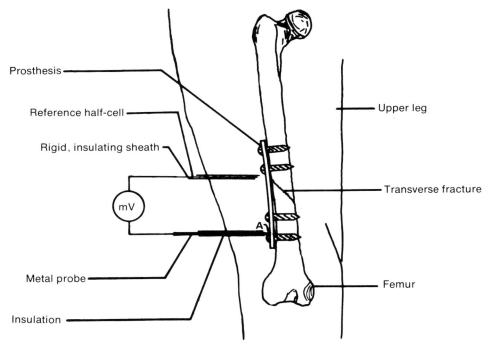

Figure 4-12. Schematic diagram of the measurement of potential of an implant *in vivo*.

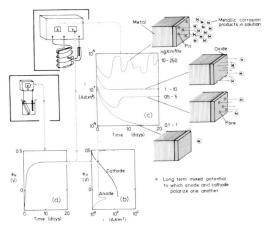

Figure 4-13. Schematic diagram of polarization method to determine long-term passive dissolution rates *in vivo*. First the mixed potential for the implant alloy *in vivo* is determined by potential/time studies, as shown in *A*. Next, a standard polarization curve for the same alloy immersed in physiological solution is portrayed, *B*. The transient dissolution rate of the metal, after brief exposure to that solution is shown by the *dot*. If the metal is controlled potentiostatically at that same potential for a prolonged period, then changes in dissolution rate with time can be revealed, *C*. Four types of current-time curve have been observed. The *top curve* with cyclic variation of current

corresponds to a metal that undergoes recurrent localized breakdown of passivity. The *second curve* represents an alloy that after a brief introductory period shows a constant, albeit minute rate of dissolution. Hence its rate of passive film formation equals the rate of film dissolution rate followed by an increase and subsequent stabilization. The *third curve* shows an initial drop of current followed by an increase and subsequently a stabilization of dissolution rate. This may represent a passive film that forms a porous structure. The fourth and lowest curve shows progressive diminution in corrosion rate for the duration of exposure of metal to solution. It represents the most desirable form of passive behavior of an alloy for implantation.

Red, anodic reactions with dissolution or passivation of metal. *Black*, cathodic reactions such as reduction of dissolved oxygen. *Green*, a combination of simultaneous anodic and cathodic reactions. Where a *red* anodic curve is superimposed on a *black* cathodic curve, the point of intersection(s) is shown as a *green dot*. Concurrent anodic and cathodic reactions polarize one another to about the same potentials. These corrosion potentials or passivation potentials are those recorded for potential/time experiments in natural environments.

rates several orders of magnitude less rapid than those measured for passive stainless steel alloys. The table also shows a comparison between dissolution rates determined potentiostatically and dissolution rates determined by spectrochemical analysis of dissolution products that accumulate in tissues around implants.[10] Regarding this discrepancy, potentiostatic measurements record passive film formation and include an initial period of film thickening, during which time the estimate of corrosion rate is unduly pessimistic. Ultimately the two processes achieve equilibrium and the film dissolves slowly, as rapidly as it forms. Once steady state conditions are achieved, the estimate is a reliable indication of dissolution rate. At this stage spectrochemical analysis of local tissues fails to account for the transport of dissolution products to such tissues as liver or kidney or for the excretion of dissolution products in urine and feces.

COMBINATIONS OF DISSIMILAR METALS

In 1791, while investigating the susceptibility of nerves to irritation, Luigi Galvani[22] showed that nervous action could be induced by electrical phenomena. Galvani discovered this phenomenon while working with a frog nerve-muscle preparation (Fig. 4-14). In one experiment a rod of brass contacted the frog's foot, while another rod of silver contacted its spinal cord. When the free ends of the rods were brought together, contraction of the leg muscles occurred. In a second experiment, a single bent rod was used to complete the circuit while the spinal cord and legs rested respectively on squares of brass and copper foil. Contraction occurred when the rod touched the two pieces of foil simultaneously.

In 1800, Volta[23] confirmed that the force which provoked the contraction of muscle was of an electrical nature. Subsequently, the electric current generated by contact of dissimilar metals immersed in an electrolyte solution has been called a galvanic current.

For over 100 years, it has been known that combinations of dissimilar metals in solutions may show rates of dissolution quite different from those of the same metals when exposed singly to the same environment. The presence of one metal might provoke more rapid dissolution of another metal as galvanic corrosion; or one metal might serve to protect the other metal and, in turn, itself dissolve more rapidly; or rarely, one metal might protect the other with-

Table 4-1

Comparison of Rate of Formation of Corrosion Products for Alloys in Hanks' solution during Current Time-Tests with Rate of Formation of Implant Corrosion Products in Rabbits

Alloy	Metal converted into compound ng cm^{-2} h^{-1}	Metal found in tissue ng cm^{-2} h^{-1}
18 Cr-10Ni-3Mo steel		
Mechanically polished	7.8	0.274
Chemically polished	230.0	–
Vitallium		
Mechanically polished	150	0.249
Commercial finish	20	–
Ti		
Mechanically polished	4.1	0.430
Chemically polished	3.5	–
Ti-16Mo	1.5	–
Ti-5Ta	0.26	–

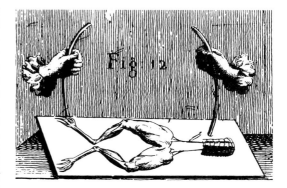

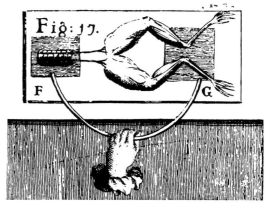

Figure 4-14. A reproduction of sketches by Luigi Galvani to show his experiments for demonstration of galvanic current.

out appreciable increase in its own rate of dissolution. Considerable practical application of this knowledge has been made, notably by cathodic protection of copper sheathing of wooden ship hulls after the observations of Sir Humphrey Davy.[24] Davy suggested that the copper sheathing on wooden ship hulls could be protected from corrosion by placing blocks of iron or zinc in contact with the copper at various sites on the hull of the ship. Corrosion would be concentrated on the iron or zinc blocks; when these corroded away they could be replaced. Similarly Michael Faraday[25] showed that while iron exposed to moderately strong nitric acid solution would undergo rapid corrosion, it could be protected by combination with platinum. On certain occasions, however, unpredictable disasters occurred. One metal, apparently protected by the presence of another metal, would, suddenly begin to dissolve far more rapidly than it would have done if immersed alone. For example, amphoteric metals such as aluminum might exhibit rapid dissolution upon excessive cathodic polarization. Such disasters created considerable skepticism toward the value of use of dissimilar metals for corrosion protection. Indeed, by the turn of this century, deleterious side effects of galvanic corrosion had been confirmed *in vivo*. Lambotte[26] used mild steel screws with magnesium plates and observed total dissolution of the magnesium before repair of the fracture had occurred. Von Baeyer[27] implanted copper plates in juxtaposition to zinc plates. When he examined the growth of connective tissue around the implants, he observed that the fibroblasts and collagen fibrils were oriented along the lines of corrosion current as determined mathematically. He hoped to show that galvanic protection could be used therapeutically to hasten tissue repair. The conclusion which had been drawn by all previous authors was that dissimilar alloys should not be used to assemble surgical implants.

In fact, the use of dissimilar alloys for implant construction has immense attraction. One might select alloys of widely different—indeed contrasting—mechanical attributes and use each material to its best advantage. For example, in the construction of a total joint replacement, a hard, wear-resistant material might be welded to a ductile material which is easily shaped for attachment to the adjacent bone. The author[28] has recently reviewed this field. It is concluded that passive alloys can be classified into a variety of types which may be combined for the construction of surgical implants. Currently avail-able electrochemical tests allow the accurate prediction of safe combinations of passive alloys. The reasons for this considerable change in view and the methods used to determine safe combinations of alloys are discussed below.

Galvanic Corrosion

As has been indicated galvanic corrosion is a mode of metallic deterioration in which two metals in contact with one another are immersed in solution and one "base" or "reactive" metal, the anode, undergoes more rapid dissolution, while the other "noble" metal, the cathode, undergoes less rapid dissolution, than the isolated specimens would exhibit when similarly immersed. Early workers[29] measured the rate of corrosion of iron in contact with numerous other materials (Table 4-2). The table shows that iron is protected by contact with a baser metal while it suffers serious corrosion by contact with a relatively noble metal. Such considerations were probably responsible for the widespread belief that the Table of Normal Potentials[30] (Table 4-3) could be used to determine dangerous or safe combinations of metals. It is well established that the EMF between two metals placed respectively in solutions that contain their salts at equivalent concentrations is obtained approximately by subtraction of the normal potential of the baser metal from that of the nobler metal. Under such conditions, the further apart the two metals stand in the Table of Normal Potentials, the larger will be the EMF of the combination. Hence, the corrosion rate of the baser metal, the anode, might be expected to increase as the difference between the two Normal Electrode Potentials becomes greater. Unfortunately, as a practical guide for prediction of the dissolution

Table 4-2

Bimetallic Corrosion of Iron and a Second Metal Immersed in 1% Sodium Chloride[29]

Corrosion of iron (mg)	Second metal	Corrosion of second metal (mg)
183.1	Copper	0.0
181.1	Nickel	0.2
171.1	Tin	2.5
183.2	Lead	3.6
176.0	Tungsten	5.2
153.1	Antimony	13.8
9.8	Aluminum	105.9
0.4	Cadmium	307.9
0.4	Zinc	688.0
0.0	Magnesium	3104.3

TABLE 4-3
Normal Potentials[30]

	Equilibrium Volt (hydrogen scale)
$Au \rightleftharpoons Au^{+++} + 3e$	+ 1.50
$Ag \rightleftharpoons Ag^{+} + e$	+ 0.7991
$2Hg \rightleftharpoons Hg_2^{++} + 2e$	+ 0.789
$Cu \rightleftharpoons Cu^{++} + 2e$	+ 0.337
$Cu \rightleftharpoons Cu^{+} + e$ (unstable)	+ 0.522
$H_2 \rightleftharpoons 2H^{+} + 2e$	0.000 (arbitrary zero)
$Pb \rightleftharpoons Pb^{++} + 2e$	− 0.126
$Sn \rightleftharpoons Sn^{++} + 2e$	− 0.136
$Ni \rightleftharpoons Ni^{++} + 2e$	− 0.250
$Cd \rightleftharpoons Cd^{++} + 2e$	− 0.403
$Fe \rightleftharpoons Fe^{++} + 2e$	− 0.440
$Zn \rightleftharpoons Zn^{++} + 2e$	− 0.763
$Al \rightleftharpoons Al^{+++} + 3e$	− 1.66[a]
$Mg \rightleftharpoons Mg^{++} + 2e$	− 2.37[a]

[a] These equilibria are not usually realized in aqueous solution owing to film formation. The numbers in such cases are calculated from thermodynamic data.

rates of combinations of metals, the Table of Normal Potentials has proved of limited value. This is not surprising, since each number in the table refers to film-free metal placed in a solution with its ions at normal activity. No alloy in present or future use in surgery is film-free when immersed in body fluids. As will be described, combinations of film-covered metals show quite different behavior. Furthermore, normal activity of metallic ions would never be encountered in physiological conditions.

As an alternative guide to the behavior of combinations of metals, engineers adopted tables of potentials obtained empirically by measurements for combinations of metals placed in sea water. This environment was selected because most serious cases of galvanic corrosion were met in marine conditions. In view of the similarity of sea water to body fluid as a corrosive environment, several workers have suggested that these tables are suitable for application in the selection of safe combinations of surgical alloys. The procedure of selection rests on the assumption that the working EMF of a bimetallic combination can be obtained by subtraction of the potential provided by one half-cell, consisting of one metal immersed in sea water in reference to a standard half-cell such as a calomel or silver chloride reference cell, from that provided by another half-cell consisting of the other metal and a reference half-cell immersed in sea water. This procedure is legitimate for reversible potentials as tabulated in Table 4-3, but incorrect for irreversible potentials as

obtained in sea water or body fluids. Furthermore, the magnitude of the EMF alone does not determine the current available for metallic dissolution. The current, and therefore the corrosion rate, is largely determined by polarization considerations. Polarization refers to changes in the driving force available in an electrochemical system that arise from: (a) differing concentrations of metallic ions in a corrosion system; (b) the activation energies of the several reactions in a corrosion system; and (c) the ohmic potential drop through the electrolyte and through the reaction product films which coat the surfaces of the electrodes. It must be emphasized that the corrosion rate will not necessarily be highest with those combinations that produce the greatest electromotive force. More recently, with the advent of the potentiostatic technique,[31] accurate methods of predicting unsafe combinations of metals have been developed. With these methods, one can rapidly screen combinations of metals and eliminate from consideration those pairs that would be liable to provoke rapid dissolution of one alloy.

There are other highly peculiar situations in which a combination of dissimilar metals may arise and thereby provoke corrosion of one of the metals.[32] A metal specimen may be exposed to a liquid which contains reducible compounds of a more cathodic metal. In hydrochloric acid solution, for example, zinc dissolves far more rapidly after the addition of a platinum salt. Similarly, Frankenthal and Pickering[33] have described the breakdown of stainless steel alloys after exposure to hydrochloric acid solutions containing platinum salts. Addition of salts of other cathodic metals such as antimony or silver may also stimulate attack. Under these conditions, the cathodic metal salts are reduced and particles of the cathodic metal are deposited on the surface of the specimen, thereby creating numerous minute galvanic cells. It is conceivable that dissolution of dental alloys could provoke similar galvanic corrosion of stainless steel implant alloys, although the author is not aware of any reported cases. Another unusual situation occurs when acceleration in the corrosion of the less noble metal is accompanied by acceleration in the corrosion of the more noble metal or alloy. This represents galvanic corrosion accompanied by corrosion of the cathode. It occurs only when the more noble metal is amphoteric such as aluminum or magnesium, or when the more noble metal undergoes hydrogen embrittlement, another unusual form of cathodic corrosion. Within the range of passive alloys currently used for surgical implants, these modes of corrosion will not be encountered.

Corrosion currents may also be generated within a single alloy which lacks homogeneity because of the presence of grain boundaries, differential grain size or orientation, differential surface treatment or surface roughness or differential mechanical strain. These factors will not be discussed.

Corrosion Control by Combinations of Alloys

Anodic Protection. Over a century ago, Schonbein and Faraday[25] studied the rates of dissolution and mechanisms of corrosion of bimetallic combinations. They observed that for iron in contact with platinum in a solution of dilute nitric acid, the platinum provoked rapid dissolution of the iron. On the other hand, in concentrated nitric acid, the platinum helped to maintain resistance of the iron to dissolution. We now know that the explanation for the altered behavior of iron in concentrated nitric acid is the formation of a passive film on the surface of the iron.[34] The platinum serves to maintain the integrity of the film by regulation of the potential of the iron within the passive range (*CD*, Fig. 4-2*B*). In the past, the principal drawback of anodic protection has been that in practice the auxillary platinum or palladium electrode could provide adequate current to *maintain* passivity but it could not provide adequate current to *produce* passivity if generalized cor-

rosion was ever provoked by some external cause (Fig. 4-2). Presently, certain stainless steels and titanium alloys are available that require so little current for passive film formation that anodic protection can be used to *provide* and to *maintain* passivity. In a recent study on anodic protection of certain stainless steel alloys, Streicher[35] reported that ruthenium was the most effective noble metal in affording protection from both chloride breakdown and active dissolution. Perhaps the greatest asset of this method of corrosion control for use in surgical alloys is that the rate of dissolution of the cathodic noble metal is *not* increased by coupling with the anodic material. Titanium-palladium alloys have been tested extensively[6] for corrosion resistance in body fluids, and the results of the tests indicate that they should perform well in the human body.

Cathodic Protection. Cathodic protection is an electrochemical method of corrosion control in which a second metal is connected to the specimen of interest and used to lower the potential that drives the corrosion process. Reference to Figure 4-2 will show that sufficient depression of the potential of a metal anode could produce a wholly inert specimen with *no* dissolution. From this point of view, the method should be of great interest to surgeons for clinical application in implant corrosion protection. Furthermore, it holds even more promise for investigations of the effect of metals on tissues without accompanying metallic dissolution. For use in surgery, the principal liability is the necessary dissolution of the auxillary or "sacrificial" anode. Even with the use of a metal whose metallic dissolution products are shown to be nontoxic by all available tests, surgeons would be concerned that prolonged accumulation of the auxillary anode's dissolution products might provoke some deleterious toxic response. Alternatively, instead of a sacrificial anode, a battery and an inert electrode can be used as a source of electrons to protect the specimen. However, for widespread use in surgery, the provision and replacement of batteries would present considerable practical problems. Hence, cathodic protection does not appear to be feasible for orthopaedic implants. It does, however, have one additional advantage for cardiovascular implants which contact the blood stream. A negative surface charge is found on blood vessels and on certain anticoagulant molecules such as heparin which resist encrustation with products of coagulation. Cathodic protection of vascular prostheses in dogs[36] has been shown to provide considerable protection from undesirable coagulation.

Combinations of Passive Alloys. There is one other situation in which certain alloys can be used in combination without liability to rapid dissolution of either metal. It is a highly peculiar situation which depends on a unique characteristic of some passive alloys. As Hoar and Mears[6] have described, it is thermodynamically impossible for certain passive alloys immersed in body fluids to undergo breakdown of passivity. This criterion is met by those alloys that conform to the polarization curve shown in Figure 4-9. Breakdown at high potential, with pitting and activity at low potential such as crevice corrosion, will both be avoided if the metal concerned has a breakdown potential more positive than the oxygen-reduction reversible potential and a passivation potential less positive than the water (or hydrogen ion) reduction reversible potential. High-potential depassivation might equally be caused by anodic oxidation of passivating oxide to soluble products known as transpassivity, not discussed here. At present, titanium and its alloys and probably some materials based on zirconium, niobium, and tantalum appear to be the only alloys that can fulfill the criterion in chloride media. These alloys may be combined with one another and they will continue to exhibit passive behavior. The slow rates of dissolution of all constituents of the combination will remain virtually unchanged.

One additional combination of passive alloys is of considerable practical importance in orthopaedic surgery. This is the combination of one truly passive metal, as defined in the previous section, with a less passive alloy, especially one that is liable to undergo crevice corrosion. From the corrosion point of view, a similar situation arises with the combination of two passive alloys, both of which are liable to crevice corrosion. The question is raised as to the likelihood of increased crevice corrosion due to the presence of the second material. In the past, many workers would have suggested that the two passive metals should be considered as a galvanic couple, wherein one, the truly passive metal, behaving as the cathode and the other less passive one behaving as the dissolving anode, so that the combination serves to accelerate the corrosion rate. In fact, for passive metals this suggestion is grossly in error. A passive metal that undergoes crevice corrosion exhibits *two* anodic dissolution processes which occur in parallel. Most of the metal surface shows an exceedingly slow rate of dissolution through the passive

oxide film, while a minute portion of the metal surface at the crevice shows rapid active dissolution. All of the metal surface apart from the minute crevice shows simultaneous cathodic reduction of oxygen. Hence, addition of a second truly passive metal in combination with the former merely serves to enlarge the surface of metal that shows passive dissolution of metal and cathodic reduction of oxygen. While the cathodic reaction on the truly passive metal might occur with much greater or lesser efficiency than occurs on the less passive alloy, this does not seem to be of practical significance within the range of alloys that are currently used for orthopaedic surgical implants. Hence, by combination of a titanium implant with a less inert stainless steel one, the liability to and rate of crevice corrosion on the stainless steel are unlikely to be diminished but are *extremely* unlikely to be increased.

Another frequently encountered clinical situation is the moving crevice, such as the junction between a screw and a plate, in which the passive oxide film may be mechanically abraded from the moving surfaces. This phenomenon is fully described for homogenous materials in Figure 4-7. Where different combinations of materials are in sliding contact, the same principles apply. If, however, one metal provides anodic protection to another, then the cathodic material must provide adequate current for *production* of passivity, as well as for *maintenance* of passivity. Scratch tests,[6] performed on combinations of metals in deoxygenated solution, must be used to show whether the electrode potential of the bimetallic couple returns immediately to that consistent with passive behavior of both alloys. The deoxygenation simulates the consumption of dissolved oxygen by continuous repassivation of the abrading surfaces in a crevice, where diffusion of oxygen from the bulk solution may be greatly hindered by the geometry of the crevice.

Past Experience in the Use of Dissimilar Metals in Orthopaedic Surgery

About 1935, when many highly corrodible metals were used for surgical implants, many observations[37] were made by surgeons of the accelerated attack on an active metal, such as mild steel, when combined with a more noble one, such as copper. Undoubtedly, these observations account for the extreme reluctance of surgeons to use mixed metals in surgery. It should be emphasized, however, that such combinations are not comparable to the combination of currently used *passive* surgical alloys. Scales,

Winter and Shirley,[38] described large numbers of orthopaedic implants after removal from human implantation. They reported the incidence of corrosion of metallic combinations of different austenitic stainless steel alloys (*e.g.,* 18% chromium-8% nickel alloy with 18% chromium-8% nickel and 2.5% molybdenum) and of combinations of austenitic stainless steel alloys with a cobalt-chromium-molybdenum alloy. The alloys in combination did not show an increased incidence of corrosion compared to their behavior when used alone. Indeed, for combinations of stainless steel alloys, mutual protection seemed to be conferred by the combination. More recently, Cohen and Wulff[39] have reported observations of the corrosion of a combination of a wrought cobalt-chromium-tungsten-nickel alloy with a cast cobalt-chromium-molybdenum alloy. Crevice attack was observed in the former alloy but not in the latter material. Laboratory tests were undertaken in which Teflon gaskets were applied to specimens of each cobalt-chromium alloy to form crevices between the metal and the polymeric material. The specimens were immersed individually in solutions of sodium chloride. Potential-time studies and metallographic observations showed that the cobalt-chromium-tungsten-nickel alloy underwent crevice attack, while the cobalt-chromium-molybdenum alloy did not undergo similar corrosion. The experiments confirm that the crevice corrosion in passive metals is provoked by the presence of a crevice on a susceptible alloy and *not* by the presence of dissimilar passive alloys.

Recently two types of total hip replacement have utilized combinations of dissimilar metals. The Müller type of total hip replacement,[40] uses a cast cobalt-chromium alloy femoral head prosthesis welded to a wrought cobalt chromium alloy intramedullary stem. More recently, the latter alloy has been replaced with a titanium alloy (Ti-6A1-4V), also welded to the cobalt-chromium femoral head prosthesis. Both combinations have performed satisfactorily. The Russin modified Sivash prosthesis[41] has combined a similar cast cobalt-chromium alloy with titanium. Again, this combination of materials has performed satisfactorily in the clinical situation. Similar observations are required for other potentially useful combinations of dissimilar surgical alloys.

Effects of Galvanic Currents on Tissues and Cells

There has been widespread speculation on the effects of corrosion currents on tissues and cells, although few facts are available. Corrosion may alter cells in at least three ways: (a) the metallic dissolution products may affect cell metabolism and thereby damage extracellular matrix; also, (b) corrosion may be accompanied by changes in the chemical environment of the cell, such as the production of hydrogen ions or hydroxyl ions or the evolution of a gas such as hydrogen, oxygen or chlorine; and (c) the corrosion currents may affect cell behavior.

The first two factors are fully reviewed in Chapter 7. For cells exposed to metals singly or in combination, toxicity would be a function of the rate of the dissolution process of a particular dissolving anode and not of the presence of combinations of metals. At present, the effects of electric currents on cell behavior are under intense scrutiny. Observations of the effects of applying direct or alternating current to cell cultures reveal a variety of potentially beneficial as well as potentially harmful actions, including induction of osteogenesis, alignment of randomly oriented collagen fibers, transformation of red cell precursor cells into fully differentiated red cells, and stimulation of neuromuscular events. While the last mentioned has received the most attention as an adverse side-effect of implanted dissimilar metals, it is most unlikely to be clinically significant for the combinations of metals recommended in this chapter because the magnitude of electric power required for neuromuscular stimulation is orders of magnitude greater than corrosion currents between the recommended combinations of implant alloys. Ultimately the toxicity of corrosion potentials between dissimilar implant alloys must be assessed in the clinical situation. In the few large studies performed to date, the author is not aware of any deleterious biological response to implantation of combinations of the alloys recommended here.

Conclusion

Even a cursory glance at present ambitious attempts to replace or repair human organs with man made devices will show the enormous advantage of the simultaneous use of a variety of alloys, each selected for its particular mechanical attributes. In many cases, nonmetallic substances will also be required. A careful review of the electrochemical and biological effects of combinations of alloys shows that a wide variety of passive alloys may be safely used together *in vivo.* Admittedly, in the absence of expert knowledge of the properties of metals and alloys, it has been considered safe practice to avoid the use of dissimilar metals for surgical implantation. Knowledge has increased, however, so that more sophisticated rules should replace this tradition. Combinations of passive alloys should be introduced into surgical practice so that materials of different mechanical properties, including those in composite form, are used in conjunction with one another. Each metal would be selected for its peculiar mechanical attributes. Also, the combination could provide improved corrosion resistance for the less inert material. Electrochemical techniques are available to test combinations of passive alloys and to classify them into the following types: (a) combinations that do not appreciably alter the corrosion resistance of any constituent; (b) combinations where the presence of one alloy improves the corrosion resistance of the other alloy by anodic protection, without deterioration of its own corrosion resistance; and (c) combinations where one alloy improves the corrosion resistance of another alloy and simultaneously undergoes more rapid corrosion itself. Such cathodic protection is unlikely to be considered useful for orthopaedic implants as the optimal method for protection of the metallic device. However, the beneficial effect of a negatively charged surface to prevent encrustation of the wall of an artificial blood vessel could conceivably be used to advantage in future orthopaedic implants. This chapter does *not* recommend indiscriminate mixture of metals but rather attempts to show that selected combinations of passive metals can be used safely with considerable advantage for all those who deal with surgical implants. The situation is analogous to the well established simultaneous application of pharmacological agents such as triple chemotherapy for tuberculosis with isoniazid, streptomycin and para-aminosalicyclic acid; or digoxin, diuretics and hypotensive agents for severe hypertensive cardiac failure; or nitrogen mustard, vincristine sulfate, procarbazine hydrochloride and prednisone for treatment of advanced Hodgkin's disease.[42] It requires a similar vigilance to avoid potentially adverse side-effects, as may occur with combined chemotherapy, with the enhanced bleeding tendency when aspirin or barbiturates are used with oral anticoagulants, or the potentiation of monamine oxidase inhibitors by sympathomimetic agents resulting in hypertensive crises. Further observations are required to confirm the author's opinion that all currently used surgical alloys can be used in combination without increased rates of corrosion in any alloy.

PAINT

One obvious method of controlling corrosion is the application of tenaciously adherent inert films to metal implants (*e.g.*, the perfect paint). For metals that lack adequate passivity, the question arises as to why industrial protective coatings have not been used to protect implants from contact with body fluids. Paint has not in fact been used because none is available which is adequately inert or adherent. In addition, the coating is likely to be damaged mechanically during implantation. Some workers have placed inert washers between areas of sliding contact on two implants such as a screw head and a plate. Unfortunately, insertion of a washer which fits snugly against a metal surface provides a susceptible site for crevice corrosion and thereby replaces one mechanism for rapid corrosion with another. Nevertheless, the image of an inert coating which grows spontaneously and which can repair itself immediately after it has sustained mechanical disruption provides considerable insight into the way in which current and future passive implant alloys might maintain their resistance to corrosion.

EFFECTS OF SUPPLEMENTARY ALLOYING ELEMENTS ON SUSCEPTIBILITY TO CORROSION

Past industrial experience has shown that the addition of small amounts of one or more elements to a metal to form an alloy may markedly alter the corrosion resistance of the base metal. On the one hand, alloying can be an effective means for improving corrosion resistance. For example, the addition of chromium to iron may stimulate passivity of iron when it would otherwise be active. Addition of a noble metal such as platinum or palladium may provide anodic protection of stainless steel, as described in the previous section. On the other hand, certain alloying elements such as carbon or nitrogen may diminish corrosion resistance. In view of the voluminous literature on this subject, the reader is referred elsewhere[43] for a detailed account. A brief description of the effects of alloying on corrosion resistance in implant alloys is given.

Stainless Steels

In 1822 Stodart and Faraday[44] published their results on the enhanced corrosion resistance of iron when additions of chromium were made. The maximum chromium content was below that required for passivity. It was not until 1911, however, that Monnartz[45] published a detailed account of the chemical properties of chromium-iron alloys, clearly describing the outstanding inertness of such alloys in which passivity was achieved with a minimum of 12% chromium. His work emphasized the need to maintain low carbon contents to maintain corrosion resistance; he also cited the beneficial effect of small quantities of alloying elements such as titanium, vanadium, molybdenum and tungsten. Subsequently Maurer and Krauss of the Krupp Steel Works revealed the corrosion resistance of the austenitic chromium-iron-nickel alloys which are used for surgical implants. Of the numerous types of stainless steel alloys described in Chapter 2, only this type has adequate inertness *in vivo*. The austenite or γ phase is a nonmagnetic alloy with a face-centered cubic structure, and is a malleable material. While γ phase is a stable structure in pure iron only between 910° and 1400°C, the additions of nickel, and to a lesser extent of manganese, cobalt, carbon and nitrogen, provide stability of the austenite when it is quenched to room temperature. Addition of molybdenum provides improved corrosion resistance in chloride-containing environments, especially in the presence of crevices. Such alloys can be cold-worked without significant change in corrosion resistance.

Intergranular Corrosion of Stainless Steels

Improper heat treatment of austenitic stainless steels stimulates intergranular attack on the alloys. The regions between adjacent crystals, the grain boundaries, show marked susceptibility to a corrosive process which produces a catastrophic reduction in mechanical strength. The specific temperatures and times that induce susceptibility to intergranular corrosion are called sensitizing heat treatments. For austenitic alloys, the sensitizing temperature range is 400°C to 900°C. The degree of damage sustained by commercial alloys by improper heat treatment depends upon the duration of exposure. A few minutes around the temperature of 750°C is equivalent to several hours at a lower or still higher temperature. Slow cooling through the sensitizing temperature range or prolonged welding operations induces susceptibility; rapid cooling avoids this susceptibility. For austenitic stainless steels, spot welding, in which the metal is rapidly heated by a momentary electric current followed by rapid cooling, does not cause sensitization. In contrast, arc welding may stimulate sensitization because the heating and cooling cycles are prolonged. Sensitizing temperatures may be attained at a distance of a few millimeters from the weld. On exposure to a corrosive environment, failure of the "weld" occurs slightly away from the weld itself. The extent of sensitization for a given temperature and time depends on carbon content. For example, an 18-8 stainless steel with 0.1% carbon may show severe sensitization after exposure at 600°C for 5 minutes. Alternatively, after similar exposure, such an alloy containing only 0.03% carbon may show no intergranular corrosion. With increased nickel content of the alloy, the time for sensitization to occur at a given temperature is decreased. The addition of molybdenum, however, increases the time for sensitization.

The mechanism of intergranular corrosion of austenitic stainless steels has been described by Uhlig.[46] At high temperatures (*e.g.,* 1050°C), carbon is uniformly dispersed throughout the alloy. Within the sensitizing temperature range, however, carbon diffuses to the grain boundaries where it combines preferentially with chromium to form carbides. The reaction depletes adjacent alloy of chromium so that the grain boundary may consist of material with less than the 12% chromium which is required for passivity. Subsequently the grain boundary may dissolve rapidly as anode while the grains constitute the cathodic areas. If the alloy is cooled rapidly through the sensitizing zone there is insufficient time for the diffusion-precipitation to occur. Alternatively, upon prolonged exposure to the sensitizing temperature, chromium diffuses into the previously depleted zones to re-establish passivity.

The addition of titanium or niobium in small amounts may reduce susceptibility to intergranular corrosion. These elements exhibit greater affinity for carbon than does chromium. Thus carbon is restrained from diffusion to grain boundaries. Furthermore, when carbon does reach the boundary, it reacts with titanium or niobium rather than with chromium.

Improvement of Corrosion Resistance of Stainless Steels by Surface Diffusion

There are several elements which, in small but significant concentration, provide marked improvements in the corrosion resistance of austenitic stainless steels. Larger concentrations of the elements in the bulk material would either reduce the stability of the γ-phase and cause loss of the good mechanical properties of the bulk metal, or would be prohibitively expensive. Hoar and Mears[6] developed a method for the improvement of corrosion resistance in stainless steel alloys by surface diffusion of molybdenum, niobium or tantalum. The air-formed film is removed from the steel with concentrated hydrochloric acid. The alloy is coated by vacuum evaporation with one of the three elements and the specimens are then heated in argon for 4 hours at 1000°C so that molybdenum, niobium or tantalum may diffuse into the surface layers of the stainless steel. Polarization measurements reveal that the diffusion process can produce improved corrosion resistance in two ways. First, the breakdown potential of a stainless steel alloy that is susceptible to chloride breakdown *in vivo* can be elevated to a value at which breakdown becomes most unlikely. Second, the rate of slow passive dissolution of the stainless steel can be decreased by up to 1000-fold. The process seems to warrant further clinical evaluation.

EFFECTS OF SURFACE FINISH ON THE DISSOLUTION OF METALS

The surface condition of an implant is a highly significant variable, because fairly simple methods of alteration may produce widely differing behavior in a material. In an earlier period when stainless steel alloys were scarcely adequate from the point of view of corrosion resistance, alteration of surface treatment might yield a material that exhibited satisfactory inertness *in vivo* or, alternatively, that showed grossly unsatisfactory performance. Hence, in an earlier work, Bechtol, Ferguson and Laing[37] emphasized stringent control of surface preparation for surgical implants. More recently this subject has been reviewed by other workers.[47, 48] For currently available alloys, including stainless steel of surgical grade, it seems that modification of this view is needed. The mechanical and chemical preparation of implant surfaces are discussed in turn.

Surface Preparation

If a metallic implant is formed on a lathe, drill, or router, its true surface area per unit area of specimen can be subsequently decreased by several orders of magnitude if it is treated with conventional techniques of mechanical and electrochemical polishing. Thus, its rate of passive dissolution *in vivo per unit area* of specimen is also diminished by several orders of magnitude. Where two metal components articulate on one

another, as in a McKee total hip joint, the rate of removal of metal by abrasion may be greatly decreased by previous application of polishing techniques. Where metal articulates against polymer, as in a Charnley total hip prosthesis, the rate of wear of the polymer may be lessened by polishing the metal surface. Apart from articulating surfaces, however, there is no evidence to show that increased surface roughness of implants provokes a clinically significant increase of corrosion rates of surgical implants. Many implants of cobalt-chromium alloys are deliberately manufactured with a roughened surface to provide improved adherence of adjacent tissues.

The question of general surface condition and scratching is also raised. Historically it has been strongly emphasized[37] that the surface of implants, especially those of stainless steel should be as smooth and undamaged as possible. There is no doubt that this caution should still apply for articular surfaces of total joint replacements. For planar surfaces, however, it needs clarification.

In the author's experience and in that of other workers, scratches on planar surfaces do not stimulate corrosion of stainless steel implants during the period of implantation. Also, Revie and Greene[47] argue that slight scratching of the implant surface subsequent to polishing but prior to service has little effect on corrosion resistance and that scratching after immersion produces only a transient decrease in the resistance. In oxygenated solution the steel may repassivate rapidly after scratching. Conceivably scratches produced on a implant by a surgical tool of dissimilar composition might cause metal transfer with subsequent galvanic corrosion. This hypothesis is discussed fully elsewhere.[50] To the author's knowledge, however, metallic transfer is not of any clinical significance as a mechanism for implant corrosion or tissue toxicity.

In conclusion, the author is in agreement with the view of Revie and Greene[47] that although the surface damage to implants should be minimized, elaborate and expensive techniques to eliminate scratching do not appear to be justified for general use. The sole exception to this view is the articular surface of total joint replacements in which special care is warranted. This situation will be described fully in Chapter 13.

Techniques for Passivation

Accelerated thickening of the oxide layer by treatment with an oxidizing agent has been recognized for many years as an effective method of improving corrosion resistance. The standard passivating medium has been nitric acid. Recently Revie and Greene[47] studied the corrosion resistance of type 316 stainless steel which had previously undergone one of several "prepassivation" treatments. Corrosion resistance was improved by immersion in either nitric acid (30% at 55°C for 30 minutes) or oxygenated isotonic saline (at 38.6°C for 150 hours), but the latter treatment was more effective. They recommended routine storage of all hospital supplies of metallic implants in oxygenated isotonic saline solution. These workers also studied the effects of sterilization on corrosion resistance.[49] Sterilization of stainless steel by either conventional steam (3 minutes at 132°C) or dry heat (2 hours at 160°C) reduced the rates of passive dissolution when the specimens were subsequently immersed in isotonic saline solution.

(In the author's experience, a widespread error in hospital sterilization technique is to fill the water receptacle in a sterilizer with isotonic saline, which is ubiquitous in hospitals for use in intravenous administration. Steam sterilization with isotonic saline provokes rapid corrosion of surgical implants, tools and sterilization equipment that are made of stainless steel alloys. Stringent safeguards are required to prevent this error.)

MECHANOCHEMICAL DETERIORATION OF METALS

In addition to the modes of deterioration, previously described metals may exhibit several deleterious phenomena which occur when mechanical abrasion, static stress or alternating stress act on a metal simultaneously exposed to a corrosive environment. Although the phenomena give rise to widely different forms of metal deterioration, they all occur by a combination of mechanical and chemical disruption of the passive oxide film on the metal.

Fretting Corrosion

When two pieces of iron are immersed in saline solution and rubbed together, they exhibit a process of rapid wear at the sliding surfaces. This process is accompanied by the formation of brownish iron oxide both as powder and as soluble dissolution product. With removal of the oxide film, further film formation follows, but the new film is neither mechanically strong nor chemically inert. If the two opposing surfaces of metal are rubbed again, the new oxide films are rapidly removed by the same mechanism. The process does not occur if the metal surfaces are rubbed together under good lubricating conditions; nor does it occur when the two pieces of metal rub together in an inert atmosphere. It is necessary to have the mechanical and chemical effect present together. This process is called fretting corrosion. Of the alloys in current use, both the stainless steel and cobalt-chromium alloys are subject to fretting corrosion, especially between screw heads and bone plates. At present, this mode of corrosion is the one most frequently encountered in clinical practice. It is rarely of clinical significance, however, as neither failure of implants nor deleterious tissue response have been related to it. Titanium and tantalum alloys may also exhibit abrasive wear at rubbing surfaces; the rate of wear, however, is not increased by immersion of the moving surfaces in body fluids. The phenomenon is strictly a mechanical one.

Metallic Transfer

Twenty years ago Bowden et al.[50] reported their observations on a similar form of deterioration which they called "metallic transfer." By the application of autoradiography to surgical tools and implants, they were able to show that insertion of a screw or bolt with a screwdriver or wrench was accompanied by the transfer of discrete particles of metal from the soft alloy to the harder one (Fig. 4-15).

Observation of metallic surfaces using the electron microscope reveals that even highly polished surfaces show an exceptionally rough terrain with many asperities and depressions. When two polished surfaces are brought into contact, the total area of contact occurs at opposing asperities which may represent less than 1/10,000 part of the total area. Inevitably the force per unit of true contact area is so immense that the opposing surfaces undergo cold-welding. If one surface slides across the other, separation occurs by fracture at the bases of peaks rather than at the welds themselves. The welding process stimulates work hardening of metal adjacent to the weld (Fig. 4-16). When the transferred metal accumulates on the surgical implant, it is subject to dissolution in vivo. If the alloys are dissimilar, a galvanic couple is created. By the Prussian blue reaction, the presence of dissolution products containing iron has been confirmed. Bowden et al.[50] hypothesized that the galvanic current generated at the site of dissimilar metals could interfere with the healing of tissue by a process of "electrolytic inflamma-

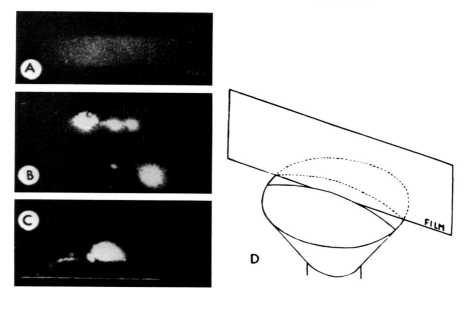

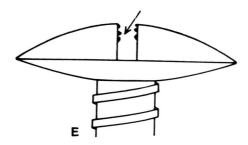

Figure 4-15. Autoradiograph and schematic diagram to show metallic transfer between a screwdriver and a screw head.

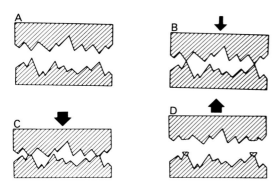

Figure 4-16. Schematic diagram to show the mechanism of metallic transfer between two metal objects.

tion." Hence, these workers concluded that implants should not be handled with tools of dissimilar composition. Subsequent investigations have failed to confirm that metallic transfer is of clinical significance as a deleterious side-effect of dissimilarity in composition between surgical tools and implants. There are several explanations for such a benign nature of metallic transfer. Usually the tips of surgical tools are made of a material, such as tungsten carbide or a high carbon steel, which is much harder than the implant alloy. Hence, transfer from the implant to the tool is the predominant process without creation of a bimetallic *implant.* Secondly, the process occurs on such a microscopic scale that the magnitude of galvanic current, created thereby is minute. Thirdly, even if an increased corrosion current is significantly larger than the corrosion current attributable to passive dissolution of the implant, within the scope of presently available knowledge of the effects of corrosion currents on healing tissues, there are as many observations to suggest that such current may *stimulate* healing as to suggest that the current may *impede* healing. It is the author's impression that "metallic transfer" is not significant and that the composition of surgical tools should be based on appropriate mechanical properties and adequate inertness.

Stress-Corrosion Cracking

When certain alloys are immersed in a corrosive environment and subjected to tensile or torsional stress, they undergo formation of minute cracks which may spread rapidly across the specimen to provoke mechanical failure. The cracks may spread between adjacent grains of metal (intergranular), as in the case of stressed brass exposed to ammoniacal liquors; alternatively, they can occur across adjacent grains (transgranular), as in the case of chromium-nickel stainless steels exposed to chloride solutions. The mechanism of stress corrosion cracking has received much attention. On a susceptible stainless steel, the process appears to begin at the site of a superficial crack or pit in the oxide surface. The base of the pit becomes an anode and the outside surface of the metal becomes a cathode (Fig. 4-17), so that a cell is established which stimulates dissolution of the base of the pit. If the metal is subjected to continuous tensile stress, the force is concentrated at the base of the pit in a direction that is approximately perpendicular to the total tensile stress. The metal in the fissure undergoes rapid yielding, so that metal atoms move parallel

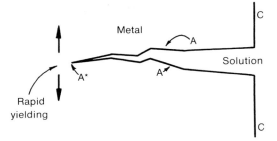

Figure 4-17. Schematic diagram of a stress corrosion crack in austenitic stainless steel. C, cathode ($^1/_2O_2$ + H_2O + 2e → 2OH$^-$); A, anode of static metal, current density ~10^{-5} A/cm^2; A^*, anode of yielding metal, current density ≥0.5 A/cm^2.

to the direction of the tensile stress. Such yielding metal may be far more chemically active than nonyielding metal. Its superficial oxide film is also mechanically disrupted by the tensile strain; thus the metal at the base of the fissure dissolves rapidly. Under experimental conditions, such a crack may propagate at rates of 0.5 to 3.0 mm/hr.[51] Susceptible alloys may be protected by cathodic protection, by altered surface preparation or specimen shape, or by change in the chemical composition. With such a variety of preventive measures available, stress corrosion cracking is rarely observed as a mode of failure in surgical implants.[52] Nevertheless, in view of its capacity to provoke rapid mechanochemical failure of implants, stress corrosion cracking merits consideration by all those who design or use surgical implants.

Corrosion Fatigue

As previously described, the process of ordinary fatigue, in which a metal undergoes disruption by cracking after subjection to many alternating cycles of stress, is not well understood. Nevertheless, it is clear that in a corrosive environment, fatigue failure of metals may occur more quickly than it does when the fatigue occurs in dry air. It is generally believed that in the corrosive environment the first effect is purely a corrosive or electrochemical one, with the production of a small pit or crack. Subsequently this site of concentration of stress provokes mechanical cracking followed by a mechanochemical process similar to the one described for stress-corrosion cracking. The detailed mechanism at the atomic scale remains obscure. Again, by careful design of surgical implants[53] to eliminate sites of concentration of stress and irregularities on the surface, corrosion fatigue can be prevented.

BACTERIAL CORROSION OF METALS

While the rapid corrosion of unprotected steel or aluminum in certain anaerobic soils has long vexed the corrosion engineer, similar examples of bacterial corrosion of surgical implants have not been reported. Nevertheless, the possibility remains that a wound infection around an orthopaedic implant might provoke more rapid dissolution of the implant. Alternatively, the presence of slowly dissolving metal and bacteria together might stimulate the formation of metabolites that would impede wound healing, thereby explaining the mystery that metal-containing orthopaedic wound infections rarely heal prior to metal removal.

In 1934 Von Wolzogen Vuhr[54] proposed the role of the sulfate reducing bacteria as depolarizing agents. For example, when iron dissolves in deaerated soil, the anode reaction can be expressed as:

$$Fe \rightarrow Fe^{2+} + 2 \text{ electrons}$$

and the cathodic reaction as:

$$2H^+ + 2 \text{ electrons} \rightarrow \uparrow H_2$$

Molecular hydrogen accumulates as gas around the cathode to inhibit the cathodic process and thereby to impede the corrosion rate. This process is called polarization. Utilization of the hydrogen by sulfate-reducing bacteria such as *Desulfovibrio desulfuricans* or *Desulfovibrio vulgaris* provides depolarization of the cathode with acceleration of the corrosion process to its uninhibited rate. Recently other explanations of this phenomenon have been suggested by Booth *et al.*[55] In practice, the bacteria may increase rates of corrosion by several phenomena[56]:

1. The production of corrosive metabolites.
2. The production of differential aeration and other concentration cells.
3. The depolarization of cathodic processes.
4. The disruption of protective layers or films.
5. The breakdown of corrosion inhibitors.

While the first four phenomena could occur *in vivo*, none have been observed. Furthermore, the types of bacteria which are of industrial concern are strict anerobes which cannot grow in the presence of oxygen. Hence they are not usually found in wound infections. Nevertheless, in view of the complication of total joint replacement surgery and of techniques for internal fixation of fractures, in which a wound infection cannot be permanently eradicated prior to metal removal, further research on the effects of bacteria on the healing of metal-containing wounds is strongly recommended.

DISSOLUTION OF NONMETALLIC IMPLANT MATERIALS

Introduction

With the proliferation of synthetic organic and inorganic materials over the past two decades, considerable research has been undertaken on the inertness of these materials. The studies of nonmetallic materials have been far more difficult than comparable ones involving metals for several reasons:

1. The results of weight change studies may be difficult to interpret because of the adsorption of water which occurs when many synthetic organic materials are immersed in aqueous solution.

2. Electrochemical tests cannot be used because the materials do not undergo electrochemical dissolution.

3. Many of the materials, particularly the polymers, are complex compounds. During their manufacture there may be incomplete reaction of their constituents so that implantation *in vivo* may lead to diffusion of the residual reactants to give much faster rates of solubilization than would occur for the fully formed compound. Furthermore many plastics contain numerous additives[57] such as catalysts, plasticizers, pigments, stabilizers, fillers and stripping agents. The additives may excite far more tissue reaction than the polymer itself even though they diffuse into extracellular fluid in minute quantities.

4. No satisfactory accelerated tests for the estimation of the rates of dissolution have been developed for nonmetallic implant materials. Hence the selection process for suitable nonmetallic materials has rested heavily on industrial experience. Laboratory tests have not accurately simulated the human environment, and therefore, biological tests of tissue reactions have been extensively used. Currently, as a general guide for the selection of untried polymers that may show favorable inertness *in vivo*, the three factors described by Atlas and Mark[58] appear to be the most useful aids: (1) the types of chemical bonds present; (2) steric hinderance and electronegativity effects produced by atoms in close proximity with these chemical bonds (*e.g.,* Cl^- or $-NH_2$ moieties provide increased inertness); and (3) supermolecular structure (*e.g.,* a crys-

talline structure is generally more inert than an amorphous one). Recently Homsy[59] has recommended a series of *in vitro* tests for screening untried polymers prior to costly evaluation by implantation in animals. The first assessment consists of the measurement of tensile, flexural and compressive strength before and after exposure to simulated body fluids. Next infrared spectrophotometric assay of migratable species is performed in simulated body fluids. The measurement is analogous to assessment of the concentration of metallic dissolution products in body fluids around metal implants. The low molecular weight mobile moieties represent degradation products of either polymeric chains, or stabilizing additives or plasticizers. Finally, tissue culture studies are performed with the polymers. The observations on cytotoxicity are compared with those obtained by infrared spectrophotometry. Homsy[59] suggests that such a comparison permits the estimation of the rate of degradation of polymers as well as an evaluation of the cytotoxicity of the polymeric dissolution products. This protocol represents one of the first concrete attempts to quantify the dissolution of polymers in a way similar to that presently available for metals. Nevertheless, there is a dearth of quantitative data on the rates of dissolution for nonmetallic materials exposed to body fluids. Under static conditions, a variety of polymers such as high density polyethylene (HDPE)[60] methylmethacrylate cement,[61] polypropylene,[62] silicone elastomers,[63] and ceramics[64] such as alumina and vitreous carbon[61] appear to show negligible rates of dissolution.

The relative inertness of these materials when exposed to dilute saline solutions of neutral pH is in marked contrast to their liability to deterioration in other environments. For example, most polymers are susceptible to the influence of heat, light, oxygen, ozone and ionizing radiation and to chemical solvents, all of which may provoke degradation by random chain, fission, depolymerization, cross-linking, bond changes and side group changes. As these phenomena have not been observed *in vivo*, they are not discussed here. The reader is referred to Chapter 8, where the effects of sterilizing agents on materials are reviewed. One exception to the general inertness of polymers to aqueous solution was the early experience with a thermoplastic, nylon. In the human environment with weight-bearing stress and wear, it showed rapid degradation, with loss of tensile strength and ultimately disintegration. The deterioration was accompanied by an intolerable tissue reaction. The nylon rapidly absorbed water and subsequently underwent hydrolysis. O'Brien[65] has since shown that the rate and depth of water penetration into polymers can be monitored by measurement of polymeric capacitance. The test represents one of the few laboratory techniques available for prediction of rates of degradation of polymers *in vivo*.

Mechanochemical Deterioration of Nonmetals

For several decades workers have reported premature mechanical failure in a variety of nonmetallic materials which occurred under the combined influence of mechanical stress and chemical effects. To the present, the underlying mechanisms of these modes of failure remain obscure.

One of the earliest forms of mechanochemical failure of polymers to be observed *in vivo* was stress-solvent crazing of acrylic Judet hip prostheses.[66]

The work of Charnley[67] stimulated great interest in the wear of polymers when exposed concurrently to abrasion and corrosive environment. During his early work on the artificial hip joint, he chose to study polytetrafluoroethylene (PTFE) as a material for the socket, because of its low frictional resistance and its reputation for chemical inertness. The standard implant alloy of stainless steel was selected for the femoral head component. A 7-year study of the wear resistance of PTFE under laboratory conditions revealed negligible wear in the plastic; hence, excellent wear resistance *in vivo* was predicted. When the measurements were repeated *in vivo* for a PTFE socket against a 22-mm diameter femoral head prosthesis, the rate of wear of PTFE was between 0.2 and 0.3 mm per *month*. No satisfactory explanation is available to account for the vast discrepancy between the results obtained in the laboratory and in clinical implantation. The wear of the plastic socket occurred as the steel ball bored into the substance of the plastic to create a cylindrical pathway of the same diameter as the steel head. The estimate of wear represents the rate of migration of the steel head into the plastic. Subsequent clinical measurements of wear in HDPE sockets with a 22.5-mm steel ball have shown variable rates of wear with typical values of 0.1 to 0.2 mm per year. These values confirm adequate longevity of the socket and insignificant pathological responses to particulate HDPE. Nevertheless all of the studies of the wear resistance of plastic against metal total hip replacements confirm that, in the human environment, currently available plastics undergo mechanochemical deterioration which is akin to fretting corrosion in metals. No satisfactory laboratory tests have been developed to provide accurate estimates of such wear *in vivo*.[68] Neither does present knowledge of the structure of polymers allow prediction of the liability of a particular material to undergo mechanochemical failure *in vivo*.

While chloride anion is the aggressive agent for passive metals, plasma proteins stimulate fatigue failure of ceramics by mechanisms which are quite unclear.[69]

The question of mechanochemical failure of silicone elastomers has been raised. Swanson[70] has subjected his finger joint spacers to flexion tests in the laboratory, where they withstand millions of flexions under simulated load without mechanical failure. Both he and other workers[71] have observed fractures of the implants after a short lifetime *in vivo* of a few thousand flexions. Swanson[70] attributes the mechanical failure to propagation of a crack from a surface imperfection since silicone rubber has poor resistance to crack propagation. Alternatively, Pierie *et al.*[72] suggest that the fractures *in vivo* represent another example of mechanochemical failure of materials. In their study on the fracture of flexible implants made of silicone rubber, these workers observed accelerated fatigue failure of implants when the joint fluid contained elevated concentration of lipid. In a recent study, however, Swanson *et al.*[73] failed to observe any relationship between fatigue failure of silastic hinges and lipid concentration in synovial fluid. There are reports in the literature[74, 75] of mechanical changes and occasional failure of silicone heart valves. After removal of these implants from patients, the silicone rubber has shown increased concentration of lipid. Hence the liability of silicone implants *in vivo* to undergo premature mechanochemical failure initiated by absorption of lipids remains unclear. In the author's experience fracture of silicone flexible joints is uncommon.

Microbial Deterioration of Plastics

While degradation of organic substances by micro-organisms has been widely observed in such industries as those related to wood, leather or wool, no similar examples of biodeterioration in nonmetallic surgical implants have been reported. Nevertheless, in view of the possibility and undesirability of this mode of potential failure of implants, it is mentioned briefly. Perhaps the most relevant example involves plasticized polyvinylchloride. While the vinyl chloride polymers are resistant to microbial attack, certain additives, notably such plasticizers as polypropylene sebacate, are vulnerable to attack by *Pseudomonas aeruginose* and *Serratia marcescens*.[76] In the main, low molecular weight polymers, such as various plasticizers or other additives, are far more susceptible to bacterial degradation than high molecular weight polymers. Similarly, high molecular weight alkanes, such as commercial waxes, are resistant to biodeterioration,[77] while low molecular weight alkanes, such as methane and propane, are susceptible to bacterial metabolism. Future clinical and laboratory studies must bear in mind the possibility of increased rates of dissolution of polymeric implants when wound infection intervenes. The possibility also exists that such polymeric dissolution products might impede the effectiveness of antimicrobial agents or the innate defense mechanisms of the body.

SUMMARY

In this chapter the mechanisms for the deterioration of materials are described. The distinction is emphasized between the liability of a material to change from a slow to a rapid rate of dissolution and the actual assessment of the rate of dissolution. Current methods for the assessment of deterioration in metals and nonmetals are reviewed. The results of such tests on currently available and several potentially superior alloys are given. Assessment of corrosion performance confirms that presently available alloys have adequate corrosion resistance, although the resistance of titanium alloys is markedly superior to that of surgical grade stainless steels. The modes of mechanochemical dissolution of alloys are discussed. Crevice corrosion remains the principal form of corrosion observed in surgical implants, although there is no evidence to confirm that it is a clinically significant problem. Stress corrosion cracking and corrosion fatigue can be prevented by appropriate selection of materials, design of implants and technique of implantation. Mechanisms of bacterial deterioration of metals and nonmetals are described as possible but unlikely causes of degradation in materials. The effects of surface preparation and of alloying elements on rates of dissolution in implant alloys are reviewed. It is concluded that the articular surfaces of total joint replacements are the only surfaces of orthopaedic implants where exceptional care is necessary to provide blemish-free surfaces.

The use of dissimilar alloys in surgery is reviewed. The author concludes that alloys can be classified into several types which can be used safely in combination *in vivo* to great advantage, since each material is selected for its peculiar mechanical attributes. In addition, the classification permits selection of alloys that can be used in juxtaposition with nonmetallic materials without significant liability to crevice corrosion.

REFERENCES

1. Emneus, H. *Acta Ortho. Scand., Suppl. 44a*:1, 1960.
2. Evans, U. R., Bannister, L. C., and Britton, S. C. *Proc. Roy. Soc., 137-A*:343, 1932.
3. Evans, U. R., and Hoar, T. P. *Proc. Roy. Soc., 137-A*:355, 1932.
4. Hoar, T. P. *J. Appl. Chem., 11*:121, 1961.
5. Hoar, T. P., Mears, D. C., and Rothwell, G. P. *Corros. Sci., 5*:279, 1965.
6. Hoar, T. P., and Mears, D. C. *Proc. Roy. Soc., 294-A*:486, 1966.
7. Pourbaix, M. *Thermodynamics of Dilute Aqueous Solutions,* Edward Arnold, London, 1949.
8. Collins, D. H. *J. Path. and Bact., 65*:109, 1953.
9. Emneus, H., Stenram, U., and Baecklund, J. *Acta Ortho. Scand., 30*:226, 1960.
10. Ferguson, A. B., Jr., Laing, P. G., and Hodge, E. S. *J. Bone and Jt. Surg., 42-A*:77, 1960.
11. Mears, D. C. *J. Bone and Jt. Surg., 48-B*:567, 1966.
12. Clarke, E. G. C., and Hickman, J. *J. Bone and Jt. Surg., 35-B*:467, 1953.
13. Edeleanu, C. *J. Iron Steel Inst., 185*:482, 1957.
14. Hoar, T. P. The anodic behavior of metals. In *Modern Aspects of Electrochemistry,* vol 2, p. 262, edited by J. O'M Bockris, Butterworths, London, 1959.
15. Young, L. *Anodic Oxide Films,* p. 227, Academic Press, London, 1961.
16. Jones, D. A., and Greene, N. D. *Corros., 22*:198, 1966.
17. Colangelo, V. J., Greene, N. D., Kettelkamp, D. B., Alexander, H., and Campbell, C. J. *J. Biomed. Mat. Res., 5*:139, 1967.
18. Prázak, M., and Barton, K. *Corros. Sci., 7*:159, 1967.
19. Stern, M., and Geary, A. L. *J. Electrochem. Soc., 104*:56, 1957.
20. Hoar, T. P. *Corros. Sci., 7*:455, 1967.
21. Hoar, T. P., and Yahalom, J. *J. Electrochem. Soc., 110*:610, 1963.
22. Galvani, L. *De Viribus electricitatis,* Modena, 1792. Translated by M. G. Foley, *Commentary on the Effects of Electricity on Muscular Motion,* Norwalk, Conn., 1953.
23. Volta, A. *Phil. Trans. Roy. Soc., 90*:39, 1800.
24. Davy, H. *Phil. Trans. Roy. Soc., 114*:151, 1824.
25. Faraday, M. *Experimental Researches in Electricity,* originally published in three volumes (1833–1835). Later the collected works were published as one volume, *Everyman's Edition,* p. 322, J. M. Dent and Sons Ltd., London, 1914.
26. Lambotte, A. *Presse med. Belge, 17*:321, 1909.
27. Von Baeyer, H. *München med. Wchnschr., 56*:2416, 1909.
28. Mears, D. C. *J. Biomed. Mat. Res., 6*:133, 1975.
29. Bauer, O., and Vogel, O. *Mitt. Mat. Prüf. Amt. Berl., 36*:114, 1918.
30. Latimer, W. M. *Oxidation States of the Elements and Their Potentials in Aqueous Solutions,* Prentice-Hall, Englewood Cliffs, N.J., 1952.
31. Edeleanu, C. E. *Metall. Manchester, 50*:113, 1954.
32. Mears, R. B., and Brown, R. H. *Indust. Eng. Chem., 33*:1001, 1941.
33. Frankenthal, R. P., and Pickering, H. W. *J. Electrochem. Soc., 112*:514, 1965.
34. Edeleanu, C. E., and Gibson, J. G. *Chem. Indust., 11*:301, 1961.
35. Streicher, M. A. *Corros., 30*:77, 1974.
36. Sawyer, P. N., and Srinivasan, S. *J. Biomed. Mater. Res., 1*:83, 1967.
37. Bechtol, C. O., Ferguson, A. B., Jr., and Laing, P. G. *Metals and Engineering in Bone and Joint Surgery,* p. 1, Williams & Wilkins Co., Baltimore, 1959.
38. Scales, J. T., Winter, G., and Shirley, H. T. *J. Bone and Jt. Surg., 41-B*:810, 1959.
39. Cohen, J., and Wulff, J. *J. Bone and Jt. Surg., 54-A*:617, 1972.
40. Semlitsch, M. *Eng. in Med., 2*:68, 1973.
41. Russin, L. A. *The Sivash Total Hip Prosthesis,* p. 3, U. S. Surgical Corp., New York, 1974. (See also Sivash, K. M. *Alloplasty of the Hip Joint,* p. 1, Medical Press, Moscow, 1967).
42. DeVita, V. T., Serpick, A. A., and Carbone, P. P. *Ann. Int. Med., 73*:881, 1970.
43. Evans, U. R. *The Corrosion and Oxidation of Metals,* Edward Arnold, London, 1961.
44. Stodart, J., and Faraday, M. *Philosoph. Trans. Roy. Soc., 112*:253, 1822.
45. Monnartz, P. *Metallurgie, 8*:161, 1911.
46. Uhlig, H. H. *Trans. Electrochem. Soc., 87*:193, 1945.
47. Revie, R. W., and Greene, N. D. *Corros. Sci., 9*:763, 1969.
48. Williams, D. F., and Roaf, F. *Implants in Surgery,* p. 164, W. B. Saunders Co. Ltd., London, 1973.
49. Revie, R. W. and Greene, N. D. *Corros. Sci., 9*:755, 1969.
50. Bowden, F. P., Williamson, J. B. P., and Laing, P. G. *Nature, 173*:520, 1954.
51. Scully, J. C. *Br. Corros. J., 1*:355, 1966.
52. Brettle, J. *Stress Corrosion Cracking of Surgical Implant Materials.* Atomic Weapons Research Establishment (Aldermaston) Report GR/44/83/73, 1971.
53. Gilbert, P. T. *Metal. Rev., 1*:379, 1956.
54. Von Wolzogen Kühr, C. A. H. and Vander Vlugst, L. S. *Water, 16*:147, 1934.
55. Booth, G. H., Elford, L., and Wakerley, D. S. *Br. Corros. J., 3*:242, 1968.
56. Menzies, I. A. *Introductory Corrosion in Microbial Aspects of Metallurgy,* edited by J. D. A. Miller, Aylesbury, Medical and Technical Publishing Co., 1970.
57. Scales, J. T. *Proc. Roy. Soc. Med., 46*:647, 1953.
58. Atlas, S. M., and Mark, H. M. Resistance of polymers to degradation. In *Plastics in Surgical Implants,* ASTM Pub. No. 386, Symposium, Indianapolis, Ind., 1964.
59. Homsy, C. A. *J. Biomed. Mater. Res., 4*:341, 1970.
60. Bloch, B., and Hastings, G. W. *Plastic Materials in Surgery,* Ed. 2, Charles C Thomas, Springfield, Ill., 1972.

61. Charnley, J. *Acrylic Cement in Orthopaedic Surgery,* E. & S. Livingstone, Edinburgh, 1970.
62. Schubert, R. J., and Cupples, A. L. Selection, characterization and biodegradation of surgical epoxies. In *Biomedical Polymers,* p. 87, edited by A. Rembaum and M. Shen, Marcel Dekker, Inc., New York, 1971.
63. Bradley, S. The chemistry and properties of the medical grade silicones. In *Biomedical Polymers,* p. 35, edited by A. Rembaum and M. Shen, Marcel Dekker, Inc., New York, 1971.
64. Klawitter, J. J., and Bhatti, N. A. *J. Biomed. Mater. Res., 8:*137, 1974.
65. O'Brien, H. C. *Indust. and Eng. Chem., 58:*45, 1966.
66. Scales, J. T., and Zarek, J. M. *Br. Med. J., 1:*1001, 1954.
67. Charnley, J. Lancet, *1:*1129, 1961.
68. Amstutz, H. C. *J. Biomed. Mater. Res., 3:*547, 1968.
69. Griss, P., Heimke, G., and von Andrian-Werburg, H. *J. Biomed. Mater. Res. 8:*956, 1974.
70. Swanson, A. B. *J. Bone Jt. Surg., 54-A:*435, 1972.

71. Weightman, B., Simon, S., Rose, R., Paul, I., and Radin, E. *J. Biomed. Mater. Res. Symp., 5:*267, 1972.
72. Pierie, W. R., Hancock, W. D., Koorigian, S., and Starr, A. *Ann. N. Y. Acad. Sci., 146:*345, 1968.
73. Swanson, A. B., Meester, W. D., Swanson, G. de G., Rangaswamy, L., and Schut, G. E. D. *Ortho. Clin. N. Am., 4:*1097, 1973.
74. Carmen, R., and Mutha, S. C. *J. Biomed. Mater. Res., 6:*327, 1972.
75. Chin, H. P., Harrison, E. C., Blankenhorn, D. H., and Moacanin, J. Circ., *43:* (Suppl.) 51, 1971.
76. Plankhorst, E. S. and Davies, J. J. Investigations into the effects of microorganisms on PVC pressure-sensitive tape and its constituents. In *Biodeterioration of Materials,* p. 302, edited by A. H. Walter and J. J. Elphick, Elsevier, Amsterdam, 1968.
77. Traxler, R. W., and Flannery, W. C. Mechanism of hydrocarbon degradation. In *Bio-deterioration of Materials,* p. 44, edited by A. H. Walters and J. J. Elphick, Elsevier, Amsterdam, 1968.

5

The Tissues of the Musculoskeletal System

Just as the carpenter, electrician or plumber must understand the structural framework, electrical circuitry or network of pipes which he would repair or replace, so the bioengineer or surgeon must comprehend the nature of the tissues which he would reconstruct. Hyaline cartilage lines the articular surfaces of the joints. These are the hard tissues which implantable materials may replace. Other essential tissues of the musculoskeletal system include the ligaments, tendons and muscles and the supportive capsule and synovial lining membrane of articular joints. There follows a brief account of the nature of musculoskeletal tissues. Their capacity to undergo regeneration is also described, since the ability of surgeons to reconstruct the various tissues is totally dependent upon the innate capacity of each tissue to undergo spontaneous repair or regeneration. Finally, the degeneration of joints is discussed relevant to the reconstruction of articular joints by the application of surgical implant techniques.

MUSCLE

The skeletal or voluntary muscles are called striated muscles because, under the microscope, they are seen to consist of long, thread-like fibers with regularly placed parallel transverse bands (Fig. 5-1).[4] A muscle fiber is the smallest independent muscle unit, 0.01 to 0.1 mm in diameter and 1 mm to 30 cm in length (*i.e.,* it traverses the entire length of a muscle). These cylindrical structures are close-packed and do not show divisions or anastomoses. Each muscle fiber consists of a multinucleate cell enclosed in a sarcolemmal membrane.[5] Within the cytoplasmic matrix, or sarcoplasm, long filamentous myofibrillae are evenly distributed and impart a regular cross-striation. The cross-striations represent alternating birefringent and monorefringent segments of two filamentous proteins, actin and myosin, which are evenly spaced at intervals of

approximately 3.0 μm in the resting fiber. With contraction, the cross-striations become narrower or crowded together. The relative amounts of sarcoplasm and myofibrillae vary in individual fibers.

Most muscles are attached to bone through the intervention of a tendon or aponeurosis of highly variable length. The capillaries of striated muscle are profuse and form a rectangular network, with branches which run longitudinally in the endomysium between the muscle fibers and are joined at short intervals by transverse anastomosing branches. The larger vessels are found only in the perimysium between the muscle fasciculi.[6] Nerves with highly specialized terminations are profusely distributed to striated muscle.

A single motor neuraxon branches at its terminus and sends a twig to each of the 5 to 200 myofibers in its group. Each twig forms a single specialized junction with a muscle fiber, the motor end plate (Fig. 5-2). The end plates are concentrated in the middle of a muscle so that excitation progresses towards both ends. The axonal terminal attaches to a synaptic trough in the sarcolemma of the motor end plate. A gap 500 to 100 Å wide separates the two plasma membranes. This synaptic gap is sufficient to prevent transmission of the signal from nerve to muscle except when a switching mechanism is activated. Within the axonal terminal are large numbers of vesicles which contain the neurotransmitter acetylcholine.[7] When the axonal terminal is depolarized, acetylcholine is discharged from the presynaptic vesicles into the synaptic gap. This mechanism requires ionic calcium. Acetylcholine is a cation and depolarizes the postsynaptic surface to initiate muscle excitation. On the postsynaptic surfaces, the enzyme cholinesterase is concentrated. It hydrolyzes the acetylcholine to terminate excitation.

For measurement of the amount of strain in

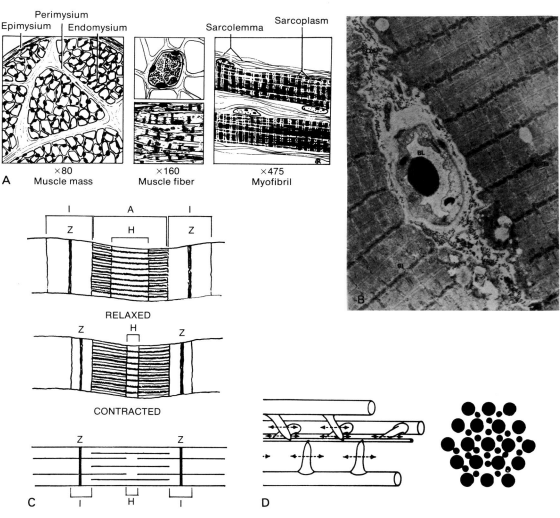

Figure 5-1. Schematic views and electron micrographs of the gross and fine structure of normal human muscle. *A.* A schematic view of muscle, of a fiber and of a myofibril. The various subunits of a muscle fiber by the epi-, peri- and endomysium with their sarcolemmal sheaths and nuclei and the sarcoplasm between the cross-striations are seen. *B.* An electron micrograph of normal muscle to show the banding, the cross-striations and mitochondria along an *I* band. *C.* A schematic view to reveal the basis for the striated appearance of muscle. According to the model of A. F. Huxley, two interdigitating sets of filaments, thick myosin filaments confined to the *A*-zone and thin actin filaments are present in the *I*-band. The latter extend into the *A*-zone as far as the *H*-band. Muscle contraction occurs with reaction between transverse bridges on actin and myosin molecules such that myosin filaments slide into the *I*-bands. In the middle figure the myofibril is contracted, with the *A*-band, which contains the myosin filament remaining constant. The *lower figure* illustrates how the actin slides between the myosin. The distance between the two *H*-zones remains constant but the widths of *I*-bands and *H*-zones varies from contraction to relaxation. *D.* A transverse section of the thicker myosin and the actin (*right*) with cross-bridging between these two protein structures. (*A,* reproduced with permission from R. B. Duthie and A. B. Ferguson, Jr.[1]; *B,* reproduced with permission from K. Hirohata and K. Morimoto[2]; *C* and *D* drawn from data of H. E. Huxley.[3])

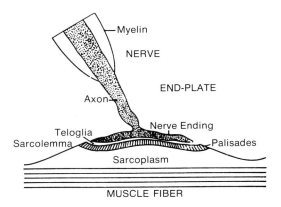

Figure 5-2. Schematic diagram of the neuromuscular junction or end plate termination of the axis cylinder. (Reproduced with permission from R. B. Duthie and A. B. Ferguson, Jr.[1])

Figure 5-3. Schematic diagram of a muscle spindle and a tendon organ. The muscle spindle, shown on the right, is attached to extrafusal muscle fibers and tendon. It consists of small diameter intrafusal muscle fibers which are largely enclosed in a connective tissue capsule. The length of the spindle approximates 50 times its width. The extrafusal muscle fibers are about 40 μm in diameter while the intrafusal fibers are of two types. Some of about 20 μm in diameter possess long fibers with spindle-shaped nuclear bags at the equator, and others of 10 μm in diameter possess short fibers with cylindrical nuclear chains at the equator. Of the group of nerve fibers, the largest fiber, marked *IA*, supplies the main primary afferent ending overlying the nuclear bags and chains. Fiber *II* goes to a secondary afferent ending on the nuclear chain fibers adjacent to the primary ending. Six small γ motor fibers of varying sizes supply motor ending on the intrafusal muscle fibers. The motor end plates on the extrafusal muscle fibers are supplied by a larger α nerve fiber. The remaining *IB* nerve fibers supply the encapsulated tendon organ on the left. Between the tendons of a group of intrafusal muscle fibers are observed branches of the afferent nerve ending. (Reproduced with permission from G. H. Bell, J. N. Davidson, and H. Scarborough.[8])

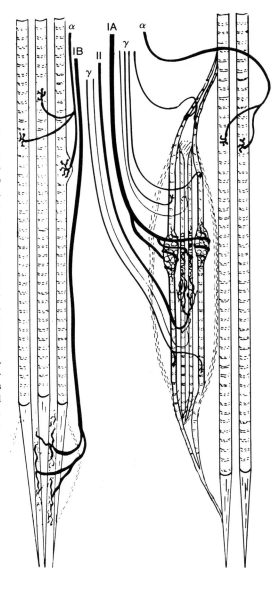

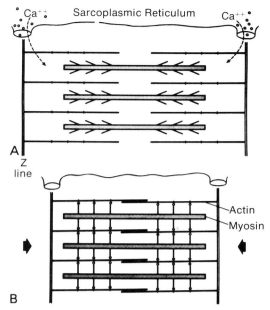

Figure 5-4. *A*. Schematic diagram of the contraction of the sarcomere and muscle fiber reveals the mediation of the reaction by calcium ions released from the sarcoplasmic reticulum. *B*. Filaments of actin slide along myosin biochemical linkage between the two molecules. (Reproduced with permission from L. Sokoloff and J. H. Bland.[10])

muscle fibers, unique encapsulated sensory organs, the muscle spindles (Fig. 5-3), are present and account for about ¹⁄₁₀ of the nerve fibers in muscle.[9] These fluid-filled capsules are 2 to 5 mm in length and contain 2 to 12 longitudinal modified muscle fibers, the intrafusal fibers. Afferent nerve endings encircle the equatorial portion of the intrafusal fibers and are stimulated when the latter are stretched. The frequency of the discharge is proportional to the velocity and the magnitude of the stretch. The afferent nerves communicate with α and γ motoneurons through interneurons in the spinal cord. The latter are small neurons that supply efferent fibers to the intrafusal fibers. A closed-loop servosystem is thereby formed which serves to maintain normal reflex control of synergistic and antagonistic muscle groups in postural and phasic activities. Similar stretch receptors are located in tendons.

Contraction of muscle is accomplished by a chemical linkage of the actin and myosin filaments at numerous minute cross-bridges (Figs. 5-1*D* and 5-4). The filaments are oriented longitudinally and partly overlap within the sarcomere. The actin filaments are attached to a noncontractile disc, the *Z-line*, which is composed of the protein tropomyosin. Contraction

represents sliding of the actin over the myosin filaments with the temporary formation of actomyosin, although the nature of the mechanochemical linkage remains unknown.

Muscle cells also possess a series of transverse tubular invaginations of the plasma membrane, the T-system, which carry electrical charges from the surface of the cells to the myofibrils in the interior. Also within the cells, calcium ion is stored by the sarcoplasmic reticulum, which is analogous to the endoplasmic reticulum of other cells. The action potential provokes release of calcium from the sarcoplasmic reticulum. The union between actin and myosin is mediated by calcium ion, which makes chelate bonds between adenosine diphosphate (ADP) and adenosine triphosphate (ATP) moieties that are attached to myosin and actin. After contraction occurs, the calcium ion is rapidly reaccumulated in the sarcoplasmic reticulum. The rapid coupling of excitation and contraction is made possible by the spatial proximity to the Z-line of the T-system of the sarcoplasmic reticulum.

The mechanical efficiency of muscle, or the proportion of energy actually converted into work against a load, is about 15%. This figure is comparable to that of moderately efficient manmade machines such as some steam turbines. The remainder of the energy appears as heat generated primarily during the process of contraction. The immediate source of energy for muscle is the hydrolysis of ATP to ADP. The energy is ultimately derived from food-stuffs which are converted into glycogen. The biochemical pathways of muscle metabolism are fully described elsewhere.[9]

Muscle fibers are derived from mesoderm. They differentiate from the mesenchyme that forms the skeleton (sclerotome) and the skin (dermatome) without neural influences. At an early stage of development the muscle cells appear to lose the ability to undergo mitotic division. Subsequently, the muscle proteins associated with contractibility may undergo rapid turnover although all of the muscle cells themselves persist throughout life. Muscle grows in length by the addition of new sarcomeres to either end of the fibers. The remarkable ability of muscle to hypertrophy represents solely an increase of myofibrils within cells rather than the formation of new cells. The liability of this mode of hypertrophy is the limited capacity of skeletal muscle to regenerate itself. After it sustains a traumatic or surgical insult, a muscle undergoes repair or replacement by scar tissue formation rather than the formation of new muscle. In fact, muscle does possess a limited capacity to undergo regeneration although the ability of the reparative procedure to form useful contractile elements remains obscure.[11, 12]

HISTOLOGICAL STRUCTURE OF CONNECTIVE TISSUES

The connective tissues include such supporting tissues as bone and cartilage. They are derived from the mesoderm of the embryo and contain large amounts of intercellular material as well as cells. The intercellular material is composed of fibers in a matrix or ground substance, which may be liquid as in tissue fluid, or gelatinous fluid, or solid as in bone and cartilage. Both the fibers and the ground substance vary according to functional requirements, and the different types of connective tissue are named according to their content of intercellular material. The cells also show specialization appropriate for each type of connective tissue. The principal cell, the fibroblast, is found in most forms of connective tissue, in which it elaborates the fibrous matrix. Closely allied cells are further specialized for the production or removal of bone and cartilage. Many other types of cells are found in connective tissue. Examples include the ubiquitous histiocyte, the phagocytic macrophages, mast cells and plasma cells. The functions of these and other cells in connective tissue are discussed elsewhere.[13, 14] The three principal types of connective tissue—fibrous tissue, bone and cartilage—are discussed here briefly, in that order.

FIBROUS TISSUE

This tissue is subdivided by its content of fibers into: (1) dense fibrous, (a) organized or (b) unorganized; (2) loose fibrous, (a) fibroelastic, (b) areolar, (c) reticular and (d) adipose.

The organized dense fibrous tissues are the tendons, aponeuroses and ligaments. The collagenous fibers are arranged in compact parallel bundles and impart a characteristic glistening, white color. They are pliable, inelastic, weak in compression and of great tensile strength in one particular direction. The unorganized dense fibrous tissues show interwoven collagen fibers. They comprise fascial membranes, the dermis of the skin, periosteum and capsules of organs. They can resist moderately strong tensile forces in many directions.

Tendons are white, glistening fibrous bands which attach the muscles to the bones. They vary in length and thickness and in cross-sectional shape from round to oblong. While of great strength (Table 5-1), they are flexible and practically inelastic. Apart from the sites of attachment, tendons possess a sheath of delicate fibroelastic connective tissue. Larger ones also show thin internal septa. They are supplied with sensory nerves whose fibers have specialized terminations, called the organs of Golgi, for mediation of a special stereognostic sensibility.

Aponeuroses are pearly white, glistening iridescent fibrous membranes which represent flattened tendons. They function as supplementary modes of skeletal attachment for voluntary muscles. They consist of close-packed parallel collagenous bundles, which differentiate them from the fibrous fascial membranes. The latter show irregularly interwoven bundles of collagen. Aponeuroses are only sparingly supplied with blood vessels.

Ligaments are strong, slightly elastic cords, bands or sheets which attach two bones to-

Table 5-1
Mechanical Properties of Human Musculoskeletal Tissues

Property	Tissue				
	Compact bone	Hyaline cartilage	Elastic ligament	Collagen	Elastin
Ultimate tensile strength, MN/m^2	1.43	0.03	0.03	0.56	0.01
Ultimate elongation, MN/m^2	0.15	1.86	100–160%		
Modulus of elasticity, MN/m^2	187.0	1.43	–	140	0.61
Ultimate compressive strength, MN/m^2	0.18	0.08	–		
Ultimate bending strength, MN/m^2	1.63	–	–		
Ultimate torsional strength, MN/m^2	0.55	–	–		
Ultimate shearing strength, MN/m^2	0.81	0.06	–		
Modulus of elasticity in torsion, MN/m^2	32.6	–	–		
Hardness					
Rockwell	40.0	–	–		
Brinell	24.0	–	–		
Vickers	26.5	–	–		

gether. Their collagenous bundles are mainly parallel, so that they favor resistance to unidirectional tensile forces. Their deep surface may form part of the synovial membrane of a joint, but their superficial surface is covered with a fibroelastic tissue which blends with adjacent connective tissue.

The term fascia refers to fibrous connective structures, such as membranous sheets, which are not otherwise specifically named and vary in thickness and density according to functional demands.

Loose fibrous connective tissue is the most pervasive structural tissue. It contains elastic fibers admixed with collagenous bundles in a loosely woven structure. It is moderately elastic and pliable. Between the fibers are interstices of variable size which may be filled with liquid ground substance or tissue fluid. One example is the capsule of organs in which the fibers are closely interwoven.

Reticular tissue is composed of delicate reticular fibers woven into a loose meshwork which surrounds individual or small groups of cells such as nerve fibers, muscle fibers or capillary blood vessels. The fibrils are made visible under the microscope by silver impregnation.

Adipose tissue refers to connective tissue cells which contain a vesicle of fat. It functions as a packing or padding material and as a reservoir of nutrients. In the latter capacity it is a well recognized source of annoyance to surgeons, as it oozes into the operative field, thereby obscuring bones or joints. In the postoperative period, it arouses the interest of resident bacteria and usually stifles the enthusiasm of the corpulent patient in his attempts to exercise the impaired limb!

Primitive animals possess a remarkable capacity to regenerate injured parts. For example, the coelenterate, hydra, may regenerate the five tentacles or its immobilizing base, the hypostome.[15] When grafted into the side of another hydra, tissue from around the base of the tentacles will induce the formation of a new individual. In the higher vertebrates, only the secondary regenerative capacity of the adult liver rivals this ability of the hydra. After resection of part of the liver, it may regenerate about ⅘ of its preinjury mass. Within the musculoskeletal system, bone possesses the greatest capacity to regenerate itself or to incorporate graft material and organize or remodel it into appropriate configuration. Other connective tissues are largely limited to sealing sites of defects by the synthesis of scar tissue. For example, a cut or tear in a ligament or joint capsule unites by the formation of a bridge of

scar tissue which joins the two opposing surfaces. The scar tissue remains as a weak point of dissimilar mechanical properties. The fully healed ligament frequently shows permanent compromise in its stabilizing ability. One of the most frequently encountered examples of this is the case of a torn medial collateral ligament of the knee.

Recent studies of the regenerative capacities of other tissues have revealed greater reparative ability than had been anticipated. In the presence of florid hypertrophy of the synovial layer which lines joints, as occurs in inflammatory conditions such as rheumatoid arthritis or chronic infective arthritis, complete synovectomy is frequently performed as part of the treatment. Following treatment, the synovial layer shows complete regeneration, a new membrane forming which may be virtually indistinguishable from the original uninflamed synovium. Similarly, in cases of total hip joint replacement of an arthritic joint where a pathologically thickened joint capsule is encountered, the surgeon may undertake total capsulectomy so that the prosthetic joint will show satisfactory range of motion, which would otherwise be excessively limited. Within a few weeks after capsulectomy, a new capsule has formed which becomes remarkably similar to a normal one.

In recent years Hunter et al.[16] and Salisbury et al.[17, 18] have studied the regenerative capacity of flexor tendons and tendon sheaths in the hand. If a flexor tendon is damaged so that it becomes scarred to its sheath, excision of both the tendon and the sheath may be necessary. A flexible silicone rubber rod may be inserted into the scarred tendon bed. Subsequently, pseudosheath formation occurs in response to the motion of the flexible rod against adjacent tissues. In experimental animals, within 5 days after insertion, mesothelial cells are aligned on the surface of the implant and within 3 weeks a well developed bursa has formed. Ultimately, a remarkably normal sheath evolves in which synovial-like fluid is secreted to facilitate gliding of the flexible rod. When the rod is replaced by a tendon graft, the sheath appears to provide nourishment and a gliding surface for the adjacent portion of the graft.

Attempts to convert such a two-stage procedure into a single stage by the application of an artificial tendon, either within an artifical sheath or without one, have failed, however, because of the limited capacity of portions of tendon to show useful regeneration or repair. Salisbury et al.[17] have studied an experimental model in which Dacron tape serves as a tendon within a thin silicone tube or sheath. The artificial tendons and tendon sheaths are implanted in chickens, and the artificial tendon is sutured to the stump of the tendon, near its musculotendinous junction, with nylon suture material. A gliding tendon system is restored, with satisfactory motion between the sheath and the tendon. At the anastomosis between the stump(s) of the tendon and the tendon graft, however, a scar of poor quality remains indefinitely. When the sutures inevitably undergo fatigue failure, the anastomosis also disintegrates. Many different types of anastomoses between artificial tendons and the stumps have been attempted unsuccessfully.

The healing ability of such cartilages as menisci in the knee is minimal. Even if scar tissue joins the torn portions of a meniscus after surgical repair, the scar fails rapidly when the knee resumes normal activity. Biochemical and histological studies of the healing processes in soft connective tissues are reviewed elsewhere.[14, 19]

BONE

The Anatomy and Physiology of Bone

Bone is a highly specialized form of connective tissue composed of interconnected cells in an intercellular composite material of collagen fibrils, the ground substance and a mineral phase. The extracellular matrix provides both the mechanical attributes of bone necessary for fulfillment of its supportive function and a storehouse of essential minerals. The inorganic portion comprises about 66% by weight. It is composed chiefly of calcium phosphate in the form of crystalline hydroxyapatite (about 58% by weight), calcium carbonate (about 7%), calcium fluoride and magnesium phosphate (from 1 to 2% each) and sodium chloride (less than 1%). These substances confer the hardness and rigidity of bone. If the minerals are removed by immersion of bone in dilute mineral acid, the bone becomes so highly flexible that a long bone can be tied into a knot.

Bone is closely related to cartilage, another specialized form of connective tissue. Most of the embryonic skeleton is deposited first as models of hyaline cartilage, the cells of which hypertrophy and undergo changes in their chemical characteristics immediately prior to their replacement by bone. After the fracture of bone, the early reparative stage of callus formation includes the appearance of cartilage and fibrocartilage.

The Structure and Physical Properties of Bone

Bone is hard, elastic and tough in both tension and compression. In cross-section, bone shows two different types of structures (Fig. 5-5A). One is hard and dense in texture, like ivory, and is termed compact or cortical bone. The other consists of slender spicules, trabeculae and lamellae, which comprise a lattice work called cancellous bone (Fig. 5-5B).[21] The exterior of a bone always is invested by a layer of compact bone, while the interior may possess additional cortical bone, as in the shaft or diaphysis, or cancellous bone, as in the metaphysis and epiphysis (Fig. 5-5C). The relative quantity of these two kinds of tissue varies in different bones and in different parts of the same bone, according to functional requirements. Upon close examination, compact bone is observed to be porous, so that the difference in structure between it and the cancellous bone depends merely upon the relative amounts of solid matter and the size and number of spaces in each.

Live bone is permeated by vessels and is enclosed, except where it is coated with articular cartilage, in a fibrous membrane, the periosteum, through which many of the vessels course to reach the hard tissue. The interior of each of the long bones of the limbs presents a cylindrical cavity filled with marrow and lined by a vascular areolar membrane called the endosteum.

Minute Anatomy

If a thin transverse slice of compact bone is examined under a microscope (Fig. 5-6) the surface is noted to possess numerous circular districts, each consisting of a central hole surrounded by a number of concentric rings. The districts are termed Haversian systems; the central hole is a Haversian canal; and the rings are layers of bony tissue arranged concentrically around the central canal and termed lamellae. On closer examination, there are numerous minute dark spots between the lamellae, the lacunae, which are interconnected to one another and to the adjacent Haversian canals by fine dark lines, called canaliculi, which radiate like spokes of a wheel. Adjacent Haversian canals are connected by cross-channels, the Volkmann's canals. Haversian canals average about 0.05 mm in diameter. Each contains one or two blood vessels, with nerve filaments and lymphatic vessels in the larger ones. The whole bone, therefore, is permeated with a complex

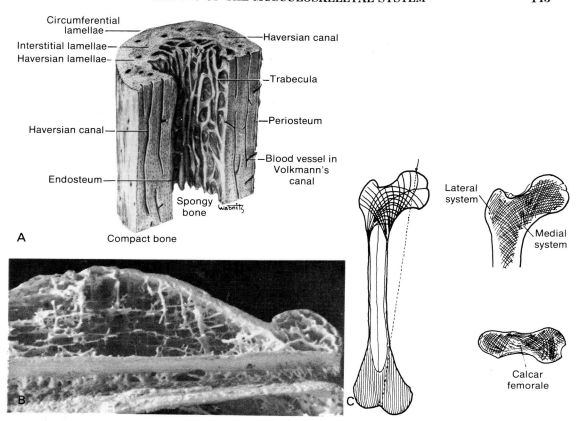

Circumferential lamellae
Interstitial lamellae
Haversian lamellae
Haversian canal
Endosteum
Spongy bone
Compact bone
Haversian canal
Trabecula
Periosteum
Blood vessel in Volkmann's canal
Wabnitz

A

B

C

Lateral system
Medial system
Calcar femorale

Figure 5-5. *A.* Schematic diagram of a phalanx in which the marrow has been removed. The dense outer ring of cortical bone is visible with a central ring of cancellous or spongy bone. *B.* A macerated specimen of bone which shows trabeculae of cancellous bone in the greater trochanter adjacent to a bony track that formed around a trifin nail. The nail track has been divided by a saw-cut in nearly a horizontal plane × 3.7 (*A*, reproduced with permission from H. Gray[20]; *B*, reproduced with permission from *J. Path. and Bact.*, 65:109, 1953). *C.* Schematic diagram of the femur. The figure on the *left* illustrates the regions of cancellous bone at its proximal and distal ends with the approximate principal alignments of the trabecular networks. The central portion or shaft consists of dense cortical bone. The figures on the *right* illustrate in greater detail the principal directions of the fibers of the cancellous bone.

network of vessels which approximate every osteogenic cell. Within the lacunae, osteocytes reside and communicate with adjacent osteocytes by processes which extend into the canaliculi. More recently, it has been shown that the lacunae possess other bone lining cells which cover the surface of bone matrix.[22, 23] These cells possess remarkably active ionic pumps in their cell membranes, which provide rapid, short-term adjustments of calcium, potassium and other ions. With advancing years they gradually disappear.

Cells of Bone

Three cellular components of bone are associated with specific functions: osteoblasts with

the formation of bone[24, 25]; osteocytes with the maintenance of bone; and osteoclasts with the resorption of bone. These specialized cells are formed from precursors which reside on the periosteum and endosteum and in the bone marrow and peripheral blood. It also seems likely that the specialized cells can alter their function from deposition to removal of bone and *vice versa*, although the relationships between the different cells remain obscure.

Osteoblasts. These cells appear on the surface of growing bone as a continuous cellular layer interconnected by thin cytoplasmic processes (Fig. 5-7). They are cuboidal in shape with a breadth of 15 to 20 μm. The cytoplasm is in-

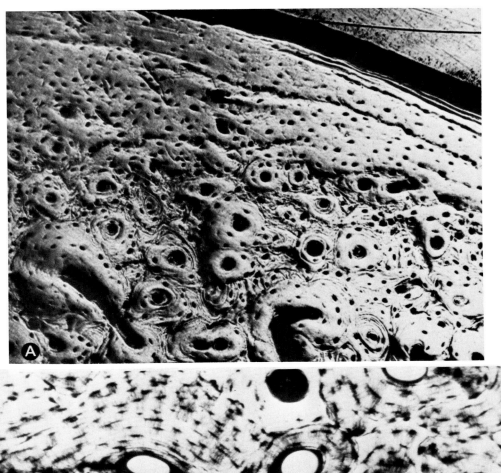

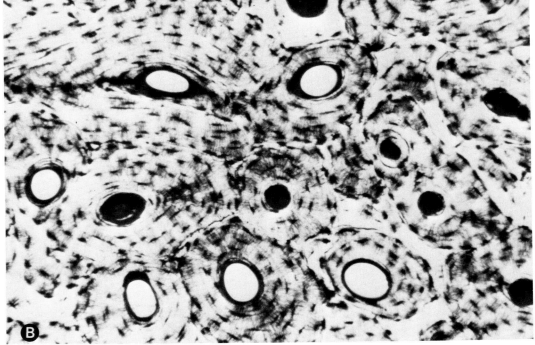

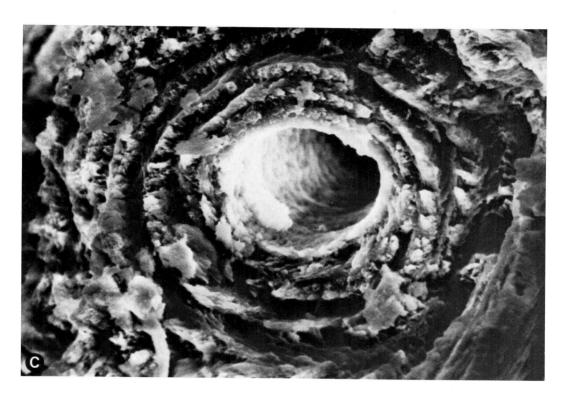

Figure 5-6. *A* and *B*. Reflected and transmission light micrographs of the surface of cortical bone. In *A* the lacunae that contain individual osteons are readily visible as depressions in the osteons. In *B* the osteons with fine striations, representative of canaliculi are observed in radial distribution around central blood vessels. *C.* A scanning electron micrograph of a deproteinized osteon. (Reproduced with permission from Dr. K. Piekarski.)

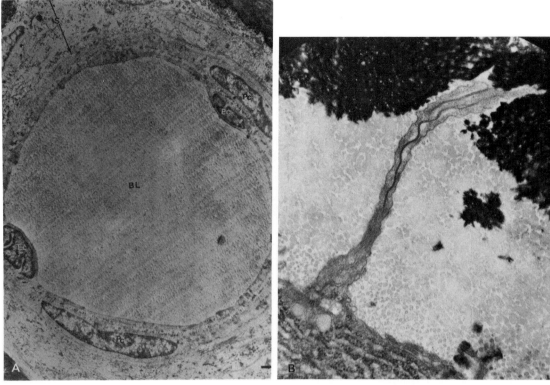

Figure 5-7. *A.* An electron micrograph of an Haversian canal with adjacent osteoblasts. The specimen represents human decalcified cancellous bone. The Haversian canal consists of two endothelial cells (*Ec*) and pericytes (*Pc*). Portions of the osteoblasts in the adjacent osteoid seams are just visible at the top and the upper left hand corner. *B.* An electron micrograph of a cellular process of an osteoblast passing through osteoid into calcified bone. Microtubules are evident within the cellular process. A well developed Golgi apparatus and numerous cisternae of rough surfaced endoplasmic reticulum are visible within the cell. ×23,000. (*A,* reproduced with permission from K. Hirohata and K. Morimoto[26]; *B,* reproduced from H. Rassmussen and P. Bordier.[27])

tensely basophilic from its high content of ribonucleic acid (RNA). With electron microscopy the principal features are seen to be: the intricate cell membrane; the endoplasmic reticulum (a highly characteristic system of canals and saclike structures, especially prominent in cells engaged in the synthesis of proteins); ribosomes (accumulations of electron-dense granules of ribonucleoprotein on the surfaces of the endoplasmic reticulum); the Golgi complex, which consists of vacuoles concentrating a secretory product, vesicles, and agranular membranes (*i.e.,* without ribosomes); lysosomes which contain hydrolytic or digestive enzymes; and mitochondria, the power plants of the cell.

Osteocytes. The osteocyte is an osteoblast that has surrounded itself with bone matrix (Figs. 5-6*C* and 5-8). The cells are enclosed within lacunae. Each cell extends minute cytoplasmic processes through apertures in the lacunae into canaliculi to connect with adjacent cells and form a syncytial network. In electron micrographs, osteocytes are similar in appearance to osteoblasts although the endoplasmic reticulum is not so profuse. From the observations of Belanger,[25] it seems that osteocytes play a significant role in the dissolution of bone mineral for the homeostatic regulation of calcium in body fluids. The recently discovered continuous layer of cells surrounding bone matrix and interposed between osteocytes and the matrix (Fig. 5-8) also serves a critical role in rapid adjustments in extracellular calcium homeostasis.[22, 23, 29]

Osteoclasts. The osteoclast is a giant cell with a variable number of nuclei, often as many as 15 or 20 (Fig. 5-9).[31, 32] The nuclei resemble those of osteoblasts or osteocytes. The cytoplasm is often foamy, and the cell has extensive processes.

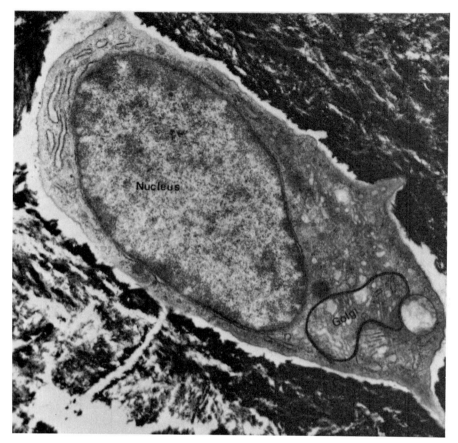

Figure 5-8. A schematic view of an osteocyte is revealed which shows a representative cell. Adjacent osteocytes are connected together by minute cytoplasmic processes to form a syncytial network. Osteocytes are separated from bone matrix by a continuous layer of cells, as described by Talmage. (Reproduced with permission from H. Rasmussen and P. Bordier.[28])

These cells may arise from precursor cells in the stroma of the bone marrow, or they may represent fused osteoblasts or fused osteocytes liberated from resorbing bone. Usually they are observed on the surface of bone at sites of active resorption, where they usually reside in shallow cavities known as Howships lacunae. In time-lapse cinemicrographs a ruffled and undulating cell membrane or "brush border," is visible on the resorbing surface, where dissolution of bone matrix proceeds. Surrounding the brush border is a rim of osteoclastic cell membrane, the "sealing point," which adheres firmly to the bone matrix and limits the extent of bone degradation. The bone matrix is digested by enzymes in the acidic secretion of the brush border. Particles of matrix are also introduced into digestive intracellular vacuoles by pinocytosis, a mechanism of

fluid transport which utilizes invagination of a cellular membrane.

Bone Matrix

Collagen. The fibrous protein network in bone is composed of collagen, which constitutes about 30% of protein in the body. Collagen comprises about 35% of the volume of bone matrix.[33] It is synthesized and secreted in soluble form from cells into the surrounding spaces where the molecules are converted into insoluble fibrils and fibers both by electrostatic forces, which yield largely reversible aggregates, and by intermolecular chemical cross-links, which provide more stable networks (Fig. 5-10A). Once deposited, collagen remains in tissues indefinitely. Inevitably, therefore, it would appear to be a natural

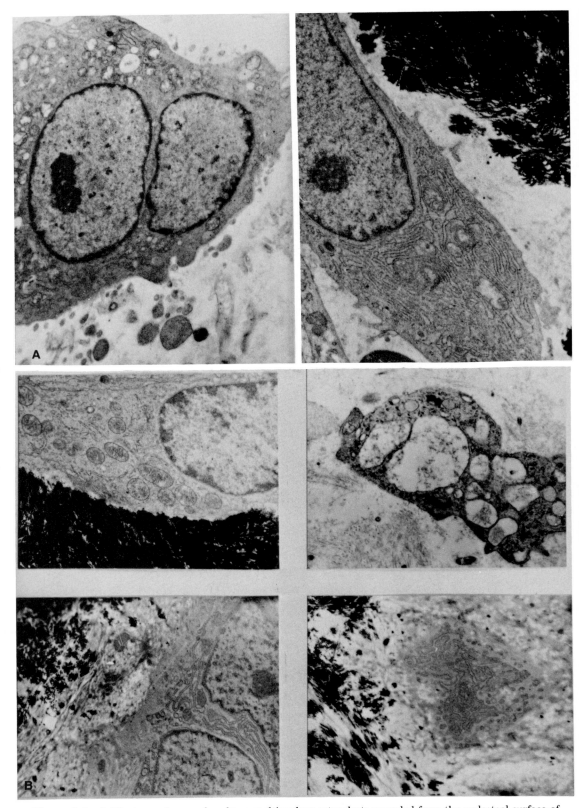

Figure 5-9. *A*. Electron micrographs of two multinuclear osteoclasts recorded from the endosteal surface of young rabbits. The syncytial nature of the cells with numerous cell processes is evident. Also many vacuoles are seen. *B*. Four electron micrographs of the features of osteoclasts. (Reproduced with permission from D. C. Mears.[30])

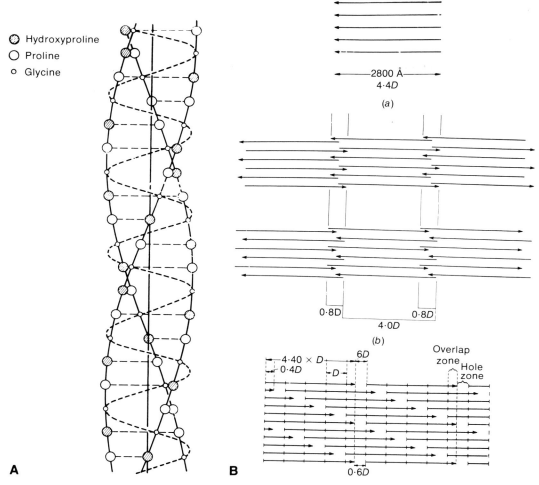

Figure 5-10. *A.* Schematic picture of the helical coiling of three polypeptide chains in the collagen molecule. *B.* Three schematic diagrams reveal the configuration of collagen molecules: (*a*), arrangement of tropocollagen molecules in segment long-spacing collagen (SLS) with isolated units 2800 Å long. SLS is believed to result from lateral aggregation of parallel tropocollagen molecules. (*b*), arrangement of tropocollagen molecules in fibrous long-spacing collagen (FLS). In FLS the molecules are thought to have an anteparallel arrangement and are able to link together to form filaments. (*c*), arrangement of tropocollagen molecules in native-type collagen fibrils are considered to have a staggered arrangement where each molecule is considered to be about 4.4 *D* long (*D* equals 640 Å). The length of a tropocollagen molecule is 4.4 *D* equals 2800 Å. Each molecule is separated from the molecule directly in front of it by 0.6 *D*, giving a distance of 5 *D* from the beginning of one molecule to the beginning of the next. (*A* and *B,* reproduced with permission from C. H. Brown.[34])

target for molecular mechanisms that constitute the phenomenon of aging.

Actually, collagen is a series of similar proteins characterized by their amino acid composition and by their arrangement into a triple helix. These proteins are synthesized mainly by connective tissue cells, fibroblasts, osteoblasts and chondroblasts.

The elementary polypeptides of collagen exist in the form of elongated strands called α-chains. The amino acid content and primary structure of α-chains vary in different tissues; but in all, every third amino acid is glycine. Two of the other amino acids, hydroxyproline and hydroxylysine, although constituting but a small proportion (14% and 1% by weight, respectively) of the total, are, with a single exception, unique in collagen and important in its molecular configuration. The α-chains are formed into three-stranded cables, united to each other by covalent, intramolecular cross-links.

Intracellular synthesis of collagen originates

on ribosomes, where a precursor, protocollagen, is formed. Protocollagen contains only hydroxy-proline or hydroxylysine rather than corresponding proline and lysine. The subsequent conversion to hydroxyproline and hydroxylysine requires ascorbic acid in addition to specific proline and lysine oxidases. In the absence of adequate amounts of ascorbic acid, a clinical condition known as scurvy ensues in which collagen formation is hampered by a failure in the oxidation of protocollagen.

The water soluble monomer of the fully formed molecule, tropocollagen (mol. wt. = 300,000), measures 3000 Å in length and 15 Å in width. Formation of microfilaments results initially from electrostatic aggregation. A progressive hierarchy of side-to-side aggregation transpires through covalent intermolecular cross-links. Fibrils are aggregates of adjacent filaments with widths of 0.01 to 0.1 μm. By contrast, fibers consist of bundles of fibrils (0.1 mm diameter) that are separated from each other by ground substance.

Collagen has a characteristic striated appearance under the electron microscope. In addition to major periods of about 640 Å in length, a series of smaller internal bands can be distinguished. The length of the major periods, 640 Å, represents approximately ¼ that of the tropocollagen molecule, 3000 Å. The "quarter-stagger" arrangement of the monomeric collagen (Fig. 5-10B) accounts for this discrepancy.[36] In this model of the fibril, the collagen molecules are aligned side-by-side so that one overlaps its neighbor by ¼ of its length. A small gap (about 400 Å) separates the actual ends of the molecules from each other. This "hole" provides a site for the nucleation of calcium salts as hydroxyapatites in the early mineralization of collagenous tissues.

Ground Substance. The components of the ground substance represent a heterogeneous group of macromolecules that, most recently, have been labeled protein polysaccharides or proteoglycans.[37] In these macromolecules, protein cores are linked covalently to special types of long-chain polysaccharides called mucopolysaccharides or glycosaminoglycans. One or two sulfate groups are fixed to each repetitive sugar unit in many mucopolysaccharides, so that they constitute strongly electronegative polyelectrolytes. Knowledge of the physicochemical properties of intact protein polysaccharides provides an insight into the function of the ground substance.

Protein polysaccharides form viscous sols with water by virtue of their large size and electrostatic properties. Their hydrodynamic size in cartilage is augmented by a noncovalent interaction with another matrix protein, link protein. While the exact nature of the interaction of ground substance with collagen remains obscure, it enables the ground substance to behave more like a gel than a sol. Accordingly it permits the ground substance to function as: a molecular sieve, to admit small molecules and to exclude large ones; an ion exchanger, to retain or exclude molecules according to their charges; and a source of oncotic pressure, to provoke turgor through imbibition of water and electrolytes. These mechanisms also enable the ground substance to regulate the transport of water and large and charged molecules throughout the body.

Mucopolysaccharides are synthesized by all types of connective tissue cells and are secreted promptly into the matrix. Unlike collagen, they turn over rapidly with degradation by lysosomal enzymes. Inherited defects in these lysosomal enzymes result in mucopolysaccharidoses, storage diseases in which the specific mucopolysaccharides accumulate within the cells.[38] The synthesis of ground substance constituents is profoundly influenced by hormones. Endocrine disorders such as acromegaly, myxedema, endocrine dwarfism and sexual dimorphism confirm this relationship.

The ground substance contains small amounts of lipid and peptides, although the functional significance of these moieties remains obscure.

Bone Mineral. At present the most logical view describes bone mineral as microcrystals of hydroxyapatite whose composition is determined largely by surface exchange and, to some unknown extent, by internal defects and substitutions.[39] The prototype for hydroxyapatite is $Ca_{10}(PO_4)_6(OH)_2$. Especially in younger animals, however, a significant portion of calcium phosphate in bone consists of an amorphous form. In any event, the mineral phase accounts for about 65% of the volume of bone matrix.

With the small size of the apatite crystal, 60 to 140 nm, it possesses a unique surface-area to volume ratio that favors exchange substitutions of ions foreign to hydroxyapatite. McLean and Urist[40] have calculated that the total surface of the area of the bone crystals in the skeleton of a man weighing 70 kg exceeds 100 acres; each gram of bone represents an area of 100 to 200 m^2.

Other Constituents of Bone

Membranes. Apart from certain locations, such as the neck of the femur, the patella and intracapsular joint surfaces, the connective tissue surrounding bones is a specialized membrane called periosteum. In young animals, especially in the regions of rapid growth, this consists of an outer dense layer of collagenous fibers and fibroblasts and an inner looser layer of osteoblasts and their precursor cells. In the quiescent state, in the adult, the periosteum serves for the attachment of tendons and conducts blood vessels,

lymphatics and nerves. The inner layer retains its osteogenic potential and in fractures is activated to form osteoblasts and new bone.

The endosteum consists of a thin layer of reticulum cells. It is a condensed peripheral, stromal layer of the bone marrow and possesses both osteogenic and hemopoietic potential. Like the periosteum, it participates actively in the healing of fractures.

Bone Marrow. The cavities within bone possess a wide variety of hemopoietic cells as well as cells which participate actively in osteogenesis.

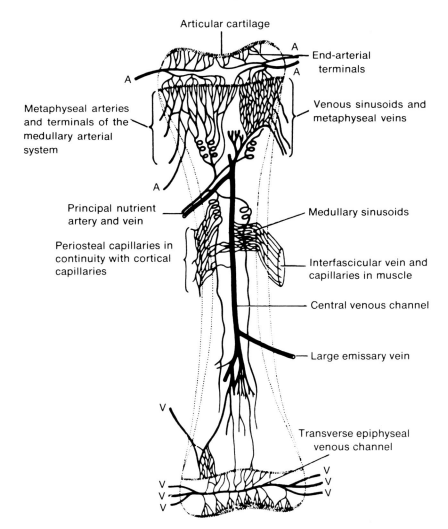

Articular cartilage

End-arterial terminals

Metaphyseal arteries and terminals of the medullary arterial system

Venous sinusoids and metaphyseal veins

Principal nutrient artery and vein

Medullary sinusoids

Periosteal capillaries in continuity with cortical capillaries

Interfascicular vein and capillaries in muscle

Central venous channel

Large emissary vein

Transverse epiphyseal venous channel

Figure 5-11. The blood supply of a long bone is shown schematically in longitudinal section after the work of Brookes and Harrison. (Reproduced with permission from M. Brookes, A. C. Elkin, R. G. Harrison and C. B. Heald.[35])

Blood Vessels. The vascular anatomy of the skeleton has a characteristic pattern closely related to the functions of bone.[41, 42] Cancellous bone has arteries that enter centripetally, branch and traverse each narrow space formed by individual trabeculae. The thin-walled capillaries, or sinuses, seen about each trabecula provide nutritive exchange. The capillaries form thin-walled intraosseous veins which enlarge and exit from the bone parallel to the arteries.

A long bone possesses three sources of blood supply (Fig. 5-11): (1) A nutrient artery perforates the midshaft cortical bone obliquely and divides into ascending and descending branches. Each branch arborizes to reach the endosteum, the metaphysis, and the epiphyseal plates. (2) A rich periosteal vascular network is concentrated at the metaphyseal ends of the bones and anastomoses with the cortical branches of the nutrient artery. (3) One to three main epiphyseal arteries course toward the center of the epiphysis, arborize and supply a portion of spongiosa and articular surface. The growth plate itself is supplied by perforating epiphyseal and metaphyseal vessels and by circumferential epiphyseal arteries.

In compact bone, virtually every Haversian canal contains one or more blood vessels. Lymphatics have also been described in some canals.

Blood Flow in Bone

The available data suggest that the rates of blood flow in various human bones are about 5 to 20 ml/min per 100 g of wet bone. The rates of flow in the entire skeleton are estimated to be 4 to 10% of the resting cardiac output. From the work of Brookes[41] and others, it seems that over ¾ of the entire blood supply reaches bone from the endosteal surface. The cortical capillary network, however, communicates not only with capillaries outside bone but also internally with the sinusoids of marrow. While blood flow usually occurs from endosteum to periosteum, it can be reversed if the bone is fractured, so that medullary arterial pressure falls. After a fracture, marked hypertrophy of the intramedullary vasculature follows to enhance the supply of nutrients. Rhinelander[43] and Rahn* have also documented the diminution of cortical blood supply beneath a rigidly applied bone plate. In subsequent weeks, the infarcted area shows gradual restoration of blood supply.

The mechanisms that control blood flow include sympathetic vasomotor nerves, hormones such as adrenaline and metabolites such as oxygen, carbon dioxide and pH, although the relative importance of each phenomenon remains obscure.

Mechanisms for the Regulation of Mineralization

The mechanism of mineralization remains a highly complex and controversial matter and is outside the scope of this book. It is well reviewed elsewhere.[23] Suffice it to say that two conflicting theories exist, with many minor variations. In one view, precipitation of crystallites occurs from a supersaturated solution of calcium and phosphorus, with "seeding" provided by another molecule of appropriate geometry and spacing.[44] While this mechanism can be confirmed for physiological solutions in beakers, its postulation raises formidable questions regarding control mechanisms to deftly regulate the calcium ion concentration of blood and other fluids as well as the inhibition of ectopic calcification on the vast stores of extraskeletal collagen in the body.[45] The alternative theories suggest that mineralization occurs in minute vesicles of about 100 to 200 nm diameter,[46] much like those documented for calcifying cartilage,[47, 48] whereby mineralization would be closely regulated by biological cells.[22, 49] While this theory is more attractive in accounting for the control of sites and rates of mineralization, it remains to be confirmed for human bone.

A complex regulatory mechanism involving the gastrointestinal tract, liver, kidney and endocrine system maintains the serum Ca^{++} level and thereby participates intimately in mineralization (Fig. 5-12).[39] A principal intermediary in calcium homeostasis is parathyroid hormone (PTH), a small polypeptide secreted by the parathyroid gland. The rate of secretion of PTH is controlled by the serum Ca^{++} concentration through a negative feed back mechanism. A fall in the Ca^{++} level directly stimulates the parathyroid glands to synthesize and promptly release PTH. Reciprocally, elevation of serum Ca^{++} reduces the PTH concentration. Little preformed hormone is stored in the parathyroid glands, and the half-life of PTH is about 10 min. Phosphate has no known direct effect on PTH secretion. PTH effects bone metabolism by stimulating osteoclastic resorption and by enhancing phosphate excretion by the kidney. Both actions are mediated at the cellular level by cyclic AMP (3:5'-adenosine monophosphate). The effect of

---

* B. Rahn, personal communication, 1975.

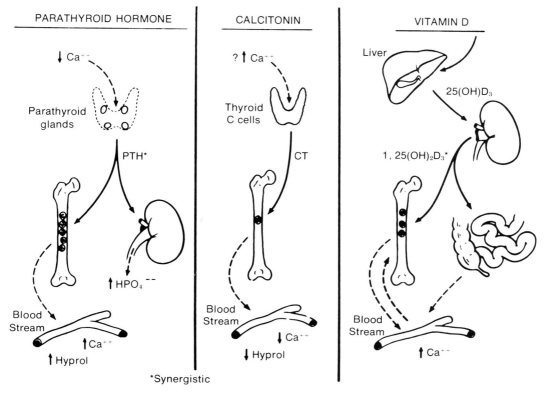

PARATHYROID HORMONE CALCITONIN VITAMIN D

$\downarrow Ca^{++}$

Parathyroid glands

PTH*

$\uparrow HPO_4^{--}$

Blood Stream

$\uparrow Ca^{++}$

$\uparrow Hyprol$

? $\uparrow Ca^{++}$

Thyroid C cells

CT

Blood Stream

$\downarrow Ca^{++}$

$\downarrow Hyprol$

Liver

$25(OH)D_3$

$1, 25(OH)_2D_3^*$

Blood Stream

$\uparrow Ca^{++}$

*Synergistic

Figure 5-12. The three-part hormonal regulation of mineralization shown by schematic view. The *hyphenated lines* indicate the movement of calcium ions. The *small circles* within the bone represent osteoclasts. PTH, parathyroid hormone; CT, calcitonin. (Reproduced with permission from L. Sokoloff and J. H. Bland.[10])

PTH on bone is to dissolve organic as well as inorganic matrix.

Calcitonin (CT) is a small peptide hormone secreted by the parafollicular C cells of the thyroid gland. It inhibits osteoclastic resorption of bone and lowers the serum Ca^{++} concentration. While its net effect counteracts PTH, CT is not simply a parathyroid antagonist.

Originally vitamin D was recognized for its antirachitic action, but it is now known to participate in calcium homeostasis over a broad spectrum of diseases.[39] Vitamin D can be synthesized from ingested plant ergosterol by ultraviolet irradiation of the skin, but it achieves maximal physiological activity by its conversion into 1,25-dihydroxycholecalciferol (1,25-$(OH)_2D_3$). In its natural form, vitamin D (*e.g.,* cholecalciferol or D_3) has one hydroxyl group added at the 25-carbon position in the liver. The final step is the addition in the kidney of a second OH at the 1-carbon. The role of PTH in regulation of the synthesis of 1,25-$(OH)_2D_3$ in

the kidney is unclear. 1,25-$(OH)_2D_3$ circulates through the blood as a hormone and regulates the transport of Ca^{++} through cells. Its role in the prevention of rickets is related to the formation of a transport protein in the intestinal epithelium which absorbs Ca^{++} from the lumen and enables it to enter the blood stream. There appears to be a close interaction between PTH and 1,25-$(OH)_2D_3$. The bone resorptive action of PTH requires that the latter be present. Both PTH and 1,25-$(OH)_2D_3$ affect a variety of cells apart from bone cells and stimulate bone resorption. The net bone accretion observed in rachitic patients treated with 1,25-$(OH)_2D_3$ results from the concurrent profound increase in serum Ca^{++} from the intestine.

A variety of other hormones (such as estrogens or growth hormone), minerals (such as fluorides), and physical agents (such as mechanical force) affect the rates of bone deposition and destruction.[51] Currently there is great interest in developing therapeutic agents to stimulate the

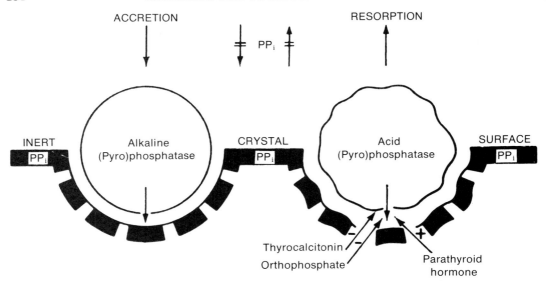

Figure 5-13. A schematic diagram shows the coating of the bone crystal surface with inorganic pyrophosphate (PP$_i$) and the possible accretion absorption mechanisms as described by Russell. (Reproduced with permission from R. G. G. Russell, S. Bisaz and H. Fleisch.[50])

healing of bone. Of the endogenous agents, only CT has gained an accepted role for the treatment of Paget's disease, where it profoundly retards the rate of bone turnover. Recent interest has focused on a series of analogues of a biological inhibitor of calcification, pyrophosphate. The small concentrations of pyrophosphate normally present in blood, urine or bone can inhibit the precipitation of calcium salts *in vitro,* in the presence of nucleating agents such as collagen. Also, pyrophosphate binds strongly to apatite crystals *in vitro* to inhibit their further growth or dissolution. Russell *et al.*[50] suggest that pyrophosphate participates vitally in calcium homeostasis by retarding the rate of dissolution of mineral at sites of resorption or by preventing the uptake of calcium by bone (Fig. 5-13). Mineralization is felt to be initiated by removal of the inhibitor, pyrophosphate. Bone cells contain at least two distinct pyrophosphatases, one with optimal activity under acid conditions and the other under alkaline conditions. Alkaline phosphatase and acid phosphatase can also function as pyrophosphatases. Indeed, with the ubiquitous presence of pyrophosphatases in bone and in the gastrointestinal tract, therapeutic applications of pyrophosphate are inevitably frustrated by its rapid degradation. It has recently been discovered that polyphosphonates, which have a P—C—P bond rather than the P—O—P bond of pyrophosphate, can act as analogues of

the latter to block bone resorption but resist enzymatic degradation by pyrophosphatases. This has provided insight into possible pharmacological methods for the treatment of metabolic bone disease and possibly for the acceleration of fracture repair. One of the diphosphonates, disodium edriodronate, has been shown clinically to greatly or completely retard the excessive bone turnover in Paget's disease.[53] Of the numerous types of diphosphonates available, some inhibit bone resorption more than bone deposition and others are likely to be discovered which will have the opposite effect. In the future, it seems likely that somewhat similar pharmacological agents may assume a significant therapeutic role to augment the rate of healing and remodeling of fractures and osteotomies.

Growth of Bones

The longitudinal growth of bones transpires primarily at highly localized sites where a disc of cartilage, the physis (also called the epiphyseal plate or growth plate [Fig. 5-14]), retains germinal cells that can divide and initiate endochondral ossification until puberty. The mechanisms of growth are described by Ham.[55] Injury to the germinal cells of the epiphyseal plate by direct trauma, circulatory loss or compression will arrest longitudinal bone growth. In Figure 5-15 a brief schematic account

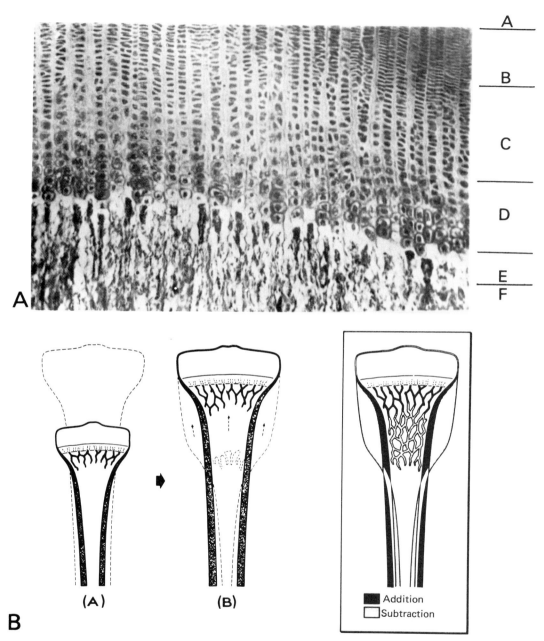

Figure 14. *A.* Photomicrograph reveals the growth plate from the upper epiphyseal cartilage of a rabbit's tibia. *A,* bone plate; *B,* zone of resting cartilage cells; *C,* zone of proliferation; *D,* zone of hypertrophy or giant cells; *E,* zone of cell degeneration or provisional calcification; *F,* a layer of bone formation. ×35 (Reproduced with permission from M. O. Tachdjian.[52]) *B.* A schematic diagram of the longitudinal growth of bone from the proximal tibial metaphysis. An intrinsic part of the growth process is removal of the peripheral portion of bone. The addition and subtraction processes are called remodeling. (Reproduced with permission from L. Sokoloff and J. H. Bland.[10])

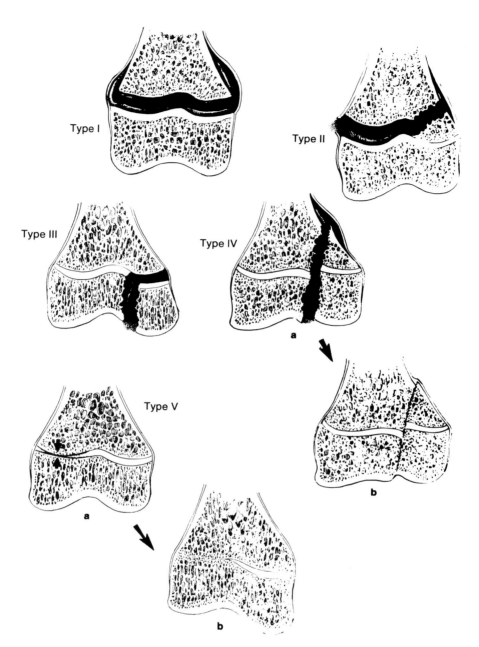

Figure 5-15. A series of schematic diagrams reveals the classification of epiphyseal plate injuries according to Salter and Harris. *Type I* represents a shearing or avulsion injury that separates epiphysis from metaphysis without any bone fragment. The plane of cleavage is through the zone of hypertrophic cells, without injury to the germinal cells of the physis remaining with the epiphysis. Growth is rarely disturbed. *Type II* represents a shearing or avulsion fracture along the hypertrophic zone of the physis to a variable distance with penetration through a portion of the metaphyseal bone. Reduction of the fracture is easy to obtain and growth is not disturbed. *Type III* is a rare injury in which interarticular shearing forces provoke cleavage along the physeal line at the weak zone of hypertrophic cells with abrupt penetration to the joint surface. Usually open surgery is necessary to restore congruity of the articular surface. With accurate reduction the prognosis for future growth is good. *Type IV* represents a fracture line from the articular surface, through the epiphysis, across the full thickness of the physis and through a segment of metaphysis. The germinal layer of the physis is split and discontinuity of the articular surface is produced. Even with accurate reduction of the articular surface, premature growth or arrest of the fracture site is likely. *Type V* represents the transmission of a severe compression force through the epiphysis to a segment of the physis with crushing of the germinal layer. The prognosis is poor in view of the likelihood of premature growth arrest. (Reproduced with permission from R. B. Salter and W. R. Harris.[54])

of the types of epiphyseal injuries is shown. A detailed account of the response of the physis to trauma is provided by Tachdjian.[57]

The management of children's fractures requires a sound knowledge of epiphyseal injuries. Where the physis is breached by the fracture, with displacement of the fragments, accurate open reduction with internal fixation usually is required. Failure to achieve accurate anatomic reduction predisposes the growth plate to initiate abnormal growth with deformity of bone. When devices for internal fixation are used in growing bones, great care is needed so that the device does not damage a physis. The center of the physis tolerates moderately well the penetration by smooth cylindrical pins of small diameter. When larger devices of irregular surface, such as a screw thread, penetrate through the growth plate, especially near its periphery, localized or generalized disturbance of growth is likely to follow. Furthermore, in the surgical approach to the metaphyseal or epiphyseal regions of growing bones or to adjacent joints, the delicate nutrient blood vessels to the sites of growth must not be disrupted. Finally, when epiphyseal injuries are treated, adequate follow-up must be provided so that deformities secondary to impaired growth of bone can be recognized promptly and treated appropriately.

The Mechanisms of Fracture Repair

Mammals have inherited from lower vertebrates an extraordinary capacity to repair injury and replace missing parts of the skeleton. The proliferative reaction is *equally* vigorous in experimental and clinical healing of fractures. A bone is not simply patched together by scar tissues, as in the healing of most other organs. Bone repair is ordinarily so thorough that it is impossible to find the area of a fracture or of a large defect 1 year after injury. New bone formation is an inevitable sequel to any form of injury in normal bone tissue, although the nature of the stimulus that initiates this response is unknown.[36, 39]

When a bone is broken, blood from ruptured medullary, periosteal and adjacent soft tissue vessels extravasates and clots, so that a hematoma or clot is formed about the fracture site. With the early phase of the immediate injury, histamine is released from most cells, platelets and other blood cells. Other permeability factors are activated, including proteases, such as kallikrein, and polypeptides, such as leukotaxine and

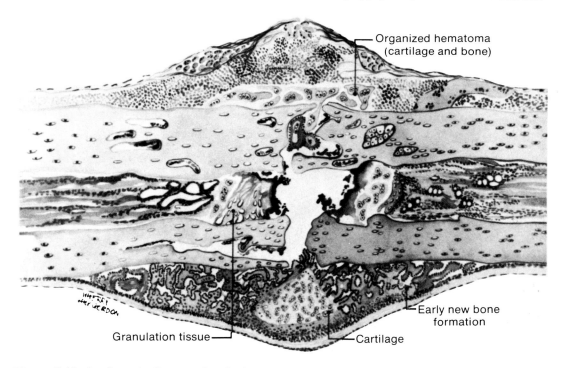

Figure 5-16. A schematic diagram of early fracture healing with callus formation is shown. The initial accumulation of hematoma beneath the periosteum and between the fracture ends has reorganized as early new bone or cartilage formation. (Reproduced from C. A. Rockwood and D. P. Green.[56])

bradykinin. These substances appear to augment small vessel permeability and cellular extravasation as well as altering the diffusion mechanisms in the ground substance. The insoluble fibrin of the clot is derived from circulating fibrinogen by the addition of two amino acids, phenylalanine and lysine, in the presence of thrombin, calcium, platelets and other clotting factors. Plasma proteins and extravasated blood cells become entangled in the fibrin framework. Subsequently the framework is invaded by reticuloendothelial cells, e.g., macrophages, round cells and histocytes; by endothelial cells, which divide to form capillaries; and finally by fibroblasts, which erect a preliminary collagenous matrix.

Concurrently, significant vascular reactions occur which augment the local blood supply. There is a rapid redistribution of blood flow through capillary channels by shunt mechanisms which are poorly defined.[58] Within the first day, there is dilation of medullary vessels; by the fourth day, periosteal vessels grow into the fracture site. Meanwhile, there is a marked invasion of inflammatory cells which initiate autolysis, phagocytosis and digestion of debris.

Within 2 to 3 days, a reconstructive proliferative stage is evident with the formation of fibrous tissue, fibrocartilage and hyaline cartilage, which seal the fragment ends together. The stimulus for this proliferation remains unclear. As the organization of this "callus" proceeds, the first new bone formation is seen subperiosteally at some distance from the fracture (Fig. 5-16). The new bone spicules are bordered by large osteoblasts, apparently derived from the inner layer of the periosteum. The new bone forms a collar around each of the fractured segments and develops toward the fracture gap. Simultaneously, endosteal bone formation develops from the cells that border the inner cortices to form an inner core of new bone, partly filling the medullary cavity and growing toward the frac-ture. The central area of cartilage tissue is replaced by bone, as the advancing osseous front reaches it, by a process similar to endochondral ossification.

The enveloping periosteal callus is usually more abundant in displaced fractures, where it acts as a scaffolding to unite the separated fragments. The preliminary callus is formed of coarse, randomly oriented fiber-bone, which is gradually replaced by more mature compact bone as the bulbous callus recedes and the new cortex and marrow cavity are formed. Fractures through cancellous bone show predominance of the endosteal phase with little subperiosteal new bone formation.

Primary Bone Healing

In 1949, on the basis of radiological evidence, Danis[60] suggested that rigidly immobilized fractures of the forearm bones underwent primary union of bone. Primary bone healing is in marked contrast to the usual secondary bone healing that is observed after external cast immobilization of fractures, in that no external ring of callus forms around the fracture. In 1964 Schenk and Willenegger[61] confirmed the phenomena of primary bone union for fractures in dogs and man which were treated by applying rigid internal fixation. Furthermore, he defined the two essential criteria for primary bone union: rigid stability and intact vascular supply of the bone. In view of their significance to techniques of internal fixation of fractures, the observations by Schenk and Willenegger[61] deserve close scrutiny (Figs. 5-17, 5-18). Initially after rigid internal fixation, hematoma fills the narrow gap between the fracture fragments. Within a few days capillaries and fibroblasts invade the gap, and in turn they are rapidly replaced by woven bone. If compression is used to attain maximal rigidity, the hematoma is in some sites replaced de novo by lamellar bone. Simultaneously, cutting cones of osteoclasts bore a cylindrical hole across the

Figure 5-17. Photomicrographs of new bone formation at a fracture site where primary bone healing is underway. A shows the initial fracture gap. B shows early bone formation at the site of the fracture gap with indirect evidence of revascularization in the form of the blackened channels. C shows a high power view of the osteoid within the fracture gap. D shows early remineralization of the osteoid at the fracture site. (Reproduced with permission from P. Gallinaro, S. Perren, M. Crova and B. Rahn.[59])

Figure 5-18. Photomicrograph reveals the vascular invasion across the fracture site with the crucial biological phenomena of primary bone healing. Cutting cones of osteoclasts bore a cylindrical hole in the bone across the fracture site with the appearance of new blood vessels and bone formation. A. Evidence of an osteotomy site with early revascularization. B. A high-powered view of a cutting cone of osteoclasts with a blood vessel across the fracture. (Reproduced with permission from P. Gallinaro, S. Perren, M. Crova and B. Rahn.[59])

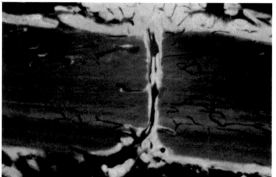

Figure 5-17A

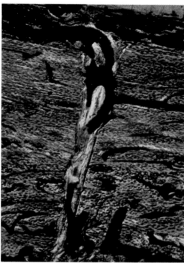

Figure 5-17B

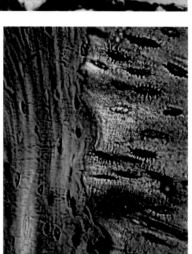

Figure 5-17C

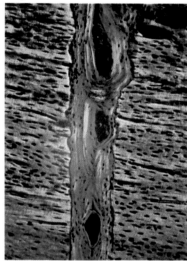

Figure 5-17D

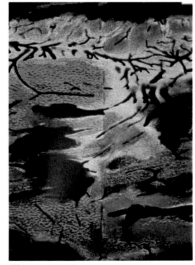

Figure 5-18A

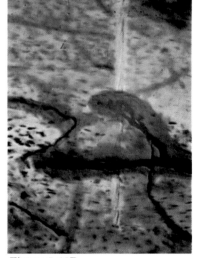

Figure 5-18B

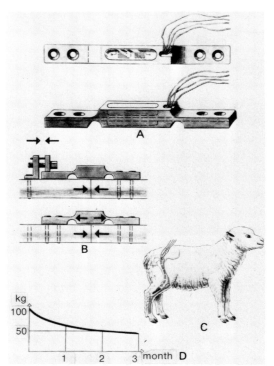

Figure 5-19. The biomechanical experiment of Perren is shown in schematic form. *A.* A unique plate fitted with strain gauges measuring up to 300 kg (± 1.5 kg) is prepared. *B.* The plate is applied to the bone with the application of a tension device. The tension in the plate is directly proportional to the compression at the fracture site. *C.* The plate is applied to the osteotomized tibia of a sheep. The leads from the gauges run subcutaneously to a point on the animal's back. *D.* A standard curve derived from numerous measurements indicates a gradual fall in pressure over a period of 4 months. (Reproduced with permission from M. E. Müller, M. Allgöwer and H. Willenegger.[62])

fracture line. Capillaries with accompanying osteoblasts invade the tunnel. The osteoblasts deposit osteoid and soon transform into concentrically arranged osteocytes.

Perren *et al.*[63] have studied the biomechanics of primary bone healing by applying force-measuring compression plates to osteotomies in such experimental animals as sheep (Fig. 5-19). Initially, compression of over 100 kg is applied to the bone. Measurements from the strain gauges in the plates reveal an early diminution of the force of compression on bone, with a gradual decrease in the rate of change in the force. About 50% of the initial force applied remains after 3 months, by which time the osteotomy has united. The early decrease in force represents

viscoelastic alteration of the bone. The subsequent gradual diminution in force represents a minute amount of resorption of bone at the osteotomy site. The resorption represents the first stage of remodeling; the new bone formed with remodeling does not maintain the compression.

It should be emphasized that the role of compression in primary bone healing is to assist in the provision of *rigid* stabilization of the fracture fragments. Compression does *not* itself enhance the rate of healing or remodeling of bone. Motion of a *stabilized* fracture or even of an *un*fractured bone appears to stimulate bone formation. When motion occurs between fracture fragments, however, primary bone healing is inhibited (Fig. 5-20). If the dynamic motion is of modest amplitude, then secondary bone healing may still occur, with external callus formation. With excessive amplitude of motion, however, even secondary bone healing is stifled and nonunion ensues. Nonunion may also be provoked by other causes, such as devascularization or irradiation of bone.

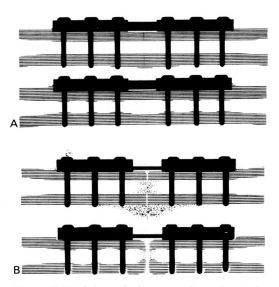

Figure 5-20. Schematic diagrams of experiments by Hutzschenruter *et al.*[63a] indicates the pattern of bone healing under rigid and flexible internal fixation. *A.* With rigid fixation, good bone healing without widening of the fracture gap and with minimal callus formation transpires over 16 weeks. *B.* With a flexible internal fixation, early callus formation is observed after 7 weeks. By 18 weeks the osteotomy gap is widened from absorption of bone induced by motion. (Reproduced with permission from S. M. Perren, P. Matter, R. Ruedi and M. Allgöwer.[64])

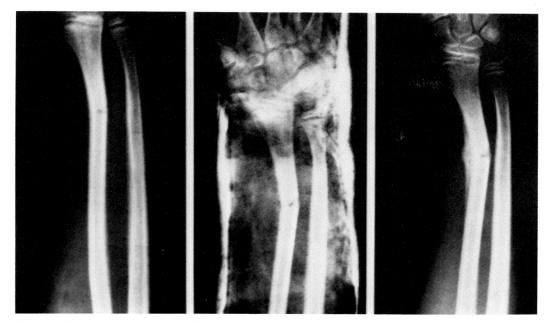

Figure 5-21. X-rays reveal a greenstick fracture of the radius with the application of a cast and subsequent formation of callus at the fracture site. Progressive loss of correction of the initial angulation deformity is observed. (Reproduced with permission from M. Rang.[65])

The Relationships between Primary and Secondary Healing of Bone

In the clinical literature, there has been considerable confusion over the relative merits of primary and secondary bone healing, as mechanisms of fracture repair. Both mechanisms may provide an equally solid union of a fracture and both require approximately the same time for completion in comparable fractures. For the treatment of any particular fracture, however, the surgeon should elect to engage one mechanism of fracture repair or the other. The choice will rest on the comparative advantages of the two systems. Rarely should one attempt initially to treat a fracture by the application of both mechanisms, for that usually evokes the liabilities of one or both techniques. Contrarily, if the application of one mechanism fails, one may have to employ the other or a combination of the two. A few illustrations are given.

If a stable, closed diaphyseal fracture of a long bone in a child is easily reduced, closed treatment with an external cast is usually preferred (Fig. 5-21). Not only does the cast provide adequate immobilization, but it prevents the risk of wound infection and the surgical devascularization of bone (especially of an adjacent physis) that might accompany internal fixation. Fur-

thermore, in the child, slight malalignment of the fracture is likely to be followed by remodeling, with anatomical restoration of shape. With the rapid healing of childrens' bones, combined with the considerable tolerance of childrens' joints to prolonged immobilization without the development of residual stiffness, casting has remarkably few liabilities.

For an elderly individual with a displaced, closed intra-articular fracture, precise open reduction of the articular fragments with rigid internal fixation is usually indicated. It provides the essential restoration of congruity of joint surfaces (Fig. 5-22). It permits early mobilization of joints when prolonged immobilization would be likely to result in residual stiffness of the joint. Attainment of these objectives hinges upon the provision of *rigid* fixation. If inadequate fixation is attained, then even a minute amount of motion at the fracture site provokes resorption of the adjacent bone ends. Simultaneously, "cloudy irritation" callus forms around the fracture site to provide a characteristic radiological feature (Fig. 5-23). With the resorption of bone, the tensile stress on the bone plate is wholly relieved and replaced by dynamic bending, and torsional stresses. Under the imposition of the latter, the plate is apt to break. With the appearance of "irritation callus," there-

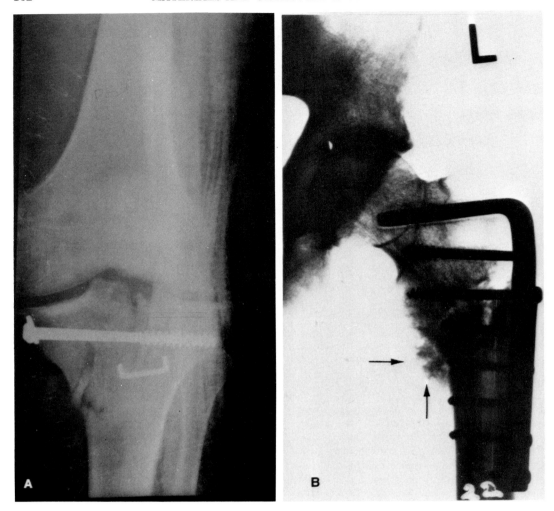

Figure 5-22. *A.* X-rays reveal evidence of a displaced interarticular fracture of the tibial plateau in which precise open reduction and internal fixation is necessary. *B.* X-rays of a fracture site after internal fixation reveal evidence of "cloudy irritation" callus. The biomechanical environment of the fracture has not been changed and subsequent mechanical failure of the plate from excessive bending forces also has occurred.

fore, the surgeon should apply external immobilization until union of the fracture is achieved.

In rare instances of complex pathological fractures or comminuted fractures, combinations of internal and external immobilization may be necessary. Usually these difficult cases merit considerable thought about the optimal biomechanics of stabilization of the fracture before any definitive treatment is initiated. The reader is referred to Chapters 9 and 10 for a description of many complex fractures.

CARTILAGE

Cartilage is a nonvascular structure which is found in various parts of the adult human, es-

pecially in the joints.[66] In the fetus, at an early period, most of the skeleton is cartilaginous. As this cartilage is subsequently replaced by bone, it is called temporary, in contrast to that which remains ossified throughout life and is called permanent. Cartilage is divided, according to the composition of its matrix, into hyaline cartilage, white fibrocartilage and yellow or elastic fibrocartilage.

Hyaline cartilage consists of a pearly bluish, resilient, slippery mass, of a firm consistency but of considerable elasticity. Except where it coats the articular ends of bones, it is covered externally with a fibrous membrane, the perichondrium. The membrane contains vessels from

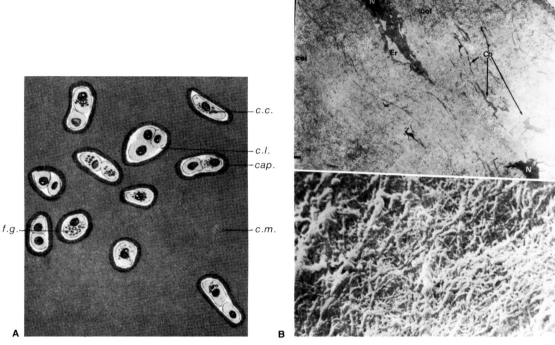

Figure 5-23. *A.* A schematic diagram of hyaline or articular cartilage. The abbreviations are: *cap.*, the capsule of the lacunae; *c.c.*, a chondrocyte or cartilage cell; *c.l.*, the cartilage lacuna; *c.m.*, cartilage matrix; *f.g.*, fat globules in a chondrocyte. ×1000. (Reproduced with permission from H. Gray.[66]) *B.* Two electron micrographs of human articular cartilage. In the superficial zone of the cartilage elongated chondrocytes are arranged tangentially to the articular surface. Their slender cellular process (*Cp*) are scattered about this zone. Intracellular matrices are composed of intertwined collagen fibers. In the lower view a scanning electron micrograph of the surface reveals the architecture of these collagen fibers with their variation in diameters. *N*, nucleus; *Js*, joint space; *Er*, rough surfaced endoplasmic reticulum. (Reproduced with permission from K. Hirohata and K. Morimoto.[2])

which the cartilage imbibes its nutritive fluids, since it is devoid of blood vessels and nerves. Under the microscope, a thin slice of cartilage shows a simple structure with groups of rounded or bluntly angular form surrounded by a granular or almost homogenous matrix (Fig. 5-23). Where the cells are clustered, they show flattened opposing surfaces with rounded free margins. The cells consist of clear transparent protoplasm in which fine interlacing filaments and minute granules are sometimes present. Within the protoplasm, one or two round nuclei are embedded. The cavities in the matrix wherein the cells reside are called cartilage lacunae; around the lacunae, the matrix is arranged in concentric lines.

The matrix is a translucent and apparently amorphous material that resembles ground glass. Upon degradation, fine fibrils are evident in the matrix. In articular cartilage, the matrix is finely granular. The cells and nuclei are small and in the superficial part are disposed parallel to the surface, while nearer to the bone they are arranged in vertical rows. Articular cartilage varies in thickness according to the shape of the articular surface on which it lies. Where this is convex, the cartilage is thickest at the center; the reverse applies for concave articular surfaces. Nutriment is derived partly from the vessels of the neighboring synovial membrane, partly from those of the subchondral bone, and partly from the synovial fluid within the joint.

White fibrocartilage consists of a mixture of white fibrous tissue arranged in bundles with cartilage cells between the bundles. To the former constituent, it owes its flexibility and toughness and to the latter, its elasticity. The white fibrocartilages are subdivided into four groups: intra-articular, connecting, circumferential and stratiform.

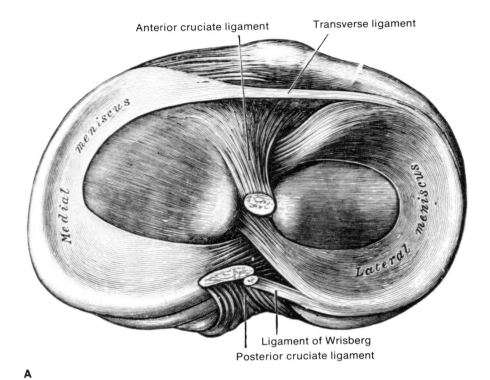

A

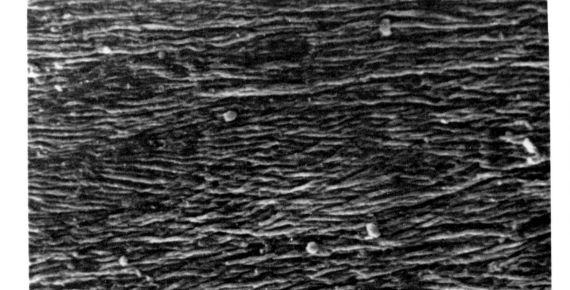

B

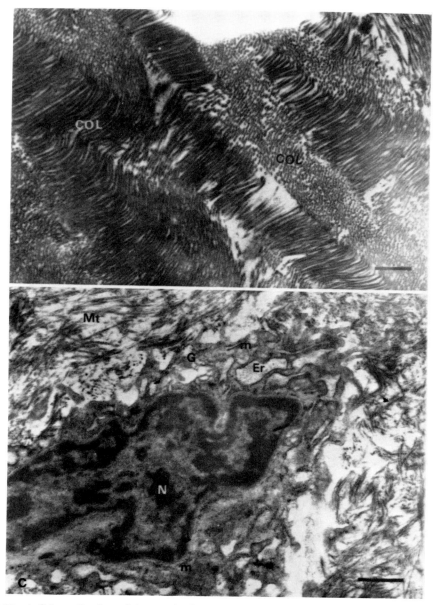

Figure 5-24. *A.* Schematic view of the proximal end of the tibia with the menisci is shown. *B.* A scanning electron micrograph of the surface of a normal meniscus. The fibrillar components are oriented regularly in parallel. *C.* Two transmission electron micrographs of meniscus. The *superior* view shows the surface of the meniscus with two dimensional orientations of collagen fibers. The *inferior* view shows the sparse population of fibroblastic cells with Golgi complex (*G*) and rough surfaced endoplasmic reticulum (*Er*). (Reproduced with permission from K. Hirohata and K. Morimoto,[2] and H. Gray.[20])

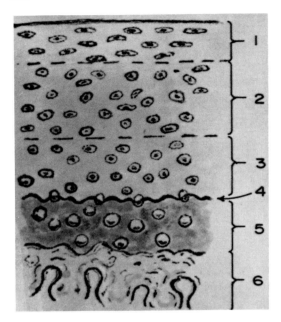

Figure 5-25. Schematic diagram of the zones of mature articular cartilage. A superficial layer of flattened cells is called the tangential zone, *1.* Beneath this is a transitional zone, *2,* in which ovoid or rounded cells are randomly distributed. Deep to this are the short, irregular columns of the radial zone, *3,* which is separated from the zone of calcified cartilage, *5,* by the "tide mark," *4.* Below the cartilage a bony end plate consists of mature cortical bone with Haversian systems. (Reproduced from H. J. Mankin.[67])

The intra-articular fibrocartilages, or menisci, are flattened plates of a round, oval, triangular or sickle-like form, interposed between the articular surfaces of certain joints (Fig. 5-24). They are free on both surfaces, usually thinner toward the center than the circumference and held in position by a peripheral attachment to surrounding ligaments. The synovial surfaces of the joints continue over them. They are found in the sternoclavicular, acromioclavicular, wrist and knee joints. They obliterate the intervals between opposing surfaces in their various motions. They facilitate gliding movements of joints, and they provide resilient shock absorbers to moderate the intensity of acute compressive forces to which the limb and joint are exposed.

The connecting fibrocartilages are interposed between the bony surfaces of those joints which show only slight mobility, as between the bodies of the vertebrae. They form discs which are closely adherent to the opposed surfaces. Each disc is composed of concentric rings of fibrous tissue with cartilaginous laminae interposed.

The former tissue predominates toward the circumference and the latter toward the center.

The circumferential fibrocartilages consist of rims of fibrocartilage which surround the margins of some of the articular cavities. An example is the glenoid labrum of the hip and the shoulder. They serve to deepen the articular cavities and to protect their edges.

The stratiform fibrocartilages comprise the coatings over osseous grooves through which the tendons of certain muscles glide. Small masses of fibrocartilage are also developed in the tendons of some muscles where they glide over bones. Examples include the tendons of the *Peroneus longus* and *Tibialis posterior.*

The Structure of Articular Cartilage

One of the notable features of articular cartilage is the structural preponderance of the extracellular materials. Even in young cartilage, the chondrocytes are sparse, while in adult cartilage the cell counts of about 2×10^5 cells/mm^3 are considerably less than the population density of many other tissues.[71]

Four distinct morphological zones are evident in adult cartilage (Fig. 5-25). Collins[71] provided the following classification: (1) a superficial or tangential zone adjacent to the joint cavity where the fibers are arranged tangentially to the surface, and the discoidal cells are aligned with their long axes parallel to the surface; (2) an intermediate or transitional zone where the coiled fibers form an interlacing meshwork, and the spheroidal cells are equally spaced; (3) a deep or radiate zone where the fibers form a tighter meshwork with a radial alignment from the articular surface, and the spheroidal cells are clustered in columns of four to eight cells; (4) a calcified zone adjacent to the subchondral bone, possessing a matrix impregnated with crystals of calcium salts and a few small, irregular cells. The last zone is delineated from the previous ones by a thin, wavy, bluish line—the "tide mark"—which is of constant photomicroscopic appearance but of uncertain significance.

While immature cartilage shows canals which carry blood vessels, adult cartilage possesses no blood vessels, nerves or lymphatics. The immediate surface layer, or "lamina" of adult cartilage contains a dense network of randomly oriented minute fibers of 40 to 120 Å in diameter and is deficient in polysaccharide as compared with deeper layers. It is believed to serve a protective function. While macroscopically it appears to be extraordinarily smooth, a microscopic view reveals the presence of pits, depressions and other

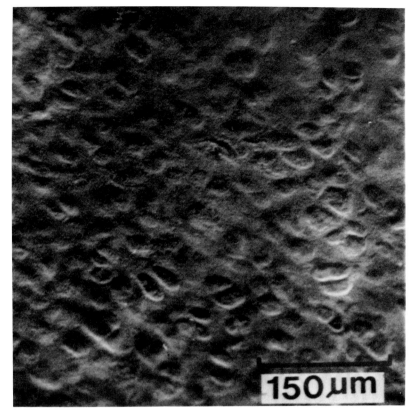

Figure 5-26. An electron micrograph of the articular surface shows bowl-shaped depressions, many of which are of the figure-8 pattern. (Reproduced with permission from M. A. R. Freeman.[68])

irregularities (Fig. 5-26). Walker *et al.*[72] believe that the irregular corregated pattern is essential for the complex system of lubrication.

For many years it has been known that the arrangement of collagen fibers in cartilage imparted considerable stiffness. In 1925, Benninghoff[73] showed histologically that the collagen fibers form bundles arranged in arcades (Fig. 5-27). The fiber bundles were considered to be anchored in the calcified zone and to course toward the joint where they curved tangentially to the surface before descent to the calcified zone. The Benninghoff arcades are visible by phase-contrast microscopy of adult cartilage. While they provide an attractive mechanical explanation of the resiliency of articular cartilage, which would function much like an innerspring mattress, recent electron micrographs have somewhat altered the concept.[74–76] Alternatively, the picture of more randomly oriented fibers possibly without continuous arcades emerges, which, nevertheless, would also help to explain the resiliency of cartilage.[77]

Chondrocytes of Articular Cartilage

In general, chondrocytes resemble other connective tissue cells. They are round, oval or flattened, depending upon the zone in which they are located; and their long axis is 15 to 20 μm in diameter. The nucleus is often eccentric, rounded and 4 to 6 μm in long diameter. The cell occupies a rounded lacuna which it probably fills *in vivo,* although it seems to shrink away from the matrix in histological sections (Fig. 5-28).

The ultrastructural characteristics of the cells vary with the zone in which they are found. A typical cell from the transitional zone shows an eccentrically placed rounded or lobulated nucleus with one or more prominent nucleoli. The nuclear membrane is well defined. The conspicuous Golgi apparatus shows close-packed granular lamellae with dilatations, small vesicles and vacuoles. A number of large vacuoles adjacent to the Golgi complex contain moderately dense amorphous material and intracellular fibrils. Also present are numerous complex cisternae.

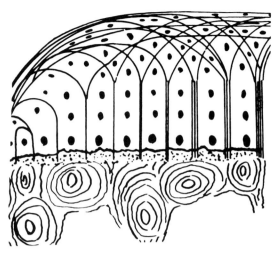

Figure 5-27. Schematic view of the Benninghoff concept of the arrangement of collagen fibers in mature articular cartilage. The fiber bundles are conceived as arcades anchored in the calcified zone that sweep jointward, run obliquely, tangentially, and then obliquely to descend in a direction perpendicular to the surface of the calcified bone. The *dots* represent cells between the arcades. (Reproduced with permission from H. J. Mankin.[70])

Small cytoplasmic pinocytic vesicles are located near the cell surface. The cytoplasm also contains many lipid droplets and aggregates of glycogen.

The well defined plasma membrane is irregular in contour although, unlike the osteocytes, it does not show long protoplasmic processes. Alternatively, there are numerous short footlike processes and indentations in a scalloped pattern that may represent vacuolar discharge. Immediately around the cell is a "halo" rich in polysaccharide and chloride and deficient in collagen.

The kinetics of chondrocyte proliferation has received considerable attention. While immature cartilage shows evidence of cell division, normal adult chondrocytes do not exhibit mitotic activity. Despite the low-friction character of mobile joints, attrition inevitably occurs, as the recent studies by Lipshitz *et al.*[79] have confirmed. It is surprising that articular cartilage does not exhibit any effective reparative process. Under certain conditions, such as osteoarthritis, mild continuous compression, lacerative injury and acromegaly, chondrocytes can undergo mitotic division. However, as Mankin[77] emphasizes, the healing process is generally feeble and ineffective.

Chemistry of Articular Cartilage

One of the striking features of articular cartilage is its degree of hydration, with 65 to 80% water content.[69] Most of the water is loosely bound to mucopolysaccharide to form a gel. This is in marked contrast to bone, where most of the water is tightly bound to collagen fibers or crystalline mineral. The water content of cartilage decreases slightly with aging, although it increases in the presence of osteoarthritis.

The concentration of electrolytes is about the same as in other intracellular and extracellular fluids, with two exceptions. In view of the concentration of sulfated polysaccharide both free and bound sulfate concentrations are high. There is also a high concentration of sodium ion, which serves as the principal cation in the polyanionic matrix.[80] Maroudas and Evans[81] record diffusion coefficients for electrolytes in cartilage of about 40% of that for an aqueous solution. The processes are almost entirely passive ones, without cellular activity.

Over 50% of the dry weight of articular cartilage, and about 90% of the protein content, is in the form of collagen. The acid mucopolysaccharides and collagen interact to form a stable complex. The other main organic solid constituents of articular cartilage—the protein polysaccharides—are viscid, hydrophilic, high molecular weight macromolecules. They consist of a protein core, to which about 60 chains of sulfated polysaccharides are attached. Schubert and his colleagues[82] have subdivided the protein polysaccharides of articular cartilage into chrondroitin-4-sulfate, chondroitin-6-sulfate and keratin sulfate. These moieties are concentrated around the chondrocytes. The protein polysaccharides possess a number of unique physical and chemical properties which are believed to contribute to the resiliency of cartilage and the provision of water for surface lubrication.

Other organic materials of lesser content in articular cartilage include sialic acid, lipids and a variety of enzymes.

Nutrition of Articular Cartilage

In view of its avascular nature, the source of nutrients in cartilage has remained a mystery. Until recently, observers had felt that diffusion of nutrients from the synovial fluid was the sole source of nutrition in adult cartilage. Recent evidence, however, suggests that at least a portion of the substrates enter articular cartilage by diffusion from the subchondral bone.[83–85] Cer-

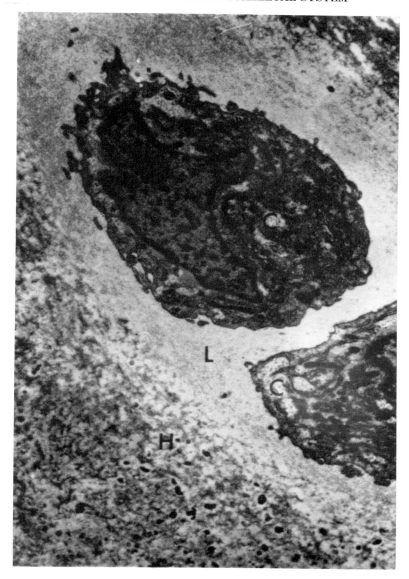

Figure 5-28. An electron micrograph of a pair of chondrocytes (*C*) surrounded by pericellular matrix (*L*) which contrasts in texture with that of the intracellular matrix (*H*). × 7500 (Reproduced with permission from M. A. R. Freeman.[68])

tainly in the immature animal the basal layers of cartilage are nourished by diffusion from the subchondral vascular buds. In the adult, where the "tide mark" shows heavy deposition of apatites in the calcified zone, diffusion of nutrients must be considerably impeded, so that virtually all nutrition is derived from the synovial fluid.[82-86] Until recently, the slow rate of nutritive exchange by diffusion was felt to be associated with a low rate of metabolism in chondrocytes.[87] Early measurements of the respiratory activity of cartilage supported this view. In fact, with the sparse cell population in cartilage, the metabolic rate of *each* cell approaches that of other cells.[88, 89] Chondrocytes show low oxygen consumption and well developed pathways of anaerobic metabolism for energy production.[90] The cells show a complex synthetic activity for the production, maintenance and degradation of the extracellular macromolecules.[69] The cells may synthesize the protein of collagen and protein polysaccharide and polysaccharide itself. Also, the cell may promote polymerization and sulfation of polysaccharide. The rates of synthesis are moderately increased by the presence of lacerative injury and by osteoarthritis.[77] Recent studies of the degradation of matrix have confirmed the presence of an active internal remodeling system.ʼ Possible functions of the rapid turnover of matrix include the maintenance of the normal high affinity of the protein polysaccharide for water, and the repair of minute notches or other defects which would predispose articular cartilage to fatigue failure.

Mechanical Properties of Articular Cartilage

When a compressive load is applied to cartilage, deformation occurs in two stages.[91] As the load is applied, an instantaneous deformation follows. This deformation results from a bulk movement of the water matrix and collagen fibers simultaneously rather than from the flow of water through the matrix. Subsequently, with the application of a constant load, the cartilage deforms increasingly with time. This behavior represents creep and seems to be related to the flow of water through the matrix and probably to the time-dependent properties of the matrix itself. The magnitude of the deformation of cartilage at a given time after application of a compressive load is governed by the magnitude of the applied force, elastic stresses in the collagen fiber mesh, the permeability of the matrix and the Donnan osmotic pressure of the proteoglycan gel in the cartilage matrix.

Several workers have determined the Young's modulus for cartilage by indentation tests.[92–94] The experimental values range from E = 0.58 MN/m^2 (85.4 lb/inch^2), 6.03 kg/cm^2, 5.8 × 10^6 dyne (cm^2) to E = 2.28 MN/m^2 (331 lb/inch^2, 23.0 kg/cm^2). The variation depends upon the thickness of the cartilage, the lack of homogeneity of cartilage and time-dependent factors. Similarly, Kempson et al.[95] record the short-term stiffness of cartilage as a creep modulus at 2 sec after the application of load. For normal cartilage on the human femoral head, he reports a stiffness of 1.96 MN/m^2 (20 kg/cm^2) to 1.44 × 10 MN/m^2 (150 kg/cm^2). If the stiffness of cartilage on the femoral head is recorded, marked variation is noted, with the highest figures observed at the superior crescentic weight-bearing portion (Fig. 5-29). Freeman[96] reports the bulk of available experimental data for tensile properties of normal articular cartilage. The maximum tensile stiffness for cartilage is 2000 kg/cm^2 for the surface layer in which the cleavage lines are oriented parallel to the direction of tension. The minimum tensile strength is 27 kg/cm^2 for the deepest layer of a transversely oriented specimen. The strength is related to the collagen content of cartilage, although it is not related to the proteoglycan content. Incidentally a comparable degree of anisotrophy of bones has been confirmed by Brown and Ferguson[96a] in their elegant finite element analysis of 2-mm cubes of femoral head, both from normal and degenerative specimens (Fig. 5-29).

It will be recalled that Poisson's ratio for any material is the ratio between the strain perpendicular to the direction of an applied load and the strain in the direction of the load. It varies between different materials and determines the change in cross-sectional area of a loaded specimen. Freeman[96] also reports the available information on determination of Poisson's ratio in cartilage with results from 0.42 to 0.48.

In life, articular cartilage is frequently subjected to cyclically applied dynamic loads. Several workers have therefore studied the response of cartilage to dynamic loads. Radin and Paul[97] evaluated the relative force alternating characteristics of cartilage, bone, periarticular soft tissues and synovial fluid in intact joints and in separate specimens. By the application of impulsive loads, these authors concluded that periarticular soft tissues play an important part in the reduction of peak transmitted loads. Bone is also important, but synovial fluid shows poor attenuation characteristics. Articular cartilage is so thin that it makes only a small contribution to the reduction of peak forces in the joint. Nevertheless cartilage seems to make an essential contribution which lowers the contact stress in the joint below a magnitude which would otherwise provoke failure of bone.

In view of the remarkably limited capacity of cartilage to show effective repair, fatigue failure would seem to be a likely factor in the initiation of degenerative processes in joints. Freeman[96] reports some preliminary observations by Weightman, in which human articular cartilage in vitro is subjected to a cyclically applied load via a cylindrical indenter with a spherical end. When a nominal compressive stress of 285 lb/inch^2 (1.97 MN/m^2) is applied on one or several occasions, microscopic examination of the cartilage after the test reveals an undamaged surface. After the application of 6 × 10^4 repetitive load cycles with the same applied force, the

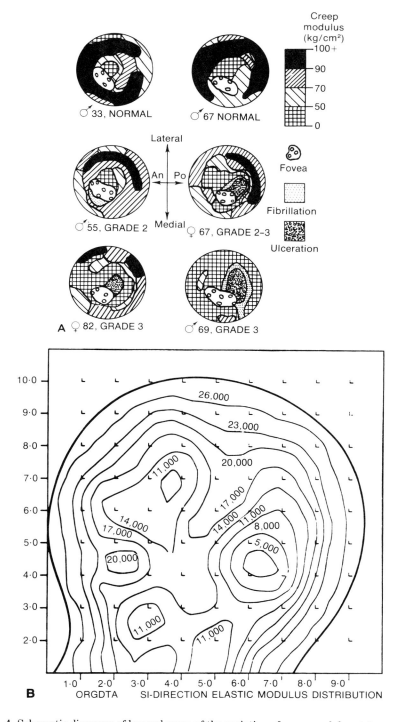

Figure 5-29. *A.* Schematic diagrams of layered maps of the variation of creep modulus at 2 sec. on the human femoral head indicate gross local variations. (Reproduced with permission from M. A. R. Freeman.[68]) *B.* Schematic diagram of local variations in the modulus of elasticity of the femoral head as determined by finite element analysis. (Reproduced with permission from Dr. T. B. Brown.)

cartilage shows evidence of microscopic fatigue fractures. Clearly, further study of the fatigue characteristics of cartilage is warranted.

Load Carriage of Articular Cartilage

Gross inspection of articular cartilage suggests that it is likely to participate in load carriage and in joint lubrication. Load carriage refers to the capacity of cartilage to sustain the loads to which it is subjected without failing mechanically and to reduce the possibility of damage to the subchondral bone from dynamic loads.

Most articular joints are subjected to loads which are rapidly applied and thereby expose the subchondral bone to high loads of short duration. Cartilage might protect the bones from these stresses if it dampened and attenuated dynamic loads, like a shock absorber, by viscoelastic deformation. With the incongruity and superficial undulations of subchondral bone, cartilage should be more deformable than bone. Also, its Poisson's ratio should favor lateral expansion of cartilage under compressive load so that the surface area of opposing articular surfaces is greater than that of the subchondral bone. If cartilage is to fulfil this role effectively in its usual environment of rapid repetitive loads, it should rapidly recover a significant proportion of its deformation in the unloaded phase, like an ideal elastic body. While there is a dearth of experimental observations and theoretical considerations, the limited information available for the hip joint indicate that normal articular cartilage is remarkably well designed for load carriage. A detailed discussion has been given by Freeman.[91]

Within cartilage, both proteoglycans and collagen contribute to load carriage. The collagen resists tensile forces within the matrix and retains proteoglycans, probably by a process of physical entanglement. The proteoglycans retain water in the matrix and regulate its flow both by osmosis and by reduction of the permeability of the cartilage. By doing so, proteoglycans prevents the collapse of cartilage under physiological loads whether rapidly or gradually applied. In unloaded cartilage, the osmotic pressure of the proteoglycans provokes imbibition of fluid which, in turn, stresses the collagen fibers of the matrix. Bulk movement of proteoglycans and water under loads of brief duration permits rapid elastic deformation of the matrix accompanied by a rise in the fluid pressure and the stresses in collagen. Under a prolonged static or dynamic load, a small amount of water is squeezed from the matrix. Both this viscous deformation and the elastic deformation of cartilage are greater than those in bone. Like other tissues of the body, cartilage appears to possess a large functional reserve. Both the stiffness and thickness of cartilage may be reduced to about 25% of normal values without materially affecting load spreading, force attenuating and damping properties of cartilage that serve to protect the subchondral bone.

While the precise nature of mechanical failure of articular cartilage is unknown, at least two causes seem plausible.[69, 91] When subjected to large tensile forces, the collagen fibers in cartilage could undergo mechanical failure with compressive deformation. In practice, this seems to occur only after severe trauma, such as central fracture dislocation of the hip, when acute cartilage necrosis often follows. Alternatively, degenerative processes may provoke depletion of proteoglycans from the cartilage, so that the matrix shows a foreshortened fatigue life or weakness in tension secondary to the associated loss of water. Also, the weakness engendered by biochemical alteration of aging articular cartilage may be related to changes in wear characteristics which will be described.

Lubrication

The other remarkable attributes of normal synovial joints are the low frictional forces and minimal erosion of the cartilaginous surfaces. In the past two decades, many workers have studied the lubrication of human joints, which is fully discussed elsewhere.[98-101] In view of the obvious relevance of biological lubrication to the replacement of human joints, a brief account follows.

In Figure 5-30A, a schematic view of a typical human joint is shown. Opposing curved surfaces of articular cartilage are bathed in synovial fluid, which is secreted by the joint lining or synovial membrane. In turn, the synovial membrane is attached to a stronger collagenous membrane or capsule, which limits the motion of the cartilaginous surfaces so that they do not dislocate spontaneously.

Measurements of static coefficients of friction in whole synovial joints and in small pieces of cartilage have been undertaken by many workers.[101, 102] Representative values would appear to be a coefficient of friction in the human hip joint of about 0.003 to 0.015, as recorded by Little.[75] For a piece of isolated articular cartilage against glass or bone, values of 0.0014 to 0.07 are reported by Walker *et al.*[102] As shown in Chapter 13, the friction in synovial joints is exceptionally

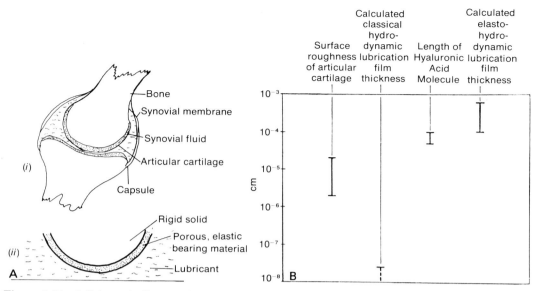

Figure 5-30. *A*. Schematic diagram of a human articular joint. *B*. The graph reveals important dimensions in a study of human joint lubrication. (Reproduced with permission from V. Wright.[78])

low by engineering standards. This is particularly true when the unfavorable biological conditions of service for human joints are considered, with low speed oscillating motion. Further studies have confirmed the presence of boundary and fluid film lubrication, although the relative contribution of each remains unclear. One solution to this problem is a mathematical analysis (Fig. 5-30*B*), which compares the surface roughness of cartilage (*e.g.*, at least 10^{-5} cm), the minimum fluid film thickness required for hydrodynamic lubrication (*e.g.*, 10^{-8} cm), the length of a hyaluronic acid molecule in synovial fluid (*e.g.*, 10^{-4} cm), and the film thickness required for elastohydrodynamic lubrication (*e.g.*, 5×10^{-3} cm).[103] From this consideration and from earlier work, it has been assumed that synovial fluid plays a major role in the lubrication of articular joints. In fact, more recent studies reveal that saline lubricates articular cartilage nearly as well as synovial fluid.[104] This and other observations have led to renewed controversy regarding the principal mode of human joint lubrication. The mechanisms of lubrication under discussion are:

Boundary Lubrication. The opposing surfaces may be deliberately contaminated with a substance chosen for its ability to be adsorbed by the surfaces, and to remain adsorbed at a range of loads and rubbing speeds, and to possess a molecular structure which offers little resistance to relative motion between the two ad-

sorbed layers (Fig. 5-31*A*).

Hydrostatic Lubrication. If the solid surfaces are completely separated by an unbroken film of fluid, the frictional forces depend upon the properties of the fluid (Fig. 5-31*B*). If the film is thick enough to prevent contact between asperities on the surfaces, but not so thick (in relation to its viscosity and other factors) as to permit turbulent motion of fluid within the film, the frictional force to be overcome results from the shearing of the fluid and depends upon the viscosity of the fluid. The frictional force is directly proportional to the relative speed of the two surfaces and to the wetted area, and inversely proportional to the film thickness. In the main, the film thickness is inversely proportional to the normal force, so that the frictional force is related to the normal force.

The previous discussion refers to a lubricant which shows a viscosity that is independent of shear rate, (*e.g.*, a Newtonian fluid). If the fluid has a viscosity that varies with the rate of shear and in particular if its viscosity is lower at high rates of shear (such as is exhibited by synovial fluid), then the behavior of the system will tend to approach that associated with boundary friction.[105, 106] To show that a bearing is lubricated hydrostatically, it is essential to show how the necessary pressure is supplied.

Squeeze-film Lubrication. If two solid surfaces are forced together with a fluid film between them, fluid will tend to flow out of the

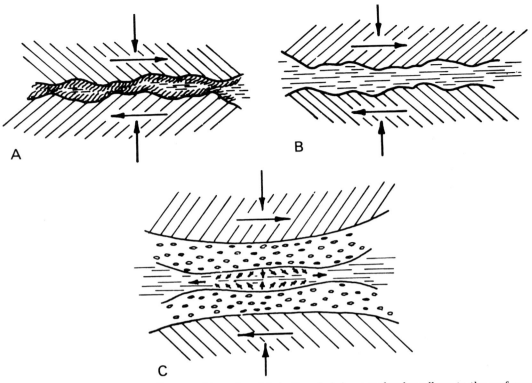

Figure 5-31. *A.* Schematic diagram of boundary lubrication. Lubricant molecules adhere to the surfaces to keep them apart. *B.* Schematic diagram of pure fluid-film lubrication. The fluid-film between the surfaces can be maintained by a hydrostatic, squeeze film or hydrodynamic mechanisms. *C.* Schematic diagram illustrates weeping squeeze-film or self-pressurized hydrostatic lubrication. As the load increases fluid is squeezed from the cartilage to provide a lubricating layer in the joint space. (*A, B,* and *C,* reproduced with permission from E. L. Radin and I. L. Paul.[100])

film (Fig. 5-31*B*). With time, the film thickness will tend to diminish under load, unless the supply of fluid under pressure is replenished continuously from an outside source. If the fluid is sufficiently viscous and if the load is applied intermittently, the fluid film may persist long enough to be useful. Upon removal of the load, expressed fluid in close proximity to the edges of the loaded region may be reimbibed. Such squeeze-film lubrication has been hypothesized to be one modality of lubrication in synovial joints.[100, 101]

Hydrodynamic Lubrication. Occasionally, a wedge-shaped film of fluid can be maintained between two sliding surfaces by the action of hydrodynamic forces in the fluid (Fig. 5-31*B*). Here the sliding surfaces must possess appropriate geometry, so that there is a wedge-shaped gap between them which contains a film of varied thickness. This type of lubricating regime occurs only when the surfaces slide at some

minimum rate. It is another possible mode of lubrication for joints in motion.

Elastohydrodynamic Lubrication. In the previously described hydrodynamic mode, considerable pressures exist in the loaded region of the fluid film, which also apply to the adjacent solid surfaces. If the adjacent solid surfaces undergo significant deformation and change in shape in comparison to the film thickness, the regime is said to be elastohydrodynamic.[102]

Self-pressurized Hydrostatic or Weeping Lubrication. When a piece of glass is pressed against articular cartilage a watery fluid "weeps" from the compressed articular cartilage and forms a lubricating layer between the two surfaces (Fig. 5-31*C*).[99, 106] The effective pore size of articulating cartilage is estimated to be about 6 nm (60 Å)[107] although occasional pores with diameters as large as 100 nm (1000 Å) have been reported.[100] The bulk of smaller pores permit only small molecules to pass while large muco-

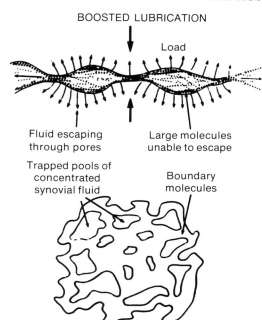

BOOSTED LUBRICATION

Load

Fluid escaping through pores

Large molecules unable to escape

Trapped pools of concentrated synovial fluid

Boundary molecules

Figure 5-32. Schematic diagram to show "boosted lubrication" with movement of water and solutes in or out of the articular cartilage. (Reproduced with permission from R. B. Duthie and A. B. Ferguson, Jr.[1])

polysaccharides are retained within the cartilage matrix and the large hyaluronate and protein molecules in the synovial fluid are blocked from entry into the cartilage. McCutchen[106] suggests that wept fluid creates the fluid film in the highly loaded joint. Such a pressed weeping or self-pressurized hydrostatic lubrication may well occur although its contribution to joint lubricating mechanisms remains unclear.

Boosted Lubrication. During the loading of a joint, the hydrostatic pressure built up in the lubricant trapped between opposing joint surfaces may extrude the fluid out of the joint space through the cartilage pores. As the fluid filters through the cartilage, the large molecules of highly viscid hyaluronate might collect on the sieve-like articular surface, especially in the depressions between the asperities. The proponents of this thesis suggest that the concentrated lakes of hyaluronate boost the effectiveness of fluid lubrication mechanisms (Fig. 5-32).[100, 108, 109]

Both the weeping and boosted mechanisms would explain the diminution of the coefficient of friction observed in animal joints that undergo increased loads. Both of them require a porosity of cartilage that impedes hyaluronate but not water. Certain confirmatory evidence indicates that experimental inhibition of the flow of water through cartilage interferes with joint lubrication. Such observations, however, do not specifically confirm the role of weeping or boosted phenomenon as significant factors in the lubrication of human joints.

Many studies have been undertaken with human and animal joints in an effort to determine the relative contributions of each of these modalities of lubrication. Useful information includes assessment of surface roughness of articular cartilage, film thickness, viscosity and other properties of the fluid, and measurements of the change in frictional forces with variation in the viscosity of the synovial fluid. While the reader is referred to the many observations available elsewhere,[101-104, 110] present evidence from frictional measurements in entire joints indicates that the predominant mode is boundary lubrication by adsorbed hyaluronate-protein, perhaps combined with fluid film lubrication by a fluid of viscosity much greater than that of synovial fluid. A principal role of the hyaluronate-protein in synovial fluid appears to be the protection of the articular surfaces from abrasive wear. Since both the matrix of cartilage and the effective lubricant in synovial fluid consist of hydrated proteoglycan gels, it is not surprising that recent work[101] has downgraded the significance of synovial fluid as an effective lubricant.

Recently, Mansour and Mow[111] published results on a mathematical and physical model of articular cartilage. The model attempts to account for both the physical properties of articular cartilage and the previous theories of joint lubrication. They observe that the permeability of articular cartilage decreases as the applied load and the resultant compressive strain increase. As the compressive strain increases fluid exudes from the cartilage into the joint space, both at the leading edge of the moving contact area and between portions of opposing cartilaginous surfaces. With further elevation of the applied load on the cartilage its permeability diminishes. With the diminution of permeability the joint fluid on the articular surface in the joint space cannot flow back into the cartilage as easily as it accumulated into the joint space. Fluid transport thereby is limited so that further fluid does not accumulate in the joint space. With removal of the applied load the cartilage recovers and shows increased permeability. In turn fluid transport is facilitated so that rehydration of cartilage ensues. The relevant mathematical model is a one-dimensional consolidation process of a porous nonlinearly permeable

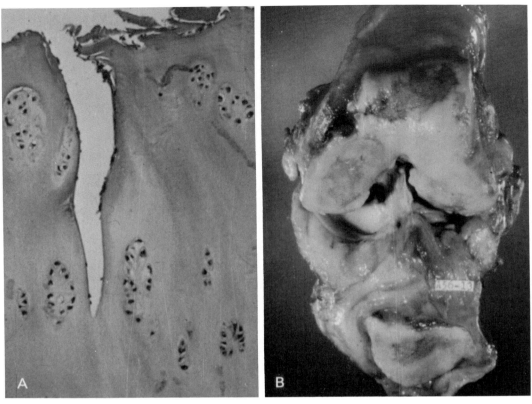

Figure 5-33. *A*. Photomicrograph of articular cartilage that has undergone early degenerative change. Deterioration of the matrix and alteration in cells is evident. *B*. A gross anatomic specimen of a knee joint with degenerative arthritis. Portions of denuded subchondral bone are evident adjacent to regions of intact articular cartilage.

layer of cartilage whose permeability varies linearly with applied load so that the permeability of cartilage is dependent on the extent to which it is deformed. Further confirmation of this work will be necessary.

Degeneration of Cartilage

With advancement in age, cartilage gradually undergoes structural change which is characterized by splitting and fraying.[112] While this asymptomatic degenerative process is very commonly observed among the general population at necropsy, it remains unclear how such fibrillation is related to primary or degenerative arthritis. Osteoarthrosis, or osteoarthritis, is a disease of synovial joints which culminates in the loss of the original articular cartilage from part or all of the joint surface, with destructive loss of the underlying bone (Figs. 5-33, 5-34).[112, 113] Beneath its denuded surface, the bone shows active remodeling, with thickening of trabeculae (osteosclerosis) and with the formation of cysts filled with nonosseous or partly liquified material. At the periphery of the joint, bony outgrowths (osteophytes) may project beyond the original joint margin. Also, new osseous or nonosseous material may spread across the peripheral articular cartilage. In many, if not most patients, no precipitating factors can be discerned. The process is therefore called primary osteoarthrosis. Alternatively, some individuals show a predilection for arthritis by the presence of: an inflammatory disorder such as infection or rheumatoid arthritis;[114] a structural abnormality such as a fracture, dislocation, Perthes' disease, or slipped epiphysis;[115] bone infarction;[112] or a metabolic disorder such as gout;[114] or ochronosis.[116] In such a case, the term secondary osteoarthrosis may be applied. Alternatively, by definition, the term rheumatoid arthritis or gouty arthritis implies that the process is a secondary phenomenon. Many workers have attempted to define the pathogenesis of primary osteoarthrosis. The most widely held view is

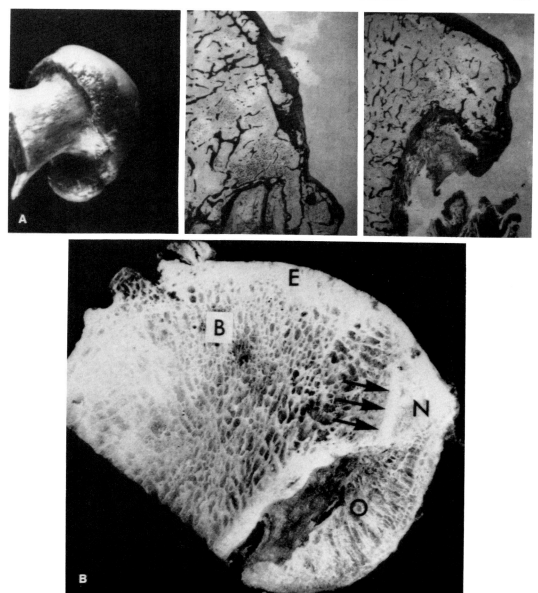

Figure 5-34. *A* and *B*. A gross specimen and cross sections of a human femoral head with evidence of degenerative arthritis. Erosion of cartilage with loss of congruity of the joint and osteophyte formation and cystic change is evident. *E,* eroded articular cartilage; *B,* subchondral bone; *N,* new bone formation; *O,* osteophyte. (Reproduced with permission from Dr. A. B. Ferguson, Jr.)

that expressed by Collins[71] and others that the first tissue affected is the articular cartilage. Other workers[113, 114] have suggested that the primary event is alteration of the blood flow in the subchondral bone. More recently, Radin and Paul[104] have suggested that the initiation arises with fatigue fractures of subchondral bone which provoke alteration of the modulus of rigidity of bone (Fig. 5-35*A, B*). With the deposition of

callus around the microfatigue fractures (Fig. 5-35*C*), the bone is believed to become more rigid, so that the overlying cartilage ceases to be well protected from dynamic impulsive loads by a resilient element of bone. Since morbid anatomical studies reveal the presence of cartilaginous abnormalities in the absence of gross pathological lesions in the adjacent bone, present evidence favors a theory of degenerative arthritis based

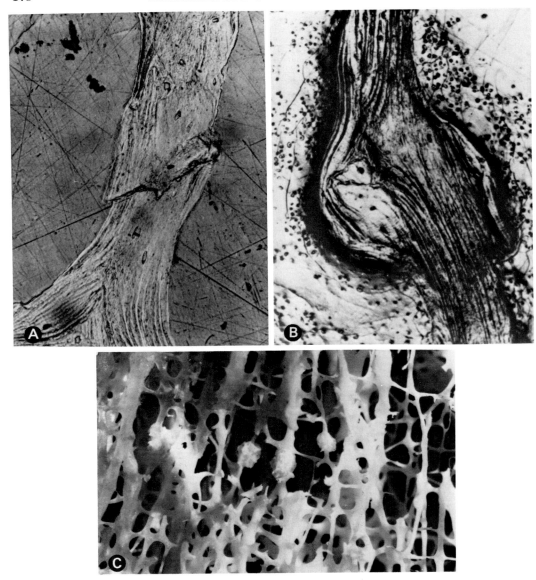

Figures 5-35. Photomicrographs of osseous microfatigue fractures in cross section are present. *A* shows a recent fracture while *B* shows a microfracture with callus formation. Specimens were prepared from rabbit femora subjected to cyclic impulsive loading. (Reproduced with kind permission from Dr. E. L. Radin.) *C.* Photomicrograph of callus formation around a healing trabecular microfatigue fracture. (Reproduced with permission from Dr. M. A. R. Freeman.)

on primary failure of articular cartilage. Nevertheless, the recent suggestions on the primary involvement of bone have provided a valuable stimulus for workers to reconsider the functional relationships of the several tissues that comprise joints.

While fibrillation appears to be the initial abnormality in a joint destined to develop pri-

mary or osteoarthritis, the immediate cause of fibrillation remains unclear. Freeman[113] speculates that it may be due to fatigue failure of the cartilage, perhaps accelerated by preliminary mechanical disruption of the superficial collagen network or possibly by a biochemical abnormality such as a glycosaminoglycans deficiency in the matrix. After the initiation of fatigue failure, propagation of the degenerative process might occur as abrasive wear of the softened and weakened cartilage. Once the degradation has occurred, mature chondrocytes have only a limited capacity to effect intrinsic repair by production of proteoglycans, but no capacity to accelerate collagen metabolism.[113] Only a modest extrinsic repair procedure with the production of nonosseous periarticular or subarticular material seems to occur.

Recent Studies on Degenerative Wear Particles

Recently Mears et al.[117] have studied synovial fluid aspirates from human joints that show evidence of degenerative arthritis. By the application of ferrographic analysis[118, 119] these workers have been able to isolate degenerative wear particles from the synovial fluid samples.[120] The observations are fully discussed in Chapter 16. In brief, they indicate that wear particles of articular cartilage, of highly specific sizes and morphologies, are shed from joint surfaces in the early stages of arthritis.[121] As the wear process evolves, the morphology of the particles changes, bony particles also begin to appear in synovial fluid. The most logical explanation for the changes in morphology of the wear particles is an antecedent change in the biochemical composition and thereby the biomechanical properties of the articular cartilage and subchondral bone. By the use of electron microscopy and electron probe microanalysis, minute particles of bone and cartilage have been observed within polymorphonuclear leukocytes isolated from synovial fluid aspirates. It seems not unlikely that biological wear particle debris of highly peculiar morphologies may be shed by articular surfaces at certain stages of degenerative arthritis. The free particles may be engulfed by ameboid white cells in the synovial fluid. Engulfment of certain types of particles may initiate lysosomal enzyme release by the phagocytes, as is known to occur in gout and pseudogout. Liberated and activated lysosomal enzymes may degrade the exposed articular surfaces and accelerate the rate of joint destruction. Such a hypothesis would account for the rapid exacerbations of joint symptoms and the precipitous deterioration of articular surfaces that has been observed in patients with longstanding degenerative arthritis. Further studies on the biochemical composition of the isolated wear particles may also shed much light on the origin of this puzzling entity.

REFERENCES

1. Duthie, R. B., and Ferguson, A. B., Jr. *Mercer's Orthopaedic Surgery,* Williams & Wilkins Co., Baltimore, 1973.
2. Hirohata, K., and Morimoto, K. *Ultrastructure of Bone and Joint Diseases,* Grune & Stratton, New York, 1971.
3. Huxley, H. E. *Brit. Med. Bull., 12:*171, 1956.
4. Bourne, G. H., editor. *The Structure and Function of Muscle,* 2nd ed., p. 14, Academic Press, New York, 1972.
5. Hirohata, K., and Morimoto, K. *Ultrastructure of Bone and Joint Diseases,* p. 21, Grune & Stratton, New York, 1971.
6. Gregg, D. E., and Coffman, J. D. Skeletal muscle circulation. In *The Physiological Basis of Medical Practice,* p. 352, edited by C. H. Best and N. B. Taylor, Williams & Wilkins Co., Baltimore, 1961.
7. Huxley, H. E. *Sci. Am. 199:*80, 1958.
8. Bell, G. H., Davidson, J. N., and Scarborough, H. *Textbook of Physiology and Biochemistry,* E. & S. Livingstone Ltd., Edinburgh, 1965.
9. Bell, G. H., Davidson, J. N., and Scarborough, H. *Textbook of Physiology and Biochemistry,* p. 807, E. & S. Livingstone Ltd., Edinburgh, 1965.
10. Sokoloff, L., and Bland, J. H. *The Musculoskeletal System,* Williams & Wilkins Co., Baltimore, 1975.
11. Carlson, B. M., Cell and tissue interactions in regenerating muscle. In *Muscle Biology,* vol. I, p. 13, edited by R. G. Cossers, Marcel Dekker, New York, 1972.
12. Sloper, J. C., Batesan, R. B., Hindle, D., and Warren, J., Muscle regeneration in man and in mouse. In *Regeneration of Striated Muscle and Myogenesis,* p. 157, edited by A. Mauro, S. A. Shafig and A. T. Milhorat, Excerpta Medica, Amsterdam, 1970.
13. Castor, C. W., The study of the connective tissue. In *Arthritis and Allied Conditions,* 8th ed., edited by J. L. Hollander and D. J. McCarty, p. 57, Lea & Febiger, Philadelphia, 1972.
14. Schubert, M., and Hamerman, D. *A Primer of Connective Tissue Chemistry,* p. 20, Lea & Febiger, Philadelphia, 1968.
15. Moment, G. B., *General Zoology,* p. 100, Riverside Press, Cambridge, Mass., 1959.
16. Hunter, J. M., Steindel, C., Salisbury, R., and Hughes, D. *J. Biomed. Mater. Res., 8:*155, 1974.
17. Salisbury, R. E., McKeel, D., Pruitt, B. A., Mason, A. D., Jr., Palermo, N., and Wade, C. W. R., *J. Biomed. Mater. Res., 8:*175, 1974.
18. Salisbury, R. E., Mason, A. D., Jr., Levine, N. S., Pruitt, B. A., and Wade, C. W. R., *J. Trauma, 14:*580, 1974.
19. Sokoloff, L., and Bland, J. H., *The Musculoskeletal System,* p. 5, Williams & Wilkins, Baltimore, 1975.
20. Gray, H. *Anatomy of the Human Body,* edited by C. M. Goss, Lea & Febiger, Philadelphia, 1975.
21. Pritchard, J. J., General histology of bone. In *The Biochemistry and Physiology of Bone,* vol. I, p. 1, edited by G. H. Bourne, Academic Press, New York, 1972.

22. Ramp, W. K., *Clin. Ortho. Rel. Res., 104:*311, 1975.

23. Talmage, R. V., Matthews, J. L., Martin, J. H., Kennedy, J. W., III, Davis, W. L., and Roycroft, J. H., Jr., in *Calcium-Regulating Hormones,* p. 284, edited by R. V. Talmadge, M. Owens and J. A. Parsons, Excerpta Medica, Amsterdam, 1975.

24. Pritchard, J. J., The osteoblast. In *The Biochemistry and Physiology of Bone,* vol. I, p. 21, edited by G. H. Bourne, Academic Press, New York, 1972.

25. Belanger, L. F., Osteocytic resorption. In *The Biochemistry and Physiology of Bone,* vol. 3, p.141, edited by G. H. Bourne, Academic Press, New York, 1972.

26. Hirohata, K., and Morimoto, K. *Ultrastructure of Bone and Joint Diseases,* p. 17, Grune & Stratton, New York, 1971.

27. Rassmussen, H., and Bordier, P. *The Physiological and Cellular Basis of Metabolic Bone Disease,* p. 32, Williams & Wilkins Co., Baltimore, 1974.

28. Rassmussen, H., and Bordier, P. *The Physiological and Cellular Basis of Metabolic Bone Disease,* p. 23, Williams & Wilkins Co., Baltimore, 1974.

29. Talmage, R. V., *Am. J. Anat., 129:*467, 1970.

30. Mears, D. C., *Endocr., 88:*1021, 1971.

31. Mears, D. C., *Ox. Med. Gaz., 22:*60, 1970.

32. Hancox, N. M., The osteoclast. In *The Biochemistry and Physiology of Bone,* vol. I., p. 45, edited by G. H. Bourne, Academic Press, New York, 1972.

33. Barnes, M. J., Biochemistry of collagens from mineralized tissues. In *Hard Tissue Growth, Repair and Remineralization,* p. 247, Excerpta Medica, Amsterdam, 1973.

34. Brown, C. H., *Structural Materials in Animals,* John Wiley & Son, New York, 1975.

35. Brookes, M., Elkin, A. C., Harrison, R. G., Heald, C. B., *Lancet, 1:*1078, 1961.

36. Vaughan, J. M., *The Physiology of Bone,* p. 66, Clarendon Press, Oxford, 1970.

37. Herring, G. M., The organic matrix of bone. In *The Biochemistry and Physiology of Bone,* vol. I., p. 148, edited by G. H. Bourne, Academic Press, New York, 1972.

38. McKusick, V. A., *Heritable Disorders of Connective Tissue,* p. 521, C. V. Mosby Co., St. Louis, 1972.

39. Omdahl, S. L., and H. F. Deluca, *Physiol. Rev. 53:*327, 1973.

40. McLean, F. C., and Urist, M. R., *Bone,* p. 72, University of Chicago Press, Chicago, 1968.

41. Brookes, M., *The Blood Supply of Bone,* p. 15, Appleton-Century-Crofts, New York, 1971.

42. Crock, H. V., *The Blood Supply of the Lower Limb Bones in Man,* p. 4, E. & S. Livingstone Ltd., Edinburgh, 1967.

43. Rhinelander, F. W., *J. Bone. Jt. Surg., 50A:*784, 1968.

44. Glimcher, M. J., and Krane, S. M., The organization and structure of bone, and the mechanism of calcification. In *A Treatise on Collagen,* vol. 2, p. 256, edited by B. S. Gould and G. N. Ramachandra, Academic Press, London, 1968.

45. Fleisch, H., *Clin. Ortho. Rel. Res., 32:*170, 1964.

46. Anderson, H. C., Calcium-accumulating vesicles in the intercellular matrix of bone. In *Hard Tissue Growth, Repair and Remineralization,* p. 213, Excerpta Medica, Amsterdam, 1973.

47. Anderson, H. C., *J. Cell Biol., 41:*59, 1969.

48. Bonucci, E., *Z. Zellforsch. Mikrosh. Anat., 103:*192, 1970.

49. Pautard, F. G. E., The molecular organization of bone, In *Modern Trends in Orthopaedics,* p. 5, edited by S. M. P. Clark, Butterworths, London, 1964.

50. Russell, R. G. G., Bisaz, S., and Fleisch, H. *Arch. Int. Med., 124:*571, 1969.

51. Harris, W. H., and Heaney, R. P., *N. Eng. J. Med., 280:*193, 253, 303, 1969.

52. Tachdjian, M. O., *Pediatric Orthopaedics,* W. B. Saunders Co., Philadelphia, 1972.

53. Smith, R., Russell, R. G. G., Bishop, M. C., Woods, C. G., and Bishop, M., *Quart. J. Med., 42:*235, 1973.

54. Salter, R. B., Harris, W. R., *J. Bone and Jt. Surg., 45A:*587, 1963.

55. Ham, A. W., *Histology,* p. 247, J. B. Lippincott Co., Philadelphia, 1965.

56. Rockwood, C. A., and Green, D. P., *Fractures,* J. B. Lippincott Co., Philadelphia, 1975.

57. Tachdjian, M. O., *Pediatric Orthopaedics,* p. 1543, W. B. Saunders Co., Philadelphia, 1972.

58. Rhinelander, F. W., Circulation in bone. In *The Biochemistry and Physiology of Bone,* vol. 2, p. 1, edited by G. H. Bourne, Academic Press, New York, 1972.

59. Gallinaro, P., Perren, S., Crova, M., and Rahn, B., *La osteosintesi con placca a compressione,* Aulo Gaggi Editore, Bologna, 1969.

60. Danis, R., *Theorie et Pratique de L'osteosynthese,* p. 3, Masson & Cie, Paris, 1949.

61. Schenk, R., and Willenegger, H., *Symp. Biol., Hung., 7:*75, 1967.

62. Müller, M. E., Allgower, M., and Willenegger, H., *Manuel of Internal Fixation,* Springer-Verlag, Berlin, 1970.

63. Perren, S. M., Huggler, A., Russenberger, M., Allgöwer, M., Mathys, R., Schenk, R., Willenegger, H., and Müller, M. E., *Acta. Ortho. Scand.,* suppl. *125:*19, 1969.

63a. Hutzschenreuter, P., Allgöwer, M., Borel, J. F., and Perren, S. M., *Experientia, 29:*103, 1973.

64. Perren, S. M., Matter, P., Ruedi, R., and Allgöwer, M., Biomechanics of fracture healing after internal fixation. In *Surgery Annual, 1975,* p. 361, edited by L. M. Nyhus, Appleton-Century-Crofts, New York, 1975.

65. Rang, M., *Children's Fractures,* J. B. Lippincott Co., Philadelphia, 1974.

66. Gray, H., *Anatomy of the Human Body,* p. 271, edited by C. M. Goss, Lea & Febiger, Philadelphia, 1975.

67. Mankin, H. J., *Bull. Rheum. Dis., 17:*447, 1967.

68. Freeman, M. A. R., editor. *Adult Articular Cartilage,* Grune & Stratton, New York, 1972.

69. Mankin, H. J., The articular cartilages. In *A.A.O.S. Instructional Course Lectures,* vol. 19, p. 204, C. V. Mosby Co., St. Louis, 1970.

70. Mankin, H. J., *A.A.O.S. Instructional Course Lectures,* vol. 19, p. 205, C. V. Mosby Co., St.

Louis, 1970.

71. Collins, D. H., *The Pathology of Articular and Spinal Disease*, p. 35, Edward Arnold, London, 1949.

72. Walker, P. S., Dowson, D., Longfield, M. D., and Wright, V., *Ann. Rheum. Dis.*, 27:512, 1968.

73. Benninghoff, A., *Z. Anat. Entwicklungsesch.*, 76:43, 1925.

74. Cameron, D. A., and Robinson, R. A., *J. Bone Jt. Surg.*, 40A:163, 1958.

75. Little, K., Pimm, L. H., and Trueta, J., *J. Bone Jt. Surg.*, 40B:123, 1958.

76. Weiss, C., Rosenberg, L., and Helfet, A. J., *J. Bone Jt. Surg.*, 50A:663, 1968.

77. Mankin, H. J., *N. Eng. J. Med.*, 291:1285, 1974.

78. Wright, V., editor. *Lubrication and Wear in Joints*, J. B. Lippincott, Philadelphia, 1969.

79. Lipshitz, H., Etheredge, R., and Glimcher, M. J., *J. Bone Jt. Surg.*, 57A:527, 1975.

80. Howell, D. S., Pita, J. C., Marquez, J. F., and Madruga, J. E., *J. Clin. Invest.*, 47:1121, 1968.

81. Maroudas, A., and Evans, H., *Connective Tiss. Res.*, 1:69, 1972.

82. Schubert, M., *Connective Tissue*, p. 119, Little, Brown & Co., Boston, 1964.

83. Ingelwork, B. E., and Saaf, J., *Acta Ortho. Scand.*, 17:303, 1948.

84. Ekholm, R., *Acta Anat., 11,* suppl. 2:1, 1951.

85. McKibben, B., and Holdsworth, F. S., *J. Bone Jt. Surg.*, 48B:793, 1966.

86. Brower, T. D., Akahoshi, Y., and Orlic, P., *J. Bone Jt. Surg.*, 44A:456, 1962.

87. Bywaters, E. C. L., *J. Path. Bact.*, 44:247, 1937.

88. Dickens, F., and Weil-Malherbe, H., *Nature, 138:*30, 1936.

89. Rosenthal, O., Bowie, M. A., and Wagoner, G., *J. Cell Physiol.*, 17:221, 1941.

90. Krane, S., Parsons, V., and Kevin, A. S., Studies of the metabolism of epiphyseal cartilage. In *Cartilage Degradation and Repair*, p. 246, edited by C. A. L. Bassett, N.A.S.N.C.R., Washington, D.C., 1967.

91. Freeman, M. A. R., editor. *Adult Articular Cartilage*, p. 238, Grune & Stratton, New York, 1973.

92. Hirsch, C., *Acta Chir. Scand., 90,* suppl. 83:9, 1944.

93. McCutchen, C. W., *Wear*, 5:1, 1962.

94. Sokoloff, L., *Fed. Proc.*, 25(3):1089, 1969.

95. Kempson, G. E., Freeman, M. A. R., and Swanson, S. A. V., *J. Biomech.*, 4:239, 1971.

96. Freeman, M. A. R., editor. *Adult Articular Cartilage*, p. 171, Grune & Stratton, New York, 1973.

96a. Brown, T. D., and Ferguson, A. B., Jr., *J. Bone Jt. Surg.*, 60A:619, 1978.

97. Radin, E. L., and Paul, I. L., *Arthr. and Rheum.*, 13:2, 139, 1970.

98. Wright, V., editor. *Lubrication and Wear in Joints*, p. 9, J. B. Lippincott Co., Philadelphia, 1969.

99. McCutchen, C. W., *Nature, 184:*1284, 1959.

100. Radin, E. L., and Paul, I. L., *J. Bone Jt. Surg.*, 54A:607, 1972.

101. Freeman, M. A. R., editor. *Adult Articular Cartilage*, p. 247, Grune & Stratton, New York, 1973.

102. Walker, P. S., Unsworth, A., Dowson, D., Sikorski, J., and Wright, V., *Ann. Rheum. Dis.*, 29(6):591, 1970.

103. Dowson, D., Wright, V., and Longfield, M. D., *Biomed. Eng.*, 4:160, 1969.

104. Radin, E. L., and Paul, I. L., *Arthr. and Rheum.*, 13:139, 1970.

105. Hamerwoke, D., and Schubert, M., *Am. J. Med.*, 33:555, 1962.

106. McCutchen, C. W., *Clin. Ortho. Rel. Res.*, 64:18, 1969.

107. McCutchen, C. W., *Wear*, 5:1017, 1962.

108. Tanner, R. I., *Phys. Med. Biol.*, 11:119, 1966.

109. Walker, P. S., Sikorski, J., Dowson, D., Longfield, M. D., *Nature*, 225:956, 1970.

110. Charnley, J., *Triangle*, 4:175, 1960.

111. Mansour, J. M., and Mow, V. C., *J. Bone Jt. Surg.*, 58A:509, 1976.

112. Duthie, R. B., and Ferguson, A. B., Jr., *Mercer's Orthopaedic Surgery*, p. 661, Williams & Wilkins Co., Baltimore, 1973.

113. Freeman, M. A. R., editor. *Adult Articular Cartilage*, p. 287, Grune & Stratton, New York, 1973.

114. Boyle, J. A., and Buchanan, W. W., *Clinical Rheumatology*, p. 74, Blackwell, Oxford, 1971.

115. Tachdjian, M. O., *Pediatric Orthopaedics*, p. 275, W. B. Saunders Co., Philadelphia, 1972.

116. McKusick, V. A., *Heritable Disorders of Connective Tissue*, p. 455, C. V. Mosby Co., St. Louis, 1972.

117. Mears, D. C., Westcott, V. C., Hanley, E. N. Jr., and Rutkowski, R., *Wear, 50:* 115, 1978.

118. Scott, D., Seifert, W. W., and Westcott, V. C., *Sci. Am.*, 230:88, 1974.

119. Scott, D., Seifert, W. W., and Westcott, V. C., *Wear*, 34:251, 1975.

120. Mears, D. C., *Ortho. Survey*, 1:64, 1977.

121. Brookes, M., and Helal, B., *J. Bone Jt. Surg.*, 50B:493, 1968.

6

The Effect of Mechanical Force on Tissues and Cells

Excessive mechanical forces applied abruptly to most musculoskeletal tissues and cells provoke disruption, of which a fracture of a bone is a representative example. When a lesser magnitude of force is applied to a tissue over a prolonged period, other changes in the tissue may ensue. Some of the changes such as elastic or plastic deformation are initiated solely by the mechanical perturbation itself. For a century, however, workers have observed that mechanical forces can initiate changes in cell metabolism.[1] One clinical example is the erosion of a syphilitic aneurysm of the thoracic aorta through the sternum and rib cage to present clinically in the subcutaneous tissues of the chest wall. The bony elements undergo resorption in response to the pulsatile flow of blood with intermittent distension of the aneurysm and impingement on the bone. Another example is the wasting of a limb, including the disuse osteoporosis of bone that follows paralysis of an extremity. As discussed in Chapter 1, early workers such as Koch[2] observed that the trabeculae in bone follow closely the lines of maximal weight-bearing stress. Mathematical analysis showed surprising agreement between the weight-bearing forces and the corresponding thickness, configuration and microstructure of bone. After 1920, Thompson[3] undertook repositional osteotomies in the long bones of experimental animals. Before and after the surgery, he studied the microstructure of the bone. He documented a marked change in the alignment of the principal columns of trabeculae as they underwent reorganization to best resist the new force pattern associated with the realignment of the limb. Glucksman[4] also recorded the changes in microstructures of embryonic tissues that were initiated by the application of various extraneous mechanical forces. Since then, numerous workers have studied the biological alterations of tissues to the imposition of sundry mechanical forces. In 1955, Fukada and Yasuda[5] recorded a minute piezoelectric potential that accompanied the mechanical deformation of bone. Other workers such as Bassett and Becker[6] confirmed the observation. The potential clinical implications of this observation were immediately apparent to scores of workers. If mechanical forces applied to bone, and presumably other musculoskeletal tissues, induced biological response such as the production or removal of extracellular matrix by a piezoelectric transducer, then therapeutic manipulation of regeneration might be undertaken by the imposition of a supplementary electric potential. Since that time many studies on the mechanisms whereby musculoskeletal tissues respond to mechanical forces have been performed. Other workers have attempted to regulate regenerative events by electrical stimulation.[7-10] While some of the independent observations are complementary, others are conflicting or confusing. In a recent review, Brighton[11] has emphasized the present degree of bewilderment in the events that intervene between mechanical deformation of tissues and metabolic responses, although virtually all of the workers in the field agree that as yet obscure relationships must exist.

In the past decade, with the widespread application of implants for internal and external fixation of fractures and for reconstructive procedures such as total joint replacements, many clinicians have noted the changes in tissues, especially bone, that seemingly are induced by the presence of the implant. With the discrepancy between the mechanical properties of the tissue and the implant the mechanical environment of the tissues is thereby altered to initiate biological remodeling. Stress-protection with osteoporosis of a segment of bone adjacent to a rigid onlay plate is the best known example.[12, 13] Such observations have encouraged workers both to alter the designs and properties of materials for surgical implants to lessen the undesirable biological side-effects or even to produce favorable biological remodeling.

At present this field is undergoing rapid

change. The underlying mechanisms which control the biological responses of tissues to mechanical forces are obscure. In view of its potential clinical significance, this chapter is an attempt to organize the present knowledge. It should be emphasized that the conclusions drawn here may be substantially altered over the course of the next decade.

THE EFFECTS OF MECHANICAL FORCES IMPOSED ON CELLS AND TISSUES IN CULTURE

It is well recognized that mechanical deformation of bone is associated with marked change in bone growth and remodeling although the precise mechanisms remain obscure. Present evidence suggests that there are two separate mechanisms, one which enables bone and cartilage to respond to static mechanical forces and another which enables these tissues to respond to dynamic load. The relationship between these two hypothetical systems is not fully known. While the studies performed on the isolated specimens of bone or cartilage under static load in tissue culture clearly indicate that isolated chondrocytes or osteocytes may show alteration in the rates of mitosis and the production of matrix, studies in vivo have failed to show any detectable alteration in cellular activity when segments of bone or cartilage are subjected to static compression or tension. In contrast, recent studies on the application of dynamic forces to bone in vivo indicate a marked alteration in osteogenic activity. The nature of the response of bone to dynamic loads has been a subject of considerable speculation. In the present discussion, the previous hypotheses are reviewed and a revised hypothesis is given. First, some available information on the mechanism for response of bone and cartilage to static load is outlined. Previous workers have studied the metabolic response or remodeling capacity of osteochondral specimens subjected to an external source of mechanical force. Tensile and compressive forces have been applied in diverse ways, including centrifugation, the application of a direct physical load and hydrostatic force. A few examples of the experimental methods follow.

The Influence of Static Mechanical Force Imposed upon Tissues

In a study on isolated specimens of chick cartilage in vitro, McMaster and Weinert[14] applied a static tensile or compressive load of 0.8 mg/cm^2 · 1.4 mg/cm^2 or 2.0 mg/cm^2 by centrifugation of the specimens. The specimens had a surface area of 1.59 mm^2, a mass of 13 mg, and a density of 1.003 g/cm^3. After 48 hours of exposure, the specimens showed enhanced numbers of mitoses of superficial cells, in comparison with control specimens. Also, the specimens showed evidence of plastic flow of cartilage. Specimens subjected to a tensile force exhibited an increase in longitudinal growth of matrix. Recently, Rodan and Rodan[15] and Norton et al.[16] have reported the reduction in the accumulation of adenosine 3′,5′-monophosphate (AMP) and guanosine 3′,5′-monophosphate (GMP) in the epiphyses of embryonic chick tibiae in vitro after the application of hydrostatic compressive force of about 60 g/cm^2 (normal weight-bearing pressure) for 15 minutes at 37°C. They observed a diminution of cyclic AMP accumulation of about 20 to 130 pmole/10^6 cells (e.g., 25 to 35% reduction). The experiments were repeated for isolated cells from the epiphyses of the chick tibiae. The results were similar to those performed on the intact specimens. When cells were extracted from the proximal, middle and distal portions of the tibiae, the results were somewhat different for the cells from the various regions of the bone. In all of the cells, however, an elevation in cyclic GMP content was observed.

Bürk et al.[17] have shown that low levels of cyclic AMP in fibroblastic cultures are correlated with growth stimulation whereas the addition of cyclic AMP inhibits growth. Previously, Rodan and Rodan[15] have shown that a hydrostatic force of 60 g/cm^2 on similar specimens of cartilage provokes a 50% reduction in glucose metabolism and augments incorporation of 14C thymidine into DNA. Carbohydrate metabolism and cell metabolism are known to be subject to the control of cellular nucleotides. In light of the more recent results by Rodan and Rodan it seems that the cyclic nucleotides may participate as messengers in the conveyance of static mechanical perturbation to the biochemical machinery of the cell to regulate cytodifferentiation and the production of extracellular matrix.[18]

After the imposition of load, cyclic AMP levels were measured in different segments of the epiphyses: (1) The distal segment rich in proliferative cells; (2) the middle segment containing growing nondividing cells; and (3) the proximal segment containing hypertrophic and bone-forming cells. In all cases the same magnitude of hydrostatic force was applied and cyclic AMP concentrations were recorded by means of radioimmunoassay techniques.

After the application of a static compressive force to the tibia, a reduction of the cyclic AMP accumulation was noted in the whole epiphyseal cartilage, whereas the cyclic AMP content of the diaphyses was not significantly different from the controls. The observations on isolated cells from the proliferative, growing and hypertrophic segments of the epiphysis revealed a statistically significant decrease in the cyclic AMP concentration of the proliferative cells exposed to pressure, when compared with their respective controls.

From these observations, Rodan et al.[15, 16] suggest that the modulation of bone remodeling initiated by mechanical stress is mediated at the cellular level by the information vehicles associated with cell membranes, cyclic nucleotides and calcium. A role for the cell membrane in differentiation has been implicated for many years. During the development of various tissues, interaction between adjacent tissues is necessary for cell differentiation to occur. For example, during odontogenesis, interaction between epithelial and mesenchymal cells is essential.[19] In certain systems, direct cellular contact is necessary while other similar events can occur through a filter.[20] In other instances, interaction of the cell membrane with extracellular matrix or with specific molecules that diffuse through the cell membrane may convey the signal. The situation is analogous to the transmission of certain hormone messages through stimulation of the membrane-bound enzyme, adenylcyclase, which in turn regulates the intracellular concentrations of cyclic 3′,5′-AMP. Parathyroid hormone (PTH), a bone remodeling agent, appears to act through this mechanism. Both PTH and calcitonin (CT), another hormone that participates in calcium homeostasis and bone remodeling, also appear to act on the cell by interaction with the cell membrane. In experiments on isolated osteoclasts from rabbits, the author[21] recorded cell membrane potentials when physiological concentrations of PTH or CT were added. The cell membranes were depolarized by PTH and repolarized by addition of CT. The observations were correlated with autoradiographic studies when the rates of RNA metabolism and the production of enzyme or matrix by the cells were estimated by the use of tritiated uridine and leucine. In brief, after the application of PTH, depolarization of the osteogenic cell membranes culminated in enhanced osteolytic activity of the osteoclasts. In contrast, the addition of CT reversed these changes. The observations are shown schematically in Figures 6-1 and 6-2.

Other evidence that PTH functions through the mediation of the adenylcyclase system has been compiled by Chase and Aurbach.[23] Involvement of the cell membrane in the control of cell proliferation via cyclic nucleotides (3′,5′-cyclic AMP and 3′,5′-cyclic GMP) has been documented in several experimental systems. While most of the studies involved the use of fibroblasts, they are likely to pertain to the behavior of osteogenic and chondrogenic cells as indicated in Figure 6-2C. The results reveal that high concentrations of cyclic AMP are inhibitory to cell proliferation. Cyclic AMP concentration is reduced by growth stimulating agents such as somatomedin,[24] serum,[25] insulin[26] or epidermal growth factor.[27] Concurrently, reciprocal changes may occur in the generation of cyclic GMP. The control mechanism may involve ionic transport such as that of calcium ion, which is known to affect the enzymes producing[27] (adenylcyclase and guanylcyclase) and destroying[28] (phosphodiesterase), the cyclic nucleotides. These changes are mediated through cell membranes and may be affected by mechanical perturbations to influence bone remodeling.

In 1953, Yasuda of Japan first described stress generated potentials in bone which he termed "piezoelectricity of bone." He also described electrically-induced bone formation. Fukada and Yasuda[5] found that mechanically stressed bone generated an electrical potential. Areas of compression were electronegative and areas of tension were electropositive. Subsequently, nu-

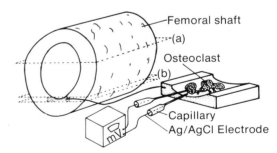

Figure 6-1. A schematic diagram of an endosteal preparation. A femur from an anesthetized newborn rabbit is removed and a sagittal section (a) is made. The marrow is teased from the medullary cavity. Small specimens are cut (b) and placed in Tyrode's solution plus 0.01% neutral red until the osteoclasts can be seen. Then the specimens are transferred to Tyrode's solution. The silver/silver chloride electrodes are placed in a micromanipulator. An osteoclast is impaled by one electrode and the membrane potential is recorded on a millivoltmeter. (Reproduced with permission of D. C. Mears[22]).

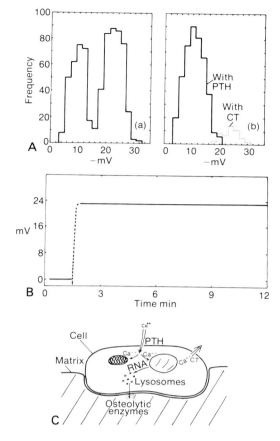

Figure 6-2. *A.* Histograms of membrane potentials recorded from osteoclasts of endosteal preparations (1190 impalements, 26 preparations). The figure on the *right* shows the bimodel distribution of membrane potentials recorded after the addition of physiological amounts of parathyroid hormone (PTH) or calcitonin (CT). *B.* Potential/time transient recorded after the impalement of a typical osteoclast. The time of im- (CT). *B.* Potential/time transient recorded after the impalement of a typical osteoclast. The time of impalement is indicated by a *short line.* The brief periods immediately preceding and the period during impalement are shown in a *broken line* as technical limitations prevented accurate recording of this part of the transient. The record shows that within approximately 10 seconds of impalement the cell membrane potential was stable for up to 10 minutes after impalement. (*A* and *B*, reproduced with permission of D. C. Mears.[21]) *C.* Schematic diagram of an osteoclast stimulated by parathyroid hormone (PTH) and calcitonin (CT). The resting osteoclast actively extrudes calcium ion. Under the influence of PTH, calcium ion rapidly enters the cell so that the intracellular concentration approaches the extracellular concentration. The enhanced calcium ion concentration in the cell promotes greater activity by mitochondria and an increased rate of ribonucleic acid (RNA) synthesis. The latter stimulates the pro-

merous other workers extended these studies. In similar investigations on viable, unstressed bones, Friedenberg and Brighton[29] observed that areas of active bone growth and repair were electronegative when compared to less active areas. Many other workers attempted to employ a great variety of alternating and direct current regimes and electromagnetic induction to influence the healing of nonunions. These observations are described shortly.

The crucial question remains: What is the nature of the events that intercede between the mechanical deformation of bone and the metabolic responses which are now well documented for osteogenic cells?

The Influence of Dynamic Mechanical Forces Imposed upon Tissues

In the previous section, the static mechanical forces imposed upon cells comprised a steady-state condition whereby the cells showed alterations of metabolism after they had been subjected to the imposed mechanical force, probably of sufficient magnitude to provide mechanical strain or deformation of the cell. After the steady-state condition is achieved, however, no additional mechanical energy is dissipated at the cell until the force is removed. In marked contrast, the specimen of bone or cartilage which undergoes a dynamic mechanical perturbation, for example, as a cyclic loading and unloading with intermittent deformation of the cell, is in an environment where mechanical energy is expended intermittently in association with the repetitive deformation of the tissue. It should be obvious that the mechanical stimulus available for tissues subjected to intermittent mechanical deformation is markedly different from that of cells subjected to continuous deformation by a mechanical force which need not expend energy during the steady-state condition.

Dynamic mechanical deformation of bone matrix is accompanied by the formation of heat, free radicals and of a piezoelectric potential, all of which have been postulated to be the principal messenger that initiates a metabolic response

duction and release of osteolytic enzymes which ultimately dissolve bone matrix around the cell. Alternatively, CT increases the rate of calcium ion extrusion from the cell and thereby impedes osteoclastic activity. Metabolic activity of other types of osteogenic cells also may be regulated by PTH- and CT-mediated adjustments of the cell membrane calcium ion "pump." (Reproduced with permission of D. C. Mears.[22])

by bone or cartilage.[30, 31] Heat seems an unlikely source of modulation because it is so rapidly dissipated in the highly vascular bone. Also, the ambient temperature of different bones, such as a femur and a distal phalanx vary considerably at any one moment. The free radical formation and other chemical derivatives of mechanical deformation of bone occur in such minute quantity that they seem unlikely to be significant. The most widely discussed possibility is the piezoelectric potential generated in mechanically deformed bone. In view of its dynamic origin only during periods of actual deformation of bone it is especially attractive.

Other observations by Pfeiffer[32] and Fukada[33] suggest that the magnitude of the piezoelectric constants increases with increasing molecular orientation of the deformed bone matrix. It seems likely that the dielectric displacement is proportional to the strain and independent of the deformation frequency. The principal liability of this hypothesis is the minute magnitude of power recorded for piezoelectric potentials in bone. For example, Cochran et al.[34] recorded the piezo-potential generated in specimens of cortical bone in vitro. The specimens were 0.6 by 2.0 by 30.0 mm. A force of 200, 500 or 100 g was applied at rates of 25 cm/sec with 0 to 8 mm vertical deformation of the specimen. Cochran et al.[34] observed the following results for deformation of dry bone:

Load applied	Piezo-potential
200 g	1 mV
500 g	2 mV
1000 g	5 mV

When wet bone was studied, the recorded piezo-potentials were smaller in magnitude because of the rapid leakage of charge from the specimens. Over the elastic limit of deformation of bone the potential showed a linear relationship to the amount of deformation. In the region of plastic deformation of bone, this relationship was not observed. In all of the experiments the electrode wick covered 2 to 4 mm^2 of bone.

In other experiments, Liboff et al.[35] have recorded the electrical resistance of bone as 2.0 to 5×10^5 ohm/cm for applied potentials of up to 1 volt. Also, they recorded values of 0.7×10^5 ohm/cm for human tibia.[36] From these studies the estimate of resistance for the specimens of bone studied by Cochran et al.[34] would be about 5×10^5 ohm. Therefore:

$$P_{piezo} = \frac{V^2}{R} = \frac{10^{-3}V^2}{5.10^5} = \frac{10^{-6}}{5.10^5} = 2 \times 10^{-12} \quad joule$$

Such a figure represents an average of values between the string electrodes. In fact, McElhaney et al.[37] reported a variable charge distribution in the human femur which correlated with the orientation of collagen fibrils. Under the imposition of a load of about 39 kg., the charge distribution varied from +1.4 to −1.6 pico coulombs/cm^2/kg./cm^2.

Suppose a piezo-potential generated by dynamic deformation of bone at a rate of 60 applied loads per minute was available to stimulate cells. From studies on other types of cells, typically a cell membrane is depolarized by an electric current of about 10^{-9} Å at $4 \times 10^{-2} = 4 \times 10^{-11}$ joules. Baud[38] estimates that a cubic millimeter of bone contains 26,000 osteocytes. The specimen of bone studied by Cochran et al.[34] would possess a volume of about 36 mm^3, which would be equivalent to about 9.4×10^5 cells. The energy required to depolarize all of the cells simultaneously would be about 3.8×10^{-5} joules if depolarization of each cell requires as much expenditure of energy as depolarization of a single isolated cell. For the electric energy generated by a single deformation of the bone matrix in the experiments by Cochran et al.[34] (e.g., 2×10^{-12} joules), there is inadequate energy produced to depolarize a single bone cell, let alone a substantial proportion of cells within the specimen.

If the piezo effect observed in mechanically deformed bone matrix is to participate in a regulatory system, one or more special provisions are necessary: (1) With localized variations of the structure of bone matrix, isolated sites of deformation might show piezo-potentials greatly in excess of the magnitude of the piezo-potential recorded for larger specimens; (2) if local conditions permit depolarization of one or more cells, the syncytial network of bone cells whereby virtually all of the cells in a particular region of bone are interconnected by junctions of low resistance, might permit depolarization of adjacent cells with a minimum additional expenditure of energy; (3) once one cell is depolarized it might be able to amplify the signal which depolarized it so that many other cells are depolarized; (4) the piezo-potential generated in bone matrix might be amplified in magnitude by a unique biological amplifier, of which two conceivable examples will be given shortly. In turn, numerous cells might be depolarized by the enlarged stimulus.

It should be understood that the cell might be stimulated by the piezo-potential through the mediation of a biochemical event rather than the electrochemical event of membrane depolarization. Current evidence suggests, however, that such biochemical stimulation requires a comparable amount of energy as an electrochemical stimulation. The problem of provision for adequate energy to stimulate a cell, therefore, is not appreciably altered if transduction of the presumed piezo-potential to a biologically useful stimulus for the cytoplasmic and nuclear apparatus of the cell occurs by means of a biochemical event rather than an electrochemical one.

For the first three possible explanations to transpire, the piezo-potential generated in deforming bone must be able to depolarize individual osteogenic cells. Conceivably, local variations in the structure of bone matrix provide local sites where much larger piezoelectric signals are generated than the values recorded over lengthy segments of bone. The energy needed to stimulate one cell is about 4×10^{-11} joules, whereas the piezo effect recorded for a single deformation of bone is about 2×10^{-12} joules. As Mascarenhas[39] has shown bone matrix is able to store modest amounts of charge (e.g., 10^{-8} C/cm^2). It is conceivable that numerous deformations of bone matrix might provide an adequate accumulative stimulus to become recognizable by one or a few cells. Piekarski and Munro[40] and Munro[41] have observed another property of bone which may participate in mechanically induced perturbations of bone. Cortical bone consists of a highly porous network with blood vessels (Haversian canals) interconnected by canaliculi with lacunae. The true porosity is probably above 20%. Bone also may be perceived as a composite material of a liquid and a solid phase. Of the constituents of the solid phase, the organic phase possesses a low elastic modulus so that it cannot contribute much to the load bearing capacity of bone, unless its displacement is restricted by the mineral phase. At high strain rates the organic phase will transmit hydrostatic forces, whereas at low strain rates it will contribute little to load-bearing capacity in view of its propensity to viscous flow.

As a model of an osteon, Piekarski and Munro[42] portray a series of concentric cylinders separated from each other by the liquid phase. An approximation of an organic mineral or organic and mineral aggregate to liquid is reasonably justified if it is recalled that the structure, mechanical properties and mechanical behavior of collagen most closely resembles the behavior of rubbery materials. For the latter, the Poissons ratio is generally assumed to be equal to 0.5 so that the application of compressive force does not initiate a change in volume. Forces transmitted through such a medium are comparable to the transmission of the hydrostatic pressure through liquids.

In their model of an osteon (Fig. 6-3), Piekarski and Munro[42] predict the hydrostatic pressure in each liquid annulus. Since each Haversian canal is interconnected with lacunae, as was shown in Chapter 5, Figure 5-6B, by the multitude of canaliculi distributed radially through all lamellae it may be assumed that after an initial increase in pressure, a flow would occur to reduce it to the normal blood pressure in the central lumen of an osteon. Thus, the total volume change for a liquid annulus is:

$$\Delta V_{total} = \Delta V_{radial} + \Delta V_{lateral} + \Delta V_{flow\ in} - \Delta V_{flow\ out}$$

The equation can be written for each liquid annulus and the resultant set of simultaneous linear algebraic equations can be solved for the unknown values of the hydrostatic pressure. The relevant assumptions of dimensions, properties of solids and liquids, the mode of flow and the resultant pressure distribution through the lamellae of an osteon are shown in Figure 6-3C.

The previous model provides another possible factor in mechanically induced remodeling of bone. The weight-bearing forces initiate transport of substantial quantities of fluid throughout a bone. The transport of liquid provides a rapid exchange of nutrients and waste products. The rapid migration of ions in the liquid phase could conceivably generate a streaming potential, thereby to influence osteogenic cells by mediation of changes in cell membrane potential.

Pfeiffer[43] has published a model to estimate the piezoelectric polarization in the osteon system. His model assumes a cylindrical symmetry in the osteon system with intervening liquid phases, similar to that described by Piekarski and Munro[40] Other assumptions of the model are: mechanical—isotropy for cortical bone; piezoelectric anisotropy according to the symmetry class C_∞ and; the absence of mechanical interaction between neighboring osteonal systems and regular alternating orientation of the mineralized collagen fibrils. He derives the charge distribution at the wall of the osteon canal, the electric field in the water-filled Haversian canal and the charge distribution near the osteocytes

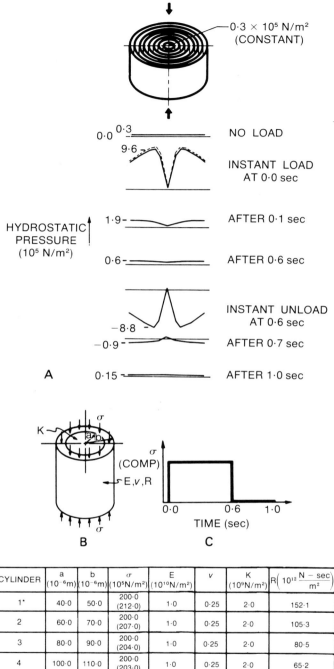

0·3 × 10⁵ N/m² (CONSTANT)

0.3×10^5 N/m² (CONSTANT)

0·0 0·3 ———————— NO LOAD

9·6 — INSTANT LOAD AT 0·0 sec

HYDROSTATIC PRESSURE (10^5 N/m²)

1·9 — AFTER 0·1 sec

0·6 — AFTER 0·6 sec

INSTANT UNLOAD AT 0·6 sec

−8·8 —

−0·9 — AFTER 0·7 sec

0·15 — AFTER 1·0 sec

A

K σ a b σ (COMP) E,ν,R σ

B

C

σ (COMP)

0·0   0·6   1·0
TIME (sec)

CYLINDER	a (10^{-6}m)	b (10^{-6}m)	σ (10^5N/m²)	E (10^{10}N/m²)	ν	K (10^9N/m²)	R ($10^{12}\frac{N-sec}{m^2}$)
1*	40·0	50·0	200·0 (212·0)	1·0	0·25	2·0	152·1
2	60·0	70·0	200·0 (207·0)	1·0	0·25	2·0	105·3
3	80·0	90·0	200·0 (204·0)	1·0	0·25	2·0	80·5
4	100·0	110·0	200·0 (203·0)	1·0	0·25	2·0	65·2
5	120·0	130·0	200·0 (202·0)	1·0	0·25	2·0	54·7
6	140·0	150·0	200·0 (201·0)	1·0	0·25	2·0	47·2
7	160·0	170·0	200·0 (200·0)	1·0	0·25	2·0	41·5
8	180·0	400·0	200·0 (200·0)	1·0	0·25	2·0	

D

*Central cylinder

Figure 6-3. Model of an osteon subjected to compressive stresses (Reproduced with permission of K. R. Piekarski and M. Munro.)[42]

for six configurations of stress. Clearly, attempts to verify the model by the use of glass microelectrodes and potential measurements near the surface of osteogenic cells adjacent to bone matrix undergoing mechanical deformation are eagerly awaited.

Inevitably, the possibility of an effective biological amplifier of the piezo effect is raised. Two possible examples of such amplifiers are presented, although, admittedly many other such possibilities must exist.

It is now known that osteocytic lacunae are lined with a unique type of cell, the "bone lining cell" which possesses the ability to respond to stimuli such as parathyroid hormone.[44] In response, the bone lining cells rapidly and actively extrude large amounts of potassium and calcium ions into the lacunae. One function of the bone lining cells is to permit rapid adjustments in the concentration of calcium ion in the blood. It is not inconceivable that the bone lining cells are stimulated by the piezoelectric effect of deforming bone matrix so that they pump calcium or other ions into the lacunae. In turn, the altered ionic concentration of the lacunae could provoke depolarization of the osteocytes. The gradual loss of bone lining cells with aging would account for progressive diminution in the rate of remodeling of bone. Although this hypothesis shifts the problem of stimulation of cells from the osteocyte to the bone lining cell, the latter cell is in intimate contact with the bone matrix. It would be in closer proximity to the site of generation of the piezo-potential.

Another possible explanation for the rectification and amplification of the piezo-potential is the electrical nature of the bone matrix and the bone cells themselves. Loewenstein[45] has described the equivalent circuit of a chain of cells (Fig. 6-4). He has shown that the measured resistance of a cell chain is proportional to the length of the chain. Resistance increases linearly with the increase in the length of the chain.

A convenient index for cell communication is the ratio of membrane voltages V_I/V_{II} in two adjacent cells that results from the flow of an electric current where:

$$\frac{V_I}{V_{II}} = 1 + \frac{2r_c}{r_p} + \frac{r_c}{r_s}\left(1 + \frac{r_c}{r_p}\right)$$

Where r_p represents the combination of cell surface membrane resistances, r_o, in cell II in parallel with the entire network to the right of cell II. Efficient communication between cells requires a high r_s and a low r_c.

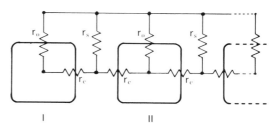

Figure 6-4. Schematic diagram of the equivalent electric circuit of a chain of cells after Loewenstein.[45] r_c, resistance of the junctional membrane $\simeq 110$ to 190 Ω/cm; r_o, resistance of the surface membrane $\simeq 10^4$ Ω/cm^2; r_s, resistance along an intercellular space $\simeq 110$ to 190 Ω/cm.

If this model of cell communication is utilized to construct a more elaborate model of osteocytes within bone matrix, the schematic representation appears as shown in Fig. 6-5.

It seems possible that such a complex network could serve to convert a piezo-potential into a useful signal for recognition by osteogenic cells, which in turn, is amplified and rectified for optimal recognition by cells. With rectification the signal might be converted into a direct current for recognition by the cells.

With the limited experimental evidence available to describe the response of biological cells to mechanical deformation of adjacent extracellular matrix, it is readily apparent that further work is needed. Such experimental work currently is in progress. Another approach is the construction of an electrical model of bone matrix with the enclosed osteogenic cells.

OBSERVATIONS ON EXPERIMENTAL ANIMALS AND MAN

From the previous account, it will be evident that current knowledge on the mechanisms by which individual mesenchymal cells respond to mechanical perturbations remains obscure. Limited observations have been made on experimental animals and man which supplement the picture. Some of the latter experiments represent attempts to develop therapeutic techniques for alteration of fracture repair. In certain instances the human experiments rest on an inaccurate understanding of present knowledge. In these cases, especially where favorable therapeutic results are reported, the reader is advised to distinguish between the therapeutic attributes of the work and its relevance to the physiological behavior of mesenchymal cells.

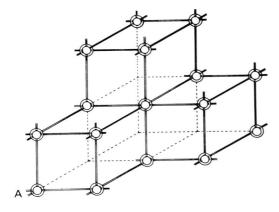

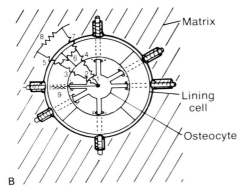

Figure 6-5. *A.* Highly schematic diagram of a syncytial network of osteocytes interspersed in bone matrix. *B.* Highly schematic diagram of typical osteocyte and its equivalent electric circuit. The numbers refer to the resistances of several structures; 1 and 2, resistance across the osteocytic surface membrane $\simeq 10^4$ Ω/cm^2; 3 and 4, resistance across the living cell surface membrane $\simeq 10^4$ Ω/cm^2; 5 and 7, resistance across the living cell outer surface membrane and the adjacent interface of bone matrix $\geq 10^4$ Ω/cm^2; 6, resistance across living cell junctional membrane $\simeq 110$ to 190 Ω/cm; 8, resistance of bone matrix $\simeq 10^5$ to 10^7 Ω/cm; 9, resistance across osteocytic junctional membrane in the cell processes ≥ 110 to 190 Ω/cm. Other pertinent information: (a) Charge distribution in loaded bone matrix $+1.4$ to -1.6 pico-coulombs/cm^2/kg/cm^2; (b) maximum storage of charge in bone 10^{-8} coul./cm^2; (c) energy required to depolarize a typical cell 4.10^{-2} V $\times$ 10^{-9} Å $= 4.10^{-11}$ J; (d) osteocytic cell concentration $26{,}000$ cells/mm^3.

The Effect of Static Compression and Tension on Internal Remodeling of Cortical Bone

In Chapters 5 and 9, a series of observations recorded by Matter *et al.*[46] on the influence of static compression and tension on cortical bone

remodeling were reviewed. These workers employed unique onlay plates with strain gauges, to document the influence of known magnitudes of compression or tension on intact and osteotomized long bones in several experimental animals, including sheep and rabbits. Static compression or tension applied *in vivo* to cortical bone is slowly diminished by remodeling of the Haversian system. The rate of Haversian bone remodeling in bones subjected to axial compression and to unstressed bones is similar. These workers conclude that the remodeling of bone adjacent to onlay plates and screws is neither the result of a foreign body effect, nor the result of the axial compression applied by means of the fixation screws.

In experimental animals in which static compressive or tensile load is applied to a plated bone, activity of the animal with the associated weight-bearing forces imposed upon the operative limb, may alter the results. If the plate is under high distractive force, weight-bearing will reduce this tension periodically, but not abolish it. The force transmission between the plate and the bone during weight-bearing remains unidirectional. If the plate is under compressive load, weight-bearing will increase compression periodically. The force transmission between the plate and the bone also remains unidirectional. If, however, the plate is under low distractive load, and compression due to weight-bearing is larger in amount than the distraction produced by the plate, periodically the plate will be under distraction and compression. The force transmission in the contact zone between the plate and the bone, therefore, periodically changes its direction. In this last group, bone resorption and loosening of the screws occurred, which was never encountered in the former two groups where the direction of force between the plate and the bone remained constant. Incidentally, these last observations confirmed the mechanism of micromotion to initiate biologically induced loosening of implants.

Stress Protection in Bone

One other observation on the influence of rigid onlay plates was made by Matter *et al.*,[46] and confirmed by others.[12, 13] After the application of a plate to bone, weight-bearing forces are transmitted in large part through the plate rather than through the adjacent segment of bone. Such stress relief of bone is accompanied by an obligatory osteoporosis of bone. In a recent study, Woo *et al.*[12] have investigated the differences in the remodeling of long bones to which plates of various bending and axial rigidity were attached. The observations were made in adult mongrel dogs in which cobalt-chromium alloy (Vitallium) plates with an elastic modulus of 248 GN/m^2, or plates made of a graphite fiber reinforced methylmethacrylate resin composite (GFMM) with elastic moduli between 10 and 39 GN/m^2, were implanted. The finite element analysis technique was employed after prolonged implantation to determine the mechanical properties in bone after the animals were sacrificed and the plates were removed. The bone, exposed to the rigid metal plates, showed a marked diminution in tensile and compressive strength, although its ultimate bending strength and flexural modulus of elasticity were not greatly different from those values recorded in normal canine femora and in the bones exposed to the less rigid plates. Histological studies on the bones confirmed the osteoporosis of the specimens.

The Mechanical Forces Exerted by Cells

In contrast to the influence that extraneous mechanical forces may have on cells and tissues, the cells themselves may impose mechanical force on adjacent surfaces. A representative example is ameboid motion, whereby a part of the cell periphery may extend beyond the bulk of the cell. The tip of the extension or pseudopodium attaches to the foreign surface, after which the residual portion of the cell advances to the site of attachment. Ameboid motion and other forms of cell behavior rest on the biological phenomenon of cell adhesion. Adherence of cells to foreign surfaces depends upon the chemical nature of the surface and the surface charge. The true surface area in the presence of microheterogeneities in the surface also influences adhesive forces. The measurement of cell adhesion, and the mechanisms involved, have been reviewed by Weiss.[47-49] In his early studies he observed that ameboid movements of cells comprised a progression of cell-substratum adhesions. When adhesions were broken, a small portion of the cell surface was observed to remain adherent to the substratum. "Clean" separations of the interfaces were rarely encountered. From this observation the author was stimulated to measure cell adhesion by various distractive techniques. He studied fibroblasts *in vitro*, after they had undergone adhesion to glass and a variety of metallic surfaces (Fig. 6-6). The cells were subjected to a moving stream of fluid, with laminar flow characteristics. The shearing force required to separate the cells was of the

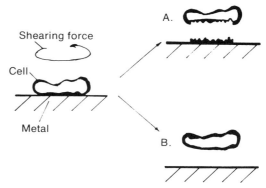

Figure 6-6. Possible conditions following the distraction of a cell from its substratum. *A.* Clean separation of the cell surface from the substratum, *i.e.,* the cohesion of the surfaces is greater than the cell/substratum adhesion. This behavior is representative of cells growing on corroding metals where the adhesive strength is affected by the dissolution products. *B.* Fracture of a cell surface resulting in cell surface material being left on the substratum, *i.e.,* the strength of adhesion of the cell to the substratum is greater than the cohesion of the cell surface. This configuration typifies the optimal mode of behavior for cells growing on inert foreign surfaces. The other possible behavior, fracture of the substratum surface where the strength of adhesion of the cell to the substratum is greater than the cohesion of the substratum surface would not be encountered with the presently available implantable materials. (Reproduced with permission L. Weiss.[49])

order of 10^5 dyn/cm^2 applied for 20 seconds. The adhesive strength also varies considerably with the rate at which the distractive force is applied. Subsequently, other workers extended the studies by a measurement of contractile force developed by fibroblasts. The clinical observation of the contraction of granulation tissue in open wounds has been noted for years. Under conditions of tissue culture James and Taylor[50] measured the force required to prevent the approximation of two small pieces of bone attached together by fibrous tissue. In the absence of applied load, the fibrous tissue interval contracts (Fig. 6-7), so that the two bony fragments approach one another. With the application of a sufficiently large load to one of the fragments, the two fragments remain in their initial positions and the width of the fibrous interval does not ultimately change.

It is not unlikely that such phenomena may occur in bone and cartilage. Their presence would substantially alter the interpretation of experiments where external mechanical forces are applied to the tissues.

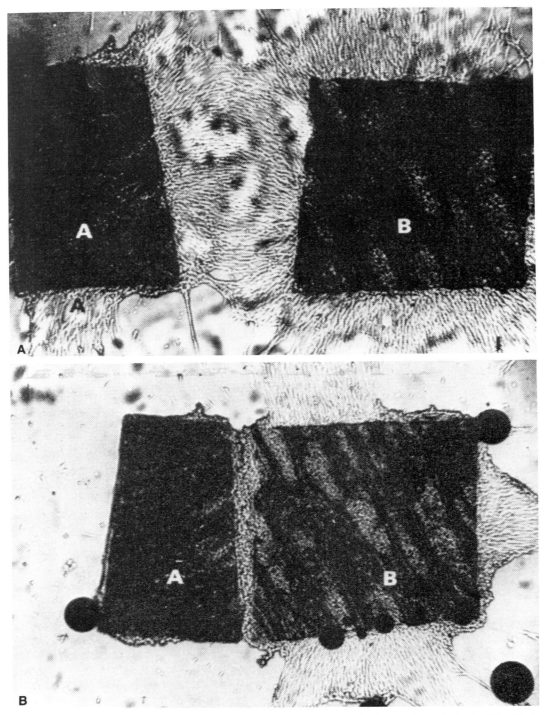

Figure 6-7. *A.* Two explants (*A* and *B*) of chick frontal bone are shown in tissue culture. A sheet of fibroblasts has grown between the explants. *B.* The explants (*A* and *B*) have been drawn toward each other by contraction of the fibroblastic sheet connecting them. (Reproduced with permission D. W. James and J. F. Taylor.[50])

The Effect of Repetitive Impulsive Loads on Cancellous Bone

Studies by Pugh et al.[51] on the response of cancellous bone to repetitive impulsive loads has provided insight into another fact of mechanical stress imposed on bone. In a previous study, these workers had studied the subchondral bone of the medial tibial plateau in 41 adult men who showed severe degenerative arthritis in the knee. Under reflective light microscopy, as has been shown in Chapter 5, microfractures of individual trabeculae were noted. Subsequently, they undertook experiments on adult male rabbits subjected to intermittent axial impulsive loads of their lower extremities. Within 8 days after the initiation of impulsive loading, remodeling of the subchondral bone in the proximal tibia of the rabbit was noted. Under the light microscope, microfatigue fractures were seen in individual trabeculae that were similar to those seen in the human specimens. Microfatigue fractures showed evidence of healing with peripheral callus formation. From these observations, the workers suggested that repetitive impulsive loads initiate stiffening of cancellous bone. The stiffening is attributed to the reparative stages of healing of the microtrabecular fractures. It is suggested that the enhanced rigidity of cancellous bone may diminish its ability to dampen impulsive loads applied to adjacent joints, thereby to augment the rate at which degenerative changes in articular cartilage progress. While the relationship of these findings to degenerative arthritis in human subjects remains unclear, there seems little doubt that the application of repetitive impulsive loads to cancellous bone provokes alteration of structure and reorganization.

CLINICAL APPLICATION OF MECHANICAL FACTORS IN TISSUES

From the observations of many workers on tissues in vitro with experimental animals and man, a number of observations can be made on the ways to influence mechanical forces imposed by implants on tissues in clinical practice.

The clinical techniques of internal fixation, with the use of screws and plates, or with external fixation in the application of percutaneous skeletal pins should insure that the bone-metal interface is subjected solely to compressive or tensile force. Where the interface is subjected to tension interspersed with compression, resorption of bone with loosening of the implant is likely to follow. One of the attributes of so-called compression plating is that the preload, undertaken at surgery, provides compression which may be augmented by weight-bearing forces. Such a system remains continuously under the imposition of compressive load and does not tend to show resorption of bone around the screws. Where a single implant fails to provide this criterion, a supplementary form of immobilization should be considered, at least for the initial postoperative period, to lessen the likelihood for reciprocal micromotion of the metalbone interface, with loosening of the device and ultimately clinical failure.

In the last decade "stress protection" of bone adjacent to rigid implants has emerged as a significant clinical problem. Initially, the AO group and others recommended the application of double plates, at right angles to one another, to stabilize highly unstable fractures of the femur and occasionally elsewhere.[52] The technique was highly satisfactory to achieve a union of bone. When both plates were removed simultaneously, however, the osteoporotic segment of bone that previously had been immobilized, was highly likely to undergo pathological fracture with minimal weight bearing. The fractures were not related to the precise sites of the previous fractures, but rather to the osteoporotic segments. After these early failures, the AO group recommended that following the use of double onlay plates with subsequent union of the bone, each plate should be removed in different procedures, separated by an interval of many months. Simultaneously, they discouraged the use of double plates unless no other technique could be undertaken.

In a somewhat similar circumstance, Wagner[53, *] employed a unique, highly rigid plate to the site of a leg-lengthening procedure. His plate possesses no holes at the site of the lengthening. After the application of the plate, osteoporosis of the adjacent segment of the bone has been a common occurrence. If the plate is removed, fracture of the osteoporotic segment is likely to ensue. Alternatively, the plate may have to be removed and replaced with a thinner, less rigid plate. Following an adaptive period of 6 to 12 months, the second plate can be removed.

In the author's experience with the application of the Hoffmann device for external fixation of fractures, stress protection also has been noted in certain cases. Many of the instances in which the Hoffmann device is used for treatment

---

* H. Wagner, personal communication, 1977.

of grossly comminuted and unstable fractures are followed by a prolonged period of relatively slow consolidation of the fracture fragments. Other workers also have confirmed this observation.† While it is unclear why fracture healing frequently progresses at a slow rate in the presence of external fixation, it seems not unlikely that the altered mechanical environment of the fracture site is a highly contributing factor.

In an effort to develop less rigid plates, many workers have studied a variety of polymeric materials, including high density polyethylene, polypropylene and others.[13], ‡ While the degree of stress protection of bone is substantially diminished, to date no polymeric plates are available which show adequate strength. Furthermore, most of the polymeric plates cannot be readily deformed plastically as with their metal counterparts. This is a substantial liability, in view of the need to shape plates during operative procedures. Nevertheless, continuing studies on composite materials may reveal some satisfactory alternatives to presently available surgical alloys.

Somewhat related to the osteoporosis, secondary to "stress protection" is the disuse osteoporosis frequently noted in the postoperative period after internal fixation of fractures. Frequently, despite the application of accepted methods of internal fixation, sufficient stability cannot be realized to make full weight bearing possible. In a study on the amount of weight bearing necessary in the lower extremity of adults to prevent disuse osteoporosis, the AO group has recommended that 25 pounds (10 kg) of force applied on the affected lower extremity in partial weight-bearing gait, is adequate.* In most instances, adequate stabilization of a fracture can be achieved, so that a force of 25 pounds, as impulsive bending or rotational load imposed by the patient will not disrupt the repair. A 4-point gait with the use of crutches and the restriction of 25 pounds weight bearing on the affected extremity greatly facilitates walking compared to the alternative of 3-point gait with complete absence of weight bearing on the affected limb. Furthermore, under the 25-pound weight restriction, the patient may undertake active motion exercises of the adjacent joints, to facilitate return or preservation of joint motion and to exercise the principal muscle groups.

The design of total joint replacements has

been influenced by the observation of stress protection and allied phenomena. In the past decade when a variety of hinge-like prostheses with long intramedullary stems were employed, numerous instances of shaft fractures of the bone adjacent to the distal portion of an intramedullary stem or its tip were noted.[54] It is likely that the site of the fractures, or perhaps even the magnitude of force required to initiate the fracture, were predetermined by the stress protection engendered by the intramedullary stem. In many cases, such as in hinge-type total knee joint and total elbow joint prostheses,[55] the constraint of motion of the hinge without the anatomical rotational component provoked loosening of the device. Reciprocal motion of the tip of the intramedullary stems was likely to initiate local resorption of bone with mechanical compromise. It is now evident that hinge-type prostheses should be used only as a last resort. With the variety of implants currently available for use in the knee and with the new multicomponent elbow joint prostheses, the hinge-type models are likely to have exceptionally limited applications in the future.

At present, isoelastic materials are undergoing intense scrutiny as a source of superior materials for total joint replacements.[56] Materials with elastic moduli that rival those of bone and cartilage would not show the alteration of force transmission otherwise anticipated at the implant tissue interface. In certain instances, the materials might dampen impulsive loads and function as shock absorbers, like their biological counterparts.

Possible applications of electrical stimulation to augment the rate of bone healing, particularly in difficult problems such as the congenital pseudarthrosis of the tibia,[8] or chronic infected nonunions, are under intense scrutiny in many clinics. Recently, the diverse methods of therapeutic technique under scrutiny have been fully reviewed elsewhere.[10, 57] Some highly encouraging results have been obtained in a few cases, although as yet there are no useful statistical surveys to reveal that these methods deserve widespread application. It should be emphasized that most of the therapeutic regimes of electrical stimulation rest on wholly empirical observations. The types and magnitudes of electromotive forces applied to the bone have little relevance to physiological events. Nevertheless, if they prove to have clinical applications, further standardization in technique and materials will follow, and no doubt the nature of these biological events will become evident.

---

† B. H. Weber, personal communication, 1977.
‡ R. Pilliar, personal communication, 1977.

REFERENCES

1. Wolff, J. *Das Gesetz Der Transformation der Knochen*, p. 3, A. Hirschwald, Berlin, 1892.
2. Koch, J. C. *Am. J. Anat., 21:*177, 1917.
3. Thompson, D. A. *On Growth and Form*, p. 997, University Press, Cambridge, 1959.
4. Glucksman, A. *Anat. Rec., 73:*39, 1939.
5. Fukada, E., and Yasuda, I. *J. Physiol. Soc. Japan, 12:*1158, 1957.
6. Bassett, C. A. L., and Becker, R. O. *Sci., 137:*1063, 1962.
7. Hassler, C. R., Rybicki, E. F., Diegle, R. B., and Clark, L. C. *Clin. Orthop., 124:*9, 1977.
8. Levine, L. S., Lustrin, I., and Shamos, M. H. *Clin. Orthop., 124:*69, 1977.
9. Becker, R. O., Spadaro, J. A., and Marino, A. A. *Clin. Orthop., 124:*75, 1977.
10. Inoue, S., Ohashi, T., Yasuda, I., and Fukada, E., *Clin. Orthop., 124:*57, 1977.
11. Brighton, C. T. *Clin. Orthop., 124:*2, 1977.
12. Woo, S. L-Y., Simon, B. R., Akeson, W. H., and McCarty, M. P., *J. Biomech., 10:*87, 1977.
13. Tonino, A. J., Davidson, C. L., Klopper, P. J., and Linclau, L. A. *J. Bone Jt. Surg., 58B:*107, 1976.
14. McMaster, J., and Weinert, C. *Clin. Orthop., 72:*308, 1970.
15. Rodan, S. B., and Rodan, G. A. *J. Biol. Chem., 249:*3068, 1974.
16. Norton, L. A., Rodan, G. A., and Bourret, L. A. *Clin. Orthop., 124:*59, 1977.
17. Bürk, R. R. *Nature, 219:*1272, 1968.
18. Rasmussen, H., and Bordier, P. *Physiological and Cellular Basis of Metabolic Bone Disease*, p. 119, Williams & Wilkins Co., Baltimore, 1974.
19. Koch, W. E., Tissue interaction during *in vitro* odontogenesis. In *Development Aspects of Oral Biology*, p. 151, edited by H. C. Slavkin and L. A. Bavetta, Academic Press Inc., 1972.
20. Wartiovaara, J., Nordling, S., Lehtonen, E., and Saxen, L. *J. Embyol. Exp. Morphol., 31:*667, 1971.
21. Mears, D. C. *Endocr., 88:*1021, 1971.
22. Mears, D. C. *Oxford Med. Gaz., 22:*60, 1970.
23. Chase, L. R., and Aurbach, G. D. *J. Biol. Chem., 245:*1520, 1970.
24. Tell, G., Cuatrecasas, P., van Wyk, J., and Hintz, R. *Sci., 108:*312, 1974.
25. Rozengurt, E., and De Asua, L. V. *Proc. Natl. Acad. Sci. USA, 70:*3609, 1973.
26. Hollenberg, M. D., and Cuatrecasas, P. *Proc. Natl. Acad. Sci. USA, 70:*2964, 1973.
27. Hardman, J. G., Robinson, G. A., and Sutherland, E. W. *Ann. Rev. Physiol., 33:*311, 1971.
28. Kakiuchi, S., Yamazaki, R., Teshima, Y., and Uenishi, K. *Proc. Natl. Acad. Sci. USA, 70:*3526, 1973.
29. Friedenberg, Z. B., and Brighton, C. T. *J. Bone Jt. Surg., 48A:*915, 1966.
30. Justus, P., and Luft, J. H. *Calcif. Tis. Res., 5:*222, 1970.
31. Bassett, C. A. L., Becker, R. O., and Pawluck, R. J. *Nature, 204:*652, 1964.
32. Pfeiffer, B. H. *J. Biomech., 10:*53, 1977.
33. Fukada, E. *Ann. N.Y. Acad. Sci., 238:*7, 1974.
34. Cochran, G. V. B., Pawluck, R. J., and Bassett, C. A. L. *Clin. Orthop., 58:*249, 1968.
35. Liboff, A. B., Rinaldi, R. A., Levine, L. S., and Shamos, M. A. *Clin. Orthop., 106:*330, 1975.
36. Moss, M. L., Lustrin, I., Shamos, M. A., Rinaldi, R., and Liboff, A. R. *Sci., 175:*1118, 1972.
37. McElhaney, J. H., Stalmaker, R., and Ballard, R. *J. Biomech., 1:*47, 1968.
38. Baud, C. A. *Excerpt. Med. Int. Congress Symp. on Calcif. Tissue*, p. 4, Excerpt. Med., Amsterdam, 1966.
39. Mascarenhas, S. *Ann. N.Y. Acad. Sci., 238:*36, 1974.
40. Piekarski, K. R., and Munro, M. *Morphology and Fracture of Bone*, p. 29, University of Waterloo, Waterloo, 1976.
41. Munro, M., Ph.D. Thesis, University of Waterloo, 1976.
42. Piekarski, K. R., and Munro, M. *Morphology and Fracture of Bone*, p. 32, University of Waterloo, Waterloo, 1976.
43. Pfeiffer, B. H., *J. Biomech., 10:*487, 1977.
44. Talmage, R. V., Whitehurst, L., and Andersen, J. J. B. *Endocrinol, 92:*136, 1973.
45. Loewenstein, W. R. *Ann. N.Y. Acad. Sci., 137:*441, 1967.
46. Matter, P., Brennwald, J., and Perren, S. M., *Helvetica Chir. Acta., Suppl. 12,* 5, 1975.
47. Weiss, L., *J. Theoret. Biol., 6:*275, 1964.
48. Weiss, L., *The Cell Periphery, Metastasis and Other Contact Phenomena*, p. 228, North Holland Publishing Co., Amsterdam, 1967.
49. Weiss, L. *Exptl. Cell Res., Suppl. 8:*141, 1961.
50. James, D. W., and Taylor, J. F. *Exptl. Cell Res., 54:*107, 1969.
51. Pugh, J. W., Rose, R. M., and Radin, E. L. *Arch. Internatl. Physiol. Biochem., 81:*27, 1973.
52. Müller, M. E., Allgöwer, M., and Willenegger, H. *Manual of Internal Fixation*, p. 48, Springer-Verlag, Berlin, 1970.
53. Wagner, H. Surgical lengthening or shortening of the femur and tibia. In *Progress in Orthopaedic Surgery #1*, p. 7, edited by N. Gschwend et al., Springer-Verlag, New York, 1977.
54. Blauth, W., Skripitz, W., and Bontemps, G. Problematics of current hinge-type artificial knee joints. In *Artificial Hip and Knee Joint Technology*, p. 374, edited by M. Schaldach and D. Hohmann, Springer-Verlag, Berlin, 1976.
55. Ewald, F. C. *Orthop. Clin. N. Am., 6:*685, 1975.
56. Morscher, E., Mathys, R., and Henche, H. R., Iso-Elastic Endoprosthesis. In *Artificial Hip and Knee Joint Technology*, p. 403, Springer-Verlag, Berlin, 1976.
57. Brighton, C. T., Friedenberg, Z. B., Mitchell, E. I., and Booth, R. E. *Clin. Orthop., 124:* 106, 1977.

7

The Biological Response to Implanted Materials

When a foreign metal specimen is placed in a human subject or an experimental animal adjacent to tissues of the musculoskeletal system, the tissues attempt to seclude the foreign material.[1] Foreign bodies are surrounded with a layer of fibrous tissue of a thickness that is proportional to the amount and toxicity of the dissolution products and to the amount of motion between the specimen and adjacent tissues. If the foreign material is exceedingly inert and immobile its enveloping fibrous layer may be less than a uniform monolayer of cells. Live cells adjacent to the metal may bond tightly to metal surfaces so that attempts to distract the cells will lead to cell disruption rather than distraction. If noxious dissolution products accumulate in sufficient concentrations, however, cellular damage occurs. Damaged or dead cells may release their "digestive" lysosomal enzymes to provoke further death of tissues.[2] The biological response of tissues to metals and other materials has been intensely scrutinized, not only to produce nonreactive metallic surfaces but also to define the attributes of certain metallic, polymeric and ceramic surfaces which could influence tissues in desirable reproducible ways.

Metals and other foreign substances may enter or depart from the body in various ways which are summarized in Figure 7-1. Some constituents of implantable materials are normal body metabolites while others serve as analogues of similar elements to influence biochemical reactions. In figure 7-2 elements of the atomic table are categorized from this aspect.

In marked contrast to the initiation of local biological phenomena, implantation of a metal or nonmetallic implant may provoke more generalized upset of the body. Hypersensitivity to metallic dissolution products is well described. Initiation of carcinogenesis by metallic ions is well known in experimental animals and has been queried in man. Also, the presence of metal implants, with or without methylmethacrylate cement, alters the host's resistance to local infection. These phenomena are described below.

Ultimately for clinicians who employ surgical implants the crucial question is the likelihood for an implant especially one composed of previously untried materials, to initiate undesirable reactions in local or distant tissues. Standards organizations and governmental agencies, who provide guidelines for new clinical methods, would like to possess data from accelerated tests that confirm the tissue tolerance of new materials. In the present chapter the available methods to study the biological responses of tissues to implanted materials are reviewed. The tests can be divided into qualitative and quantitative analyses of dissolution or wear products. The second types of tests attempt to assay the biological significance of their presence as dissolution and wear products. Finally, the currently available biological screening tests will be described.

The Response of Tissues to Inert Metal Surfaces

When a material is placed in the body, it dissolves at some finite rate. Unlike other materials, however, metals can be subjected to cathodic protection whereby they may exhibit a *zero* rate of dissolution. To learn the effect of dissolving metals on tissues the obvious starting point is to define the response of cells to inert metal. To the author's knowledge, experiments with cathodically protected specimens have not been undertaken. Nevertheless, much information is available on how cells behave under laboratory conditions when they grow on inert metal or glass substrata.[5] It is useful to start with a description of events at the cellular level and progress to the level of tissue and organ.

Perhaps the most detailed observations on the growth of living cells on foreign surfaces *in vivo* have been made by the study of specimens in rabbit ear chambers. Laboratory-Lop Rabbits[6]

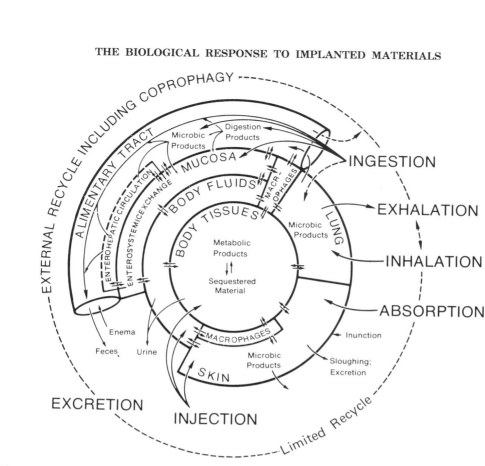

Figure 7-1. Modes of intake and excretion for metals in mammals. (Reproduced with permission of T. D. Luckey and B. Venugopal.[3])

have been bred with unusually large ears in which transparent chambers can be implanted.[7] The floor of the chamber is covered with a material of interest so that a continuous photomicrographic record of the growth of tissue over the specimen can be followed.[8] Also, minute specimens of tissue can be collected from the surface of the specimen and studied by other techniques. These observations correlate well with less detailed studies of the events that occur around implants in human subjects. Initially after implantation the floor of the chamber is covered with blood and extracellular fluid.[9] Within a few hours coagulation occurs with a subsequent invasion of inflammatory cells: fibroblasts, macrophages and polymorphonuclear leukocytes. Within 2 weeks endothelial cells cover the foreign surface although it requires an additional 8 weeks for these cells to become fully organized. The nature of the bond between the cells and foreign surfaces remains poorly understood. A detailed account of present knowledge

by Weiss[10] deserves scrutiny as the interface between organized tissues and metal implants is the most vulnerable site for failure after clinical implantation with catastrophies such as loosening, infection and metal failure.

Endothelial cells migrate from a capillary bed to an implant by ameboid motion. To initiate ameboid motion and the subsequent process of adhesion to the implant surface the cell extends minute projections.[11] For metal implants the cohesive strength of the material is always immeasurably greater than either the cohesive strength of the cell or the adhesive strength of the cell-metal interface. The improbability of true adhesional failure at an interface, as predicted by Bikerman's[12] statistical approach (Fig. 6-6) applies here. Hence cell separation is unlikely to occur cleanly over the total area of cell adhesion. In studies on fibroblasts cultured *in vitro* on a variety of substrata Weiss and Coombs[13] used an immunological technique with mixed agglutination of erythrocytes to confirm

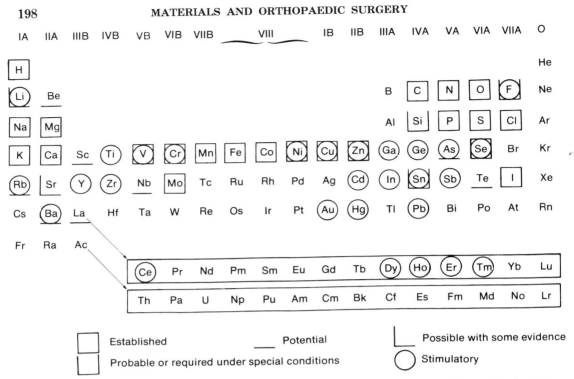

Figure 7-2. Categorization of the elements of the periodic table from the aspects of nutrition and biochemical constituents. (Reproduced with permission of T. D. Luckey and B. Venugopal.[4]

that physical distraction of cells from the surface is accompanied by surface rupture of the cells. Weiss[14] attempted to measure both the cohesive strength of the same cells and the adhesive force between the cells and a substratum of glass, stainless steel or gold. The absolute magnitude of these forces per unit of cell surface is exceedingly difficult to determine as the surface area of the cell is poorly known.[11, 15, 16]

The force of adhesion of cell to glass is estimated to be 10^5 dynes/cm^2 of cell surface presented to the substratum. Although similar data are not available for cell-metal interfaces, the previous example illustrates the likely force of adhesion. It should be emphasized, however, that in view of the net negative charge carried by all animal cells at their electrokinetic surface, and the variability of surface charge at different metallic surfaces, the forces of adhesion are expected to vary considerably for different cell-metal interfaces. Weiss[17] showed that a variety of agents affect the forces of adhesion of the cell-substratum interface and the force of cohesion of the cell including the rate of cell division, the presence of cellular enzymes and the rate of pinocytosis of the cell (*e.g.*, a form of transport

by the cell membrane). The presence of metallic dissolution products is known to affect the rate of pinocytosis of adjacent cells and it has been postulated[18] that they provoke release of cellular lysosomal enzymes. By both mechanisms corrosion products are likely to cause diminished adhesive and cohesive properties of cells on metals.

Attempts to Locate Metallic Dissolution Products

It may seem ironic that the assessment of undesirable side-effects of metallic dissolution products has become far more complex by the elimination from consideration of implantation of all rapidly dissolving metals with inexpensive and rapid corrosion tests. Only those inert alloys with minute dissolution rates require further scrutiny. In recent years, with the widespread implantation of metallic total joint replacements, which may have a desired period of function of 50 years or more, concern has arisen about side-effects of metallic wear or dissolution products that accumulate progressively. Attempts to measure the rates and sites of accumulation have been far more successful than

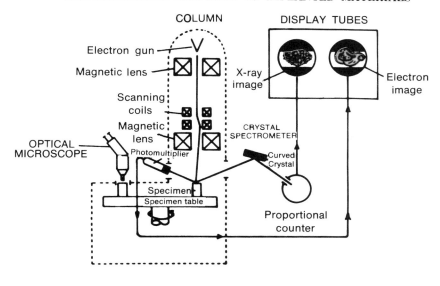

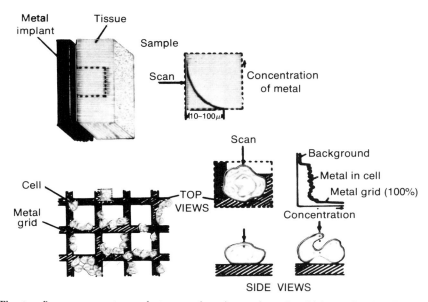

Figure 7-3. The *top figure* represents an electron probe microanalyzer in which a reflective electron image from back scattered electrons and a quantitative assessment of a specimen are made. The *bottom figure* reveals the applications of the method on tissue samples removed from the surfaces of surgical implants and of cells cultured on metal grids. The tissue specimens show a rapid diminution of metallic concentration within 10 to 100 μm of the metal surface. The method permits the resolution of metallic dissolution products although it cannot determine whether they are inside or outside of the cell, in view of the convoluted cell surface.

efforts to show the biological effects and significance of metallic dissolution products.

Frequently early workers observed the staining of tissues in juxtaposition to implants of iron-base alloys.[19] Emneus and Stenram[20] and others used the Prussian blue reaction or the Perls'

reaction to confirm the presence of metallic dissolution products in discolored tissues.

About 1960 several workers[21, 22] employed electron-probe microanalysis (Fig. 7-3) to study the location of foreign materials in tissues and to determine the amount of materials. The au-

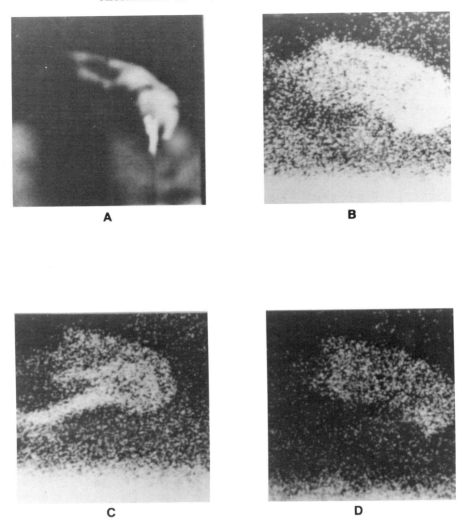

Figure 7-4. *A.* Electron image of a cell attached to a stainless steel grid (*bottom of micrograph*). Part of the cell is obscured due to shadowing effects and low depth of focus of a reflected electron image (×800). *B.* Iron X-ray image of *A* shows association of the element with the cell (×800). *C.* Chromium X-ray image of *A* (×800). *D.* Nickel X-ray image of *A* (×800). The X-ray images were recorded in the order *C, B, D* progressively and show incineration of the cell.

thor[23] has made a study of fibroblasts cultured *in vitro* on grids of gold, platinum, rhodium, nickel and stainless steel. After a few days in culture the specimens were subjected to electron probe microanalysis. Minute quantities of metallic dissolution products were recorded on the individual cells (Fig. 7-4). In view of the highly convoluted surface of the cells, especially after the dehydration associated with preparation of the specimen or with insertion into the vacuum of the microscope, it was impossible to discern whether the metallic products resided on the cell surface or within the cells.

Johannson and Hegyeli[24] used interference microscopy to study cells cultured *in vitro* on a variety of metal substrates. Their observations suggest that the metallic products are within the cells although the same difficulty of interpretation is present. Previous observations had indicated that many if not most metallic ions, dissolved in body fluid, rapidly form metalloprotein complexes.[25] These complexes were believed to bind to the surfaces of cells where they might impede the transport of nutrients or waste products across the cell membrane or they might inhibit enzyme activity. Subsequently, however,

Table 7-1

Concentrations of Elements Found in Tissues Around a Variety of Metallic Implants

Element	Alloy[a]	No. of Speci- mens	Mean Concen- tration[b]	Standard Devia- tion
Fe	Control	97	37.9	34.6
	AISI 316	61	76.8	45.7
	A 286	16	46.1	19.0
	Inconel X	14	39.3	18.0
	Hastelloy C	18	17.2	6.6
Ni	Control	132	8.0	9.3
	AISI 316	66	40.5	41.2
	A 286	16	54.9	20.2
	Inconel X	14	41.5	19.4
	Hastelloy C	18	15.7	8.2
Cr	Control	75	3.7	4.9
	AISI 316	63	76.0	55.7
	A 286	16	26.9	24.9
	Inconel X	14	7.6	1.6
	Hastelloy C	18	7.3	3.8
	Co-Cr-Mo	37	67.0	43.6
	Co-Cr-Ni-W	9	74.9	99.8
Mo	Control	124	1.8	3.2
	AISI 316	65	8.4	9.2
	A 286	19	2.6	3.2
	Hastelloy C	18	3.2	1.8
	Co-Cr-Mo	46	11.5	8.9
Co	Control	280	2.9	6.4
	Hastelloy C	18	4.7	7.6
	Co-Cr-Mo	54	76.7	45.9
	Co-Cr-Ni-W	9	63.8	77.8
Ti	Control	225	11.4	17.4
	A 286	17	27.1	32.4
	Titanium	25	236.8	168.8

[a] AISI 316; stainless steel, surgical grade; A 286, stainless steel containing Ti; Inconel X, Ni 80%, Cr 14%, Fe 6%; Hastelloy C, Mo 17%, Fe 5%, Cr 14%, W 5%, Ni bal.; Co-Cr-Mo, cast cobalt-chromium alloy; Co-Cr-Ni-W, wrought cobalt-chromium alloy.

[b] The figures give the concentration of metallic dissolution products in parts per million dry ash of the various elements found in the tissues surrounding implants of selected alloys in rabbits.

Reproduced with permission of A. B. Ferguson, Jr., P. G. Laing and E. S. Hodge.[26]

workers have clearly demonstrated that the metallic dissolution products may be concentrated within specific intracellular organelles. Koenig[18] revealed that the lysosomes of numerous types

Table 7-2

Comparison of Rates of Formation of Corrosion Products for Alloys in Hanks' Solution during Current Time Tests with Rates of Formation of Implant Corrosion Products in Rabbits[a]

Alloy	Metal converted into compound from j_a/t curve (ng cm^{-2} h^{-1})	Metal found in tissue (ng cm^{-2} h^{-1})
18Cr-10Ni-3Mo Steel		
Mechanically polished	7.8	0.274
Chemically polished	230	—
Vitallium		
Mechanically polished	150	0.249
Commercial finish	20	—
Ti		
Mechanically polished	4.1	0.430
Chemically polished	3.5	—
Ti-16Mo	1.5	—
Ti-5Ta	0.26	—

[a] The first column of figures was determined by electrochemical techniques after Hoar and Mears[29] while the second column represents the spectrochemical analyses of Ferguson et al.[26] The first data represents the amount of metallic dissolution products formed while the second indicates the amount of products that are retained in the tissues around the implant. The discrepancy in the figures may indicate the transport of products for storage elsewhere or for excretion. (Reproduced with permission of T. P. Hoar and D. C. Mears.[29])

of cells cultured in vitro could accumulate a variety of metallic ions. The possible significance of the intracellular accumulations of foreign substances are reviewed below.

More sophisticated observations were made by Ferguson, Laing et al.[26-28] who used spectrochemical analysis to record the presence of metallic dissolution products in paraspinal muscles that surrounded implants in rabbits. The concentrations of metal products stabilized in the tissues at about 4 months after implantation. Some of their results are shown in Table 7-1. Striking differences in the concentrations were observed, with a particularly high concentration of titanium and an exceptionally low concentration around several nickel-base alloys. Results for cast cobalt-chromium and AISI 316 steel were near the median.

It is of interest to compare these results by Ferguson et al.[26-28] with the results of passive dissolution rates of implantable alloys as reported by Hoar and Mears[29] (Table 7-2). From these and other estimates of the passive dissolution of titanium and titanium alloys in neutral chloride-containing solutions, the dissolution rate of titanium is much slower than the dissolution rates of surgical grade stainless steels, cobalt-chromium alloys or nickel alloys. In the experiments by Ferguson et al.[26–28] the soft tissues moved freely around the implanted specimens. In view of the liability of titanium to undergo fretting, it is quite conceivable that the titanium implants undergo mechanical erosion even when they are surrounded by soft tissues so that the titanium detected in tissues around implants represents minute particles rather than dissolution products. Also spectrochemical analysis of other organs in the rabbits were performed by Ferguson et al.[27, 28] to determine the fate of the metallic products. As seen in Tables 7-3 to 7-5, the various organs showed considerable differences in their capacity to store trace-metals. In the quantity of metal stored, the spleen showed the greatest tendency, with the lung second and liver and kidney a distant third

and fourth. While muscles in juxtaposition to the implant showed modest accumulation, other muscles did not show this tendency. The spleen tended to store chromium, cobalt, titanium, nickel, iron, aluminum and zirconium. The lung and kidney tended to accumulate cobalt and nickel. From these and other similar studies one may understand the dynamic migration of metallic dissolution products from the site of formation to other tissues, notably of the splenic reticuloendothelial system where they are concentrated. In addition some of the products are excreted.

A variety of other sophisticated analytic techniques are available for quantitative assessment of metals. The analytic limits for the measurement of small amounts of metals by several methods are shown in Table 7-6. Spark-source mass spectrometry and electron probe microanalysis are the most sensitive in detection levels. For the latter the detection limits for many elements in biological tissues is about 100 to 800 ppm. Since the tissue analyzed measures only a few cubic microns in volume, the absolute amounts detected range from 10^{-2} to 10^{-17} g.

Table 7-3

316 Stainless Steel Concentrations of Trace Metallic Dissolution Products in Parts per Million Dry Ash of Designated Tissues[a]

316 SS (Cr 17.8   Ni 13.4   Mo 2.3   Cu 0.23   Fe 66.27)

	Surrounding Muscle		Liver		Kidney		Spleen		Lung		Control Muscle	
	6 wks	16 wks	6 wks	16 wks	6 wks	16 wks	6 wks	16 wks	6 wks	16 wks	6 wks	16 wks
Cr	145/67	115/295	<2/7	<2/3	<2/2	4/3	4/5	<2/22	2/5	24/7	20/2	7/3
Co	<2/2	10/—	<2/18	12/—	5/11	17/113	<2/5	16/1300	2/3	—/250	<2/—	—/90
Ni	14/52	68/200	21/21	2/96	4/14	14/14	6/17	64/1000	19/220	23/46	13/3	5/5
Ti	19/8	24/11	<2/9	4/6	<2/7	67/4	<2/6	8/49	<2/13	6/6	6/11	7/9
Mo	3/9	11/35	9/76	63/48	9/84	80/73	<2/8	13/150	<2/14	5/5	2/<2	<2/<2
Fe	70/87	117/210	260/600	535/575	125/265	210/250	230/510	600/300	140/290	185/355	29/13	15/12
Al	78	116/97	120	36/68	77	58/44	84	35/82	135	53/72	73	38/26

[a] The composition is shown by the figures in parentheses. Each number represents the mean result of two determinations on each of the designated tissues. The spleen showed an occasional tendency to retain dissolution products such as nickel at 16 weeks. Minimal elevation of molybdenum was evident in the liver and kidney. In general, the concentrations of dissolution products in tissues were low. (Reproduced with permission of A. B. Ferguson, Jr. et al.[27])

Table 7-4
Vitallium Concentrations of Trace Metallic Dissolution Products in Parts per Million Dry Ash of Designated Tissues[a]

Vitallium (Co$_{61.9}$ Cr$_{28\text{-}34}$ Mo$_{4.73}$ Ni$_{1.52}$ Fe$_{0.61}$)

	Surrounding Muscle		Liver		Kidney		Spleen		Lung		Control Muscle	
	6 wks	16 wks	6 wks	16 wks	6 wks	16 wks	6 wks	16 wks	6 wks	16 wks	6 wks	16 wks
Cr	24 32	16	<2 4	<2.5 <2.5 7	<2 3	<2.5 3 6	<2 6	<2.5 <2.5 6	<2 10	<2.5 <2.5 5	2 2	5
Co	24 47	28	<2 8	<2.5 <2.5 5	— 105	3 5 71	— 21	<2.5 <2.5 <300	— <300	10 <2.5 9	— 48	7
Ni	19 37	5	2 8	3 — 82	5 109	5 4 28	4 205	5 <2.5 <1000	<2 40	3 — 46	3 6	5
Ti	5 9	13	<2 5	— 7	2 8	— 3 9	3 4	<2.5 — 18	6	— 17	8	7
Mo	4 5	3	14 80	12 11 73	24 51	17 20 74	2 13	<2.5 — 6	2 12	3 5 6	— <2	—
Fe	37 80	63	217 <600	166 190 59	90 220	124 139 36	280 345	320 310 52	110 460	126 119 30	11 26	19
Al	69	90	80	50	38	64	46	38	160	52	44	37

[a] The composition is shown by the figures in parentheses. Each number represents the mean result of two determinations on each of the designated tissues. Cobalt and nickel were elevated in the kidney, spleen and lung in some animals. The elevations appeared to be related to individual variations of the animals. There was also a relative elevation of these elements in the surrounding muscle at 6 weeks, as compared with 16 weeks. (Reproduced with permission of A. B. Ferguson, Jr. et al.[27])

Table 7-5
Titanium Concentrations of Trace Metallic Dissolution Products in Parts per Million Dry Ash of Designated Tissues[a]

Titanium (Ti$_{99.7}$ Fe$_{0.25}$ N$_{0.04}$)

	Surrounding Muscle		Liver		Kidney		Spleen		Lung		Control Muscle	
	6 wks	16 wks	6 wks	16 wks	6 wks	16 wks	6 wks	16 wks	6 wks	16 wks	6 wks	16 wks
Cr	3 3	7 25	<2 <2.5	6 <2	<2 3	5 4	<2 13	8 13	2 4	6 4	3 <2.5	2 2
Co	— —	— 8	— —	— 4	4 2	16 12	— 5	— 64	— —	— —	— —	— —
Ni	16 5	5 8	>100 4	175 7	6 6	32 19	4 11	25 37	5 40	9 9	— —	5 5
Ti	27 47	235 230	3 <2.5	7 <2	— 17	4 7	3 900	12 14	<2 <105	10 6	7 8	10 12
Mo	<2.5	5	13 15	75 47	16 13	34 59	2 5	9 9	<2 3	5 8	<2.5	—
Fe	28 26	47 70	250 150	>600 530	115 105	300 >500	180 540	>600 >600	75 105	300 320	14 10	19 14
Al		74 98		74 23		42 70		115 150		60 63		34 56

[a] The composition is shown by the figures in parentheses. Each number represents the mean result of two determinations on each of the designated tissues. There was a high concentration of titanium in the surrounding muscle but no storage tendency elsewhere, except in the spleen and lung of one animal. (Reproduced with permission of A. B. Ferguson, Jr. et al.[27])

Table 7-6
Analytic Limits for Metals in Various Techniques[a]

Metal	GLC	Atomic absorption	Neutron activation	Emission spectroscopy	Spark-source mass spectrometry
Be	6×10^{-14}	1×10^{-8}		2×10^{-10}	8×10^{-12}
Cd		5×10^{-9}	1×10^{-10}	2×10^{-6}	
Hg		5×10^{-7}	1×10^{-8}	2×10^{-8}	
Ga		7×10^{-8}	1×10^{-10}	1×10^{-8}	
In		5×10^{-8}	3×10^{-12}	2×10^{-9}	
Tl		2×10^{-7}	———	2×10^{-8}	
Sc		1×10^{-7}	1×10^{-9}	3×10^{-8}	
Ge		1×10^{-6}	3×10^{-9}	5×10^{-7}	
Pb		3×10^{-8}	———	2×10^{-7}	
Ti		1×10^{-7}	1×10^{-9}	2×10^{-7}	
Zr		5×10^{-6}	5×10^{-7}	3×10^{-6}	
As		2×10^{-7}	2×10^{-10}	———	
Sb		1×10^{-7}	2×10^{-10}	———	
V		2×10^{-8}	1×10^{-11}	1×10^{-8}	
Nb		3×10^{-6}	———	1×10^{-6}	
Se	4×10^{-9}	5×10^{-6}	2×10^{-9}	———	1×10^{-6}
Te		3×10^{-7}	2×10^{-9}	———	
Cr	2×10^{-14}	2×10^{-9}	1×10^{-6}	1×10^{-9}	5×10^{-11}
Mo		3×10^{-8}	1×10^{-9}	1×10^{-7}	
W		3×10^{-6}	2×10^{-10}	5×10^{-7}	
Mn		2×10^{-9}	4×10^{-12}	5×10^{-9}	
Fc		5×10^{-9}	1×10^{-5}	5×10^{-8}	
Co	1×10^{-11}	2×10^{-9}	5×10^{-10}	5×10^{-8}	5×10^{-11}
Ni		5×10^{-9}	2×10^{-8}	3×10^{-8}	
Pd		2×10^{-8}	2×10^{-9}	5×10^{-8}	
Pt		1×10^{-7}	1×10^{-8}	2×10^{-6}	

[a] Limits expressed in g metal/g sample.
[b] Reproduced with permission of T. D. Luckey and B. Venugopal.[30]

Gas-liquid chromatography (GLC) is the next most sensitive method. The techniques are described fully elsewhere.[25] Radiochemical separation techniques were performed by Coleman et al.[31] on the blood, urine and hair of patients who had total hip joint replacements made of cobalt-chromium alloys. For patients with metal-to-metal joints the concentration of cobalt in the blood and hair was usually raised by a factor of 10 to 20, and in the urine by a factor of 10 to 50 compared with preoperative levels. The chromium levels were also raised. It was predicted that the average increase in concentration of cobalt in liver and kidney was about twice the normal levels for these organs. Jones et al.[32] have confirmed the results of Coleman et al.[31] Also they have discovered minute quantities of metallic wear products in many other tissues from similar total joint replacements that are significantly higher than normal variations. The limited data on the metal-to-plastic joints re- vealed no detectable elevation of cobalt and chromium in the body.

The Kinetics of Metal Ion Transport in Tissues

Recently Perkins[33] has investigated the binding of trivalent metal ions with transferrin, the iron transporting protein of the vascular system. Chromium, manganese, cobalt and nickel bind with transferrin although they do not appear to block iron in its complex formation with transferrin. Most of these elements appear to be excreted by the fecal route, with much less urinary excretion, and only chromium excretion *via* the biliary tree. Taylor[34] has described the relationship for a given rate of continuous release of corrosion products, R/day. The increase in an organ or the total body content of a metal can be calculated from the expression:

$$Qt = Q_0 + R(1 - e^{-kt})/k$$

where Q_0 is the normal metal content, Qt the content at time t days and k is the fractional rate of excretion of the metal. When the rate of excretion balances the rate of release of the metal into the circulation, the total body content of the metal is given by the expression:

$$QE = Q_o + \frac{R}{K}$$

Values of k can be derived from data contained in publications no. 2 and 10 of the International Commission on Radiological Protection. For any given corrosion rate the value of the QE may be calculated.

Maroudas[35] has studied the distribution of metallic ions between connective tissue and extracellular fluids. The extracellular component of connective tissue consists of collagen fibers embedded in a gel of acid glycosaminoglycans and water. The glycosaminoglycans possess fixed negatively charged groups. The distribution of mobile ions between connective tissue and extracellular fluids, therefore, is unequal. The concentration of cations in the tissue is always higher than their concentration in the extracellular fluids, while that of the anions is lower. Studies on articular cartilage reveal that the distribution of ions obeys, quantitatively, the ideal Donnan equilibrium:

$$\frac{\bar{m}_A}{m_A} z_B = \frac{\bar{m}_B}{m_B} z_A$$

where

$\bar{m}_A$ and $\bar{m}_B$ = molal concentrations of ions A and B in solution;

m_A and m_B = molal concentrations of ions A and B in tissue;

z_A and z_B = valencies of ions A and B.

For monovalent cations the ratio $\bar{m}_A/m_A$ is always greater than unity whereas for anions it is always less than unity since z is negative. If there are both monovalent and bivalent cations in solution, the distribution coefficient of the divalent ion would be equal to the square of that for the monovalent ion. The Donnan equilibrium, therefore, favors the concentration of divalent cations in tissues that possess a large number of negatively charged groups. Clearly it promotes unequal distribution of metallic ions in different tissues and fluids. In addition there are specific interactions between some ions and some constituents of tissue matrix. For example copper and iron are strongly and irreversibly absorbed by cartilage.

THE TOXICITY OF IMPLANTABLE METALS

In the previous century, when iron nails, copper screws or brass plates were implanted, fulminant destruction of adjacent tissues was not an uncommon observation.[19] Concomitant wound infection, either before or after the onset of rapid corrosion, was encountered frequently. In 1913 Lane[36] published the first useful report on the influence of corrosion in tissues around vanadium steel plates in which the infection rate was sufficiently low so that the significance of corrosion could be distinguished from that of chronic infection. Adjacent tissues were heavily stained with corrosion products. In marked contrast, the results of the vast survey by Scales,[37] on 2518 components of various orthopaedic implants for the stabilization of fractures and composed of AISI 316 steel, cobalt-chromium-molybdenum alloy and titanium showed no relationship between visible corrosion or erosion of the implant and the incidence of inflammation or sepsis of adjacent tissues. Several less dramatic side-effects follow the use of metal implants, however, especially where large articulated implants are used for prolonged periods. It appears likely that these side-effects are manifestations of toxicity from small concentrations of dissolution products and other attributes of metallic corrosion. Confirmation of this suspicion, however, remains a formidable task. Recent efforts in this direction are described below.

Histological Studies. One approach to assay toxicity has been gross photomicroscopy of tissues that grow around implants. Several decades ago Collins,[1] reported the presence of appositional bone formation around moderately inert stainless steel implants for the fixation of hip fractures. Conversely, around similar devices that were composed of low-grade stainless steels, thick fibrous tissue enveloped the implant. More recently Laing et al.[28] attempted to correlate the concentration of metallic contaminants with the thickness of fibrous tissue sheathes around a great variety of different alloys embedded in rabbits. They observed a crude correlation between the thickness of sheaths and the concentrations of metallic products (Figs. 7-5 and 7-6). In all of their studies motion between the implant and the surrounding soft tissues may have augmented the formation of thicker fibrous tissue capsules although the amount of motion should have been constant in all of their experiments. With closer scrutiny of the tissue response to metallic contaminants they observed

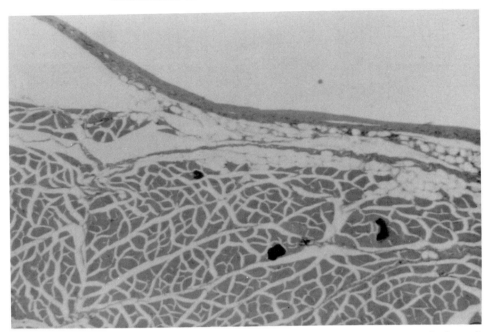

Figure 7-5. Fibrous tissue response to the presence of implants embedded in rabbit paravertebral muscle. The photomicrograph reveals a thin investing membrane in response to an inert material, cobalt-chromium alloy. Compare with Figure 7-6. (Reproduced with permission of Dr. P. G. Laing.)

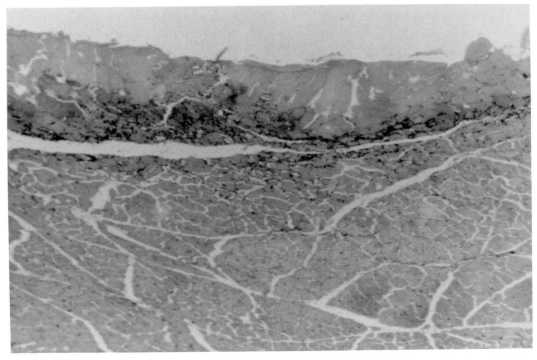

Figure 7-6. Fibrous tissue response to the presence of implants embedded in rabbit paravertebral muscle. The photomicrograph shows the thick fibrous layer around a less inert alloy, AISI 302 stainless steel. (Compare with Figure 7-5.) (Reproduced with permission of Dr. P. G. Laing.)

two zones: (1) In juxtaposition to the implant was a collection of cells aligned as a pseudomembrane. In favorable cases the cells were mostly fibroblasts. In unfavorable instances polymorphs, small round cells and macrophages were present. In markedly unfavorable reactions, necrotic or dead tissue was present. (2) Further away from the metal was an area of replacement of muscle with connective tissue and fat.

These workers believed the observations were similar to the actual occurrence in human implantation. Again it is emphasized that these attributes of metallic implantation with presently available materials have not been shown to be detrimental. The proliferation of a fibrous layer of up to 2 mm thickness is still encountered, principally with the use of stainless steel implants. The significance of the layer is related to the slippery, nonadherent nature of the surfaces which oppose the implant. The lack of a firm union may be advantageous or disadvantageous. Where rigid fixation between implant and tissue is sought, the fibrotic response to a metal is obviously detrimental. Where ease of removal of the implant is desired, as with many skeletal traction pins, fibrosis may be beneficial. As discussed below, the presence of fibrosis represents one predisposition to infection at the implant-tissue interface.

The assessment of fibrosis around surgical materials has been widely employed as a biological screening procedure. It has the merits of a simple experimental technique and the potential for at least a crude quantitative assessment for determining the thickness of the fibrous envelope. It is now evident that the amount of motion between the specimen and adjacent tissues participates heavily in the biological response. In retrospect the nature and the amount of motion around the specimens of Laing et al.[28] may have varied substantially. Other workers have recommended that the implantable specimens should possess a recess or other irregularity in shape which tends to anchor the material after tissues regenerate around it. Alternatively, where the tissue under scrutiny is bone or cartilage, the implant should be anchored rigidly to its surface or secured in a drill hole. The studies by Pilliar et al.[38] provide an application of the latter technique.

A simplified version of such histological assessment has been used by Homsy[39] as a rapid indication of biocompatibility. Cells are cultured in vitro on metallic surfaces and changes in the appearance of the cells are used to rate the toxicity of the metal from 0 to 4 where:

0   = excellent outgrowth with normal cell morphology;
+1   = excellent outgrowth but minor vacuolation of cells;
+2   = diminished outgrowth and major vacuolation of cells;
+3   = severe inhibition of growth;
+4   = total inhibition of growth, possibly with cell death.

While such rapid, inexpensive screening techniques may be of use for the selection of polymers, they are of limited value for the selection of new alloys as the more rapid and precise electrochemical tests permit exclusion from consideration of all but the most corrosion-resistant metals. For inert alloys the results of such crude histological studies would be unlikely to provide further discrimination, unless more precise biophysical measurements, such as the strength of adhesion between the cells and metals, are made.

The principal mechanisms whereby metallic dissolution products may damage cells are inhibition of enzymes, prevention of diffusion through the cell membranes or at the periphery of the cell, and breakdown of lysosomes.[40] In recent years, attention has focused on the last event. Weiss and Dingle[41] have shown that heavy metals may activate lysosomes to release their acid hydrolases, one of the principal intracellular digestive enzymes. These workers also have shown that lysosomal enzymes may be activated by changes in the outer cell membranes.[42] Furthermore, Fell and Weiss[2] have demonstrated in vitro that such release of lysosomal enzymes will cause enzymatic degradation of the intercellular matrix of embryonic bones. Also Dingle[43] has shown that lysosomes may cause connective tissue disease. It seems possible that such lytic processes may occur around metallic implants and contribute to tissue resorption.

In Figure 7-7 a schematic diagram indicates the sequence of events that might follow the uptake of metallic corrosion products by local mesenchymal cells. The corrosion products are stored in lysosomes, which after accumulation of a certain amount of the foreign material, undergo release and activation of the digestive enzymes. In turn, the enzymes lyse adjacent cells which release further activated lysosomal enzymes to initiate a self-stimulating process. The enzymes could degrade extracellular matrix, as well as cells to provoke loosening of an implant. Further studies on the significance of lysosomes in the toxicity of implant dissolution products are clearly needed.

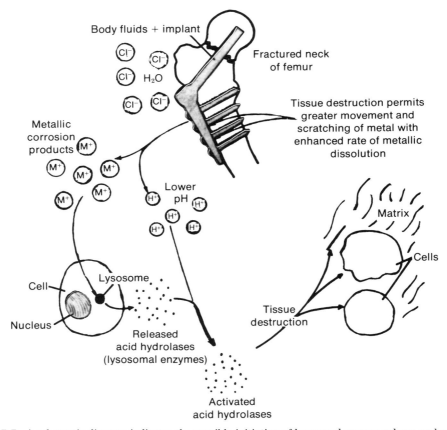

Figure 7-7. A schematic diagram indicates the possible initiation of lysosomal enzyme release and activation by metallic dissolution products that might lead to tissue destruction and loosening of the implant.

The Effect of Metallic Wear Particles on Isolated Cells

One of the cells that participates in the removal of foreign particulate matter from tissues is the macrophage. Tissues surrounding total joint replacements often show an inflammatory response with variable numbers of macrophages as well as lymphocytes, neutrophils, giant cells and wear particles. Rats given intramuscular injections of particulate cobalt-chromium alloy show a steady removal of the alloy to the regional lymph nodes where it is observed only in macrophages.[44] Necrosis and regeneration of muscle fibers have also been observed. In a recent study Rae[45] observed the effects of a variety of wear particles on the behavior of macrophages. Mouse peritoneal macrophages were grown in monolayer cultures. The cells were exposed to particulate cobalt-chromium alloy, nickel, cobalt-chromium, molybdenum, or titanium. Morphological changes in the cells

(Fig. 7-8) have been compared with changes in intracellular enzymes. Lactic dehydrogenase (LDH) and glucose-6-phosphate dehydrogenase (G6PD). LDH is located in the soluble cell fraction so that damage to the cell membrane initiates a release of enzyme into the surrounding tissue culture medium. Assessment of LDH, therefore, can be used as a marker of the integrity of the cell membrane. In contrast, G6PD is required for the synthesis of nucleic acids and lipids and its activity is needed during phagocytosis.

In Figure 7-9 the changes in LDH activity after exposure of macrophages to the different alloys are shown. Extracellular LDH starts to increase above the control values at about 3 hours and continues to rise and reaches a plateau at about 25 hours. Control cultures, however, show smaller amounts of LDH release. The increase toward the end of the culture period is characteristic of cells maintained in cultures. Figure 7-8, *D* and *E*, are photomicrographs of

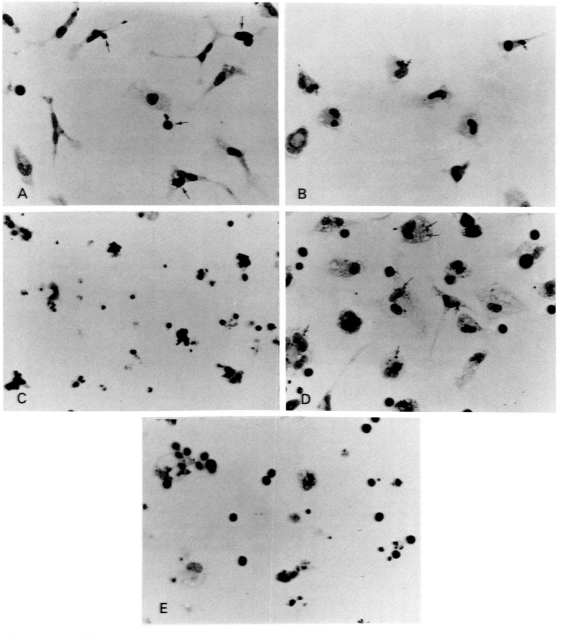

Figure 7-8. *A.* Photomicrographs of macrophages 6 hours after the addition of particulate chromium (*arrowed*). Cells are about 20 μm in length (methyl green and pyronin). (Reproduced with permission of T. Rae.[46] *B.* Macrophages 29 hours after the addition of molybdenum in particulate form (*arrowed*) (methyl green and pyronin). *C.* After 48 hours exposure to particulate cobalt the macrophages have been damaged as shown by cytoplasmic debris, shrunken cytoplasm and pyknotic nuclei (methyl green and pyronin). *D.* Particulate cobalt-chromium alloy (*arrowed*) has been present for 2 hours and has been ingested by the macrophages which show cytoplasmic vacuolization (methyl green and pyronin). *E.* After 48 hours exposure to particulate cobalt-chromium alloy the cells show shrunken cytoplasm and pyknotic nuclei (methyl green and pyronin). (*B, C, D,* and *E,* reproduced with permission of T. Rae.[46])

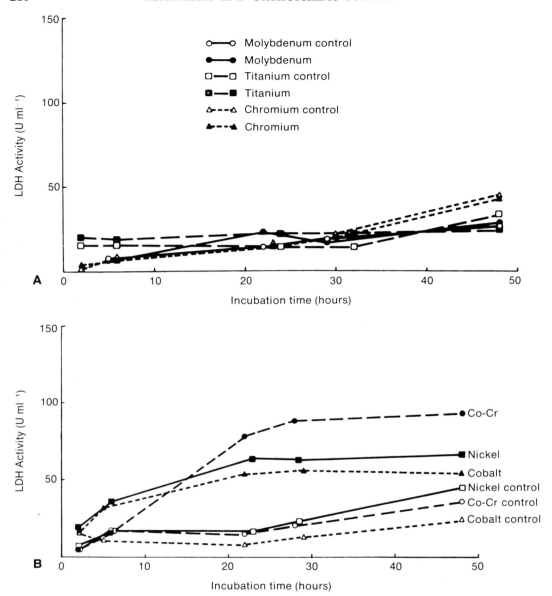

Figure 7-9. *A.* Lactic dehydrogenase (LDH) activity and supernatant of monolayer cultures exposed to particulate material. *B.* Lactic dehydrogenase (LDH) activity and supernatant of monolayer cultures exposed to particulate material. (*A* and *B,* reproduced with permission of T. Rae.[47])

macrophages in contact with the cobalt-chromium alloy for 2 and 48 hours respectively. After 2 hours metal is in close contact with the cells which look healthy. After 48 hours, however, the cells have withdrawn their cytoplasmic processes and some nuclei have become pyknotic. These changes are consistent with the leakage of LDH. In contrast, the metals molybdenum, titanium and chromium in particulate form do not produce any increase in extracellular LDH

above the control values. The macrophages shown in Figure 7-8*A* have been in contact with particulate chromium for 48 hours. The cells remain well spread and appear to be viable.

In comparable experiments to record the influence of metallic particles on G6PD activity, particulate titanium, molybdenum and chromium appear to have no demonstrable effect on the intracellular activity of the enzyme Fig. 7-10*A*) In contrast, particulate cobalt-chromium

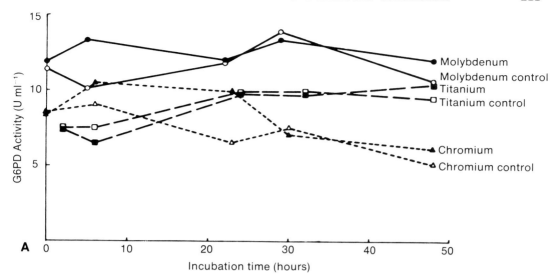

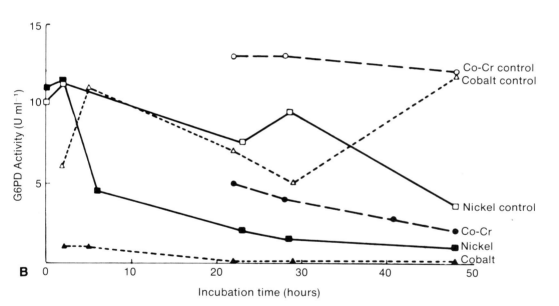

Figure 7-10. *A.* Glucose-6-phosphate dehydrogenase (G6PD) activity in lysate of cells exposed to particulate material. *B.* Glucose-6-phosphate dehydrogenase (G6PD) activity in lysate of cells exposed to particulate material. (*A* and *B,* reproduced with permission of T. Rae.[47])

alloy, cobalt or nickel show a marked decrease in their activity of G6PD as seen in Figure 7-10*B*. After 25 hours no activity was detectable in cobalt-treated cultures whereas those treated with nickel and cobalt-chromium alloys showed a reduction in enzyme activity of about 80% and 60% respectively. At 48 hours all three treated cultures showed a marked decrease in enzyme activity. Again, morphological changes in the cells could be correlated with the changes in enzyme distribution.

The results indicate that particulate cobalt is highly toxic to murine macrophages whereas particulate chromium and molybdenum are well tolerated under the experimental conditions. The difference between the result of cobalt and cobalt-chromium alloy is probably referable to the high solubility of pure cobalt in biological solution. Despite its relatively low solubility in a tissue culture medium, nickel was observed to be toxic to the macrophages. Whether the results observed here refer to the effect of the physical presence of the metallic particles or of the soluble dissolution products from the particles is not clear. Certainly soluble metallic dissolution products can have harmful effects on tissues although, as will be shown shortly, variation in particulate size also plays an important part in determining harmful biological effects of a material.

The alteration in the concentration of G6PD encountered with macrophages exposed to cobalt, nickel, or cobalt-chromium alloy suggests one of the possible deleterious side-effects of the metal on intracellular activity. It is the first enzyme in the hexose monophosphate shunt and its key role in phagocytosis is summarized in Figure 7-11. Any diminution in the activity of the enzyme is likely to decrease the phagocytic capacity of the cell. With the critical role of phagocytosis of bacteria by macrophages, a hindrance of their phagocytic capacity could conceivably help to explain late infections around total joint replacements. Further studies comparable to that by Rae[45] are greatly needed to reveal the biochemical alterations in intracellular organelles initiated by corrosion or dissolution products.

Quantitative and Morphological Analysis of the Tissue Reaction to Implants in Experimental Animals and Man

Many recent studies have attempted to correlate the reaction of connective tissues around metal implants with the amount of metallic dissolution product that can be recorded in the tissues. Scanning electron microscopy with electron probe microanalysis provides a useful tool for the quantitative assessment which can be correlated with photo and electron microscopy. In one recent study by Riede et al.[48] a series of dynamic compression plates (DCP)* applied to long bones of sheep were subjected to such an analysis. In some studies the implants consisted of the conventional stainless steel alloy while in others pure titanium was employed. The tissues at the site of the screw-plate junction were felt to be of particular interest in view of the likely motion with fretting corrosion and enhanced concentrations of metallic dissolution and wear products. The connective tissues surrounding the steel implants contained demonstrable quan-

_____
* Synthes North America, Wayne, Penn.

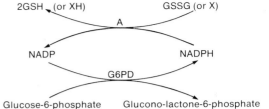

Figure 7-11. The critical role of G6PD in phagocytosis is indicated. G6PD generates NADPH from NADP. NADPH is one factor required to maintain glutathione in a reduced state which is essential for a functional intact cell membrane. NADPH is also required by enzymes dissolved in the phagocytic process. The abbreviations are: G6PD, glucose-6-phosphate dehydrogenase; GSSG, oxidized glutathione; GSH, reduced glutathione; A, glutathione reductase or enzymes stimulated by the attachment of particles to cell membranes. For example $X = O_2$ and $XH = H_2O_2$ a reaction catalyzed by NADPH oxidase. (Reproduced with permission of T. Rae.[47])

tities of iron and chromium while the titanium implants were surrounded by fibrous tissue in which titanium dissolution products were recorded. In the histological preparations of the connective tissue around the implants, larger numbers of inflammatory cells were encountered adjacent to the steel implants than were found adjacent to the titanium ones. These workers also attempted to correlate the number of giant cells in tissue. In this assessment it was felt that the steel implants provoked a greater cell response with more giant cells than the titanium implants.

A somewhat similar study was reported by Winter[49] who studied the tissue response to metallic wear and corrosion products in tissue biopsies removed with surgical implants. Samples of tissue were taken from around plates, screws, nails and wires and tissues adjacent to joint replacements. The tissue samples were subjected to routine histological preparation with conventional stains. Some specimens were prepared for electron microscopy while others were employed for electron defraction studies and for X-ray spectrographic analyses. Tissues from over 700 patients with surgical implants were observed with light microscopy. Among the different specimens the whole gamut of histopathological reactions were seen, including acute inflammation, granulation tissue, fibrosis, hyaline and acellular collagen and necrosis. In some instances the cell reactions were mainly polymorphonuclear while in others they were lymphocytic with plasma cells or with macrophages, giant cells or fibroblasts. Some of the tissue disturbance undoubtedly represented infection or blunt trauma to the tissues at surgery while in other instances the response might represent some underlying pathological condition of the patient, such as rheumatoid arthritis. The problem for the histopathologist was to elucidate the specific histological features attributable to the presence of the implant.

Many of the specimens contained frank metallic particles, or in the case of total joint replacements, of polyethylene or polymethylmethacrylate. Forty-four patients had cobalt-chromium alloy implants removed, of which 38 comprised total joint replacements. There were foreign-body particles and abnormal numbers of macrophages in 27 of the tissue samples from these 44 patients. The nature of the tissue reaction depended upon the number of foreign particles in the tissue. In the presence of scanty numbers of particles the macrophages appeared mainly around blood vessels and possessed phagocytosed particles in their cytoplasm. In these instances there are often no other cell reactions and the surrounding fibrous tissue appears to be normal. When the tissue was necrotic there were particles deposited among acellular collagen in linear array. It appeared that the particles had been engulfed by phagocytic cells prior to the death of the tissues. Where the tissue contained large numbers of particles it consisted of a granuloma (Fig. 7-12A) composed of a mass of contiguous large macrophages and a few multinucleate giant cells. Such granulomatous reactions were seen in 13 of the 44 patients.

Some macrophages carried few visible foreign particles but were stained gray in color, apparently indicative of numerous submicroscopic particles in their cytoplasm. In many cases the phagocytes were filled with optically dense particles of irregular shape and size, a few as large as 2 μm but most were 0.1 μm and smaller and numbering in the hundreds per cell (Fig. 7-12B). In the electron micrographs corresponding electron opaque particles, 0.1 μm to 50 μm, were embedded in electron dense material in numerous phagosomes which together often occupied up to about one half of the volume of the cytoplasm (Fig 7-13A).

Thin sections of tissue studied from a 57-year-old patient who had an all cobalt-chromium total hip prosthesis for 1 year prior to fracture and removal of the device, were particularly interesting. Small fragments of highly crystalline material were identified in the transmission electron micrographs. The Debye-Scherrer defraction pattern indicated that the particles were unchanged cobalt-chromium alloy. The local tissue reaction consisted of a granulomatous nodule with a well defined border and the presence of numerous macrophages (Fig. 7-13A). Tissues from two other patients characterized by massive macrophage reactions were studied from a patient who had had a knee prosthesis for 3 years and 6 months and another who had had an elbow prosthesis for 1 year and 4 months. Electron micrographs (Fig. 7-13B) revealed agglomerates of numerous minute acicular particles. Electron defraction studies showed these to be carbides of chromium, $Cr_{23}C_6$ and Cr_7C_3 and cobalt carbide Co_2C and other phases which were present but not identified. A consistent histological feature of tissues near worn cobalt-chromium joint prostheses is the numerous, minute particles in macrophages which, as yet, have not been positively identified. These macrophages are typically large cells, frequently clumped together and fused to form giant cells with many nuclei (Fig. 7-14A). The frequency of bizarre-shaped nuclei and pyknotic nuclei suggest that the material ingested by the phagocytes is cytotoxic.

Tissues removed from a cobalt-chromium knee prosthesis which had been in place for 1 year and 4 months were studied by X-ray fluorescent spectroscopy. Cobalt-chromium, molybdenum and nickel were identified in approximately the proportions specified for the cast cobalt-chromium alloy used for surgical implants.

In tissues adjacent to implants manufactured from stainless steel, three types of foreign material are recognized in the optical microscope: type I deposit—opaque small, irregular shaped particles, 0.3 mm to 0.1 μm; type II deposit—large platelets sometimes green, 5.0 mm to 0.5 mm of variable size and morphology; and type III deposit—yellow-brown granules mainly spherical "hemosiderin" 3 μm to 0.1 μm. Where the implant has undergone substantial wear as with a stainless steel knee joint replacement, the tissues are densely impregnated with a type I deposit (Fig. 7-14B). It seems likely that the opaque particles represent fragments of alloy abraded from the bearing surfaces. When examined in reflected light at high magnification, the particles show a grain structure indicative of a metal alloy. By the use of electron microscopy and electron defraction, the particles have been identified as austenite (face-centered cubic, a_0 = 3.60 Å) and a small amount of α-iron (body-centered cubic, a_0 = 2.88 Å). The smaller alloy

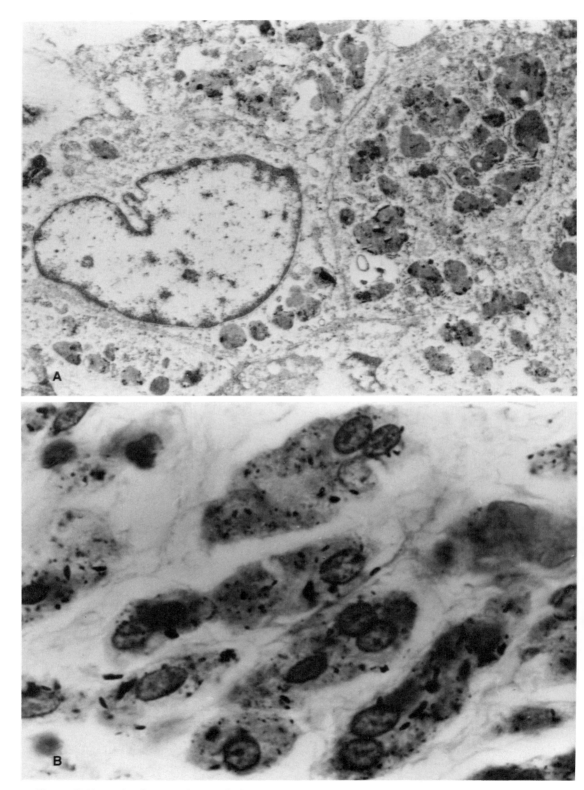

Figure 7-12. *A.* An electron micrograph shows a macrophage in a granuloma characteristic of the reaction to wear particles generated in cobalt-chromium joint replacements. Minute foreign-body fragments are visible in phagosomes (×4300). *B.* Phagocytes containing fragments of alloy in tissue from around a cobalt-chromium elbow joint prosthesis removed after 1 year, 4 months (H & E, ×865). (*A* and *B*, reproduced with permission of G. D. Winter.[50])

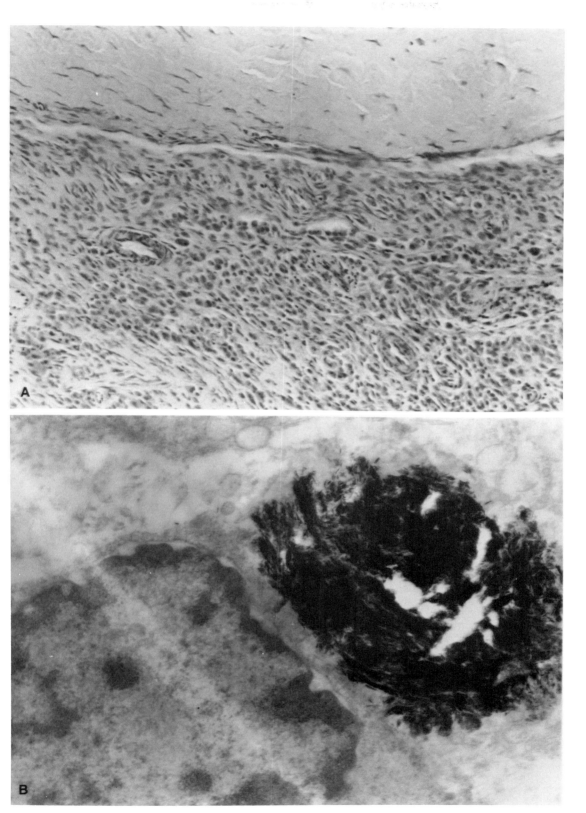

Figure 7-13. *A*. Edge of a granuloma containing macrophages in tissue from around the cobalt-chromium hip prosthesis in a 57-year-old patient. The prosthesis was removed after 1 year (H & E, ×88). *B*. Electron micrograph shows an agglomerate of minute acicular particles embedded in the cytoplasm of a macrophage and tissue from around a cobalt-chromium elbow joint prosthesis. Electron defraction pattern obtained from this material showed it to consist of mixed carbides of chromium and cobalt (×15,900). (*A* and *B*, reproduced with permission of G. D. Winter.[50])

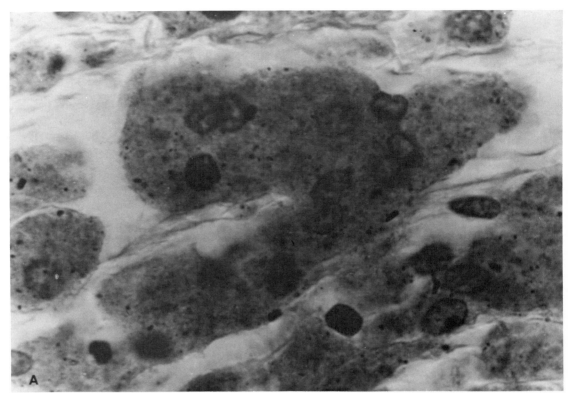

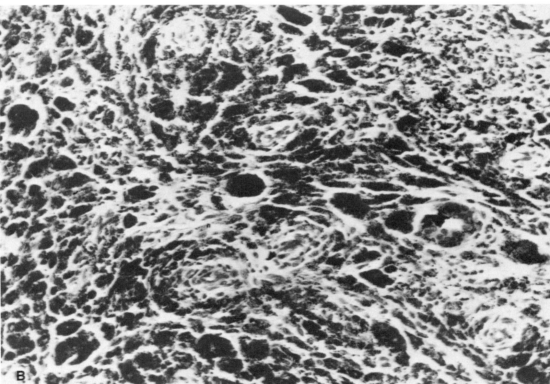

Figure 7-14. *A.* Cells from a granuloma in the tissue around a unique cobalt-chromium total hip joint prosthesis used in the treatment of osteoclastoma in a 34-year-old patient was removed after 4 years, 5 months when the implant broke. Photomicrograph shows typical clumping of macrophages which contain particles of foreign material (H & E, ×865). *B.* Tissue from around an austenitic stainless steel knee joint prosthesis used in a 49-year-old patient in the treatment of rheumatoid arthritis. The implant was removed after 6 years when the hinge pin fractured. The tissue contains massive amounts of debris from the worn alloy (H & E, ×138). (*A* and *B,* reproduced with permission of G. D. Winter.[50])

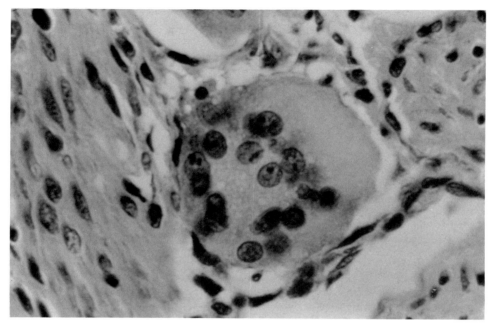

Figure 7-15. Tissue from around a stainless steel nail-plate device shows the presence of a typical giant cell reaction and fibrosis (H & E, ×400). (Reproduced with permission of P. G. Laing.)

particles were observed mostly in macrophages while the larger particles were surrounded by multinucleate giant cells. There was no granulomatous reaction and the impregnated fibrous tissue appeared to be normal despite the large amount of foreign material present.

Type II and III deposits were frequently observed together. The type II deposits were not seen in tissues from around cobalt-chromium implants but they were present in 11 of the 44 tissue specimens sampled from stainless steel implants. Often the material has the appearance of an amorphous film although occasionally a fibrous nature is evident. It is normally pale green in hematoxylin and eosin stained sections. While it has not been positively identified from electron defraction patterns, it is believed to represent an insoluble corrosion product of the alloy. It invariably provokes a vigorous foreign body giant cell reaction with fibrosis (Fig. 7-15). Frequently tissues impregnated with type II deposits consist of relatively acellular collagen or frankly necrotic tissue (Fig. 7-16A).

The type III deposit (Fig. 7-16B) closely resembles the hemosiderin pigment of classical histopathology, the residue of previous hemorrhage. Abnormally large quantities of "hemosiderin" are frequently evident in tissues adjacent to stainless steel implants. In an attempt to quantify the hemosiderin content, Winter[49] observed far more of the material around stainless steel implants than around cobalt-chromium implants. This worker felt that the hemosiderin-like granules were a feature of tissues around stainless steel implants. It is conceivable that iron released by corrosion of stainless steel is processed by the same pathophysiological processes which handle iron from effete erythrocytes.

Tissues studied from a stainless steel nail-plate assembly removed after 2 years of implantation because of persistent pain were of particular interest. The metallurgical examination revealed corrosion pits in the countersink surfaces of the screws and the holes of the plate. Numerous granules of iron-containing material were present in the tissues with a characteristic morphology seen in Figure 7-16B. The granules appear roughly spherical often about 1 μm in diameter although highly variable in size. They are most often observed in macrophages although others seem to be lying free in the tissue. In electron micrographs spherical shaped electron dense particles of highly variable size were embedded in a less dense material within phagosomes bounded usually by double membranes. Frequently the phagocytes laden with the particles show excessively vacuolated cytoplasm and bizarre distorted nuclei. Even when the

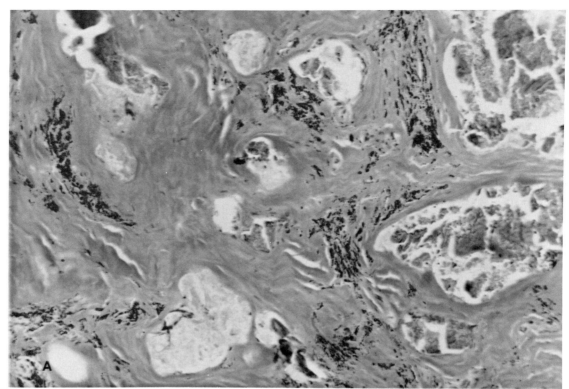

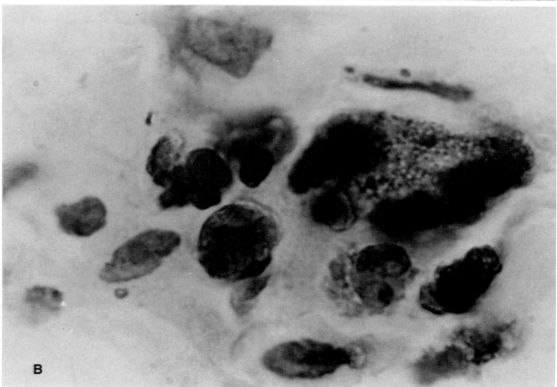

Figure 7-16. *A.* Tissue from around an austenitic stainless steel nail-plate removed from a 13-year-old patient after 4 years, 4 months because of persistent pain. Necrotic tissue around a type II deposit and hemosiderin-like material are observed (H & E, ×194). *B.* Typical morphology of hemosiderin-like (type III) particles of tissue around a corroded stainless steel nail-plate removed after 11 months (×1380). (*A* and *B,* reproduced with permission of G. D. Winter.[50])

tissue was heavily impregnated with type III iron-containing granules there was no associated granulomatous reaction as seen in juxtaposition to particles derived from cobalt-chromium implants. Where there were few particles in the tissue there was no recognizable tissue disturbance. Where contamination was heavy, several abnormalities were seen including the evidence of cytotoxicity, previously mentioned, and fibrosis or necrosis. Thin sections of tissue containing type III deposits were examined by selected area electron diffraction. The areas contained mixtures of two or more of the iron oxides, αFe_2O_3 and γFe_2O_3 and the hydrated iron oxides $\alpha Fe_2O_3 \cdot H_2O$ (geotite) and $\gamma Fe_2O_3 \cdot H_2O$ (lepidocrocite).

The tissue reactions to metallic wear documented by Winter[49,50] are described in great detail because they represent that type of information which is essential as a baseline for future studies. The careful histological record defines the unique cell responses to the presence of various alloys and their corrosion products or wear particles. Precise characterization of the nature of the wear particles or metallic dissolution products are sorely needed so that the causal relationships between particular types of metallic dissolution products and pathological cell response can be defined. Around cobalt-chromium implants that undergo wear with the evolution of numerous minute particles, tissues show an intense macrophage reaction. Granulomatous foci are encountered in areas where wear particles are particularly dense. The presence of cobalt and chromium carbides may indicate that inclusions in the chrome-cobalt casting were liberated as wear progressed.

Despite the elaborate details reported here the clinical significance of the adverse tissue reactions remains obscure. Most of the patients from whom the implants were removed or most of the thousands of other patients who have similar implants *in situ* have no symptoms referable to such tissue reactions. Most of the failures that provoke removal of the implants represent errors in surgical technique, mechanical faults in the implants, infection or loosening, none of which, at least at the present time, can be attributed to the pathological events described here.

Most studies on pathological effects on particulate foreign material have been related to silica, asbestos, coal dust and comparable particles in the lung. The particles vary greatly in their toxic potential depending upon their size and chemical nature. Particles which react with or alter the permeability of membranes surrounding phagosomes may provoke liberation of lysosomal enzymes and initiate macrophage cell death in a self-stimulating manner as described previously. Macrophages which phagocytose foreign particles may interact with fibrocytes and provoke excessive fibrosis. While such reactions may compromise substantially the function of the lung or liver they may be of much less functional significance in tissues around joints. For example, around worn stainless steel implants, massive amounts of metallic particles were frequently observed in the tissues although the particles did not appear to provoke severe tissue reactions.

Winter[49] has discussed the possible significance of tissue reactions to stainless steel implants. The characteristic tissue reaction to stainless steel implants, cytosiderosis, represents the terminal degradation of stainless steel *in vivo* as an insoluble mineral similar to hemosiderin which is a normal storage form of excess iron in the body. The cytological response is a local accumulation of macrophages.

The metabolism of iron and other heavy metals have been documented in detail elsewhere.[25] About 26% of total body iron (4 to 5 g in adult man) is normally stored as ferritin and hemosiderin. The former consists of a protein, apoferritin in which micelles, 50 Å in diameter, of a ferric-hydroxide-phosphate complex are embedded. Hemosiderin appears to possess a similar chemical composition to ferritin but is insoluble. Both have a high content of iron. Hemosiderin stores appear to be slowly transformed from an amorphous to a crystalline state. In contrast, geotite provides a fairly inert store of iron that is unavailable for further synthetic reactions. In the study by Winter[49] geotite was identified in the type III deposits around stainless steel implants. The formation of geotite may represent a protective detoxication mechanism for the removal of potentially dangerous iron salts that would otherwise represent a source of toxic ferrous ions.

Excessive iron storage in the body comprises hemosiderosis. Iron storage diseases, hemosiderosis and hemochromatosis, are caused by an accumulative excess of 20 to 60 g of body iron. For a conventional nail-plate assembly used for treatment of a proximal femoral fracture complete biodegradation of 2 to 6 mg of alloy per day could provide such accumulative excess of iron after about 40 years of deterioration. In fact, as Winter[49,50] emphasizes, it is most unlikely that any stainless steel alloy in present or future use would ever corrode to that extent so that iron storage disease initiated by stainless steel implants is most unlikely. Nevertheless, the observations of dying cells, acellular collagen and tissue necrosis around type II and type III deposits in some specimens suggest that localized tissue toxicity does occur around some worn and corroded stainless steel implants. While the tissues show an unnatural appearance the significance of these changes remains obscure.

The Reaction of Tissues to Metal and Polymeric Total Joint Replacements

Most total joint replacements currently in use consist of a cobalt-chromium alloy or stainless alloy component articulating against a polyethylene unit in which anchorage of both components is realized by use of methylmethacrylate. A number of workers have studied the tissue response to such implants after total hip and knee joint replacement. Willert and Semlitsch[51] have studied tissue specimens from 123 reoperated total joint replacements. The application of routine histological preparation with photomicroscopy and by the use of polarized light permits both a distinction of polyethylene or in certain instances of polyester wear particles from the total joint replacements from those of the polymethylmethacrylate cement. Under polarized light, polyester and polymethylmethacrylate show widely differing birefringence which is revealed in the subsequent subsection on ferrographic analyses. In metal-on-polymeric total joint replacements few metallic wear particles are encountered in the surrounding tissues, while large amounts of high density polyethylene wear particles are observed. Both a giant cell foreign body reaction and a histocytic response can be observed. Willert and Semlitsch[51] believe that the particles initiate a marked tendency for fibrosis. They have observed highly variable numbers of polymethylmethacrylate particles probably depending upon surgical technique. The particles initiate a giant cell histocytic foreign body reaction but little tendency to fibrosis. In implants where polyester (polyethylene terephthalate) is employed large numbers of wear particles have been encountered in the tissues with a predominantly histocytic foreign body reaction, marked granulomata formation and a tendency toward necrosis. Frequently lymphoplasma cellular infiltrates have been observed in proliferative granulation tissue. They feel that the histological response has culminated in massive bone resorption especially around the acetabular component with loosening of the prosthesis. Their conception of these events is shown schematically in Figure 7-17. From their study they concluded that polyethylene terephthalate is unsatisfactory for clinical application. The tissue response to metallic components, high density polyethylene and methylmethacrylate cement was not considered to be a contraindication to their application.

Another extensive study on the histology of joint tissues around total joint replacements has been reported by Mirra et al.[53] Their clinical material comprised 24 hip and 12 knee prosthetic failures in patients who underwent surgical revision. Synovial and capsular biopsies were taken from the sites of the implants. The tissues were examined for acute and chronic inflammatory and histocytic cells and for metallic and polymeric particles. An attempt was made to quantify the numbers of inflammatory cells and wear particles and to correlate clinical, radiological and pathological data.

Fifteen of the patients had clinical and bacteriological evidence of infected joint replacements. Histological specimens from this group revealed evidence of polymorphonuclear leukocytes, and in the cases of chronic infection, of accumulations of lymphocytes, lymphoid follicles and plasma cells. In the remaining 21 tissue biopsies, polymorphs were not observed, even though variable amounts of metal, polyethylene and acrylic wear particles were documented. Twenty-eight biopsies, including 15 joint infections, showed substantial numbers of mononuclear histiocytes. Usually, these cells were associated with polyethylene and acrylic particles, which usually were found within their cytoplasm or surrounding cells. Giant cells were consistently seen in association with the presence of modest accumulations of polyethylene, acrylic or metallic wear particles. They are also present in some of the infected specimens. In the noninfected cases, the giant cells either contained the wear particles within their cytoplasm or surrounded particles greater than 100 μm in diameter.

Under the light microscope, the metallic debris appeared in the tissues as small, black spheres, or irregular particles of 1 to 4 μm in length. Care must be taken to distinguish them from the usually nonrefractile and larger golden-brown hemosiderin pigment. Metal in large quantities stains joint tissues and joint fluid jet black, while in moderate quantities, various shades of gray. When small amounts of metal were present, it was found mostly extracellularly or in mononuclear histiocytes. In the presence

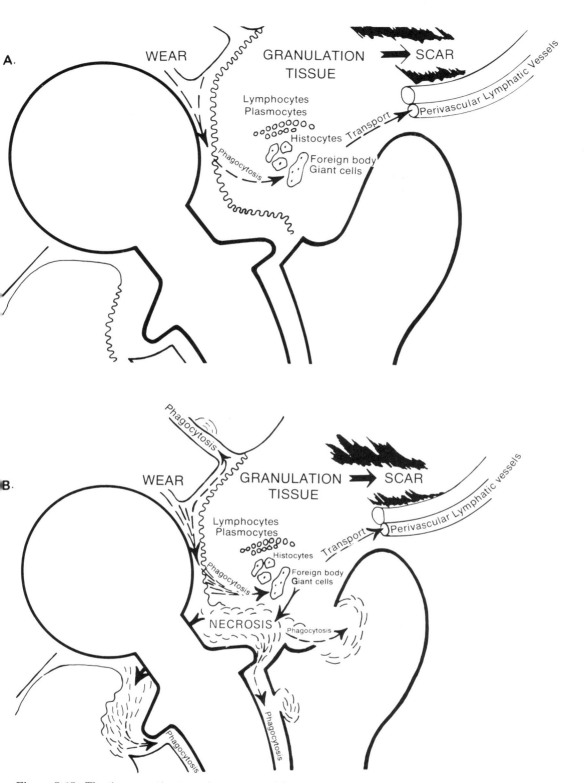

Figure 7-17. The tissue reaction to noxious wear particles such as those of polyester initiates a series of events which may culminate in loosening of the total joint replacement. *A.* Small amounts of the wear particles can be removed without overloading the transport mechanisms. In the presence of excessive release of wear particles, however, the transport system is overwhelmed and the local concentration of wear particles increases. *B.* In turn, granulation tissue within the articular capsule becomes necrotic. The bone marrow and the connective tissue membrane along the bone-cement interface participates in the storage of particles and thereby in the foreign body reaction. (Reproduced with permission of H. D. Willert and M. Semlitsch.[52])

221

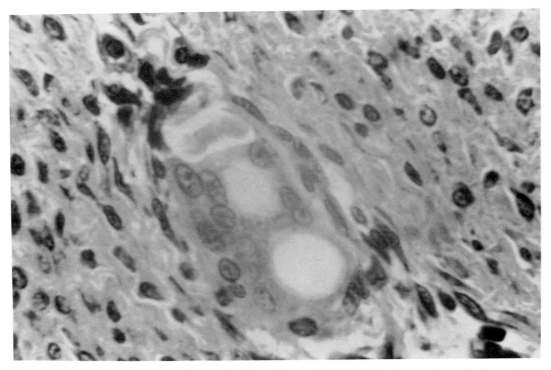

Figure 7-18. A photomicrograph of a capsular biopsy from a total hip joint replacement reveals the presence of spaces which previously housed polymethylmethacrylate particles. With the application of xylene solvent during routine histological processing the acrylic is dissolved from the sections. A residual space of about 100 μm or more in diameter is surrounded by multinucleate giant cells, histocytes and fibroblasts. (Reproduced with permission of P. G. Laing.)

of greater amounts of metal, it was associated with mononuclear histiocytes in ever greater quantities. Histiocytes with numerous metallic inclusions were also found in one patient in a subcapsular lymph node.

Some metallic wear particles were observed in all of the patients. Of 29 biopsies of tissues surrounding metal on plastic prostheses left in place for an average of 7 months, 26 showed small amounts of metallic particles. Polyethylene wear particles were observed in all 29 biopsies with a polyethylene component. Usually, it appeared as fibers with smooth borders from 5 to 40 μm in length and 2 to 5 μm in width. Occasionally, the fibers were smooth or irregularly fibrillated and over 100 μm in length by 5 to 10 μm in width. Rarely, large flakes of up to 1 mm in size were seen. Polyethylene fibers stimulated the most proliferative histocytic reaction. Fibers less than 40 μm were usually contained within mononuclear histiocytes and occasionally multinucleated histiocytes. Larger fibers were surrounded by mononuclear or multinuclear histiocytes or within the cytoplasm of multinuclear histiocytes. The appearance of

polymethylmethacrylate is altered by routine histological processing when xylene solvent dissolves acrylic out of the sections. A residual round or oval space remains in the tissue of approximately 100 μm in diameter to 1 mm or more. An example is seen in Figure 7–18. In most of these cases where barium sulfate was added to the acrylic as a radiological contrast material, polarizable granules of 1 to 2 μm in diameter were visible at the edges of the tissue abutting on the acrylic spaces or arranged in a circular distribution. Each circle had an average diameter of 10 to 30 μm indicative of the 10- to 30-μm diameter spheres of acrylic present in acrylic powder. Photographs of the unaltered acrylic spheres are shown below in the subsection on the use of Ferrography. Acrylic spaces in joint tissues were usually surrounded by 1 to 4 layers of multinucleate giant cells, or spindle-shaped histiocytes and fibroblasts. Of the 30 biopsies in which acrylic was used to stabilize the implants, 13 possessed the material in the tissues. In 9 out of 10 biopsies, there was a strong positive correlation between substantial amounts of acrylic in the tissues and radiological or surgical evidence of a loose implant.

The study of Mirra et al.[53] confirms the strong correlation between the presence of polymorphonuclear leukocytes and bacterial infection. There is a striking absence of polymorphs in aseptic cases in which even substantial quantities of metallic, polyethylene or acrylic wear particles are present. At the rate at which the wear particles are normally shed, they do not seem to stimulate an acute inflammatory response. Admittedly, previous observations by Cohen[54] in which pulverized metallic particles were injected into the flanks of rats showed an early polymorphonuclear response followed by histiocytes, and finally fibrosis. Within 1 week after injection of cobalt-chromium particles, the polymorph response had dissipated, while the polymorphs persisted for 2 weeks after injection of stainless steel powder, and for more than 5 weeks with mild steel and silica. The observations of Cohen,[54] however, should be referable only to experiments where large numbers of particles are released acutely into tissues.

Mirra et al.[53] attempted to correlate the pathological response of failed implants and the clinical cause of failure. The best correlation is the presence of polymorphs and bacterial infection. Large amounts of metallic particles were mainly encountered where metal on metal prostheses were employed. Large amounts of polyethylene wear particles were suggestive of excessive wear usually secondary to subluxation of a component or impingement. They were much more common in failed total knee prostheses than in total hip prostheses. Polyethylene stimulated the most vigorous mononuclear and giant cell histocytic tissue reaction. Large numbers of acrylic particles were suggestive of a loose component.

Walker and Bullough[54a] have presented another comparable study on the tissue reaction to wear debris generated from total hip joint replacements. His findings are primarily in accordance with those reported here, although he reports strongly birefringent polymethylmethacrylate particles in the tissues. The presence of the acrylic indicates that xylene was not employed in tissue preparation. Again, in the subsection below on the use of ferrographic analyses, the author has observed strongly birefringent acrylic particles.

Despite the plethora of observations documented by the previous workers, the significance of the diverse types of chronic inflammatory response to wear particles and dissolution products can not be closely correlated with the failures of surgical procedures, other than those that become infected.

The Histological Response of Bone to Implantable Materials

Perhaps the first useful observation on the response of bone to foreign material was undertaken by Collins,[1] who published cross-sections of proximal femora in which triflanged nails had been extracted. A fairly uniform layer of moderately dense bone was deposited around the nail. From his and other observations, it was clear that smooth implants with chemically polished surfaces showed a layer of fibrous tissue between the implant and the bone. Early workers such as Laing et al.[28] suggested that the fibrosis was indicative of a slow but significant rate of dissolution of the metal. The corrosion products were believed to excite the fibrosis. More recently, other workers have employed implants which are rigidly stabilized in bone. Pöhler* imbedded sandblasted titanium specimens in bone and noted close approximation of bone to the metallic surface without any intervening tissue. Many other workers such as Pilliar et al.[55] have confirmed this observation. Porous implants, described in Chapter 16, are particularly representative of this finding, probably in view of the enormous surface area of the bone-metal interface and the excellent interdigitation and mechanical bond. Other workers have studied a variety of ceramics and bioglasses imbedded in bone. Again, the typical response of the bone to the presence of any inert and rigidly stabilized foreign body, is to deposit bone matrix around the specimen without any intervening substance. If the interface between a rigid metal implant and bone is subjected to repetitive impulsive loads or to other mechanical perturbation, however, a secondary remodeling process may ensue, as described in Chapter 6.

One special case is the interface between bone and glasses. Hench[56] and Hench and Paschall[57] studied a series of bioglasses that undergo slow but progressive biodegradation with the evolution of degradation products that can be utilized by bone for the elaboration of organic matrix. The various bioglasses show considerable variation in their surface reactivity. Bone tends to grow and bond with the surface of the bioglass, as seen in Figures 7–19 and 7–20. If the bioglass undergoes degradation with excessive rapidity, the surface reactivity tends to kill osteogenic cells. Where the bioglass shows insufficient surface reactivity, it does not induce bonding with the bone. The rate of reactivity of the bioglass can be altered by the preparation of the glass. The dissolution rate of the glass can be con-

* O. Pöhler, personal communication, 1977.

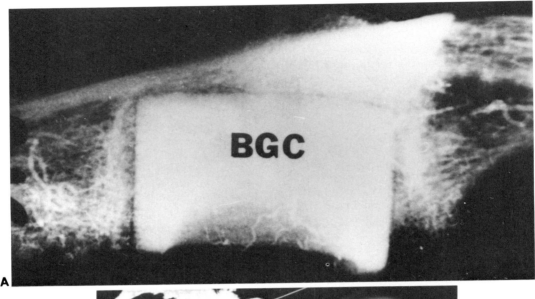

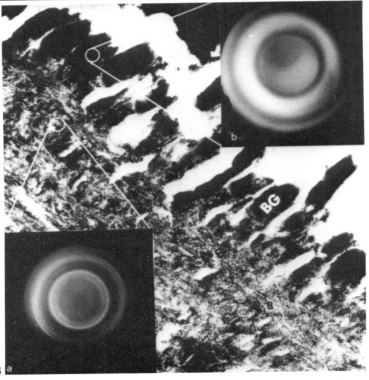

Figure 7-19. *A.* An X-ray reveals the acetabular cup of a total hip prosthesis consisting of bioglass-coated fully dense Al₂O₃ ceramic (*BGC*) after 3 months in an adult sheep. The bioglass coating provides the fixation of the bone by forming an interfacial bond. (Reproduced with permission of P. Griss *et al.*[58]) *B.* A transmission electron micrograph shows the formation of a contiguous chemical bond between bioglass (*BG*) in well mineralized bone in a rat femur at 6 weeks. The dark, electron opaque bioglass shows a fracture artifact due to chipping of the bioglass by the diamond knife. The interface of the bioglass bone, however, is maintained. Insert *a* is a defraction pattern of bone while insert *b* is a defraction pattern of bioglass. (Reproduced with permission of L. L. Hench *et al.*[59])

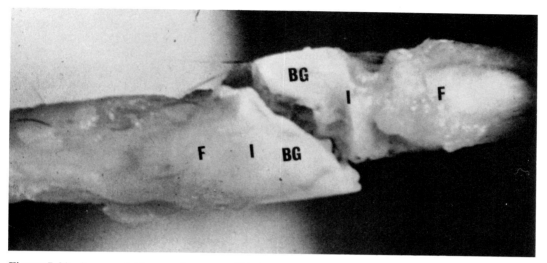

Figure 7-20. A segmental bone replacement of bioglass ceramic (*BG*) implanted in a monkey femur (*F*) for 6 months. The ends of the femur were subjected to a torsional implant loading. The bioglass segment failed at a stress approximately two-thirds that of the contralateral control femur. The interface (*I*) did not fail. (Reproduced with permission of G. Pitorowski *et al.*[60])

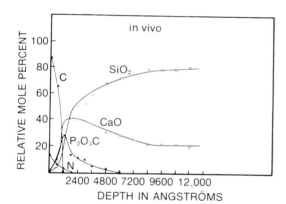

Figure 7-21. A chemical composition profile of the surface of a bioglass implant 1 hour after its removal from a rat femur. After argon ion beam milling an Auger electron spectroscope was used to obtain the data. The profile shows deposition of a calcium-phosphate layer on the bioglass which has incorporated an organic face, probably mucopolysaccharides containing carbon and nitrogen ions. (Reproduced with permission of C. G. Pantano, Jr., A. E. Clark, Jr., and L. L. Hench.[62])

trolled by the temperature of formation, the pH and the glass composition.

Carlisle[61] has studied the silicon content of bone at the mineralization front. In a study of the mineralization in murine bone by the use of electron probe microanalysis, she showed a relative abundance of silicon in the region of bone immediately ahead of the mineralization front (Fig. 7-21). She suggested that silicon may be an important constituent of bone to initiate mineralization. Most bioglasses show a silicon-containing gel on their surface. The gel also contains calcium and phosphorus and may thereby replicate the surface of bone in which osteogenesis proceeds. The replication of bone surface by bioglasses could explain their initiation of mineralization with incipient union of the two materials.

CURRENT METHODS OF ASSESSMENT OF TOXICITY FOR PREVIOUSLY UNTRIED MATERIALS

The previous discussions have indicated the types of reaction that wear or dissolution products of implantable materials may provoke to adjacent tissues. They have indicated that despite the complex methods of study presented here, the responses of tissues to an implantable material are not well understood, even when tissues can be studied *in vivo* after many years of exposure to a foreign material. Despite this dearth of knowledge, new materials continue to appear which must be assessed within the limitations of available methods. A variety of experimental approaches have been tried, all of which have severe shortcomings. Most new materials that would be employed in the future, and certainly all newer metals and alloys, should undergo tests for inertness in body fluids or simulated body fluids, prior to a biological assessment. Especially for metals where a variety of electrochemical assessments of corrosion can be employed, all but the most inert materials can be eliminated from consideration prior to initiation of costly biological tests. The tests are designed to be an "accelerated" short-term assessment of the anticipated toxicity of an untried material if it were exposed to the body for a prolonged period, usually of 2 to 50 years. From practical and economic considerations, the duration of the tests must be limited to periods of a few weeks to 2 years. Most of the tests are designed for studies *in vitro,* in view of the great reduction in cost compared to those observations performed in experimental animals. Ultimately, tests in rodents, and finally in large experimental animals, such as dogs, pigs or sheep, must be undertaken, where specimens are implanted in bone and soft tissues. For the large animals, implants which simulate their human counterparts should be employed. A recent review by Luckey and Venugopal,[25] provides an excellent documentation on the physiological and chemical basis for metal toxicity. Somewhat similar studies are also available on polymeric[63] and other materials.[64] Several of the available tests are now described.

ACUTE TOXICITY TESTS

Rabbit Muscle Test. This method appears in the *United States Pharmacopeia*[65] and represents one of the simplest biological tests for detection of leachable components of a polymeric material. It has been fully described by Turner *et al.*[66] A test material is shaped into thin cylinders or rectangles measuring approximately 1.5 cm by 1 mm. A specimen is placed into the beveled point of a 15 G trocar needle 4 cm long. The needle is inserted into the paravertebral muscle of a rabbit. Then it is withdrawn to leave the material implanted in the muscle. Two animals are used for each type of material under investigation. A positive control of a known toxic polymer and a negative control of a nontoxic material are also implanted in the animals. After 1 week the animal is sacrificed and the sites of the implants are compared with positive and negative controls. The microscopic examination of the implant sites is scored from 0 (nonreactive) to 3 (marked reaction). A questionable response is scored as ±. Histopathological assessment is also performed on the excised tissue around the implant. Autian[67] recommends 12 histological criteria to describe the tissue response. They include: (1) necrosis; (2) inflammation; (3) polymorphonuclear leukocytes; (4) macrophages; (5) lymphocytes; (6) plasma cells; (7) giant cells; (8) foreign body debris; (9) fibroplasia; (10) fibrosis; (11) fatty infiltrates; (12) relative size of involved areas.

Each of these criteria is then scored as follows:

0 = item not present;
1 = item occasionally not present;
2 = item present to a mild degree;
3 = item present to a marked degree.

From these 12 items an overall toxicity rating of the test samples is assigned as follows:

0 = nontoxic;
1 = very slightly toxic reaction;
2 = mild toxic reaction;
3 = moderate toxic reaction;
4 = marked toxic reaction.

Tissue Culture-Agar Overlay. This assay was described by Guess *et al.*[68] and is designed to detect the response of a mammalian monolayer cell culture to readily diffusible components from materials or test solutions applied to the surface of an agar layer overlying the monolayer. A 24-hour confluent monolayer is propagated in the bottom of a Petri dish. The liquid medium is aspirated and replaced by a standard layer of agar containing the minimum nutrient requirements of the cells. The monolayer is stained with a vital dye, neutral red, by the application of a standard quantity of the dye to the surface of the agar. After a standard period of time excessive dye is aspirated from the agar surface. Solid test samples approximately 1 cm^2 are placed on the surface of the agar. Each Petri dish receives two test samples plus one positive control (a known toxic material) and one negative control (a nontoxic material). For powder specimens 100 mg of material is applied directly to the agar surface to cover an area of approximately 1 cm^2. Extracts or other liquid samples are tested by imbibing 0.2 ml of the test liquid in a 1-cm diameter cellulose assay disc and applying it to the agar as previously described. After application of the test samples the Petri dishes are placed in a 37°C incubator for 24 hours with a 5% carbon dioxide atmosphere. The response of the cell monolayer is evaluated with respect to the extent of decolorization of the red stained monolayer under and around the sample when the Petri dish is viewed against a white background. Loss of color of the stained cells is considered to be a pathologically significant reaction of the cells. The extent of decolorization is confirmed by examination of the monolayer on an inverted microscope. Also the extent of lysis of the cells within the decolorized zone is estimated. Typically decolorization of cells precedes lysis as manifested by a region of decolorized cells between a normal fully stained region and a region showing lysis. A sample is reported as "cytotoxic" only if lysis is observed. The magnitude of the response of the monolayer may be reported in terms of a "Response Index".

RESPONSE INDEX = ZONE INDEX/LYSIS INDEX

Where the Zone Index is related to the size of the decolorized zone and the Lysis Index is related to the extent of lysis within the zone as outlined below:

Zone Index	Description of Zone
0	No detectable zone around or under sample.
1	Zone limited to area under sample.
2	Zone not greater than 0.5 cm in extension from sample.
3	Zone not greater than 1 cm in extension from sample.
4	Zone greater than 1 cm in extension from sample but not involving the entire plate.
5	Zone involving entire plate.

Lysis Index	Description of Extent of Lysis by Light Microscopy
0	No observable lysis.
1	Less than 20% of the zone lysed.
2	Less than 40% of the zone lysed.
3	Less than 60% of the zone lysed.
4	Less than 80% of the zone lysed.
5	Greater than 80% lysed within the zone.

The test method is a useful and sensitive procedure to detect diffusible biologically active constituents from polymeric materials. It correlates well with the *United States Pharmacopeia* rabbit implant procedure[65] but is more sensitive. It is possible, therefore, to report a negative response in the rabbit muscle while recording a cytotoxic response in the cell culture method. The Zone Index is related to leachability or diffusibility while the Lysis Index is related to acute toxicity. Should greater sensitivity be desired the test samples can be placed directly on the cells without the use of agar. In this case the material test sample must be stabilized to prevent movement during incubation and evaluation. Liquids, powders and fine fibers are not suitable for this procedure.

Biological Tests on Extracts. As part of a biological assessment of polymeric materials a variety of extracting media including sodium chloride solution, cotton seed oil, 5% ethyl alcohol in sodium chloride solution and polyethylene glycol 400 have been employed. The extraction is conducted at 121°C in an autoclave for 1 hour and the resultant extracts are set aside for biological testing. The tests are initiated with a 24-hour period for completing the extraction procedure. For the "inhibition" of cell growth assay (ICG) distilled water is used as the extracting medium. Alternatively, the procedure described by Guess *et al.*[68] for tissue culture may be employed except that 0.2 ml of the extract is placed on the surface of sterile paper discs which have been previously placed on the agar. Two plates are used for each extract and for each plate two paper discs with the extract are included. The negative control with solvent alone is also included in each plate as well as a positive toxic control. The remainder of the procedure is exactly as that described in "Tissue Culture-Agar Overlay."

Sensitization Tests. Special tests have been devised to determine the antigenic potential of various polymeric extracts. The test is based upon the work of Magnusson and Kligman[69] and will not be discussed in detail here. It requires approximately 6 weeks from initiation to completion with the use of guinea pigs as the test animal.

Histochemical Assessment of Toxicity

In a somewhat similar way, several workers[18, 41] have attempted to develop histochemical methods as sensitive indices of the capacity of dissolution productions to disrupt certain enzymatic reactions in cells *in vitro*. While the method would seem to be one of great promise, to date the results have been disappointing. For example the author studied the metabolism of alkaline phosphatase of cells cultured on a variety of metals by the application of the Gomori stain technique. The results did not provide any useful distinction among alloys of markedly dissimilar toxic potential.

TOXICITY ASSESSED BY THE USE OF CELL CULTURE

In addition, one other qualitative assay of the toxicity of metal particles to cells in culture has been reported by several workers who recorded rates of cell growth and mitoses as well as cellular degeneration. The metals under study have included a variety of implantable stainless steel and cobalt-chromium alloys. Again the results are of questionable relevance to clinical implantation of metal implants, both because of their insensitivity and because of the discrepancy between the results of the tests and clinical experience. More recently, Pappas and Cohen,[70] developed a quantitative assessment of cellular proliferation around metallic powders in tissue culture. A variety of surgical grade stainless steel and cobalt-chromium alloys were ground to a diameter of about 0.1 to 0.01 μm with acicular shape. Standardized amounts of metallic particles were added to a predetermined number of cells in culture. The cells under scrutiny, basal cell carcinoma, KB, a derivative of a human cell line, and P1534, a murine leukemic cell, were selected because of their predictable rates of cellular growth and for their availability. A variety of other cell lines, such as HeLa cells also were studied. Then the effect of a particular dose of metallic powder on the rate of proliferation of the cells was recorded. All of the metallic particles were toxic for the cultures and differences between the relative toxicity of various concentrations of stainless steel or cobalt-chromium alloy particles were reproducible. In contrast, the addition of similar amounts of glass particles did not influence the rates of cell proliferation in comparison with the control specimens. The addition of a unit weight of cobalt-chromium particles was more inhibitive to cell proliferation than a 100-fold addition of stainless steel particles. Cytological studies on the cultures revealed no significant morphological alterations except for collections of brown granules within the cytoplasm. Lamentably, even the results of this careful study are of questionable relevance to clinical implantation. Whether observations for such established cells lines are comparable to the effects of similar concentrations of wear particles on human tissues *in vivo* is unknown. As Swanson *et al.*[71] have emphasized, the size of wear particles is a critical factor in the nature of the cellular response to the particles. As will be described shortly, particles of 0.1 μm diameter may stimulate a markedly different response than particles of 2 or 3 μm diameter. With a change in particulate size, both the physical-chemical behavior of the particles and the mechanism for cellular transport and metabolism of the particles may alter greatly. Within the confines of present knowledge, such accelerated tests of the toxicity of wear particles are of questionable value.

In a similar way, the histological assessment described by Homsy[72] is of limited value. Cells are cultured *in vitro* on metallic surfaces and changes in the appearance of the cells are used to evaluate the toxicity of the metal from 0 to 4 where:

0 = excellent outgrowth with normal cell morphology;

+1 = excellent outgrowth but minor vacuolation of cells;

+2 = diminished outgrowth and major vacuolation of cells;

+3 = severe inhibition of growth;

+4 = total inhibition of growth, possibly with cell death.

While such morphological changes in cells *in vitro* are easily quantified, again, their correlation with observations on tissues around specimens *in vivo* is not reliable. Other workers[73] have reported the toxicity of metallic ions of known concentration on embryonic bones in tissue culture. In the presence of cobalt or other ions diminution in growth of bone is readily observed although the significance of this toxicity *in vitro* for tissues adjacent to implants is unknown. In summary, the effects of metallic dissolution products and wear particles on tissues have been widely studied. Many empirical observations are available although their relevance to clinical implantation remains obscure. Nevertheless, in view of the urgent need for accurate accelerated indications of tissue toxicity and of the need for precise knowledge on the influence of implantable materials on subcellular events within cells, further work is needed.

SUBACUTE TOXICITY TESTS

Twelve-week Implantation Test in Rabbits. After implantation of the cylinder specimens the animals are sacrificed serially starting at 3 days and then at 1 week and each week thereafter for 12 weeks. The implant sites are extricated and prepared for histopathological examination. Fifteen histological features are used to evaluate the material with each feature being scored as to its intensity. The test reveals pathological changes *vs.* time and the liability of a particular biological environment to degrade a given material.

Thirty-day Systemic Toxicity of Saline Extract. The saline extract of a given material is prepared as was described in the previous subsection, "Acute Toxicity Tests". The extract is administered intraperitoneally into a group of rats on each day for 30 days. The general health

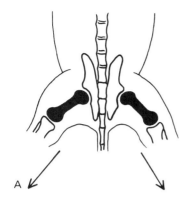

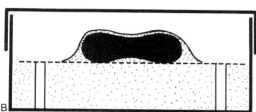

Figure 7-22. *A.* Assessment of tissue tolerance of corrosion products by organ culture. Embryonic rat femora are carefully dissected by microsurgical techniques. *B.* Schematic diagram shows the technique for organ culture of embryonic rat femora on plastic grids. (*A* and *B*, reproduced with permission of H. Gerber, *et al.*[73])

of the animals is observed over this period of time. Weight gain or loss and food consumption are reported. At the end of the 30 days blood samples are subjected to hematological evaluation. The animals are sacrificed, autopsied and examined for gross pathological changes. Selected tissues and organs also are removed and prepared for histopathological assessment.

Tissue Tolerance of Corrosion Products by Organ Culture. Gerber *et al.*[73] have devised a quantitative assessment of tissue tolerance to soluble corrosion products exposed to organ cultures. Pregnant rats were sacrificed 17 days after a limited mating period and the embryos were surgically removed. The embryonic femora were carefully dissected free by mirosurgical techniques (Fig. 7-22*A*) The remainder of the embryos were homogenized and diluted with Hanks' solution to provide an embryonic extract. The organ culture was performed with a modification of the technique originated by Fell and Weiss.[2] Plastic grids were employed *in lieu* of metal grids. The femora were cultured for 10 days with periodic renewal of the culture medium (Fig. 7-22*B*). Metallic chlorides were added to provide various concentrations of

$CrCl_3$, $FeCl_3$, $TiCl_3$, $CoCl_2$ and $NiCl_2$ in logarithmically calculated concentrations between 10^{-2} and 10^{-5} M. The contralateral femur was used as a control. At the end of the test period some of the specimens were subjected to routine histological preparation. Other femora were weighed after 48 hours of drying in a desiccator. Of the 106 femora under study, 44 were used for histological examination while the remaining 62 were examined by dry weight.

In the preliminary study the effect of addition of different metal chlorides to permit 10^{-3} M solutions on the growth of embryonic rat femora was investigated. Only the addition of $NiCl_2$ and $CoCl_2$ had a significant deleterious effect on growth (Fig. 7-23). In the histological sections of cobalt chloride and nickel chloride groups the cells appeared smaller and more numerous than the controls and most of the nuclei seemed pyknotic. In the histological sections from the titanium chloride, chromium chloride and ferric chloride the cells appeared to be normal in size and number with only a small number of pyknotic nuclei.

In the remaining experiments with 11 different concentrations of cobalt chloride and nickel chloride, the following observations on measurements of wet weight were made: in $3.16 \cdot 10^{-5}$ to $2 \cdot 10^{-4}$ M $NiCl_2$ a distinct but weak inhibition of growth occurred and from $5 \cdot 10^{-4}$ M solutions to higher concentrations total inhibition of growth occurred. The value of the 50% inhibition was found to be $3.5 \cdot 10^{-4}$ M.

In 10^{-5} to 10^{-4} M solutions of $CoCl_2$, no significant inhibition of growth occurred and from $5 \cdot 10^{-5}$ M solution upward a virtually total inhibition of growth occurred. The value of a 50% inhibition was found to be $4.2 \cdot 10^{-4}$ M.

Histologically with increasing concentration of $NiCl_2$, the cells were observed to be smaller, more numerous and with more pyknotic nuclei. A definite increase in pyknotic nuclei in the

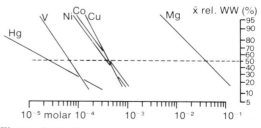

Figure 7-23. Dose response curve of influence of different metal chlorides on the growth of rat femora and tissue culture is shown. (Reproduced with permission of H. Gerber, *et al.*[73])

nickel chloride solution was first seen at a concentration of 10^{-4} M and in a cobalt chloride solution in a concentration of $5.62 \cdot 10^{-4}$ M. At the highest concentration, however, a few apparently normal nuclei were found. In the intermediate concentrations many lysed nuclei appeared.

From these observations the growth of embryonic rat femora in organ culture provides a useful determination of *in vitro* tissue toxicity. In 10^{-3} M metallic chlorides of chromium, iron, titanium, nickel and cobalt appear to be nontoxic while those of nickel and cobalt are toxic. In the latter instances a dose-effect curve can be made and the alterations in cellular structure, size and number correlate well with the concentration of the chloride. Somewhat similar experiments could also be undertaken with an *in vivo* technique although some metallic ions are constantly eliminated from the surrounding tissues. In an attempt to correlate a disturbance of growth of the bones with the presence of varying amounts of metallic chlorides, a large variation in the data did not permit reliable or useful correlation. This method was applicable only to soluble metallic salts.

In order to determine the influence of solid metallic specimens a second experimental technique was devised by Gerber et al.[73] Metallic wires of 0.1 mm to 0.125 mm in diameter and approximately 3 mm in length were inserted into the distal epiphysis of the femora at the onset of the *in vitro* culture (Fig. 7–24). The control femora did not receive implants. The growth of the embryonic bones was measured at the end of a 7-day period. The wet weight and dimensions of the femora and the histological appearance around the wire was studied. The gross determination of the inhibition of growth by the metals could be determined by the differences between the wet weight of the experimental and the control specimens. From the overall length and the distance from the midshaft of the epiphysis, the relative inhibitions of growth initiated by the presence of different wires could be assessed, as shown in Figure 7-25.

Histological studies revealed that stainless steel 316L, titanium and cobalt-chromium alloy wires were well tolerated. Specimens were surrounded by cartilage cells of normal appearance. In contrast the cells around implants of cobalt, nickel, copper and iron showed abnormalities such as pyknotic nuclei and pleomorphism. Depending upon the nature of the metal at various

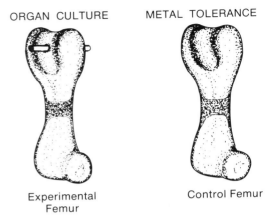

ORGAN CULTURE   METAL TOLERANCE

Experimental   Control Femur
Femur

Figure 7-24. The experimental technique of H. Gerber *et al.* for an assessment of embryonic rat femora in organ culture to metal wires is shown. A small metallic wire is inserted into the distal epiphysis of the femur at the onset of the culture. (Reproduced with permission of H. Gerber.)

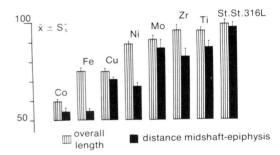

Figure 7-25. A histogram shows a comparison of the inhibition of growth of rat femora initiated by the presence of various types of metallic wire. (Reproduced with permission of H. Gerber.)

distances remote from the implant a sharp borderline was observed between the damaged and the undamaged cells (Fig. 7–26).

These workers cite several limitations of the experimental technique. The organ cultures lack a blood supply which might appreciably alter the tissue reaction to a foreign material. Lack of blood supply also limits the duration of the experiment. In order to overcome the latter limitation another experimental technique was employed to study the reaction of tissues to metallic cylinders implanted subcutaneously in the cervical spine of adult mice. Each animal received one cylindrical specimen 10 mm in length and the animals were sacrificed after 1, 3 and 9 weeks. The specimen including the surrounding

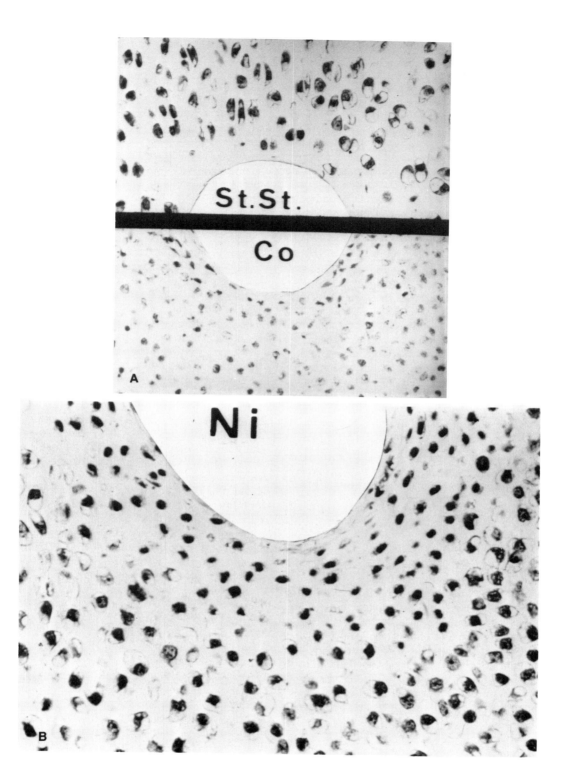

Figure 7-26. Histological preparations of embryonic rat femora impaled by metallic wires show the presence of the chondrocytes adjacent to various types of metallic wire. *A.* The cells adjacent to a 316L stainless steel wire are apparently normal chondrocytes. A similar picture is seen adjacent to titanium and cobalt-chromium alloy wires. In marked contrast is the histological picture adjacent to the pure cobalt wire below. Many small nonuniform cells with pyknotic nuclei are seen. The zone of abnormal cells extends for a considerable distance away from the wire. *B.* The histological picture adjacent to a nickel wire reveals a narrow zone of pleomorphic cells beyond which the chondrocytes are of normal appearance. (Reproduced with premission of H. Gerber.)

tissues was embedded in methylmethacrylate for histological examination. A quantitative evaluation of round cells and foreign body giant cells near and remote from the implant was undertaken. Cobalt specimens displayed a marked reaction to the metal with necrotic round cells and fibrosis near the cylinder. After 1 week of implantation, vanadium showed a round cell reaction which intensified over the following weeks. At 9 weeks all of the animals had died. Even after 9 weeks of implantation a thin cell layer invested and confirmed the inertness, and innocuous nature of the titanium cylinders metal.

These techniques provide an elegant assessment of tissue tolerance at the celluar level. Their principal limitation is the inability to distinguish the types of cellular response that would be likely to appear around new implantable materials in man. Presently available corrosion tests would eliminate from consideration metals such as cobalt or vanadium which show rapid dissolution and marked toxicity. In contrast, surgical grade stainless steel, titanium or cobalt-chromium alloys show favorable results as would alloys of titanium, tantalum or niobium.

LEUKOCYTE MIGRATION INHIBITION TEST FOR METAL SENSITIVITY

The assessment of contact dermatitis by patch tests with metal salts applied topically to the skin, provokes a complex of metal salts with the skin proteins of allergic patients. As part of the allergic reaction, T-lymphocytes respond to the antigen to produce a number of lymphokines, one of which is the migration inhibition factor (MIF) which prevents the migration of leukocytes. Since there is a risk of sensitizing patients by skin testing, an *in vitro* test for metal sensitivity has been developed which tests the production of MIF in response to metal salts complexed with the patient's own serum proteins. The test protocol has been described in detail, along with the results of clinical applications by Brown et al.[74]

THE REACTION OF TISSUES TO SILICONE RUBBER

Medical grade silicone elastomer has been widely employed as a spacer to replace carpal bones and the articulating surfaces of smaller long bones such as the proximal radius or the distal ulna or the proximal trapezius. Its applications are described in Chapters 14 and 15. The biological response of tissues to silicone rubber has been described in detail by Swanson et al.[75] In most applications the material is employed at sites where soft tissues move in repetitive fashion across the surface of the implant. Indeed the functions of the silicone spacer include restoration and maintenance of motion without loss of stability. The implants are rapidly surrounded by a fibrous tissue capsule which replicates that observed around a normal joint. Studies by Swanson on hundreds of joints have failed to document deleterious histological responses. Where silicone rubber articulates with hyaline cartilage the latter surface appears to tolerate remarkably well the foreign body without undergoing deleterious changes. In one report by Apker et al.[76] a foreign body reaction to silicone rubber was documented around a finger joint implant. The patient was a 63-year-old woman with seropositive rheumatoid arthritis who had undergone Swanson metacarpophalangeal joint arthroplasties. Prior to surgery the patient had had marked radial deviation which was corrected at the time of surgery. In the 3 years after surgery the radial deviation recurred in the index finger and culminated in a painful proximal joint with marked synovial proliferation. At that time surgical exploration was undertaken when a broken implant was found. The mechanical failure occurred at the junction of the phalangeal portion of the implant with the hinge. The surface of the implant showed superficial pits. The capsular tissue beside the implant was biopsied and subjected to routine histological analysis. Photomicroscopy revealed silastic shards with a foreign body giant cell reaction in the capsule. The shards were colorless, refractile bodies with irregular contours of variable diameter from 10 to 100 μm. Most of the shards were enveloped by hyaline fibrotic tissue with minimal cellular infiltrate. Few chronic inflammatory cells with foreign body giant cells were seen. Other portions of the capsular biopsy revealed evidence of chronic inflammatory change consistent with the diagnosis of rheumatoid arthritis.

While the significance of the previous observations remains unclear, most mechanical failures of silastic proximal joint arthroplasties occur when the surgeon does not undertake an adequate reconstructive procedure with the soft tissues to correct the ulnar deviation deformity. After mechanical failure of the silicone rubber spacer, repetitive motion of the fracture surfaces is likely to produce wear particles similar to the shards. The tissue response appears to reflect the presence of the silastic wear particles which under normal use are not encountered.

HYPERSENSITIVITY AND METAL IMPLANTS

In addition to the direct damage to cells that toxic metallic dissolution products may provoke, tissues may be harmed indirectly by the presence of metal products that stimulate a hypersensitivity response by the immune defenses. In recent years evidence has accumulated that such metal sensitivity may have several manifestations. Hicks[77] has described aseptic necrosis of skin with an eczematous reaction superficial to stainless steel plates on tibial fractures. It is likely that this undesirable side-effect was far more common with previous surgical grades of stainless steel alloys. Certainly, it appears to be distinctly uncommon when AISI 316 steel is used. For many years skin sensitivity to nickel-plated fasteners on undergarments[77] and surgical instruments has been well understood. More recently, urticaria after insertion of a Smith-Petersen cobalt-chromium nail was reported by McKenzie et al.[78] Subsequently Evans et al.[79] queried whether metal sensitivity might be a cause of bone necrosis and loosening of prostheses after total joint replacement. While loosening may occur as a result of improper surgical technique and/or trauma and infection in the tissues adjacent to the implant, there are many cases of loosening where none of these factors appears to be involved. The application of neutron activation analysis and atomic absorption spectrophotometry of tissues adjacent to all cobalt-chromium total joint prostheses showed that both cobalt and chromium levels were considerably elevated. Increases of cobalt compared with controls, ranged from 300- to 6000-fold while increases of chromium ranged from 30- to 100-fold. Skin tests for sensitivity to cobalt, chromium and nickel in patients with loose prostheses showed a strong association between metal sensitivity and loosening of prostheses composed entirely of cobalt-chromium alloy. Finally, they undertook histopathological studies on the bone and soft tissues adjacent to loose prostheses in patients who exhibited skin sensitivity to cobalt. From the study they conclude that release of metal products from a prosthesis to which the tissues are sensitive may produce changes in local blood vessels leading to interruption of the blood supply and subsequent necrosis of bone and soft tissues. The dead bone appears to undergo fibrous replacement and possibly fatigue fracture so that a combination of osteolysis and fracture is radiologically evident in these patients. It should be emphasized that the results of this small study refer solely to implants where metal rubs against itself, the situation wherein the greatest quantity of metallic wear and dissolution products are released.[80]

Recently Elves[81] has undertaken patch tests to assess the cutaneous hypersensitivity of patients with both metal-on-metal and metal-on-plastic arthroplastic joints. Forty-three per cent of the patients with metal-on-metal prostheses demonstrated sensitivity to cobalt, chromium or nickel; only 27% of the sensitized patients had a previous history of metal sensitivity. In those patients on whom the prosthesis had failed, the incidence of metal sensitivity was 60%. In this group the predominant sensitivity was cobalt. Of the patients treated with metal-on-plastic total joint replacement, 17% had evidence of hypersensitivity to metal. Of the 11 sensitized patients in this group only 1 had a previous history compatible with the pre-existing state of metal hypersensitivity. The most commonly encountered reaction in this group was against nickel. For patients with failed metal-on-plastic joint replacements 20% gave a positive skin reaction to metallic salts. The results of the study by Elves are rendered somewhat more difficult to interpret in view of the fact that most of the patients with metal-on-metal total joint replacements had undergone surgery more than 4 years prior to the study while those patients with metal-on-plastic prostheses had had the reconstructive surgery undertaken in the most recent 2-year period.

In Elves' study the patients were subjected to a cutaneous patch test on their back prior to total joint replacement. In his study 5.8% of the preoperative patients have shown a positive result upon exposure to cobalt, whereas in a comparable study by Goodwin and Benson[82] 5.1% of the patients showed a positive preoperative result. In the former study, upon failure of McKee-Farrar metal-on-metal total joint replacements 18% of the patients showed positive cutaneous tests. Whether the sensitivity is a cause or a result of the failure remains unclear. A few patients with titanium implants have undergone the cutaneous patch test although none have given a positive result. Apparently titanium is a poor allergen.

The use of cutaneous patch tests should not be undertaken indiscriminantly. The tests themselves can provoke hypersensitivity to the material in question. Goodwin and Benson[82] report that the value of the metal ion applied to the skin for the patch test is an important factor in the rate of diffusion of the substance through the skin although the valence is not known to be directly related to the liability of the material to provoke hypersensitivity.

The role of metal ions in hypersensitivity has been reviewed by Abraham.[83] The metal ions in question are of such small size that they cannot themselves stimulate the production of antibodies although they do react specifically with antibodies that can be formed against them when they are conjugated with a protein. Such a substance is termed a hapten after the work of Landsteiner.[83] Although a conventional antigen and antibody reaction initiates the formation of the precipitate this is not generally observed when a free hapten, such as a metallic ion, combines with its corresponding antibody. Nevertheless, the combination of the free hapten with its corresponding antibody can be readily demonstrated for when a hapten has combined with an antibody the latter no longer forms a precipitate upon the addition of homologous hapten-protein antigen. There is a specific inhibition of precipitation observed for the antibody. These reactions can be written as follows:

rial, clinical signs of superficial inflammation of the skin may appear, usually with a vesiculation restricted to the area of contact with the exciting substance. The pathological process comprises a superficial chronic inflammation of the local area of the skin with swelling of epithelial cells, vesicle formation and perivascular infiltration of the dermis with mononuclear cells. The lesion is similar to that of other forms of delayed hypersensitivity. The sensitization requires contact with the skin or injection of the agent into the skin. Provocation by other parenteral routes or by feeding the provocative agent does not yield the same response. Sensitization develops 8 to 21 days after exposure with a local reaction at the patch site. Typically delayed reaction appears 24 hours after the most recent exposure to the provocative material. The sensitizing agent such as a metal may possess other toxic manifestations when it is applied to the skin in much larger concentrations. Alternatively it may provoke toxicity in other tissues upon other modes of exposure. For example, the Quebec epidemic of poisoning by beer that occurred in 1965 and 1966 illustrated the high toxicity of cobalt chloride when ingested.[84]

$$hapten\text{-}protein + antibody = hapten\text{-}protein\ antibody\ precipitate$$
$$hapten + antibody = hapten\text{-}antibody\ complex$$
$$hapten\text{-}protein + hapten\text{-}antibody\ complex = no\ precipitate.$$

When a hapten is conjugated with a protein it can largely determine the antigenic properties of the complex and combines specifically with antibodies formed against it.

At present Elves[81] and others are attempting to develop more sophisticated and sensitive ways to assess the role of hypersensitivity in the pathogenesis of wear particles from surgical implants. A lymphocyte transformation test appears to provide a much more accurate and convenient method than the cutaneous patch test. The changes in the lymphocyte indicate that the cutaneous hypersensitivity observed for metallic ions is in fact a systemic phenomenon and therefore has possible implications for pathological changes in many other tissues.

The Significance of a Positive Patch Test. A positive cutaneous patch test indicates that a material provokes a contact dermatitis. This manifestation of hypersensitivity represents a drug allergy of the delayed type and is usually initiated by chemical substances of low molecular weight such as metallic ions. Upon prolonged or repetitive exposure to the provocative mate-

There are other delayed types of drug sensitivities which may be encountered as a response to wear debris from total joint replacements. The serum sickness type of sensitivity occurs after prolonged parenteral administration. The manifestations may include urticarial rashes, angioneurotic edema, arthropathies, and arteritis including renal involvement culminating in renal failure. There may be no past history of contact with the provocative agent. McKenzie *et al.*[78] have reported generalized urticaria with pruritus that developed 1 day after the insertion of a Smith-Peterson cobalt-chromium nail. Cutaneous patch testing with cobalt-chromium alloy initiated an eczematous response which was followed, about 48 hours later, by severe noneczematous periorbital edema. A positive transfer (Prausnitz-Küstner) test performed on a volunteer was positive. Once the fracture of the femoral neck had healed the nail was removed under local anesthesia. Within 24 hours the urticaria resolved spontaneously although dermographism persisted and remained a clinical problem for 1 year after removal of the nail. Urticarial rashes also have been reported by Calnan[85] and Stoddart[86] for a series of patients sensitive to nickel.

Several workers have observed painful, aseptic failures after McKee-Farrar hip arthroplasty. McKee[87] described two patients in whom symptoms occurred $3\frac{1}{2}$ and $4\frac{1}{2}$ years after arthroplasty. In both cases a sterile necrotic material was obtained from the affected joint at exploration. Charosky et al.[88] described 18 McKee-Farrar arthroplasties that failed, 10 of which were not associated with infection. These workers found a considerable quantity of metallic debris in the tissues surrounding the prosthesis. The particles had initiated a nonspecific inflammatory response. More recently Jones et al.[80] have observed seven patients in whom McKee-Farrar arthroplasties became painful after a variable period. The pain was accompanied by a feeling of instability and, in two cases, spontaneous dislocation. On patch testing, six of the patients were cobalt-positive but nickel and chromium negative. Radiological features included bone resorption in the pelvis and proximal femur, acetabular fracture and loosening and dislocation of the prosthesis. Upon surgical exploration, macroscopic and histological necrosis of bone, muscle and joint capsule around the prosthesis were observed in five patients. By the use of atomic absorption spectrophotometry substantial elevations in cobalt concentrations were observed in the urine of four patients and in a variety of tissues in one patient. The elevations of urinary cobalt levels is consistent with the previous observations by Coleman et al.[31]

Jones et al.[80] concluded that the cobalt wear and dissolution products provide the undesirable side-effects by hypersensitivity. In support of their view, the histological changes indicate an avascular phenomenon such as the endarteritis of small vessels seen in certain types of hypersensitivity reactions. Hypersensitivity also would account for the relatively low incidence of the condition. The observations by Jones et al.[80] as well as those of Evans et al.[79] clearly indicate that patients with McKee-Farrar hip arthroplasties who develop pain at their arthroplastic hip should undergo cutaneous patch testing with cobalt.

Less frequently encountered manifestations of delayed-type drug sensitivities include thrombocytopenic purpura, hemolytic anemia and agranulocytosis. The author is not aware of any reported cases of patients who have presented with these serious problems after exposure to surgical implants.

Clearly, further work in this field is indicated to reveal the clinical significance of metal sensitivity.

Assessment of Toxicity by Ferrographic Analysis

Previous clinical studies on the wear of total joint replacements and on the influence of the resultant wear particles on musculoskeletal tissues have been undertaken in fairly independent efforts. In Chapter 3 the recent change in assessment of wear with the application of Ferrography,* was mentioned. Whereas, previous analyses of wear had focused attention on the appearance of the worn bearing surfaces, Ferrography provides a superior index of the mechanism of wear and the anticipated rate of future wear of a machine by the study of the by-products of wear. Ferrography provides a method for the orderly magnetic separation and study of wear particles from small samples of lubricant. With this technique, as devised by Seifert, Scott and Westcott[89-91] the wear mode of a machine can be characterized by the number, shape and size of the particulate wear matter present in a small sample of lubricant. The particles characteristic of different modes are identified and studied by various microscopic techniques. The method provides a practical and accurate means for serial determinations of the mechanisms and rates of wear and facilitates prognostication of the future performance of such machines. Recently, the author and associates[92] have employed Ferrography for the analysis of wear particles from surgical joint replacements and from human arthritic joints. In combination with other techniques of synovial fluid analyses the method provides a nondestructive repetitive assessment of the rates of wear of surgical joint replacements of human arthritic joints. It provides insight into the pathological responses to the wear particles and it seems not unlikely that it may provide considerable new knowledge on the pathogenesis of reconstructive joints where autogenous cartilage transplants are employed, as described in Chapters 15 and 16. To date over 400 degenerative and arthroplastic joints have been studied by the technique described below.

Wear Particle Analysis in Surgical Joint Replacements

Synovial fluid is obtained by sterile needle aspiration from symptomatic joints after hemi- or total arthroplasty. To eliminate artifactual debris, needles and containers are washed prior

---

* Foxboro Analytical, Inc., Burlington, Mass.

to collection of specimens. The synovial fluid is subjected to ferrographic and histological analysis.

With the Ferrograph analyzer 2 ml of the synovial fluid are pumped across a glass microscope slide subjected to a magnetic field (Fig. 3-17). Small, weakly magnetic or paramagnetic particles in the fluid, often a fraction of a micron in size, are precipitated according to their volumetric magnetic moment. Larger particles are deposited near the entry end of the substrate. Further along the flow path progressively smaller particles are differentially deposited. After preparation of the Ferrogram the deposited particles are examined by a bichromatic microscope which employs simultaneously transmitted green light and direct red light (Fig. 3-18). Metallic particles are readily identified by their appearance due to their attenuation of the green transmitted light and their reflection of the red direct light. Nonmetallic compounds appear to be green, yellow or pink depending upon their density and thickness. Surface conditions are distinguished by the intensity of the light that the particles reflect. Polarized light microscopy permits characterization of birefringent compounds such as the high density polyethylene and the polymethylmethacrylate commonly used in orthopaedic implants.

To assess the inflammatory changes within the arthroplastic joints we examined the cytological characteristics of the aspirated synovial fluid. A clot was induced in a portion of the liquid specimen and the resultant coagulum subjected to routine histological preparation and staining (Fig. 7-27). The method permits excellent resolution of the intra-articular inflammatory response.

Specimens of synovial fluid, synovium, and implants were obtained at operation from 60 patients in whom surgical revision was necessary after implantation periods of 2 to 10 years. Synovial tissue was prepared for histological analysis in routine fashion. Alternatively, the synovial surfaces were washed in methanol to release superficial cells and associated particles and the washings then were used to prepare a Ferrogram. After removal, implants were examined macroscopically and microscopically for evidence of wear.

The composition of the implants and of the metallic wear particles was confirmed by scanning electron microscopy (SEM) energy dispersion X-ray analysis. In separate studies, standard scissors, disposable needles, and scalpel blades were examined microscopically. Washings from

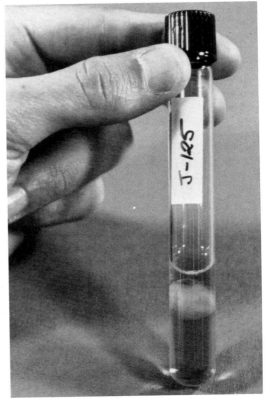

Figure 7-27. A photograph reveals a clot induced in a portion of synovial aspirate. The coagulant facilitates routine histological preparation and staining of the free cells in synovial fluid.

the tools were analyzed ferrographically. Subsequently the chemical elements of the metallic particles were identified with the SEM X-ray apparatus.

Our study reveals that after surgical joint replacement with metallic articular implants, metallic particles always are identifiable in the synovial fluid; larger numbers of particles are evident when both articular surfaces are composed of metal. With metal on polyethylene joint replacements, most of the wear particles are polyethylene although analysis with polarized light usually reveals particulate polymethylmethacrylate cement. The number and the morphology of the particles in the specimen appear to correlate with the rates of wear and the nature of the mechanism of wear in the implants.

The metallic particles identified range in size from less than 0.25 μm to 5.0 μm in specimens from joint replacements experiencing a relatively small amount of wear (Fig. 7-28). In in-

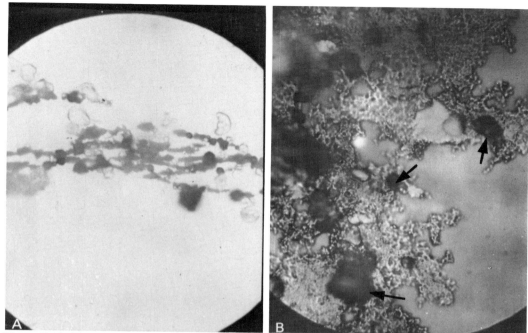

Figure 7-28. Two photomicrographs of Ferrograms are seen. *A.* Linear arrays of wear particles abraded from a surgical hemostat are seen. *B.* Wear particles in cellular debris aspirated from a patient with a geometric total knee replacement are shown. In practice metallic particles appear to be red and the largest are about 5 μm in major dimension.

stances where evidence of abrasive or fatigue wear is found, particles from several hundred microns to 1 mm in length are seen. Where implants of cobalt or titanium base alloys have been studied, synovial fluid analysis reveals wear particles from both the implant and from stainless steel surgical tools. Separate studies show that most of the wear particles from surgical tools originate in those which undergo repetitive use, such as hemostats, scissors, and osteotomes. A small quantity of metallic debris arises from disposable needles and scalpel blades. The needles are relatively free of particles if flushed prior to use.

Polyethylene, most often in the form of shredded fibers, is seen in a variety of sizes, ranging in diameter from 1 to 10 μm and up to several hundred microns in length (Fig. 7-29A). Polymethylmethacrylate particles generally have the appearance of irregular granular chunks with a larger variation in size (Fig. 7-29B). The diameter is less than 1 μm in the case of identifiable granules and up to 1 mm or more in the larger pieces. This acrylic cement is found in large quantities in the knee joint replacements which have been studied and sometimes is noted to be adherent to metallic fragments.

Cytological examination of synovial fluid re-veals the presence of inflammatory cells, macrophages, sheets of synovial cells, and in the presense of hemi-arthroplasties, free chondrocytes. In addition, cartilaginous and bony fragments have been identified in the latter cases. The wide variety of cells seen in synovial fluid after surgical joint replacement approximates the spectrum of cells found in many different human joint diseases; it follows no pattern distinctive of any heretofore described disease process. The quantity of cells appears to correspond with the degree of inflammation noted in the synovial tissue obtained from these same joints. This description refers solely to cases where no evidence of infection, either by clinical findings or culture has been present.

Specimens of synovium reveal the presence of particles of comparable composition and morphology to those found in samples of joint synovial fluid (Figs. 7-30 and 7-31).

Observations on removed implants show that conditions of abrasive wear engender significant acceleration in the rates of wear of the components with wear particles of characteristic morphology. Abrasive wear is found with metal-on-metal implants, and in instances where particulate polymethylmethacrylate or bone erodes polyethylene.

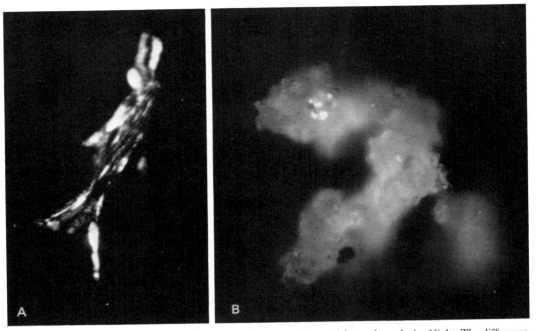

Figure 7-29. *A* and *B*. Polyethylene and polymethylmethacrylate particles under polarized light. The difference in their appearance is clearly evident. The greater degree of crystallographic orientation of polyethylene is manifest as a large refraction of polarized light. The particles are about 10 μm in length. (Reproduced with permission of D. C. Mears.[94])

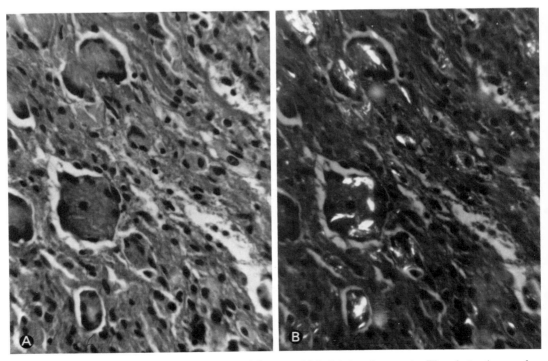

Figure 7-30. *A* and *B*. Synovial biopsies excised from total hip joint replacements. The photomicrographs show tissue removed from a metal on polyethylene total hip joint replacement. *B*, polarized light is used to reveal the polymeric material which is not readily distinguished in the same preparation, seen in *A*.

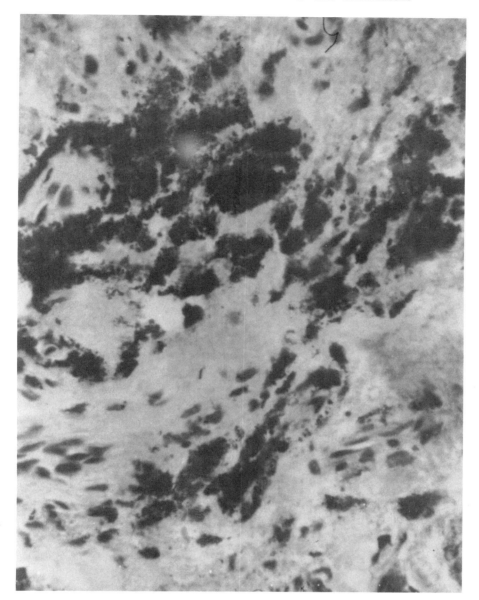

Figure 7-31. A synovial biopsy from a McKee-Ferrar total hip arthroplasty. The photomicrograph was taken with reflective red light and green transmitted light. All of the dark particles and agglomerates of particles represent cobalt-chromium wear particles in and around synovial cells.

Wear Particle Analysis in Degenerative Arthritis

Synovial fluid is aspirated from degenerative joints of patients by routine sterile technique. The biological wear particles of cartilage, bone, synovial tissue and meniscus are diamagnetic. Under the influence of the magnetic field of the Ferrograph analyzer the particles would be repelled to the periphery of the glass microscope slide. To obviate this difficulty a proprietary solution of magnetic erbium ions is added to the synovial fluid. The magnetic ions bind to the biological wear particles and induce them to behave in a paramagnetic fashion. Subsequently, Ferrograms can be prepared in the routine way.

Bichromatic and SEM microscopy of the Ferrograms reveals the presence of cartilaginous, osseous, meniscal, and synovial particles of unique optical properties and morphological

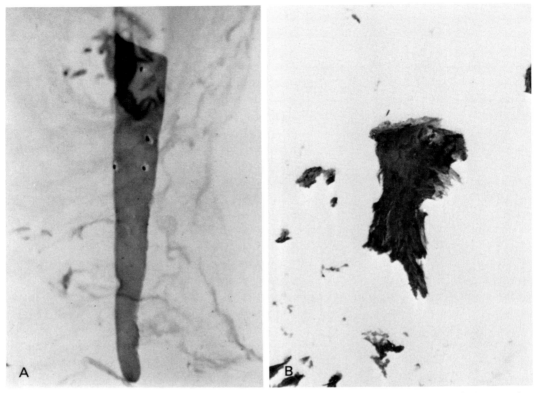

Figure 7-32. Photomicrographs of wear particles seen in the synovial aspirates of patients with degenerative arthritis are shown. *A.* The highly characteristic polygonal shape of a cartilaginous particle. Five chondrocytes can be seen in the lacunae each with a major diameter of about 15 μm. *B.* An osseous particle of subchondral bone in a patient with more severe degenerative change. The highly irregular surface is evident. The particle is about 30 μm in length.

characteristics (Figs. 7-32 and 7-33). The volume of the cartilaginous and bony particles appears to be directly related to the severity of the degenerative process. More than seven different types of particles have been identified in aspirates from degenerative joints. They include a filamentous particle abraided from the articular surface, a polygonal particle that appears to flake from the subarticular zone, osteochondral particles from the region of the interface between cartilage and bone, and osseous fragments from subchondral bone. Also, cuboidal and spherical cartilaginous particles, and others with strikingly beautiful flagellations have been documented although they are of unclear origin. Numerous sizes and shapes of osseous particles are seen although an irregularly surfaced chunk predominates. The geometry of each type of particle appears to reflect its mechanical properties and corresponding wear mode as well as its biochemical composition at the time of its production. Meniscal and synovial tissue fragments vary greatly in quantity in different synovial specimens. No single morphological pattern has been identified although large sheets of synovial cells are common in specimens from joints with a proliferative synovitis.

Significance of Wear Particles in Human Joints

Ferrography and allied techniques of synovial fluid analyses permit serial assessment of the wear of surgical joint replacements and prognostication concerning their future function. The methods permit a correlation between the mechanisms and rates of wear of the implants with the biological responses of the adjacent tissues. It is conceivable that different wear modes may stimulate unique pathological reactions. Our ability to monitor wear in presently available surgical joint replacements may provide information that will assist in the selection of future implantable materials and in the design of superior articular replacements.

Ferrographic analysis of human degenerative joints provides a way to study the site of articular cartilage or bone which has undergone the primary deterioration. An assessment of wear of

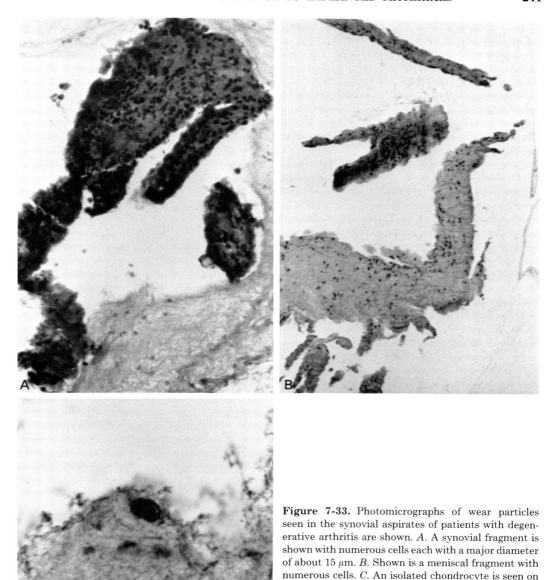

Figure 7-33. Photomicrographs of wear particles seen in the synovial aspirates of patients with degenerative arthritis are shown. *A.* A synovial fragment is shown with numerous cells each with a major diameter of about 15 μm. *B.* Shown is a meniscal fragment with numerous cells. *C.* An isolated chondrocyte is seen on the edge of proteinic film (H & E).

porous implants with autogenous articular cartilaginous surfaces described in Chapter 16, also, is under scrutiny by ferrographic analysis in our laboratories. It enables future studies to shift their attention from the bulk cartilage which may not as yet have undergone the critical biochemical and biomechanical alteration to that site of maximal degeneration. Currently we have initiated biochemical characterization of the wear particles. With further scrutiny of degenerative joints a wide variety of shapes and sizes of cartilaginous and osseous wear particles presumably of unique biochemical compositions, ultimately may permit the recognition of several degenerative processes of peculiar biochemical origin, initiation and progression.

It is conceivable that the biological wear particles may contribute to the pathogenesis of degenerative arthritis. The biochemical composition of some of the osseous particles and possibly certain cartilagenous particles is comparable to the pyrophosphate crystals encountered in pseudogout.[93] It is plausible that the particles created by degenerative wear may undergo phagocytosis, with the activation and release of lysosomal enzymes or that they may initiate numerous other cellular or humoral responses that could serve to augment joint destruction. In transmission micrographs of ultrathin sections of polymorphonuclear leukocytes (Fig. 7-34) observed in the clotted specimens of joint fluid aspirated from degenerative joints, we have observed large numbers of vacuoles which appear to contain minute fragments of cartilage and bone, as seen in Figure 7-35.

Irrespective of its conceivable implications for the pathogenesis of degenerative arthritis, Ferrography and allied techniques of synovial fluid analysis appear to be a useful clinical method for repetitive nonsurgical assessment of the rates and mechanisms of wear of both arthroplastic and degenerative joints and of the pathological responses to wear particles.

CARCINOGENESIS OF METALS

In the past decade perhaps the most widely speculated risk of prolonged exposure to metal or other implants has been the origin of malignant tumors. The speculation arose from two observations:

1. Individuals with prolonged chronic exposure, usually of 15 to 20 years, to a variety of industrial noxious agents have developed tumors. For example, workers with chronic exposure to nickel carbonyl, beryllium and certain chromates, have a greatly enhanced incidence of carcinoma of the lung.[95] Similarly and better known, is the high incidence of carcinoma of the bladder among workers in the analine dye and rubber industry, after exposure to β-naphthalene and benzidine and of carcinoma of the lung, pleura, pericardium and peritoneum in workers who are exposed to particles of asbestos.[96]

2. The second observation was the high incidence of malignancy in certain species of animals that arises after they are exposed to metal products. Oppenheimer et al.[97] have shown that both AISI 316 and cobalt-chromium-molybdenum implants in rats may be carcinogenic. Particles of cobalt[98] and soluble chromates[99] have been implicated in the carcinogenicity of other animals.

In Table 7-7, a list of metals that have initiated carcinogenesis in experimental animals are tabulated. For many years Heath[103] studied the production of malignant tumors in rats given intramuscular injections of pure cobalt metal powder. Tumors occurred at the injection sites in 17 out of 30 rats over a period ranging from 5 to 12 months after the injections. Of the 17 tumors, 13 contained a malignant component derived from muscle. Malignant connective tissue elements were also present in some of the 13. In the remaining 4 tumors the malignant process appeared to have arisen predominantly in the connective tissue. The tumors were rhabdomyosarcomata, rhabdomyofibrosarcomata, pleomorphic and fibrosarcomata. Heath[103] has documented with histological studies the progression of changes in the rat skeletal muscle tissue, after the injection of powered cobalt, up to the stage of frank malignancy. Several of stages are revealed in Figure 7-36.

Two processes were observed in all of the rats that underwent malignant transformation. There was evidence of regeneration and repair in the muscle after the mechanical injury produced by the injection of the metallic granules. Concurrently, the regenerative and repair process was modified by the chemical action of the cobalt presumably by slow dissolution of cobalt with the liberation of cobalt dissolution products into the tissues or by direct catalysis at the surface of the metallic particles.

The first response of the muscle to the injection appears at day one as an infiltration of leukocytes into the spaces between the muscle bundles and fibers in the regions near the primary injury (Fig. 7-36A). While this infiltrate remains visible at 4 days by this time fibroblasts have invaded the region. Large aggregates of cobalt particles are observed in intimate contact with intact muscle which sometimes shows no evidence of damage (Fig. 7-36B) whereas at sites distant from the cobalt some muscle fibers contain a greatly increased population of nuclei (Fig. 7-36C). In other damaged muscle fibers both nuclei and striations have disappeared to yield a homogenous hyaline material.

The muscle continues to regenerate and at 7 days necrotic, unstriated bundles often lie between bundles of normal striated fibers (Fig. 7-37A). Further deterioration of the hyaline substance into amorphous granular residue appears. The zones between adjacent muscle fibers are invaded by a variety of cells including leukocytes, fibroblasts and characteristic fusiform cells. The last are mononucleates or multinucleates with two to five nuclei. Their cytoplasm is basophilic and stains with pyronin. They appear to be myoblasts possibly derived from the injured muscle fibers. Another cell type is the multinucleate cell tube (of Waldemeyer) (Fig. 7-37B) in which the cytoplasm is poorly stained with pyronin. The cell tubes represent collapse of muscle fibers.

Extensive areas of degeneration are still present at 12 days with increasing amounts of the amorphous granular material although regeneration is well underway. In some zones many long multinucleate basophilic or striated muscle straps are seen which may be continuous with damaged muscle bundles. Collagen fibers appear sometimes interspersed with mast cells. So far the reparative stages are similar to those seen in the repair of infarcted muscle.

Between 2 and 3 weeks after the injection of cobalt, however, the tissue response begins to differ from that previously described by Godman[104] for infarcted muscle. Whereas in muscle infarction, undifferentiated myoblastic elements diminish in number after 16 weeks, in the cobalt-treated material they continue to increase. At 4 weeks changes initiated by the presence of cobalt have spread further from the metal deposit to more distant regions of the muscle (Fig. 7-37C). The cobalt granules, still present, are usually surrounded by a narrow band of necrotic degenerate muscle. Two or three cell widths away there is a broad zone of viable cells of various types mainly leukocytes and fibroblasts beyond which viable muscle fibers are seen. Signs of "dedifferentiation" of mature muscle fibers continue to appear under the influence of cobalt. Free myoblasts appear in the zones near the cobalt injection. At 6 weeks these cells are larger than in the initial stages of the tissue response and assume more abnormal forms usually with basophilic cytoplasm and large deeply stained nuclei. They may be present between the existing muscle bundles and their residual necrotic material and in masses of collagen.

At 8 to 10 weeks free myoblasts are abundant. Numerous mytoses are seen in various cell types. At 14 weeks, giant cells (Fig. 7-38A) appear in increasing numbers along with the myoblasts with peculiar cross-striations (Fig. 7-38B). At 16 weeks, further deterioration of muscle into pigmented granular masses is evident along with large numbers of mytoses. By 20 weeks, tumor nodules become discernible (Fig. 7-38C).

The elegant documentation by Heath[103] is described in the detail in view of its possible implications for the development of tumors in man secondary to the presence of implantable materials.

Recently, Heath et al.[105] have implanted wear particles from cobalt-chromium total hip prostheses into rats and observed a high incidence (e.g., 24%) of carcinogenesis. A representative sample is seen in Figure 7-39. The wear products were generated in a laboratory simulator and were of much smaller diameter than those encountered in the erosion of total joint replacements in man. The particles which Heath employed in this study showed a diameter of 0.1 μm whereas those encountered in man are mostly of size 2 to 3 μm. In more recent tests Swanson et al.[106] have studied the mode of transport of particles of various sizes around the body. They report that the larger particles show a different mode of transport than the smaller wear particles and that the former are not such potent initiators of tumors.

Carcinogenesis and Polymeric, Ceramic and Graphite Implants

In consideration of the polymeric materials currently employed in orthopaedic implants there is scanty evidence to suggest they have any role in the initiation of malignant transformation. Autian[107] has reported the experiments undertaken by Oppenheimers et al.[97] in which the insertion of plastic foils around the kidneys provoked the formation of granulomata and ultimately of neoplasia at the sites of implantation. Bischoff and Bryson[108] extended this work by the study of comparable implants of various metals as well as a variety of polymers. These workers concluded that the chemical composition of the material was relatively unimportant. The important factors were the size, shape and surface finish of the specimen. Smooth surfaces were more effective in initiating carcinogenesis than rough or perforated surfaces. The neoplastic change became evident after a long latent period of greater than 1 year. The precise mechanism of action of the implant was unknown and no human counterparts of this observation have ever been documented. In a few instances sarcomas have appeared in juxtaposition to vascular grafts in man although the number of cases is insufficient to make any useful observation. Bering et al.[109] observed the pathogenesis of neoplastic changes around pure polyethylene, polystyrene and cellophane specimens in rats. After implantation of any of the materials, they observed a "latent period." Removal of the polymer prior to this duration of exposure inhibited tumor formation. Removal of the specimen after implantation for this period might or might not be followed by the subsequent development of a tumor, typically 6 months later. Abatement of

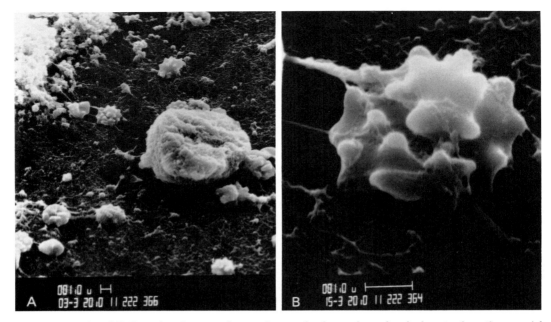

Figure 7-34. *A* and *B*. Scanning electron micrographs reveal polymorphonuclear leukocytes from the synovial fluid aspirate of a patient with degenerative arthritis. The highly convoluted surface of the cell is a characteristic morphological feature. *B*. A higher power view of a single cell is shown.

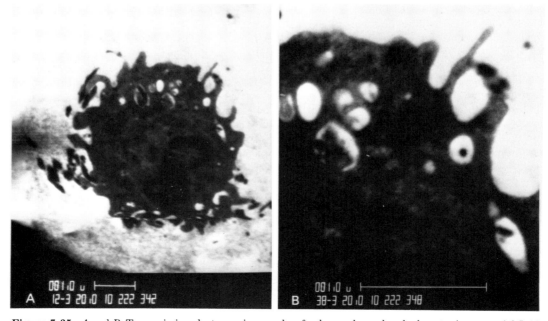

Figure 7-35. *A* and *B*. Transmission electron micrographs of polymorphonuclear leukocytes in a synovial fluid aspirate from a patient with degenerative arthritis. Vacuoles are visible in low and high magnification. In the vacuoles particulate matter is apparent which, from other studies, is identified as osteochondral wear particles. (Reproduced with permission of D. C. Mears.[94])

Table 7-7
Metal Carcinogenesis in Experimental Animals[a]

Metal	Compound	Species	Route	Type of tumor
Cd	CdS, CdO, CdCl$_2$, CdSO$_4$, Cd powder	Rats, mice	SC, IM	Sarcomas Leydigiomas
Cr	metallic Cr	Rabbits	Intraosseous	Sarcomas
	roasted chromite ore	Rats, mice	IM, IP, SC	Sarcomas
	CaCrO$_4$, CrO$_3$, Na$_2$Cr$_2$O$_7$ Cr$_2$O$_3$		Intrapleural	Squamous cell carcinoma
	CaCrO$_4$	Rats	Intrabronchial	Squamous cell carcinoma and adenocarcinoma
Co	Metallic Co, Co powder	Rats, rabbits	SC, IM	Sarcomas
	CoO, CoS		Intraosseous	
Fe	Fe-carbohydrate complexes	Rats, mice, rabbits	IM, SC	Sarcomas
Ni	Ni dust, Ni(CO)$_4$	Guinea pig, rats	Inhalation	Anaplastic and adenocarcinoma
	Ni dust, Ni$_3$S$_2$ dust	Rats	IM, SC	Sarcomas
	NiO dust, Ni pellets			
	Ni$_3$S$_2$	Cats	Nasal sinus Implantation	Squamous cell and adenocarcinoma
Zn	ZnCl$_2$	Rats	Intratesticular	Leydigiomas, serminoma
	ZnSO$_4$, ZnCl$_2$	Chickens	Intratesticular	Chorioepithelioma
Ti	Titanocene	Rats, mice	IM	Fibrosarcoma, hepatomas
Al	Al foil	Rats	Implantation	Sarcomas
Ag	Ag foil	Rats	Implantation	Fibrosarcomas

[a] A. Furst and R. T. Haro[100] and F. W. Sunderman, Jr.[101, 102]

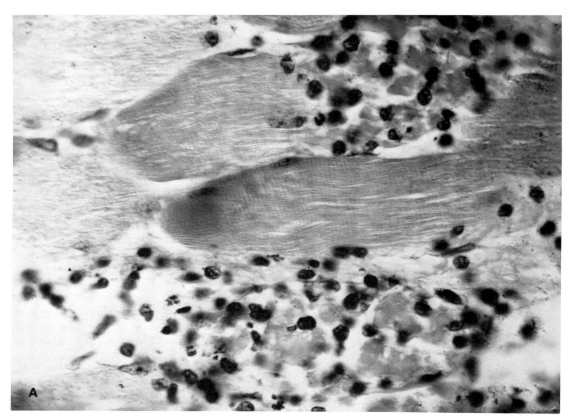

Figure 7-36. Photomicrographs of several of the stages in tumor induction by cobalt are shown. *A.* Infiltration of leukocytes into the space between muscle bundles and fibers, 1 day after injection of cobalt (methyl green and pyronin, × 390). *B.* Grains of cobalt metal are seen in intimate contact with apparently undamaged muscle, 4 days after injection of cobalt (methyl green and pyronin, ×390). *C.* Increased numbers of nuclei at a site different from the injected cobalt but in the same muscle are apparent, 4 days after injection of cobalt (methyl green and pyronin, ×390). (*A, B,* and *C,* reproduced with permission from J. C. Heath.[103])

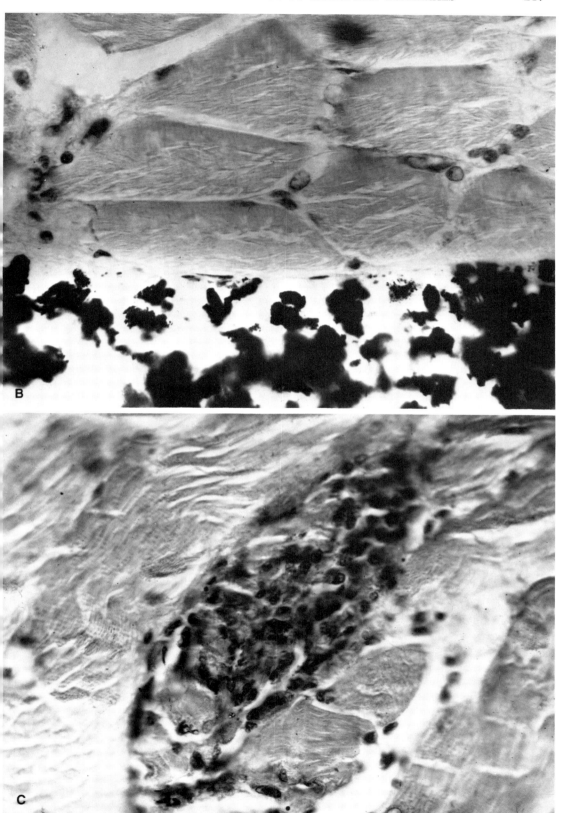

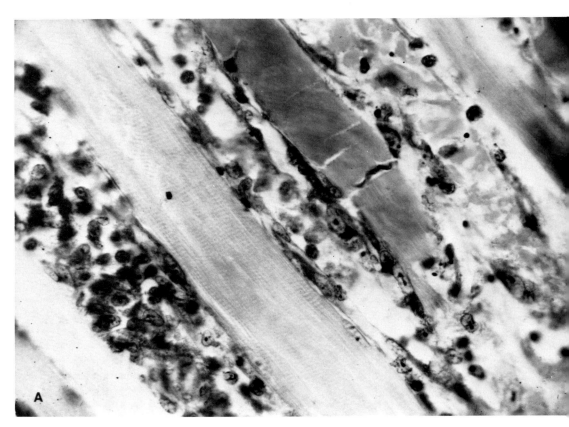

Figure 7-37. Photomicrographs of several of the stages in tumor induction by cobalt are shown. *A.* A damaged muscle fiber with its hyaline, almost homogenous nature is evident in contrast with a neighboring undamaged fiber, 7 days after injection of cobalt (methyl green and pyronin, ×390). *B.* Multinucleate cell tubes in which the cytoplasm scarcely stains with pyronin, 7 days after injection of cobalt (methyl green and pyronin, ×390). *C.* A damaged muscle fiber with a chain of nuclei disturbing the regular pattern of striations. The nuclei and nucleoli are larger than normal and stained much more deeply, 4 weeks after injection of cobalt (Azan, ×820). (*A, B,* and *C,* reproduced with permission of J. C. Heath.[103])

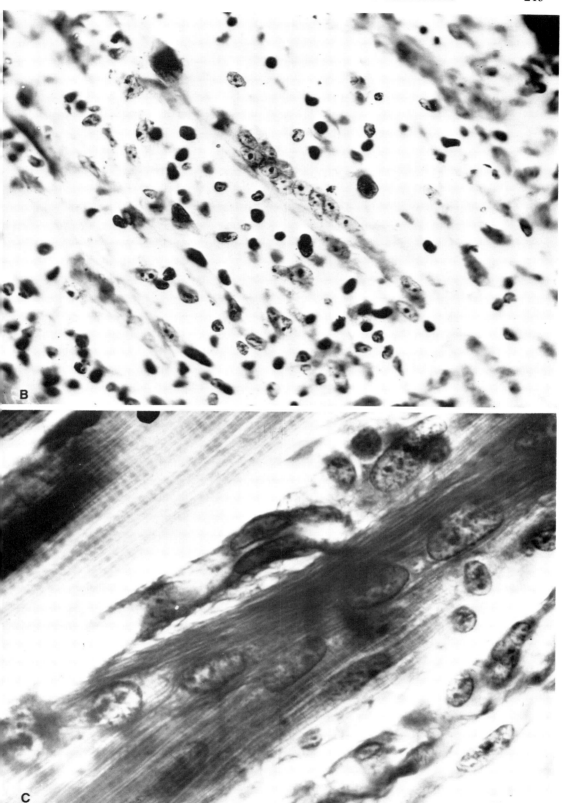

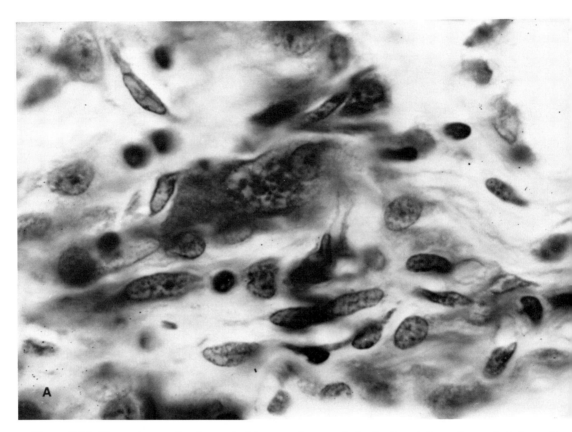

Figure 7-38. Photomicrographs of several of the stages in tumor induction by cobalt are shown. *A*. A giant cell similar to those found in the established cobalt-induced tumors is seen, 14 weeks after injection of cobalt (methyl green and pyronin, ×810). *B*. Binucleate myoblasts and a mitosis, 10 weeks after injection of cobalt (methyl green and pyronin, ×810). *C*. Mitoses in giant cells in an early tumor nodule is evident. By this stage there is much necrotic material and degenerative muscle substance with granular pigmented deposits, 20 weeks after injection of cobalt (methyl green and pyronin, ×810). (*A, B,* and *C,* reproduced with permission of J. C. Heath.[103])

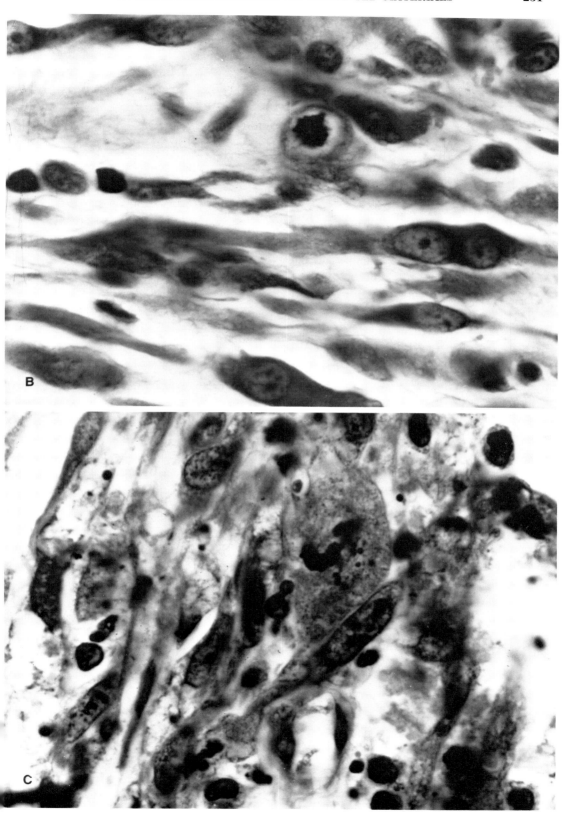

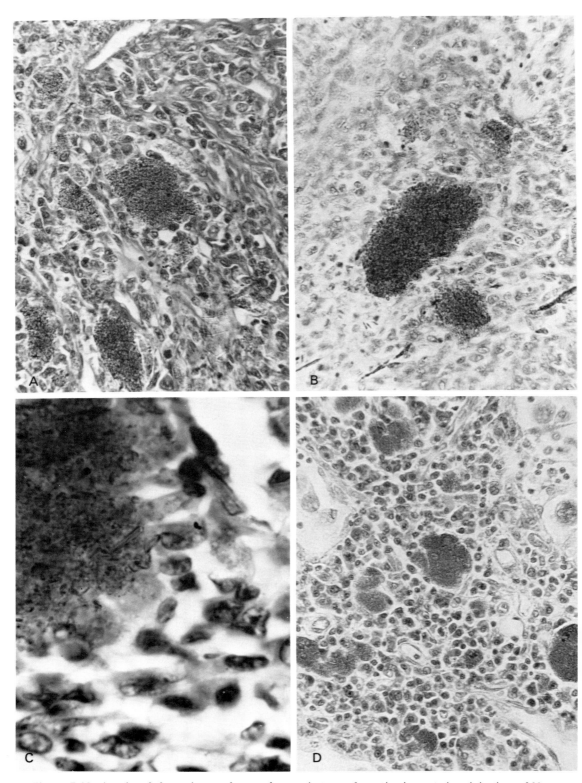

Figure 7-39. A series of photomicrographs reveal stages in tumor formation in a rat given injections of 28 mg of cobalt-chromium alloy wear particles into the muscle of the right thigh. After 16 weeks the tumor developed at the injection site. The experimental technique was otherwise similar to that previously described by Heath.[103] *A* and *B* show a cellular sarcoma with giant cells. (*A,* Azan; *B,* methyl green and pyronin, ×280). *C.* Wear particles within the cellular sarcoma are seen along with an as yet unidentified crystalline material (periodic acid-Schiff, ×580). *D.* A prevertebral lumbar lymph node and numerous wear particles and crystalline material in multinucleate macrophages. No tumor metastasis is present (methyl green and pyronin, ×280). (*A–D,* reproduced with permission of J. C. Heath.[103])

tumor formation after the critical minimum period was realized by excision of the tissue pocket that previously had surrounded the specimen. Polymeric powders are much more potent imitators of tumor formation than solid specimens.[110]

Numerous observations on the initiation of tumors in rats by the presence of a variety of polymeric materials have been documented in detail and are fully described elsewhere.[111-115] While many of the observations, such as those by Brand et al.[111] provide a critical analysis of tumor formation in rats, their relevance to the initiation of tumor formation in man after surgical implantation remains unclear.

A few cases of augmentation mammoplasty in humans with the use of synthetic materials such as Ivalon, polyurethane or silicone sponge, liquid or gel, have been followed by the presentation of carcinoma of the breast.[108] The intervals between implantation and observation of a tumor have varied between 2 months and 6 years. Out of the 40,000 or more of the augmentation mammoplasties performed less than a dozen cases of neoplastic change have been reported. The few cases are statistically insignificant in view of the 5.5% incidence of carcinoma of breast in all women.

The Significance of Experimental Studies on Animals

To date there have been few recorded cases where malignant tumors were observed to arise in juxtaposition to implants in man. Indeed the number of recorded cases is far less than statistical likelihood would predict.[108] It must be emphasized that different tissues show great differences in their predilections to malignant tumor formation. The lung, stomach, large bowel, breast and uterus show a high incidence in Western adult population while muscle and bone show a low incidence of primary neoplastic change. Bone, however, is a frequent site of metastatic spread from many primary tumors. One would not expect, therefore, to observe tumors around implants in the sites where the latter are most frequently used. Furthermore when metallic implants are used to stabilize pathological fractures of bone at the sites of metastatic deposits of tumor, they do not appear to alter the behavior of the tumor.

Observations on experimental animals, notably the rat, suggest that some species of animals have an inherent liability to tumor formation after exposure to soluble metal species or to small metal particles; this has not been observed

in man. From all presently available evidence, carcinogenesis is not a significant risk associated with the use of metal, polymeric, ceramic or graphite implants in man.

SPECIAL PROBLEMS WITH THE USE OF POLYMETHYLMETHACRYLATE CEMENT

With the widespread application of polymethylmethacrylate cement in reconstructive orthopaedic surgery, considerable interest has focused on the possible deleterious side-effects associated with its use. Charnley et al.[115, 116] have documented the local histological response to solid polymethylmethacrylate which is discussed elsewhere. During the admixture of the liquid and powder components of the cement considerable evolution of heat is observed over a period of about 5 to 10 minutes. This temperature depends upon the size of the bolus of cement, as well as other factors. Various workers disagreed on whether the temperature realized is adequate to coagulate proteins.[117] It seems that with a sufficient volume of cement a high temperature can be realized although it probably does not occur frequently in clinical applications.

During the injection of a mixed cement into bone, systemic hypotension has been recorded by many workers.[118, 119] Volatile monomer which enters the systemic circulation appears to be the insulting agent. Several explanations for its effect have been suggested. It is possible that it has a direct effect on the lung[120, 121] or alternatively that it provokes peripheral vasodilatation.[122] The fall in blood pressure is usually transient and rarely persists for more than 3 to 5 minutes. At the time when this side-effect was first noted, several fatalities were reported. Several precautionary measures have been recommended which appear to eliminate the problem. The liquid and powder constituents should be thoroughly mixed to eliminate the residual volatile monomer. This side-effect is largely avoided if the cement is not applied until it is of firm dough-like consistency as the content of free monomer in the mixture varies with its hardness.[115] Prior to the insertion of cement the anesthesiologist should be informed so that an early tendency toward hypotension may be corrected promptly. Patients with a particular risk from transient hypotension, including hypertensive, arteriosclerotic patients and elderly individuals, can be identified so that prophylactic measures can be undertaken.

The substantial evolution of heat during the solidification process of the cement may provoke damage to a variety of soft tissues especially neurovascular structures.[117] For example during the insertion of total hip joint components particularly in patients with an abnormal pelvis such as those treated for congenital dislocation of the hip, particular care is necessary to prevent the cement from oozing into the vicinity of the femoral artery. When drill holes are made through the pelvis, the cement may ooze into the vicinity of the femoral vein unless cement restrictors are used to occlude large parts of the drill holes.

More recently cutaneous sensitization to cement has been reported mostly by surgeons with prolonged irregular exposure to cement.[123] Many surgeons, therefore, recommend that two pairs of surgical gloves be worn simultaneously whenever the cement is handled to diminish the risk of cutaneous exposure through a leak in a glove. Two other possible hazards in the use of cement have been suggested but never confirmed. Systemic sensitivity reactions in patients with implants secured by cement have been proposed as a cause of a painful joint replacement. As Charnley[115] mentions, many patients who have cement in two or more sites have complained at one site but a systemic sensitivity reaction would provoke a hypersensitive reaction at all sites of cement. Hence, the evidence is weak that hypersensitivity to cement provokes loosening. Other workers have suggested that constituents of the cement might contain infective agents but this has not been confirmed.

THE INFLUENCE OF SURGICAL IMPLANTS ON WOUND INFECTION

One of the most disturbing aspects of the application of surgical implants is the increased risk of both early and late postoperative wound infections. Also, after the development of a deep wound infection adjacent to an implant, total irradication of the infection is rarely achieved by any measure unless it includes removal of the entire implant.[124] Many possible reasons for this deleterious side-effect of implants have been proposed although the specific role of the implant, in most cases, remains obscure. Implantation of a contaminated prosthesis is the simplest explanation although with modern sterilization techniques this hazard should be exceptionally uncommon. When the implant shows rapid corrosion or wear the metallic products may stimulate the formation of a thick barrier of fibrous tissue.[26] The barrier shows less vascularity than bone or skeletal mus-

cles so that it may be a particularly susceptible site for proliferation of bacteria. In a somewhat similar way, the application of bone cement, with its capacity to produce enough heat to kill surrounding tissue, may provide a susceptible site for bacterial innoculation and proliferation.[125] Also, irregularities of the surface of the implant may provide nooks wherein bacteria can lodge and proliferate without spread to the body's defense mechanisms. A laboratory test could verify the significance of fibrous tissue sheaths as a susceptible site for bacterial growth. If this is a significant problem it could be lessened by the selection of more inert alloys or by the application of cathodic protection to implants in the bone. Also the superficial temperature of solidifying cement and the temperature of the adjacent tissues can be minimized if the surgeon applies chilled saline solution to the wound.[126]

Metallic corrosion may be accompanied by hydrogen ion production and increased consumption of dissolved oxygen. A local decrease in pH or oxygen concentration may damage or kill surrounding cells to lessen bacterial resistance. The electropotential gradient across the metal-extracellular fluid boundary may discourage the presence of neutrophils, macrophages and lymphocytes[127] and may attract bacteria.[128] There is abundant evidence of the role of surface charge and cell behavior, attachment and migration.[129-131]

A recent study by Barranco et al.,[132] however, suggests that weak anodic or cathodic currents are inhibitory to the growth of Staphylococcus aureus. The significance of these aspects of metallic dissolution or wear of the degradation of other implantable materials with their possible deleterious side-effects to reconstructive procedures is obscure and further studies are needed.

SUMMARY

From the previous discussion it should be evident that surgical implants have the potential to initiate a wide spectrum of deleterious responses by tissues. In view of the numbers of implants that are employed and of the considerable limitations of presently available techniques to evaluate the potential toxic manifestations of previously untried materials, it is surprising how few clinically significant deleterious biological reactions have been documented in which presently available materials were shown to be culpable. Perhaps the greatest concern at present is the role of apparently inert materials *in vivo* to alter locally the resistance of tissues to bacterial infections. In the future much greater attention should be focused on this problem.

REFERENCES

1. Collins, D. H. *J. Pathol. Bacteriol., 65:*109, 1953.
2. Fell, H. B., and Weiss, L. *J. Exp. Med., 121:*551, 1965.
3. Luckey, T. D., and Venugopal, B. *Metal Toxicity in Mammals*, p.40, Plenum Press, New York, 1977.
4. Luckey, T. D., and Venugopal, B. *Metal Toxicity in Mammals*, p. 8, Plenum Press, New York, 1977.
5. Weiss, L. *The Cell Periphery, Metastasis and Other Contact Phenomena*, p. 75, North Holland Publishing Co., Amsterdam, 1967.
6. Wood, S., Lewis, R., Mulholland, J. H., and Knaack, J. *Bull. Johns Hopkins Hosp., 119:*1, 1966.
7. Williams, R. G. *Int. Rev. Cytol., Vol. B.,* p. 359, edited by G. H. Bourne and J. F. Danielli, Academic Press, New York, 1954.
8. Williams, R. G. *Anat. Rec., 137:*107, 1960.
9. Pugatch, E. M. *J. Proc. Roy. Soc., 160B:*412, 1964.
10. Weiss, L. *The Cell Periphery, Metastasis and Other Contact Phenomena*, p. 239, North Holland Publishing Co., Amsterdam, 1967.
11. Weiss, L. *J. Theor. Biol., 6:*275, 1964.
12. Bikerman, J. J. *Colloid Sci., 2:*163, 1947.
13. Weiss, L., and Coombs, R. R. A. *Exp. Cell Res., 30:*331, 1963.
14. Weiss, L. *Exp. Cell Res., suppl.* 8, 141, 1961.
15. Pappas, G. D. *Ann. N.Y. Acad. Sci., 78:*448, 1959.
16. Ambrose, E. J. *Exp. Cell Res., suppl.* 8, 54, 1961.
17. Weiss, L. *The Cell Periphery, Metastasis and Other Contact Phenomena*, p. 200, North Holland Publishing Co., Amsterdam, 1967.
18. Koenig, H. *J. Histochem. Cytochem., 11:*120, 1963.
19. Von Baeyer, H. *Beitr. Klin. Chir., 58:*1, 1908.
20. Emneus, H., and Stenram, U. *Acta Orthop. Scand., 36:*115, 1965.
21. Mellors, R. C., and Carroll, K. G. *Nature, 192:*1090, 1961.
22. Tousmis, A. J. *ISA Proc., 8:*53, 1962.
23. Mears, D. C. *J. Bone Jt. Surg., 48B:*567, 1966.
24. Johannson, R. I., and Hegyeli, A. F. *Ann. N.Y. Acad. Sci., 146:*66, 1968.
25. Luckey, T. D., and Venugopal, B. *Metal Toxicity in Mammals*, p. 42, Plenum Press, New York, 1977.
26. Ferguson, A. B., Jr., Laing, P. G., and Hodge, E. S. *J. Bone Jt. Surg., 42A:*77, 1960.
27. Ferguson, A. B., Jr., Laing, P. G., Hodge, E. S., and Akahoshi, Y. *J. Bone Jt. Surg., 44A:*317, 1962.
28. Laing, P. G., Ferguson, A. B., Jr., and Hodge, E. S. *J. Biomed. Mater. Res., 1:*135, 1967.
29. Hoar, T. P., and Mears, D. C. *Proc. Roy. Soc., 294A:*486, 1966.
30. Luckey, T. D., and Venugopal, B. *Metal Toxicity in Mammals*, p. 36, Plenum Press, New York, 1977.
31. Coleman, R. G., Herrington, J., and Scales, J. T.

*Br. Med. J., 1:*527, 1973.
32. Jones, D. A., Lucas, H. K., O'Driscoll, M., Priet, C. H. G., and Wibberle, B. *J. Bone Jt. Surg., 57B:*289, 1975.
33. Perkins, D. J. *J. Bone Jt. Surg., 55B:*423, 1973.
34. Taylor, D. M. *J. Bone Jt. Surg., 55B:*424, 1973.
35. Maroudas, A. *J. Bone Jt. Surg., 55B:*424, 1973.
36. Lane, W. A. *The Operative Treatment of Fractures*, p. 10, Medical Publishing Co., London, 1914.
37. Scales, J. T. *J. Bone Jt. Surg., 53B:*344, 1971.
38. Pilliar, R. M., Cameron, H. U., and MacNab, I. *Biomed. Eng., 35:*126, 1975.
39. Homsy, C. A. *J. Biomed. Mater. Res., 4:*341, 1960.
40. Passow, H., Rothstein, A., and Clarkson, T. W. *Pharmacol. Rev., 13:*185, 1961.
41. Weiss, L., and Dingle, J. T. *Am. Rheum. Dis., 23:*57, 1964.
42. Weiss, L. *The Cell Periphery, Metastasis and Other Contact Phenomena*, p. 97, North Holland Publishing Co., Amsterdam, 1967.
43. Dingle, J. T. Nuffield Foundation Conference on the Causes and Treatment of Rheumatic Diseases, Ashridge College, 1962.
44. Heath, J. C. Freeman, M. A. R., and Swanson, S. A. V. *Lancet, 1:*564, 1971.
45. Rae, T. *J. Bone Jt. Surg., 57B:*444, 1975.
46. Rae, T. *J. Bone Jt. Surg., 57B:*447, 1975.
47. Rae, T. *J. Bone Jt. Surg., 57B:*446, 1975.
48. Riede, U. N., Ruedi, T., Rohner, Y. L. E., Perren, S., and Guggenheim, R. *Arch. Orthop. Unfall-Chir., 78:*199, 1974.
49. Winter, G. D. *J. Biomed. Mater. Res., 8(3):*11, 1974.
50. Winter, G. D. *J. Biomed. Mater. Res., 8(3):*15, 1974.
51. Willert, H. G., and Semlitsch, M. *Reaction of the Articular Capsule to Plastic and Metallic Wear Products from Joint Endoprostheses*, Congress of Dutch-Swiss Orthopaedic Societies, Lausanne, 1974.
52. Willert, H. D., and Semlitsch, M. Problems associated with cement anchorage of artificial joints. In *Artificial Hip and Knee Joint Technology*, p. 342, edited by M. Schaldach and D. Hohmann, Springer-Verlag, Berlin, 1976.
53. Mirra, J. M., Amstutz, H. C., Matos, M., and Gold, R. *Clin. Orthop., 117:*221, 1976.
54. Cohen, J. *J. Bone Jt. Surg., 41A:*152, 1959.
54a. Walker, P. S., and Bullough, P. G. *Orthop. Clin. North Am., 4:*2, 275, 1973.
55. Pilliar, R. M., Cameron, H. U., and MacNab, I. *Biomed. Eng., 12:*126, 1975.
56. Hench, L. L. *Ann. Rev. Mater. Sci., 5:*279, 1975.
57. Hench, L. L., and Paschall, H. A. *J. Biomed. Mater. Res., 8:*49, 1974.
58. Griss, P., Greenspan, D. C., Heimke, G., Krempien, B., Buchinger, R., Hench, L. L., and Jentschura, G. Evaluation of a bioglass coated Al_2O_3 total hip prosthesis in sheep. *J. Biomed. Mater. Res. Symp.*, 1975.
59. Hench, L. L., Splinter, R. J., Greenle, T. K., and Allen, W. C. *J. Biomed. Mater. Res., 1:*117, 1971.
60. Pitorowski, G., Hench, L. L., Allen, W. C., and Miller, G. J. *J. Biomed. Mater. Res. Symp., 9:*6, 47, 1975.
61. Carlisle, E. M. *Sci., 167:*9, 1970.

62. Pantano, C. G., Jr., Clark, A. E., Jr., and Hench, L. L. *J. Am. Cer. Soc.*, *57*:412, 1974.

63. Rigdon, R. H. Tissue reactions to foreign materials. In *Critical Rev. Toxicol.*, *3*:435, 1975.

64. Klaassen, C. D. Absorption, distribution and excretion of toxicants. In *Toxicology*, p. 26, edited by W. Casarett and J. Doull, Macmillan Company, New York, 1976.

65. *The United States Pharmacopeia XIX.* Biological Tests-Plastic Containers, p. 644, Mack Publishing Co., Easton, Pa. 1975.

66. Turner, J. E., Lawrence, W. H., and Autian, J. *J. Biomed. Mater. Res.*, *7*:39, 1973.

67. Autian, J. *CRC Critical Rev. in Toxicol.*, *2*:1, 1973.

68. Guess, W. L., Rosenbluth, S. A., Schmidt, B., and Autian, J. *J. Pharm. Sci.*, *54*:156, 1965.

69. Magnusson, B., and Kligman, A. M. *J. Invest. Derm.*, *52*:268, 1969.

70. Pappas, A. M., and Cohen, J. *J. Bone Jt. Surg.*, *50A*:535, 1968.

71. Swanson, S. A. V., Freeman, M. A. R., and Heath, J. C. *J. Bone Jt. Surg.*, *55B*:427, 1973.

72. Homsy, C. A. *J. Biomed. Mater. Res.*, *4*:341, 1970.

73. Gerber, H., Burge, M., Cordey, J., Ziegler, W., and Perren, S. M. *Proc. ESAO*, *1*:29, 1974.

74. Brown, S. A., Mayor, M. B., and Merritt, K. Leukocyte migration inhibition test for metal sensitivity. *Second Conference on Materials for Use in Medicine and Biology*, Brunel University, London, Sept. 1976.

75. Swanson, A. B., Meester, W. D., Swanson, G. deG., Rangaswamy, L., and Schut, G. E. D. *Ortho. Clin. N. Am.*, *4(4)*:1097, 1973.

76. Apker, R. G., Davie, J. M., and Cattell, H. S. *Clin. Orthop.*, *98*:231, 1974.

77. Hicks, J. H. Pathological effects from surgical metal. In *Modern Trends in Surgical Materials*, p. 29, edited by H. Gillis, Butterworth & Co., London, 1958.

78. McKenzie, A. W., Aitken, C. V. E., and Ridsdell-Smith, R. *Br. Med. J.*, *4*:36, 1967.

79. Evans, E. M., Freeman, M. A. R., Miller, A. J., and Vernon-Roberts, B. *J. Bone Jt. Surg.*, *56B*:626, 1974.

80. Jones, D. A., Lucas, H. K., O'Driscoll, M., Price, C. H. G., and Wibberley, B. *J. Bone Jt. Surg.*, *57B*:289, 1975.

81. Elves, M. Hypersensitivity to metals in patients with orthopaedic prostheses. *Second Conference on Materials for Use in Medicine and Biology*, Brunel University, London, Sept. 1976.

82. Goodwin, P. G., and Benson, M. K. D. The incidence and significance of acquired metal sensitivity in patients with joint replacement arthroplasties. *Second Conference on Materials for Use in Medicine and Biology*, Brunel University, London, Sept. 1976.

83. Abraham, E. P. The nature of antigens and antibodies. In *General Pathology*, p. 932, edited by H. W. Florey, Lloyd-Luke Medical Books Ltd., London, 1970.

84. Sullivan, J. F., George, R., Bluvas, R., and Egan, J. D. *Ann. Int. Med.*, *70*:277, 1969.

85. Calnan, C. D. *Br. J. Derm.*, *68*:229, 1956.

86. Stoddart, J. C. *Lancet*, *2*:741, 1960.

87. McKee, G. K. McKee-Farrar total prostetic replacement of the hip. In *Total Hip Replace-* *ment*, p. 47, edited by M. Jayson, Sector Publishers Ltd., London, 1971.

88. Charosky, C. B., Bullough, P. G., and Wilson, P. D., Jr. *J. Bone Jt. Surg.*, *55A*:49, 1973.

89. Seifert, W. W., and Westcott, V. C. *Wear*, *21*:27, 1972; *23*:239, 1973.

90. Scott, D., Seifert, W. W., and Westcott, V. C. *Sci. Am.*, *230*:88, 1974.

91. Scott, D., Seifert, W. W., and Westcott, V. C. *Wear*, *34*:251, 1975.

92. Mears, D. C., Westcott, V. C., Hanley, E., and Rutkowski, R. *Wear*, *50*:115, 1978.

93. McCarty, D. J. *Arthritis and Allied Conditions*, ed. 8, p. 1140, edited by J. L. Hollander, Lea & Febiger, Philadelphia, 1972.

94. Mears, D. C. *Ortho. Survey*, *1*:64, 1977.

95. Browning, E. *Toxicity of Industrial Metals*, ed. 2, p. 119, Butterworths, London, 1969.

96. Walter, J. B., and Israel, M. S. *General Pathology*, p. 577, Little and Brown, Boston, 1965.

97. Oppenheimer, B. S., Oppenheimer, F. T., Danishefsky, I., and Storet, A. P. *Cancer Res.*, *16*:439, 1956.

98. Heath, J. C., Webb, M. and Caffrey, M. *Br. J. Cancer*, *23*:153, 1969.

99. Hamilton, A., and Hardy, H. L. *Industrial Toxicology*, p. 73, Publishers Science Group, Acton, Mass., 1974.

100. Furst, A., and Haro, R. T. *Prog. Exp. Tumor Res.*, *11*:102, 1969.

101. Sunderman, F. W., Jr. *Fed. Cosmet. Toxicol.*, *9*:105, 1971.

102. Sunderman, F. W., Jr. Nickel poisoning. In *Laboratory Diagnoses of Diseases Caused by Toxic Agents*, p. 389, edited by F. W. Sunderman and F. W. Sunderman, Jr., Warren Green, Inc., St. Louis, 1971.

103. Heath, J. C. *Br. J. Cancer*, *14*:478, 1960.

104. Godman, G. C. *J. Morph.*, *100*:27, 1957.

105. Heath, J. C., Freeman, M. A. R., and Swanson, S. A. V. *Lancet*, *1*:564, 1971.

106. Swanson, S. A. V., Freeman, M. A. R., and Heath, J. C. *J. Bone Jt. Surg.*, *55B*:759, 1973.

107. Autian, J. Toxicological problems and untoward effects from plastic devices used in medical applications. In *Essays in Toxicology*, p. 1, edited by W. J. Hayes, Jr., Academic Press, New York, 1975.

108. Bischoff, F., and Bryson, G. *Progr. Exp. Tumor Res.*, *5*:85, 1964.

109. Bering, E. A., McLaurin, R. C., Lloyd, J. B., and Ingraham, F. D. *Cancer Res.*, *15*:300, 1955.

110. Carter, R. L., and Roe, F. J. C. *Br. J. Cancer*, *23*:401, 1969.

111. Brand, K. G., Busen, L. C., and Brand, I. *J. Nat. Cancer Inst.*, *39*:663, 1967.

112. Hueper, W. C. *Pathol. Microbiol.*, *24*:77, 1961.

113. Bates, R. R., and Klein, M. *J. Nat. Cancer Inst.*, *37*:145, 1966.

114. Hueper, W. C. *J. Nat. Cancer Inst.*, *33*:1005, 1964.

115. Charnley, J. *Acrylic Cement in Orthopaedic Surgery*, p. 10, Livingstone, Edinburgh, 1970.

116. Charnley, J., Murphy, J. C. M., and Pitkeathly, D. A. *Br. Med. J.*, *3*:474, 1971.

117. Jefferiss, C. D., Lee, A. J. C., and Ling, R. S. M. *J. Bone Jt. Surg.*, *57B*:511, 1975.

118. Peebles, D. J., Ellis, R. H., Stride, S. D. K., and Simpson, B. R. J. *Br. Med. J.*, *1*:349, 1972.

119. Bayne, S. C., Lautenschlager, E. P., Greener, E. H., and Meyer, P. R. *J. Biomed. Mater. Res., 11*:859, 1977.

120. Homsy, C. A., Tullos, H. S., and King, J. W. *Clin. Orthop., 67*:169, 1969.

121. McLaughlin, R. E., DiFazio, C. A., Hakala, M., Abbott, B., MacPhail, J. A., Mack, W. P., and Sweet, D. E. *J. Bone Jt. Surg., 55A*:1621, 1973.

122. Thomas, T. A., Sutherland, I. C., and Waterhouse, T. O. *Anaesthesia, 26*:298, 1971.

123. Fries, I. B., Fisher, A. A., and Salvati, E. A. *J. Bone Jt. Surg., 57A*:547, 1975.

124. Scales, J. T. *J. Bone Jt. Surg., 53B*:344, 1971.

125. Charnley, J. *J. Bone Jt. Surg., 52B*:340, 1970.

126. Lee, A. J. C., and Ling, R. S. M. *Clin. Ortho., 106*:122, 1975.

127. Weiss, L. *The Cell Periphery, Metastasis and Other Contact Phenomena*, p. 228, North Holland Publishing Co., Amsterdam, 1967.

128. Cieszynski, T. *Arch. Immun. Ther. Exper., 12*:269, 1964.

129. Lowenstein, W. R. *Ann. N.Y. Acad. Sci., 137*:441, 1967.

130. Scott, B. I. H. *Proc Soc. Exp. Biol. Med., 113*:337, 1963.

131. Weiss, L. *The Cell Periphery, Metastasis and Other Contact Phenomena*, pp. 104, 164, North Holland Publishing Co., Amsterdam, 1967.

132. Barranco, S. D., Spadaro, J. A., Berger, T. J., and Becker, R. O. *Clin. Orthop., 100*:250, 1974.

8.

The Design, Use and Care of Implants

A surgical implant undergoes a moderately consistent life which starts with its conception and proceeds with its design and manufacture. Subsequently, it is packaged, sterilized and stored prior to its application in the human body. It may be removed after a variable period when its role has been completed or, alternatively, it may remain in the body for an indefinite period. Each sequence in the story is considered here, in an effort to mold the information provided in previous chapters into a practical account of the use and care of implants.

IMPLANT DESIGN

The initial idea for a novel implant may present itself as a minor adaptation of an existing design or as a wholly new concept. Particularly in reconstructive surgery, the design may be an attempt to replicate a structure provided by nature. The crucial question arises on the desirability of a design for a novel implant to conform in principle and detail to the natural component to be reconstructed. As an alternative, the design might attempt to operate by a completely different mechanism with a different geometry or location. While there is no single answer to this question, on the basis of previous successes and failures in the development of orthopaedic implants, certain guidelines may be useful. When an inert man-made material of appropriate mechanical properties exists from which to design and fabricate an exact replica of a biological tissue, the use of such a material appears to be the most likely solution that will provide long term success. Where the implant serves a limited period of function, a radically different geometry or mechanical property may still be consistent with satisfactory function. For many applications where prolonged service *in vivo* is essential and where the available inert materials show widely differing mechanical properties, the designer may have to design a radically different structure from its anatomic counterpart. One example is the development of the total hip joint replacement by Charnley, which he rightly called an arthroplasty in view of its unique attributes of design. In such an instance, particular caution is required in the predictions of the successful duration of anticipated function. In this instance it becomes particularly important that the first clinical trials are undertaken in those individuals of short life expectancy or generally limited functional capacity, such as many rheumatoid arthritic patients.

General Principles of Design

At the time of the inception of a novel idea for a surgical implant, the designer requires detailed analysis of the human environment and the functional attributes of the part of the body to be repaired or replaced. In many instances such knowledge is not available when the novel problem or design is first approached. Before the optimal design can be achieved, an exacting analysis of the physiological conditions found in the body at the relevant site must be clarified. Recent advances in biomechanics of the locomotor system have greatly facilitated the development of joint replacements, artificial tendons and other implants.[1-3] The design of an implant is constrained by the need for inert materials of appropriate mechanical properties as well as anatomical and surgical constraints. For devices that are expected to function for prolonged periods, simplicity in design becomes essential. Methods to attach implants to the skeletal system, with rigid fixation to the appropriate location and without the likelihood of migration or loosening, remain elusive.[4, 5] For widespread acceptance of a technique, the reconstructive procedure should involve simplicity in the surgical procedure itself. Where the method requires rigid adherence to an intricate format, such as a cup arthroplasty, the chances of substantial failures by other surgeons are great and prolonged acceptance of the technique is considerably jeopardized unless it represents an extraordinary advance in the method of treatment.

Principles of Design. Williams and Roaf[6] have provided an excellent detailed account on the engineering principles of design to which the interested reader is recommended. The present discussion is a much abbreviated account which discusses many of their ideas. It will be understood that implants inserted into the human body must withstand the loads to which they are exposed without breaking, distorting or deforming, and without undergoing other forms of deterioration. Certain objectives of the design must be considered if this goal is to be realized. Common examples of the various types of loading are shown in Figure 8-1.

Design for Rigidity. In certain orthopaedic applications, rigidity is as important as the strength of an implant, where strength refers to the stress at which a structure ceases to deform elastically and starts to break or deform plastically. In contrast, rigidity refers to the amount of deformation induced in a structure by stress before the elastic limit is reached. Rigidity defines how much alteration of shape occurs when the device is stressed below the point at which it would deform plastically. In an ideal model where a pure tensile force acts upon a uniform rod of a material, the amount of elastic deformation induced by the force is dependent solely upon the Young's modulus, the magnitude of the force and the cross-sectional area. Resistance to deformation can be augmented by the use of a material of a high modulus, a rod of large cross-sectional area, or both. In most practical applications, however, the structure is generally stressed not only in tension, but it is also subjected to bending and nonaxial compression. Rigidity in bending is fully described elsewhere.[7] Whereas previous workers believe that optimal design was realized by the application of implants that were much more rigid than the adjacent column of bone, most recent workers have agreed that future implants for anchorage or immobilization of bone should possess a rigidity comparable to the relevant segment of bone. This concept is described in more detail in Chapters 6, 9 and 13.

The Design of Nails for Use in the Femoral Neck. One orthopaedic implant of widespread application, the solid nail-plate device for fixation of femoral neck fractures, provides a particularly useful example of beams subjected to bending moments. While the human stress analysis would be complex, it is useful to consider an idealized homogeneous structure (Fig. 8-2A) with a fracture plane AA', where the purpose of a fixation device is to minimize motion in this plane in the direction Y under the influence of a force W transmitted through the hip. The device is attached to the femoral shaft by sufficient screws to stabilize point B, so that the force transmitted to the device is contained solely in the section BB', which is assumed to be uniform along its length. With B rigidly immobilized, the reference axes are AA' (the Y axis) and BB' (the X axis) with an initial load W assumed to be concentrated at the origin O of these axes. In this simple cantilever arrangement the component of the force acting in the direction Y is $W \cos \theta$, where θ is the angle between the line of action of W and the AA' plane. If the total length is L and the distance BO is l, then the deflection y_B at B is:

$$y_B = \frac{W \cos \theta \cdot l^2}{2\,EI} (L - \tfrac{1}{3}l)$$

Types of Loading

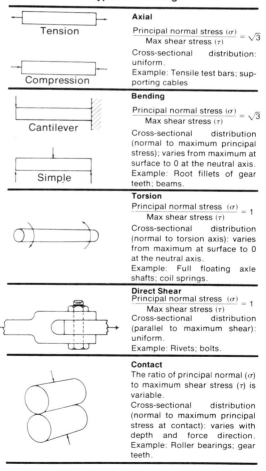

Tension	**Axial**
	$\dfrac{\text{Principal normal stress } (\sigma)}{\text{Max shear stress } (\tau)} = \sqrt{3}$
Compression	Cross-sectional distribution: uniform. Example: Tensile test bars; supporting cables
Cantilever	**Bending**
	$\dfrac{\text{Principal normal stress } (\sigma)}{\text{Max shear stress } (\tau)} = \sqrt{3}$
Simple	Cross-sectional distribution (normal to maximum principal stress); varies from maximum at surface to 0 at the neutral axis. Example: Root fillets of gear teeth; beams.
	Torsion
	$\dfrac{\text{Principal normal stress } (\sigma)}{\text{Max shear stress } (\tau)} = 1$
	Cross-sectional distribution (normal to torsion axis): varies from maximum at surface to 0 at the neutral axis. Example: Full floating axle shafts; coil springs.
	Direct Shear
	$\dfrac{\text{Principal normal stress } (\sigma)}{\text{Max shear stress } (\tau)} = 1$
	Cross-sectional distribution (parallel to maximum shear): uniform. Example: Rivets; bolts.
	Contact
	The ratio of principal normal (σ) to maximum shear stress (τ) is variable. Cross-sectional distribution (normal to maximum principal stress at contact): varies with depth and force direction. Example: Roller bearings; gear teeth.

Figure 8-1. Schematic diagrams reveal the types of loading which are imposed upon surgical implants.

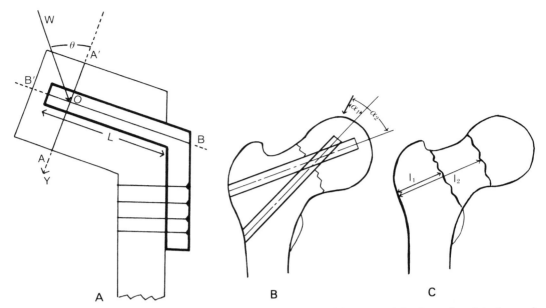

Figure 8-2. *A.* An idealized structure of a device for the fixation of fractures of the femoral neck is shown. A description is provided in the text. (Reproduced with permission of D. F. Williams and R. Roaf.[8]) *B.* The relationship between the alignment of a femoral nail and the direction of the resultant force is indicated. The component of the force to provoke bending will be greater for angle α_2 and α_1. *C.* The relationship between the site of the fracture in the femoral neck and the appropriate length of the femoral nail is shown. The deflection tends to be greater for the length l_2 than l_1. (Reproduced with permission of D. F. Williams and R. Roaf.[9])

and the deflection y_o at O is:

$$y_o = \frac{W \cos \theta \cdot l^3}{3\,EI}$$

For a given load W, therefore, the following are the criteria for a minimum deflection: $\cos \theta$ should be small and θ should be large; l should be small; E should be large; and I should be large. While the present example is somewhat oversimplified and thereby contains a few minor inaccuracies, it reveals the design criteria that would be applicable for a much more complex analysis. Namely, a rigid beam must be manufactured of a material with a large elastic modulus. It will be self-evident that the angle θ should be large since the direction of the principal weight-bearing forces are fixed. A resultant force more nearly approximating the axis of the device is realized if the device is inserted as far distal as possible in the lateral cortex of the femoral shaft (Fig. 8-2B). Such a distal insertion, however, affects another variable in the equation, the length (l) of the nail which appears in the equation as l^3. Slight increases in l will produce proportionately much larger increases in the deflection. With the more distal insertion

technique, the distance from the fracture surface to the fixed point may be considerably increased. On the other hand, with the more oblique approach, the weight-bearing forces tend to provoke optimal impaction of the fracture surfaces so that weight-bearing forces are transmitted to a greater degree directly across the fractured surfaces of bone with an equivalent relief of bending moments that otherwise would be imposed upon the nail.

The other attribute of the nail which influences its rigidity is its cross-sectional shape and area. As discussed in Chapter 9, the rigidity increases as the mass of material is moved away from the neutral axis. For a given amount of material, a cylinder will show the greatest resistance to bending moments.[6] Of the open designs which permit vascularization of adjacent bone, the I-beam and the H-beam augment rigidity, in comparison with a rectangular beam, along a somewhat similar principle.

Combined Bending and Direct Stress. Many practical situations possess more complex effects such as a combination of bending and direct stress. One example is shown in Figure 8-3, where a vertical column is subjected to a force

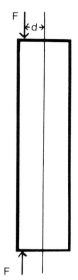

Figure 8-3. A vertical column is subjected to a force, *F*, displaced a distance, *d*, from the axis of the column. (Reproduced with permission of D. F. Williams and R. Roaf.[10])

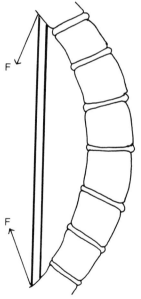

Figure 8-4. A spinal distraction rod is frequently exposed to a nonaxial compressive force. (Reproduced with permission of D. F. Williams and R. Roaf.[11])

(*F*) displaced a distance (*d*) from the axis of the column. At any point in the column the material of the beam will be subjected to a stress which is a summation of a bending and a direct stress. In a uniform structure the direct stress component will be constant and equivalent to *F/A*. The bending stress component will be variable

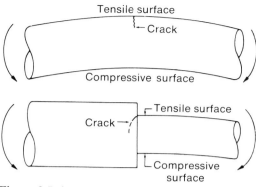

Figure 8-5. An example of a bending stress applied to a beam is shown. The stress is tensile on one surface and compressive on the opposite one. For most metals, mechanical failure will tend to occur on the tensile aspect.

over the section, whereas in the state of pure tension or compression the nature of the cross-section would have no influence on the elastic behavior of the structure. Under the imposition of nonaxial loading the dimensions of the section have a crucial bearing on rigidity. One practical example of an implant exposed to a combination of bending and direct stress is the distraction rod employed for spinal correction as seen in Figure 8-4. The forces applied to such a rod may be approximately parallel to the rod but not necessarily axial.

Designing against Excessive Plastic Deformation

Under the imposition of a pure tensile load, a structure composed of a material which displays a yield point, undergoes negligible plastic deformation if the applied tensile force (*F*) does not exceed $\sigma_s \cdot A$ where the yield stress is σ_s and the cross-sectional area is *A*. Alternatively, for a given force either the yield stress of the material must be greater than *F/A* or the cross-sectional area must be greater than F/σ_s, depending upon which factor is fixed. Where the material has a diffuse yield point the situation is more complex and beyond the limits of discussion here.[7]

For consideration of a bending stress in a beam, the stress σ_y at a point *y* from the neutral axis is given by:

$$\frac{\sigma_y}{y} = \frac{M}{I} = \frac{E}{R}$$

During bending, the stress in a beam is maximal at its surface. The stress is compressive on one surface and tensile on the opposite one, as seen in Figure 8-5. While the optimal design of the beam which resists plastic deformation involves many factors, the yield point of the material and the second moment of area of the beam section are the critical ones. The maximum stress, σ_{max}, may be written as:

$$\sigma_{max} = \frac{yM}{I}$$

where y is the distance from the surface to the neutral plane. If the choice of the material is limited to one of yield stress σ_s, then σ_s must be greater than σ_{max}, which means that for a given bending moment, y/I should be minimized Since the term y will be incorporated in the expression for the second moment of area where it will be raised to the power three or more, depending upon the nature of the section, this does not imply that the beam should be as thin as possible. It is the second moment of area that is the dominant factor.

While the yield point of a material controls plastic instability, the elastic modulus regulates elastic instability. In the selection of an alloy for an implant that possesses a limitation of elastic deformation, stainless steel or conventional surgical grades of cobalt-based alloys show a clear advantage over titanium and its alloys. Where avoidance of plastic deformation is critical, then the age-hardened titanium alloys or the multi-phased cobalt and nickel-based alloys are perhaps marginally superior to the conventional stainless steel and cobalt-based alloys or pure titanium.

Designing Against Fracture

As a general observation, fracture of an implant while it is in service within the body is highly undesirable for the patient, the surgeon, the company which manufactured the implant, and the primary producer of the alloy itself, albeit for different reasons. Admittedly, after the fracture has united, breakage, loosening, migration, or instability of a fixation device usually is of little significance apart from the difficulty of extraction of certain parts of the broken implants. Nevertheless, it should be self-evident that most implants must be designed to avoid fracture in service. In the following discussion, ductile failure, brittle failure and fatigue failure are reviewed briefly. Again, for a more detailed account the reader is referred to a discussion by Williams and Roaf.[6]

Ductile Failure. Since ductile failure represents the conclusion of plastic deformation, design to circumvent ductile failure comprises an extension of design against excessive plastic deformation. The ultimate stress, however, is used as the criterion instead of the yield or proof stress. Where negligible plastic deformation is essential, the yield stress also will satisfy the criterion for fracture. In view of the hazard of loading a component with a magnitude of stress that rivals the ultimate stress, it is usual to introduce a factor of safety so that

$$\text{working stress} = \frac{\text{ultimate stress}}{\text{factor of safety}}$$

The value chosen for this factor will depend upon the type of loading, the accuracy with which the imposed forces can be determined or estimated, the environment of the component, the degree of accuracy to which the component can be manufactured, the permissible magnitude of deformation and the nature of the material itself. Under optimal conditions a safety factor of 2 might be applied while the presence of various unknowns, especially of the mechanical forces imposed upon the device, may elevate the factor to a value of 10.

Sometimes the yield stress is employed, in which case the safety factor is usually not less than 1.5. The design stress is equivalent to the yield stress divided by the safety factor and is never more than two-thirds of the yield stress.

Brittle Failure. The alternative form of mechanical failure under static load without plastic deformation, brittle failure, should be rarely encountered in surgical implants. While brittle materials, such as the early cobalt-chromium alloys or the solid form of polymethylmethacrylate used in the Judet hip prosthesis were first employed, the materials used in the recent past have been selected in large part for their ductility. Recently, many workers have expressed much interest in the application of ceramics[12-14] or vitreous carbon[15] which are also inherently brittle. While the former material is currently undergoing clinical application for use in total hip joint replacements, it seems quite unsatisfactory to the author, unless some novel solution is used to circumvent the highly likely possibility of brittle fracture which already has been documented in certain of these implants. Figure 8-6 shows the primary difference displayed by brittle and ductile materials during a tensile test. In most cases the actual ultimate tensile strength (UTS) of a brittle material may exceed that of a ductile one. The problem of brittleness arises because brittle materials are extraordinarily sensitive to flaws in their structure, especially under the influence of multiaxial stresses. As elabo-

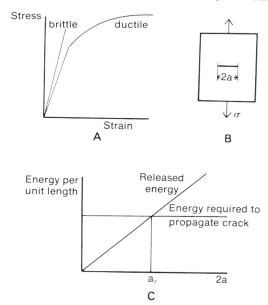

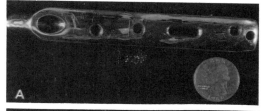

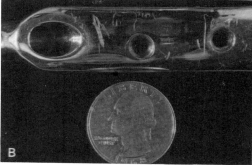

Figure 8-6. Stress-strain curves for a ductile and a brittle material are shown.

Figure 8-7. *A* and *B*. The photographs of a hip screw after routine application and removal reveal the superficial flaws produced by conventional surgical maneuvers. Several defects are enlarged in the close-up, *B*. For use in internal fixation an implant must be ductile to eliminate the possibility for the propagation of a superficial defect. Ultimately a fracture may ensue in such a brittle substance.

rated in Chapters 2 and 3, the application of a static load to a ductile structure with superficial flaws or cracks has little influence on the fracture mechanism other than reducing the cross-sectional area. The material is able to deform plastically around the cracks so that they do not become catastrophically self-propagating. In contrast, a flaw on the surface of a truly brittle solid greatly compromises the effective strength displayed by the material. If a brittle solid is to be safely employed, it must tolerate, without significant compromise to its mechanical properties, the initiation of flaws in the surface that might occur during surgical implantation or clinical exposure. Also, the inherent features of the design must eliminate features which could serve as stress raisers. Figure 8-7 reveals the defects on the surface of a hip screw noted at the time of its removal. The defects are indicative of those observed on most devices for internal fixation after their period of use. Admittedly, some of the blemishes arise during the removal itself. Nevertheless, the surgical procedures for the application of many orthopaedic implants necessitates the use of tools and maneuvers that causes superficial damage to the implants. In these instances, the application of brittle materials with their notch sensitivity conceivably might culminate in fracture of the implant.

Fatigue Failure. For orthopaedic applications of surgical implants, fatigue failure is probably the primary concern. The failures arise by prop-

agation of a crack from stress concentrations produced at superficial irregularities. The irregularities may consist of holes, grooves, abrupt change in cross-section, recesses, machine marks or corrosion pits. A review will be found in Chapters 3, 4 and 13.

Factors in Stress Concentration

A stress concentration arises in a material where a change of shape interrupts the lines of stress. For a uniform rod under a state of uniform tensile stress, $\sigma_{(average)}$, a notch in the surface of the specimen introduces a peak stress at the notch root, $\sigma_{(peak)}$, given by:

$$\sigma_{(peak)} = K_t \times \sigma_{(average)}$$

where K_t is the theoretical stress concentration factor in what is assumed to be an elastic mode of behavior.[16] The value of the factor may increase to 3 where it becomes highly significant. Abrupt changes in the cross-sectional area of a specimen or the presence of small radii of curvature in the transitional zone between two adjacent sections of an implant may severely compromise fatigue resistance. Figure 8-8 reveals how the stress concentration factor varies with the radius of curvature of the "fillet", as this

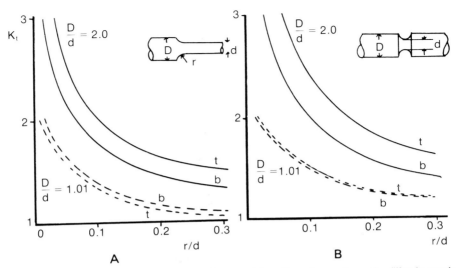

Figure 8-8. *A.* Variation of stress concentration factors with radius of curvature of a fillet in tension, *t,* and bending, *b. B.* Variations of stress concentration factors with geometry of circumferential groove in tension, *t,* and bending, *b.* (Reproduced with permission of C. Ruiz and F. Koenigsberger.[17])

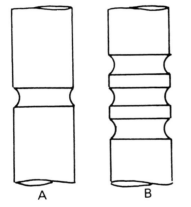

Figure 8-9. Relief grooving is illustrated. (Reproduced with permission of C. Ruiz and F. Koenigsberger.[17]

zone is called. With a large fillet the factor approaches zero. Where design constraints inhibit the presence of a generous fillet, an internal fillet may be employed. Where a circumferential groove is necessary in the surface of a shaft, the groove should show the maximal radius of curvature. Where the groove must have a small radius of curvature, the associated stress concentration may be minimized by the presence of adjacent grooves on either side of the former.[18] This method, shown in Figure 8-9, is called relief grooving.

A hole in the surface of a bone plate is another example of a stress concentration. Where the diameter of a hole is less than one-fifth of the width of the plate, then the maximum stress adjacent to the hole will be 3 times greater than the average stress in the material. This factor diminishes as the hole enlarges, with respect to the width of the plate, and approaches 2 in the limiting case. If the hole is elliptical, the maximum stress at the ends of a horizontal axis of the hole will be:

$$\sigma_{max} = \sigma_{av} \, (1 + 2 \; c/h)$$

where $2c$ and $2h$ are the major and minor axes respectively. For holes perpendicular to the direction of the tensile stress, the stress concentration factor enlarges dramatically, since as σ_{max}/σ_{av} increases so c/h increases. For small circular holes in a plate the actual size does not affect the stress concentration greatly until the diameter of the hole approaches 20% of the width of the plate. Elliptical holes present a more formidable problem where the stress system is complex or unknown and where high tensile stresses might be established perpendicular to the hole. For present designs of self-compression plates, such as the Dynamic Compression plate,* the possibility of substantial stress concentration initiated by the elliptical holes should be considered.

The fatigue strength reduction factor K_f is a useful index of the degree to which a given material is sensitive to superficial notches or

---

* Synthes Corp., Wayne, Pa.

other irregularities. The fatigue limit of a material without stress concentration is determined, after which the measurement is repeated when a specific notch is introduced into the test specimen. The ratio of the former to the latter value is known as the fatigue strength reduction factor, or K_f. As a first approximation $K_f \simeq K_t$, but with certain exceptions. A notch sensitivity factor Q, may be defined as

$$Q = \frac{K_f - 1}{K_t - 1}.$$

It provides a measure of the effect of stress concentrations on the fatigue properties of the material. A stress concentration is most significant when $K_f = K_t$ and therefore $Q = 1$. The material is then said to be completely notch sensitive. In contrast, K_t may be equal to 1, whereupon there is no reduction in the fatigue strength in the presence of a notch, and Q is equal to 0. When conditions dictate the need for stress concentrations in the design, a material with a low value of Q, compatible with other requirements, should be selected.

Fatigue in Implants with Multiple Components. Many hip nails and other fixation devices consist of multiple components secured together. The mating surfaces, however, are liable to undergo fretting with micromotion, thereby to accelerate fatigue damage. The severity of the fretting can be diminished in several ways. Certain materials such as cobalt-based alloys should be employed instead of others, such as titanium alloys, that possess a greater tendency to fret. The design of the interface should permit a high, uniform pressure to be exerted between the surfaces, without any areas of contact that do not share the uniform compressive load.[18] The tension in the retention bolt should be maximized, although below the yield point of the material. Over tightening could impose high tensile and sheer stresses in a bolt, which might thereby undergo premature failure in service, when additional stresses were imposed. Nevertheless, adequate tightening of the components with respect to each other is also essential to reduce both fretting at the interface and the magnitude of the stress cycle that is established in the retention bolt.

In many applications the risk of fatigue failure can be minimized by appropriate preparation of the metallic surface. Fatigue usually initiates at a stress concentration on the surface. Prevention in the early growth of the fatigue crack might be undertaken by the application of a uniform compressive stress on the surface to prevent micro

fatigue cracks from yawning. While commercial methods such as shot-peening or cold rolling might be beneficial from this point of view, they are contraindicated because they compromise corrosion resistance. Unfortunately the exceptionally smooth electropolished surfaces of most surgical implants do not possess optimal resistance to fatigue.

Designing Against Corrosion

The influence of design features on corrosion was elaborated in Chapter 4. In summary, fretting corrosion is best avoided by appropriate selection of resistant materials. Crevice corrosion can be diminished by the selection of highly resistant alloys, such as titanium, or by the elimination of unnecessary crevices with appropriate design of interfaces. Stress corrosion and corrosion fatigue are avoided by the selection of resistant alloys such as titanium or by alteration of design to avoid stress risers. While galvanic corrosion has been cited as a problem by previous workers,[19] the author is unaware of its presence when any two of the available passive alloys are employed in juxtaposition to one another.[20] Nevertheless, such materials may still undergo crevice corrosion[21] or fretting corrosion, which are different mechanisms.

DESIGN AND MANUFACTURING

An implant design must be consistent with available techniques of fabrication from suitable materials at a realistic cost. At present, economic considerations are highly influential in the production of surgical implants and they must be taken into account. Metallic components can be fabricated by casting, forging and machining. Casting is widely employed in the preparation of cobalt-based alloys. The design should permit molten metal to flow freely within the mold and to avoid differential cooling rates in various parts of the component which might provoke porosity and blow holes. Abrupt changes of shape and sharp corners influence the flow of metal and the homogeneity of the crystal structure. Upon removal of the cast from the mold, X-ray analysis of the implants is necessary to insure homogeneity of the structure. Forged implants usually require a simple shape without protrusions, such as flanges or bosses. While machine-assisted forging permits more complex shapes, it is expensive and consistent only with the production of fairly large numbers of implants.

Machining permits greater variety in design features since the method of fabrication does not significantly influence the material qualities of the product. Necessarily strict tolerances in the specifications and intricacies of shape add to the difficulty and the cost of preparation. Optimal design should minimize these factors.

Production of Plastic Components. Injection molded thermoplastics are widely employed. During the molding process, shrinkage of heavy sections may give rise to internal voids or surface shrink markings that initiate internal stresses and warpage. Unnecessary irregularities should be avoided or where possible, radii and fillets may be employed to equalize the distribution of stresses and to facilitate the molding procedure. Plastic flow is facilitated by smooth corners and surfaces without undercuts. A minute taper, even as small as 1 degree may facilitate removal of the device from the mold. Extrusion of molten plastic at the clearance between part of the mold frequently gives rise to flash lines which may be deleterious from functional and esthetic points of view. Flash lines should be avoided on articular surfaces of joint replacements and other critical surfaces.

MANUFACTURING AND PACKAGING

Some manufacturers of metal implants purchase the raw materials from a primary supplier, while others prepare their own alloys. In recent years many manufacturers of surgical implants have had difficulties in purchasing the small amounts of a high grade alloy that they require. This is not surprising when one considers the minute amounts of material that are employed for surgical implants in contrast to the needs of many other basic industries. When a batch of metal is procured, a certified spectrographic analysis or another document of quality control should certify the composition of the alloy.

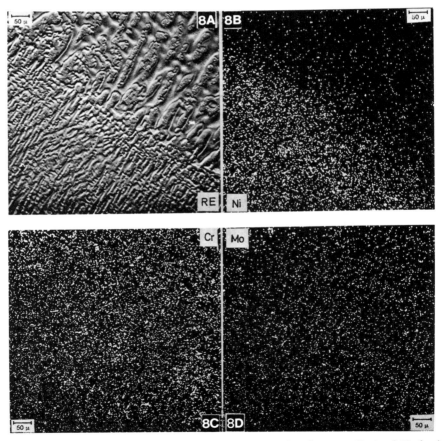

Figure 8-10. A scanning electron micrograph of a welded joint between Protasul-10 forging alloy (Co35Ni35Cr20Mo10) and Protasul-2 casting alloy (Co65Cr30Mo5) reveals an intimate fusion of the alloys at the weld site (×300). *B.-D.* Elemental distribution surfaces analyses of nickel, chromium and molybdenum of the welded zone are shown. In all of the illustrations, Protasul-10 is on the left diagonal half. (Reproduced with permission of M. Semlitsch, Sulzer Bros., Winterthur, Switzerland).

When manufacturers make their own alloys by the preparation of small melts, comparable methods must be undertaken to insure consistent composition. Where implants are cast, each implant must undergo scrutiny, such as X-ray analysis, to insure the absence of internal defects.

Automated techniques of machining are now available whereby extraordinarily stringent tolerances in the dimensions of implants may be maintained. Previously, welding of implants was discouraged in view of the likelihood of cracks or cavities at the weld site and of diminished corrosion resistance at the site of the welded junction.[19] More recently, welding techniques have improved immensely, so that sophisticated processes such as electron beam welding can be recommended.[22] Figure 8-10 is a scanning electron micrograph which shows the microstructure of the welded combination of fine grained forging alloy, Protasul-10 (CoNiCrMo), with the casting alloy, Protasul-2 (CoCrMo). The welded combination is subjected to stress relieving and

homogenation treatment under vacuum. Its microstructure reveals an exceptional degree of fusion between the two cobalt-base alloys. The benefit of welding and allied techniques is that materials of dissimilar mechanical properties can be combined to provide an implant composed of the materials of optimal mechanical properties for each portion of the device.

Surface Finish. The final preparation of many implants includes specific treatment of their surfaces. The removal of metal burrs or other irregularities is essential. Degreasing is necessary if supplementary procedures are to be undertaken. Chemical or electrochemical polishing may be undertaken in oxidizing solutions to provide a regular surface with a thick oxide barrier film. Such a highly polished surface is generally employed on stainless steel and titanium implants, although implants prepared from cobalt-base alloys are usually treated to provide a rough satin-like surface. From a clinical aspect, a highly polished surface inhibits tissue adherence and facilitates removal of the implant, whereas

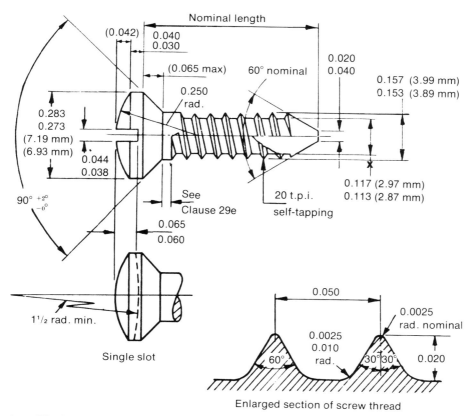

Figure 8-11. The British Standards specification for a 4-mm surgical bone screw is shown. (Reproduced with permission of British Standards Institution, London).

the rougher surface encourages adherence of adjacent tissues.

The American Society for Testing Materials (ASTM)[23] and the British Standards Committee[24] have provided elaborate formulae for the specifications of virtually all presently available surgical implants. The specifications define the materials that may be employed, the dimensions and tolerances of various portions of the implants, the necessary types of surface finishes and the standards for packaging. Figures 8-11 and 8-12 present two typical standard specifications for British implants. Supplementary standards for marking permit electric spark for electrolytic etching or the application of a dye provided that excessive deformation of the surface of the implant does not occur.

The ASTM designation for stainless steel bars and wires states that bars may be furnished in the annealed, or annealed and cold-drawn condition. Wire may be furnished as specified in either annealed, bright-annealed or annealed and cold-drawn condition. Surface finishes may include: pickled, ground, or ground and polished, for bar; and bright-annealed, pickled, ground or ground and polished for wire. Mechanical specifications for the purchased materials are detailed. An implant manufacturer may choose to specify the grain size of stainless steel sheet and strip for use in surgical implants. The steel should be made by electric-arc or electric-induction or other process suitable for manufacture. Vacuum induction or consumable electrode vacuum melting also may be employed. A wide

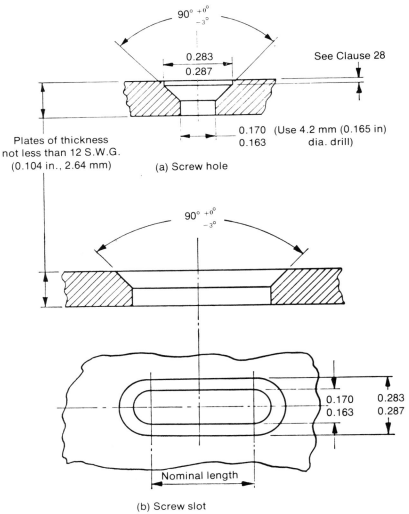

Figure 8-12. The British Standard for holes and slots in bone plates for surgical screws of 4 mm nominal size is shown. (Reproduced with permission of British Standards Institution, London.)

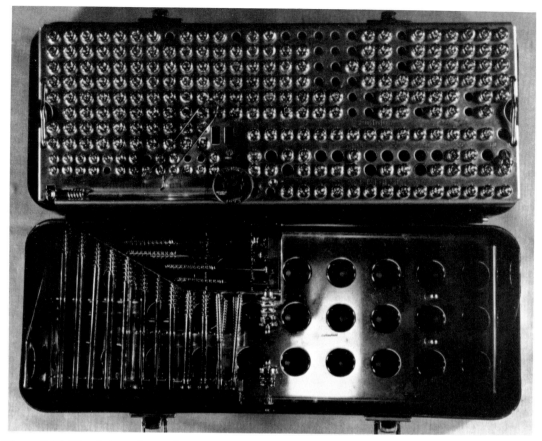

Figure 8-13. The photograph reveals the storage of a variety of AO screws in the special metal box. At surgery, the surgeon may rapidly select the appropriate screws from a wide variety.

range of surface finishes may be purchased, including a range from dull, satin finish to high luster or mirror finish. Tensile, bending and hardness tests should be made on specimens taken from each coil for which recommended specifications are published.

Packaging. Implants manufactured of diverse materials, and those prepared for different applications show widely differing needs for packaging. Implants with articular surfaces, such as total joint replacements, require careful envelopment in separate soft packages that will prevent superficial scratching. Certain other implants such as the spacers and joint replacements manufactured from silicone rubber, require isolation in soft packages for a similar reason. In contrast, most metallic implants used for fixation of fractures may be housed in larger metal containers that may include a whole set of fixation apparatus, such as a series of screws, plates or intramedullary nails. An example is shown in Figure 8-13. In the latter examples,

there is no evidence that individual packaging (Fig. 8-14*A*) provides superior resistance to metallic failure *in vivo*. The surgeon is greatly facilitated at the time of the operation if he has a complete range of screws of assorted lengths and thread patterns from which he can make a rapid selection. The principal problem is a method of display which enables the operating room or scrub nurses and surgeons to see virtually all of the implants for a rapid selection process. Also, a proper display expedites the replacement of particular items after they have been used in previous operations. Recently, manufacturers such as the former Samson Corporation* have provided metallic boxes lined with an impervious plastic coating. This is an excellent technique provided that exceptionally tough and adherent coatings are available. It

---

* At present, a division of 3-M Company, 3-M Center, St. Paul, Minn.

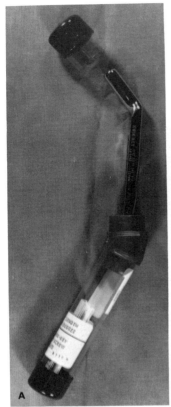
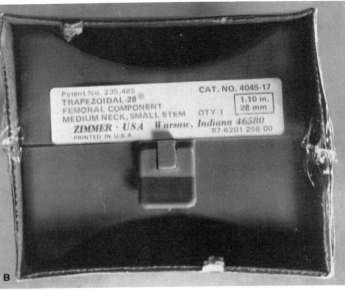

Figure 8-14. *A.* The photograph shows part of a hip screw in a separate plastic container. *B.* The femoral stem of a total hip joint replacement is stored in a protective plastic container with a cellophane wrapper.

permits the box to be color coded in different portions to assist in rapid identification of individual components.

Storage of Implants. Many of the total joint replacements and silicone rubber implants must be stored in the package provided by the manufacturer (Fig. 8-14*B*). Usually, the instructions for recommended method of storage are printed in bold letters on the wrapper. Once the wrapper on the package has been opened, as in the case of high density polyethylene acetabular components, the presterilized implant must be used immediately or discarded. Alternatively, many metallic implants such as the simulated models of total joint replacements can be stored in cloth holders that hold a full range of implants of various sizes. Two examples are shown in Figure 8-15. The implants can be packed by the operating room staff and autoclaved in the suitable wrapping. Each implant is protected from contact with another device and its size can be specified on the cloth wrapper. For the various

sets of internal fixation apparatus such as screws, nails or plates, storage in a metal box is virtually essential so that the screws provided by one manufacturer are not confused with those provided by another. As previously mentioned, a full complement of screws is necessary to facilitate the surgeon during the operating procedure. During the operation, such sets should be handled only by the scrub nurse with clean gloves so that the unused implants are not soiled by the surgeon.

Once an implant has been used, it should be discarded. If certain costly devices such as the metallic components of total joint replacements are inadvertently placed on the operative field but not used in view of incorrect size or other problems, they may be returned to the manufacturer who can repeat the surface finishing technique and undertake appropriate methods of analysis to insure that the implant can be safely resterilized and repackaged for subsequent application.

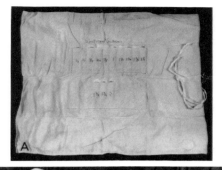

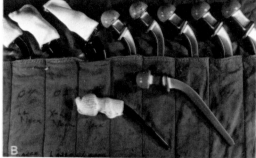

Figure 8-15. *A* and *B*. Implants stored in cloth holders permit the individual protection of each implant but the rapid availability of several sizes of the device. *A*. The redundant superior and inferior portions of the wrapper permit complete protection of the implants. *B*. A series of trial and implantable femoral stems are shown in assorted sizes. The highly polished articular surfaces of the implantable models are covered with a supplementary cloth wrapper.

Methods of Handling Implants at Surgery

In the predecessor of this book,[25] great emphasis was placed on the need to handle metallic implants with rubber shod tools so that the implant would neither be scratched nor subjected to the possibility of metallic transfer from the tool to the implant.[25] In the past 20 years, metallic transfer has failed to emerge as a clinical problem. Similarly, the superficial scratches frequently observed on the surfaces of implants (Fig. 8-7), have not been implicated as initiators of clinical failures. It would appear that implants can be handled safely by the application of the surgeon's gloved hands or by the appropriate surgical tools, such as screwdrivers and forceps. The AO screw set is supplied with a small pair of metallic forceps (Fig. 8-13) that are designed to handle the screws. The author has encountered no deleterious side-effects from this practice. Further recommendations in regard to the handling of fixation devices and of reconstruc-

tive implants are given in Chapters 10 and 14, respectively.

Sterilization of Surgical Tools and Implants. Prior to application, surgical implants must be rendered free of bacteria or other potentially pathogenic organisms including their spores. Sterilization refers to the physical or chemical destruction of micro-organisms, including those in the sporing state. Disinfection refers solely to the destruction of bacteria in the vegetative state, and usually implies the use of chemical agents.[26] Spores consist of resistant, dormant forms of bacteria which are generally produced under adverse conditions. Spores multiply and grow within bacteria until the bacteria disappear to leave the sessile spores. When environmental conditions subside to a less adverse state, the spores reproduce the original form of bacteria, which is called the vegetative state. Spores possess a much greater resistance to adverse environmental conditions than the vegetative form, and are therefore, more difficult to irradicate.

Sterilization of implantable materials may be undertaken by the application of moist heat, dry heat, radiation or chemical agents. When applied appropriately, all of these methods provide effective bactericidal conditions, although any of them may be unsuitable for application with certain materials which are damaged by a particular agent.

Steam Sterilization. The most widely employed process of sterilization is by the application of moist heat. Under moist conditions, the thermal denaturation of the bacterial proteins readily transpires.

Steam sterilization can be achieved at lower temperatures and shorter periods of exposure than with the application of dry heat. Moist heat sterilization is conventionally performed in an autoclave where steam is generated under pressure. The Medical Research Council of the United Kingdom has published recommendations for routine procedures of steam sterilization.[27] A widely employed regime is the use of a pressure of 15 lb./inch^2 when the steam is produced at 120°C. Exposure for 15 minutes at this temperature kills all but the most heat-resistant spores. Further elevation of pressure results in higher temperatures and more efficient sterilization. Other representative temperatures and pressures of sterilization are 126°C at 20 lb./inch^2 for 10 minutes and 135°C at 30 lb./inch^2 for 3 minutes. Steam sterilization is effective only if the steam reaches all parts of the article under treatment. For this to happen, air must be removed from all the surfaces with which steam has to come in contact. Temperatures of air and steam mixtures are lower than those of steam by itself. If the air is not removed, residual air tends to form an insulating film which delays heat transfer. In the current designs for autoclaves, arrangements for proper removal of air are of paramount importance. The design and use of autoclaves is fully discussed by Williams et al.[27]

Dry Heat. Dry heat also may be employed for sterilization which initiates thermal oxidation of the bacteria. The temperatures involved vary from 160°C to 190°C. The Medical Research Council recommends 45 minutes duration at 160°C, 18 minutes at 170°C, 7.5 minutes at 180°C or 1.5 minutes at 190°C for effective sterilization.[27]

Ionizing Radiation. Sterilization can be achieved by the use of particulate high energy electrons produced from a linear accelerator or from γ-rays emitted from a radioactive element, usually cobalt-60. γ-Rays are uncharged and resemble short wavelength X-rays.[28] They possess much greater penetrative ability than electron radiation. Ionizing radiation achieves sterilization either by the direct action of the radiation on the nucleic acids of the bacteria, especially deoxyribonucleic acid (DNA) or by the interaction between the radiation and the constituent molecule of the bacteria which liberates various free radicals and molecules which themselves initiate the actions in the nucleic acids.[29] With the techniques in current use there is no risk that sterilized articles will be radioactive. The articles may, however, show deterioration, such as discoloration or loss of tensile strength. Radiation offers safe sterilization for vast numbers of articles such as plastic devices which would be damaged by heat. In view of their size, expense and need for skilled manipulation, radiation plants are generally associated with large commercial enterprises rather than hospitals. It is a particularly useful method of sterilization for disposable articles. The radiation dosage necessary for sterilization is generally accepted as 2.5 Mrads, where 1 Mrad is the dosage corresponding to the absorption of energy of magnitude 10^{-2} J/kg of the material irradiated.[30] In certain unusual cases, however, bacteria may require lethal doses up to 6 Mrads. While γ-rays have greater penetrating capacity than electrons and can be generated with lower energies, both types of radiation are otherwise equally effective.

Chemical Agents. Numerous antibacterial chemical agents have been studied and employed for various applications, although the sterilization achieved by chemicals is a much more complex subject than sterilization by heat. A full account of the various chemical agents available for sterilization is provided by Williams et al.[27] The most common chemical sterilants are formaldehyde and ethylene oxide. Formaldehyde is particularly effective in destroying all forms of microbial life, including spores, although it may require from 2 to 24 hours of exposure. It possesses an exceptionally limited penetrating power since the gas condenses on specific areas. Humidity, therefore, is an important controlling factor. The penetration capacity may be improved by the use of formaldehyde in conjunction with steam generated at low temperatures (60 to 80°C) within a partial vacuum. Its main objection to use is its irritating vapor, which is both unpleasant and likely to induce a cutaneous sensitization.

The gaseous disinfectant, ethylene oxide, possesses certain advantages over formaldehyde, particularly in its ability to adhere to surfaces and to destroy all micro-organisms, including spores. Unfortunately, it forms explosive mixtures with air, is inflammable and toxic to man. While it possesses excellent penetrating power, the gas is retained by certain materials such as silicone rubber and released at later stages. In view of its toxicity to man, ethylene oxide is substantially compromised for application with surgical implants that show a subsequent slow release of the agent. Other chemical sterilants, including ozone, propylene oxide, and β-propriolactone are fully reviewed elsewhere.[26, 27]

The conventional form of sterilization is by the use of pressurized steam in an autoclave. Where materials are affected by moist heat, dry heat may be preferred. If the material has inferior thermal properties, radiation sterilization should be considered. If the material is damaged by radiation, or if the appropriate facilities are unavailable, chemical methods such as ethylene oxide or formaldehyde may have to be employed.

In view of the effects of a variety of methods of sterilization on medical plastics which do not occur with metallic implants, a brief description of these techniques is given which summarizes a recent article by Plester.[31] Of the commonly employed medical plastics, only polytetrafluoroethylene and silicone rubber can be sterilized by the use of dry heat in the accepted range of 160°C to 190°C. At this range of temperature, polypropylene and polyethylene would undergo softening or deformation while nylon 66 would undergo oxidation. At the range of temperature involved in steam sterilization, 120°C to 134°C, polypropylene can be autoclaved safely. Polyethylene, however, continues to undergo softening or deformation while molded polyvinylchloride suffers from creep or distortion under the influence of residual stresses within the material. Polyacetals undergo distortion due to water absorption.

γ-Radiation can be employed safely for sterilization of polyethylene, polystyrene, nylon and polyvinylchloride as well as thermosetting resins. Other polymers such as polypropylene may suffer radiation damage in the dose range normally employed for sterilization. Such plastics undergo cross-linkage with radiation after which they show a slight improvement in tensile and shear strengths and elastic moduli but a substantial drop in impact strength and ductility so that they become brittle. Other polymers such as polytetrafluoroethylene undergo chain scission with a concomitant loss of most mechanical properties.

Chemical sterilants are widely employed to prepare polymers. The major problems associated with chemical sterilants are the concentrations of the agents required to produce effective sterilization and the removal of all traces of the chemicals prior to implantation to avoid deleterious tissue reactions. Occasionally, the chemical sterilants such as ethylene oxide may react chemically with polymers such as polyurethane and polyesters. This problem does not appear to arise with polymers currently employed in orthopædic implants.

CLEAN AIR AND THE OPERATING ROOM

One of the principal concerns in all applications of surgical implants is the risk of postoperative wound infection. Particularly for reconstructive procedures such as total joint replacements, postoperative wound infection represents one of the greatest catastrophies which almost inevitably necessitates subsequent removal of the implant and culminates in surgical failure. More than any other single individual, Charnley[32] rekindled interest in the need for rigorous asepsis in the operating room. In the past 20 years, great thought has been given to the optimal design of the operating room suite and the particular portion of the operating room that houses the patient and the surgical staff. These two aspects of the operating room are discussed below.

The Medical Research Council of the United Kingdom has published guidelines for the basic requirements to control infection in operating rooms.[33] They make six recommendations:

1. The operating suite should be independent of the general traffic and air movement in the rest of the hospital.

2. The rooms of the suite should be arranged so that there is a continuous progression from the entrance of the suite, through zones that increasingly approach sterility, to the operating and sterilizing rooms.

3. People working within the suite should be able to move from one "clean" area to another without having to pass through unprotected or general traffic areas. After the surgeon has changed into his operating suit, he should be able to move into the scrub room without passing through the entrance lobby.

4. It should be possible to remove dirty materials from the suite without passing through a clean area.

5. The directions of air-flow within the suite should always be from the cleaner to the less clean areas.

6. The heating and ventilating system should insure safe and comfortable climatic conditions for the patient, surgeons and staff.

Previously, operating rooms in large hospitals were situated close to the wards which they served. Often they were dispersed throughout the hospital so that each floor or region of the hospital had its own suite. More recently, most operating suites have been centralized to provide simplification of the administration, staffing, discipline, supplies, disposal, cleansing and maintenance. While the centralization has so many advantages that it is almost inevitable, it appears to have one great liability. Grossly contaminated wounds are treated surgically in the same region of the hospital where procedures requiring great precautionary measures, such as total joint replacement, will be undertaken. As Duthie and his staff* at the Nuffield Orthopaedic Centre in Oxford have recommended and practiced, grossly contaminated procedures are best performed in a separate operating room which is wholly isolated from the principal operating room as well as from the postoperative recovery rooms and from the wards. At the Nuffield Orthopaedic Centre, a "one way traffic flow" concept has been put into practice, whereby all of the patients for routine admission, other than

---

* R. B. Duthie, personal communication, 1977.

those with open wounds or chronic infections, are admitted to a specific admitting ward. Immediately prior to surgery, they are taken into an annex adjacent to the operating room suite where their preoperative surgical gown is replaced by a clean garment. The nurses and other ancillary staff from the admitting ward are not allowed beyond this barrier. The patient is taken from the annex into the operating room suite by attendants who work solely within that complex. After surgery, they are taken to a postoperative recovery room and subsequently transferred to another annex. The operating room personnel are not allowed beyond the second annex. Nurses and attendants from separate postoperative wards collect the patient and take him to one of the series of wards that are remote from the admitting ward so that there is minimal risk of cross-contamination between preoperative and postoperative patients. Patients with known infections are admitted through a separate ward and undergo surgery in a wholly separate operating room. Afterwards, they are managed in a ward that is distant from the "clean" wards. While a statistical survey of infection rates is still under way, the early data suggests that this system is an effective method to limit rates of infection. It is self-evident, however, that this system would be difficult to incorporate into many existing hospitals. Nevertheless, existing facilities could make substantial improvements in their attempt to limit the opportunities for cross-contamination between clean and infected patients which are well described by Williams *et al.*[33]

Clean Air. By 1966, Charnley[32] had defined the various ways in which the opportunities for contamination of wounds at surgery could be diminished. The previous concept of cleansing air in an operating room to eradicate bacteria was to install a high quality "plenum" ventilation system which raised the number of air changes per hour to 2 or 3 times. The air was passed through filters to remove particles of any size. In fact, the air-born particles which are most likely to contaminate a wound are those which are sufficiently heavy to settle in less than an hour. Dust particles of this type are usually greater than 10 μm in size and they may carry clusters of organisms. Particles as small as 1 μm, the size of a bacteria or a spore, remain suspended in the air by "Brownian" motion. It is not entirely clear whether bacteria are ever really suspended in the air without being carried on particles of dust. Charnley reasoned that the installation and running costs in an air filtration

unit for a surgical operating room could be minimized without sacrificing efficiency by filtration of the air to particle sizes no smaller than 1 μm.

Charnley[32] also became concerned about the source of the dust particles which carry bacteria within the operating room during the course of an operation. Most infected dust particles represent epithelial scales shed from the skin of the whole surface of the bodies of the personnel in the operating room, and they do not originate merely from exposed parts such as the face or the nasopharynx. The generation of infected dust inside a conventional operating room is not controlled by its ventilating system. It is self-evident that the greater the number of persons in the operating room, the greater the rate of emission of infected particles. Charnley assumed that the number of infected particles in the air around the patient's wound could be minimized if the surgical personnel in direct relation to the operating room were isolated from the ancillary staff such as the anesthesiologist and observers. The surgical team in direct relation to an open wound is rarely more than four persons. The rest of the ancillary personnel in the operating room can be outside the ultraclean zone. The rate of emission of clean air to the clean air enclosure is augmented to yield a positive movement of air in a predetermined direction when the same amount of air admitted in an open operating room would not influence the normal turbulence from thermal convection. Charnley hoped to realize "laminar" air flow from the ceiling to, or even through, the floor. This objective is thwarted by the turbulence that is generated at air speeds over 80 feet per minute when the air flow strikes irregular surfaces, such as the bodies of the surgical teams and the patients. The higher the speed of air flow, the more dangerous does turbulence become by abetting the entrapment of dust particles with the possibility for their forceful injection into the open wound. Fast air streams also may provoke excessive cooling of the wound by evaporation and desiccation of moist tissue. To further reduce the numbers of contaminated dust particles, Charnley[34] conceived of the idea of elaborate operating gowns with helmets so that a vacuum could be used to extract expired air and dust particles from within the operating gowns. With this supplementary procedure, it became possible to economize in the number of air changes per hour and to enhance the effect of existing air changes. While the special gowns with helmet provide a substantial source of heat retention, the vacuum extraction within the

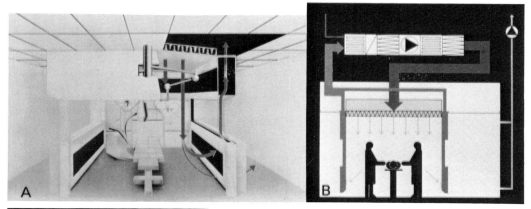

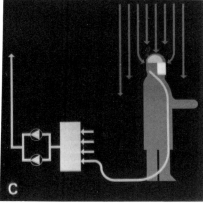

Figure 8-16. *A, B,* and *C.* Figures *A* and *B* show schematic diagrams of a clean air cabin with a vertical air supply. The *arrows* denote the direction of air flow through the clean air cabin. *C.* A protective clothing system for the operating staff is shown. The sterile clothing consists of a hood with a transparent visor and an overcoat. A quantity of air several times greater than that exhaled by the staff member is extracted from inside the helmet through an outlet tube. The air is extracted by means of an exhaust pump. A replacement of air is permitted by slots in the anterior of the helmet. (Reproduced with permission of ALLO PRO AG, Baar/Zug, Switzerland).

gowns provides a method to improve the exchange. The temperature within the operating room is maintained at 65°F, which is 10° lower than customary in operating rooms. The rapid circulation of 65° air through the total investing helmets and gowns provides a comfortable ambient temperature for the surgeons. Charnley's operating room enclosure and gowns are described in detail elsewhere.[34] Figure 8-16 shows pictures of a similar commercially available system.

At the time these special operating room enclosures were introduced at Wrightington by Charnley,[34] other changes in sterile techniques were being made. While a substantial diminution in infection rate was observed, the statistical analysis did not permit a ready distinction of the principal factor responsible for the improvement. Charnley feels that the principal contribution was provided by the clean air and allied techniques. Other workers,[35] however, have questioned the value of the highly expensive clean air enclosure with unidirectional air flow. There is no doubt that clean air flow has im-

mense theoretical and practical attractions. It provides an absolute barrier whereby nonparticipants of surgical procedures may be close at hand without providing any remote possible source of contamination. Discipline among the surgical team is spontaneously improved for a similar reason. As Nelson[36] has emphasized, it cannot be harmful to eliminate all possible sources of bacterial contamination. On the other hand, the system is immensely expensive and the gowns, particularly with the helmets, are found to be unpleasant to wear by many surgeons. An electronic communication system is needed so that the operative team may communicate. To date, statistical studies have not been able to confirm the benefit of routine application of clean air flow systems. Perhaps the largest ongoing study is underway in England under the auspices of the Medical Research Council where numerous hospitals are involved in a double-blind survey. Preliminary results made available to the author have failed to show a statistically significant improvement in infection rate in the operations performed under

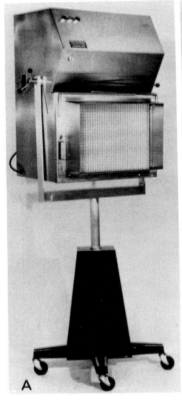

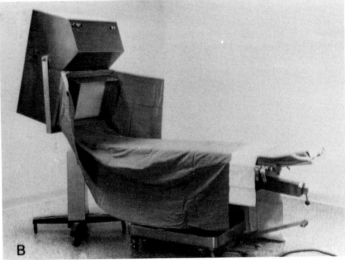

Figure 8-17. *A* and *B*. A portable air filtration unit for use in hospital operating rooms is shown. A source of locally directed clean air is provided by a unit seen in *A* which is conventionally placed at the end of the operating table, near the patient's feet *B*. (Reproduced with permission of W. E. Anspach, Jr., and M. Bakels.[42])

clean air conditions.* Again, interested readers are referred to several other discussions to enhance their knowledge.[35, 37-40]

A somewhat less expensive form of clean air technique has been the local air blanket protection of surgical wounds during operative procedures.[41, 42] A source of laminar flow bacteria-free air is placed close to the wound to direct an intense flow of clean air across the surgical wound. The air is passed through a prefilter to remove large particles of lint and dust, after which it is forced through a finer filter which removes 99.9% of all particles, 0.3 μm in diameter and larger. The exhausted air flows with a smooth stream line or laminar flow profile, having a Reynolds number less than 2000. A cubicle unit with a maximum design capacity of 2000 cubic feet per minute is shown in Figure 8-17. In an average operating room the air theoretically could be filtered in 1 minute, although actually, part of the air would be recirculating so that the probability would be that in a 2000-cubic-foot

operating room, 50% would have passed through the operating room in 1 minute and 90% would have been exchanged in approximately 10 minutes. Studies by Ansbach and Bakels[42] suggest that the provision of true laminar flow across the room is an effective barrier to prevent particles dropping into or reaching the wound. Particulate matter generated by the surgical team is entrapped in the flow and may be deposited on the open instrument tables unless special protective measures are undertaken. Their studies indicate that this much less expensive system may be nearly as effective as the much more elaborate clean air system.

Nevertheless, it should be emphasized that clean air systems have yet to show statistically valid results that confirm conclusively the superiority of these methods to provide a significant decrease in the rates of postoperative wound infections. A variety of other methods to reduce intraoperative contamination of wounds are under consideration such as the use of ultraviolet light[43] and antibiotic chemotherapy.[44, 45] These are reviewed in Chapter 13.

---

* R. B. Duthie, personal communication, 1977.

SUMMARY

In summary, optimal implant design demands a detailed knowledge of the anticipated function of the device in man, a precise characterization of the mechanical environment *in vivo*, assessment of the mechanical properties of available materials and awareness of the principles of mechanical design. Standards specifications are available which outline acceptable methods of procurement of raw materials, manufacturing techniques, labeling and packaging of implants. Procedures for the storage of implants vary with the functions of the devices and the nature of the implantable material. Certain reconstructive implants require careful protection of fragile surfaces while others, such as screws and plates for internal fixation of fractures, should be stored in a rigid sterilizable container which permits the display of numerous complementary devices of various sizes and shapes to facilitate the selection process at surgery. Several techniques of sterilization are available to prepare the many implantable materials despite the limited tolerance of many materials to heat, steam, chemical agents or radiation. With the renewed interest in rigorous aseptic surgical techniques, diverse methods to limit bacterial contamination of open wounds at surgery have been studied including the design of the operating room, unidirectional traffic flow, clean air techniques, ultraviolet light and antibiotics. While marked improvements in postoperative wound infection rates have been realized, the relative contributions provided by each of the supplementary methods remain unclear.

REFERENCES

1. Mow, J. C., and Mansour, J. M. *J. Biomech.*, 10:31, 1977.
2. Jurist, J. M., and Foltz, A. S. *J. Biomech.*, 10:455, 1977.
3. Berme, N., Mengi, Y., and Inger, E. *J. Biomech.*, 10:643, 1977.
4. Klawitter, J. J., Weinstein, A. M., Hulbert, S. F., and Sauer, B. W. Tissue ingrowth and mechanical locking for anchorage of prostheses in the locomotor system. In *Artificial Hip and Knee Joint Technology,* p. 422, (edited by M. Schaldach and D. Hohmann, Springer-Verlag, Berlin, 1976.
5. Fernie, G. R., Kostuik, J., Lobb, R. J., Pilliar, R. M., Wong, E., and Binnington, A. G. *J. Biomed. Mater. Res.*, 11:883, 1977.
6. Williams, D. F., and Roaf, R. *Implants in Surgery*, p. 364, W. B. Saunders Co., London, 1973.
7. Minns, R. J., Bremble, G. R., and Campbell, J. *J. Biomech.*, 10:569, 1977.
8. Williams, D. F., and Roaf, R. *Implants in Surgery*, p. 370, W. B. Saunders, Co., London, 1973.
9. Williams, D. F., and Roaf, R. *Implants in Surgery*, p. 371, W. B. Saunders Co., London, 1973.
10. Williams, D. F., and Roaf, R. *Implants in Surgery*, p. 373, W. B. Saunders Co., London, 1973.
11. Williams, D. F., and Roaf, R. *Implants in Surgery*, p. 374, W. B. Saunders Co., London, 1973.
12. Hench, L. L. *Ann. Rev. Mater. Sci.*, 5:279, 1975.
13. Semlitsch, M., Lehmann, M., Weber, H., Doerre, E., and Willert, H. G. *J. Biomed. Mater. Res.*, 11:537, 1977.
14. Hulbert, S. F., and Klawitter, J. J. Ceramics for artificial joints. In *Advances in Artificial Hip and Knee Joint Technology*, p. 287, edited by M. Schaldach and D. Hohmann, Springer-Verlag, Berlin, 1976.
15. Lemons, J. E. *J. Biomed. Mater. Res.*, 9:9, 1975.
16. Ruiz, C., and Koenigsberger, F. *Designs for Strength and Production*, p. 31, Macmillan Co., London, 1970.
17. Ruiz, C., and Koenigsberger, F. *Designs for Strength and Production*, Macmillan Co., London, 1970.
18. Redford, G. D. *Mechanical Engineering Design*, p. 42, Macmillan Co., London, 1966.
19. Bechtol, C. O., Ferguson, A. B., Jr., and Laing, P. G. *Metals and Engineering in Bone and Joint Surgery*, p. 96, Williams and Wilkins Co., Baltimore, 1959.
20. Mears D. C. *J. Biomed. Mater. Res.*, 6:133, 1975.
21. Levine, D. L., and Staehle, R. W. *J. Biomed. Mater. Res.*, 11:553, 1977.
22. Semlitsch, M. *Reconstr. Surg. Traumat.*, 15:82, 1976.
23. Annual Book of ASTM Standards, Part. 46, p. 387, ASTM, Philadelphia, 1975.
24. British Standard 3531: 1962 and 1968, *Specification for Metal Implants and Tools Used for Bone Surgery*, p. 2. British Standards Institution, London, 1968.
25. Bechtol, C. O., Ferguson, A. B., Jr., and Laing, P. G. *Metals and Engineering in Bone and Joint Surgery*, p. 77, Williams & Wilkins, Baltimore, 1959.
26. Lawrence, C. A., and Block, S. C. S. *Disinfection, Sterilization and Preservation*, p. 17, Lea & Febiger, Philadelphia, 1968.
27. Williams, R. E. O., Blowers, R., Garrod, L. P., and Shooter, R. A. *Hospital Infection*, p. 291, Lloyd-Luke, London, 1966.
28. McLaughlin, W. L., and Holm, N. W. Physical characteristics of ionizing radiation. In *Manual of Radiation Sterilization of Medical and Biological Materials*, p. 5, International Atomic Energy Agency, Vienna, 1973.
29. Ley, F. J. The effect of ionizing radiation on Bacteria. In *Manual of Radiation Sterilization of Medical and Biological Materials*, p. 37, International Atomic Energy Agency, Vienna, 1973.
30. Holm, N. W. Dosimetry. In *Manual of Radiation Sterilization of Medical and Biological Materials*, p. 99, International Atomic Energy Agency, Vienna, 1973.
31. Plester, D. W. *Bio-Medical Eng.*, 5:443, 1970.
32. Charnley, J. *Cleveland Clin. Quartr.*, 40:99, 1973.
33. Williams, R. E. O., Blowers, R., Garrod, L. P., and

Shooter, R. A. *Hospital Infection*, p. 197, Lloyd-Luke, London, 1966.

34. Charnley, J. *Clin. Orthop.*, 87: 167, 1972.
35. Dixon, R. E. *Cleveland Clin. Quartr.*, *40*:115, 1973.
36. Nelson, J. P. *Instructional Course Lectures, A.A.O.S.*, *26*:52, 1977.
37. Nelson, C. L. *Ortho. Clin. N. Am.*, *4*:2, 533, 1973.
38. Nelson, C. L. *Contemp Surg.*, *6*:44, 1975.
39. Amstutz, H. C. *Cleveland Clin. Quartr.*, *40*:125, 1973.
40. Anspach, W. E. *Instructional Course Lectures, A.A.O.S.*, *26*:47, 1977.
41. Nelson, J. P., Glassburn, A. R., Talbott, R. D., and McElhinney, J. P. *Cleveland Clin. Quartr.*, *40*:191, 1973.
42. Anspach, W. E., and Bakels, M. *Cleveland Clin. Quartr.*, *40*:229, 1973.
43. Lowell, J. D., Kundsin, R. B. *Instructional Course Lectures, A.A.O.S.*, *26*:58, 1977.
44. Bowers, W. H. *Instructional Course Lectures, A.A.O.S.*, *26*:30, 1977.
45. Hill, J., Klenerman, L. Trustey, S., and Blowers, R. *J. Bone Jt. Surg.*, *59B*:197, 1977.

9.

Fractures and Methods of Internal Fixation

Until the development of X-ray, aseptic surgery and general anesthetics, the management of fractures in a systematic fashion was impossible. Previously, surgeons made a diagnosis of a fracture or dislocation by the use of inaccurate clinical evaluation and their knowledge of anatomy. Open methods of fracture treatment, then, were associated with intolerable and uncontrollable pain and wound infections.

The chronology of innovations leading to the modern method of fracture treatment began with the introduction of general anesthetics in 1846. Then, in 1867, Lister introduced antiseptic surgery and subsequently its offspring, aseptic technique. Concurrently, the plaster of Paris bandage, as first described by Mathysen in 1852[1] gained popularity for immobilization of fractures. The first widespread use of this technique appears to have been by Pirogoff[2] in 1854 during the Crimean War.

In 1870, during the Franco-Prussian War, Louis Ollier, the French orthopaedic surgeon, introduced the technique of complete immobilization of fractured limbs in a plaster of Paris cast.

In 1895, the discovery of X-rays was announced by Roentgen and in February 1896, the first clinical diagnostic application of X-rays was performed.

The discovery of antiseptic surgery, anesthetics and X-rays opened the way for the sound management of closed and simple fractures. It was not until 1935, however, when corrosion resistant surgical alloys were introduced, that surgeons possessed adequate materials to be able to manage complex fractures, such as the femoral neck, and displaced interarticular fractures.

Subsequently, numerous surgeons have introduced novel implants for clinical application on various diverse fractures. Concurrently, other workers attempted to improve the closed methods of fracture treatment with casts, braces and cast-braces. Still other surgeons focused attention on external fixation devices which immobi-

lized fracture fragments with stainless steel percutaneous pins.

With the enormous volume of publications presently available on the management of fractures, the clinical practitioner of orthopaedic surgery frequently is puzzled by conflicting reports on the relative merits of closed or operative treatment for a particular fracture. The authors of some reference textbooks on fracture treatment have distorted the relative merits of open or closed treatment by a simplistic approach. Such authors generally recommend closed or open treatment for all classifications of fractures unless their favored method is specifically contraindicated on a particular injury by established practice. Most of the English or American authors generally favored the use of closed methods.[3] In 1969, a Swiss group, known as AO* or ASIF†, published its recommendations on methods for the internal fixation of fractures.[4] They attempted to provide a systematic outline for open fracture treatment wherein the specific indications and the optimal methods of application for screws, plates, wires and nails were described. Many of the implants were redesigned and improved by their advocates. The AO group advertized its manual as a compendium of the optimal methods for open treatment for use by a surgeon who has previously elected to undertake open reduction and internal fixation. It is unfortunate that these recommendations have been misinterpreted by many workers as a general recommendation to operate on most all fractures.

At present, orthopaedic surgeons possess three methods for the treatment of fractures: (1) with a cast or cast-brace; (2) open methods with a wide variety of implants; and (3) with transfixing pins and external fixation (Fig. 9-1). Some fractures clearly respond best to only one of

---

* Arbeitsgemeinschaft für Osteosynthesefragen.

† (Swiss) Association for the Study of Internal Fixation.

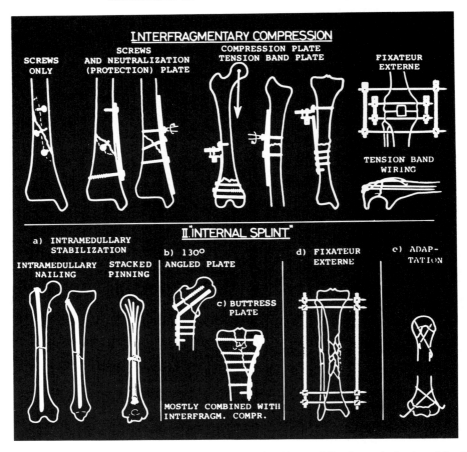

Figure 9-1. A schematic diagram shows the various methods of internal fixation and of external fixation with percutaneous transfixing pins. (Reproduced with permission of Dr. H. Willenegger.)

these approaches. In other cases two or more of the methods should be considered equally to supplement one another (Fig. 9-2). For the treatment of still other fractures a surgeon may be advised to combine two or more approaches. A thorough background in all three methods of treatment gives a surgeon the training necessary to manage satisfactorily an enormous variety of fracture problems, including closed pediatric and geriatric fractures of long bones, interarticular fractures, open, comminuted and infected fractures, pelvic fractures and complex 3-plane corrective osteotomies. In all of these cases the goal of treatment remains total or optimal restoration of function of the limb.

The next four chapters describe the various approaches in the management of fractures and osteotomies. Chapter 9 provides a background for the use of internal fixation while Chapter 10 discusses clinical methods of internal fixation for specific fracture problems. In Chapter 11 the use

of external fixation, especially for the stabilization of open or infected fractures and joints is presented. The special considerations of stabilization of the spine are discussed in Chapter 12.

CLASSIFICATION OF FRACTURES

A fracture may be one complete break in the continuity of a bone, many breaks or an incomplete break or crack. Fractures may be subdivided into 3 broad groups: (1) fractures caused solely by the application of overwhelming mechanical forces which provoke sudden injury; (2) fatigue or stress fractures; and (3) pathological fractures.

Fractures Caused Solely by Violent Trauma

Fractures caused by trauma constitute the overwhelming majority so that the term, "fracture", if unqualified, usually refers to this type

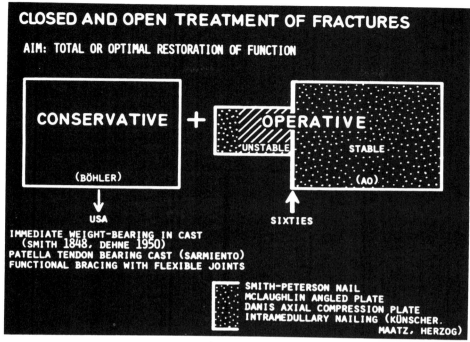

Figure 9-2. The relationships between conservative, or closed, and operative, or open, methods of treatment are shown with the workers who developed the principal methods. (Reproduced with permission of Dr. H. Willenegger.)

of injury. A fracture may be caused by direct violence, as when a phalanx is fractured by a heavy weight dropped on a toe. Other traumatic fractures may be caused by indirect forces transmitted along the body, as when a clavicle is fractured in a fall on the outstretched hand.

A fracture is termed "closed" or simple when there is no communication between the site of the fracture and the exterior of the body (Fig. 9-3A). A fracture is called "open" or compound when there is a wound on the surface of the skin that extends to the site of the fracture and thereby provides a pathway for infection of bone (Fig. 9-3B). Cutaneous lacerations or abrasions may be present superficially to a fracture although they do not necessarily communicate with it. These injuries do not constitute an open fracture. The liability of infection after an open fracture or after surgical intervention on a closed fracture has an important bearing on the clinical management of the fracture.

Patterns of Fracture

Fractures are often designated by descriptive terms which denote the shape or pattern of the fracture surfaces (Fig. 9-3C). The following terms are in general use: transverse fractures; oblique fractures; spiral fractures; comminuted fractures with two or more fragments; compression or crush fractures; and greenstick fractures with incomplete breaks as observed in the resilient bones of children. Impacted fractures are those in which the bone fragments are driven firmly together; they become interlocked with an inhibition of motion between them.

The patterns of fractures are of great practical interest to the surgeon. They may indicate the nature of the causative violence and may provide insight to the simplest method of treatment. For instance, a transverse fracture through a long bone is usually caused by lateral bending or angulatory force, while a spiral fracture is caused by a torsional stress.

The patterns of fractures observed in a single X-ray of a portion of a bone may indicate to the surgeon a likelihood of other injuries which are not made visible by the X-ray. For example, a spiral fracture of the distal tibia, observed on an X-ray of the ankle joint, may be accompanied by a similar fracture of the proximal fibula. (In Fig. 9-4. a schematic diagram of a skeleton indicates the accepted names of bones and joints.)

The patterns of fractures may indicate the likely stability of the fragments after reduction.

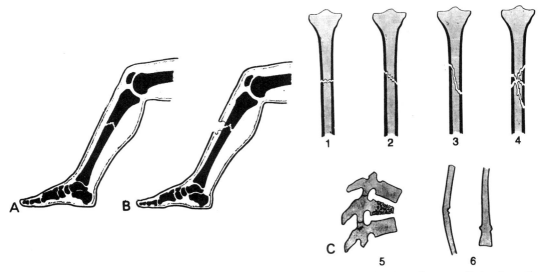

Figure 9-3. *A.* A diagram of a closed fracture. *B.* A schematic diagram of an open fracture. *C.* A schematic diagram illustrates the various fracture types including transverse, oblique, spiral, comminuted, compression, greenstick and impacted. (*A–C,* reproduced with permission of J. C. Adams.[5])

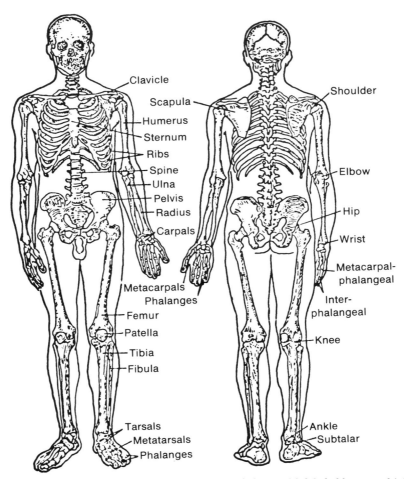

Figure 9-4. A schematic diagram shows the human skeleton with labeled bones and joints.

Thus a transverse fracture is less likely to become redisplaced after reduction, whereas an oblique or spiral fracture is prone to redisplacement unless projecting spikes of bone can be locked into notches in the opposing surface (Fig.

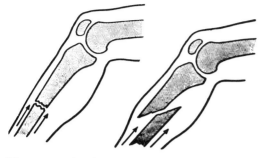

Figure 9-5. A schematic diagram illustrates the inherent stability of a transverse fracture and the instability of an oblique fracture. (Reproduced with permission of J. C. Adams.[5])

9-5). A compression fracture does not generally permit anatomical reduction because the spongy bone substance is crushed, with diminution of the volume of the segment of bone involved so that the segment cannot be restored fully to its original trabecular form.

Fatigue Fractures

Fatigue or stress fractures occur by the application of repetitive small stresses to bone so that any single stress is inadequate to provoke mechanical failure.[6] Stress fractures are observed primarily in the lower extremities of young adults who undertake prolonged vigorous activity such as is encountered in marathon runners, army recruits in basic training camps, and more recently, the enthusiastic suburban joggers who pound the city streets for several miles each day (Fig. 9-6). While the mechanisms of initiation and propagation of stress fractures in bone are

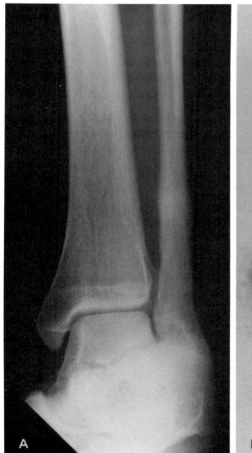

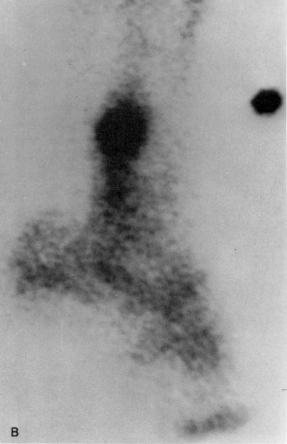

Figure 9-6. X-rays (*A*) and a bone scan (*B*) of a stress fracture in the distal fibula. The bone scan indicates the diagnostic feature of enhanced isotopic labeling of the fracture site. (Reproduced with permission of Dr. E. Hanley.)

poorly understood,[6] to the author it seems likely that they are similar to the phenomena observed in fatigue failure of metals. Observations by Freeman et al.[7] on the human femoral neck and by Simon et al.[8] on experimental animals reveal that under conditions of dynamic impulsive loads, bones undergo isolated fatigue fractures of individual trabeculae. Photomicrographs of the microfatigue fractures and the possible role of microfatigue fractures in the initiation of degenerative arthritis were presented in Chapter 5. As the minute trabecular fractures heal with the deposition of a dense ring of mineralized calcium hydroxyapatite, the modulus of elasticity of that segment of bone is increased so that it becomes more rigid. With continued exposure to fatigue forces, the rate of propagation of trabecular fractures may outstrip the maximal rate of bone healing. Certainly gross mechanical failure of bone may occur ultimately. Fatigue fractures, also, are notable for their slow rate of

healing. Such fractures show negligible bleeding into the fracture site. In the absence of bleeding the initiation of fracture repair mechanisms is greatly retarded. Delayed union represents a serious problem in the management of stress fractures, especially of large bones such as the femur.

Pathological Fractures

The term "pathological" denotes a fracture through a bone already weakened by disease.[9] Often the bone gives way from trivial violence or even spontaneously. Local diseases of bone that are associated with pathological fractures include: infections of bone, or osteomyelitis; benign and malignant tumors of bone; and a wide variety of miscellaneous causes such as paralytic bone atrophy, brittle failure induced by irradiation of bone and certain obscure inflammatory conditions such as monostotic fibrous dysplasia

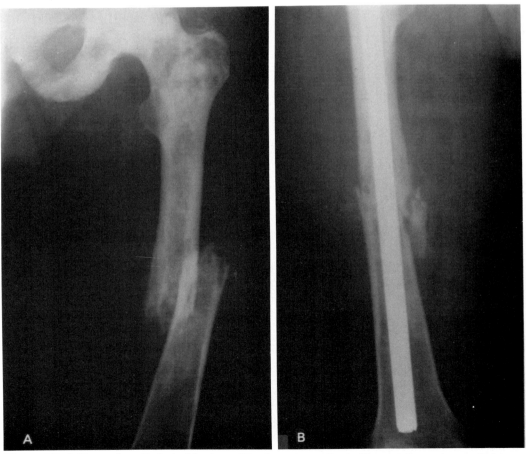

Figure 9-7. A. X-ray of a pathological fracture of the femur in a patient with prostatic carcinoma. B. A second X-ray taken after the insertion of an intramedullary nail for internal fixation.

and eosinophilic granuloma. An example is shown in Fig. 9-7. A great variety of general afflictions of the skeleton also may be associated with pathological fractures, such as osteoporosis, osteomalacia, Paget's disease, disseminated tumors such as multiple myeloma, rare congenital disorders such as osteogenesis imperfecta, and polystotic fibrous dysplasia. With the combination of extensive destruction of a localized segment of bone and of serious impairment of reparative processes, union of the fracture may be particularly difficult to achieve. Recent clinical advances in the management of difficult pathological fractures, such as malignant tumors of bone, are described in Chapter 10.

METHODS OF INTERNAL FIXATION

The general indications for the use of internal fixation are: the treatment of recent fractures including surgically created fractures (osteotomies); the treatment of ununited fractures (nonunions or pseudarthroses); and the fixation of joints where elimination of motion with the production of bony ankylosis or arthrodesis is sought. The types of implants available include: screws and pins, both for the fixation of diaphyseal fractures of cortical bone and for the fixation of metaphyseal and epiphyseal fractures of cancellous bone; onlay plates with screws for the fixation of shaft fractures; blade plates or nail plates for the fixation of fractures near the ends of weight-bearing bones; the application of intramedullary nails for shaft fractures of long bones; wires for tension band wiring of bone fragments or, rarely, circumferential cerclage for comminuted or unstable shaft fractures; and external clamp fixation with skeletal pins for fusion of joints and open fractures or infected nonunions (Fig. 9-1). These devices are described in sequence, except for external fixation which is presented in Chapter 11.

The Screw

Screws are a highly satisfactory form of internal fixation of fractures, both as the sole method of fixation and in combination with onlay plates. The screws must be capable of relatively easy insertion and removal. They must obtain a good purchase on the bone so that they do not loosen or pull out. They must be strong enough to withstand the tensile, torsional and shearing stresses associated with insertion, removal and use. Internal fixation will be considered in terms of the biomechanics of the screw, the response of the bone to the screw and, subsequently, the surgical techniques of the application of screws.

The Biomechanics of the Screw

A wide variety of types of screws have been developed for use in bone surgery. At present four styles (Fig. 9-8) account for most applications: (a) a self-tapping cortical bone screw with a cross-slotted head and a thread diameter of 4 mm; (b) a non-self-tapping cortical bone screw with a hexagonal socket or recess and a thread diameter of 4.5 mm and a core diameter of 3 mm; (c) a cancellous screw with a hexagonal recess and a thread diameter of 6.5 mm; and (d) a self-tapping malleolar screw with a hexagonal recess. The latter three designs represent screws developed by the AO group which are fully

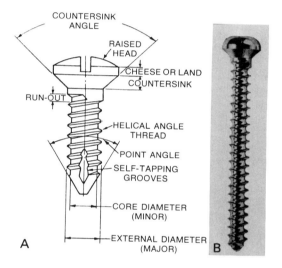

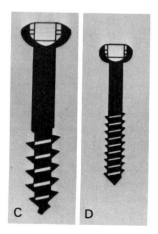

Figure 9-8. Schematic views and photographs show three types of screws: *A*, 4-mm self-tapping screw; *B*, 4.5-mm AO cortical screw; *C*, 6.5-mm cancellous screw; and *D*, a self-tapping malleolar screw.

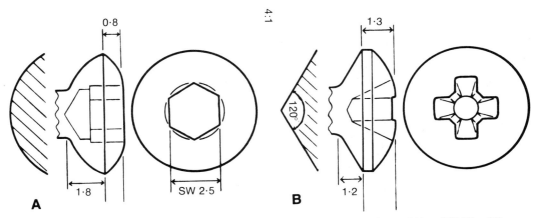

Figure 9-9. Schematic views show the screw heads of AO sunken hexagonal type (*A*) and Phillips (*B*).

described elsewhere.[4] They are available in a variety of smaller diameters.

The discrepancies in design arise from consideration of three functional portions of a screw: (a) the driving head requires a recess which provides firm grip for the screwdriver without excessive bulk; (b) the threaded shaft of the screw requires maximal fixation in dense cortical bone or the more coarsely woven, less dense cancellous bone; and (c) the tip of the screw requires appropriate shape for either self-tapping or tapping conditions. These three portions of a screw are described in turn.

The Screw Head. During insertion or removal of a screw, firm purchase of the screwdriver on the screw head is essential. If the screwdriver suddenly disengages under load, it may cause considerable trauma to surrounding tissues. Also, with disengagement, excessive force may be applied to a part of the recess in the screw head, which may become distorted. Such damage to the screw head may greatly hinder subsequent attempts to remove the screw. Clearly, single slots have no place in the heads of bone screws. For many years the Phillips or Woodruff type cross-slots have been popular. The Phillips type (Fig. 9-9*B*) has been especially popular for small screws as it is compatible with a tiny screw head. Mechanical erosion of the Phillips head, however, has been a considerable problem. More recently the AO group has popularized the hexagonal recess which the author believes to be a superior design (Fig. 9-9*A*). It provides excellent grip with the screwdriver so that a screw engaged on the screwdriver need not be held by the surgeon. This frees a most valuable second hand. While there are special designs of cross-slotted screwdrivers with attachments that temporarily secure the screw to the screwdriver, all

are cumbersome compared to the hexagonal recess. The liability of the hexagonal recess is that it requires a larger screw head. Until recently, small AO bone screws were not available with this type of head; fortunately this has been rectified.[10]

The Screw Shaft. Considerable research has been undertaken on the optimal diameter of bone screw, as well as the preferred size and shape of screw thread. Reports by Hughes and Jordan,[11] Ansell and Scales,[12] Bechtol *et al.,*[13] and Müller *et al.*[4] deserve scrutiny. The essence of screw performance is the generation of compression between the screw head and bone, or between a bone plate and bone, by means of a tensile stress in the screw.

To drive a screw into a pilot hole, a clockwise torsional force (*i.e.,* "torque") and an axial compressive load are transmitted from the screwdriver to the screw (Fig. 9-10). While in theory a purely compressive stress would be induced in the screw by the axial load, in practice the load usually is applied at an angle to the axis of the screw, so that bending and shear stresses may be introduced into the screw. The stresses can be large at the start of insertion when most of the length of the screw is unsupported. (In theory, the insertional stresses depend upon the eccentricity of loading although in practice it is strongly influenced by the initial instability of the unsupported screw.)

The tensile stress in the screw is derived from the torque applied to the screw head. The efficiency with which applied torque is converted into tension in the screw depends upon the forces required to cut threads in bone and to overcome friction between screw threads and the bone. Both of these losses are greater with self-tapping screws. With the final "screwing-home", torque

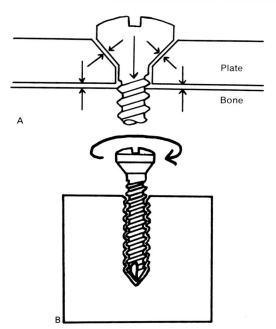

A

B

Figure 9-10. The compressive and torsional force applied to a screw during its insertion are shown schematically in *A* and *B*, respectively.

is lost to friction at the countersink of the screw where it contacts bone or a plate.

If a screw is stressed sufficiently in tension or in torsion ultimately it breaks. A fracture stress can be defined as that stress which ultimately provokes breakage of the screw. If a screw is subjected to both a torsional shear stress and a tensile stress, it will fail at a tensile stress which is less than the previously determined tensile fracture stress. Thus, in clinical practice if a screw is under high tensile stress, then the additional application of a small shear stress may provoke failure; conversely if a screw is under a high shear stress, addition of a small tensile stress may cause fracture. In the latter case, breakage of the screw may occur before rigid immobilization of the bone has been achieved.

For a cylindrical specimen it can be shown[11] that

$$\lambda = \frac{16 \, Mt}{\pi \, d^3}$$

where

λ = torsional shear stress, which occurs at the outer surface

Mt = torsional moment producing the shear stress

d = diameter of cylinder.

Similarly,

$$\sigma = \frac{4L}{d^2}$$

where

σ = tensile stress, uniform across the cross section

L = applied tensile load (lb).

Although a screw does not have the geometry of a cylinder it may be inferred from the previous relationships that the ultimate torsional shear strength of a screw is related to the cube of its diameter while its ultimate tensile strength is related to the square of its diameter. A screw has two diameters, but it is the minor or core diameter to which strength can be directly related. Optimal screw strength is attained by application of the largest core diameter of screw which can be used. The limit to the size of screw which can be used is the obvious anatomical consideration. Bechtol *et al.*[13] recommended a maximal core diameter of 0.116 ± 0.002 inch (2.95 mm) for screws inserted into an adult femur, if the risk of fracture at the drill hole is to be avoided. The British Standards Institution[14] recommends a 4 mm (0.156 inch) external diameter with a core diameter of 3.0 mm (0.118 inch). The standard AO cortical screw has an external diameter of 4.5 mm with a core diameter of 3.1 mm. Lindahl[15] has compared the strength of a standard self-tapping screw with external diameter of 3.7 mm and a core diameter of 2.7 mm with that of the standard AO 4.5-mm screw. The mean tensile force for fracture of the former is 409 kg and of the latter is 511 kg. In contrast, the mean strength of anchorage of the screw in cortical bone (*e.g.*, the stripping strength) is 178 kg for the former and 232 kg for the latter. These figures demonstrate primarily that the holding power of a screw depends largely upon the strength of the bone. Secondly, they reveal the superiority of the 4.5-mm AO screw. It is common engineering practice to specify a safety factor of three. If a screw should withstand forces three times greater than the strength of the anchorage, then the AO screw is satisfactory and the standard self -tapping screw is of inadequate strength.

The Screw Tip

The holding power of a screw is reduced slightly by the presence of self-tapping flutes, by reduction of the effective number of threads engaged, and by decrease in the width of the *thread crest* which reduces the effective *shear-*

Table 9-1

Comparison of Critical Resolved Shear Stress of 4-mm Bone Screws[a]

Screw material	Mean maximum critical resolved shear stress	Relative strength in arbitrary units
	$Kg\ cm^2$	
AISI 316 stainless steel	8.4×10^3	100
Cast Co-Cr-Mo alloy	7.0×10^3	80
Pure titanium (160 alloy)	5.4×10^3	65
Ti-6Al-4V alloy	9.0×10^3	100

[a] From Hughes and Jordan.[11]

ing length of the *pitch* of the screw. Ideal geometry of the thread crest represents a compromise between an excessively sharp design, when the thread tip is likely to bend, and an unduly flat tip or large radius of curvature, with a reduced shearing length. The radius of curvature of 0.0025 inch (0.064 mm) recommended by British Standard 3531 of 1962[14] appears to be a reasonable figure.

Other factors which affect the performance of screws are the nature of the screw material and the size of the drill hole. In a comparison of the critical resolved shear stress of 4-mm bone screws, Hughes and Jordan[11] reported mean values as shown in Table 9-1. The superiority of the stainless steel and the titanium alloy screws, especially over a pure titanium screw, is evident. Hughes and Jordan also have shown that the use of a drill hole with the largest practical diameter will greatly diminish the shear stress on the screw. For a 4-mm screw they advise a drill hole of 3.45 mm. Under optimal conditions they estimate that about 65% of applied torque may be usefully employed to induce tension.

For extraction of 4-mm bone screws, Ansell and Scales[12] showed that the size of the drill holes within the range of 2.87 and 3.17 mm (0.113 to 0.125 inch) had little effect on the mean extraction force from cadaveric specimens. What is more influential is the cutting flute of a self-tapping thread, which is filled by new bone and greatly resists the force of extraction.

One other attribute of a screw which determines its holding power is the shape and size of the threads. Bechtol *et al.*[13] have reported a study on a variety of threads for use in cortical bone. A variety of the sharp threads associated with self-tapping screws showed a 5 to 10% decrease in holding power compared to non-self-tapping screws. Other considerable variations in thread geometry appear to yield remarkably little variation in holding power. The present thread designs also appeared to be satisfactory. More recently, Müller *et al.*[4] studied the optimal thread pattern for cancellous screws. The preferred threads possess large flutes on screws of large core diameter.

The Holding Power of Bone Screws in Vivo

The previous evaluation of bone screws refers to traditional studies on screws in the laboratory where cadaveric bones or synthetic bone-like materials have been used. Most workers have been aware that in living bone the holding power of a screw is largely a function of the bone adjacent to the screw. Inevitably the trauma to the bone from insertion of the screw, the reaction of the bone to the metallic implant and the remodeling of the bone with healing must be crucial factors in the holding power of screws. Until recently, the significance of these biological factors could only be conjectured. In a series of papers, Schatzker *et al.*[16, 17] reported their observations on the response of living bone to the insertion of screws into the intact femora of dogs. A variety of self-tapping and non-self-tapping screws of AISI 316 stainless steel or cast Co-Cr-Mo alloy with external diameters from 3.5 to 4.5 mm was inserted into the foreleg. After a variable period of implantation, the dogs were sacrificed and the pull-out strength of the bone around each screw was recorded (Fig. 9-11). The

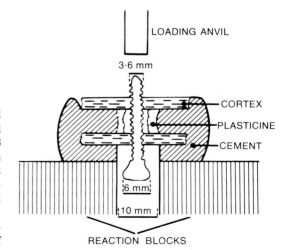

Figure 9-11. Schematic diagram illustrates the experimental method for measurement of the pull-out strength of the screw. (Reproduced with permission of J. Schatzker, R. Sanderson, and J. P. Murnaghan.[16])

results confirm that immediately after insertion of the screw, the diameter of the screw thread is the dominant factor in determination of the holding power of the screw. The thread profile, the manner of insertion (self-tapping *versus* non-self-tapping) and the ratio of the drill hole to the external diameter of the screw appear to play minor roles. Further experiments were performed on the response of bone to the trauma of drilling, with microvascular or thermal damage, and of self-tapping or of inserting a non-self-tapping screw. The results indicate that with normal care on insertion for all screw types tested, the tissue reaction to an unloaded screw in bone does not diminish the holding power of the screw during the initial 12-week period. The same degree of bone death was observed after insertion of self-tapping or non-self-tapping screws. Neither the dead bone nor its subsequent replacement by living bone provoked a deterioration of holding power, below the zero-time holding power.

Additional experiments on the effect of motion of screws within the living canine bone were performed. The histological observations clearly reveal that movement between screw threads and bone inhibits bone formation, revascularization and remodeling of dead bone. Movement provokes fibrous tissue proliferation around the screw so that all holding power is lost. Radio-

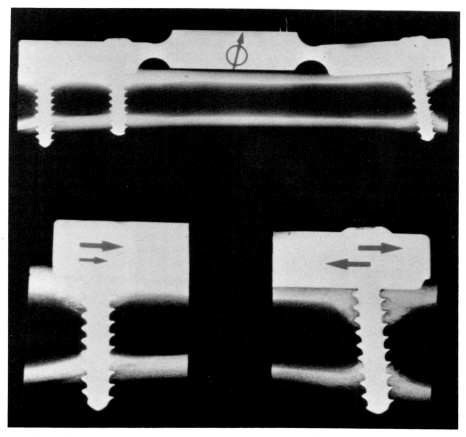

Figure 9-12. The influence of oscillating motion, as intermittent compression and as alternate compression and tension, on the remodeling of bone at the interface with screws is shown. The experimental model employed on sheep femora *in vivo* is shown. A special dynamic compression plate (DCP) with a load-measuring cell is attached to bone with 4.5 mm cortical screws. On the end of the plate where two screws are used, the more central screw is inserted in a round hole while the more peripheral screw is inserted in a loading position of a DCP hole. The two screws exert a compressive force in the intervening bone which varies in magnitude with activity of the animal. The single screw at the other end of the plate imposes a compressive force on the adjacent bone with periodic reversal of the stress. The two different stress patterns are shown schematically with the *arrows* on the two lower drawings. (See also Fig. 9-13.) (Reproduced with permission of S. M. Perren and M. Allgöwer.[18])

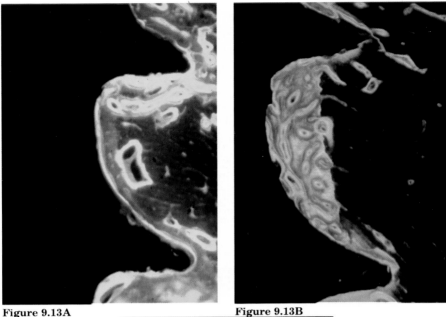

Figure 9.13A   Figure 9.13B

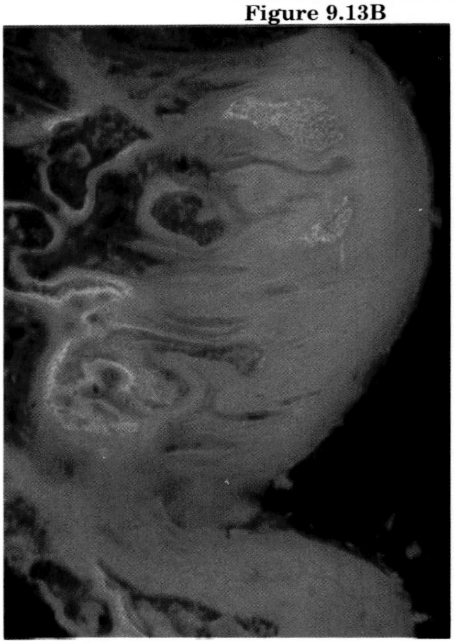

Figure 9.13C

Figure 9-13. The influence of oscillating motion, as intermittent compression and as alternate compression and tension, on the remodeling of bone at the interface with screws is shown. *A.* A photomicrograph of a fluorescent histological preparation of the bone adjacent to the peripheral screw on the left side of the plate. As in the other histological preparations the animal was sacrificed 8 weeks after insertion of the plate and 4 weeks after sequential tetracycline labeling of bone. Bone deposition and remodeling within the screw threads is evident with close approximation of bone to the entire screw thread. The *black area* on the left is indicative of the screw. *B.* A similar histological preparation is evident wherein the experimental technique was altered by a slightly eccentric insertion of the screw into the drill hole. In this situation enlarged gaps between the screw and the adjacent bone were thereby created. The labeled bone reveals the deposition to fill the gaps. Since the bone completely fills the gaps, the mechanical stability of the screw insertion is confirmed. *C.* The histological preparation obtained from the bone adjacent to the screw positioned on the right side of the plate is seen. Under the imposition of cyclic load callus formation with islands of fibrocartilage is apparent. The reparative tissue does not closely approximate the surface of the screw. With its resilient nature the tissue fails to rigidly stabilize the screw. (See also Fig. 9-12.) (*A, B* and *C*, sequential labeling with tetracycline; magnification: each screw thread has a width of 0.75 mm and a pitch of 1.75 mm.) (*A, B* and *C*, reproduced with permission of S. M. Perren and M. Allgöwer.[18])

graphically the process of loosening produced a pathognomonic sign, a radiolucent "halo" about the screw (Figs. 9-12 and 9-13 A–C).

Next, the experiments were repeated with the application of compressive load on the cortical bone by the screw threads. With a torque-measuring screwdriver, a force of 180 kp was applied, which represents 80% of the torque-out value of the screw. Histological sections of the cortical bone adjacent to the screw threads reveals the presence of dead bone along surfaces under compression. At these sites there is no evidence of resorption or remodeling of bone. Along portions of screw thread where the bone is not under compression, intense remodeling of bone is in evidence. As the healing period progresses, the area of remodeling bone extends gradually toward the adjacent regions under compression. The dead bone under compression is replaced by creeping substitution. Once all of the dead bone under compression is replaced by new bone, the compression at the interface falls to zero. The loss of compression would be anticipated by the observations of Perren et al.[19] who showed that interfragmentary compression of bone diminishes primarily with the gradual remodeling of bone and not as a result of bone resorption. The histological evidence and the biomechanical data indicates that cortical bone around screws that are tightly inserted do not resorb to provoke loosening of the screws. After insertion into cortical bone fragments with considerable compressive load, the screws remain rigidly anchored in the bone. In contrast, moderately loose screws induce local resorption of bone so that further loosening of the screws ensues. The clinical significance of the results is that screws which generate compression at the interface of their threads with bone can be expected to provide adequate fixation until bone union occurs.

Somewhat similar observations have been reported by Wagner[20] for studies of cancellous bone under compression by screw threads. While resorption of the cancellous bone does not occur, hypertrophy and realignment of the trabeculae in line with the force of compression ensues. Again, with remodeling of the trabeculae the compression gradually is relieved.

The Clinical Application of Bone Screws

The recommendations by the AO group for techniques of insertion of bone screws currently are unexcelled. The AO methods are summarized below.

To achieve rigid internal fixation, screws must apply compression to the fracture surfaces. Interfragmental compression is achieved by the application of the lag technique, whereby a gliding hole is drilled into the proximal fragment. As the screw is tightened the screw head approximates the distal fragment. The technique can be applied to virtually all types of screws. For the cortical bone of diaphyseal or shaft fractures, cortical screws are applied; for the cancellous bone of epiphyseal or metaphyseal fractures, cancellous screws are employed.

Cortical Screws. The cortical screw behaves as a lag screw only when it obtains a grip on the distal cortex and not on the proximal cortex. For insertion of an AO 4.5-mm cortical screw (Fig. 9-14), first the fracture is reduced, without minimal stripping of soft tissue and devascularization of bone. Then a 4.5-mm drill is used to prepare the hole in the proximal cortex. A 4.5-mm tap sleeve is used to provide a drill guide and to prevent soft tissue entanglement in the drill. Next, a special drill sleeve with an outer diameter of 4.5 mm and an inner diameter of 3.2 mm is inserted into the drill hole. Insertion of the 3.2 mm drill into this drill guide insures accurate placement of the distal hole. After the distal cortex is drilled, the depth gauge measures the required length of screw. Now the thread is tapped and a countersink is bored in the proximal cortex for the screw. Finally the screw is inserted. Satisfactory variations in the method of insertion of cortical screws are show in Figures 9-15 and 9-16. Adherence to this procedure provides the surgeon with a rapid and precise technique for insertion of cortical screws. Where cortical screws are the sole method of fixation, two or more screws must be applied to achieve rotational stability. The direction of each screw is critical. In a spiral or lengthy oblique fracture at least one screw should be inserted at right angles to the shaft of the bone to prevent overriding of the fragments. Another screw should be positioned at right angles to the fracture surfaces to provide maximal compression of the fragments. Other screws may be aligned as a compromise between these two goals. The screws should not be tightened until all of them have been inserted.

For stabilization of comminuted segments with screws, first accurate reduction of the fracture is essential. The reduction is maintained with bone holding forceps (Fig. 9-17 A) and, where necessary, with temporary Kirschner wire fixation. With the lag technique, the fragments are immobilized (Fig. 9-17 B). Where possible at

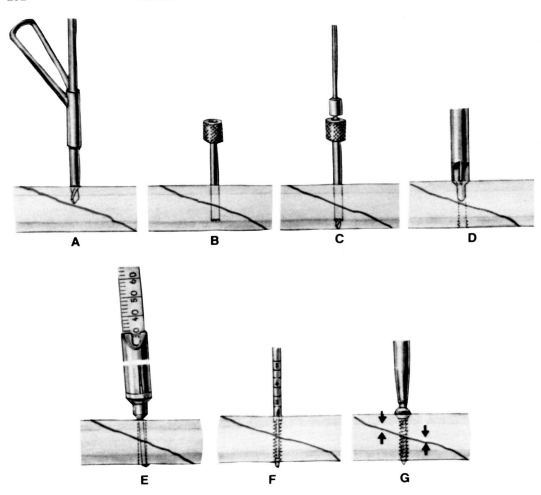

Figure 9-14. A schematic diagram illustrates the standard method to use cortical screws with the lag technique. *A*. The proximal cortex is drilled with a 4.5-mm drill inserted into a 4.5-mm tap sleeve. *B*. A special drill sleeve with an outer diameter of 4.5 mm and an inner diameter of 3.2 mm is inserted into the drill hole until it meets the opposite cortex. The drill sleeve permits an accurate hole to be drilled through the far cortex. *C*. The far cortex is drilled with 3.2-mm drill, fitted with a stop. *D*. With a countersink the near cortex is beveled for the screw hole. *E*. With a depth gauge the required screw length is measured. *F*. A thread is prepared in the distal cortex with the short 4.5-mm cortical tap. *G*. With the screwdriver the screw is inserted until loose approximation of bone is observed. After all the screws have been inserted they are tightened securely. Where a cortical screw is anchored into a single bone fragment the lag technique is not necessary. Alternatively, a drill hole of 3.2 mm is made in both cortices. The special drill sleeve is needed to protect soft tissues from the rotating drill. With the short 4.5-mm cortical tap both cortices are threaded. Then the screw is introduced into the drill hole.

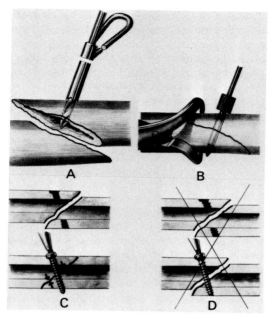

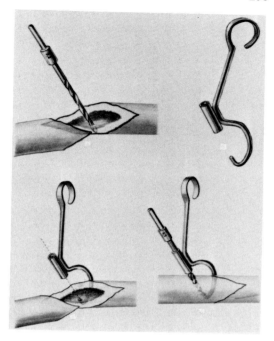

Figure 9-15. A correct method for insertion of a screw positioned obliquely across a spiral or oblique fracture is shown. The proximal screw hole is drilled (*A*) and the fracture is secured with bone holding forceps in an anatomical alignment (*B*). Two diagrams show the correct (*C*) and incorrect (*D*) methods of screw insertion. The fracture has to be reduced prior to drilling the distal cortical hole or accurate coadaptation of the fracture surfaces is not achieved.

Figure 9-16. A modified technique of screw insertion is shown. A thread hole of 3.2 mm is drilled into the distal cortex prior to reduction. After the drill hole is made the fracture is reduced and a gliding hole is prepared with a 4.5-mm drill. Screw fixation is completed as described in Figure 9-14.

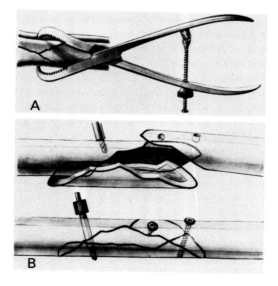

Figure 9-17. Schematic diagrams illustrate the method of insertion of cortical screws in a spiral fracture. *A.* First the fracture is accurately reduced and secured with bone holding forceps. If necessary, provisional stability can be augmented by the use of Kirschner wires. *B.* With the lag technique, screws are inserted across the fracture. Only the proximal gliding holes can be made before the fracture is reduced. (See also Fig. 9-18.)

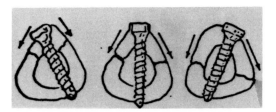

Figure 9-18. Schematic cross-sectional views of cortical screws in a spiral fracture show the appropriate oblique orientations of the screws. (See also Fig. 9-17.)

least one screw should secure the two main fracture fragments. As shown in Figure 9-18, the rotational alignment of the screws varies from one region of the fracture to another, depending upon the orientation of the fracture.

In the preparation of a drill hole for any type of screw, the use of a power drill is essential. The hand drill is likely to wobble and to yield an eccentric hole, with the pressure exerted by the surgeon on the drill. Either the reduction of the fracture is apt to be lost, or the pointed drill may slip from the curved surface of bone to impale adjacent soft tissues. The power instrument also facilitates the attempt to position the hole in the midaxis of the bone.

How Tight Is Tight Enough? For the carpenter or surgeon who inserts screws, the problem inevitably arises of when to cease tightening a screw. The balance between adequate fixation and the application of excessive force, with stripping of the threads from failure of the bone around the screw or by mechanical failure of the screw itself, is a narrow margin. The question of the surgeon's capacity to judge the correct torque by "feel" is raised. Most surgeons, naturally would claim to be adept in this "feel", as it is a frequent experience in their operative practice. In a previous study, Ansell and Scales[12] suggested that judgement of torque by "feel" was exceptionally difficult; they advised the introduction of torque-limiting screwdrivers. None have been invented which tolerate repeated sterilization without lubrication.

Recently, at a Swiss AO course on "Techniques of Internal Fixation," which the author attended, Perren *et al.*[21] used torque-measuring screwdrivers to judge the ability of several hundred surgeons from all parts of the world, to "feel" torque correctly during insertion of AO 4.5-mm cortical screws into cadaveric bone. Each surgeon was asked to tighten a screw into the threaded hole until optimal tightness was achieved; then the torque was recorded. Next, the surgeon proceeded to tighten the screw until the bony threads were stripped or the screw

fractured. Admittedly a few of the surgeons tightened their screws with the optimal force that is about 20% below the force needed to break the screw or to strip the osseous thread. Nevertheless the results for the surgeons revealed a variation in applied screw torque between 20 and 200 kp and about 20% of the surgeons failed to apply any significant compression to their screw fixations. A few surgeons fractured their screws. While some surgeons possess a remarkably accurate ability to estimate the optimal torque for insertion of bone screws, most surgeons lack this attribute and would profit greatly by the use of a torque-measuring screw driver.

Cancellous Screws. The AO cancellous screws are lag screws which possess a threadless proximal shaft which is larger than the inner or core diameter. Provided that the proximal fragment does not engage the screw threads, the screw threads do not cross the fracture line. The screw will compress the fragments by the lag principle. For insertion of a cancellous screw, the fracture is first reduced. Where precise anatomical alignment is essential, as in an interarticular fracture or where the fracture is inherently unstable, temporary fixation with Kirschner wires may be needed. Next, a hole is drilled and the depth gauge is applied for measurement of the length of screw. Afterwards the thread is cut with a cancellous tap and the screw is inserted. In osteoporotic bone either the smaller 3.2-mm cortical tap or no tap may be preferred. Where the bone is so soft that the screw head may sink into bone, a washer is applied. For rotational stabilization, a second screw or a Kirschner wire may be added. Alternatively, in pure cancellous bone such as the malleoli, a malleolar screw may be inserted without predrilling or tapping. A few clinical examples are shown in Figure 9-17 *B*, 9-18 and 9-19.

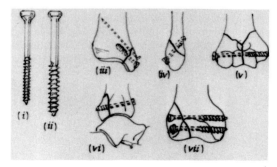

Figure 9-19. Several applications of cancellous screws including malleolar screws are demonstrated. (Reproduced with permission of M. E. Müller, M. Allgöwer and H. Willenegger.[22])

A Comparison of Self-tapping and Non-self-tapping Screws

Self-tapping screws are widely used in bone surgery in view of their rapid insertion. Inevitably the question of the need for the additional step of tapping is raised. All of the biomechanical studies reported in the previous sections show narrow but measurable superiority of the AO 4.5-mm non-self-tapping screw over its 4.0-mm self-tapping rivals. As mentioned, much of this benefit is derived from the larger core diameter of the non-self-tapping screw. Wagner[20] compared the histological reaction of the epiphysis of a growing canine tibia to the presence of self-tapping and non-self-tapping screws. The screws were inserted across the epiphysis and into the metaphysis. The continued growth of the epiphyseal plate produced a constant tensile force on the screw. Wagner observed the remodeling of bone with the production of cortical lamellar bone at the sites of compression across the bone screw interface. From the histological pattern of bone surrounding the screw thread it is evident that a non-self-tapping screw possesses a much larger surface area of bone under compression than a self-tapping screw. Close scrutiny of the thread design of a non-self-tapping screw reveals that the thread approximates a right angle to the core, thereby to minimize the shear forces at the screw bone interface under compression. In contrast, the thread on the self-tapping design presents an acute angle to the core which is consistent with much larger shear forces at the screw bone interface under compression. In the latter situation the elevated shearing forces are more likely to initiate premature mechanical failure of the bone or the screw with loss of stability at the interface. Precutting the channel in bone for the screw also permits a closer approximation of the entire screw thread to the adjacent bone. Also, it allows the use of a thread design in which the threads penetrate more deeply into the bone to provide a larger area of contact between the thread and the bone than would be possible with a self-tapping screw.

Another relative advantage of the use of non-self-tapping screws is their ease of insertion. After the use of a tap, the screw can be threaded into bone with minimal force, to reduce the likelihood of loss of reduction of the fracture. The extra time required for insertion of the tap is recovered with the foreshortened time of insertion of the screw. Also the non-self-tapping screw is readily removed. The self-tapping screw is more difficult to remove because bone grows into the cutting flute of the screw. Ultimately the AO non-self-tapping screws are superior because they are part of a very complete system that includes a wide variety of screws, each of unique attribute, and numerous designs of plates and blade plates. In many clinical applications, the combination of a variety of AO cortical and cancellous screws permits the surgeon to achieve a rigid fixation that could not be replicated by the use of the conventional self-tapping screws with other implants.

Fixation with Plates and Screws

While historically a great variety of onlay bone plates have been designed and employed clinically, the biomechanical studies and clinical experience of the AO group have profoundly enhanced the biomechanical knowledge and techniques for application of plates.

Early in the present century, surgeons such as Lane,[23] applied plates merely to fix two bone fragments in approximate alignment. More ambitious goals were hampered by mechanical failure of the screws or plates. Many minor improvements were made in the design of the implants to make them stronger. In 1949 Danis[24] reported the use of interfragmentary compression with plates applied under tension along the longitudinal axis of the bone. His plate incorporated a compression device (Fig. 9-20 A). Subsequently, Müller[4] designed the ASIF compression plate with a removable tension device; clearly there was no advantage in leaving the tension device in place after surgery (Fig. 9-20 B). Also, Eggers[25] exploited the compression effect attained by the use of elongated holes (Fig. 9-21 A and B). Eccentric placement of screws with conical shoulders which engage one end of the elongated hole and thereby achieve compression is an established principle in carpentry. By the application of the same principle, Bagby and Janes[26]

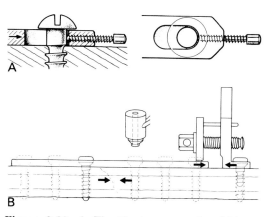

Figure 9-20. *A.* The Danis compression device is shown schematically. *B.* Schematic diagram of Müller compression device applied to one end of an AO plate.

designed a plate in which compression in the long axis of bone is achieved as the screws are driven home. In his design, the screws possess a conical shoulder which glides down the edge of an oval screw hole. Many other designs, such as the AO semitubular plate, employ a similar concept (Fig. 9-21 C and D). Most recently Perren et al.[27] described a self-compression plate where spherical geometry permits a congruent fit be-

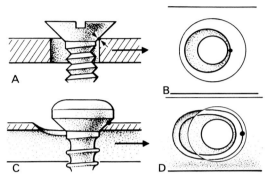

Figure 9-21. *A* and *B.* The use of an eccentrically placed screw with a conical shoulder is a widely applied method to achieve compression. The Eggers plate modified this method by the use of oval shaped holes in the plate. *C* and *D.* Schematic view of the oval hole in an AO semitubular plate. The conical geometry of the screw should facilitate the application of compression.

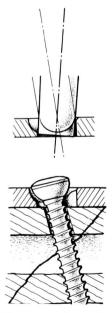

Figure 9-22. Diagram illustrates the complex geometry of a hole in a dynamic compression plate. Not only does the hole permit the application of self-compression, but it permits a screw to be inserted in an oblique direction.

tween screw and plate, in any position along the screw hole even with a certain degree of tilt between the screw and plate (Fig. 9-22). In addition to longitudinal compression of the fracture, it enables the surgeon to insert a lag screw through the plate and across the fracture to greatly augment stability. Previously this dynamic compression plate (DCP) was made of pure titanium. In view of the somewhat smaller ultimate tensile strength of titanium (80 kp/mm$_2$) when compared to that of the AISI 316 L stainless steel of the regular AO compression plate (90 kp/mm^2) the DCP showed a larger cross-section. The Young's modulus of titanium (11,000 kp/mm^2) is markedly lower than that of surgical stainless steel or cobalt-chromium alloys. This attribute permitted the combination of rigid internal fixation of the fracture with a limited dynamic flexion of the plate bone so that osteoporosis of bone is less than that observed in bone where rigid plates dampen the physiological strain in adjacent bone. In view of manufacturing problems and of breakage of some titanium screws, the titanium alloy has been replaced by AISI 316L stainless steel. Before clinical consideration is presented, the mechanical and biomechanical bases of the use of compression plates will be discussed.

The Mechanical Basis of Compression Plating

When a plate is applied to two fracture fragments without the application of interfragmentary compression, physiological activities inevitably produce motion between the fracture fragments. The motion stimulates resorption of bone at the opposing ends of the fragments. With

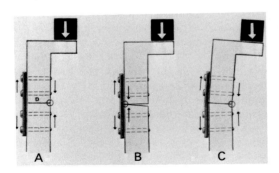

Figure 9-23. A schematic diagram (*A*) illustrates an unstable fracture treated with plate fixation. As the accompanying diagrams show, activity of the patient provokes micromotion at the fracture site with resorption of adjacent bone (*B*). Enhanced instability of the fracture site provokes increased bending moments on the plate which ultimately undergoes fatigue failure (*C*).

shortening of the fragments, further mechanical instability is assured. As described in Chapter 3, metal plates are especially liable to fatigue failure from bending and torque. The mechanical failure is particularly likely to occur if shortening of bone produces a loss of bony contact and support as shown in Figure 9-23. When the X-rays of cases where clinical failure of presently available bone plates are reviewed, the vast majority of cases confirm bony instability as the cause of fatigue failure of the implant, a situation which could have been predicted *and prevented* before the implant failed.

In the first instance, static compression of the fragments provides interfragmentary friction to oppose physiological shearing forces which would otherwise induce large bending moments and torque on the plate.[28] Next, the application of tensile forces on the plate enables it to show optimal resistance to bending forces and to torque. Finally, by restoration of the anatomical continuity of the fracture fragments, either by anatomical reduction of the fracture or by the use of bone grafts or other means, the fractured bone may be restored as a rigid support to relieve greatly the stresses which arise in the plate with postoperative activity of the patient.

Another essential consideration in the application of onlay plates is the comparison of bending moments that arise in intact limbs and the mechanical properties of the implants. While biomechanical measurements *in vivo* have lagged behind the clinical application of bone plates, nevertheless consideration of the physical environment of implants is obviously essential if mechanical failures are to be avoided.

Lawrence *et al.*[29] have studied the loads sustained by the human tibia. They find that at the moment of toe-off in normal walking, the longitudinal compressive force in the tibia may reach 4 times body weight. With a single bone plate offset by 2 cm from the line of action of this force, a bending moment of about 54 newton-meters arises with a body weight of 670 newtons. Unresisted straight leg raising produces a bending moment in the tibia of about 10 newton-meters. With complex postural adjustments, torsional moments of 13.7 to 18.4 newton-meters might be encountered. Lawrence *et al.* and Lindahl[15] also have reported the rigidity of bone plates. In bending, all of the devices show elastic followed by plastic deformation. Using an arbitrary criterion that a maximum of 5% of angular deformation is permissible, the weakest plate (Venables) can withstand a bending moment of only 7 newton-meters, while the strongest plate can withstand a bending mement of 24 newton-

meters. With a more stringent criterion of restriction of deformation to the elastic range, the moments that the plates can withstand are considerably less. When torsional moments are considered, the overall inadequacy of single onlay plates is equally apparent.

When a plate is used to immobilize a fracture, anatomical considerations govern the permissible thickness of the plate. The essential transverse curvature of plate must match the contour of the cylindrical shaft of the long bone. Nevertheless, the application of more than 1 plate placed perpendicularly to another merits consideration despite the associated increased risk of devascularization and of "stress protection" induced osteoporosis of the bone fragments. For the Venables plate the bending moment needed to produce 5° angulation with 2 plates is 40 newton-meters compared to 7 newton-meters for the single plate. In fact, as Frankel and Burstein[28] emphasize, the bending rigidity depends upon the configuration of the plate or plates, as shown in Table 9-2. This table indicates why the surgeon should select carefully the site on a bone where he secures the plate, so that optimal stabilization is achieved. Clinical examples of optimal plate position are shown in Chapter 10.

The final mechanical consideration with the use of plates is the number, size and shape of screws. On the basis of extensive clinical experience, the AO group has published recommendations on the minimum number of screws for use in plates on particular fractures which are reviewed in the next section. Clearly, each screw hole is a site of weakness of both the plate and the corresponding drill hole in the bone. For example, as Lawrence *et al.*[29] reported, when a bending moment of 13 newton-meters is applied to similar fracture plates with variable diameter of screw holes, the degrees of angular deformation produced in plates with holes of 6 mm, 8 mm, 9 mm, and 10 mm are 9°, 11°, 20° and 27° respectively. The presence of a screw in the hole lessens this effect. With imperfections in the surface finish of the drill holes, further deterioration in rigidity and strength of the plates would be recorded.

Biomechanical Basis of Internal Fixation

The application of compression to achieve rigid internal fixation hinges completely on the nature of the biological response of bone to compression. If, as many previous authors have suggested, the application of compression to bone provoked bone resorption, then *rigid* internal fixation of fractures would be impossible to maintain. It should be emphasized that forces

Table 9-2
The Relative Rigidity of a Fracture after the Application of One or Two Onlay Plates is Shown for Various Configurations of the Plate

Configuration	Bending moment	Rigidity relative to (a)
(a)		1
(b)		200
(c)		60
(d)		35
(e)		218
(f)		235

of compression of at least 200 kp (*i.e.*, kiloponds or kilograms force) may be applied without harmful effect. Rather, the effect of application of clinically useful magnitudes of static compression on bone is to rapidly provoke a minute amount of viscoelastic shortening. Static compression, by itself, does not cause any significant change in the mechanism or rate of bone remodeling or repair. Alternatively dynamic relative motion of the fracture, even on a minute scale, greatly influences the mechanisms of fracture repair. Where internal fixation is applied, the influence of motion is wholly detrimental, both by its initiation of bone and by its retardation of vascularization of bone. These liabilities of micromotion of a fracture treated by internal fixation are not necessarily liabilities if conservative treatment is applied.

In Chapter 5 a detailed account of primary bone healing was given. The observations on dogs and man by Schenk and Willenegger[30] and Gallinaro *et al.*[31] showed that primary bone healing could occur if certain biomechanical conditions prevailed and if each of the fracture fragments possessed intact blood supply. After rigid fixation, living bone fragments undergo resorption and bone formation simultaneously. The study of a transverse osteotomy of a canine radius rigidly stabilized with compression plates indicates that bone is able to withstand high

static loads without undergoing significant resorption at the fracture site. The histological features of the experiments are shown in Figure 9-24. After fixation of the radius, scrutiny of the osteotomy gap reveals that the gap is considerably wider at the cortex opposite from the plate (Fig. 9-24*A*). Initially the osteotomized surfaces show irregular zones of necrosis. Eight days after surgery the narrow gap (*b'*) is unchanged while the wider gap in the opposite cortex (b″) contains blood vessels that have invaded from the periosteum and the intramedullary cavity (Fig. 9-24*B*). In the third stage of repair (Fig. 9-24*C*) (8 to 10 weeks) revascularization of the necrotic fragments occurs in two ways. In the narrow cortical defect near the plate, the vessels invade from the widened Haversian canals. In the opposite cortical defect vessels invade from the Haversian canals and from the outside. The narrow osteotomy gap on the compressed side of the osteotomy does not permit the invasion of blood vessels from the periosteum or endosteum. In the wider opposite gap the vessels invade from the periosteum and endosteum. Close examination of a capillary bed within a Haversian canal that is undergoing remodeling, shows that bone resorption is followed immediately by bone formation (Fig. 9-24*D*). At the head of the cylindrical column of penetrating cells, multinucleated giant cells or osteoclasts

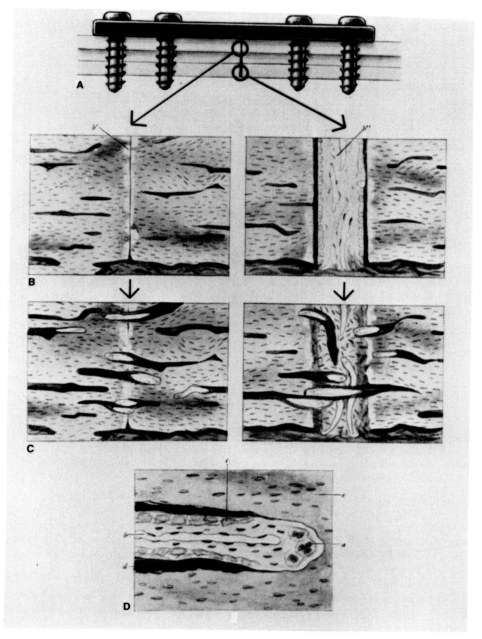

Figure 9-24. Schematic views reveal the histological stages of primary bone healing as described by Schenk and Willenegger.[30] (A) After a transverse osteotomy is made on a canine radius and a compression plate is applied, a wider gap is observed in the distal fracture site than the proximal fracture site. (B) One week after surgery the narrow gap shows little change while the wider gap shows an ingrowth of vessels from the periosteum and endosteum. Osteoblasts have migrated from the vessels and deposited osteoid on the necrotic edges of the fragment to rejoin them. (C) At 2 weeks the narrow gap is observed to have an ingrowth of vessels from the widened Haversian canals. At the wider cortical gap the vessels come from the Haversian canals as well as from the periosteum. Both gaps, however, heal by primary vascular bone formation. In D, an enlargement of a capillary bud arising from the Haversian canal reveals a cutting cone of multinucleated osteoclasts followed by an ingrowth. (Reproduced with permission of M. E. Müller, M. Allgöwer, and H. Willenegger.[34])

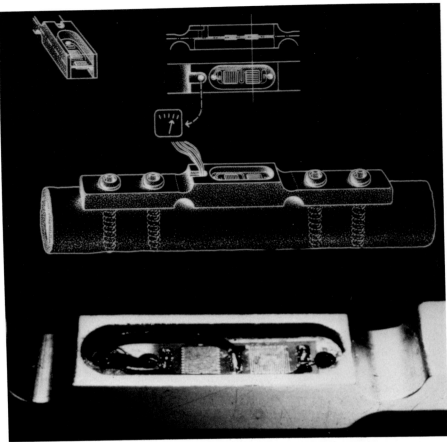

Figure 9-25. Shown are schematic views of a special compression plate designed by Perren which contains strain gauges to measure tensile forces in the plate as an index of compression at an osteotomy site. (Reproduced with permission of S. M. Perren.)

(*a*) resorb necrotic bone (*e*) and provide room for capillaries. Simultaneously osteoblasts deposit osteoid (*d*) and convert into concentrically aligned osteocytes.

Perren performed osteotomies on the tibia and metatarsals of rabbits and sheep which were stabilized with unique compression plates[32] (Fig. 9-25). The plates contained strain gauges which could measure up to 300 ± 1.5 kg. Daily records of the prevalent compression in bone reveal that an initial compression of over 100 kg rapidly decreases by a small amount because of the viscoelastic properties of bone. Over the subsequent 2 month period further diminution of compression occurs until about 50% of the initial value remains. The decrease in compression is related to remodeling of bone and not to resorption. If resorption of bone occurred, foreshortening of the osteotomy site by about 8 μm would totally relieve the initial compression at the fracture site. In the presence of dynamic motion

at the osteotomy site a different histological pattern is seen (Fig. 9-26). Resorption of bone rapidly ensues at the osteotomy gap so that progressive loss of the initial (and inadequate) stability provided by the plate is lost.

The Clinical Application of Bone Plates

As the AO group[33] has stressed, a plate applied to a stable fracture should convert tensile forces into axial compressive forces on the bone. The original AO compression plate is placed under tension with the tension device. It must be applied, however, to the tensile side of the bone. If it were placed on the compression side of bone it could not function as a tension band to immobilize the fracture; it would be unduly liable to fatigue failure from the immense bending forces encountered *in vivo*. Since long bones are subject to eccentric loading, the surgeon must know the proper side of the bone for application of the plate. In practice, a tension plate must be

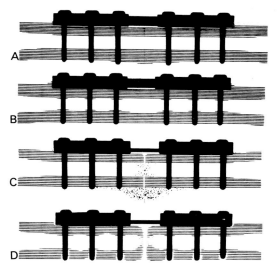

Figure 9-26. In *A*, an osteotomy is immobilized with a rigid plate and primary bone healing ensues (*B*). In *C*, the osteotomy is immobilized with a special plate of thin cross-section at the osteotomy site. In the presence of micromotion, callus appears on the osteotomy site opposite the plate, about 1 month after surgery. About 1 month later, resorption of the osteotomized surfaces is seen as in *D*. (Reproduced with permission of S. M. Perren).

applied to the convex or lateral side of the femur. Similarly for a nonunion of the tibia, the plate would be placed on the convex side of the bone. In fresh fractures of the tibial shaft where internal fixation is felt to be necessary a side of the bone subject primarily to axial forces is rarely present. Hence the bending or torsional forces must be neutralized by lag screws before the plate is applied, as described in the next section. In the upper limbs, the side under tension is determined by the arrangement of the muscles. Transverse midshaft fractures of the humerus, radius and ulna may be adequately immobilized solely by tension band plates. In the forearm the plates are applied on the convex, posterior surface.

For the application of a straight tension band plate, the fracture is reduced and the plate is attached to one fragment (Fig. 9-29). Next, the compressor is secured to the second fragment and axial compression of up to 150 kg is applied. The residual screws are attached and the compressor is removed.

Tension Band Fixation with Self-compression Plates. Especially in the forearm, there is inadequate room to apply the tension device without excessive risk to soft tissues, in this case, the posterior interosseous nerve (*e.g.,* deep ra-

dial nerve) adjacent to the proximal radius. Previously, the semitubular plate was widely applied to stabilize forearm fractures. Provided that the reduction is perfect, the oval holes enable the plate to be placed under tension by insertion of the screws eccentrically in the oval holes. As the conical head of the screw engages the plate, it places the plate under tension. As the two lateral margins of the plate engage the cortex they provide further resistance to rotation. While the semitubular plate functions satisfactorily for stable fractures it has inadequate resistance to bending or torsion for application on unstable fractures. Its chief indications are for fractures of the radius, the proximal ulna, the lateral malleolus, metacarpals and metatarsals. Other applications have vanished with the introduction of the DCP. In fact, the DCP suffices for all forearm fractures where previously a semitubular plate would have been used.

The Dynamic Compression Plate (DCP). In the past decade since its clinical introduction, the applications of this unique plate have gradually increased so that, for the AO surgeons, it has virtually replaced all of its predecessors.[32] It possesses the mechanical strength and the rigidity of the standard AO plate. It can be used with the external compressor or solely with the application of its self-compressive action. The geometry of the screw holes and screws permits a congruent fit even when the screws are tilted. The spherical geometry also inhibits the generation of undersirable bending moments in the plate. Rather than become wedged between the countersink or the hole in the plate, the screw readily shifts into a more desirable alignment. Both cancellous and cortical screws can be applied. The plate is available in AISI 316 L stainless steel.

Application of this plate is similar to that of the semitubular plate (Fig. 9-27). The fracture is reduced and the plate is contoured and applied to the bone (Fig. 9-27*A*). Whenever possible it is placed on the tension side of the bone, the opposite side from the strongest group of muscles which act on the bone. A drill guide is used to prepare a drill hole next to the fracture. The hole should be directed away from comminuted regions (Fig. 9-27*B*). The hole is tapped with the appropriate tap. The plate is attached to the bone fragment with a screw that is tightened until the plate barely contacts the bone. The plate is pulled until the screw is situated eccentrically in the hole. A second hole is drilled in the other bone fragment and a special drill guide ("load" guide) is used to position the hole eccen-

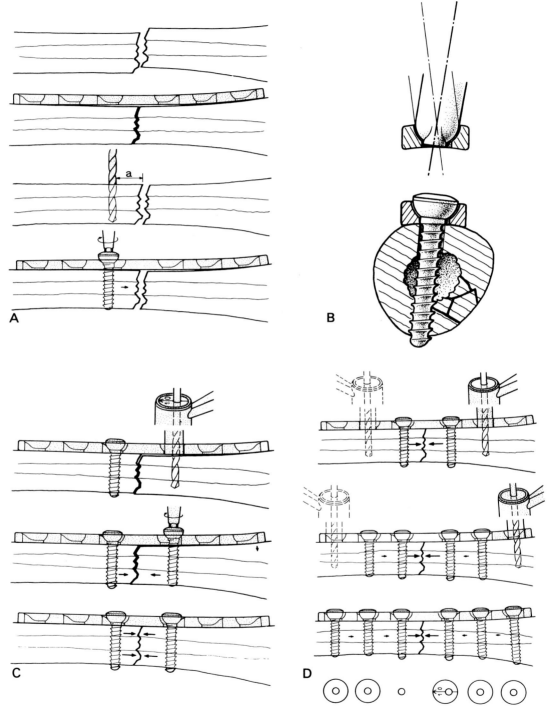

Figure 9-27. *A–D*. Diagrams show the method of application of a dynamic compression plate (DCP). (Reproduced with permission of Synthes Ltd., U.S.A.).

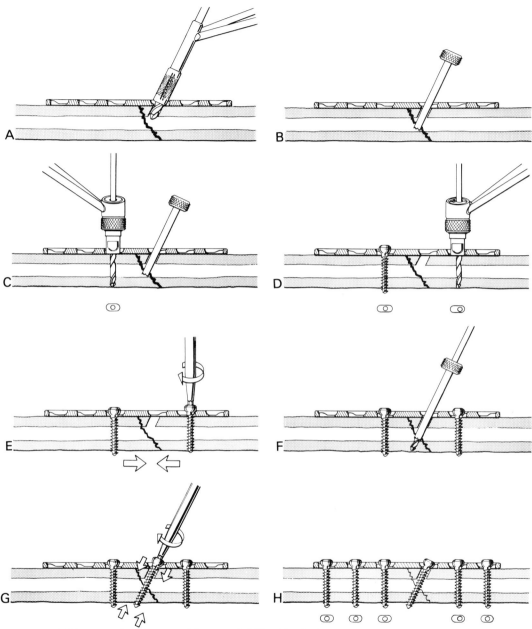

Figure 9-28. Diagrams show the use of the several drill guides during the application of a dynamic compression plate (DCP) with the use of the 4.5-mm drill guide for the proximal cortex (*A*), and a 3.2-mm drill guide for the distal cortex (*B*). An obliquely situated lag screw can be used to achieve interfragmentary compression across the fracture site. Subsequently the neutral drill guide is used for a screw in the other fracture fragment (*C*). As shown in *D* and *E*, a load guide conventionally is used to achieve compression with the DCP. After the three central screws are inserted the oblique lag screw is tightened (*F* and *G*). Subsequently the other screws are inserted with the use of the neutral drill guide (*H*). (Reproduced with permission of Synthes Ltd., U.S.A.).

trically in the oval hole of the plate as far as possible from the fracture (Fig. 9-27C). The hole is tapped and a screw is inserted. As the screws are tightened, compression is applied to the fracture as the edge of the oval holes in the plate push the screws together (Fig. 9-27D). By proper use of the load guide and with good approximation of the fracture fragments, 60 kp compression is obtained. Figure 9-28 shows the drill guides in use. After the two screws closest to the fracture have been inserted, the subsequent drill holes can be positioned in the center of the plate holes by the use of another special drill guide ("neutral" guide). Alternatively the compression applied to the fracture can be increased if the subsequent holes are positioned eccentrically, and as far as possible from the fracture site. During the insertion of the screws the previous screws must be loosened. When all of the screws have been inserted, they are tightened. Whenever possible, a screw through the plate is used as a lag screw to achieve optimal stability by interfragmentary compression perpendicular to the fracture line. This obliquely positioned screw also prevents over-riding or buckling of bone fragments (Fig. 9-28) at an oblique fracture.

In the forearm, with the small diameter of the radius and ulna, however, the lag screw must be positioned with sufficient obliquity so that it does not penetrate a narrow apex of the distal fragment. Otherwise the screw may damage the major blood supply to the apical segment. The avascular portion of bone undergoes resorption and the initial stabilization achieved by the use of the plate is lost.

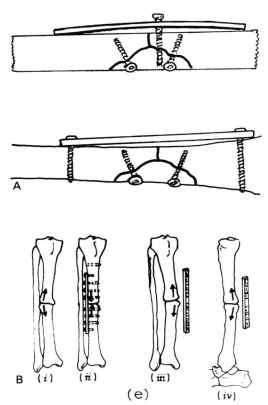

Figure 9-30. Diagrams show the appropriate contour for a dynamic compression plate to provide a relatively uniform distribution of compression on the proximal and distal cortices. A. Two ways are shown in which the plate may be applied with a convexity greater than that of the adjacent bone so that the force of compression at the fracture site is distributed uniformly across the two cortices. In both cases the maximal gap between the plate and the bone should be 1.0 to 1.5 mm. B. Plates are applied to the convex surfaces of nonunion sites so that the angular deformity is corrected and optimal distribution of compression across the fracture surfaces is achieved. (Reproduced with permission of M. E. Müller, M. Allgöwer and H. Willenegger.[34])

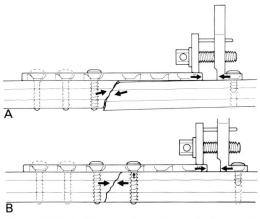

Figure 9-29. A. Diagram shows the method of application of a dynamic compression plate to an oblique fracture. A screw loosely placed near to the fracture site on the side of the tension device (B) prevents over-riding of the fracture. ((Reproduced with permission of Synthes Ltd., U.S.A.).

Previously, for use on the forearm a 4- to 6-hole plate was considered to provide adequate stabilization. During the past 5 years it has become evident that the use of a 4-hole plate results in a substantial incidence of delayed union or nonunion from loosening of the screws and loss of stability. A 6- or 7-hole plate is recommended as the minimal length. For the femur or tibia, an 8- or 10-hole plate is the minimal acceptable length. In the lower extremity the terminal screws in the plates should penetrate a single cortex so that the stress relief

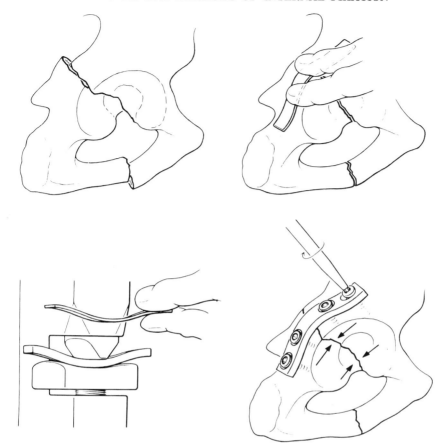

Figure 9-31. Schematic diagram shows the use of a bending press to shape a dynamic compression plate for application to a pelvic fracture. (Reproduced with permission of M. Allgöwer, P. Matter, S. M. Perren and T. Rüedi.[35])

provided by the plate to the adjacent segment of bone is gradually terminated.

The outside surfaces of most bones show complex curves. For the application of an onlay plate, usually the plate must be contoured to fit the surface of the bone. Alternatively, the contour of the plate may require a greater radius of curvature than that of the adjacent surface of bone (Fig. 9-30). The greater convexity of the plate permits the application of a moderately uniform compressive force across the entire width of the fracture site. In either situation an exacting technique must be available to make precise angulations and torsional bends in the plate. A bending press is essential to produce a gentle bend in the plate (Fig. 9-31). While the plate is gripped in a bending press, it can be grasped with bending irons to twist the plate.

The recommendations on bending plates represent a considerable change of view from that

expressed in the previous edition.[36] Twenty years ago, onlay plates were manufactured of a rigid material, either of a stainless steel alloy or a cast cobalt-chromium alloy. The rigid material was difficult to deform with gradual bends. Frequently, sharp indentations were formed along the edges of the plate. With the combination of the work hardening at the acute bend and the sharp indentations or notches, the fatigue forces, to which the plate was exposed *in vivo*, were likely to provoke the propagation of a fatigue crack from the superficial notch (Fig. 9-32). With this knowledge, some authors[36] discouraged the bending of plates except where it was absolutely unavoidable. The presently available AO plates, of stainless steel possess a lower modulus of elasticity and tolerate gradual deformations.

With the combination of improved surgical alloys and tools for bending plates and of superior clinical methods for the application of plates

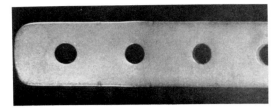

Figure 9-32. Cracks are apparent in the onlay plate at the site where it was deformed acutely with bending irons. (Reproduced with permission of C. O. Bechtol, A. B. Ferguson, Jr. and P. G. Laing.[37])

that require the surgeon to bend many, if not most, plates immediately prior to their application, the recommendations on the bending of plates have altered greatly. Highly deformable templates of the same dimensions as the AO plates are a prerequisite for the bending technique (Fig. 9-31). A template of appropriate length is applied to the surface of the bone. It is readily deformed by hand to prepare a replica of the bony surface. The appropriate plate is secured in the bending press with the template held beside it. Finally, the plate is deformed to match the shape of the template. For the application of plates to highly curved surfaces, such as the proximal and distal tibia and the pelvis (Fig. 9-31) considerable practice is necessary before the bending technique is mastered. For sites of complex anatomical contour of bone, the DCP is unexcelled. It tolerates the complex contours, as well as the application of compression across adjacent fracture surfaces, including segmental fractures. The DCP also permits the insertion of lag screws obliquely across spiral or oblique fractures.

Where a fracture is comminuted, interfragmentary compression with lag screws is the foremost method of stabilization. Frequently, a segment of bone stabilized by lag screws cannot adequately withstand bending movements and torsional shearing forces. The screw fixation should, therefore, be protected by the application of a plate which is not under tension. When a plate is simply applied to a fracture without the use of supplementary compression, it is called a neutralization (or protection) plate. It neutralizes the comminuted segment that was previously stabilized with interfragmentary compression. It conducts forces from one main bone fragment to the other main fragment while primary bone healing occurs. For most applications of neutralization, a DCP is employed.

In certain instances a neutralization plate can be placed under tension. This apparent contradiction is associated with the somewhat imprecise meaning which the AO group has attached to the word "neutralization". It is a recurrent source of confusion to surgeons unfamiliar with the AO method. Figure 9-30*A* shows a plate placed under tension without the use of a tension device and without eccentric placement of drill holes. The plate is contoured so that its central portion is 1 mm away from the surface of adjacent bone. When the screws are tightened, as on this butterfly fracture in which the two main fragments previously have been stabilized with lag screws, axial compression is applied to the transverse component of the fracture. This technique is applicable *only* for comminuted fractures that possess transverse elements. If the fracture is oblique, the application of this technique provokes angulation. If the same butterfly fracture with a transverse component exists in a straight bone, the plate is contoured with a minor convexity at the fracture. The plate is attached to the bone with one screw close to the fracture line. This screw is tightened until the plate approximates the bone. The plate is now placed under tension by the use of the tension device on the opposite side of the fracture from the first screw. The rigidity of the fixation is, hereby, greatly augmented.

The T-plate. The T-plate may provide an unsurpassed buttress for difficult fractures of the anatomical or surgical neck of the humerus (Fig. 9-33), the distal radius or for the tibial plateau (Fig. 9-34). It should be applied with the tension device and with cancellous screws in the segments of cancellous bone. If the cancellous bone at the fracture site is compressed from the initial injury so that a void is present, the void must be filled with cancellous bone graft to restore a continuous column of bone, which can be stabilized by interfragmentary compression. One example is a typical tibial plateau fracture in which the medial cortex or metaphysis has been comminuted. Unless the defect in the comminuted region is filled with bone graft, the healing process will be complicated by the appearance of a varus deformity. Even in the presence of a buttress plate, such an ungrafted plateau fracture would possess substantial bending moments; ultimately fatigue failure of the plate would occur. The plate is of satisfactory tensile strength for stabilization of a fracture with interfragmental compression. The anatomical constraints on the thickness of the plate preclude its tolerance of large bending, torsional or shearing forces. Alternatively for certain tibial plateau fractures,

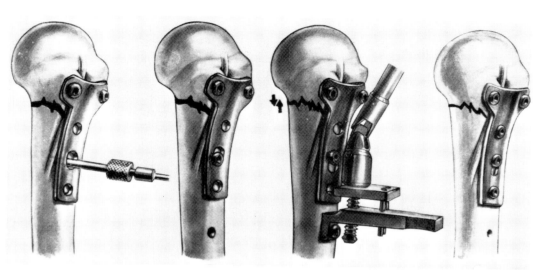

Figure 9-33. Schematic diagrams illustrate the method of application of a T- or buttress plate to a proximal humeral fracture. (Reproduced with permission of M. E. Müller, M. Allgöwer and H. Willenegger.[34])

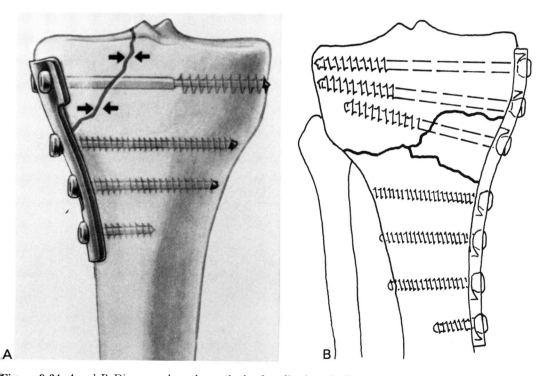

A

B

Figure 9-34. *A* and *B*. Diagrams show the methods of application of a T-plate and of a dynamic compression plate respectively to buttress tibial plateau fractures. (*A* and *B* reproduced with permission of M. Allgöwer, P. Matter, S. M. Perren and T. Rüedi.[35])

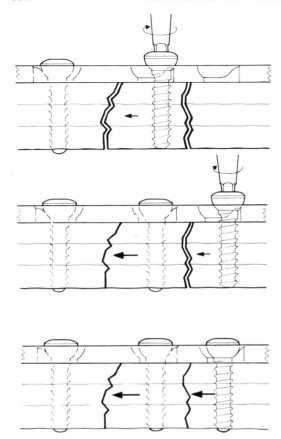

Figure 9-35. A dynamic compression plate is applied to a segmental fracture. The diagrams show how the plate may be used to compress one and subsequently the other fracture. (Reproduced with permission of Synthes Ltd., U.S.A.).

the DCP may provide the optimal form of buttress (Fig. 9-34B).

The Application of Plates to Comminuted Fractures and Other Unstable Fractures

For these complex fractures supplementary screw fixation must be applied prior to plating so that bending and torsional forces may be neutralized. Otherwise, miscroscopic motion between the fragments is inevitable. With motion, bone resorption, delayed union and eventually fatigue fracture of the plate are likely to follow. Again, where the integrity of the cortex has been breached, a bone graft should be applied. For segmental fractures, the DCP is particularly valuable. It permits the simultaneous compression of each fracture to lessen considerably the otherwise high risk of development of a nonunion at one site (Fig. 9-35).

The Use of Nail-plate and Blade-plate Assemblies in Cancellous Bone

The provision of stable fixation in the cancellous portions of weight-bearing bones has been one of the greatest challenges in fracture treatment. The classic problems are fractures of the proximal and the distal femur and the proximal tibia. First the biomechanics of the fractures and available instrumentation will be described. In Chapter 10, the clinical approach to the treatment of these fractures is given.

The Biomechanics of Stabilization in Weight-bearing Cancellous Bone. For the fixation of weight-bearing cancellous bone the central problem is stabilization of the fragments in the mechanically weak trabecular bone, which is frequently further compromised by the trauma and by senile osteoporosis. Ideally, a large surface area of implant should contact the cancellous bone to provide a large interface with low force per unit area. The area of the implant, however, is limited severely both by anatomical considerations of the size of available bone stock and by the location of certain vital intramedullary blood vessels. Both the fragile cancellous bone fragments and the stabilizing implant are liable to mechanical failure.

A precise account on the chronological development of hip nails is extremely difficult and it illustrates a much wider problem in the cataloging of progress. As Tronzo[38] relates, many of the inventions were never formally reported. Others are available in the files of patent offices but are not widely disseminated. In a letter which Watson-Jones sent to Tronzo, the former states that Hey-Groves used 4-flanged and 3-flanged nails in about 1906, approximately 30 years prior to the widely publicized "inventions" of the same devices by Smith-Petersen and McLaughlin.

In 1879 von Langenbeck[39] reported the first open reduction and internal fixation for a fractured hip. The first account of the use of a screw for fixation was published by Senn[40] in 1881. Subsequently a number of workers described a variety of crude procedures in which the use of wood screws or nails and bone grafts for femoral neck fractures were used. In view of the great risk of postoperative infection, and the highly corrosive nature of the implants, the common method of treatment remained the application of a body cast with the hip held in abduction and internal rotation, as taught by Whitman.[41]

In 1931 Smith-Petersen *et al.*[42] reported his experience with a precise anatomical approach to the hip, and the introduction of the triflanged stainless steel nail (Fig. 9-36). Johannson[38] ad-

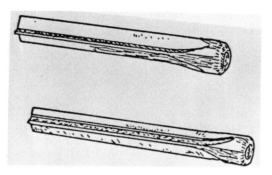

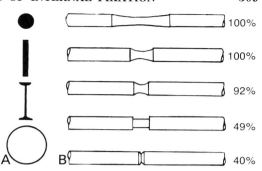

Figure 9-36. A schematic diagram shows the original Smith-Petersen nail (*top*) and the Johannson cannulated variety (*bottom*).

Figure 9-37. *A.* Diagram shows the relative strength of a solid bar, a simple beam, an I-beam and a cylinder all made of the same amount of material. If the cylinder is considered to be 100%, the resistance to bending of the solid bar in a vertical direction is 350%, the I-beam is 588%, and the cylinder is 533%. The cylinder, however, will resist bending uniformly well in any direction while the simple beam and the I-beam are weak in lateral bending. *B.* Schematic diagram shows a series of rods each with a notch of the same depth but of different shape and the strength of each rod. (Reproduced with permission of C. O. Bechtol, A. B. Ferguson, Jr. and P. G. Laing.[37]).

vised cannulation of the triflanged nail. With his technique, the fracture was reduced by the nonoperative Leadbetter maneuver. Then it was stabilized by the use of guide pins over which the cannulated nail was inserted. His "closed nailing" technique represented an attempt to reduce the incidence of nonunion and avascular necrosis by minimizing damage to local circulation.

While the innovation of the cannulated triflanged nail was one of the great advances in orthopaedic surgery, there remained a high incidence of failure of the procedure because of breakage of the nail or the surrounding bone. Such failures stimulated surgeons to devise an extraordinarily diverse group of implants.[38] The proliferation of devices attests to the difficulties of this surgery and to the modest degree of success that has been achieved by the application of any available implant. The principal criterion is the mechanical stabilization of the femoral head against the forces of shear and rotation with respect to the remainder of the femur. Frequently, union of the fracture is not achieved for 3 to 6 months; premature loosening or mechanical failure of the implant is apt to impede or prevent satisfactory healing. For stabilization, numerous types of nail cross-sections have been applied. The bending rigidity varies proportionately with the moment of the area of the section.[36] For equivalent cross-sectional areas, a tube, therefore, is more rigid than a solid rod (Fig. 9-37). While a tube would be the optimal design for mechanical criteria, it is excluded by anatomical considerations. For rectangular sections, rigidity is enhanced when the long side is parallel to the bending force, rather than perpendicular to it. The H-beam as proposed by Laing and O'Donnell[43] is the most rigid, although it is bulky.

In contrast to bending moments, rotational forces would not be stabilized by a circular cross-section which offers poor resistance to rotation. Radial rather than tangential surfaces are essential. With its three radial flanges, the classic Smith-Petersen nail provided considerable resistance to rotation.[28] Of the numerous other cross-sections, including the 4-flange, U, V, I and H, the last is superior in rotational stability. An alternative approach was undertaken by Deyerle,[44] who argues that greater resistance would be achieved by peripheral fixation rather than central fixation. He devised a series of ⅛-inch diameter pins which are inserted into the neck of the femur. The proximal parts of the pins are threaded while the distal parts are secured to a plate screwed to the shaft. Deyerle claims that with ideal positioning of seven pins, up to 20 times the resistance of a Smith-Petersen nail can be achieved. Deyerle's argument assumes a homogeneity of bone which is in marked contrast to the heterogenous, anisotropic structure of the human femoral neck.[45] With the great variation in bone structure, one or two pins are likely to assume most of the structural support and to encounter forces that are greater than their strength can resist. It has been argued, therefore, that the radial pins may fail like a "row of dominoes", as each pin, in turn, assumes the principal weight-bearing role, fails and thereby

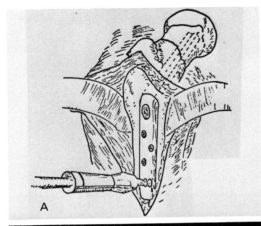

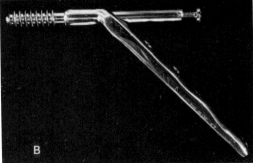

Figure 9-38. A schematic diagram shows a Jewett nail (*A*) and a photograph illustrates a Richards hip screw (*B*).

shifts that responsibility to another inadequate pin. In any event, the Deyerle device has not achieved wide popularity.

Another concept in the femoral neck fixation is the application of a large screw, as originally popularized by Lorenzo,[46] and more recently by Charnley, the Richard's Company[38] and others. During insertion, provisional rotary stability must be provided by additional pins. After insertion, the compression between the fragments induced by the lag technique appears to provide adequate rotation stability.

In clinical practice the refined models of tri-flanged nails have shown adequate strength and greatest popularity among American surgeons. Most designs have a central cannulation so that a preliminary wire of small diameter can be inserted and X-rayed to confirm correct alignment of the fracture and position of the wire before a large amount of bone is disrupted by the insertion of the nail. Presently available nails of AISI 316 stainless steel, cobalt-chromium alloys and titanium, appear to show a low incidence of fracture, considerably less than 1%. Corrosion is limited to crevice corrosion of the

stainless steel and the cobalt-chromium alloys and is of no apparent clinical significance. Where breakage occurs it usually involves fatigue failure and is almost invariably attributable to a technical error by the surgeon when he fails to achieve a mechanically stable reduction of the fracture, especially of the strong medial buttress of the femoral neck and proximal femoral shaft, called the calcar. A recent review by Sönstegard *et al.*[47] confirms that two of the most popular fixation devices, the Jewett nail and the Richard's compression screw (Fig. 9-38) provide adequate biomechanical stability if the surgeon achieves continuity of the principal fracture fragments.

In North America and Great Britain the "closed pinning" of fractured hips remains the most popular method of operative treatment.[48] It is a more rapid surgical procedure than open reduction with internal fixation especially with the use of image intensification, and it does lessen the magnitude of operative exposure. There is, however, no evidence to show that the preservation of the intact capsule of the hip reduces the incidence of nonunion, avascular necrosis or wound infection.

The concept of "closed pinning" has been strongly criticized by the AO group[33] who maintain that many comminuted and unstable fractures of the hip joint are not recognized and adequately stabilized by surgeons who perform the "closed technique". The AO group recommend a precise open reduction and stable osseous reconstruction so that the role of the hip nail is lessened to that of an ancillary stabilizing and aligning device. A glance at the evolution of the hip nails used by advocates of the "closed" and "open" techniques reveals the marked difference in the structural demands on the relevant devices. To avoid breakage of implants after closed reduction, where a minute amount of motion at the fracture is likely to occur, progressively larger devices, such as the heavy duty version of Jewett nail[38] and the Holt[49] and Sampson nails have evolved. Alternatively, after open reduction with precise reconstruction of the fracture, the smaller AO nail plates are adequate. Nevertheless, the larger implants, such as the Jewett nail, permit a margin of technical error by the surgeon who fails to attain an accurate reduction that is not provided by the comparable AO hip nails.

Penetration of the Nail. One of the most persistent problems with the use of nails has been penetration of the nail through the femoral head and into or across the hip joint. With a sharp cutting edge located on the proximal tip of the nail, advancement of the nail into the osteoporotic bone of the typical geriatric bone is not surprising. Penetration occurs because most nails are secured to a plate; with impaction of the femoral neck during postoperative weight bearing, the femoral neck shortens. To prevent this provocation of hip pain, stiffness and premature onset of arthritis, nails have been devised by Massie,[50] Pugh[51] and the Richards Company and others,[38] which slide out of the femoral neck during impaction. Not only do sliding nails prevent penetration of the femoral articular surface, they also encourage impaction to assist the healing process.

The Nail-plate Junction. It is rare for femoral neck fractures to be treated solely by a nail. Usually the nail is attached to a plate which is secured to the shaft of the femur to provide additional stability. Design considerations of the plate are the same as those discussed previously for onlay plates. The site of attachment of the nail to the plate is the crucial feature of the implant in regard to strength and stability. Early attempts to secure a triflanged nail to a side plate with nuts and bolts failed, frequently by loosening, mechanical failure or corrosion. Subsequent designs incorporated washers, counterthreaded lock screws and other interfaces which provided several undesirable stress concentrations as sites of weakness and numerous crevices with predisposition to corrosion. Also, as the assembly grew in size, painful bursitis, superficial to the nail-plate junction, became a frequent complaint by the patients. A variety of implants with the nail welded to the plate, therefore, were devised. Initially, weld or bulk metal failure at the junction was not uncommon in the 1-piece nail plates despite the superiority of their stress distribution.[52] Also, a welded assembly is necessarily of a fixed angle, which makes introduction of the nail more difficult and greatly restricts the surgeon's ability to make last minute minor adjustments in reduction or positioning of the fracture fragments.[53, 54] Furthermore, it requires the hospital storeroom to stock implants with a wide variety of nail-plate angles as well as various lengths of nail and plate.

Despite improvements in design, both 1-piece and 2-piece designs have limitations. For presently available 1-piece configurations, such as the Jewett nail, strength is adequate provided that mechanical stability of the fracture fragments is achieved.[47] The other limitations of the 1-piece design, however, are unchanged. Many of the 2-piece designs continue to show poor

engineering considerations. In particular, the features of the assembly that permit the nail to be secured in any desired position within a slot in the plate predispose to stress concentrations (Fig. 9-39). In the author's opinion, the Richards compression hip screw is the best compromise for the provision of mechanical stability and versatility (Fig. 9-38B). This unique design embodies a tube welded to the side plate, of fixed angle. A screw replaces the conventional nail and enables the surgeon to apply compression to the fracture fragments. The screw slides in a grooved track in the plate assembly which permits spontaneous impaction. In addition to sound engineering design, the implant is supplied with several tools for insertion which show equally good features of design.

Despite intense clinical research, treatment of fractures of the femoral neck remains a great problem. Indeed, statistics on the rate of nonunion of the fractures have shown little improvement over the past 40 years. In certain fractures, especially with severe comminution and osteoporosis of the femoral neck, primary replacement of the femoral head and neck with an implant may be the preferred treatment.[55, 56] Another frequent complication of femoral neck fractures in the elderly is the death of the proximal femoral head fragment, or avascular necrosis.[50, 57] Other continuing problems, especially in institutional geriatric patients, are postoperative wound infections,[58, 59] anesthetic complications[60] and thromboembolism.[61] The alternative mode of treatment for femoral neck fractures, prosthetic femoral head replacement, has not provided the outstanding results that were anticipated. Rates of wound infections are high[62, 63] (*e.g.,* up to 40% in some series of geriatric patients), and the prosthesis may loosen or provoke excessive wear of the opposing acetabular articular cartilage. Also, in nonambulatory institutional patients who sit continually with marked flexion of hips and knees, late postoperative, and usually irreducible, dislocation of the prosthesis is not uncommon.

When femoral neck fractures also involve the adjacent subtrochanteric region, then the altered biomechanical characteristics of the region may dictate the need for larger fixation devices, often of a unique design.[64, 65] The Zickel device incorporates an intramedullary femoral nail with a second nail in the femoral neck and head which slides through a hole in the former nail (Fig. 9-40A). It is inserted without difficulty and provides excellent stability for most simple subtrochanteric fractures. More recently the Sampson

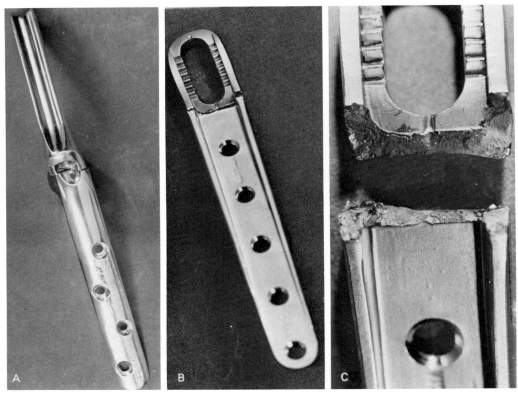

Figure 9-39. Photographs illustrate two failed hip nails. *A.* A device is shown that has failed in the slot of the plate while in *B* and *C*, the device that has failed near the slot is shown. (Reproduced with permission of C. O. Bechtol, A. B. Ferguson, Jr. and P. G. Laing.[37])

Corporation has marketed a strong fluted rod for use with subtrochanteric fractures that would appear to be highly satisfactory (Fig. 9-40*B*).

Osteotomy, or surgical fracture of the proximal femur, is a widely performed procedure both for the treatment of early arthritis of the hip[33, 66] and for realignment of traumatic deformity. There are also numerous applications in children, including certain clinical stages of congenital dislocation of the hips, Perthes' disease and slipped capital femoral epiphysis.[67, 68] In addition to the application of the appliances previously described, a variety of novel implants have been designed. In many of these procedures, the shaft of the femur is displaced medially with respect to the femoral neck and head at the site of division. The complex geometry renders fixation difficult. Two widely used implants embody markedly different features of design (Fig. 9-41). One device of historic interest, the Wainwright spline,[69] provides a straight blade plate or spline of simple design, in which the blade is inserted into the inferior surface of the greater trochan-

ter, through the osteotomy site. In contrast, the angled nail plates of Müller and Harris (Fig. 9-41) incorporate rather complex shape, and certainly an imaginative mechanical design.[33, 70] After the application of compression with an AO removable compressor on the distal end of the plate, rigid stabilization is achieved.

The Use of Intramedullary Nails

Intramedullary nail fixation, especially for the fractured femur, has achieved a secure position in the management of fractures. This is not surprising when the theoretical superiority of this form of fixation for shaft fractures, in respect to bending forces, is considered. In their work on the tibia, Lawrence *et al.*[29] report that the bending moment required to produce an angular deflection of 5° in a fixed tibia is 50 newton-meters with a 13-mm intramedulary nail compared to 8, 17 and 22 newton-meters respectively in the same onlay plates. The attested clinical success of intramedullary nails indicates that torsion is unlikely to be significant for unstable simple fractures near the midshaft of long bones.

Two types of large intramedullary nails have emerged. The first was designed by Küntscher,[71] who used a flexible, hollow stainless steel tube of clover-leaf cross-section. More recently, a variety of solid rigid nails have become available. The markedly dissimilar biomechanical concepts which these two types of nail employ, are described in turn.

The clover-leaf nail provides rigid fixation in bone by a novel technique which Küntscher likens to the elastic compression that retains a carpenter's nail in a piece of wood (Fig. 9-42). Whereas the carpenter's nail achieves rigidity by the elastic compression of the wood, the clover-leaf nail achieves stability by its own elastic compression. With the inevitable micromotion between the nail and the bone, resorption of bone ensues. Stability is maintained, however, both because of the elastic recoil of the nail and because of the conformity of the shape of the nail to that of the intramedullary cavity. Other features of the nail are a wedge-shaped tip to achieve effective compression and a proximal notch to permit extraction of the nail by engagement with a hook-shaped extractor.

The AO group has undertaken minor adaptations of Küntscher's design.[73] Extraction and insertion are achieved by threaded adaptors, which is a considerable improvement. The nail is more elastic and is curved to conform to the physiological anterior bow of the femur. It possesses an anterior longitudinal slit, instead of its predecessor's posterior slit, to prevent jamming of the nail during insertion. It also possesses several small slits which permit the insertion of small nails or screws to augment rotational stability of the fracture. The distal end of the nail shows a convex anterior curvature so that it does not bite into the cortex during insertion.[74]

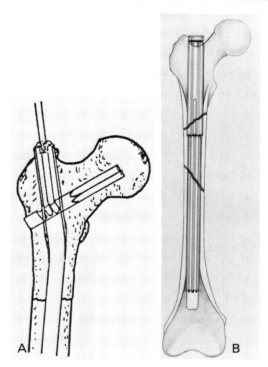

Figure 9-40. *A.* Schematic diagram shows a Zickel nail. *B.* Schematic diagram shows a Sampson subtrochanteric fluted nail.

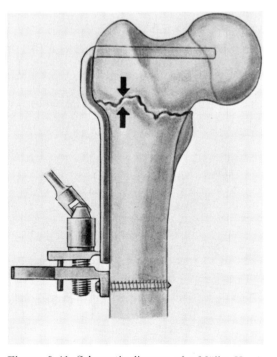

Figure 9-41. Schematic diagram of a Müller-Harris nail plate applied with tension device.

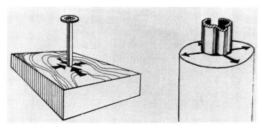

Figure 9-42. Schematic diagram shows the method by which an intramedullary nail anchors the surrounding bone in an analgous way to the fixation of a nail in a block of wood. (Reproduced with permission of G. Küntscher.[72])

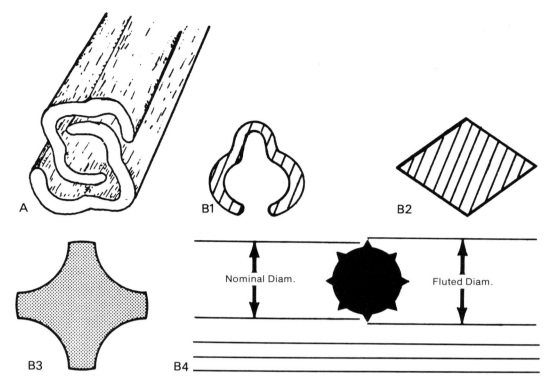

Figure 9-43. *A.* A schematic view shows two "stacked" or "nested" Küntscher nails. *B.* Diagram shows the cross-sectional shape of a variety of intramedullary nails: (*1*) Küntscher or "clover leaf"; (*2*) Hansen-Street or "diamond"; (*3*) Schneider; and (*4*) Sampson fluted intramedullary nail system, upper extremity series titanium fluted nails (type Ti-6 Al-4V; ASTM F-136).

Reaming

Küntscher, himself, emphasized the need for reaming the intramedullary cavity prior to insertion of the nail. Reaming provides a way to enlarge the narrowest portions of the bone so that an approximately cylindrical cavity is available to receive the largest diameter of nail for a given diameter of cavity. Additional reaming permits the insertion of a nail that is still larger in diameter and correspondingly stronger. If one compares the bending strength of the intramedullary nail and the intact femur or tibia, where the strength of the intact bone is definite as 100%, nails of the following diameters provide a bending strength as shown below*:

Diameter of nail	9 mm	11 mm	13 mm	15 mm
Bending strength (% of intact bone)	7%	15%	30%	50%

The comparable bending strength provided

by one AO broad plate is about 15% of that of an intact long bone. The figures indicate the value of reaming and the application of the largest diameter of nail if stable fixation is desired. Excessive reaming is a considerable hazard, however, if the guidelines expressed in Chapter 10 are not carefully followed.

Another method for effective enlargement of the size of a clover-leaf type nail is to interlock, or "stack" two nails (Fig. 9-43A) and insert them simultaneously.[75] Charts are available which tabulate the largest outside diameter of different sized nails in various combinations. The charts also state the appropriate size of reamer to be used. If a surgeon possesses a complete set of nails of different diameters, he should insert one large nail rather than two stacked nails of lesser diameters.

Several types of the solid nails are available. Their cross-sectional configurations are shown in Figure 9-43B. Both the design by Schneider[76] and the diamond-shaped nail by Hansen and Street[77] possess self-cutting broaches to obviate the technical difficulties of intramedullary ream-

---

* F. Straumann and O. Pöhler, personal communication, 1977.

Table 9-3

Comparison of the Relative Torsional and Bending Strengths of the Intact Femur and an Appropriate Size of Closed- or Open-section Intramedullary Nail

Specimen	Torsional rigidity (per unit length)	Bending strength[a]
Average femoral shaft	$2.0 \pm 0.5 \times 10^5$ kg cm^2	780 to 880 kg cm
Clover-leaf nail (open-section)	1.6×10^3 kg cm^2	290 to 350 kg cm
Diamond-section nail (closed-section)	1.2×10^4 kg cm^2	210 kg cm[b]
		250 kg cm[c]
Schneider nail	1.5×10^4 kg cm^2	285 to 400 kg cm
Sampson fluted nail	4.8×10^4 kg cm^2	700 to 900 kg cm

[a] Bending strength is defined as the moment required to produce permanent deformation.
[b] The bending axis is through the long diagonal.
[c] The bending axis is through the short diagonal.

ing. The solid nails are much more rigid than the clover-leaf design; for example, the diamond-shape design is about 7 times stiffer than the clover-leaf nail.

Frankel and Burstein[78] have published a comparison between the torsional rigidity and the bending strength of the intact human femur and an appropriate size of closed- or open-section intramedullary nail (Table 9-3). The open-section nail is about 1/100 as rigid as the bone. The closed-section nails are 10 times more rigid than the open-sectioned nails and about 1/10 as rigid as the bone which they support. In bending, the weight-bearing load is readily transmitted to the nail so that the bending strength of the system is comparable to that of the nail itself. The nature of the cross-section of the nail and especially the area moment of inertia determines the strength of the system in any particular bending direction. In bending strength the closed- or open-sectioned nails are 1/4 to 1/2 as strong as the intact femoral shaft. In compressive loading the bone itself bears most of the load and the nail provides geometric alignment.

In fact, extreme rigidity of a nail is probably a disadvantage during the functional life of the implant when the rigidity provides "stress-protection" of the bone, which in turn provokes osteoporosis. It is certainly a disadvantage after union of the fracture occurs. As Frankel and Burstein[78] have emphasized, after union of bone the implant should possess comparable rigidity to that of bone, lest it assume the principal weight-bearing role. As previously mentioned, with the formidable fatigue conditions imposed upon the human femur, mechanical failure of a weight-bearing nail is extremely likely if it remains *in situ* for many years.

With advancing age the femur shows progression of the anterior bow. In the presence of various metabolic diseases such as Paget's dis-ease, marked anterior bow is frequently encountered.[79] Insertion of a straight rigid nail into the curved femur is likely to provoke further, often extensive, fracture of the bone. Recently, the Sampson Corporation has marketed a fluted design by Burstein which is available in straight and curved models of two radii of curvature. Before surgery, the appropriate nail is selected by scrutiny of lateral X-rays of the intact femur. The flutes provide superior rotatory stability to any previous nail. The nail is designed to be inserted into the femur after the intramedullary cavity has been reamed 0.5 mm larger in diameter than the outside diameter of the nail. After reaming, a fluted nail may be inserted to achieve a rigidity of the fractured bone which rivals that of the intact femoral shaft.

Intramedullary nails have also been designed for application to tibial fractures.[73, 80] The tibial nails show a proximal posterior curve to permit insertion of the nail through the anterior wall of the proximal tibia, distal to the knee joint. Rotatory stability is a much greater problem with tibial fractures than with comparable midshaft femoral fractures; additional modes of fixation may be required. Large intramedullary nails are not generally advised for treatment of shaft fractures in the upper extremity although a few workers have reported excellent results with them. Rotational stability has been difficult to achieve; also damage to the wrist, elbow and shoulder have been a frequent complication of the insertional procedure.[81] More recently a fluted nail has become available for treatment of these fractures, which provides excellent rotatory stabilization. The long-term results of clinical trials are eagerly awaited. In the author's limited experience, the fluted nails are difficult to insert into the radius and ulna.

Another concept in intramedullary nail fixation was provided by Rush[82] with his flexible

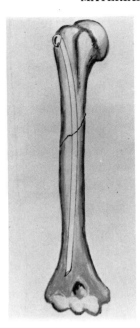

Figure 9-44. Schematic diagram illustrates the insertion of a Rush rod for treatment of a humeral shaft fracture. (Reproduced with permission from L. V. Rush.[83])

nail or rod, similar to Hackenthal's contribution in Europe. In 1938 Rush described a method of dynamic, 3-point fixation in which one or two resilient curved thin rods are introduced through small incisions into the intramedullary cavity of the fractured bone (Fig. 9-44). In 1968 he reported 30 years' experience with this method[84]; for the 190 closed fractures of the femoral shaft treated with his rods, he observed two instances of nonunion and no primary infections. Other workers[85] have not been able to duplicate his good results, especially for the treatment of the femur. Migration of the rod and unacceptable motion between the fracture fragments are frequent complications. The method remains in widespread application for immobilization of fractures of the distal fibula and the midshaft humerus, radius and ulna.

Condylocephalic Nail Fixation for Trochanteric Fractures of the Femur

The condylocephalic nail for the intramedullary fixation of trochanteric fractures of the femur was developed by Küntscher[86] who reported it in 1966. He modified a procedure originally conceived by Lezius and Herzer who used a short curved intramedullary nail that extended from the medial cortex of the superior third of the femoral shaft to the center of the femoral head. Küntscher's modifications lowered the operative risk by alteration of the wound on the midthigh to the medial femoral condyle. The condylocephalic nail has a clover-leaf cross-section of standard diameter 10 mm and lengths of about 34 to 44 cm. Recently, Herrero *et al.*[87] reported generally favorable results on nearly 500 cases. In a few instances spontaneous protrusion of the nail into the hip joint or under the skin of the knee occurred.

In a recent embodiment by Ender,[88] the closed insertion of multiple flexible intramedullary nails, under image intensification and with the patient positioned on a special operating table, has been developed for the treatment of proximal femoral fractures. The nails are inserted in the distal femur, usually in the region of the adductor tubercle (Fig. 9-45A). With the absence of significant tissue trauma or blood loss, and with its capacity to stabilize pertrochanteric and subtrochanteric fractures, the method appears to be particularly useful for application in the geriatric population. Ender suggests that the use of flexible nails provides a more favorable mechanical situation than does a nail-plate device because the former is situated a short distance from the compression vector of the femur (Fig. 9-45B). The points of the nails are dispersed in

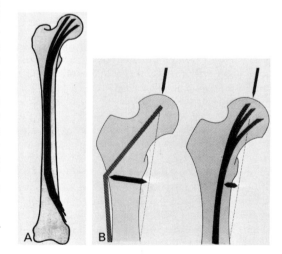

Figure 9-45. *A.* Schematic diagram illustrates the technique of insertion of an Ender's nail with reduction of an intertrochanteric fracture. *B.* Schematic diagram shows the biomechanical basis for fixation of an intertrochanteric fracture with an Ender's nail and a conventional nail plate device is shown.

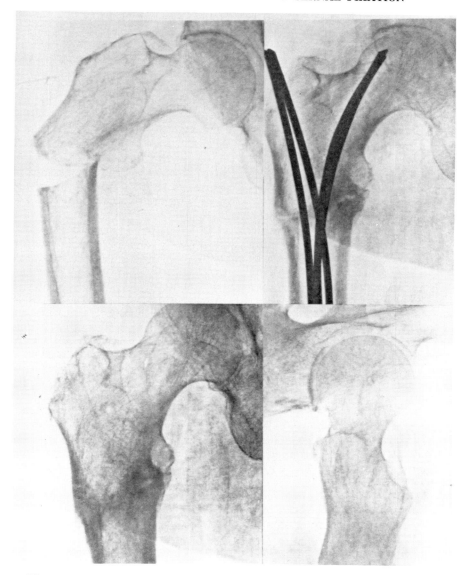

Figure 9-46. X-rays show an intertrochanteric fracture treated with an Ender's nail.

the cancellous region of the femoral head to provide firm fixation and rotational stability (Fig. 9-46). Upon weight bearing, the nails distribute the forces uniformly along the entire length of the lateral femoral cortex. Ender also suggests that the flexibility of the nails during their insertion permits manipulation of the impaled proximal femoral fragment to facilitate reduction of the fracture. His instructions for reduction of comminuted fractures should be studied thoroughly prior to the application of his technique.

The Biological Response of Bone to the Insertion of Intramedullary Nails

As mentioned in a previous section, the principal blood supply of long bones occurs *via* the intramedullary vessels, with a centrifugal distribution of blood to the periphery.[89, 90] Insertion of an intramedullary nail must be accompanied by a preliminary disruption of the primary blood supply of the bone. Many opponents of the intramedullary nail have argued strongly against the nail on the grounds of this iatrogenic trauma. More recently several workers, especially Rhinelander,[91] have studied the effect of insertion of intramedullary nails on the blood supply of long bones in experimental animals, particularly mature dogs. In the intact femur, about 65% of the blood supply of the shaft is derived from endosteal vessels in the intramedullary cavity. After a shaft fracture of the femur or tibia, the main intramedullary vessels may be undamaged from the trauma if the fracture does not show significant angular deformity. With marked angular deformity, significant intramedullary vascular damage is inevitable. Upon fracture, by mechanisms which remain unknown, hypertrophy of all the intraosseous vessels is initiated which is particularly prominent in the intramedullary diaphyseal vessels. If the intramedullary cavity is reamed immediately prior to insertion of the nail, the diaphyseal vessels are destroyed. Nevertheless, histological studies performed on specimens 1 week after surgery reveal the presence of newly formed medullary vessels. Two weeks after surgery, the vessels have spread to the fracture site. Six weeks after surgery the fracture has healed and the cortex is again nourished primarily by medullary vessels. The rapid restoration of the intramedullary blood supply after femoral reaming would appear to support the recommendation by the AO group, that the patient with an appropriate fracture of a femur or tibia should undergo insertion of an intramedullary nail as soon as his general medical condition permits. The previous suggestion by Charnley[92] that a delayed fixation enabled provisional revascularization of the bone fragments that shortened the total healing time, does not seem to be tenable.

If the intramedullary nail fails to provide adequate stability however, the histological picture is altered. The unstable sections of bone do not regain a good medullary vascular supply. If bacterial contamination should occur, the devascularized bone provides a nidus for infection. In summary, intramedullary reaming and insertion of a nail produce a temporary risk to the viability of adjacent bone, although the bone usually recovers completely and rapidly.

Technical Features of Intramedullary Nail Insertion

Two aspects of insertion merit further consideration. The first concerns the execution of nailing by open or closed techniques. As originally described by Küntscher, the femoral shaft fracture is reduced under X-ray control without open manipulation. Next a small incision is made over the greater trochanter and a guide wire is inserted with continuation of X-ray control. A flexible stainless steel reamer is inserted over the guide wire and the intramedullary cavity is enlarged. Then a nail of adequate length and diameter is carefully inserted. Böhler[93] and Clawson et al.[94] have presented extensive reviews of this method, in which infection rates of about 1.7% and a rate of union of 100% have been achieved. The liabilities of the method are the requirement of a special operating table, X-ray image intensification and considerable skill by the surgeon.[95] Where the fracture is comminuted, this technique becomes difficult or impossible. Also, during insertion of the nail, clinically invisible cracks may develop into displaced fractures. The technical problems of closed nailing are especially great for the treatment of tibial shaft fractures.

As an alternative, the open method of insertion is widely applied.[33] The fracture is approached and the fragments may be reamed, preferably as previously described, or alternatively, by the insertion of rigid reamers into the fracture ends. With or without reaming, the nail is inserted in a retrograde fashion into the proximal fragment. Its proximal end is brought through the skin at the greater trochanter until the distal end of the nail lies flush with the end of the proximal fragment. The fracture is reduced and the nail is advanced into the distal fragment until about 1 inch of nail remains exposed at the greater trochanter.

The advantages of the open technique include the ease and speed of reduction of the fracture and insertion of the nail, and the lack of requirement for special operating table or X-ray equipment. Also, under direct observation, insertion of the rod across the fracture site may be performed more safely and in the presence of minor comminution of the fracture ends. One considerable liability, however, may be a higher infection rate. In contrast to the closed method, open reduction is accompanied by infection rates in various series, that range between 2 and 10%. When either method is applied to open fractures, the infection rate increases further. When open reduction and insertion of the nail are performed within 48 hours after the time of injury it is greater than 10%.[96] Intramedullary nails, therefore, should not be inserted in fresh open fractures. The other major liability is that open reduction necessitates further damage to the periosteal blood supply of the fracture site as well as to the medullary vessels. Presumably the

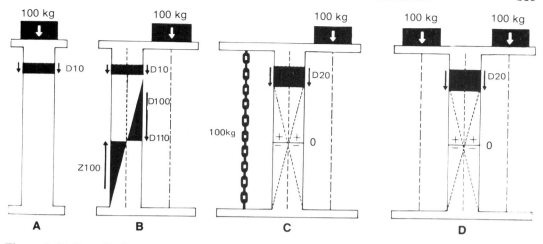

Figure 9-47. Pauwel's diagram illustrates the tension band principle. *A*, A column is loaded with a central weight so that only compressive stresses arise within the column (D = 10). *B*, When the weight is applied eccentrically a bending moment is introduced. This introduces additional compressive stresses (D = 100 and equal and opposite tensile stresses Z = 10). *C* and *D*, The additional bending stresses produced by eccentric loading are neutralized by use of a tension band, shown as a chain in *C*. The neutralization of the bending stresses could also be achieved by the application of a second weight (*D*) placed at an equal distance from the center of the axis of the column but on the opposite side. In either *C* or *D* the total stress is reduced to 20 kg/cm² because the bending stresses are completely neutralized. (Reproduced with permission of M. E. Müller, M. Allgöwer and H. Willenegger.[34])

extensive devascularization helps to explain the higher risk of infection observed in patients with open fractures.

The Application of Wire for Internal Fixation

Pauwels[97] was the first surgeon to employ surgical wire with the application of the tension band principle, borrowed from engineers. His diagram (Fig. 9-47) merits scrutiny so that the concept of tension band wiring is grasped. If a column is loaded so that a weight is positioned in its midaxis, then only compressive stress arises within the column (*e.g.*, stress D = 10). If the weight is applied eccentrically, then in addition to the same compressive stresses, a bending moment is introduced. This produces additional compressive stresses (D = 100) and equal and opposite tensile stresses (Z = 100). As in Figure 9-47*C*, the additional bending stresses provoked by eccentric loading can be neutralized by means of a tension band, which is represented diagrammatically by a chain. This neutralization of the bending stresses acts as if an additional compression were exerted by a second weight (Fig. 9-47*D*) placed at an equal distance from the center of the axis of the column, but on the opposite side. Although the load is increased (D = 200 kg) the total stress is reduced to a fifth

(20 kg/cm²) because the bending stresses are completely neutralized.

An example from Pauwels' work illustrates the clinical application of the tension band in internal fixation. If, as in Figure 9-48*A*, a cerclage wire is placed posteriorly to the center of the patella, then the fragments must open up anteriorly. If, however, the wire is placed anteriorly, as shown in *A'*, then tensile stress in the wire is converted into compressive stress at the fracture site. The same principles are observed when tension band wiring is utilized for fixation of fractures of the olecranon, greater trochanter and medial malleolus (Fig. 9-49). In these cases, Kirschner wires may be added to augment rotatory stability.

Another application of wire has been "cerclage" or circumferential stabilization of long bones (Fig. 9-50). For example, it may be used to control a butterfly fragment of a midshaft femoral fracture that is primarily stabilized by an intramedullary nail. Cerclage wiring has largely fallen into ill-repute because it was alleged to strangulate the periosteal blood supply and to lead to infarction of bone. A recent review by Böhler[98] suggests that the deleterious side-effects of cerclage wiring may be overstated. He believes that the avascular necrosis of bone associated with cerclage is due to excessive soft

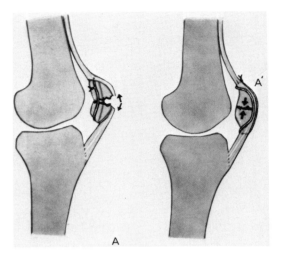

Figure 9-48. The use of a tension band wire in internal fixation of a patellar fracture is shown, as originally described by Pauwels. If a cerclage wire is placed posteriorly to the central axis of the patella the fragments separate anteriorly. If, however, the wire is placed anteriorly (A') the tensile stress in the wire is converted into a compressive stress at the fracture site. (Reproduced with permission of M. E. Müller, M. Allgöwer and H. Willenegger.[34])

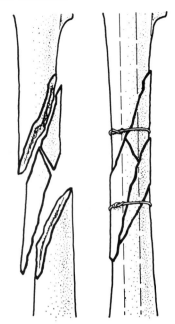

Figure 9-50. The application of a cerclage wire as supplementary fixation to a femoral shaft fracture treated with an intramedullary rod is shown.

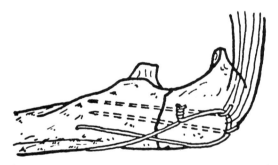

Figure 9-49. Schematic diagram illustrates the use of tension band wires for a fracture of the olecranon.

tissue stripping. He recommends the use of cerclage by itself, or in combination with an intramedullary nail for the treatment of spiral fractures of the tibia.

Schatzker* has emphasized that a moderately comminuted midshaft femoral fracture, treated by intramedullary nail fixation is best supplemented by an onlay plate. The plate is applied to the large posterior ridge, the linea aspera, so that the screws do not violate the intramedullary cavity and block the reamer or the nail. A DCP

* J. Schatzker, personal communication, 1977.

provides much better stabilization than a cerclage wire and it permits interfragmentary compression.

FAILURE OF IMPLANTS FOR INTERNAL FIXATION

In a useful review Schatzker[74] has described the common conditions which lead to implant failure. If the goal of rigid fixation is born in mind then the necessity for the presence of strong bone should be recalled. The application of a thick strong plate to reinforce an excessively osteoporotic bone will not provide a more satisfactory fixation than the application of a thin weak plate. Secondly, absolutely accurate anatomical reduction is essential to provide the transmission of primary weight-bearing forces through the column of bone across the fracture site. The goal should be the minimal transmission of force from bone to metal and again from metal to bone at the other side of the fracture. Figure 9-51 illustrates the ideal mechanical situation in the typical eccentrically loaded bone which has a tensile side and a side that is under compressive load. A tension band plate has been applied to the tensile side of the bone so that the fracture surfaces tend to separate on this side. Alternatively, on the compressive side of

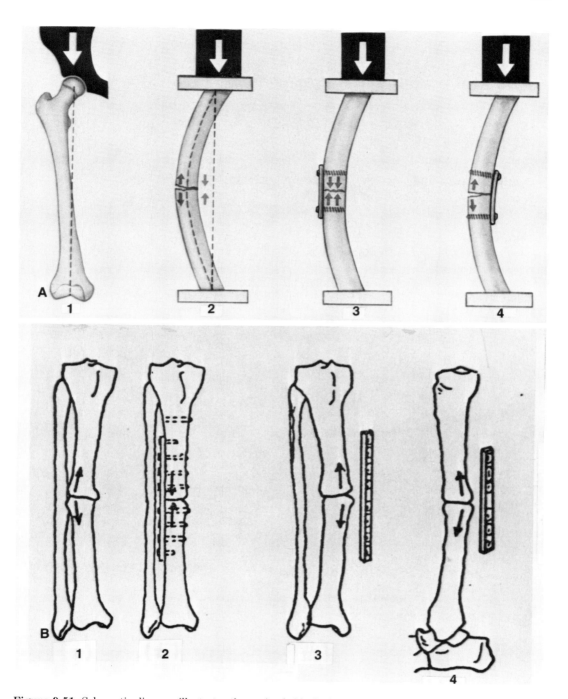

Figure 9-51. Schematic diagram illustrates the optimal side for location of a plate on the tensile side of the bone (*A*). In the intact musculoskeletal system the compression side of the bone is the one with the larger and more powerful muscle groups. At a site of a tibial nonunion (*B*), the tensile side possesses the convex aspect of the deformity.

the bone the fracture surfaces are approximated. The fulcrum is on the compressive side. By the application of greater load the bone is subjected to greater compressive forces across the fracture site. If, however, there is a minute defect of bone on the compressive side the application of initial load shifts the fulcrum to the plate. The gap in bone on its compressive side closes and the plate is subjected to bending forces. If the defect is minute the fulcrum rapidly shifts to the compressive cortex and the ideal situation is re-established. While metal has great resistance to tensile forces, it readily undergoes fatigue failure when subjected to cyclic bending elements. The third example shows predictable failure of the implant if there is no medial buttress of bone. In this instance the force is borne completely by the plate which is subject to large bending moments. With recurrent contractions of muscles, the dynamic load associated with weight bearing, the plate undergoes cyclic loading until fatigue failure ensues. The mechanical failure of a plate subjected to such an environment of fatigue forces is wholly predictable. When applied to the lower extremity conventional stainless steel plates will tolerate about 2 to 3 million cycles of loading before they undergo fatigue failure. Such surgical mistakes can be avoided if, at the time of surgery, a solid column of bone is restored on the surface or cortex opposite to the plate. The buttress of bone may be intact cortex, fracture fragments, or in the form of bone graft.

Some manufacturers have attempted to overcome this problem by the provision of thick onlay plates. There are several liabilities of such rigid plates, however. They provoke osteoporosis in the cortex directly beneath the plate with the so called "stress protection" phenomenon. When they are applied incorrectly so that a gap remains at the fracture site, they prevent apposition of bone and thereby establish conditions for a delay or nonunion. A few clinical examples are given below.

Mechanical failure of the over 40 types of internal fixation devices used in the proximal femur probably occurs more frequently than mechanical failure of devices that are applied to any other parts of the skeleton. Black[99] has classified the clinical failures into three principal categories: (1) Functional failures may occur in which the wrong device is used for a particular surgical problem. The device may be applied incorrectly; postoperative infection may necessitate premature removal; or inadequacies of postoperative management may provoke loosening or dislocation. (2) Material failures may

occur secondary to corrosion or to tissue reaction to corrosion or hypersensitivity. (3) True mechanical failures may be associated with errors in implant design. Also intra-operative deformation of the implant may occur so that the yield point of the material is exceeded and permanent change in shape and mechanical properties ensues. In his useful review Black[99] has tabulated the incidence of mechanical failures of hip fixation devices for a total of 1290 cases in which 77 mechanical failures occurred. The numbers of failure observed in various anatomical patterns of fractures are described in Table 9-4.

The individual cases in which failure occurred were further analyzed. Most of the failures occurred because the surgeon failed to achieve full stability of bone across the fracture site at the time of surgery. Subsequently, the early onset of weight bearing provoked excessive mechanical forces on the implant with ultimate mechanical failure. Other cases of implant corrosion and limitations of design were cited. More recently a study group at Carnegie-Mellon University[100] has confirmed these findings which further em-

Table 9-4

Clinical Incidences of Mechanical Failures of Hip Fixation Devices[a]

Type of fracture	Failure	Total
All cases	77	1290
Femoral neck	23	194
Intertrochanteric	33	814
Subtrochanteric	17	162
Other	4	130

[a] After Black[99].

Table 9-5

Failures after Internal Fixation and Their Causes

I. Instability—Main cause
    Inadequate implants
    Incorrect position of implants
    Insufficient bone support
        Inadequate interfragmentary compression
        Inadequate reduction
        Remaining defects
        Absence of cancellous bone graft
        Weak bone (*e.g.,* osteoporosis, osteomalacia *etc.*)
    Bone necrosis
    Inadequate postoperative treatment
II. Complications
    Local: Skin necrosis, wound infection
    General: *e.g.,* Thromboembolism

phasize that for presently available implants most of the mechanical failures occur secondary to technical failures at the time of surgery. Most failures represent examples of comminuted, unstable proximal femoral fractures in which the surgeon attempts a closed reduction and internal fixation in which the fracture fragments are not restored into appositional alignment with or without the use of supplementary bone graft.

A tabulation of failures of internal fixation by Willenegger amplifies the causes which are not directly related to the implant (Table 9-5). Avascular necrosis of bone secondary to faulty surgical technique, wound infections and thromboembolism are significant contributors to failures in which the implant cannot be directly implicated.

Clinical Examples of Failed Internal Fixation

One of the greatest contributions by recent collaborative efforts between mechanical engineers and orthopaedic surgeons has been an analysis of failed internal fixations. Perhaps the most effective study has been that organized through the AO Documentation Center and the Straumann Institute in Waldenburg, Switzerland.[4]

The first example, shown in Fig. 9-52, is a broken cancellous screw that was inserted across the highly mobile interface between the distal fibula and tibia. Fracture occurred 18 weeks after surgery during a postoperative course in which the patient remained fully weight bearing. In view of the well documented motion between the fibula and tibia, the mechanical failure could have been predicted and prevented by the application of a non-weight-bearing postoperative course for the patient.

In the second example, the application of a long DCP to a comminuted midshaft femoral fracture is shown in Figure 9-53. In the postoperative X-rays a gap at the fracture site on the medial femoral cortex opposite the plate is readily visible. As described previously the presence of such a gap indicates a strong likelihood that fatigue failure of the plate will ensue unless the surgeon alters his postoperative course. In the postoperative X-ray taken 4 weeks after surgery, enlargement of the gap is clearly visible. Even at this late date the surgeon still has the opportunity to alter the incipient failure of the plate. Either he may elect to provide some sort of external immobilization or he can drastically reduce the amount of activity and weight bearing by the patient. Alternatively, he can elect to

undertake a second operation for the application of bone graft to the gap or, by other means, eliminate it. Another possibility would be to revise the method of internal fixation. In the absence of such changes in management, failure of the plate was detected in the 7th postoperative week. At that time the surgeon reoperated and applied cancellous bone graft. Twelve weeks later radiological evidence of union was visible.

Figure 9-54 illustrates another example of unsatisfactory application of an onlay plate. A young woman of 21 years sustained an oblique distal tibial fracture which was initially treated by the application of a long leg cast. Three weeks later the surgeon elected to revise his management in view of the unstable nature of the fracture. He applied a 4-hole plate to the undisplaced fracture without provision of an anatomical reduction. The postoperative X-rays reveal evidence of faulty application of internal fixation. The plate is of inadequate length and it is malpositioned. It has not been contoured to approximate the surface of bone. The fracture has not been reduced and a gap is visible at the fracture site on the opposite cortex from the implant. Bending moments imposed upon the plate are likely to provoke mechanical failure of the implant. In the race to achieve union of the fracture, failure of the plate is likely to win because the fracture surfaces are distracted by the implant. When the surgeon recognized his error he elected to apply a long leg cast to the extremity. The patient developed a nonunion which required further surgical intervention. By this time the patient had been subjected to the liabilities associated with a cast and to those associated with internal fixation.

In Figure 9-55, a pertrochanteric fracture in a woman of 65 who was treated by the application of an H-beam nail and McLaughlin side plate is shown. Close scrutiny of the postoperative X-rays reveals evidence of a gap at the fracture site which is particularly noticeable on the lateral view at the region of the lesser trochanter. Three months later radiological evidence of fracture of the retaining screw was visible. The proximal femur had shifted into a varus malalignment. The subsequent X-ray shows a postoperative view after surgical revision when a Richards screw device was applied and the implant was realigned into a valgus position. Unfortunately the lateral X-ray continues to show poor apposition of bone in the region of the lesser trochanter. At this stage the surgeon elected to apply a hip spica cast to prevent the likelihood of further "failure of the implant". The second surgical

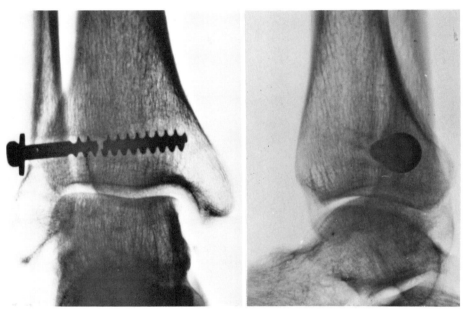

Figure 9-52. Two X-rays show a broken cancellous bone screw 18 weeks after surgery. (Reproduced with permission of Miss O. Pöhler.)

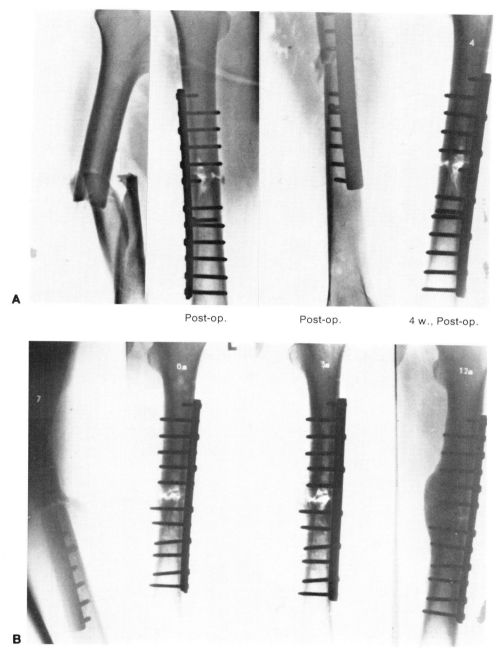

Post-op.   Post-op.   4 w., Post-op.

Figure 9-53. A series of X-rays shows a femoral fracture treated with a dynamic compression plate. *A.* The postoperative X-ray reveals evidence of a gap on the cortex opposite the plate. In an X-ray taken 4 weeks after surgery the gap has widened. *B.* Seven weeks after surgery an X-ray shows the broken plate. At that time a new plate was applied with the application of cancellous bone graft. Three weeks after the second operation the cancellous bone has begun to consolidate while 12 weeks after the second procedure the fracture has healed. (Reproduced with permission of Miss O. Pöhler.)

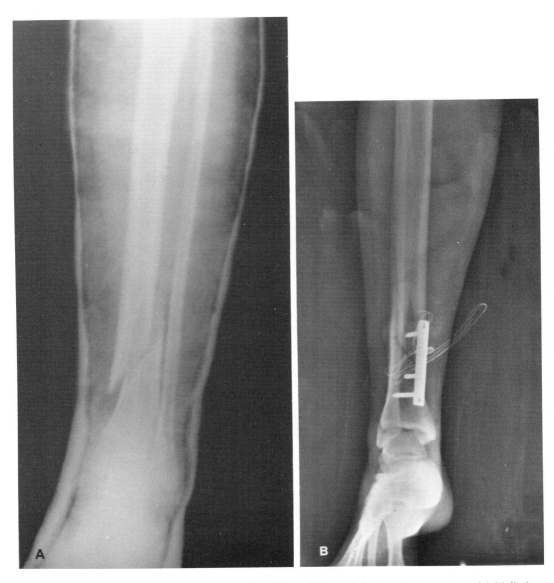

Figure 9-54. A series of X-rays show an unstable oblique tibial shaft fracture that was treated initially by a long leg cast (*A* and *B*). Four weeks later the surgeon elected to operate. Postoperative X-rays show poor reduction of the fracture with inadequate screw fixation (*C* and *D*). In the absence of supplementary external fixation and limitation of weight bearing by the patient, fracture of the plate is extremely likely. Even if the appropriate restrictions in activity and supplementary immobilization are undertaken a delayed union or nonunion is likely because the plate distracts the fracture surfaces.

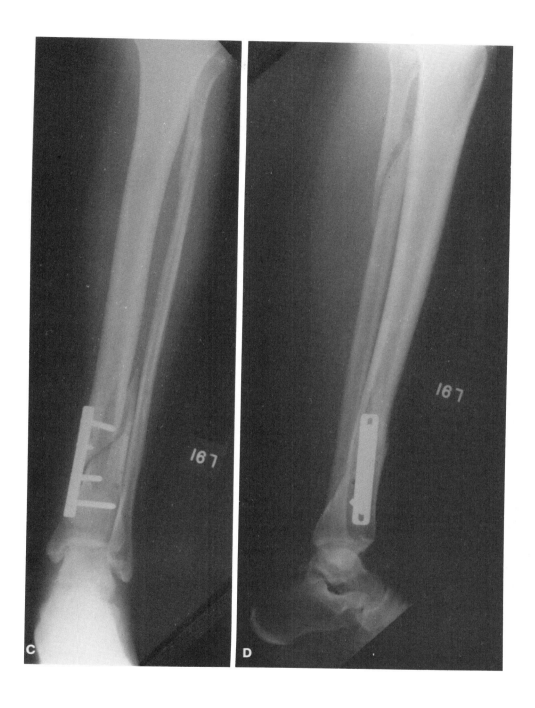

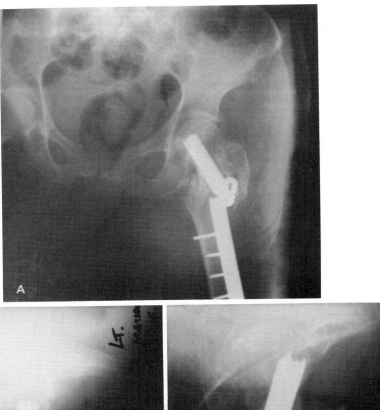

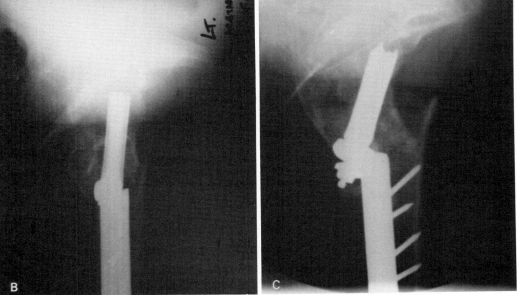

Figure 9-55. The treatment of a comminuted pertrochanteric fracture by two unsuccessful attempts at internal fixation is shown. The initial postoperative anterior-posterior X-ray seems to show adequate reduction and restoration of a column of bone at the fracture (A). On the lateral X-ray, however, a large posterior defect is evident at the fracture site (B). An X-ray taken 6 weeks later shows that the retaining screw has loosened (C). Twelve weeks after surgery an X-ray reveals separation of the nail plate device and varus deformity of the fracture with nonunion (D). At reoperation another attempt is made to perform a stable valgus nailing but postoperative X-rays show a similar posterior defect (E and F). At this stage the surgeon elected to treat the patient with the use of a hip spica cast.

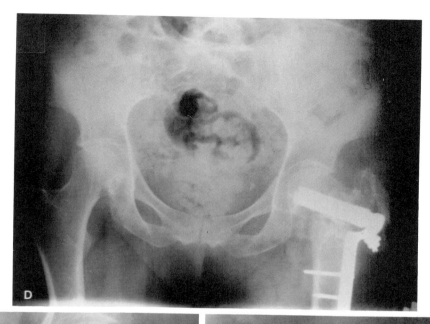

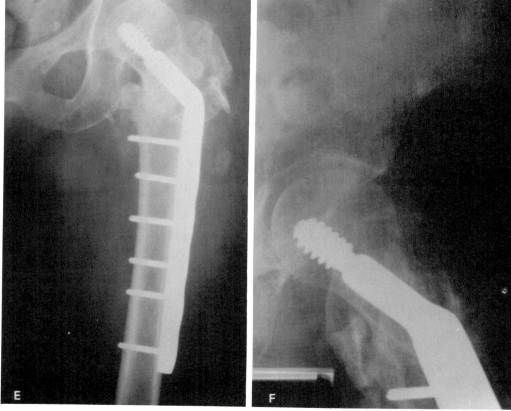

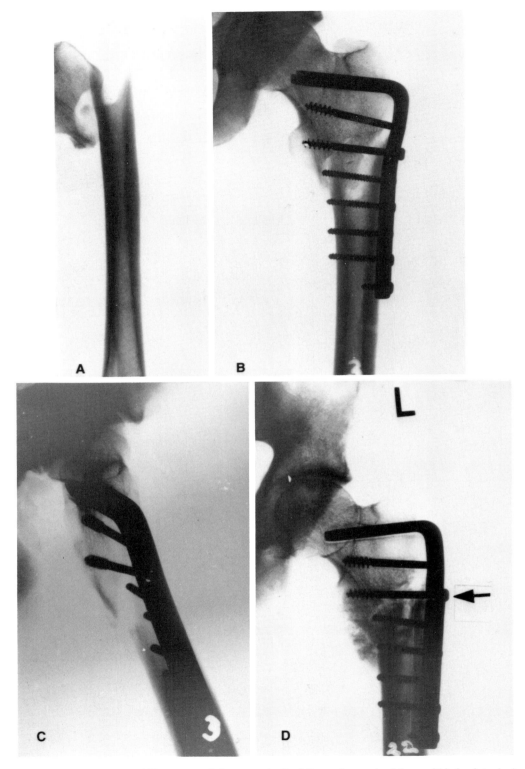

Figure 9-56. *A–D.* A series of X-rays reveal the stages in the failure of a proximal femoral blade plate device. A comminuted oblique subtrochanteric fracture is treated with internal fixation. X-rays taken 3 weeks after surgery reveal the presence of a large gap at the fracture site. Twenty-two weeks after surgery X-rays reveal the presence of a fractured plate at the site of the second screw hole. A radiolucent linear defect in the proximal fragment immediately under the blade in the femoral head reveals evidence of motion of the metal within the bone. (Reproduced with permission from Miss O. Pöhler.)

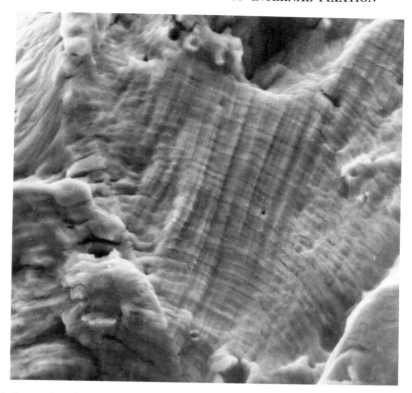

Figure 9-57. A scanning electron micrograph shows the fatigue fracture surface with striations of the broken implant shown in Figure 9-56. The implant is made of 316 L stainless steel. (× 2200) (Reproduced with permission of Miss O. Pöhler.)

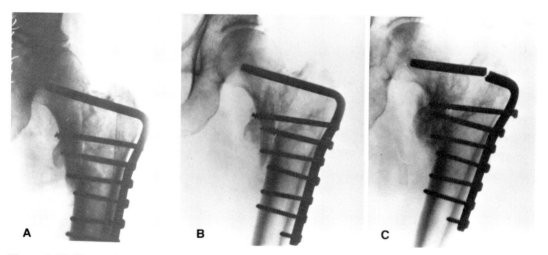

A   B   C

Figure 9-58. X-rays show a highly unstable fracture of the base of the femoral neck treated with a blade plate device. In the postoperative X-ray (A) and another X-ray taken 9 weeks after surgery (B), a large gap is observed in the crucial weight-bearing region at the base of the femoral neck. Also the latter X-ray shows deformation of the first screw. In a third X-ray taken 20 weeks after surgery fracture of the blade is evident (C). (Reproduced with permission of Miss O. Pöhler.)

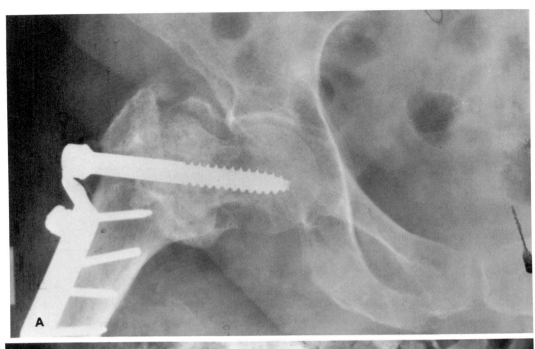

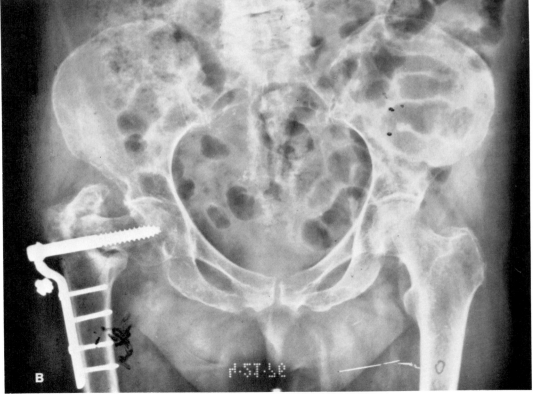

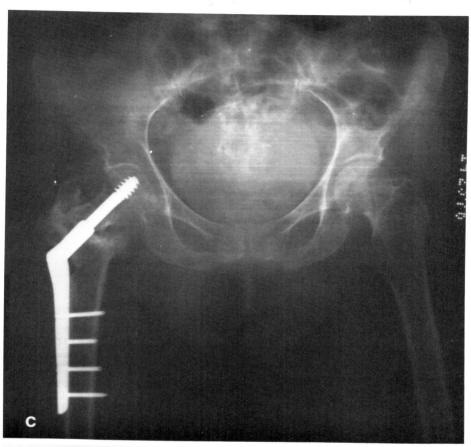

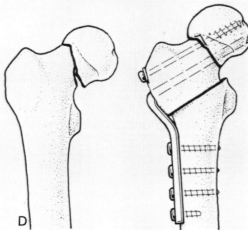

Figure 9-59. Another radiological example of an unstable Pauwel's type III fracture of the femoral neck treated with internal fixation is shown (*A*). The surgeon did not achieve a stable reduction in the initial surgery. With the large bending moments to which the Lorenzo screw is subjected, failure of the device can be predicted unless changes in early postoperative management are made. The second X-ray reveals evidence of failure of the device with marked varus deformity of the femoral head (*B*). In the third X-ray surgical revision has been performed (*C*). A valgus osteotomy is visible in the intertrochanteric region. Now the fracture site has been converted into a relatively stable geometry where it is immobilized with a Richards screw device. The osteotomy is shown schematically in *D*. (*D* Reproduced with permission from M. E. Müller, M. Allgöwer, and H. Willenegger.)

procedure might have had a more favorable outcome if cancellous bone graft had been applied to the region of the lesser trochanter to restore a continuous column of bone.

Figure 9-56 shows the series of X-rays in which a comminuted oblique subtrochanteric fracture was treated by the application of a blade plate device. Two X-rays taken 3 weeks after surgery reveal evidence of marked distraction at the fracture site which is particularly apparent on the oblique view. At 22 weeks fracture of the plate was evident at a screw hole. Figure 9-57, a scanning electron micrograph of the broken implant, shows the surface of the fatigue fracture with the characteristic striations. When the distraction of the fracture became visible in the postoperative film, alteration of the previous postoperative plan was essential if this clinical failure, attributed to an implant, was to be prevented. At the time of recognition, reoperation with reduction of the fracture site and possibly with the application of bone graft should have been undertaken. Otherwise this surgical error was highly predictable.

In Figure 9-58, a highly unstable, vertical fracture of the femoral neck was treated by the application of a blade-plate device. In the postoperative X-ray the unstable reduction is readily apparent which provokes large shearing forces on the screws and bending moments on the blade. In an X-ray taken 9 weeks after surgery, distraction of the inferior aspect of the fracture fragments is readily apparent. At this time the surgeon can prevent the otherwise anticipated mechanical failure if surgical intervention is undertaken to realign the proximal fracture fragment in a valgus configuration. Figure 9-59 shows radiological views and a schematic illustration of a similar subcapital fracture and vertical neck fracture (Pauwels type III) in which a 30° trochanteric valgus osteotomy has been performed. The osteotomy realigns the fracture site to a more favorable position. Simultaneously, the superior cortex of the proximal fragment has been impaled on the superior cortex of the femoral neck of the distal fracture fragment. Interfragmenteric compression of the fracture site is applied by the use of the cancellous lag screw.

Figure 9-60 shows a comminuted tibial shaft fracture that has been treated by the application of a Küntscher nail. The postoperative X-ray shows the unstable fixation with gaps visible at the segmental fractures. X-rays taken 25 weeks later reveal evidence of the fractured intramedullary nail and the unstable bone at the site of the metal failure. In the early postoperative period the likelihood of implant failure could have been predicted and prevented by application of a long leg cast, a non-weight-bearing gait or by surgical revision.

The next clinical example, shown in Figure 9-61, presents the X-rays of a patient who sustained a highly comminuted distal femoral fracture with interarticular components (Fig. 9-61A). Initially a blade plate was applied in combination with interfragmentary screws. The postoperative X-rays reveal that the nail has protruded into the joint space (Fig. 9-61 B and C). Also, separation between the metaphyseal and diaphyseal fragments on the medial femoral cortex is evident. In an X-ray taken 12 weeks later (Fig. 9-61D), fracture of the device is evident. During this period the patient had undertaken full weight-bearing gait. Under this mechanical environment, failure of the device could have been predicted. Subsequently the device was removed and a Charnley external fixation device was applied in combination with a cylinder cast. Ultimately, union was achieved but with an angular and rotational deformity of the distal femur.

Infection in the Presence of Internal Fixation

The risk of infection after the application of internal fixation and the complications of this catastrophe have continued to be a major factor in the role of internal fixation of fractures. The surgical approach to the fracture, the death of soft tissue and bone from the initial trauma or the operation, and the diminution of body defenses at the site of an implant all enhance the growth and spread of infection. Even in the presence of infection, however, a fracture can heal under favorable biomechanical conditions. The role of the biomechanical response of bone to a local infection are of great interest both for the treatment of fresh fractures where infection follows the application of internal fixation and for the treatment of infected nonunions of bone by the use of surgical implants. Recently Rittmann and Perren,[101] and Burri[102] have reviewed the biomechanical factors as well as clinical and therapeutic considerations of bone infection. A brief synopsis of their observations is given.

The incidence of bone infections after operative treatment of fractures varies greatly in reported literature.[103, 104] For closed fractures an incidence of about 0.5 to 6.5% has been cited while for open fractures figures from 3 to 15% are available. The significance of infections

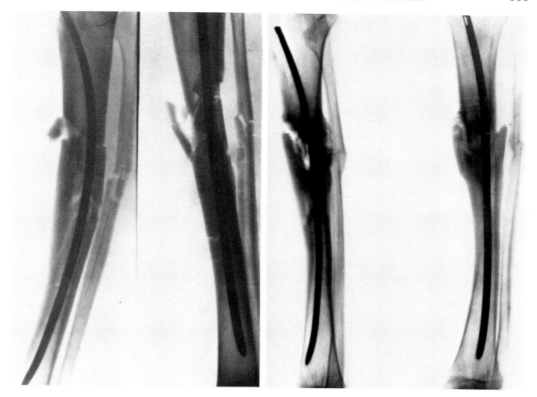

Figure 9-60. X-rays show the presence of an unstable fixation of the tibial shaft with the Küntschner nail. In the postoperative X-ray a large anterior defect in the tibia is evident. Unless supplementary fixation or limitation of weight bearing is initiated failure of the rod can be predicted. An X-ray taken at 24 weeks reveals the presence of a fatigue fracture in the rod. (Reproduced with permission of Miss O. Pöhler.)

arises both from the onset of chronic and lifelong osteomyelitis as well as a significant incidence of subsequent amputation. Various authors have reported an amputation rate as the culmination of an infected nonunion of the tibia ranging between 0.5% and 9%. The bacteria most frequently implicated in most traumatic osteomyelitis is *Staphlococcus aureus* in 54% to 93% of the infections.

The first surgeon to recognize the infectious origin of tissue reactions after the application of onlay plates was Lane.[23] Subsequently the treatment of such infections has evolved to include the use of systemic antibiotics, both in the postoperative period and as a systemic chemoprophylaxis and intra-operative topical agents. The surgical management of the infections, however, has remained controversial. Some authors recommend the removal of all metal as soon as the infection is clinically apparent. Other authors favor the removal of the bulk of the implant although they would accept that one or two screws might be left in place until union occurs. Other workers have emphasized the critical stabilizing function of the implant and recommend leaving the implant in place at the site of the infection until bony union has occurred.[104, 105] The last authors accept the presence of a prolonged period of soft tissue infection in return for the advantage of bone healing. There is, however, unanimous agreement that implants which no longer offer stability must be removed.

Recently Rittmann and Perren[101] examined the role of biomechanical factors in the healing process of infected fractures. From their past experience these workers raised several questions. How long would stability, engendered by an implant, persist in the presence of local infection? Would infection produce bone resorption with loss of initial fragmentary compression? Would primary bone healing occur under conditions of infection? To study these and other problems the authors performed transverse osteotomies of the tibia in sheep and stabilized

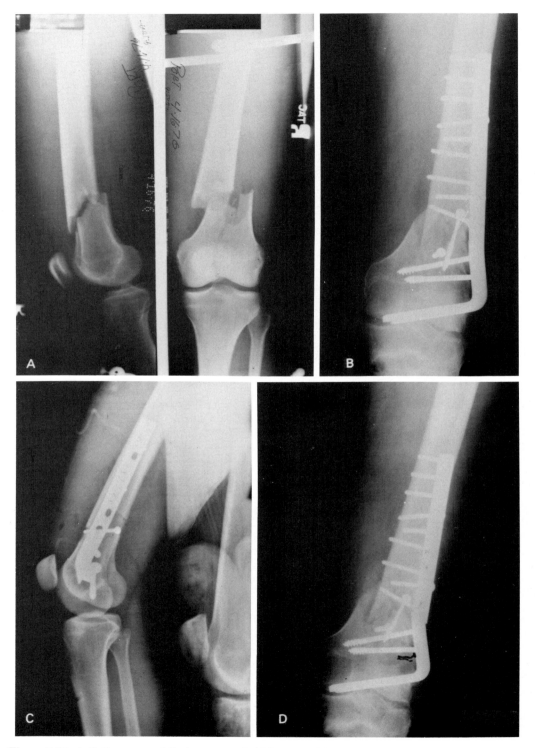

Figure 9-61. *A–D.* X-rays reveal the treatment of a T-fracture of the distal end of the femur by the application of a blade plate device and supplementary screws. The postoperative X-ray shows obvious malalignment of the fracture with interarticular penetration of the nail. Nevertheless, the patient is committed to undertake early weight bearing. Twenty weeks after surgery a repetitive X-ray reveals evidence of a fracture in the plate with further loss of alignment.

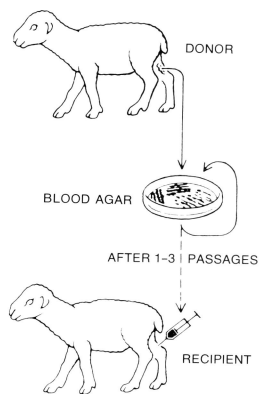

Figure 9-62. Schematic diagram illustrates the innoculation of the tibial osteotomy in sheep after the use of internal fixation to create an infected wound. (Reproduced with permission of Dr. S. M. Perren.)

them with a variety of implants (Fig. 9-62). The steps in the experiment are listed in Table 9-6. After one week staphylococci were injected into the osteotomy site. Local bacterial examinations were made twice between the 2nd and the 6th postoperative weeks. In a few cases with negative or only slightly positive bacterial cultures of staphylococci, repetitive injections of bacteria were undertaken. Loading of the postoperative extremity was tested clinically and by electronic apparatus (Fig. 9-63). Interfragmentary compression was measured during and after surgery. At the termination of the experiments in the 9th week, bacteriological examinations were repeated prior to filling the vessels of the extremity with contrast media. The measurements of compression were repeated at the time of implant extraction. Subsequently histological studies were undertaken.

Injection of the human-pathogenic staphylococci produced chronic bony infection with fistulae, sequestrum formation, bone destruction and callus apposition similar to osteomyelitis in

human subjects. After 8 weeks, 18 of the 19 osteotomies showed histological and angiographic patterns of bony union including features of primary bone healing (Figs. 9-64 and 9-65). *In vivo* measurements of interfragmentary compression were somewhat different from the pattern previously described for noninfected osteotomies (Fig. 9-66). Where resorption and sequestrum formation were extensive, a rapid pressure decrease was observed between the 4th and the 8th week. Measurements of interfragmentary compression showed a good correlation between the stability of the fixation and the type of nonhealing.

These workers also studied the histological pattern of secondary bone under comparable conditions of osseous infection. Figures 9-67A and B show a comparison of the gross pathological response of bone which has undergone primary and secondary bone healing. In conditions of primary bone healing the infected bone heals with minimal callus formation. After secondary bone healing, marked periosteal callus formation is evident and surrounds dead cortical or sequestrum formation. The dead bone persists as a chronic source of infection.

From the results of their study it becomes evident that rigid fixation of bone fragments offers favorable conditions for the healing of an infected nonunion. Implants which provide stable fixation of an infected nonunion should be left in place. If the implants become unstable then they should be removed and other devices should be implanted to provide absolute stability. In the presence of an infected nonunion, primary bone healing is preferable to secondary bone healing because it provides conditions where minimal sequestration is likely to occur. The advantage of the stabilizing effect of implants far outweighs the disadvantage of the implant as a foreign body. Radiographic appearance of callus after internal fixation and infection is not necessarily a sign of instability. Alternatively, the callus participates in fracture healing in infected nonunions. The clinical implications

Table 9-6

Steps in the Experiment

1.	Osteotomy
2.	Internal fixation
3.	Injection of staphylococci
4.	Measurement of compression
5.	Polychrome labeling
6.	X-rays
7.	Measurement of forces during gait
8.	Angiography, microradiography, histology

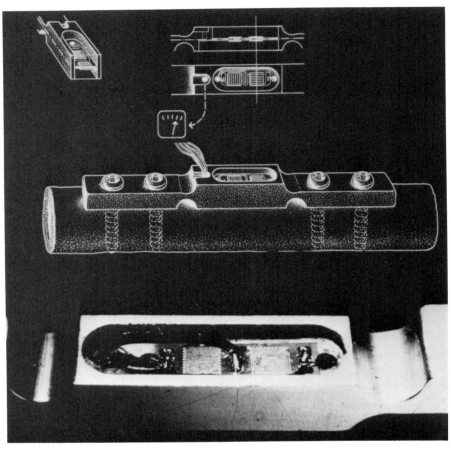

Figure 9-63. Schematic diagram reveals the special force measuring plate applied to the osteotomy in the sheep's tibia. (Reproduced with permission from Dr. S. M. Perren.)

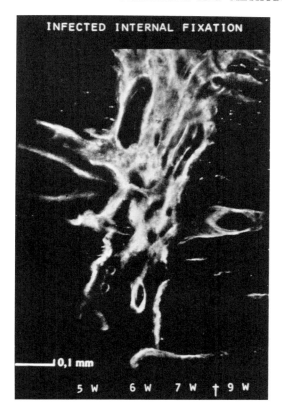

Figure 9-64. A photomicrograph reveals evidence of primary bone healing at the site of an infected non-union. The green and yellow fluoroscent vital stain reveal evidence of active bone remodeling. (Reproduced with permission of Dr. W. W. Rittmann.)

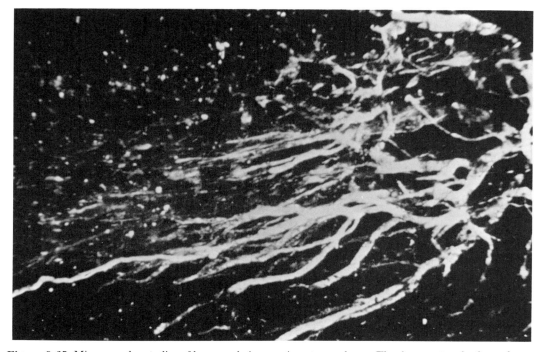

Figure 9-65. Microvascular studies of bone made in experiments are shown. The dense network of vessels are indicative of the active resorption phase of remodeling. (Reproduced with permission from Dr. W. W. Rittmann.)

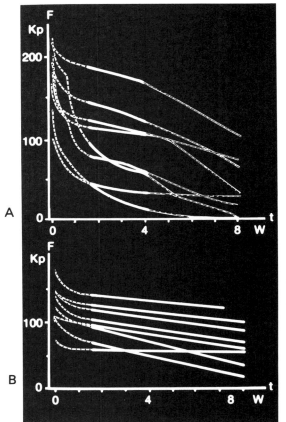

Figure 9-66. *A*. The three phases of the interfragmentary compression curves observed during the healing process of an infected bone are shown. After an initial pressure drop (*dotted line*) a phase of slower reduction is seen (*broken line*). Following these two phases which resemble the curves obtained under noninfected conditions, a third phase of accelerated pressure drop is often seen (*solid line*). It starts after the 4th week and is specific for infection. *B*. The two phases of the pressure curve seen during the healing process of infected osteotomies are shown. After an initial decrease in pressure (*dotted line*) a phase of slower additional decrease is seen (*broken line*) which persists for the duration of the experiment. (Reproduced with permission from Dr. S. M. Perren.)

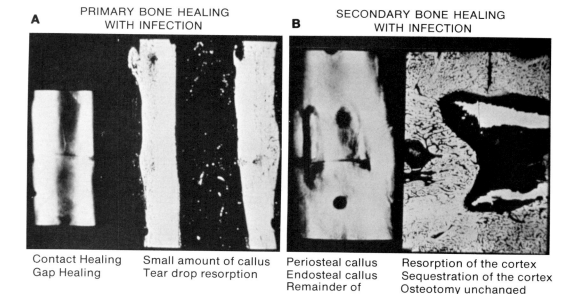

Figure 9-67. A comparison of the healing pattern of primary and secondary bone healing with infection is shown. In *A*, primary bone healing occurs with minimal callus formation and minimal sequestrum. In *B*, secondary bone healing within infection reveals substantial periosteal and endosteal callus. Resorption of cortex with sequestration formation is evident along with large area of persistent osteotomy gap. (Reproduced with permission of Dr. S. M. Perren.)

of these studies are enlarged in Chapter 10. One clinical factor, however, should be borne in mind.[105] The potentially satisfactory results of treatment of infected nonunions by the use of internal fixation is realized only if *absolutely* stable fixation is achieved. Otherwise the presence of the implant aggravates the infection. If the surgeon lacks sufficient skill, appropriate bone stock, or the necessary implants to provide rigid internal fixation of an osteoporotic segment of an infected nonunion, he should consider strongly the use of other methods of treatment. For example, by the use of external fixation (Chapter 11) the metallic foreign body can be inserted at a distance from the infection and still provide compression. The latter method does not require the presence of an unfavorable foreign body at the fracture site.

REFERENCES

1. Trueta, J. Principles and Practice of War Surgery, p. 30, C. V. Mosby Co., St. Louis, 1943.
2. Pirogoff, N. I. *Voyenno-Med. J., St. Petersburg, 63:*83, 1854.
3. Charnley, J. The Closed Treatment of Common Fractures, p. 10, Vol. 19, Churchill-Livingstone, London, 1972.
4. Müller, M. E., Allgöwer, M., and Willenegger, H. *Manual of Internal Fixation,* p. 12. Springer-Verlag, Berlin, 1970.
5. Adams, J. C. *Outline of Fractures, Including Joint Injuries,* ed. 5, E. & S. Livingstone, Edinburgh, 1968.
6. Devas, M. Stress Fractures, p. 21 Churchill-Livingstone, Edinburgh, 1975.
7. Freeman, M. A. R., Todd, R. C., and Pirie, C. J. *J. Bone Jt. Surg., 56B:*698, 1974.
8. Simon, S. R., Radin, E. L., Paul, R. L. and Rose, R. M. *J. Biomechan., 5:*267, 1972.
9. Sim, F. H., Daugherty, T. W., and Ivins, J. C. *J. Bone Jt. Surg., 56A:*40, 1974.
10. Heim, U., and Pfeiffer, K. M. *Small Fragment Set Manual,* p. 13, Springer-Verlag, New York, 1974.
11. Hughes, A. N. and Jordan, B. A. *The Mechanical Properties of Surgical Bone Screws,* p. 18, A. W. R. E. GRO/44/83/84/, Aldermaston, Berks, 1971.
12. Ansell, R. H., and Scales, J. T. *J. Biomech., 2:*279, 1968.
13. Bechtol, C. O., Ferguson, A. B., Jr., and Laing, P. G. *Metals and Engineering in Bone and Joint Surgery,* p. 100, Williams & Wilkins, Baltimore, 1959.
14. British Standard 3531, 1962 and 1968. *Specification for Bone Surgery,* p. 2, British Standards Institution, London, 1968.
15. Lindahl, O. *Acta. Orthop. Scand., 38:*101, 1967.
16. Schatzker, J., Sanderson, R., and Murnaghan, J. P. *Clin. Ortho. Rel. Res., 108:*115, 1975.
17. Schatzker, J., Horne, J. G., and Summer-Smith, G. *Clin. Ortho. Rel. Res., 111:*257, 1975.
18. Perren, S. M. and Allgöwer, M. *Nova Acta Leopoldina, 44:*223, 61, 1976.
19. Perren, S. M., Matter, P., Rüedi, T., and Allgöwer, M. Biomechanics of fracture healing after internal fixation. In *Surg. Ann. 1975,* p. 361, edited by L. M. Nyhus, Appleton-Century Crofts, New York, 1975.,
20. Wagner, H. *Verh. Dtsch. Ortho. Ges.,* 49, Kong. 1961, p. 418, 1962.
21. Perren, S. M., Rahn, B., and Allgöwer, M. in Press, 1977.
22. Müller, M. E., Allgöwer, M., and Willenegger, H. *Manual of Internal Fixation,* Springer-Verlag, Berlin, 1970.
23. Lane, A. W. *The Operative Treatment of Fractures,* p. 10, Medical Publishing Co., London, 1914.
24. Danis, R. *Theorie et pratique de l'osteosynthese,* p. 25; Masson, Paris, 1949.
25. Eggers, G. W. N. *N. Bone Jt. Surg., 30A:*40, 1948.
26. Bagby, G. W., and Janes, J. M. *Am. J. Surg., 95:*761, 1958.
27. Perren, S. M., Huggler, A., Russenberger, M., Straumann, F., Müller, M. E. and Allgöwer, M. *Acta. Ortho. Scand.,* suppl. *125:*7, 1969.
28. Frankel, V. H., and Burstein, A. H. *Orthopaedic Biomechanics,* p. 118, Lea Febiger, Philadelphia, 1970.
29. Lawrence, M., Freeman, M. A. R., and Swanson, S. A. V. *J. Bone Jt. Surg., 51B:*754, 1969.
30. Schenk, R., and Willenegger, H. *Symp. Biol. Hung., 7:*75, 1975.
31. Gallinaro, P., Perren, S. M., Crova, M., and Rahn, B. La Osteosinte con Placca a Compressione. In *Moderni Orientamenti nelle Osteosini della Fratture Diafisarie,* p. 21, edited by F. Roaesenda and G. L. Lorenzi, Aulo Gaggi, Editore, Bologna, 1969.
32. Allgöwer, M., Matter, P., Perren, S. M., and Rüedi, T. *The Dynamic Compression Plate,* p. 7, Springer-Verlag, Berlin, 1973.
33. Müller, M. E., Allgöwer, M., and Willenegger, H. *Manual of Internal Fixation,* p. 102, Springer-Verlag, Berlin, 1970.
34. Müller, M. E., Allgöwer, M., and Willenegger, H. *Manual of Internal* Fixation, Springer-Verlag, Berlin, 1970.
35. Allgöwer, M., Matter, P., Perren, S. M., and Rüedi, T. *The Dynamic Compression Plate,* Springer-Verlag, New York, 1973.
36. Bechtol, C. O., Ferguson, A. B., and Laing, P. G. *Metals and Engineering in Bone and Joint Surgery,* p. 117, Williams & Wilkins Co., Baltimore, 1959.
37. Bechtol, C. O., Ferguson, A. B., Jr., and Laing, P. G. *Metals in Engineering in Bone and Joint Surgery,* Williams & Wilkins Co., Baltimore, 1958.
38. Tronzo, R. G. *Ortho. Clin. N. Am., 5:*479, 1974.
39. von Langenbeck, B. *Verh. Dtsch. Ges. Chir., 7:*92, 1878.
40. Senn, N. *Trans. Am. Surg. Assn., 1:*333, 1881.
41. Whitman, R. *Med. Rec., 65:*441, 1904.
42. Smith-Petersen, M. N., Cave, E. F., and van Gorder, W. *Arch. Surg., 23:* 1931.
43. Laing, P. G., and O'Donnell, J. M. *Surg. Gyne. Obstet., 112:*567, 1961.
44. Deyerle, W. M. *Ortho. Clin. N. Am., 5:*3, 615, 1974.
45. Yamada, H. Strength of Biological Materials, p.

19, edited by F. G. Evans, Williams & Wilkins Co., Baltimore, 1970.

46. Stewart, W. G., Jr. *Ortho. Clin. N. Am.*, *5*:933, 1974.
47. Sönstegard, D. A., Kaufer, H., and Matthews, L. S. *Ortho. Clin. N. Am.*, *5*:551, 1974.
48. Barnes, R., Brown, J. T., and Garden, R. S. *J. Bone Jt. Surg.*, *58B*:1, 1976.
49. Holt, E. P. *Ortho. Clin. N. Am., 5:3*, 601, 1974.
50. Massie, W. K. *Clin. Orthop.*, *92*:16, 1973.
51. Pugh, W. L. *J. Bone Jt. Surg.*, *37A*: 1085, 1955.
52. Mears, D. C. *Ortho. Survey 1*:64, 1977.
53. Gorden, R. S. *Ortho. Clin. North Am.*, *5*:683, 1974.
54. Dimon, J. H. *Clin. Ortho.*, *92*:100, 1973.
55. Salvati, E. A., Artz, T., Aghetti, P., Asnis, S. E. *Orthop. Clin. N. Am.*, *5*:757, 1974.
56. Tronzo, R. G. *Surgery of the Hip Joint* p. 512, Lea and Febiger, Philadelphia, 1973.
57. Coleman, S. S. *Ortho. Clin. N. Am.*, *5*:819, 1974.
58. Niemann, K. M. W., and Mankin, H. J. *J. Bone Jt. Surg.*, *50A*:1327, 1968.
59. Barr, J. S. *Ortho. Clin. N. Am.*, *5*:847, 1974.
60. Ellison N., and Mull, T. D. *Ortho. Clin. N. Am.*, *5*:493, 1974.
61. Rogers, P. H., and Morder, V. J. *Ortho. Clin. N. Am.*, *5*:509, 1974.
62. Hunter, G. A. *Br. J. Surg.*, *56*:229, 1969.
63. Greer, R. B., and Niemann, K. M. W. *Geriatrics*, *26*:86, 1971.
64. Fielding, J. W., Cochran, G. V. B., and Zickel, R. E. *Ortho. Clin. N. Am., 5:3*, 629, 1974.
65. Cech, O., and Sosna, A. *Ortho. Clin. N. Am., 5:3*, 651, 1974.
66. Harris, N. H. *Proc. Roy. Soc. Med.*, *58*:879, 1965.
67. Sharrard, W. J. W. *Paediatric Orthopaedics and Fractures*, p. 190, Blackwell Scientific Publications, Oxford, 1973.
68. Tachdjian, M. O. *Paediatric Orthopaedics,* p. 476, W. B. Saunders Co., Philadelphia, 1972.
69. Goldstein, L. A., and Dickerson, R. C. *Atlas of Orthopaedic Surgery*, p. 522, C. V. Mosby Co., St. Louis, 1974.
70. Goldstein, L. A., and Dickerson, R. C. *Atlas of Orthopaedic Surgery,* p. 628, C. V. Mosby Co., St. Louis, 1974.
71. Küntscher, G. *The Practice of Intra-medullary Nailing"*, p. 2, Charles C Thomas, Springfield, Ill., 1967.
72. Küntscher, G. *The Practice of Intra-medullary Nailing,* Charles C Thomas, Springfield, Ill., 1967.
73. Müller, M. E., Allgöwer, M., and Willenegger, H. *Manual of Internal Fixation,* p. 80, Springer-Verlag, Berlin, 1970.
74. Schatzker, J. *A Primer on the AO/ASIF Method of Internal Fixation,* p. 31, University of Toronto, Toronto, 1974.
75. Goldstein, L. A., and Dickerson, R. C. *Atlas of Orthopaedic Surgery*, p. 634, C. V. Mosby, St. Louis, 1974.
76. Schneider, H. W. *Clin. Ortho. Rel. Res.*, *60*:29, 1968.

77. Street, D. M. *J. Bone Jt. Surg.*, *33A*:659, 1951.
78. Frankel, V. H., and Burstein, A. H. *Orthopaedic Biomechanics*, p. 161, Lea & Febiger, Philadelphia, 1970.
79. Aegerter, E., and Kirkpatrick, J. A. *Orthopaedic Diseases*, p. 407, W. B. Saunders Co., Philadelphia, 1975.
80. Lottes, J. O. *Clin. Ortho. Rel. Res.*, *105*:253, 1974.
81. Epps, C. H. Fractures of the shaft of the humerus. In *Fractures*, p. 564, (edited by C. A. Rockwood and D. P. Green) J. B. Lippincott Co., Philadelphia, 1975.
82. Rush, L. V. *Atlas of Rush Pin Techniques*, p. 5, Berivon Co., Meridian, Miss., 1955.
83. Rush, L. V. *Atlas of Rush Pin Techniques,* Berivon Co., Meridian, Miss., 1955.
84. Rush L. V. *Clin. Ortho.*, *60*:21, 1968.
85. Goldstein, L. A., and Dickerson, R. C. *Atlas of Orthopaedic Surgery,* p. 78, C. V. Mosby, St. Louis, 1974.
86. Kuntscher, G. *Proc. Roy. Soc. Med.*, *63*:1120, 1966.
87. Herrero, F. C., Brichs, J. V., and Beltran, J. E. *Ortho. Clin. N. Am.*, *5*:669, 1974.
88. Ender, H. G. *Treatment of Per- and Sub-trochanteric Fractures with Ender's Flexible Intramedullary Pins,* p. 2, de Kostendrukkers, Schiedam, Holland, 1976.
89. Rhinelander, F. W. *Effects of Medullary Nailing on the Normal Blood Supply of Diaphyseal Cortex, Instructional Course Lectures, A.A.O.S.*, p. 161, C. V. Mosby Co., St. Louis, 1973.
90. Brookes, M. *The Blood Supply of Bone*, p. 73 Butterworth's, London, 1971.
91. Rhinelander, F. W. *Clin. Ortho. Rel. Res.*, *105*:34, 1974.
92. Charnley, J. "Closed Treatment of Common Fractures", p. 9, Williams & Wilkins Co., Baltimore, 1971.
93. Böhler, J. *J. Trauma,* *5*:150, 1965.
94. Clawson, D. K., Smith. R. F. and Hansen, S. D. *J. Bone Jt. Surg.*, *53A*:681, 1971.
95. Rascher, J. J., Nahigian, S. H., Macys, J. R., and Brown, J. E. *J. Bone Jt. Surg.*, *54A*:534, 1972.
96. Rüedi, T., and Allgöwer, M. in Press, 1979.
97. Pauwels, F. *Der Schenkelhalsbruch, em mechanisches Problem,* p. 25, Enke, Stuttgart, 1935.
98. Böhler, J. *Clin. Ortho. Rel. Res.*, *105*:276, 1974.
99. Black, J. *Ortho. Clin. N. Am.*, *5:4*, 833, 1974.
100. Piehler, H. *Regulation of Orthopaedic Surgical Implants,* p. 71, Carnegie-Mellon University, Pittsburgh, 1976.
101. Rittmann, W. W., and Perren, S. M. *Cortical Bone Healing after Internal Fixation and Infection,* p. 18, Springer-Verlag, Berlin, 1974.
102. Burri, C. *Posttraumatic Osteomyelitis,* p. 129, Huber, Vienna, 1975.
103. Hicks, J. H. *Lancet,* *1*:86, 1963.
104. Meyer, S., Weiland, A. J. and Willenegger, H. *J. Bone Jt. Surg.*, *57A*:836, 1975.
105. Willenegger, H., and Mears, D. C. in Press, 1979.

10

Clinical Methods of Fracture Treatment

The immense variety of fractures plus the varying shape, consistency, strength and other properties of bone have resulted in an enormous number of designs of apparatus to immobilize fractures and joints. For each fracture the surgeon must review the advantages and disadvantages of open as opposed to closed treatment. The general applications for open techniques of internal fixation on recent fractures are: (1) The provision for early mobilization of the patient either in the interests of his general condition or for the preservation of mobility of joints. (2) The restoration and maintenance of satisfactory alignment of fractures that cannot be reduced or maintained in acceptable positions by the application of closed methods. Intra-articular fractures and epiphyseal fractures in growing children are outstanding examples where open methods frequently are required. (3) Where injuries of skin, blood vessels or nerves occur in juxtaposition to the fracture, internal osseous stabilization may be a prerequisite to satisfactorily treat soft tissue injuries. (4) With multiple fractures in one extremity, internal fixation may provide superior reduction of the fractures, early return of motion to adjacent joints and a great reduction in the rate of delayed or nonunion. (5) With multiple trauma to several extremities and to other organs, internal fixation of one or more bones may facilitate nursing care and the management of other problems, e.g., thoracic, abdominal or intracranial injuries. (6) Occasionally indications may include social, psychological and cosmetic considerations. Also, the economic stimulus of rapid discharge from the hospital, hopefully with equally rapid return to work, becomes ever more urgent.

Inexperienced fracture surgeons should establish a system of fracture management that rests upon a firm understanding of: the biomechanics of fractures and the techniques for closed and open stabilization; the devices for internal fixation; and the clinical aspects of closed and open methods. A systematic approach to closed methods is well taught in most English-speaking teaching hospitals but frequently a systematic approach to open methods is absent. For rapid acquisition of the latter formidable goal, the author has found the AO * technique of internal fixation to be superior, mainly because it does represent an integrated *system,* founded on biomechanical knowledge on the pathophysiology of fracture repair and on metallurgical considerations of surgical tools and implants. While an intensive study of the AO methods provides a sound background for internal fixation, it is not intended to provide training in the use of closed methods. In the present discussion, both closed and open methods of treatment are described so that the reader may better appreciate their relative merits and the indications and techniques for each. For the fracture surgeon it represents an effort to mold his armamentarium for fracture treatment so that it contains an organized complement of closed and open techniques. To extend this armamentarium and to present many recent advances, techniques of percutaneous transfixing pins with external fixation are discussed in Chapter 11.

For a more extensive presentation of open or closed methods of treatment of fractures, the reader is advised to consult other sources.[1-7]

Some Criteria for Techniques of Internal Fixation

Once a surgeon has elected to apply a technique of internal fixation then he should plan the operation and postoperative management in an attempt to meet certain standards which the AO group has recommended.[3] An incision and surgical exposure should be selected which enables the surgeon to preserve the blood supply to all of the living fracture fragments. A devitalized fragment possesses no intrinsic capacity to heal and it functions as a foreign body and a nidus

---

* Arbeitsgemeinschaft für Osteosynthesefragen or ASIF (Swiss) Association for the Study of Internal Fixation.

for infection. Throughout the procedure, compulsive attention to the soft tissues is essential. Soft tissues should be handled as little as possible. When a large amount of blood will accumulate after surgery, suction drainage should be inserted. The wound should be closed with great care. Especially for wounds with a tenuous blood supply, such as the anterior lower leg, simple, interrupted sutures should be placed with minimal tension on the edges of the wound. Alternatively the AO group favors the Donati technique of mattress suture which penetrates the epidermis on one side of the wound. In the forearm and lower leg, subcutaneous sutures are rarely necessary or beneficial.

The Goals of Internal Fixation

Once a surgeon has elected to apply a technique of internal fixation, certain technical goals and postoperative criteria should be maintained. The need for rigid stabilization of the fracture from the point of view of biomechanical considerations was described in Chapter 9. In the absence of rigid fixation, bending moments on an unstable fracture site are likely to provoke mechanical failure of the implant and loss of stability of the fracture. The need for rigid stabilization, however, also extends into the postoperative period when the results of a satisfactory internal fixation should enable the patient to undertake a rehabilitation program with early return of function of the relevant extremity. The therapy program requires exercises for adjacent muscle groups and mobility of adjacent joints. The exercise program may permit the patient to regain the optimal range of motion of joints and function of muscles. In addition to the physical factors, the psychological advantages of a rapid postoperative return of function are enormous. With the augmented mobility, an earlier discharge from the hospital may be possible. Ultimately, however, the principal advantage of the early postoperative return of function is a superior clinical result for the patient. As Schatzker[8] has documented for a series of patients who sustained comminuted interarticular fractures of the distal femur treated by accurate open reduction and internal fixation followed by early postoperative mobilization of the knee, the clinical results recorded as range of motion of the knee and return to previous activity is markedly improved over previous conservative or operative approaches.

Bone Grafting and Internal Fixation

Many fracture and reconstructive problems are accompanied by the loss of bone substance and osseous stability. Bone graft may be applied to fill osseous defects both as a mechanical support and as a source of osteogenic potential. The pathophysiology of bone grafting has been fully reviewed elsewhere.[9-11] A few pertinent clinical observations follow.

Previously, cortical bone graft was widely applied to osseous defects for mechanical stability as well as osteogenic potential. It is apparent that cortical grafts provide neither the rigid stabilization of good internal or external fixation nor the osteogenic stimulus that is created by the presence of cancellous bone. Cortical bone grafts remain as a highly satisfactory source for stabilization of the cervical spine after discectomy and occasionally for use in small segmental defects in the smaller bones. In the presence of an infected nonunion, after thorough debridement of the infected and dead bone, autogenous cancellous bone can be placed in a previously stabilized pseudarthrosis. The graft will be incorporated into the fracture fragments. Alternatively, cortical bone would remain as a sequestrum and stimulate the spread of the infection. A variety of homologous or heterologous sources of bone graft have been widely applied, especially in children where the available stores of graft bone are limited. For 2 years the author has successfully applied freeze-dried autologous bone* in such difficult pediatric problems.

The donor site for autologous cancellous bone graft depends upon the quantity of bone that is required and upon the operative site. The conventional donor and recipient sites are shown in Figure 10-1. When a large quantity of bone is needed, the posterior iliac crest is the preferred site. At the level of the posterior inferior spine and lateral to the sacroiliac joint the thickest portion of cancellous bone is encountered. The second largest donor site is the anterior iliac crest. The bone graft can be obtained through the superficial or the deep cortex. When the greater trochanter is used for a graft site, the graft should be taken from the same limb as the recipient site. In this way the mechanical integrity of a single lower extremity is violated and full weight bearing may be undertaken without the risk of propagation of a crack from the greater trochanteric graft site.

Prior to a brief systematic review of fracture treatment a few special fracture problems are discussed.

---

* Courtesy of Lt. Comdr. Gary E. Friedlaender, M.D., MC, USNR,

Naval Medical Research Institute, Bethesda, Md.

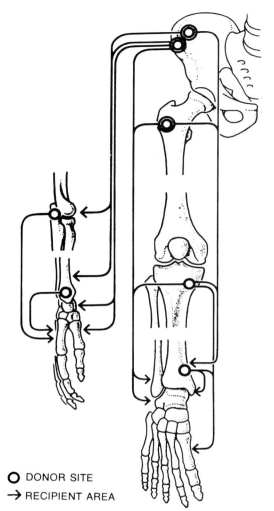

○ DONOR SITE

→ RECIPIENT AREA

Figure 10-1. The principal donor site and recipient areas for autogenous bone grafting are shown. The main donor sites are the iliac crest and the iliac fossa. Occasional donor sites are the olecranon, the distal radius, the greater trochanter and the proximal and distal tibia. (Reproduced with permission of U. Heim and K. M. Pfeiffer.[12])

OPEN FRACTURES

An open fracture always demands urgent attention to minimize the risk of infection from contaminating organisms. The objectives of treatment are cleansing the wound, removal of all dead and devitalized tissue and stabilization of the fracture. The extent of the operation depends upon the size and nature of the wound. Open fractures may be classified as follows:

Grade I. Open from within by a spike of bone which punctures the skin. About 60% of open fractures are of this type where the extent of soft tissue death and destruction, as well as bacterial contamination, usually is small.

Grade II. Open from without with contusion of skin and muscle. About 30% of open fractures are of this type. With the more extensive exposure of denuded bone, and frequently contamination by foreign bodies such as gravel, and disruption of soft tissues, these injuries constitute a moderately grave risk of infection.

Grade III. Extensive damage to skin and muscle with comminuted fractures and often with associated injuries to vessels or nerves. About 10% of open fractures are of this type which are frequently encountered in motorcycle accidents or shotgun injuries. With the extensive disruption and death of soft tissues and denuded bone fragments, these injuries are particularly vulnerable to infection, including gas gangrene (*Clostridium welchii*).

Principles of Treatment

Grade I Open Fractures. The puncture wound is thoroughly irrigated with saline or antibiotic solution. If necessary the cutaneous wound is enlarged for a clear display of the extent of soft tissue damage. As in all open wounds a careful scrutiny for foreign bodies must be performed so that all contamination is removed. The wound is left open. The fracture is immobilized by conventional means, although there should be greater reluctance to use internal fixation. In open fractures the application of an intramedullary nail is associated with a particularly high rate of infection. Rëudi and Allgöwer[13] report greater than a 10% infection rate for open tibial shaft fractures treated with intramedullary rods. Where operative treatment is indicated they advise that such open tibial fractures should be stabilized by an onlay plate that is inserted through untraumatized soft tissues.

Grades II and III Open Fractures. First, careful debridement with a thorough cleansing and removal of dead tissue, but not a drastic excision of viable tissues, is performed. Small detached bone fragments may be removed but larger fragments with soft tissue attachment should be carefully preserved. Damage to a major blood vessel is treated as circumstances dictate, by ligation, suture or grafting. The ends of severed nerves are marked with sutures and approximated to facilitate definitive repair.

With few exceptions primary closure of skin should not be attempted. For extensive wounds delayed secondary closure or the delayed application of split thickness skin grafts to a clean granulating bed are preferred.

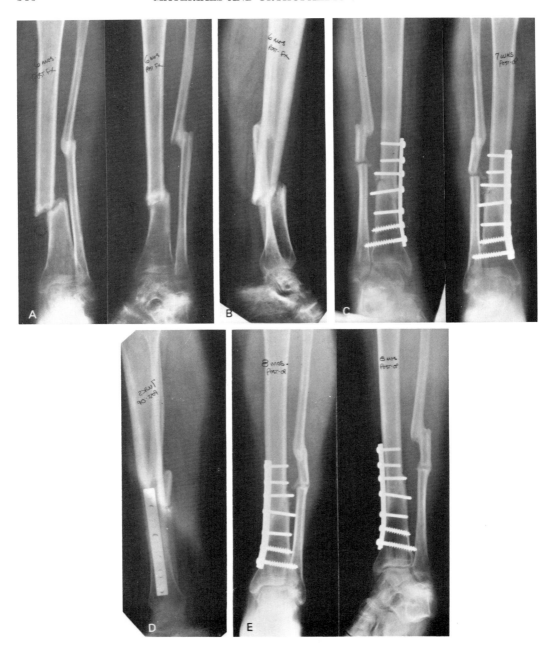

Figure 10-2. A series of X-rays shows a male patient of 18 years who presented 6 months after a distal tibial shaft fracture with a nonunion and malunion, as seen in *A* and *B*. In *C* and *D*, the postoperative X-rays show the fracture after open reduction and internal fixation with the application of a dynamic compression plate (DCP) and cortical and cancellous screws. The surgical procedure was much more difficult because of the prolonged period between the presentation and the internal fixation. The malalignment could have been corrected easily by open reduction in the first postoperative months. In *E*, the extremity is shown 8 months after surgery when the fracture had healed. In *F* through *J* radiological views are shown of an infected nonunion

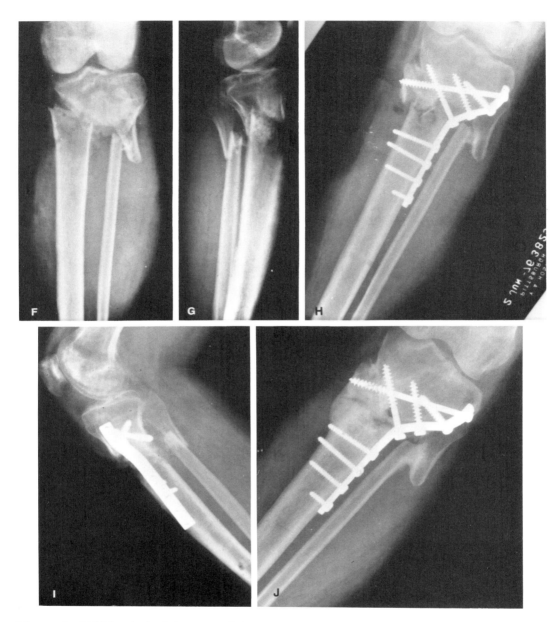

of the proximal tibial metaphysis in a man of 30 years treated with open reduction and internal fixation. Six months after the open fracture occurred closed treatment with a cast was abandoned and the draining unstable fracture was debrided, reduced and a DCP with cancellous and cortical screws was applied (h, I). As shown by X-rays 2 months later (J), the fracture line was largely obliterated. A small sinus tract persisted. Once the infected nonunion was converted into an infected union, the implant was removed and a further debridement performed for irradication of the infection.

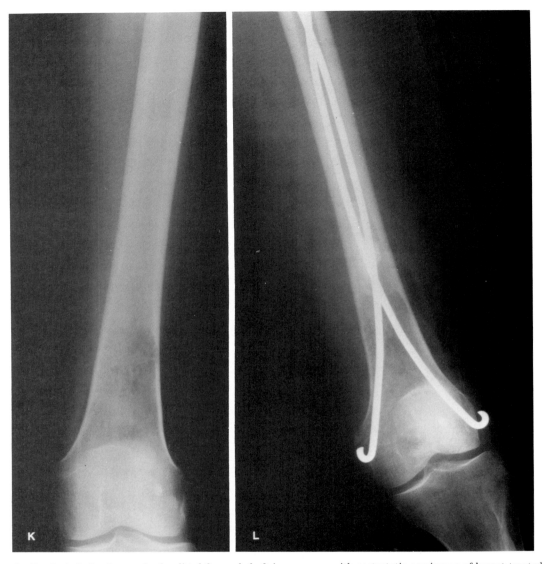

In *K*, a lytic lesion is seen in the distal femoral shaft in a woman with metastatic carcinoma of breast treated with Rush rods and cement (*L*).

While stabilization of the fracture is essential, internal fixation should be avoided if possible. Alternatively, external fixation with the use of percutaneous transfixing pins, such as the Hoffmann device, provides a highly satisfactory alternative especially where segmental bone loss has occurred. After soft tissue healing has transpired, the deficiency of bone may be restored by the application of cancellous bone graft. This excellent method is fully discussed in Chapter 11.

THE TREATMENT OF NONUNIONS

The classical "elephant-foot" type of nonunion comprises 85 to 90% of pseudarthroses which develop in fractures treated by closed methods. X-rays reveal a proliferative bone reaction which represents well vascularized bone. With the application of rigid immobilization, by a straight compression plate or an intramedullary nail after intramedullary reaming, these nonunions will heal. The interposed fibrous tissue and cartilage rapidly ossify. Figure 10-2 *A* to *E* shows an example of a tibial nonunion treated by plate fixation.

When nonunion ensues after the application of rigid internal fixation of a diaphyseal fracture, a different radiological picture is observed. X-rays reveal minimal bone reaction and the fracture gap is poorly vascularized. Treatment must include extensive decortication and the application of both autogenous cancellous bone graft and rigid internal fixation with a compression plate or an intramedullary nail.

In metaphyseal nonunions, broad, close contact of the fracture fragments must be achieved before rigid internal fixation is applied. The implants inevitably are different from those applied for diaphyseal nonunions. A nonunion of the proximal humerus is immobilized with a T-plate. In the distal humerus and proximal tibia, double plates may be employed while in the proximal and distal femur, condylar blade plates may be used. In nonunions of the femoral neck, healing depends upon the angle of the nonunion relative to the resultant forces acting upon the femoral head. Where the femoral head is viable a subtrochanteric valgus osteotomy may improve the mechanics of the pseudarthrosis so that conditions for union are favored. Recently, Weber and Cech[14] have provided a detailed account of pseudarthroses and their management.

The Treatment of Infected Ununited Fractures

All fracture surgeons should be well prepared to cope with infected nonunions, a most difficult complication of open fractures or operative fracture treatment. First, the infection is characterized by the extent of the active cellulitis, the extent of dead and infected bone and the nature of the nonunion.

In the presence of a fulminant soft tissue infection with septicemia, at the very least, immediate drainage of the abscess and systemic antibiotics are indicated. In most cases with more localized soft tissue infection, a formal elective debridement of the wound is indicated. All devitalized bone and soft tissues are excised. At the same procedure stabilization of bone is achieved. In most cases, external fixation, such as the Hoffmann device, is the optimal method (see Chapter 11). It enables the surgeon to achieve rigid fixation without the insertion of a metallic foreign body into the focal point of the infection. The transfixing pins can be inserted into a remote portion of the same bone or, in the presence of extensive osteomyelitis, into adjacent bones. External fixation greatly facilitates the management of the open wounds. In many cases, especially with extensive loss of skin coverage, the wounds are packed open. Alternatively, when good cutaneous coverage is available, as with many cases of proximal femoral infection, a system of continuous irrigation with inflow and outflow tubes may be preferred. Either method is readily managed with external fixation and is cumbersome when windowed casts are applied. Elevation of the involved limb in the early postoperative period is essential.

Within 1 to 2 weeks after the debridement, usually the acute infection has defervesced. Occasionally secondary minor debridement procedures are necessary. Once the infection is controlled, reconstitution of the osseous segment at the nonunion site can be initiated. For cases in which an external fixation device is used and where the fracture gap is small, the device can be adjusted to shorten the bone and obliterate the fracture gap. For similar cases, but with a lengthy fracture gap, strips of autogenous iliac crest cancellous bone are applied to bridge the gap.[15] Prior to the insertion of bone graft the external fixation device is adjusted to lengthen the limb. After insertion, the device is adjusted to shorten the bone and compress the graft to reform a continuous osseous column.

In certain instances after control of the infection has been achieved, the surgeon may elect to replace the cast or an external fixation device with internal fixation. Most previous workers[5, 7] have discouraged this practice. According to them, the implant functioned as a foreign body to excite the infection. Recently, Rittmann and Perren[16] studied the healing response of an experimental infected nonunion in the sheep tibia in the presence of conditions appropriate for primary or secondary fracture repair. As fully described in Chapter 9, when healing occurs by primary repair achieved by the use of a compression plate, minimal callus sequestrum formation is observed. After union is achieved, the likelihood of chronic osteomyelitis, thereby, is greatly diminished. When the healing occurs by secondary repair, the proliferative callus formation is associated with enhanced sequestrum formation and a greater incidence of chronic osteomyelitis. Recently Burri *et al.*[17] and Meyer *et al.*[18] have reported an impressive series of cases of infected nonunions of long bones that were treated with debridement, rigid stabilization with internal or external fixation and, where indicated, the application of cancellous bone graft. In view of the excellent results achieved by these workers, careful scrutiny of their method is recommended. In Figure 10-2 *F* to *J,* the treatment by internal fixation of an infected nonunion and malunion of the proximal tibia is shown. Particularly in cases of infected nonunion of the forearm, internal fixation is a valuable method. It permits early return of pronation and supination as well as elbow and wrist flexion. Alternatively, an external fixation device may restrict motion of several of these joints for the prolonged period needed for union to occur, after which full return of joint mobility is unlikely. If the transfixing pins of the external device penetrate the flexor or extensor muscle masses of the forearm, serious compromise of strength and mobility of the hand are likely to ensue. Admittedly, full skin coverage over the plates may not be achieved until union of the fracture and metal removal have occurred. This temporary absence of complete cutaneous coverage is easily managed.

Where a fracture treated by rigid internal fixation becomes infected, incision and drainage or debridement are indicated, depending upon the extent of the infection. If the implant maintains rigid fixation, however, it should *not* be removed. An unstable infected nonunion is a much more difficult problem than a stable one for the stability is essential to achieve control of the infection. Alternatively, if an implant is present in an unstable fracture it is removed and replaced with rigid internal or external fixation.

An explanation for the altered role of internal fixation in the treatment of infected nonunions is readily apparent. The previous workers who discouraged the use of internal fixation did not possess satisfactory implants for the provision of rigid stability. They did not have clinical experience with truly stable infected nonunions. The recent improvement in fixation devices has greatly altered this situation. The use of cancellous bone screws and self-compression plates permits the stabilization of moderately osteoporotic, infected bone. Where the bone is markedly osteoporotic, however, stable internal fixation may be impossible. The surgeon who elects to use internal fixation must decide whether he can obtain rigid stabilization. If he cannot, he must alter his plan and apply another method.

Despite the recent improvements in the treatment of infected nonunions, this complication remains a challenging problem often attended by prolonged hospital admissions. A recent detailed account by Burri *et al.*[17] is recommended.

PATHOLOGICAL FRACTURES

When bones have been weakened by the presence of osteoporosis, tumor or other destructive process, spontaneous fractures may occur with minimal trauma. While osteoporosis secondary to paralysis may be consistent with rapid healing of bone, malignancy of bone may stifle reparative phenomena. Open intervention may be indicated from several considerations. In paralytic osteoporosis, such as occurs with traumatic paraplegia or with myelomeningocele, where long bones in the lower extremities show more than one fracture per year, prophylactic intramedullary rod fixation of both femora and tibiae is recommended. The Sampson fluted rods are particularly useful both because of the excellent strength and torsional rigidity exhibited by the rod and because of the screw thread at the proximal end of the rod which enables the surgeon to lengthen the rod with growth of the bone. Similar principles of management may be applied to children with severe forms of osteogenesis imperfecta.[19] Where the fragile bones show deformity, multiple corrective osteotomies may be required at the time of insertion of the intramedullary rods.[20]

In contrast, treatment of many malignant bone tumors, with pathological fracture, usually occurs in a different clinical setting. Most of the patients are middle-aged or older and have a limited life expectancy. Prolonged immobilization in bed is contraindicated both by the foreshortened life expectancy and by the likely ill-effects of bed rest on the patient's general condition. The objectives of surgery are excision of the tumor and reconstitution of the site with a combination of bone graft, implants, and/or methylmethacrylate.[21, 22] An example is seen in Figure 10-2 *K, L.* Mechanical stability is provided by the application of metal implants. As Sim *et al.*[23] have emphasized, adherence to sound mechanical principles is essential for these complex reconstructive procedures. Also, the nature of the specific tumor should be understood prior to surgery because it determines the anticipated extent of bony healing. Certain metastatic deposits, such as carcinoma of the breast, may show proliferative callus formation. Others, such as renal cell carcinoma, may not be accompanied by effective remodeling of bone. In the latter situation reconstruction may include the application of titanium or Vitallium mesh reinforced with methylmethacrylate. Alternatively, where the tumor involves bone adjacent to an articular surface, a hemijoint replacement such as a Moore prosthesis may be cemented in place. For the treatment of some extensive tumors with pathological fractures, Burrows et al.[24] report successful massive replacement of segments of bone, often with entire joints.

Such aggressive surgery requires careful planning. Should the patient survive longer than anticipated, the reconstruction would have to withstand exacting fatigue conditions. Wound infections are a formidable and frequent complication because of the massive size of the implant and cement and because of decreased host resistance to infection engendered by ancillary treatment such as local irradiation and systemic antitumor chemotherapy.

Prophylactic Internal Fixation

Some types of primary malignant tumors are recognized to have a predilection to metastasize to bone. These are carcinomas of the breast (about 30%), prostate, thyroid, kidney and lung. Medical management of such tumor patients should include consideration of the possible development of large lytic lesions in bone.[24-27] Most of the lesions occur in the shafts of the femur or humerus or the neck of the femur. When radiological assessment indicates that the lesions approach one-half the diameter of the bone, prophylactic internal fixation should be performed to prevent the greater discomfort and morbidity associated with a pathological fracture. A lesion in the shaft of a long bone should be stabilized by the insertion of an intramedullary rod under image intensification. Supplementary stabilization with methylmethacrylate cement may be helpful as shown in Figure 10-2 K, L. For lesions in the neck of the femur a nail-plate device such as a compression hip screw is recommended. Following internal fixation the area is irradiated.

PELVIC FRACTURES

Fractures of the pelvis usually result from violent trauma. Frequently they are accompanied by associated injuries to the pelvic or abdominal viscera, the hip joint and femoral shaft and by injuries to the chest, head and neck and extremities. One-third of patients with multiple pelvic fractures die as a result of local hemorrhage. Early management must include a rapid but thorough physical examination especially for signs of accompanying injuries to the bladder, urethra, bowel and lumbosacral plexus, and treatment for shock.

Numerally most pelvic fractures can be treated by bed rest or by closed reduction and other conservative means. For a full discussion the reader is referred elsewhere.[4, 28-31] The concise analysis of pelvic fractures and their management by Judet et al.[31] is particularly useful. Open intervention should be considered for displaced acetabular fractures, and for fractures with gross disruption of the pelvic ring or marked displacement of the sacroiliac joint.

Acetabular Fractures

Prior to surgical intervention, accurate documentation of the type of fracture is necessary by the application of three special X-ray projections (Fig. 10-3), the anterior-posterior and two oblique views. For descriptive purposes the acetabulum is divided into its three embryonic columns, the ilium, the ischium and the pubis. The iliopubic segment becomes the anterior column and the ilioischial segment becomes the posterior column.

Simple and combinations of acetabular fractures have been classified by Judet and Le-Tournel as shown in Figure 10-4: (1) The simple posterior lip fracture with posterior-lateral subluxation or dislocation of the femoral head. (2) The simple posterior column fracture with posterior-medial subluxation or dislocation of the femoral head. (3) The simple anterior column fracture with anterior-medial subluxation or dislocation of the femoral head. (4) The simple transverse fracture of the acetabulum with inward displacement of the femoral head. (5) Combinations of fractures include: (a) Transverse fractures with fracture of the upper and posterior acetabular rim; (b) fractures of both columns; (c) fracture of one column with a transverse fracture of the others; (d) more complex combinations.

Next, the surgical approach (Fig. 10-5) is carefully planned to enable the surgeon to visualize all of the fracture. The posterior-lateral, or Gibson, approach provides optimal exposure of the roof and posterior lip of the acetabulum, and the ilioischial column, distal to the ischial tuberosity. The direct lateral approach with osteotomy of the greater trochanter and upward reflection of the abductors provides optimal exposure of the roof of the acetabulum and the hip joint. The iliocrural approach of Smith-Petersen provides optimal exposure of the iliopubic column, the wing of the ilium and the anterior rim of the acetabulum as far as the iliopectinal eminence. The ilioinguinal approach of Judet and Le-Tournel provides optimal exposure of the entire

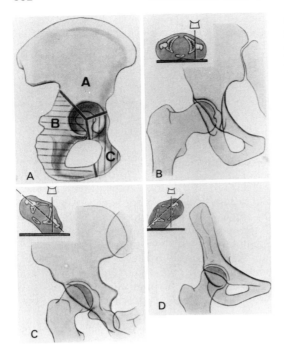

Figure 10-3. *A.* A schematic diagram shows a hemipelvis with the acetabulum. A Y-shaped intersection of three columns of bones is shown in the center of the acetabulum. The ilium (*A*) is superior and provides the roof of the acetabulum. The ischium (*B*) forms the posterior lip of the acetabulum. The pubis (*C*) provides the anterior lip of the acetabulum. Three special X-ray projections are necessary to study the acetabulum. A standard anteroposterior projection of the pelvis is seen in *B*. Two oblique views of the affected hip were taken with the patient rolled through a 45° arc. One oblique view (*C*) was taken with the patient turned toward the affected side. This view shows the posterior edge of the ilium, the sciatic notch and the anterior lip of the acetabulum. In the other view the patient was turned away from the affected side. This last view shows the obturator foramen with the medial border of the iliac fossa and the posterior lip of the acetabulum and acetabular roof. (Reproduced with permission of M. E. Müller, M. Allgöwer and H. Willenegger.[32])

iliopubic column, the floor of the acetabulum and the inner aspect of the pelvis and superior pubic ramus.

The priorities of operative technique must follow biomechanical considerations. The AO group[33] suggests that the roof and dorsal lip of the acetabulum should be reduced and immobilized first. Fractures of the posterior lip larger than simple capsular avulsions are reduced and secured with cancellous or malleolar screws. Fractures of the posterior column are reduced

with respect to the acetabular surface and fixed rigidly with a contoured dynamic compression plate (DCP).[34] Fractures of the anterior column are accurately reduced and fixed with a contoured DCP attached to the medial border of the iliac fossa. Combined fractures are carefully analyzed; subsequently each component is reduced individually and secured. Examples are shown in Figure 10-6. Many of the more comminuted varieties are best treated by the application of external fixation, as described in Chapter 11.

In view of the considerable exertion by large muscles on the fracture fragments and of the inability of the surgeon to apply adequate leverage on the fragments, accurate reduction can be a formidable undertaking. Similarly, early operative intervention on pelvic fractures may be accompanied by significant blood loss. While the surgeon must be prepared for these difficulties they should not deter him from intervening when open reduction is clearly indicated otherwise. External fixation is a particularly useful way to reduce grossly displaced fractures. The percutaneous pins are inserted into the ilium

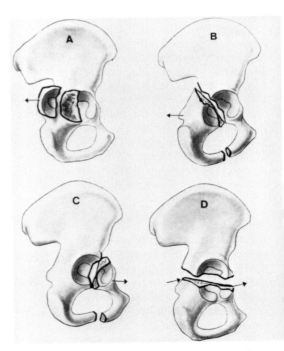

Figure 10-4. The classification of acetabular fractures by Judet and Letournel[31] is presented: *A*, fracture of the posterior lip; *B*, fracture of the posterior column; *C*, fracture of the anterior column; *D*, transverse fracture of the acetabulum. (Reproduced with permission of M. E. Müller, M. Allgöwer and H. Willenegger.[32])

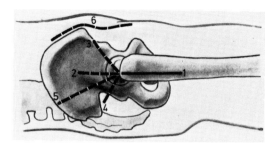

Figure 10-5. Schematic view presents six approaches to the hip joint. The lateral incision (*1*) runs distal from the lip of the greater trochanter. The fascia lata is incised in a longitudinal plane and the insertion of the vastus lateralis is divided transversely with anterior reflection of the muscle. It is employed for intertrochanteric fractures and osteotomies. The lateral incision can be extended in a superior direction (*2*) for a lateral approach to the pelvis, osteotomy of the greater trochanter and arthrodesis or arthroplasty of the hip. An anterior lateral approach to the hip (*3*), a modified Watson-Jones approach, is useful for open reduction of subcapital fractures and arthroplasty of the hip. Moore's posterior approach (*4*) (Southern) requires a split in the plane of the fibers of the gluteus maximus with division of the short external rotators of the hip near their insertion. Alternatively, the Gibson approach (*5*) between the gluteus maximus and minimus can also be used for insertion of a femoral head prosthesis, a total joint replacement or for exposure of a posterior acetabular fracture. A Judet-Letournel incision (*6*) courses from the middle of the iliac crest along the upper pubic ramus to the symphysis pubis. Alternatively the Smith-Petersen approach, also, permits good exposure of the anterior acetabulum and pelvis. (Reproduced with permission of M. E. Müller, M. Allgöwer and H. Willenegger.[32])

and the distal femoral shaft and enable the surgeon to obtain a firm grasp on the major fracture fragments. The external frame provides the necessary mechanical advantage to achieve and maintain precise reduction of the displaced fractures. In the presence of pelvic ring and central acetabular fractures, a combination of external and internal fixation may be advisable. The pelvic ring is reduced and stabilized by external fixation. Then, the femoral head is reduced from its malposition, with intrapelvic displacement, by manipulations of the external device which spans the ilium to the femoral shaft. Finally, open reduction and internal fixation of the central acetabular fracture is performed (see Chapter 11). The surgeon should undertake open reduction of the acetabulum only if relatively large fracture fragments are visualized by X-ray and if his surgical skills are adequate to achieve this formidable undertaking. Otherwise,

surgery may not provide a satisfactory reconstruction of the acetabulum. Postoperative wound infection is of great concern because it would probably preclude the subsequent insertion of a total hip joint replacement, an operation that otherwise might be anticipated to provide an excellent result for a painful hip with traumatic arthritis.[35]

After internal fixation of a pelvic fracture is undertaken, suction drainage is advised for 24 to 48 hours. Three to four days after surgery, active movements of the hip joint may be started in bed. Within 2 to 3 weeks, non-weight-bearing exercises may begin. After 3 to 4 months, the fractures should be united and full weight bearing may be resumed.

With severely displaced pelvic fractures where marked disruption of the pelvic ring or superior migration of a hemipelvis occurs, surgical intervention should be considered. The objectives include restoration of the equivalent height and alignment of the acetabuli with correction of

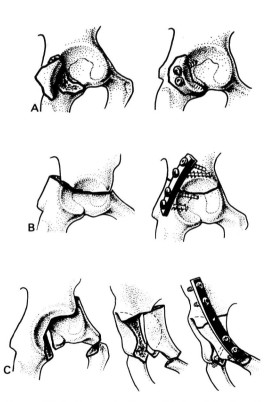

Figure 10-6. Open reduction and internal fixation of three acetabular fractures is shown. *A* shows a posterior lip fracture; *B*, a transverse fracture of the acetabulum; and *C*, a fracture of the anterior column. (Reproduced with permission of M. E. Müller, M. Allgöwer and H. Willenegger.[32])

apparent leg length discrepancy and of rotational malalignment of the hip joint. In young female patients it may achieve restoration of the pelvic outlet to permit vaginal delivery of children. In the past, many authors[29, 36–38] have argued against open intervention both because of the frequency of moderate hemorrhage and because of the technical complexities involved. These workers have applied closed techniques such as a pelvic sling, skeletal traction and plaster casts. In the author's experience, severely comminuted pelvic fractures treated in these ways progress to a moderately high incidence of nonunion of the pelvic ring and malunion of the pelvic ring and acetabulum. Admittedly, the pelvic nonunions can be treated moderately well by reconstructive procedures. The malunions culminate in gross apparent leg length discrepancy, rotational deformity of the hip and cephalopelvic disproportion in female patients. In recent years, the AO group has recommended a more aggressive approach to these injuries. Internal fixation is achieved by the use of cancellous screws and contoured DCPs.[33, 34] Even the AO group, however, emphasizes the formidable nature of such operations and the need for considerable technical skill by the surgeon if the procedures are to be undertaken with adequate likelihood for success and without unwarranted risk of complications. For this challenging category of injuries, the use of external fixation[39, 40] with or without subsequent internal reconstruction of the acetabulum appears to be the optimal method of treatment. It enables surgeons of moderate technical skills to achieve highly satisfactory reductions and fixations of grossly displaced pelvic fragments that would otherwise require a technical exercise in internal fixation of much greater complexity and potential morbidity.

FRACTURES IN THE LOWER EXTREMITY

Fractures of the Femur

Fractures of the Proximal Femur

Fractures of the proximal femur continue to represent a formidable challenge to the surgeon. In some series reporting on geriatric patients,[41] the mortality of such patients both in hospital and during the subsequent 3-month period has reached 25%. Such a high figure is explained, at least in part, by the relatively short anticipated life expectancy of such groups of geriatric patients as predicted by actuarial charts. Most of the patients are more than 60 years of age and

do not tolerate well the immobility provoked by the pain that accompanies motion of the fracture fragments. Previous workers reported high mortality after conservative management.[42] In the absence of antibiotics and other therapeutic measures, patients succumbed from chest infections, urinary tract infections, thromboembolic disease and other intervening medical problems. With modern methods of management, the closed treatment of intertrochanteric fractures does not possess such a fearful mortality and, as will be described, it has a real place in the treatment of severely comminuted fractures in markedly osteoporotic bone. Nevertheless, even in the feeble geriatric patient who has several chronic diseases, early operative treatment is usually recommended, both for early mobilization of the patient and for relief of pain. A recent review on this extensive topic merits scrutiny.[43]

Femoral Neck Fractures

While such fractures usually occur in the elderly, occasionally they occur in young adults or children when severe trauma is involved. In the elderly the fractures usually occur with a fall. Frequently, however, the history suggests that

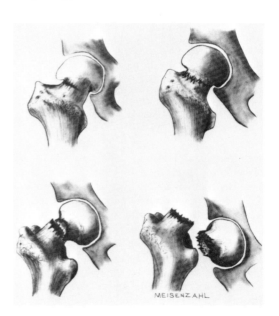

Figure 10-7. The classification of femoral neck fractures by Garden according to displacement and comminution is shown: Type I, incomplete fractures (*upper left*); type II, complete fractures without displacement (*upper right*); type III, partially displaced fractures (*lower left*); type IV, complete displacement (*lower left*). (Reproduced with permission of F. T. Hoaglund and R. B. Duthie.[45])

the fracture occurred from torque in weakened, osteoporotic bone, while the patient was standing or walking, so that the patient fell as the fractured femoral neck displaced.

Garden[44] has classified femoral neck fractures according to displacement and comminution (Fig. 10-7). Type I fractures are incomplete, type II are complete fractures without displacement, type III are partially displaced fractures, and type IV are completely displaced. The classification is useful to evaluate therapy, since displaced fractures have a higher rate of nonunion and avascular necrosis. In adults, the blood supply to the femoral head is *via* metaphyseal vessels (which are disrupted by the fracture), the artery of the ligamentum teres, and the lateral epiphyseal vessels. The location of a fracture site high on the neck with associated displacement or of a poorly placed surgical incision may damage the lateral epiphyseal vessels. If the artery of the ligamentum teres provides insufficient circulation, avascular necrosis may ensue. Furthermore, the periosteum on the neck has no cambium layer so that external callus does not develop. The absence of external callus and the precarious circulation contribute heavily to the high incidence of nonunion. Massie[46] has shown that early reduction and adequate immobilization of the fracture site can overcome these difficulties.

Treatment of Impacted Femoral Neck Fractures. Opinions vary on the optimal method of treatment of type I (Garden) or impacted type II subcapital fractures. In fact, some patients who present with this fracture will have walked on it for several days since the injury occurred. Crawford[47] argues in favor of conservative management with limited weight bearing. He observes that the few late displacements occur within the first 10 days. At that time closed reduction and internal fixation still are readily achieved. In contrast, Bentley[48] recommends internal fixation for these fractures so that subsequent displacement of the fracture, nonunion and avascular necrosis of the femoral head are minimized. The author supports this thesis because internal fixation through a small lateral incision is so rapidly and easily achieved under local or general anesthesia. Five to seven threaded Steinemann pins or preferably Neufeld pins are inserted under image intensification.[43] Complications of the procedures are uncommon and late displacements with possible avascular necrosis and nonunion are unlikely to occur.

Displaced Fractures of the Femoral Neck. The severe pain associated with the patient's spontaneous immobilization, after he sustains the injury, favors a rapid deterioration of the patient's general medical condition. Internal fixation, therefore, should be performed within 1 or 2 days. For patients in congestive heart failure, dehydration or diabetic ketoacidosis, 24 hours of intensive medical management should provide an adequate period for sufficient correction of these problems so that surgery may be performed. Further delay usually is accompanied by complications such as pneumonia, pulmonary emboli, decubitus ulcer or urinary tract infections.

Method. Under general or spinal anesthesia the patient is transferred to a standard fracture table equipped for intraoperative anterior-posterior and lateral X-rays or image intensification. Closed manipulative reduction is performed[41, 43] and check X-rays are taken. When a satisfactory reduction is achieved with the femoral head positioned in a few degrees of valgus and with the proximal fracture surface displaced 1 or 2 mm lateral to the calcar, internal fixation is performed through a lateral incision (Fig. 10-5). Of the many devices available, the author favors the application of a compression hip screw (Fig. 8-7) as discussed in Chapter 9. The surgical technique for its insertion is shown in Figure 10-8 and is described below.

After a lateral incision down to subperiosteal level is completed, a reference point, the tuberosity on the lateral aspect of the greater trochanter, is identified. If a drill track is started 1 inch below this point and aimed proximally and medially at 135° it will pass directly through the femoral neck and head. If a drill track is started 2 inches below this point and aimed proximally and medially at 150° it will pass along the calcar femorale into the center of the femoral head. For subcapital and base of neck fractures a 150° compression screw is inserted by use of the more distal guide point. A 6.3-mm pilot hole is drilled and a preliminary guide wire is inserted through an angled protractor. Biplane X-rays are taken to confirm satisfactory alignment and depth of the guide wire. A second guide wire is drilled through the greater trochanter, neck and into the femoral head to provide rotatory stability. Next, an adjustable 8.7-mm reamer is passed over the preliminary guide wire. The movable stop is set so that the reamer may be advanced to the medial third of the femoral head. The reamer is removed and a 13-mm reamer of fixed length is used to enlarge the most lateral portion of the drill track. A compression lag screw which is 12.7 mm (½ inch) shorter than the length of

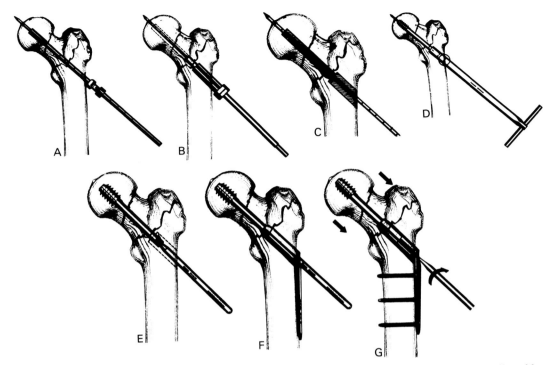

Figure 10-8. The principal stage in the insertion of a compression hip screw is seen. In *A*, the adjustable reamer is inserted over the intramedullary guide pin. In *B*, the preset cortical reamer is inserted. *C* shows a shaded area representative of the reamed channels prepared for insertion of a screw shaft and plate barrel. *D* presents the insertion of the hip screw with a screw wrench. Two calibration lines are visible on the wrench. The first shows that the screw is entering the femoral head. The second (*circled area*) indicates that the screw tip has reached the center of the femoral head. In *E*, the guide wire is removed and the barrel guide is threaded into the end of the screw. The barrel guide assures concentric alignment of the plate barrel with the hip screw. In *F*, the plate barrel is slipped over the barrel guide. In *G*, the plate has been screwed to the shaft of the femur. Subsequently the impacting screw is inserted so that the fracture fragments are compressed together. (Reproduced with permission of R. G. Tronzo.[42])

the original 8.7-mm hole is inserted over the preliminary guide wire. Correct depth is ascertained when the second alignment mark on the screw inserter is opposite the lateral femoral cortex. The inserter is removed and the compression tube and plate assembly is inserted over the lag screw. An aligning device is available which attaches to the lag screw and ensures that the compression tube is aligned concentrically with the lag screw. Insertion of the compression tube over the lag screw follows rapidly and easily. The entire interlocked unit is adjusted until the side plate parallels the femur. The guide wires are removed and the side plate is secured to the femoral shaft with bone screws. Traction is released and the set screw is inserted into the base of the lag screw until moderate resistance is felt. The wound is closed and dressed in conventional manner.

In the author's experience the one shortcom-

ing of the compression hip screw is that a perfectly positioned compression screw may cut out through a markedly osteoporotic femoral head. This complication could be prevented if the otherwise complete set of instruments included a simple type of torque measuring screw driver. If an essential and predetermined amount of resistance was not provided by the porotic bone for the compression screw, then the procedure could be abandoned and primary femoral head replacement could be completed.

In the presence of severe osteoporosis, two surgical alternatives remain. The surgeon may reposition the proximal fragment into a valgus position so that the predominant forces of weight bearing are compressive loads.[33] The osteoporotic bone resists compression moderately well or it undergoes impaction at the fracture site which does not detract from fracture healing. Alternatively, the surgeon may inject methylmethacrylate into the center of the femoral head and neck to augment the strength of the bone.[48] This method has greater application for pertrochanteric fractures.

For displaced fractures of the femoral neck, some classification of the inherent biomechanical stability of the fracture is helpful. Pauwels' classification[50] gives such information, although it refers to the fracture *after* reduction has been achieved.

Pauwels classified the obliquity of the femoral neck into three categories: Type I showed a fracture of 30° with respect to the femoral neck; type II, a fracture of 50°; and type III, 70°. Initially Pauwels designed his classification as a prognostication for the ultimate fate of the fracture. While that objective may be of questionable use, knowledge of the inherent stability of a fracture is of considerable practical significance for the surgeon. One cannot decide on the angle that the fracture line makes with the horizontal in the unreduced fracture because the X-ray of all types of subcapital fractures appear to be unstable, vertical, Pauwels type III. Garden's classification of subcapital fractures is also useful because it reflects the biological aspect of the hip in relationship to its blood supply. For all but the minimally displaced and stable fractures, a combination of Pauwels and Garden's classification is the optimal approach.[48]

Considerable controversy has continued in the literature over the relative merits of anatomical reduction of the fracture and realignment of unstable fracture fragments into an inherently stable position.[48] Advocates of the former method suggest that anatomical reduction provides the optimal nutritive condition for regeneration of essential intramedullary blood vessels and subsequent union of the fracture without avascular necrosis of the femoral head. While this approach might possess certain theoretical attraction in clinical practice, it does not rest on a sound biomechanical basis. Either stable fixation of the fracture is achieved or subsequent mechanical failure of the implant or of the bone at the fracture site is excessively likely. Several clinical examples of such failure were described in Chapter 9. For the unstable Pauwels type III fracture, an intertrochanteric displacement osteotomy should accompany the internal fixation so that the unstable fracture is converted into a highly stable Pauwels type I fracture. As the AO group has emphasized,[50] the implant should serve primarily as an aligning device to maintain the fragments in stable bony configuration, possibly with a supplementary role of interfragmentary compression. The implant, however, should *not* in itself provide the principal stability against rotational and bending moments. Admittedly excessive valgus correction should be avoided as it may be associated with avascular necrosis of the femoral head, probably as a result of interference with the blood supply in the ligamentum teres.[48] Alternatively an intertrochanteric osteotomy may be performed to convert the fracture into a stable Pauwels type I, as seen in Figure 10-9A.

In the presence of an unstable femoral neck fracture accompanied by posterior comminution of the neck (*e.g.*, Garden type IV fracture), an additional displacement procedure is necessary if stable reduction is to be realized. As the AO group has described, the valgus correction previously mentioned, is accompanied by anterior displacement and anteversion of the femoral head (Fig. 10-9B). A capsular incision is made parallel to the femoral neck. For displacement, the leg is manipulated and the fracture is impacted. The internal fixation merely buttresses the impacted reduction.

Prosthetic Femoral Head Replacement. For patients of short life expectancy (*e.g.*, less than 10 years), who sustain markedly displaced femoral neck fractures, primary femoral head replacement is recommended.[51] In the presence of osteoarthritis of the hip, total hip replacement is a better procedure. Recent novel designs of femoral prosthesis such as Bateman's design,[52] permit rapid replacement of the articular surface at a later operation so that a primary femoral head replacement can be converted easily into a total hip replacement.

Technique. The author prefers a posterior lateral incision of the proximal half of the Gibson approach (Fig. 10-5). With the patient in a lateral position, the incision is extended down to the border between the gluteus medius and gluteus maximus. The latter is bluntly divided after which the short external rotators, pyriformis, gemellus and obturator internus are divided just proximal to their insertion on the femur. The superior portion of the quadratus femoris also may be incised. A T-shaped incision with a proximal base, is made in the hip capsule and the detached femoral head is gently levered from the joint. The neck is fashioned to accept the Moore prosthesis and the intramedullary cavity is reamed with a Moore rasp. Care must be taken to correctly orient the rasp in the proper position of 20° anteversion and to seat the prosthesis sufficiently laterally. The diameter of the excised femoral head is carefully measured. An

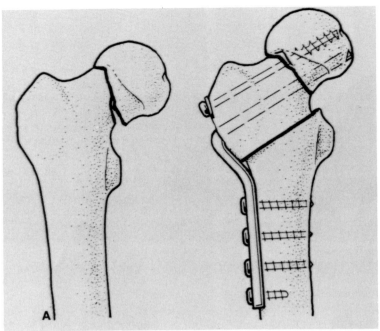

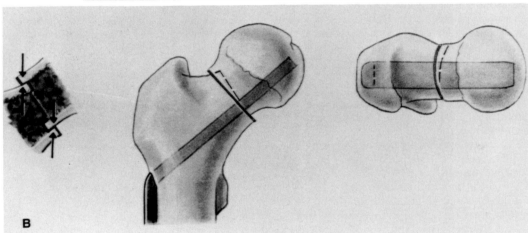

Figure 10-9. *A.* A schematic diagram shows a vertical subcapital femoral neck fracture of highly unstable mechanical configuration that is treated by a repositioning intertrochanteric osteotomy and internal fixation. The osteotomy converts the unstable fracture into a much more stable configuration. *B.* An unstable subcapital femoral neck fracture with comminution of the posterior portion of the neck is reduced with slight valgus and, as seen in the axial projection, slight overcorrection into anteversion. The cortices of bone may be interlocked, as seen in the view on the far left. (*A* and *B,* reproduced with permission of M. E. Müller, M. Allgöwer and H. Willenegger.[32])

equivalent Moore prosthesis is securely driven into the femoral shaft and the prosthesis is located in the acetabulum. The prosthesis should be positioned with slight varus alignment of the stem so that the inferior border of the proximal stem rests firmly on the thick buttress of calcar and the lateral border of the distal stem rests on the lateral femoral cortex. A trial range of motion of the hip should be performed to confirm the stability of the prosthesis. Then the wound is closed in conventional manner. Nursing care must prevent adduction, flexion and internal rotation, the positions which predispose to dislocation of the prosthesis. The day after surgery the patient is allowed out of bed and may start weight bearing to tolerance.

Especially in the institutionalized geriatric patient with a femoral neck fracture, the relative technical ease of prosthetic femoral head replacement should not detract the surgeon from the liabilities of this method. In the institutionalized geriatric patients, wound infections are high (up to 40%) and are associated with considerable morbidity and mortality. In the confused bedridden patient, spontaneous, painful postoperative dislocation is not uncommon. In the more active patient postoperative hip pain from loosening of the implant or excessive wear of the opposing acetabular articular cartilage is likely to occur within 5 to 10 years after surgery. Whenever the surgeon can undertake a stable internal fixation with satisfactory alignment, the restoration of a living hip joint should be seriously considered in favor of prosthetic femoral head replacement.

Femoral Neck Fractures in Children. Such fractures require violent trauma whereupon the primary medical care may focus on another concurrent injury. Frequently satisfactory closed reduction can be obtained and maintained by early Russell's or Buck's traction followed by the application of a hip spica for the duration of healing. If closed reduction is unsatisfactory, usually with varus deformity, operative internal fixation is indicated.[53] The fracture is reduced and approached as in an adult. Fixation is achieved by three threaded pins or with small nail-plate assemblies. The author prefers a tiny fluted Sampson nail with attached side plate as seen in Figure 10-10. Careful positioning of the pins or nail under X-ray control is essential to limit the otherwise high incidence of avascular necrosis of the femoral neck and head in children who sustain displaced fractures.[54] The fluted pediatric nail is an excellent design for reconstructive osteotomies of the proximal femur. For example, a varus osteotomy, for treatment in congenital dislocation of the hip, Perthes disease or cerebral palsy, can be undertaken with a precise angulatory or rotational correction by application of the technique described by Makley *et al.*[55] Alternatively, the AO pediatric nail is a highly satisfactory implant (Fig. 10-10B).

Intertrochanteric Fractures

These fractures are encountered frequently in the elderly after a direct fall onto the hip and in young adults after violent trauma. Instability of the fracture is a common feature. In virtually all of the elderly patients and in most of the young adults, internal fixation is necessary for relief of pain, and stabilization with satisfactory alignment.

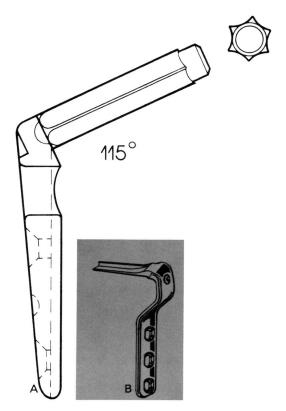

Figure 10-10. *A.* A Sampson pediatric fluted hip nail for a varus osteotomy is shown. The small cross-sectional view on the right shows the fluted nail which provides rotational stability. *B.* Schematic diagram shows the AO pediatric hip nail. (*B*, reproduced with permission of Synthes Ltd. (U.S.A.).)

Technique. The crucial features of operative management are the provisions for bony stability with a continuous medial buttress of cortical bone and the application of a strong fixation device.[56] A variety of techniques (Fig. 10-11) have been classified by Tronzo,[58] Dimon and Hughston,[59] and by the AO group[60] for achievement of this goal: (a) For simple minimal displaced pertrochanteric fractures with an intact calcar, roughly anatomical reconstruction with minor valgus displacement may be undertaken as shown in Figures 10-11A and 12; (b) for comminuted fractures where the calcar consists of a sturdy spike attached to the proximal fragment, valgus displacement with impalement of the intramedullary cavity of the distal fragment by the spike of calcar may be performed (Fig. 10-11C); (c) for comminuted fractures where the calcar, as well as the greater and lesser trochanters are comminuted, the proximal fragment may be rotated into marked valgus alignment

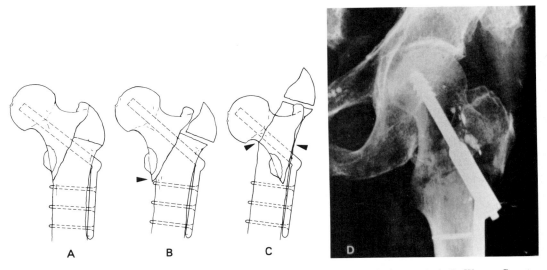

Figure 10-11. Three methods of intertrochanteric reduction are shown. *A*, Anatomical. *B*, Wayne County, with medial displacement of the proximal fragment and impingement of the calcar femoralis of the proximal fragment on the medial cortex of the shaft. *C*, Hughston-Dimon in which the intertrochanteric portion of the proximal fragment is embedded into the distal fragment. (*A, B* and *C*, reproduced with permission of D. A. Sonstegard, H. Kaufer and L. S. Matthews.[57]) *D*. A radiological view shows an unstable pertrochanteric fracture with comminution of the lesser and greater trochanters and the proximal calcar femoralis. Stability of the fracture and anatomical length of the proximal femur are regained by marked valgus displacement of the proximal femoral fracture and fixation with a compression hip screw.

(160°) both to provide osseous stability and to restore length in the proximal femur (Fig. 10-11*D*) and (d) in young adults with a comminuted fracture through normal solid bone, roughly anatomical alignment, perhaps with minor valgus displacement, may be achieved by the application of lag screw reconstruction of the fragments followed by a nail-plate assembly (Fig. 10-12*B*). In the typical osteoporotic elderly patient, this technique is unsatisfactory because the implants do not encounter adequate resistance in the fragile bone.

At surgery the patient is placed supine on a regular operating table that permits the placement of an X-ray plate under the hip. A small bolster may be placed under the hip. The entire leg is prepared completely free without applied traction. The conventional lateral approach to the hip is used. The vastus lateralis is reflected downward and forward and the front of the intertrochanteric area is approached. The fracture is visualized and reduced under direct vision. Disimpaction is achieved by flexion and adduction to disimpact; then traction, abduction, internal rotation and lastly extension are applied to realize reduction. Provisional stabilization of the fracture is achieved by the use of Steinmann wires. Alternatively, for uncomminuted fractures with minor displacement, the

patient may be placed on a fracture table and closed reduction of the fracture may be performed by manipulation of the hip as previously described. After X-rays confirm satisfactory reduction, lateral exposure of the proximal femoral shaft is undertaken. Whenever marked displacement or comminution are present, the open reduction is preferable to ensure close approximation of bone fragments, particularly in the region of the lesser trochanter.

Of the numerous fixation devices available, the author favors the compression hip screw.[61] The adaptability of the former to conform to the multiple types of fractures and techniques of stabilization as well as its excellent assortment of accessory tools is the reason for this choice. The techniques of closed reduction and surgical approach are similar to the previous account. For anatomical reductions or minor valgus displacements a 135° device is selected. For marked valgus displacements, a 150° appliance is used as seen in Figure 10-12*C*. With the 150° device, the technique of insertion is simplified because the angle of the device approximates the reconstructed neck-shaft angle. Bending moments on the implant, also, are considerably reduced compared to those that would be imposed upon a 135° device applied to the same fracture. Several examples are shown in Figures 10-11 and 10-12.

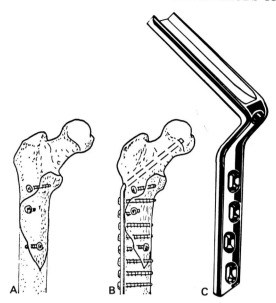

Figure 10-12. *A* and *B.* A comminuted fracture of the upper femur is treated with interfragmental compression by means of screws and the application of a blade plate. If anatomical reconstitution is excessively difficult, the proximal fragment should be slightly overcorrected into valgus rather than into a varus position. (*A* and *B,* reproduced with permission of M. E. Müller, M. Allgöwer and H. Willenegger.[32]) *C.* A schematic diagram shows a condylar blade plate with a 150° angle between the blade and the plate. (*C,* reproduced with permission of Synthes Ltd. (U.S.A.).)

The application of autologous bone graft may be necessary for reconstruction of a comminuted medial cortex. Postoperative mobilization may be retarded if rigid internal fixation is not achieved. Stability of the fracture should be checked by the surgeon before he closes the wound and in biplane postoperative X-rays.

In geriatric patients with severely comminuted pertrochanteric fractures through markedly osteoporotic bone, endoprosthetic replacement, possibly with the use of methylmethacrylate, may provide the optimal solution for rapid mobilization of the patient.[23] A long stem Moore or Thompson prosthesis is required as the prosthesis protrudes above the end of the fractured lateral cortex. Cement has to be built up around the proximal end of the femur to fill the void left by the comminution of the greater trochanter. Alternatively, as Schatzker[48] has recommended, methylmethacrylate may be injected into the intramedullary cavity of the proximal femoral shaft, the trochanteric region and the femoral neck. Subsequently, excellent purchase of the lag screw and the screws that anchor

the plate is observed. Whenever it is technically feasible, the more biological reconstructive method with preservation of the femoral head is preferred.

Subtrochanteric Fractures

These uncommon fractures pose a particularly challenging problem which is fully described elsewhere.[62] In the author's experience, the best available method for the essential operative stabilization is the Zickel device (Fig. 10-13*A*). As described in Chapter 9, it consists of an intramedullary rod with a second nail for anchorage of the femoral neck and head. After insertion of the intramedullary rod, an aligning jig is applied and the nail is inserted through a hole in the proximal end of the rod. Finally a stabilizing screw is added. The principal liability of the Zickel device is the small diameter of the intramedullary rod which limits rotational stability, especially in patients who show a large diameter of femoral shaft, or pathological fractures secondary to Paget's disease or metastatic bone tumors. Such patients may require injection of methylmethacrylate into the intramedullary

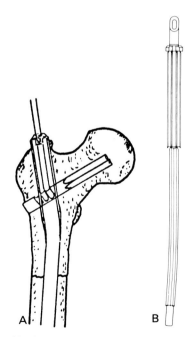

Figure 10-13. *A.* A schematic diagram shows a Zickel device for stabilization of a transverse subtrochanteric or a proximal femoral shaft fracture. *B.* A Sampson fluted intramedullary rod for application on subtrochanteric fractures is shown. The proximal portion of the rod has a larger diameter than the distal portion for stabilization in the trochanteric region.

canal immediately prior to insertion of the intra-medullary rod.

More recently, a fluted subtrochanteric device has been developed which provides a simple method for rigid stabilization of simple subtrochanteric fractures. An example is shown in Figure 10-13B. For comminuted fractures, especially those which extend into the intertrochanteric region, supplementary stabilization, however, would be necessary. For comminuted subtrochanteric fractures a nail-plate device such as a Jewett nail with a long side plate may be necessary. The surgeon must ensure that bony stability of the proximal femur is attained or fatigue fracture of the implant is likely to occur. The Ender's condylocephalic nail[63] provides a more satisfactory biomechanical solution, although a special operating table and image intensification are required. In comminuted fractures, through structurally sound bone, especially in young adults, preliminary lag screw fixation of major fragments possibly with the application of autologous bone graft may be necessary.

Fractures of the Femoral Shaft

In recent years considerable, and as yet unresolved, controversy has focused on the optimal method of management of these major fractures. The central question is the extent of indications for internal fixation. Closed and open methods are described with the author's indications. Interested readers may study detailed accounts of particular methods elsewhere.[64–66]

Closed Methods of Treatment. Femoral shaft fractures in children are treated almost exclusively by closed methods.[67] Internal fixation is contraindicated because of potential damage to the epiphyseal plate and growth disturbances of the femur. Anatomical reduction is not required because of the child's ability to correct certain malalignment with growth and remodeling. Over-riding of 1 cm may be completely corrected by the epiphyseal stimulation of the fracture to encourage longitudinal growth. Angular deformity near the distal metaphysis and in line with the axis of motion of the knee joint is moderately well corrected with growth. Transverse angular deformity, especially at the level of midshaft, or rotatory deformity is poorly corrected. Stable fractures may be provisionally treated with nonskeletal traction followed by the application of a hip spica after radiological evidence of callus appears, usually within 10 to 20 days. Unstable fractures are provisionally treated by skeletal traction with a Steinmann

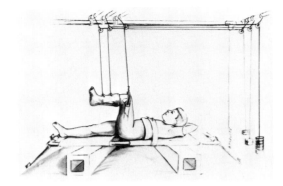

Figure 10-14. Schematic view shows a child treated in skeletal traction for a fracture femur. The hip and knee are flexed to 90° and a short leg cast is applied. (Reproduced with permission of M. O. Tachdjian.[68])

pin inserted into the distal femur or proximal tibia. Management is greatly simplified if the hip and knee joints are maintained at 90° in traction (Fig. 10-14). When radiological evidence of callus appears, a hip spica is applied.

In young adults, similar provisional management of simple femoral shaft fractures is widely used. Skeletal traction usually is applied in balanced suspension since the weights required to maintain 90° of hip and knee flexion are large. In the absence of skeletal traction, large distractive forces would have to be applied by the application of cutaneous traction, with considerable likelihood of ischemia and possibly necrosis of the skin. Balanced suspension requires frequent, time consuming adjustments to counter postural movements; the adjustments must be performed by someone who is knowledgeable in the method. When provisional callus is seen in X-rays, a hip spica or cast-brace may be applied. While the application of a cast-brace requires considerable technical skill, it comprises a significant advance in fracture treatment which merits close scrutiny.

Technique of Cast-brace Application. An elastic spandex socket is placed over the thigh and surrounded by one layer of webril. Elastic plaster followed by standard plaster is applied to the thigh as a well molded quadrilateral cast. Alternatively, plastic sockets can be purchased commercially for incorporation into the cast. The proximal rim is fashioned with an adjustable plastic rim or by conventional technique. An elastic bandage is applied to the knee and a well molded short leg cast is secured with the ankle at 90° and the foot in a neutral position. When the casts have dried, single axis or preferably polycentric knee joint hinges are applied medi-

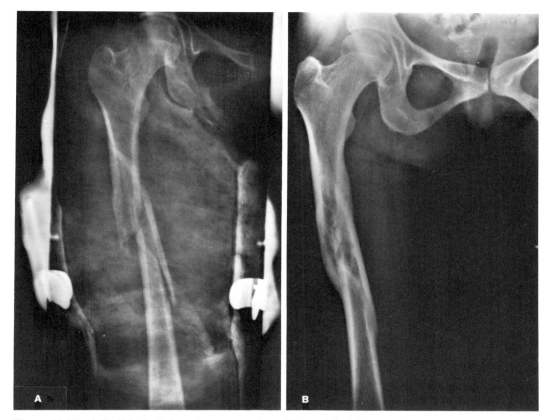

Figure 10-15. *A.* Radiological views show a comminuted femoral shaft fracture in a woman of 22 years that is treated with a cast-brace. Within a month after sustaining the fracture this patient, a secretary, was able to walk to work in the cast-brace. *B.* The radiological view is shown 5 months after injury when the fracture had united in satisfactory alignment.

ally and laterally to adjoin the two plasters. The knee hinges must correspond to the anatomical axis of motion.

The patient is instructed in quadriceps exercises, active knee motion exercises and gait training with progressive weight bearing to tolerance. Usually the cast-brace can be discontinued in 6 to 8 weeks. Mooney *et al.*[69] report a mean healing time of 14½ weeks after the use of provisional skeletal traction and subsequent cast-bracing for distal femoral shaft fractures. The incidence of nonunions is small, just as after treatment with hip spicas and early weight bearing. Unlike treatment with a hip spica, however, the cast-brace is not often associated with residual restriction of knee motion. For simple fractures of the middle and distal third of the femoral shaft, cast-bracing is ideal. For simple fractures of the proximal third or comminuted but well aligned fractures of any portion of the femoral shaft, provisional skeletal traction followed by the application of a hip spica is indicated. As the

surgeon's technical skill with the use of the cast-brace improves, he may apply it, after a shorter period of skeletal traction, to more proximal or more comminuted fractures. A radiological example is shown in Figure 10-15. If delayed union occurs, internal fixation with the application of autologous bone graft may be necessary.

One of the principal liabilities of cast-bracing is the great technical difficulty in the application of a well molded cast to a grossly obese patient. In the presence of comminuted femoral shaft fractures, obesity may preclude the satisfactory application of a cast-brace until provisional callus formation has occurred. Obesity, also, greatly hampers the application of all alternative methods of fracture treatment!

Internal Fixation of Femoral Fractures. *Application of the Intramedullary Rod.* The best form of internal fixation for simple transverse or short oblique fractures of the proximal or middle third of the femoral shaft is an intramedullary rod. When inserted by the closed

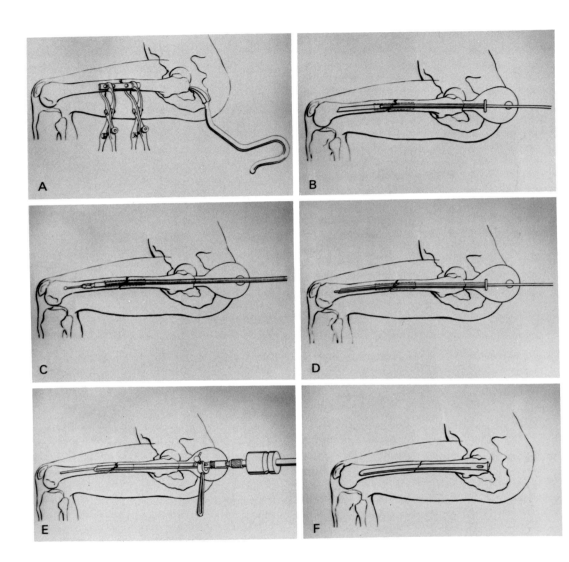

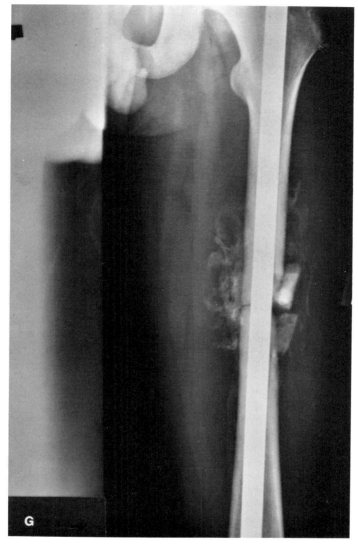

Figure 10-16. Schematic views present the insertion of an intramedullary rod into the femur by the open or closed technique. *A.* By application of the open technique, the fracture is exposed and the guide rod is inserted through the greater trochanter and advanced until it appears at the fracture. The deformity is increased until the fragments are almost at 90° to each other. The tip of a small Hohmann retractor is introduced into the medullary canal of the distal fragment. Leverage on the retractor permits reduction of the fracture. The guide rod is advanced into the distal fragment and the fracture is temporarily stabilized with a semitubular plate. For application of the closed method (*B*), the fracture is reduced on the special fracture table and the guide rod is inserted through the greater trochanter *C.* Reaming is undertaken with graduated flexible reamers. *D.* A polyethylene medullary tube is inserted over the 3-mm ball-ended guide rod which subsequently is replaced with a solid guide rod. Prior to insertion of the latter, the medullary cavity is irrigated with saline solution. *E.* The medullary nail is carefully advanced over a special guide rod. For the insertion of the conventional Küntscher nail, the slot in the nail faces posterior-medially. For insertion of the newer AO medullary nail, the slot faces anteriorly. *F.* The rod is shown in its optimal position. *G.* A radiological view of a transverse and slightly comminuted midshaft femoral fracture with intramedullary rod fixation is shown. The minute fragments of bone collected from the reaming procedure were carefully packed into the comminuted region and have begun to heal with visible callus formation. (*A,* reproduced with permission of M. E. Müller, M. Allgöwer and H. Willenegger.[32]; *B–D,* reproduced with permission of Synthes, Ltd., (U.S.A.).)

method under X-ray image intensification, infection rates of less than 1% may be achieved. In contrast, the open method is associated with an infection rate of perhaps about 1 to 5%. The sequelae of infection frequently includes 3 to 4 years of treatment, (mostly in the hospital), residual stiffness of adjacent joints and possibly chronic osteomyelitis. When the surgical team possesses the necessary skill, the expensive image intensification and special operating table, the closed method of Küntscher[70-72] should be applied. Otherwise the open technique is preferred.[73, 74] The intramedullary cavity should be reamed so that a nail of at least 15 mm is inserted. A few other technical aspects must be emphasized.

For closed nailing the patient is positioned on the special operating table and skeletal traction is applied to the leg. Alignment of the fracture is confirmed with image intensification. Alternatively, for open nailing of the femur, the patient is placed on the contralateral side. The leg and the gluteal region are exposed in the prepared region. For application of the open or the closed techniques initially exposure of the greater trochanter is undertaken through a vertical incision, splitting the underlying glutei, for accurate placement of the reaming guide in the superior-lateral aspect of the greater trochanter (see Fig. 10-16). A more medial location, directly cephalad to the femoral shaft is undesirable because: (a) the more medial placement may sever vessels to the femoral head; (b) more medial placement provides a stress riser for the femoral neck; and (c) if osteomyelitis occurs more medial placement may provide an intracapsular pathway so that the infection spreads to the hip joint. Starting with a 9-mm reamer, reaming is undertaken in graduated 0.5-mm increments with a minimum length of reaming of 5 cm on either side of the fracture. For application of a Küntscher nail, the intramedullary cavity is reamed 1 mm larger in diameter than the diameter of the nail. After completion of reaming, a Teflon tube is inserted into the intramedullary cavity for irrigation. A nail guide is inserted and the tube is withdrawn. A nail of at least 15 mm in diameter is carefully inserted.

The length of the nail is measured prior to surgery from an X-ray of the normal femur and is confirmed from the guide rod. The nail should extend from the top of the greater trochanter to the adductor tubercle. For the insertion of an AO nail a threaded impacting and extracting device is attached to the rod which greatly facilitates insertion or withdrawal, in contrast to the difficulties previously encountered with comparable procedures with the original design of a Küntscher rod. Other manufacturers, also, have improved the devices for insertion and withdrawal of the rod. Insertion of the nail should be undertaken with gentle taps of a weighted impactor. If resistance is encountered, the nail should be withdrawn and reaming should be repeated. Occasionally a smaller size of nail may be needed. If the nail becomes lodged, the femoral shaft may be split on the lateral cortex, at the site where the tip of the nail is lodged, by the use of a power oscillating saw. If the tip of the nail impinges upon the tip of the distal bone fragment, it may distract the fracture or split the bone. Close attention to the insertion procedure is necessary to ensure uncomplicated internal fixation with the intramedullary nail. After the nail is inserted, an X-ray should be taken to confirm satisfactory alignment of the fracture and the nail. Adjustments should be made with radiological confirmation of a satisfactory result prior to closure of the wound.

Where minor comminution or segmentation of the fracture is present, an intramedullary rod still may be applied although considerable technical skill and experience with the method are essential. Additional stabilization frequently is essential. The application of autogenous bone graft frequently is necessary. Previously, the AO group favored cerclage wires for augmentation of rotatory stability. In view of the complication of segmental avascular necrosis, cerclage has been replaced by the use of a 4-hole DCP on the linea aspera where the thick ridge of bone permits insertion of screws without violation of the intramedullary canal. After 3 months the plate is removed to limit excessive stress protection of the femur.

After surgery the leg is positioned with 90° of flexion of the hip and knee for about 2 to 5 days. The position may be maintained by balanced traction or by the use of a splint. On the day after surgery the patient initiates quadriceps exercises and active extension of the knee. Subsequently, the patient undertakes gait training with the use of crutches. The amount of weight bearing is ascertained by the degree of stability of the fracture as observed at surgery and by scrutiny of the postoperative X-rays. In the presence of comminution of the fracture, minimal early weight bearing is permitted. The nail is not removed until radiological appearance of the femoral cortex at the fracture site appears to be normal. Usually the nail is not removed prior to 18 to 24 months after its insertion. While insertion of an intramedullary nail provides a method for rapid rehabilitation and weight bearing of a patient with a simple transverse or short oblique midshaft fracture of the femur, it should not be undertaken without careful consideration and technical preparation by the surgeon. The technical complications of nail insertion, such as gross comminution of the femur can be disastrous. When the femoral shaft is comminuted, only surgeons with extensive training in the use of intramedullary rods should proceed with this technique.

Markedly comminuted femoral shaft fractures pose formidable technical problems with attempts to undertake internal fixation. Nevertheless, the alternatives, especially for segmental fractures where the rates of nonunion are high,

may be poor. A few examples are shown in Figures 10-12 and 10-17. A lateral compression plate is the preferred method of fixation. If the buttress effect of the medial cortex has been disrupted by comminution, then cancellous bone graft should be added. Supplementary lag screw fixation of the fragments frequently is required prior to stabilization with the plate. For severely comminuted fractures a second shorter anterior plate may be necessary if rigid stabilization is to be achieved. After surgery, supplementary external immobilization may be necessary.

When a considerable delay occurs between the time of the fracture and the internal fixation, or when an established delayed or nonunion is treated by internal fixation, over-riding of the fracture fragments, as seen in Figure 10-17*B*,

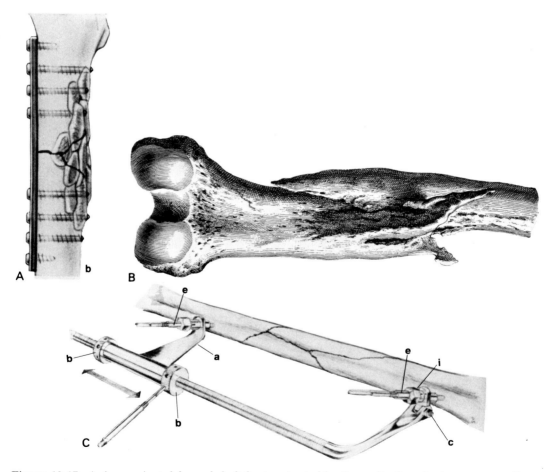

Figure 10-17. *A*. A comminuted femoral shaft fracture treated by the application of autogenous cancellous bone graft and a lateral dynamic compression plate with screws is shown. The crucial weight-bearing portion of the medial femoral cortex is carefully restored. *B* and *C*. A schematic view shows a nonunion of the femoral shaft with marked over-riding of the fragments (*B*), which is realigned by the application of the AO distraction device (*C*). (*A* and *C*, reproduced with permission of Synthes Ltd. (U.S.A.).)

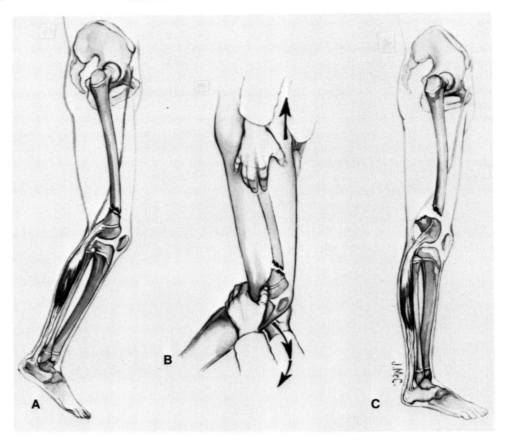

Figure 10-18. (*A*). A simple supracondylar femoral fracture treated by closed reduction with the knee in flexion (*B*), and the application of a long leg cast is shown. If the flexed position is not employed, a malunion, as indicated in *C*, would ensue. (Reproduced with permission of M. O. Tachdjian.[68])

may pose a considerable problem. Restoration of length is highly desirable to irradicate the leg length discrepancy that otherwise would occur. Recently the AO group has developed a distraction device, shown in Figure 10-17C. With the apparatus, the surgeon possesses suitable mechanical advantage so that he may correct and temporarily maintain anatomical alignment, until the internal fixation is completed. Alternatively the author also has used external fixation (see Chapter 12) to restore leg length.

Fractures of the Distal Femur

Supracondylar fractures of the femur and Y- or T-intracondylar fractures occur from violent trauma in all age groups. With their communication with the suprapatellar pouch of the knee, these intra-articular fractures provide scarring of the pouch with subsequent limitation in knee motion.[76]

The supracondylar fragment is angulated posteriorly from the pull of the gastrocnemius muscle while the quadriceps and hamstrings produce posterior angulation as seen in Figure 10-18. Exertion of the adductors on the proximal fragment may yield a valgus deformity. In T- or Y-fractures, the proximal fragment tends to become wedged between the condylar fragments. Until recently, treatment by closed or open techniques has been discouraging. With optimal treatment, one-third of patients showed marked residual limitations of knee motion. For simple supracondylar fractures, closed treatment appeared to provide better results.[76, 77] Initially, after failed closed reduction, further closed treatment was undertaken by insertion of a Steinmann pin through the tibial tuberosity for the application of skeletal traction. If persistent posterior angulation persists, a trans-supracondylar pin is inserted for traction at right angles to the shaft of the femur. If the fracture is stable, a cast-brace is applied when radiological evidence of callus is present.[69] Otherwise, skeletal traction with concurrent quadriceps exercises is undertaken until clinical stability is achieved at about 6 weeks.

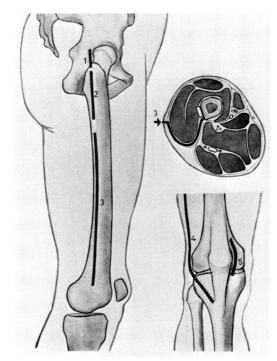

Figure 10-19. Surgical approaches to the femur are seen. *1.* A small longitudinal incision centered over the greater trochanter is used for intramedullary nailing. *2.* A lateral trochanteric approach is used for trochanteric fractures or for intertrochanteric osteotomies. The vastus lateralis is reflected forward and downward. *3.* The lateral approach to the femur is undertaken posterior to the vastus lateralis, as seen in the upper transverse incision of the thigh. The plate is applied anterior to the linear aspera. *4.* The distal femoral condyles are approached through a curvilinear incision which permits inspection of the intra-articular surfaces. *5.* A medial parapatellar incision permits inspection of the medial femoral condyle. (Reproduced with permission of M. E. Müller, M. Allgöwer and H. Willenegger.[32])

For isolated displaced condylar fractures or for displaced Y- or T-fractures, open reduction and internal fixation are essential if restoration of a functional knee is to be achieved. The AO technique provides a satisfactory biomechanical solution. Recently, Schatzker* has reported the experience of a group of surgeons in Toronto who undertook careful anatomical reconstruction with the AO techniques.[73] By assessment of knee motion and gait, the results provide a new superior standard not previously attained by the use of closed or open methods. The AO technique is briefly reviewed.

---

* J. Schatzker, personal communication, 1977.

Technique for Fixation of Y- or T-Fractures. A lateral incision at the level of the knee joint is extended distally and medially to the tibial tubercle (Fig. 10-19). The joint is entered in front of the lateral collateral ligament and the knee is flexed to 90°. This exposure provides the essential good visualization of the femoral condyles. Accurate reduction of the condyles is undertaken and secured provisionally with Kirschner wires. Next, a series of Kirschner wires is introduced to identify, in turn, the axis of the knee joint, the center of the patella in a transverse plane and the plane of the articular surfaces of the femoral condyles. The last defines the site for the blade of the condylar plate. Subsequently, the condyles are secured with cancellous lag screws which must be positioned anterior or posterior to the site for the blade plate. A hole is chiseled in the distal lateral femur, parallel to the surface of the condyles, for introduction of the blade. Next the blade is inserted by use of a mallet. The plate is attached to the lateral femur with the tension device and the plate is placed under tension. Additional screws are inserted into the femur. If impaction of cancellous bone has occurred to leave a defect at the fracture site, the defect should be filled with autologous cancellous bone.

Two types of fractures and examples of appropriate internal fixation are shown in Figure 10-20. As an alternative fixation device a modification of the Richards compression screw is available. The compression screw is satisfactory for simple oblique fractures of a distal femoral condyle. Where a comminuted T- or Y-fracture is present, preliminary fixation of the femoral condyles with cancellous screws is essential. After intra-articular reconstruction is completed, the distal femoral metaphysis and shaft are immobilized with the compression screw device.

After surgery the hip and knee are supported at 90° flexion. Immediate active-assisted knee motion is begun. Six days after surgery the patient is encouraged to sit and to undertake partial weight-bearing gait, not to exceed 10 to 15 kg, for 2 to 3 months. Metal removal is deferred for at least 18 months and until X-rays confirm homogenous cortical structure.

With severely comminuted fractures of the femoral condyles, or similarly for the tibial plateau, anatomical restoration of the articular surfaces may be an unrealistic goal. In such instances, closed treatment with intensive physical therapy for quadriceps strengthening and active knee motion may be undertaken. While rapid traumatic arthritis of the irregular and/or incongruous articular surfaces may be inevitable,

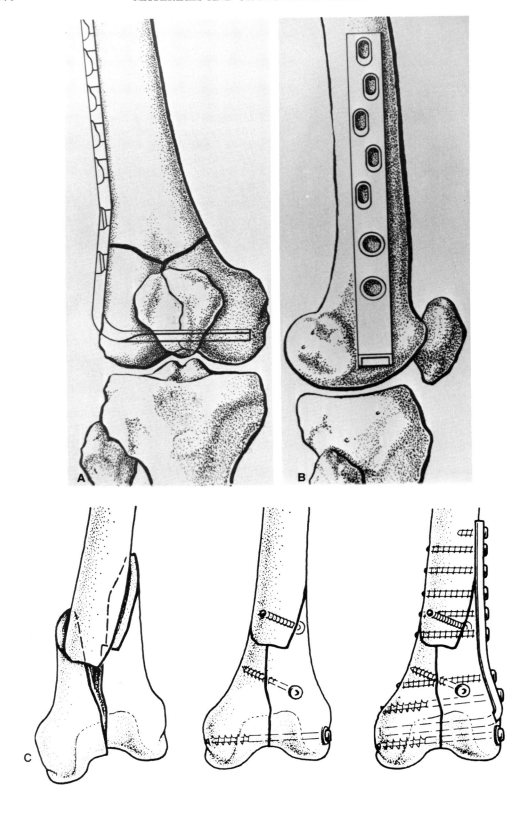

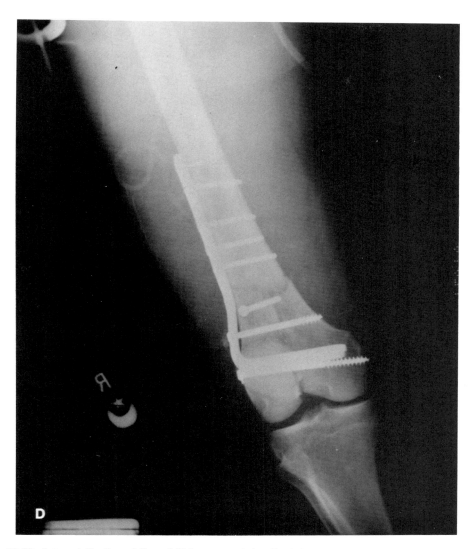

Figure 10-20. Internal fixation of T- and Y-fractures of the distal femur are shown. *A* and *B*. The correct placement of an AO angled blade plate is seen. The articular fragments are reconstructed with cancellous lag screws prior to the insertion of the plate. *C*. The views show the stages in the reconstruction of a Y-fracture with interfragmentary lag screws followed by the application of the blade plate. *D*. A radiological view shows the reconstruction of a similar fracture. (Reproduced with permission of Synthes Ltd. (U.S.A.).)

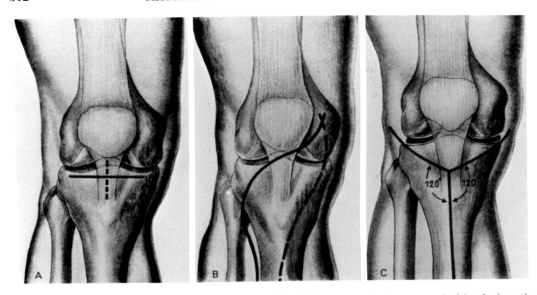

Figure 10-21. Surgical approaches to the upper end of the tibia are seen. *A.* A transverse incision for insertion of a tibial intramedullary nail is present. The patellar tendon can be split for insertion of the nail. Alternatively, the nail can be placed on either side of the patellar tendon. *B.* A curvilinear incision permits exposure of the medial or the lateral tibial plateau. *C.* A triradiate incision with 120° between each limb provides good access to both tibial plateaus. The incision is centered over the patellar tendon. The articular surfaces are observed deep to the menisci. Upon closure the medial ligament of each meniscus is repaired. (Reproduced with permission of M. E. Müller, M. Allgöwer and H. Willenegger.[32])

prosthetic replacement of the surfaces can be performed. In the absence of previous surgical scarring, and especially of postsurgical pyogenic arthritis, total knee replacement may provide a highly functional result.

When the distal femoral shaft and metaphysis are severely comminuted but with simple intra-articular fractures, a combination of external fixation, with a Hoffmann device may be undertaken with intra-articular reconstruction with cancellous screws. The supplementation with external fixation is described in Chapter 11. The combination may permit the surgeon to stabilize a comminuted segment that would be impossible for him to undertake satisfactorily by the use of internal fixation.

Fractures of the Patella

Fractures of the patella occur in all age groups from direct trauma to the knee.[73, 77]

Undisplaced patellar fractures in children or young adults are satisfactorily treated by the use of a cylinder cast for 6 weeks, after which full knee motion is rapidly restored. Possibly in the elderly with undisplaced transverse fractures and certainly all displaced simple fractures, tension band wiring is preferred.

Technique. Through a transverse cutaneous incision, the fracture is exposed (Fig. 10-21). Accurate reduction is undertaken and secured with a towel clip. A wire is passed deep to the insertion of the quadriceps and patellar tendon (Fig. 10-22*A*). A second wire lies more superficially. After slight over-correction the wires are tightened and tied on the anterior surface of the patella. On knee flexion, the over-correction vanishes and the fracture surfaces are compressed. The tension band wire may be augmented by parallel Kirschner wires which provide lateral rotational stability. Large comminuted fragments may be reduced and attached to the residual bone by the use of cancellous lag screws (Fig. 10-22*B*). Smaller comminuted fragments may require excision. In the presence of a rupture of the patellar tendon or a fracture of the inferior pole, a second tension band wire is inserted into the patella and around a transverse screw through the tibial tubercle (Fig. 10-22*C*). The second wire protects the more fragile repair of the patellar mechanism.

The wound is closed in conventional fashion. After surgery the knee is managed in 90° of flexion. Quadriceps exercises and active knee motion are started immediately.

Markedly comminuted patellar fractures may require patellectomy as realignment and fixation of small fragments may be impossible.

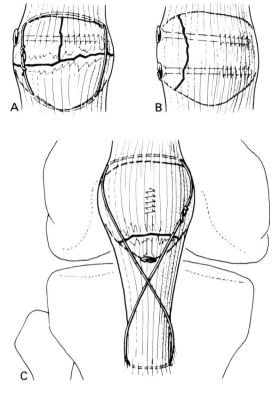

Figure 10-22. Internal fixations of three types of patellar fractures are shown. *A.* A longitudinal fracture is secured with cancellous lag screws. *B.* A T-fracture is restored with a cancellous lag screw and a tension band wire. *C.* A transverse fracture of the distal pole is secured with cancellous lag screw. Subsequently the patellar tendon is protected with a figure-of-8 wire that extends from the quadriceps tendon to the anterior tibial tubercle. (Reproduced with permission of Synthes Ltd. (U.S.A.).)

Fractures of the Tibia

The tibia is the most frequently fractured long bone. Both at the time of injury and afterward, complications commonly occur, especially when high velocity accidents with high energy of impact have transpired.

As in previous discussions, tibial fractures are considered in anatomical sequence as the management of the tibial plateau, the shaft and the malleoli. As Brown,[78] Watson-Jones[79] and others[80, 81] have confirmed, the indications for open reduction and internal fixation include: irreducible intra-articular fractures; irreducible epiphyseal injuries in growing children; concomitant neurovascular injury where emergency intervention and osseous stabilization is necessary;

certain unstable or comminuted metaphyseal and diaphyseal fractures; and nonunions. Together these indications still represent a small portion of all tibial fractures. The development of cast-bracing for tibial shaft fractures has led to further improvements in the results of closed management.[80] Nevertheless, when open intervention is necessary it requires the application of gentle handling of the fragile pretibial skin and subcutaneous tissues, a sound biomechanical appreciation of the principles of internal stabilization and deft surgical technique. Whenever surgical intervention is deemed necessary, the principles of surgery management defined by the AO group should be carefully considered. For a detailed account of the management of tibial fractures, the reader should consult elsewhere.[82]

Surgical Approaches to the Tibia. The incision must be placed so that the final scar does not lie over the metal implant or isolated screws. The position of the implant(s), therefore, must be decided before the incision is made. In the diaphyseal region longitudinal incisions should not coincide with the subcutaneous anterior border.

In Figure 10-21, examples of surgical approaches to the proximal tibia are shown. S-shaped incisions or gently curved parapatellar incisions are satisfactory for exposure of the medial or lateral plateau. A triradiate incision (120° between each branch) provides excellent visualization of both tibial plateaus and the intercondylar eminence, especially if the patellar tendon with a distal bone block is retracted in a superior direction. The incision should not meet over the tibial tubercle but over the patellar tendon. To visualize the periphery of the articular surface, it may be necessary to go deep to the menisci. A transverse incision over the patellar tendon, midway between the inferior pole of the patella and the tibial tubercle, is satisfactory for the insertion of an intramedullary nail. The patellar tendon is split lengthwise and held apart. The knee is bent to 40° and the intramedullary cavity is entered with an awl. Shaft fractures of the tibia are approached through longitudinal incisions at least 1 cm medial or lateral to the anterior border, usually on the lateral side. The incisions may be extended in curvilinear fashion to reach the malleoli.

Fractures of the Tibial Plateau

While these fractures may be present at any age, they are especially common in middle-aged and elderly people. Fractures of the lateral pla-

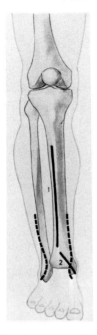

Figure 10-23. Surgical approaches to the tibia are shown. *1.* Fractures of the tibial shaft are exposed through a longitudinal incision 1 cm away from the anterior crest of the tibia, usually on the lateral aspect of the bone. *2.* Curvilinear approaches to the distal tibia and malleoli are shown. (Reproduced with permission of M. E. Müller, M. Allgöwer and H. Willenegger.[32])

teau occur when a forced valgus stress is applied to the knee joint and may be accompanied by rupture of the medial collateral ligament. Common causes include automobile bumper accidents with direct trauma to the knee and falls from heights. The fractures are classified as: (a) a simple split fracture of the lateral or less often of the medial tibial plateau; (b) severely comminuted fractures of one or both plateaus; and (c) impacted fractures which involve the medial eminence as well as the condyles. These complex injuries are fully reviewed elsewhere.[83–85] Careful clinical assessment of the knee joint is essential for prompt recognition and treatment of ligamentous and meniscal injuries which often accompany tibial plateau fractures.

Treatment. Most stable, minimally displaced fractures can be treated by the closed method of Weissman and Herold.[86] In the first week the knee is splinted or the extremity is placed in Buck's traction. During this period quadriceps exercises are initiated. When control of the limb is regained, active knee flexion is encouraged. If moderate comminution is present, flexion may

be deferred for 4 weeks, and the extremity may be placed in a cylinder or long leg cast. Non-weight-bearing activity is continued for 6 to 8 weeks and full weight bearing is deferred for 12 weeks to prevent crushing the subcondral trabecular bone. Despite the apparent severity of these fractures as seen by X-rays, good results may be achieved.

Where irreducible displacement of the fracture is observed, open intervention is necessary. A few types of internal fixation are shown in Figure 10-24. Simple shear fractures in young patients with strong cancellous bone may be fixed with cancellous screws and washers. Where the bone is osteoporotic, a buttress plate is necessary in addition to the screws. Impacted fractures with depression of the tibial plateau should be elevated from below. A large drill hole is made about 5 to 6 cm below the tibia joint surface. A broad punch is inserted and the plateaus are gently elevated slightly above their anatomical site to allow for sinkage. The underlying metaphyseal defect is filled with cancellous graft. Long cancellous screws and a buttress T-plate or a DCP may supplement the fixation.

Severely comminuted fractures provide formidable technical problems. Wide exposure, fre-

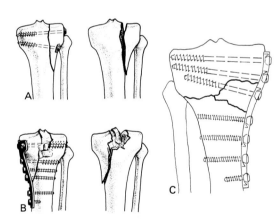

Figure 10-24. Schematic views show methods of internal fixation for tibial plateau fractures and fractures of the proximal tibial metaphysis. *A.* A shear fracture of the lateral tibial plateau is reduced and immobilized with cancellous lag screws and washers. *B.* A comminuted tibial plateau fracture is secured with a buttress T-plate, cancellous lag screws and autogenous bone graft. *C.* A comminuted fracture of the tibial metaphysis is reduced and a dynamic compression plate is used to buttress the medial cortex. Cancellous and cortical screws are applied; frequently bone graft must be added to a metaphyseal region. (*A, B* and *C,* reproduced with permission of Synthes Ltd. (U.S.A.).)

quently of both plateaus and the medial eminence may be necessary. Reduction may be facilitated by the application of cerclage wires, taking care in the popliteal fossa, that no neurovascular structures are compromised by the wire. Fixation is achieved with bilateral T-plates or DCPs, and frequently cancellous screws or nuts and bolts. Some of the severely comminuted fractures are technically impossible to accurately reconstruct. Rather than devitalize tissues extensively around the knee, with numerous scars and abundant soft tissue stripping or retraction, a more modest and possibly closed approach should be considered so that the late resurfacing potential of total knee replacement is not lost by a surgical wound infection.

Within a day or two after surgery, quadriceps exercises are initiated. When control of the leg is regained, active knee flexion is resumed. Again, as with closed treatment, partial weight bearing is restricted for 6 to 8 weeks and full weight bearing is not introduced for 12 weeks.

Shaft Fractures of the Tibia

Fractures of the tibial shaft occur at any age from direct or indirect trauma. About 70% of such fractures are closed and 30% are open. While numerous patterns of tibial fractures are seen, the rate of healing correlates with the severity of the trauma, especially to the surrounding soft tissues, rather than to the location of the fracture or to the plane of the fracture surface.

Considerable controversy on the optimal method of treatment, and especially on the indications for open intervention has continued to the present. Recently Leach[82] has provided an excellent review of the subject. As he indicates, a comparison of the results obtained for closed treatment of this fracture in the 1930s and in the 1960s has shown dramatic approvement. For one series from St. Michael's Hospital in Toronto published in 1942, there were 54 tibial fractures which culminated in 4 deaths, 2 amputations and 1 nonunion.[87] In contrast, Weissman and Herold,[88] in 1966, reported on 140 consecutive adult closed tibial fractures in which there were no deaths, no amputations, no infections, 1 nonunion and 24 delayed unions where the fracture took longer than 6 months to unite. Similarly, in 1942, Singer and Norman[89] reported on 231 open fractures of the tibia of which 21 became infected, 31 failed to unite and 11 required amputation. In 1969, Brown and Urban[90] reported 63 open fractures of which all united, none required amputation and 4 showed chronic drainage. In

57 of the 63 patients completely normal function was re-established. These and other surveys[80, 81] clearly indicate the excellent results that can be anticipated from the correct method of application of closed techniques of treatment for many types of tibial fractures.

Nevertheless there are some advantages of open methods of treatment. With rigid internal fixation, the loss of position or foreshortening ceases to be a major concern in the healing period. With precise intraoperative anatomical alignment, there should be no postoperative deformity. This may be of particular value in those cases when satisfactory closed reduction is difficult or impossible. With rigid internal fixation, adjacent joints can be mobilized in the early postoperative period so that there is less stiffness. Also, exercises of muscles may be encouraged to lessen wasting of muscles. Where both tibias are fractured, earlier resumption of walking may be feasible. Advocates state that even with single tibial fractures earlier resumption of full weight bearing and return to work are observed. In fact, the statistics of the AO group[91] do not support either point. In their experience, patients are rarely able to return to work until the fracture has healed.

The overwhelming disadvantage of internal fixation is the liability of wound infection with osteomyelitis that usually entails months or years of treatment in the hospital. The great morbidity of osteomyelitis of a long bone secondary to internal fixation provides insight into a marked difference in the treatment of femoral fractures and tibial fractures. For femoral fractures, in the absence of rigid internal fixation and especially if the patient is unable to have early application of a cast-brace or hip spica, a prolonged and expensive stay in the hospital is inevitable. While internal fixation may greatly foreshorten the duration of hospital admission, even an infection rate of 1 or 2% will erase the financial savings of the other 98 or 99 uncomplicated cases.[18] In contrast to femoral fractures, most tibial fractures treated by nonoperative methods require a short admission to the hospital, usually of less than a week. In most cases, for all but severely comminuted fractures, operative intervention and internal fixation will be associated with a prolongation of hospital stay compared to closed treatment of the same fracture. If the internal fixation is followed by infection, again appropriate treatment is likely to require a much more prolonged course of hospital admission. Admittedly, the AO group has greatly improved their methods for treating infections that accompany internal fixation.[17, 18] Their emphasis on the need to maintain *rigid* fixation in the presence of infection is crucial. The rigid stabilization promotes soft tissue healing and, as Rittmann and Perren[16] have demonstrated, it permits healing of the fracture with minimal formation of sequestrum.

Internal fixation can be accompanied by other complications, especially avascular necrosis of bone from excessive stripping of soft tissues from bony fragments and by damage to skin and subcutaneous tissues. With careful surgical technique these complications should be rarely encountered.

Whereas for internal fixation of closed tibial shaft fractures several authors have reported infection rates of from about 1 to 4%, for open fractures the reported infection rates vary from about 10 to 20%. With insertion of intramedullary rods the infection rate seems to be considerably greater than it is with the application of onlay plates, especially if the plates are inserted through untraumatized skin and muscle away from the open wound.[91] Intramedullary rods do not provide absolute rotational stability. They also compromise at least temporarily the extensive intramedullary blood supply to a long bone. The micromotion and the diminution in vascular supply of a contaminated open fracture, treated with an intramedullary nail probably account for the high postoperative infection rate observed in these injuries.

Some proponents of internal fixation suggest that such stabilization of open tibial fractures may provide immobilization of adjacent soft tissues so that they show optimal rate and quality of repair. While absolute immobilization *does* augment soft tissue healing, it rests on the assumption that the surgeon possesses the technical skill to achieve absolute stability. If the surgeon lacks the skill or if the open fracture is extensively comminuted so that absolute stability cannot be achieved by the use of internal fixation, then the surgeon is much more likely to achieve a satisfactory result by the use of external fixation[92, 93] such as the Hoffmann device (see Chapter 11). With external fixation, the possibility of an unstable implant at the fracture site serving as a nidus for infection is eliminated.

Also, the proponents of internal fixation argue that the application of closed methods with prolonged immobilization culminates frequently with profound stiffness and swelling of adjacent joints. In the author's experience the application of the cast-brace with early weight bearing and exercise programs has largely eliminated such soft tissue problems. As Leach[82] has stated, the residual stiffness of joints after cast-bracing reflects in large part the after effects of the initial traumatic injury and is of comparable magnitude to that encountered after recourse to internal fixation.

The best indications for internal fixation of tibial shaft fractures are the presence of neurovascular injuries, segmental or other unstable fractures and failure of closed reduction. Surgical repair of a major vessel or nerve demands previous stabilization of the limb for which internal fixation is generally the most convenient method. In the presence of severe contamination with grave risk of infection, stabilization should be achieved by the insertion of skeletal pins with external clamp fixation. When a segmental fracture is treated by the application of a cast or a cast-brace, one of the fractures is especially likely to progress to a nonunion. As will be shown, the use of a DCP is ideal as each fracture fragment can be immobilized rigidly to the adjacent fragment(s).[94]

There is one other highly significant indication for internal fixation of tibial shaft fractures that numerically accounts for a large percentage of such injuries that are best treated by operative techniques. Many open or closed tibial shaft fractures possess moderate instability of which the simple oblique fracture is an example. In the early post-traumatic period, treatment with a cast usually will be undertaken. As the soft tissue swelling in the injured extremity diminishes, satisfactory alignment of the fracture may prove to be difficult to maintain. For the first 4 weeks after injury, the surgeon may elect to revise the reduction and the cast on several occasions. If, at the end of the 4-week period, the reduction is still inadequate, then the surgeon should elect to undertake open reduction and internal fixation. At that time the anatomical landmarks are still evident. They have not as yet become obscured by provisional callus. The soft tissues have not become rigorously adherent in the foreshortened, angulated or malrotated position. The goal of the surgeon to achieve anatomical reduction remains realistic. If, however, the surgeon defers the internal fixation, several factors change so that subsequently the principal goals of early internal fixation are rarely realized. As the patient progresses to a malunion or nonunion, anatomical reduction becomes impossible. Further wasting of the surrounding muscles and stiffness of the adjacent joints is inevitable in view of the prolonged immobilization with the conservative period of treatment, and the subsequent surgical course. In Figures 10-2 and 10-25 three clinical examples reveal the formidable technical difficulties that arise if internal fixation of a malunion is postponed beyond the early post-traumatic period.

Treatment. Closed tibial shaft fractures are best treated by closed conservative methods. By the application of plaster or plastic casts or braces and early weight bearing, Sarmiento,[80] Dehne[81] and others have reported rapid union without infection and a low incidence of delayed union. For reduction of the fracture the patient is placed supine with the involved extremity flexed at the knee with the lower leg dangling off the table. Most tibial shaft fractures can be realigned by gentle manipulation. The opposite leg is used as a guide to determine correction of rotation and deformity. After reduction, most fractures are stable and a long leg cast is applied with the knee placed in extension for a partial or full weight-bearing gait. For wholly unstable fractures, the knee is flexed to about 80° to assist in non-weight-bearing gait with crutches. Occasionally skeletal pins may be inserted above and below the fracture to control rotation, angulation and over-riding. Whenever instability of the fracture is so great that it cannot be controlled by a cast, the surgeon should seriously consider another method of treatment, such as rigid external fixation or the use of internal fixation. Patients with straight leg casts are allowed to start to walk with weight bearing to tolerance when they are comfortable and can actively control the affected extremity. At 3 to 4 weeks, the cast may be replaced by a patellar tendon bearing (PTB) model, as described by Sarmiento[80] with rotation controlled by molding about the tibial condyles and the patellar tendon. The average time for removal of the cast is 13 weeks. The weight-bearing treatment usually provokes about 0.5 cm of tibial shortening.

Open fractures require immediate debridement followed by immobilization. The wounds should not be closed primarily, although the surgeon should attempt to cover denuded bone with soft tissue such as muscle. Secondary closure may be performed or the wound may be left to granulate under the cast. Antibiotics are given until the wound has healed or until clean granulation tissue is present.

Open Treatment. While the indications for internal fixation of tibial shaft fractures are limited, when they arise, meticulous technique is essential. For the treatment of closed transverse or short oblique midshaft fractures, many workers advise the insertion of an intramedullary nail. The narrow intramedullary canal is reamed so that a larger rod may be inserted. A rod of at least 11 to 13 mm is necessary if it is to possess adequate strength and rotatory stabilization in adults. The risk of operative infection is minimized if closed reduction of the fracture is followed by insertion of the rod under image intensification.[95, 96] If satisfactory closed reduction cannot be obtained or if the surgeon lacks the considerable technical skill and the essential apparatus for image intensification, open reduction of the fracture may be undertaken. Most comminuted fractures, however, require the application of preliminary cortical lag screws followed by a supplementary DCP. Prior to stabilization of the tibia with a plate, the fibula should be reconstructed as it provides a strut for rotational alignment and restoration of length. Usually, fibular stabilization is readily achieved by the use of lag screws, a compression plate or a small intramedullary rod. Where the tibial fracture is accompanied by shortening of the bone, reconstruction of the fibula will create a gap between the tibial fracture fragments. Either the gap must be filled with cancellous graft or the fibula must be shortened to provide continuity of the tibia. Whenever possible the former method is preferred because it prevents the formation of a residual leg length discrepancy. Three examples of tibial reconstruction are shown in Figure 10-25. Where marked segmental comminution is observed, two plates, one applied to the anterior border and the other to the medial border of the tibia, may be needed.[97] Any bony defect should be filled with autologous cancellous bone graft. Segmental fractures are best treated with a DCP which permits compression at each fracture level.

The application of double plates should not be undertaken unless the surgeon cannot restore stability by the use of interfragmentary lag screws and a single neutralization plate. The use of double plates necessitates a substantial loss of periosteal blood supply. It provides substantial "stress-protection" to the adjacent segment of bone so that marked osteoporosis occurs. The likelihood for pathological fracture of bone is likely to occur if, after union of the fracture, both plates are removed simultaneously. At least a year should separate the removal of the first and second plates. During this period, partial restitution of the bone matrix occurs spontaneously.

After surgery, early elevation is followed by rapid restoration of quadriceps exercises and active motion exercises of adjacent joints. Partial

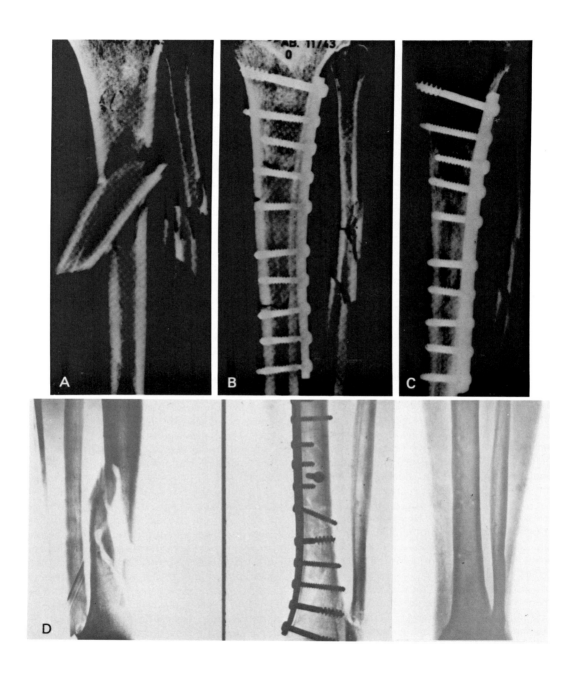

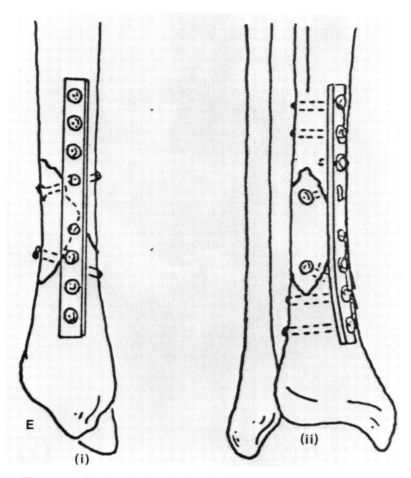

Figure 10-25. Three examples of comminuted tibial shaft fractures treated with internal fixation are shown. *A* to *C.* A segmental fracture with comminution is treated with a dynamic compression plate (DCP) and screws. The distal tibial metaphysis is anchored with a cancellous screw. In 4 months time (*C*) the fracture lines are largely obliterated. *D.* A markedly comminuted tibial shaft fracture is treated with a DCP and screws and supplementary interfragmentary lag screws. In the view on the far right taken 1 year after injury, the metal has been removed. (Reproduced with permission of Miss O. Pöhler.) *E.* An example of a tibial shaft fracture with a butterfly fragment is shown schematically in which interfragmentary lag screws and a neutralization plate are applied. (Reproduced with permission of Synthes Ltd. (U.S.A.).)

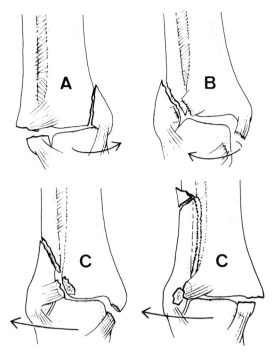

Figure 10-26. A schematic classification of malleolar fractures is shown. *Type A.* Fracture of the fibula at the level of, or distal to, the ankle joint, including a rupture of the lateral collateral ligament, has occurred with or without a shear fracture of the medial malleolus. If the lateral collateral ligament is ruptured, a stress film is necessary to make the diagnosis. The syndesmosis, the interosseous membrane and the deltoid ligament are intact. *Type B.* A spiral fracture of the fibula at the level of the syndesmosis with or without an avulsion fracture of the medial malleolus or equivalent rupture of the deltoid ligament are present. Usually disruption of the anterior syndesmosis or its avulsion has occurred. *Type C.* A fracture of the fibula above the syndesmosis or even in the proximal fibula (Maisoneuve's fracture) has occurred. In addition the deltoid ligament is ruptured or an avulsion fracture of the medial malleolus is present. Total disruption of the syndesmosis is inevitably present with varying degrees of damage to the interosseous membrane. (Reproduced with permission of U. Heim and K. M. Pfeiffer.[12])

weight-bearing gait is restricted for 4 to 12 weeks depending upon the radiological evidence of healing. Alternatively, many surgeons prefer to apply a cast in the early postoperative period so that the patient may begin a partial weight-bearing gait. This may be of particular value after intramedullary rod fixation where, frequently, rotatory stabilization is poor.

Ankle Fractures

Fractures of the ankle present one of the most difficult challenges to surgeons. The role of surgical intervention has remained in dispute to the present time.

Open Techniques. Where open intervention is indicated, either the surgery must be performed within 6 hours after the time of injury or it must be deferred until the soft tissue swelling incurred from the injury has resolved. During this period the leg is elevated and observed closely for evidence of a compartmental syndrome which could dictate immediate fasciotomy. Also, if fracture blisters appear on the skin, surgery must be deferred, usually 1 to 2 weeks, until they have healed. Again, the AO group has provided useful guidelines for surgery.[98]

The initial problem for these intra-articular fractures is to classify them. Watson-Jones,[99] Lauge-Hansen[100] and others[77, 78, *] have made elaborate classifications which correlate the mechanism of injury with the anatomical structures. From the therapeutic aspect, these classifications have two liabilities. Their reference to the precise mechanism of injury is a needless complexity which often is unobtainable since the patient may not recall details of the accident. Furthermore, the great complexity of these classifications is of little therapeutic importance and lends unnecessary confusion for the surgeon who elects to perform internal fixation. Schatzker[48] has reclassified ankle fractures into two broad categories as shown in Figure 10-26. The first type of injury is sustained by forceful adduction, inversion and internal rotation. The distinct radiological features include a transverse fracture of the fibula at or below the joint line or a rupture of the lateral collateral ligament. Also, a shear fracture of the medial malleolus shows an oblique, spiral or vertical course. A posterior malleolar fracture may complete a triad although this injury is on the medial aspect of the ankle. There is never a diastasis. The central problem with the injury is the likelihood for trauma to the medial corner of the talus and for comminution at the site of the medial malleolar fracture. Residual deformities with internal rotation, varus and posterior displacement are not uncommon. Nevertheless, many of these injuries can be treated satisfactorily by the use of a long leg cast. Whenever there is a suspicion of comminuted intra-articular fragments, the fracture

---

* J. Schatzker, personal communication, 1977.

should be opened to remove the loose bodies. Concurrently, internal fixation may be performed.

The second broad classification of ankle fractures are much more sinister and occur from deforming forces that provoke adduction, external rotation and eversion. Any one direction of force may predominate. There may be a rupture of the deltoid ligament or a transverse fracture of the medial malleolus, associated with a shear, oblique or spiral fracture of the lateral malleolus. A diastasis, secondary to rupture of the syndesmotic ligament, may be present. About 50% of the injuries have a rupture of the anterior tibiofibular ligament but with an intact posterior tibiofibular ligament. In these patients diastasis does *not* occur. Another fracture pattern, however, does include a diastasis. The fracture of the lateral malleolus occurs proximal to the insertion of the anterior and posterior syndesmotic ligaments and the interosseous membrane is damaged. Alternatively, the fibular fracture may occur at the proximal end or fibular neck or the

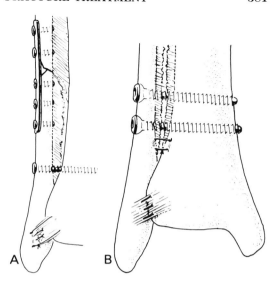

A   B

Figure 10-28. Two examples of transfixion of the fibula and the tibia for the repair of type C fractures are shown. In *A*, the fibular fracture has been stabilized with a plate and a separate, more distal, transfixion screw has been inserted. In *B*, where a Maisoneuve's fracture of the proximal fibula has occurred two 4.5-mm transfixing screws are applied which engage both cortices of the fibula and the tibia. The supplementary ligamentous repairs are evident. (Reproduced with permission of U. Heim and K. M. Pfeiffer.[12])

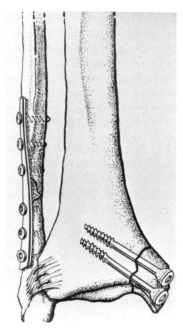

Figure 10-27. A type C bimalleolar fracture with rupture of the anterior syndesmotic ligament has been repaired by the application of a plate to the fibula and cancellous screws in the medial malleolus. Alternatively malleolar screws might have been employed. The anterior syndesmotic ligament, also, has been repaired. (Reproduced with permission of Synthes Ltd. (U.S.A.).)

proximal fibula may dislocate from the tibia. Where a diastasis is in question, stress views of the ankle may confirm the diagnosis. If a diastasis occurs, anatomical reconstruction of the fibula is essential. The distal fibula possesses a complex radius of curvature that enlarges and subsequently decreases. The maximal diameter opposes a "fibular notch" in the distal tibia and the corresponding curves on the lateral talus. If the fibula is not restored to its anatomical length the complex curves on the opposing surfaces of the tibia, fibula and talus cease to fit properly.[101] A permanent deformity with residual diastasis becomes inevitable. Incongruity of the ankle mortice ensues, and with the considerable reciprocal motion of the fibula during gait,[102] a great predilection for traumatic arthritis follows.

Fibula fractures may be stabilized by screws, wires, semitubular plates or intramedullary rods (see Figs. 10-27 and 10-28). Tibiofibular diastasis is restored by direct suturing of the torn syndesmosis. Where the whole interrosseous membrane has been disrupted and direct repair is not feasible, then two positional screws may be se-

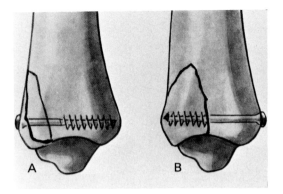

Figure 10-29. Internal fixation of a posterior lip fracture of the tibia is shown. Where the fragment is medial, adjacent to the medial malleolus (type A injury), it is screwed directly from back to front (A). Where the fragment approximates the lateral malleolus (type B and type C injuries), it is screwed from front to back by the insertion of a cancellous screw introduced at right angles to the axis of the tibia (*B*). (Reproduced with permission of M. E. Müller, M. Allgöwer and H. Willenegger.[32])

cured (Fig. 10-28). These should be removed at 6 weeks.

For surgical exposure of the lateral malleolus, the use of the classic approaches, by a posterior malleolar curved incision is likely to culminate with necrosis of the anterior skin flap unless forces of retraction are minimized. Alternatively, the ankle may be approached through a recurrent curved incision (Fig. 10-23) which provides excellent exposure of the anterior syndesmotic ligament and anterior surfaces of the ankle joint.[98] Similarly, a recurrent curved incision for the medial malleolus is also preferred (Fig. 10-23). The saphenous vein and nerve must be protected. In the presence of a posterior malleolar fracture a postero-medial hockey stick incision is preferred. Exposure should remain anterior to the posterior tibial tendon to prevent damage to the neurovascular bundle. Where exploration of the posterior ankle joint is necessary, a longitudinal posterior lateral incision on the lateral aspect of the tendoachillis is made.

For internal fixation of isolated malleolar fractures, usually a malleolar screw introduced with a lag technique, approximately perpendicular to the fracture surfaces and engaging the distal cortex, provides excellent fixation. If the bone is softer with osteoporosis, small cancellous lag screws may be preferred. An example is shown in Figure 10-27. A precise aim is necessary for each screw as the limited bone stock inhibits repeated attempts to insert the screw.

Where the malleolar fracture violates the ankle joint, as it usually does, the ankle joint may have to be opened to remove small fracture fragments and ensure anatomical reduction of the principal fragments. A more proximal transverse fracture of the fibular shaft is readily stabilized by the use of a small semitubular plate (Figs. 10-27 and 10-28) or, alternatively, with a smooth intramedullary nail. The nail or rod must be bent to conform to the curved pathway within the bone. If there is comminution of cancellous bone with loss of volume, bone graft should be applied.

For adduction fractures of the medial malleolus, two malleolar screws are inserted in a horizontal axis so that shearing forces do not produce postoperative displacement. Large avulsion fractures can be secured with two Kirschner wires or by tension band wiring. A posterior lip fragment greater than one-third of the joint surface is immobilized with a lag screw introduced from the anterior medial direction (Fig. 10-29). When the syndesmotic ligament is ruptured, the repair is protected with a screw that secures the distal fibula to the tibia. The screw is not a lag screw so that all four cortices are tapped, as seen in Figure 10-28*B*; it provides the anatomical spacing between the two bones.

In the presence of marked comminution of the articular surface of the ankle, the surgeon may be unable to provide accurate reconstruction of the joint surfaces. Inevitably, in extreme cases, the role for primary ankle fusion is self-evident. In other less comminuted cases, however, preliminary skeletal traction with an os calcis pin, followed by the application of a cast and a nonweight-bearing course may culminate in the restoration of a surprisingly acceptable ankle with a modest degree of motion. Where traumatic arthritis ensues, total joint replacement may provide a suitable means for reconstruction.

When ankle fractures result from high velocity accidents, the distal tibia may be grossly comminuted. These exceptionally difficult fractures have not responded well to previous methods of nonoperative or operative treatment. Malunion of the distal tibia and of the ankle mortice was common. Frequently the distal tibial metaphysis progressed to delayed or nonunion. The AO group has had extensive experience in the management of this fracture in downhill skiers as a result of which they have considerably improved the standard of operative treatment. First the fibular fracture is reduced and a semitubular or a DCP is applied, as in Figure 10-30 so that the length of the limb is restored. Restoration of the fibula correctly positions a large lateral intra-articular fragment of the distal tibia. The residual articular fragments of the distal tibia are reduced with respect to the previously men-tioned lateral fragment. Preliminary stabilization with Kirschner wires is supplanted by malleolar or cancellous screws. After the reconstruction of the ankle mortice, the distal tibial metaphysis is reconstructed. Again, provisional stabilization with wires is helpful. A defect of bone becomes apparent at the central portion of the metaphysis. It is filled with autogenous cancellous bone graft. A buttress plate is applied to the medial surface of the tibia (Fig. 10-30). A DCP (see Fig. 10-31) or clover-leaf plate may be applied; in either case the plate is carefully contoured to match the surface of the bone. After surgery the ankle joint is immobilized in a U-shaped splint to encourage early resumption of active ankle motion. Alternatively a patellar tendon-bearing cast or caliper may be applied. In either case, weight bearing is restricted for 2 to 4 months.

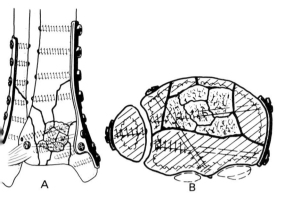

Figure 10-30. *A.* A grossly comminuted distal tibial fracture and fibular fracture (so called Pilon fracture) is treated by the application of a semitubular plate on the fibula, a clover-leaf buttress plate on the tibia, ancillary interfragmentary screws and a bone graft in the distal tibial metaphysis. *B.* A schematic cross-section of the internal fixation is shown to reveal the precise positioning of each screw so that the appropriate fragments are stabilized and the articular surfaces are not violated. (*A* and *B*, reproduced with permission of Synthes Ltd. (U.S.A.).)

In a recent series of severe distal tibial fractures treated by Allgöwer and Rüedi,[91] of the AO group in Basel, 75 patients showed excellent anatomical restoration and good ankle motion, 3 patients developed osteomyelitis, 7 patients ultimately required ankle fusions, of which 5 patients showed traumatic arthritis of the ankle, 5 patients required a late corrective osteotomy and 1 patient had a nonunion. It should be emphasized that all of these were severe fractures where conservative methods probably

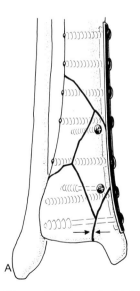
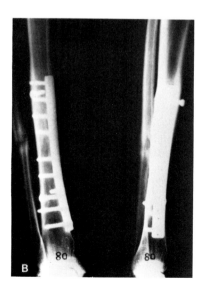
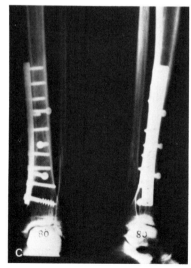

Figure 10-31. *A.* A distal tibial shaft fracture combined with a fracture of the medial malleolus is stabilized with a semitubular neutralization plate. The distal cancellous screw is inserted parallel to the articular surface to compress the intra-articular fracture. *B* and *C.* Radiological views of similar comminuted distal tibial shaft fractures are shown with the application of dynamic compression neutralization plates and screws. (*A*, reproduced with permission of U. Heim and K. M. Pfeiffer[12]; *B*, reproduced with permission of Synthes Ltd. (U.S.A.).)

would have yielded a high incidence of post-traumatic arthritis, spontaneous fusion of the ankle or malalignment.

When a surgeon is presented with such a complex comminuted tibial fracture, however, he should assess carefully the degree of soft tissue damage, comminution of bone, the severity of osteoporosis and his technical skills before he attempts to undertake internal fixation. In some cases, conservative treatment, or primary fusion of the ankle may be the optimal method.

Fractures and Fracture Dislocations of the Foot

Osseous injuries to the foot follow the principles which have been described previously. A more detailed account may be consulted elsewhere.[103–105]

Fractures and Dislocations of the Talus

Numerically most talar fractures represent chip or flake fractures with avulsion of ligaments that can be managed as ligamentous injuries, usually with below-knee cast immobilization for 3 or 4 weeks. The much more serious shear fractures usually occur through the neck, and less often in the body. Fractures of the neck occur from forced dorsiflexion of the foot, so that the neck is driven against the anterior margin of the tibia. With a coincidental vertical force, subtalar dislocation also may occur. With still greater force, in addition, the body of the talus may undergo posterior displacement from the ankle joint. Inversion injuries, also may provoke dislocation of the talus from the ankle joint. With fractures of the neck of the talus or with fracture dislocations, avascular necrosis of the body may follow. In the series by Dunne et al.[106] avascular necrosis developed in 69% of neck fracture dislocations and 50% of body fractures.

Treatment. Fractures of the body or head or displaced fracture dislocations are treated by closed reduction and cast immobilization until union is evident (3 months or longer). Complete talar or subtalar dislocations are reduced by placing the foot in maximal inversion. With direct pressure over the talus, the calcaneus and forefoot are brought into eversion and a cast is applied. Where accurate closed reduction is impossible, open reduction through a lateral approach is indicated. Small cancellous screws or Kirschner wires are used for internal fixation. If a defect of bone is evident cancellous bone graft should be applied. For severe compression fractures, primary tibial-talar fusion may be advisable. Alternatively for open fractures with sub-stantial loss of bone, external fixation is preferred (Chapter 11).

Avascular necrosis, which occurs with many of these injuries, does not dictate a poor result provided that immobilization is continued until union is achieved and that weight bearing is prevented until revascularization occurs.

Fractures of the Calcaneus

Most calcaneal fractures occur from falls in which the patient lands on his plantar surfaces. The type of fracture depends upon the position of the subtalar joint at the time of impact. A classification of the fractures by Dart and Graham[107] is useful. In the severe injuries that accompany falls from considerable height, early treatment focuses on the injuries to the soft tissues, principally with elevation and occasionally with the application of compression dressings.

Treatment. The minimally displaced fractures are treated with a below-knee cast. Moderately displaced transverse fractures require open reduction and insertion of a Steinmann pin through the posterior fragment which is forcibly depressed until the angle formed by the axis of the subtalar joint and the superior surface of the tuberosity is restored. The foot with a protruding pin is immobilized in plaster for 6 weeks. Where open reduction is planned, a precise knowledge of the normal anatomy of the calcaneus and highly skillful reduction is essential if the surgery is to be of any benefit.[104, 105] Otherwise, closed treatment and early mobilization are likely to provide a superior result.[108]

The grossly comminuted and depressed fractures may be treated in one of two ways. A recent series presented by Hall* reveals that remarkably good results may follow accurate open reduction and internal fixation with the application of autogenous cancellous bone graft. Hall has described a medial approach to the os calcis which enables the surgeon to visualize most of the displaced subtalar surfaces. In some cases a second lateral approach through the sinus tarsi permits restoration of the articular surfaces at the calcaneocuboid joint. As Hall relates, fractures of the calcaneus can be visualized as a sudden impact force applied to a hollow box. The sides of the box are distracted while the superior surface of the box approximates the inferior surface. The central core of cancellous bone is crushed with marked diminution in its volume. The surgical reconstruction through the

---

*H. Hall, personal communication, 1977.

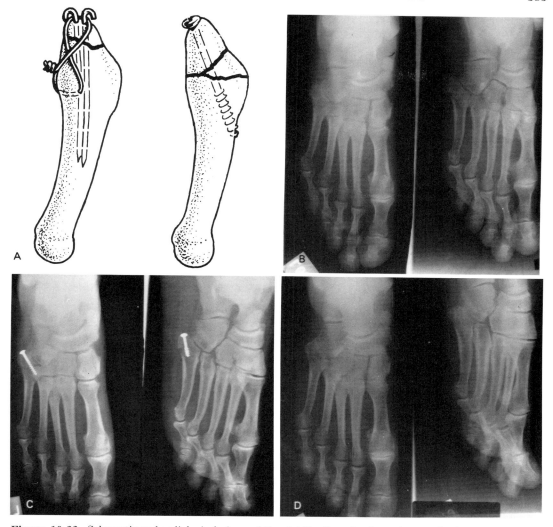

Figure 10-32. Schematic and radiological views of the stabilization of a Jones fracture in the proximal fifth metatarsal are shown. In *A*, either a lag screw or a tension band wire is employed. *B–D*. Radiological views are presented of a nonunion of the proximal fifth metatarsal (*B*) that is treated with a small cancellous lag screw (*C*). Six months later the fracture is united and the screw has been removed, as in *D*. (*A*, reproduced with permission of U. Heim and K. M. Pfeiffer.[12])

medial approach necessitates elevation of the superior calcaneal surface with accurate restoration of the subtalar joint. The sides of the calcaneus are approximated with fixation by cancellous screws. The hollow central portion of the calcaneus is filled with the bone graft. A non-weight-bearing course is essential for 8 to 12 weeks, although early active motion of the ankle and subtalar joints are encouraged.

In some instances, after violent trauma, primary triple arthrodesis (*e.g.,* fusion of the subtalar, talonavicular and calcaneocuboid joints) of a grossly comminuted subtalar joint may provide the most rapid and realistic solution.

For avulsion fractures of the insertion of the Achilles tendon, open reduction with cancellous screw fixation is advised through a posterior-lateral longitudinal incision

Metatarsal Fractures

The commonest type, fracture of the base of the fifth metatarsal, is an inversion injury that responds to symptomatic treatment, usually with a below-knee cast for 4 to 6 weeks. Rarely a painful nonunion ensues which is readily treated with a lag screw (Fig. 10-32). Multiple metatarsal shaft fractures may occur with severe trauma. Usually closed reduction and cast immobilization is adequate. With severe displacement of multiple metatarsal shaft fractures, Kirschner wire fixation may be necessary. More elaborate methods are rarely required. For the exceptional severely comminuted or grossly contaminated open fracture, external fixation may be preferred (Chapter 11).

Phalangeal Fractures

Fractures of the phalanges of the toes occur at any age from direct trauma to the forefoot. Common causes are the dropping of heavy objects upon the toes and striking the toes against a door. While comminution of a phalanx is common, satisfactory general alignment is preserved. With malalignment, dislocation of interphalangeal joints should be anticipated. Open reduction with pin fixation is advised. Usually the treatment for minimally displaced fractures is symptomatic with weight-bearing to tolerance.

FRACTURES OF THE UPPER EXTREMITY

Scapular Fractures

The uncommon fractures of the scapula, including the acromion, respond satisfactorily to conservative treatment except for lip fractures of the glenoid. Such fractures may provoke instability of the shoulder joint and should be treated with small cancellous lag screws

Clavicular Fractures

Fractures and fracture dislocations of the clavicle occur in all ages from direct falls to the shoulder region and indirectly by falls onto the outstretched hand. The indications for internal fixation of these injuries are very limited. Simple midclavicular fractures are best treated symptomatically by the application of a sling and swathe. They inevitably heal provided that open intervention is *not* applied; with internal fixation they may culminate in a painful nonunion. There are two indications however, for rapid open intervention of clavicular fractures.[109] With posterior dislocations or fracture dislocations of the proximal end of the clavicle, mediastinal

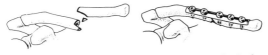

Figure 10-33. A comminuted midshaft clavicular fracture is treated by the application of a semitubular plate. (Reproduced with permission of Synthes Ltd. (U.S.A.).)

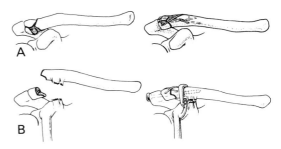

Figure 10-34. Schematic diagrams present the stabilization of distal clavicular fractures with or without disruption of the coracoclavicular ligaments. In *A*, a distal clavicular fracture is stabilized with a tension band wire. In *b*, a similar fracture is stabilized and the coracoclavicular ligaments are reconstructed the coracobrachialis tendon. The author prefers to supplement the tendonous repair with a 6 or 8 mm diameter woven Dacron vascular graft. (Reproduced with permission of M. E. Müller, M. Allgöwer and H. Willenegger.[32])

compression, or rarely injury to major vascular trunks may occur. While closed reduction of such dislocations is usually possible, with life threatening vascular or mediastinal injuries, urgent operative intervention is required. Similarly depressed midclavicular fractures may be complicated by injuries to the brachial artery, vein or plexus for which emergency surgery is indicated. Usually the approach to the neurovascular structures includes resection of the middle third of the clavicle. In fact, most portions of the clavicle can be resected without marked deleterious side-effects. Rarely internal fixation is necessary; fixation with a semitubular plate is shown in Figure 10-33.

For acromioclavicular dislocations or for fractures of the distal clavicle a variety of fixation pins have been used for internal fixation. In view of the major neurovascular structures that reside in close proximity to this region, it is not surprising that insertion of the pins and postsurgical migration of pins have been accompanied by major neurovascular complications. Breakage of pins that are left *in situ* is common due to the unfavorable fatigue conditions. For immobilization of displaced distal fractures, short threaded pins or screws and/or a figure-of-8 tension band wire may be inserted under direct vision or under X-ray control (Fig. 10-34A). For the stabilization of acute acromioclavicular dislocations, reconstruction of the coracoclavicular ligaments (*e.g.,* conoid and trapezoid) is recommended. Of the numerous procedures that have been described, the author favors a dual approach. A Gortex or woven Dacron vascular graft of 6 to 8 mm diameter, is passed deep to the coracoid process and secured around the midshaft clavicle or through a clavicular drill hole. The graft provides immediate stabilization and it permits fibrous ingrowth for a long term regenerative ligament. Late failures of the vascular grafts have been observed by many workers. At surgery, therefore, supplementary stabilization with a biological structure is recommended. The author prefers to use the tendonous portion of coraco brachialis. The tendon is detached from its musculotendonous junction. The free end is threaded through a drill hole in the clavicle as seen in Figure 10-34B.

Fractures of the Humerus

Humeral fractures can be divided into those of the proximal and distal ends and of the shaft. Those of the proximal end may involve surgical or anatomical necks, the tuberosities and the articular surface. The useful classification by Neer[110] relates the type of fracture(s) or dislocation of the glenohumeral joint to the likelihood of an avascular proximal, articular fragment. Where the risk is high (e.g., fracture dislocations with fractures of the humeral neck and both tuberosities), replacement of the proximal humerus with a Neer prosthesis is the preferred primary treatment. The technique is reviewed

in Chapter 14. Where less severe injuries occur, open reduction may be required to realign the articular fragment which is acceptable in view of the vast range of motion of the shoulder. Fractures through the cancellous bone of the proximal humerus heal with minimal risk of nonunion, despite the modest degree of stabilization provided solely by external immobilization of a sling and swathe. Proximal fractures that extend distally into the cortical bone of the humeral shaft, however, have a significant rate of nonunion when treated by closed methods. Thus, when such fractures are accompanied by unacceptable malalignment that cannot be reduced by closed methods they should be treated by open intervention. The application of an AO buttress T-plate (Figure 10-35) or, alternatively, of a small Jewett nail is preferred. With less extensive comminuted fractures, especially in younger patients who possess less porotic bone, cancellous screws may be adequate. Still other workers remain highly satisfied with intramedullary fixation. Either multiple Rush rods[111] or Hackenthall rods, or, more recently, a fluted Sampson rod, may provide adequate fixation.

Shaft fractures of the humerus remain a source of difficulty. For stable transverse or short oblique fractures, closed techniques of immobilization such as U-shaped plaster splints around the sides of the upper arm and elbow or

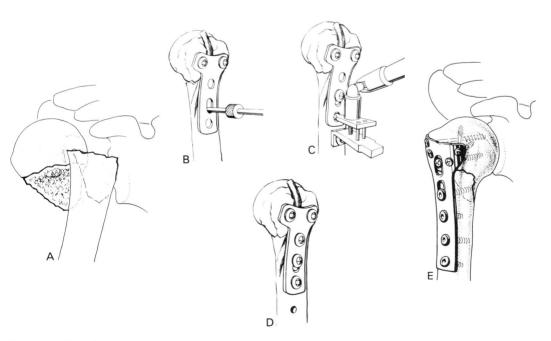

Figure 10-35. A fracture of the surgical neck of the humerus (A) is stabilized by the application of a cloverleaf plate and screws. (Reproduced with permission of Synthes Ltd. (U.S.A.).)

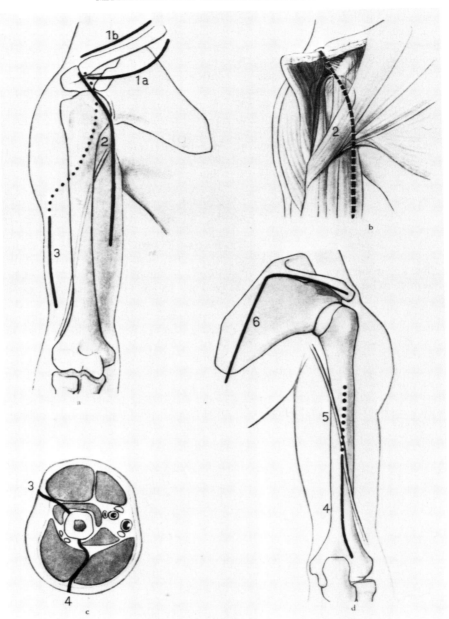

Figure 10-36. The surgical approaches to the shoulder joint and humerus are shown. *Incision 1.* Exposure of the clavicle through a curved or straight incision is possible although the superior straight incision provides a superior cosmetic result. *Incision 2.* A curved incision from the lateral acromion across the tip of the coracoid provides excellent exposure of the humeral head and proximal third of the humeral shaft. For visualization of the humeral head, the anterior third or half of the origin of deltoid is reflected. Neer's method of osteotomizing flakes of clavicle attached to the muscle is preferred so that the muscle is not disrupted. *Incision 3.* Exposure of the midshaft humerus is approached along the lateral edge of biceps and extended through the ventral substance of the brachialis. The radial nerve is identified. The cross-section of the arm in the lower left-hand corner expedites this approach. *Incision 4.* Exposure of the distal humerus through a dorsal incision is shown. *Incision 5.* Dorsal exposure of the midshaft humerus provides exposure of the long-head and lateral head of the triceps which are reflected away from one another. The radial nerve is identified as it spirals around the humerus. *Incision 6.* Exposure of the scapula and the dorsal aspect of the shoulder joint may be undertaken by reflection of infraspinatus from the scapula. (Reproduced with permission of M. E. Müller, M. Allgöwer and H. Willenegger.[32])

the hanging cast technique may be employed.[112] Moderate deformity or shortening may be accepted since the highly mobile shoulder joint allows great accommodation and since arm length inequality is not a problem as it is in the lower extremity. Many comminuted shaft fractures in satisfactory alignment also may be treated in this manner. Furthermore, radial nerve palsy, a common complication, is not an indication for open intervention because most of the nerve injuries that accompany humeral shaft fractures are neuropraxias that resolve spontaneously.

A small percentage of humeral shaft fractures treated with conservative methods progress to nonunion. Subsequently, even by the application of rigid internal fixation, with or without the use of bone grafts, union of the fracture can be difficult to achieve. Other indications for internal fixation of these fractures include: double fractures of the humeral shaft; associated fractures through the elbow; associated neurovascular injuries where urgent intervention is required on a stable extremity; multiple rib fractures and Parkinsonism or other neuromuscular disturbance. Occasionally open fractures and pathological fractures warrant open intervention. Management of the latter problem is discussed in a subsequent section.

Approaches to the humeral shaft are shown in Figure 10-36. Unstable fractures may be immobilized by the use of a self-compression plate, with or without additional lag screws and bone graft. Careful exposure of the radial nerve is essential. Since nerve damage is more likely with removal of the plate, metal removal should not be undertaken routinely. The plate resides under a thick cover of muscles and is secured to a non-weight-bearing bone. Transverse fractures of the midshaft region are adequately stabilized by the insertion of two 2.5- to 3-mm Kirschner wires, or Rush rods after the techniques of Hackenthal

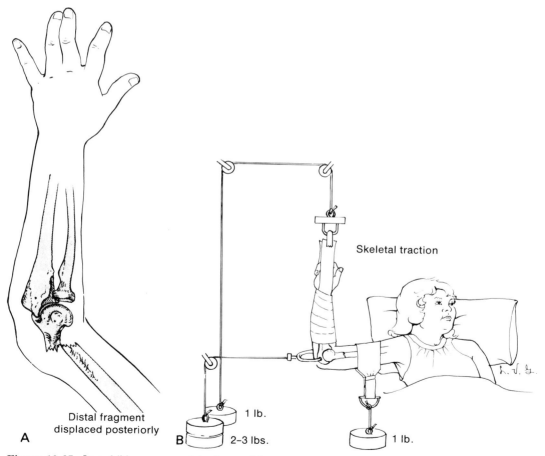

Figure 10-37. In a child, a supracondylar humeral fracture with posterior displacement (*A*) is treated by the application of skeletal traction and an olecranon transfixing pin as shown in *B*. (Reproduced with permission of M. O. Tachdjian.[68])

or Rush as was shown in Chapter 9. Usually this procedure can be performed blindly under X-ray control. More recently the Sampson fluted rod has provided a way to achieve rotational as well as angular stability.

Fractures of the distal humerus occur in all age groups but are especially common in children. Usually they occur indirectly as a result of falls onto the outstretched hand. Children with displaced supracondylar fractures frequently are treated by closed reduction and preliminary skeletal traction[113] (Fig. 10-37). When provisional callus appears by X-ray, the traction is replaced by a long arm cast. For displaced fractures, however, the author prefers closed reduction with the insertion of Steinmann pins under image intensification. Prior to this undertaking the surgeon should review carefully the anatomy of the elbow to preclude accidental insertion of a percutaneous pin into the radial or ulnar nerve or accompanying vessels. After internal fixation, the elbow can be extended to confirm anatomical alignment and a full range of motion of the elbow joint. Also, rapid discharge from the hospital is possible. Unstable distal humeral fractures, or ones that involve displacement of joints or growing epiphyses, frequently require internal fixation. Concomitant neurovascular injury and compartmental syndromes that arise as a result of soft tissue swelling from trauma, must be carefully excluded prior to surgery. Full discussion of these infrequent but severe complications should be reviewed elsewhere.[114]

Technique. A medial or lateral approach is usually preferred, as dictated by the site of the fracture; occasionally a wide posterior approach is necessary (Fig. 10-38). Isolated medial or lateral condylar fractures require precise anatomical reduction followed by provisional immobilization with Kirschner wires. Then rigid fixation can be achieved with malleolar screws. After fixation, full passive motion of the elbow joint and restoration of the anatomical carrying angle of the upper extremity should be confirmed.

Isolated fractures of the medial epicondyle frequently are malrotated by about 90°. Dislodgement of the fragment from the joint and accurate selection of the anatomical site for reduction require patience, care and skill. A hole is carefully drilled in the fragment and the fragment is threaded on to a lag screw, like a washer, to attach it to the humerus.[115] The screw should penetrate the opposite cortex.

A displaced fracture of the trochlea is repaired with open reduction and the insertion of two small lag screws. Grossly displaced fractures of

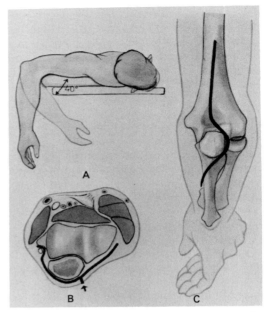

Figure 10-38. An extensile surgical approach to the elbow is presented. The patient is placed prone with the elbow flexed over a support (*A*). A dorsal curvilinear incision is made as shown in *B* and *C*. The ulnar nerve may be identified in the approach. Lateral exposure of the elbow joint preserves the olecranon bursa. The triceps aponeurosis is incised to form a tongue base distally which is reflected along the forearm. With the elbow flexed to 40° the trochlea and capitellum are completely exposed. The radial nerve must be protected at the superior extent of the incision. (Reproduced with permission of M. E. Müller, M. Allgöwer and H. Willenegger.[32])

the medial epicondyle may be treated in a similar way.

Prior to open reduction and internal fixation of comminuted elbow fractures the surgeon should make a careful assessment of his ability to achieve rigid stability of the fractures so that early active motion of the elbow can be encouraged. If the severe comminution or other technical limitations such as gross osteoporosis preclude this goal, then a nonoperative approach may provide a superior result.[116]

Many of the fractures of the intra-articular surface of the distal humerus are of complex nature and require unobscured visualization of the entire articular surface. Optimal exposure necessitates placing the patient in a prone position with his elbow flexed over an arm table. The surgeons may sit around the exposure. As shown in Figure 10-39*A*, an osteotomy of the olecranon permits an unexcelled view of the distal humerus. If the fracture extends in a prox-

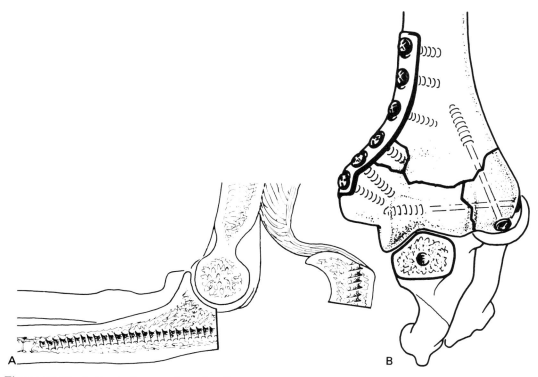

Figure 10-39. *A.* Surgical approach to the elbow joint may be facilitated by osteotomy of the olecranon as shown schematically. Prior to the osteotomy a drill hole is made and tapped so that anatomical reconstruction is assured. In certain cases the olecranon may be osteotomized without violation of the articular surface although the exposure of the capitellum and trochlea is limited somewhat. *B.* A comminuted fracture of the distal humerus is stabilized with a semitubular plate and supplementary small cancellous or malleolar screws. The osteotomy of the olecranon is apparent in the lower end of the exposure. (*A* and *B*, reproduced with permission of U. Heim and K. M. Pfeiffer.[12])

imal direction, the triceps muscle may be split. Prior to osteotomy of the olecranon a 3.2-mm drill hole is made in the olecranon so that, subsequently, anatomical reduction of the osteotomy site is ensured.

When the surgeon elects to perform internal fixation of a simple Y-fracture of the distal humerus, provisional reduction and stabilization with Kirschner wires is undertaken. The capitellum is reduced with respect to the trochlea. It may be helpful to drill the 3.2-mm hole in the capitellum prior to the reduction. Malleolar screws are used with a lag technique. Afterward the restored articular fragment is attached to the residual humeral shaft. Ideally, the small fragment set is employed with small DC or semitubular plates and 3.5-mm cortical screws. When possible interfragmental compression of the fragments is achieved by the use of 3.6-mm drill holes in the proximal fragment, deep to the plate. In the presence of gross comminution of the metaphyseal region, cancellous bone graft

may be needed. An example of internal fixation of a comminuted fracture is shown in Figure 10-39*B*. In the presence of fractures of the trochlea and the capitellum with comminution in the intervening region, cancellous bone graft may also be needed to fill this gap. Subsequently, a cortical screw is inserted through a 3.2-mm tapped drill hole. The lag technique is thereby avoided as it would cause excessive approximation of the trochlea to the capitellum.

Fractures of the Radius and Ulna

Fractures of the Proximal Radius and Ulna

Surgical approaches to the forearm are shown in Figure 10-40. A schematic representation of the types of fractures in the radius and ulna is presented in Figure 10-41.

Fractures of the Olecranon

For simple displaced fractures of the olecranon the use of the tension band principle is the

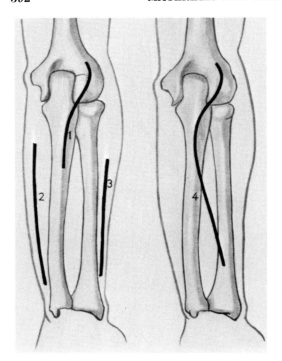

Figure 10-40. Surgical approaches to the forearm are shown. For exposure of the Monteggia fracture, or where both bones of the forearm are fractured, the patient should be placed in a prone position with the elbow supported on sand bags and flexed to about 90°. Most other exposures can be made with the patient placed in a supine position. *Incision 1.* Boyd's approach for a Monteggia fracture is seen. The radio-humeral joint is usually approached from the ulnar side without incision of the anconeus. *Incision 2.* Exposure of the middle and distal third of ulna for the application of a 6-hole dynamic compression plate on the posterior surface of the bone. *Incision 3.* The longitudinal incision permits exposure of the middle and distal third of the radius. Extension of the wound in a proximal direction, however, is hazardous to the posterior interosseous nerve which divides into four branches as it courses through supinator muscle. *Incison 4.* Thompson's approach provides exposure of both forearm bones, both proximally and distally. It is especially indicated in markedly comminuted fractures. Its proximal end is similar to Boyd's approach. More distally it dissects between the extensor carpi radialis brevis and the extensor digitorum communus. (Reproduced with permission of M. E. Müller, M. Allgöwer and H. Willenegger.[32])

optimal solution which enables the patient to initiate active motion of the elbow on the second or third postoperative day and to resume full elbow motion within a week or two. Two parallel, straight Kirschner wires are inserted in the long axis of the ulna after precise reduction of

the fracture. The wires must be parallel and properly aligned to permit subsequent interfragmentary compression. A transverse drill hole is made in the distal fragment with adequate purchase on the bone so that the tension band wire will not erode through the bone. The tension band wire passes deep to the triceps tendon and the ends of the Kirschner wires are bent over the tension band wire. At the end of the operation, the bent Kirschner wires are hammered into the olecranon. The tension band wire follows a figure-of-8 course (Fig. 10-42). Its free ends are tightened; simultaneously a loop is created in the opposite intact side of the wire so that both sides of the figure-of-8 may be tightened simultaneously. Where the fracture fragment is small, primary excision and rapid restoration of active elbow motion provides the optimal functional result. If a comminuted fracture fragment extends distal to the coronoid fossa, a tension band plate is the optimal method of fixation. If the fracture is unstable a DCP is preferred, as seen in Figure 10-43, while stable fractures subject to interfragmentary compression can be treated with the smaller semitubular plate. Screws should be carefully positioned to avoid the elbow joint. Fractures of the coronoid process require a similar technique; to lessen the likelihood of recurrent subluxation of the elbow, large fragments should be accurately reduced and secured with cancellous screws. Small fragments may require primary excision.

Simple undisplaced or minimally displaced

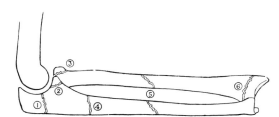

Figure 10-41. A schematic diagram of the forearm shows the common sites of ulnar and radial fractures. *1.* An olecranon fracture; *2.* fracture of the coronoid process; *3.* fracture of the radial head; *4.* fracture of the proximal ulnar shaft; *5.* midshaft fractures of the forearm. Alternatively, a fracture of the midshaft ulna may occur in association with a dislocation of the radial head (Monteggia's fracture) or a fracture of the midshaft radius may be accompanied by subluxation of the distal ulna; either situation provides a complex reconstructive problem. *6.* Fracture of the distal radius which may be combined with comparable injuries to the distal ulna. (Reproduced with permission of Synthes Ltd. (U.S.A.).)

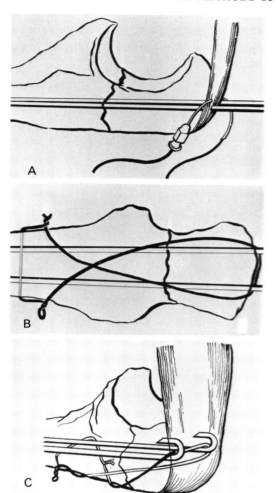

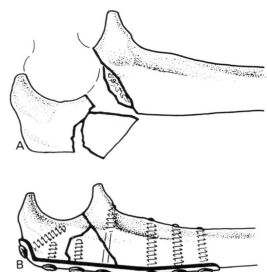

Figure 10-43. A comminuted olecranon fracture, seen schematically in *A*, is stabilized with a semitubular plate and screws. The single cancellous screw, seen in *B*, provides interfragmentary compression between two of the fragments. (Reproduced with permission of U. Heim and K. M. Pfeiffer.[12])

Figure 10-42. Internal fixation of a simple olecranon fracture is shown. *A*. The fracture is exposed and stabilized with two straight parallel Kirschner wires. A 1.2-mm stainless steel wire is passed around the protruding ends of the Kirschner wires, deep to the triceps tendon. A wire passer is helpful for this maneuver. *B*. The tension band wire is passed through a drill hole made transversely through the posterior cortex of the ulna, distal to the fracture. The wire is tightened and tied in a figure-of-8 fashion. Opposite to the twist in the two free ends of wire, a loop is fashioned so that the wire can be tightened in a symmetrical fashion. *C*. The free ends of the Kirschner wire are shortened and bent to form U-shaped hooks which are hammered into the bones over the tension band wire. (Reproduced with permission of Synthes Ltd. (U.S.A.).)

fractures of the radial head are best treated by plaster immobilization for 3 weeks, followed by active motion exercises. With significant displacement of a large fragment, open accurate reduction and lag screw fixation is indicated. When, as frequently occurs, gross comminution and displacement are present, primary resection of the radial head may be indicated.

A Monteggia fracture may be treated by Boyd's approach. The proximal ulna is approached and the fragments are reduced carefully prior to fixation with a 6-hole DCP applied posteriorily. No attempt should be made to repair the annular ligament as the repair increases the likelihood of myositis ossificans. If the ulnar fracture is reconstructed accurately, subsequent displacement of the radial head is unlikely. A long arm cast is applied with the elbow at 90°. At about 4 weeks after surgery, mobilization can begin.

Fractures of the Midshaft Radius and Ulna

Midshaft fractures of the radius and ulna require accurate reduction for satisfactory ranges of pronation and supination to be recovered.[117, 118] In the adult, the application of open reduction and rigid internal fixation is usually necessary if this goal is to be realized. Both the upper and lower extremities distal to the elbow and knee respectively are surrounded by a thick inelastic sheath of subcutaneous fascia. As such there is often difficulty in closing the wounds unless surgery is performed within 6 hours after the

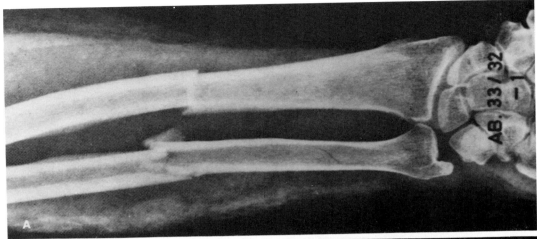

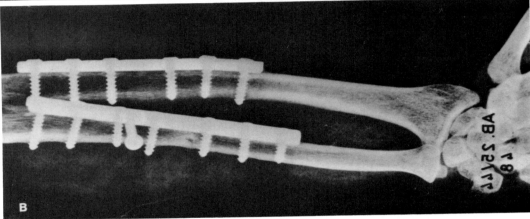

Figure 10-44. Radiological views show fractures of the midshaft forearm (*A*), treated by the application of dynamic compression tension band plates and one supplementary screw. Whenever possible a screw through the plate is inserted to provide interfragmentary compression between the two separate fracture fragments. (Reproduced with permission of Synthes Ltd. (U.S.A.).)

injury, before significant post-traumatic edema has occurred, or after a delay of several days by which time the swelling has subsided. A delay of more than 2 weeks is inadvisable as restoration of length becomes difficult. The fractures usually are approached through separate incisions although they may be visualized through a single incision (Fig. 10-40). Both fractures are exposed and examined. Next, the ulna is reduced because it is easier than the radius. A DCP is attached to the shorter principal fragment and the fracture is immobilized provisionally by clamping the plate to the other fragment (Fig. 10-44). The radius is reduced. Frequently the ulnar reduction must be released and reapplied in order that simultaneous anatomical reduction of both fractures may be obtained in full supination. Then the radius is fixed with a DCP or semitubular

plate and two screws. The reduction of the ulna is checked and pronation and supination are tested. If satisfactory, all of the rest of the screws in both plates are inserted. The shortest satisfactory length of plate is 6 holes; at least five cortices in each fracture fragment must be secured by screws.

When rigid fixation with compression is achieved, active motion of the forearm may be undertaken 48 hours after surgery. In many comminuted fractures rigid fixation cannot be realized. Then a long arm cast is applied for 3 to 4 weeks. Alternatively, irresponsible patients with stable fixation also may require supplementary cast fixation.

A variety of workers[119, 120] have reported favorable results after intramedullary fixation of forearm fractures. In Figure 10-45 an example is

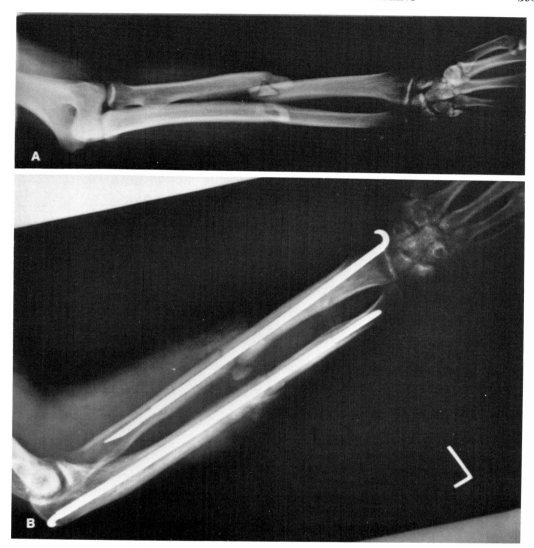

Figure 10-45. Radiological views present fractures of the midshaft radius and ulna (*A*), treated by the insertion of a Sampson fluted rod into each bone. The ulnar rod is inserted through the olecranon while the radial rod is inserted through the distal end of the radius (*B*). (Reproduced with permission of the Sampson Corporation.)

shown in which Sampson fluted rods were inserted by the application of a closed technique and image intensification. In the author's experience, intramedullary fixation of the forearm is particularly difficult and hazardous. The intramedullary cavity in the radius is curved so that advancement of the rod is likely to provoke comminution of the bones or malalignment of the fracture.

Isolated fractures of the midshaft of the radius or ulna deserve particular consideration for rigid internal fixation. The intact bone provides dis-

traction of the fracture ends so that the rate of nonunion is high with cast immobilization

Fractures and Fracture Dislocations of the Distal Radius and Ulna

Fractures of the distal radius and ulna are especially common at the two extremes of age. This distribution appears to be related to the frequency of falls in small children and the weakness of sites of cancellous bone, especially the distal radius, the femoral neck and the vertebral bodies, in the elderly. As Nordin[121] and others have shown, senile osteoporosis is primarily a disease of cancellous bone so that about three-quarters of its bone resorption affects trabecular bone. While the trabeculae undergo continuous remodeling to provide more strength and rigidity with an ever decreasing volume of bone, there comes a time when further resorption of bone provokes rapid decline in strength. Osteoporosis of cortical bone is accompanied by slowly progressive enlargement of the diameter of shafts of long bones, apparently as a similar biological adaptation whereby the strength of bone is not significantly altered by the loss of bone substance, at least within certain limits.

In children, most fractures of the distal radius and ulna can be treated satisfactorily by closed reduction with the application of a long arm cast for 6 weeks[122] In geriatric patients the opinions vary as to the optimal method of treatment for uncomplicated distal radial fractures, with or without a fracture of the ulnar styloid. At the time of injury the volume of trabecular bone of the distal radius is markedly decreased. After closed reduction, even if the anatomical length of the distal radius is restored, the application of a short or long cast is accompanied by significant shortening of the distal radius. As such, the distal ulna extends beyond the radius and behaves as a block to limit motion of the wrist. Internal fixation of the fragile osteoporotic fragments is nearly impossible. Incorporation of skeletal pins, that transfix the shafts of the metacarpals and radius into the plaster cast will impede considerably the shortening of the radius. As Sarmiento et al.[123] reported, however, such rigid immobilization of the geriatric upper extremity in a long arm cast is followed by pronounced stiffness of the wrist and elbow which may be largely irreversible. He has advised closed reduction followed by the application of a short arm cast or brace for 3 weeks. Afterward, vigorous active motion exercises of the wrist and pronation and supination are pursued. He reports excellent functional results despite the frequent presence of foreshortening and angular deformity of the distal radius. Alternatively for grossly comminuted fractures through osteoporotic bone, external fixation may be applied (Chapter 11), possibly with open reduction of the intra-articular surfaces.

The indications for internal fixation of fractures and fracture dislocations around the distal radial-ulnar joint are greater in children and especially in young adults where such fractures often occur with much more violent trauma.[122] Especially in the latter group, the presence of certain soft tissue injuries, certain patterns of fractures or the presence of a compartmental syndrome may dictate the need for surgical intervention. Specifically, the indications for open management include: displaced epiphyseal and intra-articular fractures, where acceptable closed reduction has failed; unstable fractures; and fractures accompanied by injuries to soft tissues such as neurovascular structures which require urgent surgical intervention. An example is shown in Figure 10-46. The application of pins or cancellous screws usually provides adequate stability. With comminution of the distal radius a small T-plate may be helpful. Where a defect has arisen from crushing of trabeculae, an autologous bone graft may be advisable.

In Galeazzi fractures, the radius can be repaired with a semitubular plate or a DCP. The styloid process of the distal ulna often is avulsed but the fibrocartilogenous disc usually is intact. While the AO group recommends internal fixation of the ulnar styloid process, in the author's experience this is unnecessary.

Fractures in the Hand

In view of the complexity of the hand, it is not surprising that injuries including fractures of the hand occur with countless variety. In view of the complexity and close proximity of the soft tissues adjacent to bones in the hand, special skill and care is required by the surgeon. Furthermore, techniques of external immobilization and physical therapy for the hand are more exacting than comparable care required for other injuries. The interested reader is referred elsewhere.[124, 125] The present discussion is limited to a few examples where open reduction and internal fixation of the hand frequently are indicated.

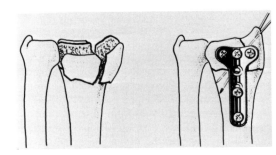

Figure 10-46. Schematic views show the fixation of a comminuted interarticular fracture of the distal radius that is stabilized by the application of a T-plate. Preliminary fixation with Kirschner wires (*right*) is essential. (Reproduced with permission of U. Heim and K. M. Pfeiffer.[12])

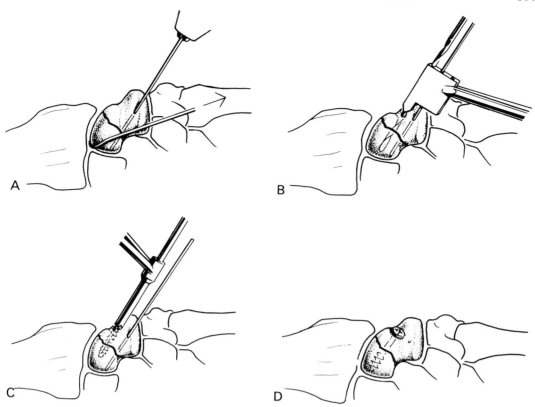

Figure 10-47. Schematic views of the stages of internal fixation of a fracture of the scaphoid are shown. The fracture is exposed through the radial aspect of the distal radius and carpus (Matti-Russe approach). A fine Kirschner wire transfixes the reduced fracture and anatomical alignment is confirmed by X-ray (*A*). A drill guide is used to position a drill hole parallel to the guide wire (*B*). The hole is tapped (*C*) for insertion of the lag screw (*D*) and the Kirschner wire is removed. (Reproduced with permission of U. Heim and K. M. Pfeiffer.[125])

Fractures of the Carpal Bones

Young adults who fall and land on the outstretched hand frequently fracture the scaphoid against an unyielding anterior radial carpal ligament. Most of the injuries show minimal displacement of the fragments in which case optimal treatment is provided by a plaster thumb spica cast. Immobilization for 8 to 16 weeks may be necessary. In the few displaced fractures where closed reduction is impossible, open reduction and the insertion of a small lag screw is advisable. Figure 10-47 shows the insertion of a lag screw as treatment of a displaced scaphoid fracture. If open intervention is deferred until after a trial of cast immobilization, nonunion is more likely.[126] Furthermore, with immobilization, osteoporosis of the fragments ensues so that delayed screw fixation becomes excessively difficult; the screw will not find adequate resist-

ance in the porotic bone. Displaced scaphoid fractures are especially common in combination with dislocations of the lunate. Early closed, or if necessary, open reduction of the lunate is essential to diminish the likelihood of avascular necrosis of the bone.

Avascular necrosis often with nonunion of the scaphoid is not uncommon. The arterial supply enters the distal third of the bone and courses in a retrograde fashion to the proximal end. Fractures of the waist or proximal third may interrupt the circulation to the proximal fragment. When a late nonunion with avascular necrosis presents itself the quality of the bone determines the optimal form of treatment. If the bone is of solid consistency, a lag screw can be applied.[125] If the bone has become markedly osteoporotic, the screw will not achieve fixation in the bone. In this situation, the application of autologous bone graft, as an internal stabilizing strut across the reduced fracture fragments is recommended.

Another uncommon injury of the carpus which may require open intervention is a comminuted or longitudinal fracture of the greater multangular[127]. Usually this injury is accompanied by a Bennett's fracture of the proximal end of the first metacarpal, which is discussed below. For the former fracture, open reduction and fixation with Kirschner wires or small screws is undertaken.

Fractures of the Metacarpals and Phalanges

Metacarpal fractures commonly occur from direct violence to the hand, especially by striking the hand against an opponent. Rotational deformity of the fracture is determined clinically. When flexed individually into the palm, each finger points to the scaphoid; deviation from this direction represents rotational deformity of the finger or adjacent metacarpal shaft. Alternatively, Milford[128] recommends a comparison of the rotational angle of the fingernails of both hands. This method of alignment eliminates the need to flex the injured finger. Angular deformity is recorded by X-ray. Most acute fractures of metacarpals are treated by closed manipulation with the application of a splint for 2 or 6 weeks depending on whether the fracture involves cancellous or cortical bone. Midshaft fractures of

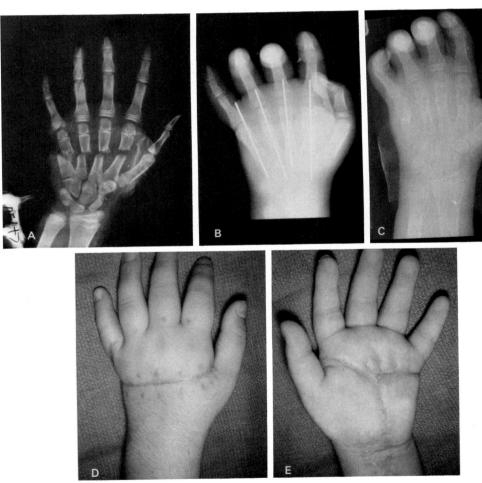

Figure 10-48. Radiological views and photographs present a boy of 9 years who sustained a traumatic amputation through the level of the midshaft metacarpals when the blade from a rotary power saw separated from its shaft. *A* shows the radiological view prior to microsurgical vascular anastomosis. *B* shows an X-ray of the hand after stabilization with Kirschner wire fixation of the metacarpal fractures and microvascular repair. *C* shows the hand 6 weeks after injury when the fractures have healed and the pins have been removed. *D* and *E* show the hand 2 months after injury.

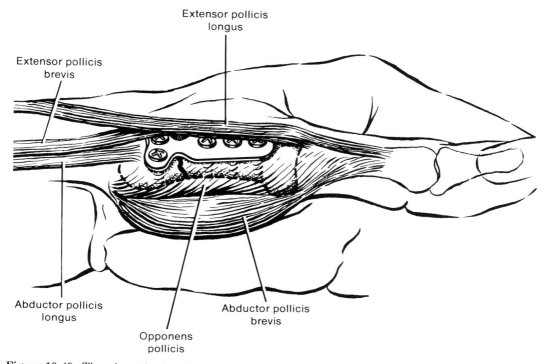

Extensor pollicis
longus

Extensor pollicis
brevis

Abductor pollicis
longus

Opponens
pollicis

Abductor pollicis
brevis

Figure 10-49. The schematic view shows an extra-articular fracture of the first metacarpal that is stabilized with internal fixation. An AO finger T-plate is attached to the proximal fragment and used as a lever to achieve the reduction. Additional screws are inserted. (Reproduced with permission of U. Heim and K. M. Pfeiffer.[12])

the metacarpals frequently show dorsal angulation and instability provoked by the pull of both the intrinsic muscles and the powerful long flexors. The insertion of a longitudinal Kirschner wire, in retrograde fashion, provides leverage on the distal fragment for accurate reduction. Further insertion of the wire immobilizes the fracture. Additional rotatory stability may be achieved by insertion of a second wire, either obliquely across the fracture site or transversely through the distal fragment and an adjacent metacarpal.

Other indications for internal fixation of metacarpal fractures include multiple metacarpal shaft fractures and comminuted shaft fractures.

Replantation of the hand, or digits, after clean guillotine-type amputation is a special indication for Kirschner wire fixation. A clinical example is shown in Figure 10-48. The wires can be inserted rapidly so that minimal time is diverted from the critical task of microvascular repair of severed arteries and veins of 1 to 2 mm diameter. The reader is referred elsewhere for a more complete account.[129, 130] For the latter especially, the application of small finger plates (Fig. 10-49) may be necessary.[125] Another peculiar intra-ar-

ticular metacarpal fracture, first described by Bennett,[131] involves the first carpometacarpal joint. As the result of forced abduction of the thumb, an oblique, unstable fracture of the base of the metacarpal transects the articular surface. If unreduced the fracture would lead to marked diminution in carpometacarpal joint motion and abduction of the thumb. When, as frequently occurs, satisfactory closed reduction[126] is unsuccessful, a Kirschner wire may be inserted under X-ray control. If this fails, open reduction and screw or wire fixation is performed (Fig. 10-50).

Most fractures of phalangeal shafts show little or no displacement so that closed reduction and splint fixation is advisable. Small minimally displaced chip fractures of the interphalangel joints also may be treated in this way. The frequently encountered comminuted fractures of the tip of distal phalanges, secondary to a crushed finger tip, are treated similarly with drainage of a subungual hematoma. Indications for open treatment include displaced avulsion fractures of insertions of the extensor or flexor mechanisms of the volar plate, displaced intra-articular fractures and unstable diaphyseal fractures. Such fractures require precise reduction and

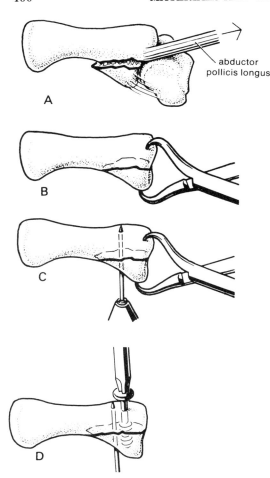

Figure 10-50. The stages of internal fixation of a Bennett's fracture of the first metacarpal are shown schematically. The intra-articular fracture seen in *A* is exposed by Gedda-Moberg's approach. The fracture is reduced with forceps (*B*) and temporary stabilization with a Kirschner wire is performed from the volar aspect (*C*) A small cancellous lag screw is inserted through a dorsal approach (*D*). (Reproduced with permission of U. Heim and K. M. Pfeiffer.[12])

wire or small lag screw fixation[125, 132] (Fig. 10-51). Markedly displaced open fractures of a distal phalanx especially near-complete amputation are best handled by Kirschner wire fixation.

Another common indication for internal fixation of metacarpals and phalanges is the immobilization of joint fusions by the use of wires. The general principles of the fixation are similar to techniques previously described. The reader is referred elsewhere for technical details of the operations.[124, 125, 128, 131]

FUSION OF JOINTS

Another surgical procedure for which a variety of special implants have been devised is arthrodesis or fusion of joint.[133] Perhaps the best example is hip fusion. The AO group has devised a unique cobra plate, which, combined with the appropriate operative technique, permits immediate postoperative weight bearing without external immobilization. The implant and the operative technique are shown schematically in Figure 10-52. An osteotomy of the pelvis accompanies the fusion to provide stable opposing surfaces of bone. Arthrodesis of the knee can be achieved by the use of double, right-angle, compression plates or by the application of external fixation (see Chapter 11). Similarly arthrodesis of the ankle can be achieved by internal or external fixation. Arthrodesis in the foot is usually achieved by the use of screws or wires and the application of a plaster cast. In the upper extremity, conventional plates and screws are generally employed for internal fixation. Alternatively, when infected joints are fused, external fixation is preferable.

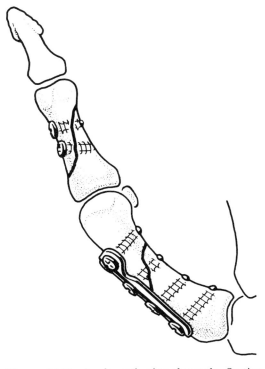

Figure 10-51. A schematic view shows the fixation of unstable fractures in the thumb by the application of screws or a small T-plate and screws. (Reproduced with permission of U. Heim and K. M. Pfeiffer.[12])

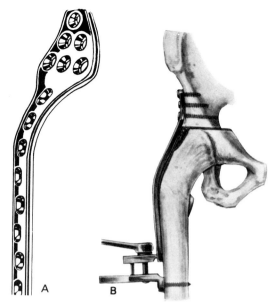

Figure 10-52. *A.* A schematic diagram shows a Cobra plate for the stabilization of a fusion of the hip. *B.* A schematic view shows the application of the plate to the hip. A transverse osteotomy through the pelvis with medial displacement of the distal fragment is evident. The plate is attached with screws to the superior pelvic fragment and an external compression device secures the distal end of the plate to the femoral shaft. Compression is applied to the hip joint and the osteotomy site after which additional screws are inserted. (Reproduced with permission of Synthes Ltd. (U.S.A.).)

REFERENCES

1. Charnley, J. *The Closed Treatment of Common Fractures,* p. 10, E. & S. Livingstone, London, 1971.
2. Rockwood, C. A., and Green, D. P. editors. *Fractures,* p. 25, J. B. Lippincott, Philadelphia, 1975.
3. Müller, M. E., Allgöwer, M., Willenegger, H. *Manual of Internal Fixation,* p. 16, Springer-Verlag, Berlin, 1970.
4. Hoaglund, F. J., and Duthie, R. B. Fractures and joint injuries. In *Principles of Surgery,* p. 1791, edited by S. I. Schwartz, McGraw-Hill, New York, 1974.
5. Watson-Jones, R. *Fractures and Joint Injuries,* p. 53, Williams & Wilkins Co., Baltimore, 1960.
6. Apley, A. G. *A System of Orthopaedics and Fractures,* p. 77, Butterworths, London, 1968.
7. Rang, M. *Children's Fractures,* p. 1, J. B. Lippincott, Philadelphia, 1974.
8. Schatzker, J. In Press, 1978.
9. Burwell, R. G. The fate of bone grafts. In *Recent Advances in Orthopaedics,* p. 115, edited by A. G. Apley, Williams & Wilkins Co., Baltimore, 1969.
10. Goldstein, L. A., and Dickerson, R. C. *Atlas of Orthopaedic Surgery,* p. 450, C. V. Mosby Co., St. Louis, 1974.
11. Bassett, C. A. L. *Clin. Ortho. Rel. Res., 87:* 49, 1972.
12. Heim, U., and Pfeiffer, K. M. *Small Fragment Set Manual,* Springer-Verlag, Berlin, 1974.
13. Rëudi, T., and Allgöwer, M. In Press, 1977.
14. Weber, B. G., and Cech, O. *Pseudarthrosis: Pathophysiology, Biomechanics, Therapy, Results,* p. 12, Grune & Stratton, New York, 1976.
15. Burri, C., Fridrich, R., Hell, K., and Schenk, R. *European Surg. Res., 3:*166, 1969.
16. Rittmann, W. W., and Perren, S. M. *Cortical Bone Healing after Internal Fixation and Infection,* p. 19, Springer-Verlag, Berlin, 1974.
17. Burri, C., Willenegger, H., *et al. Post-traumatic Osteomyelitis,* p. 30, Hans Huber, Bern, 1975.
18. Meyer, S., Weiland, A. J., and Willenegger, H. *J. Bone Jt. Surg., 57A:*836, 1975.
19. Tachdjian, M. O. *Pediatric Orthopedics,* p. 303, W. B. Saunders Co., Philadelphia, 1972.
20. Sofield, H. A., and Miller, E. A. *J. Bone Jt. Surg., 41A:*1371, 1959.
21. Murray, J. A., and Parrish, F. F. *Ortho. Clin. N. Am., 5:*887, 1974.
22. Harrington, K. D. *J. Bone Jt. Surg., 57A:*744, 1975.
23. Sim, F. H., Daugherty, T. W., and Ivins, J. C. *J. Bone Jt. Surg., 56A:* 40, 1974.
24. Burrows, H. J., Wilson, J. N., and Scales, J. T. *J. Bone Jt. Surg., 57B:*148, 1975.
25. Johnstone, A. D. *Clin. Ortho. Rel. Res., 73:*8, 1970.
26. Craig, F. S. *Clin. Ortho. Rel. Res., 73:*33, 1970.
27. MacAusland, W. R., and Wyman, E. T. *Clin. Ortho. Rel. Res., 73:* 39, 1970.
28. Kane, W. J. Fractures of the pelvis. In *Fractures,* p. 905, edited by C. A. Rockwood and D. P. Green, J. B. Lippincott, Philadelphia, 1975.
29. Watson-Jones, R. *Fractures and Joint Injuries,* p. 934, Williams & Wilkins Co., Baltimore, 1955.
30. Holdsworth, F. W. *J. Bone Jt. Surg., 30B:*461, 1948.
31. Judet, R., Judet, J., and Letournel E. *J. Bone Jt. Surg., 46A:*1615, 1964.
32. Müller, M. E., Allgöwer, M., and Willenegger, H. *Manual of Internal Fixation,* Springer-Verlag, Berlin, 1970.
33. Müller, M. E., Allgöwer, M., and Willenegger, H. *Manual of Internal Fixation,* p. 144, Springer-Verlag, Berlin, 1970.
34. Allgöwer, M., Matter, P., Perren, S. M., and Rüedi, T. *The Dynamic Compression-Plate,* p. 38, Springer-Verlag, Berlin, 1973.
35. Beck, H. Hip joint replacement in trauma therapy. In *Advances in Artificial Hip and Knee Joint Technology,* p. 81, edited by M. Schaldach and D. Hohmann, Springer-Verlag, Berlin, 1976.
36. Peltier, L. F. *J. Bone Jt. Surg., 47A:*1060, 1965.
37. Froman, C., and Stein, A. *J. Bone Jt. Surg., 49B:*24, 1967.
38. Worland, R. L., and Keim, H. A. *Clin. Ortho. Rel. Res., 112:*215, 1975.
39. Hoffmann, R. *Acta. Chir. Scand., 107:*72, 1954.
40. Vidal, J., Rabischang, P., Bonnel, F., and Adrey, J. *Montpellier Chir., 16:*53, 1970.

41. Niemann, K. M. W., and Mankin, H. J. *J. Bone Jt. Surg., 50A:*1327, 1968.
42. Tronzo, R. G. *Surgery of the Hip Joint,* p. 512, Lea & Febiger, Philadelphia, 1973.
43. Tronzo, R. G. *Ortho. Clin. N. Am., 5:*679, 1974.
44. Garden, R. S. *J. Bone Jt. Surg., 46B:*630, 1964.
45. Hoaglund, F. T., and Duthie, R. B. Fractures and Joint Injuries. In *Principles of Surgery,* edited by S. I. Schwartz, McGraw-Hill, New York, 1974.
46. Massie, W. K. *J. Bone Jt. Surg., 48A:*784, 1966.
47. Crawford, H. B. *J. Bone Jt. Surg., 42A:*47, 1960.
48. Schatzker, J. *A Primer on the AO/ASIF Method of Internal Fixation,* p. 24, University of Toronto, Toronto, 1974.
49. Tronzo, R. G. *Surgery of the Hip Joint,* Lea & Febiger, Philadelphia, 1973.
50. Müller, M. E. Allgöwer, M., and Willenegger, H. *Manual of Internal Fixation,* p. 142, Springer-Verlag, Berlin, 1970.
51. Hinchey, J. J., and Day, P. L. *J. Bone Jt. Surg., 46A:*223, 1964.
52. Bateman, J. E. *Ortho. Digest, 9:*15, 1974.
53. Ratcliff, A. H. C. *Ortho. Clin. N. Am., 5:*903, 1974.
54. Tachdjian, M. O. *Pediatric Orthopaedics,* p. 1671, W. B. Saunders Co., Philadelphia, 1972.
55. Makley, J. T., Heiple, K. G., Jackman, K. V., and Burstein, A. H. Varus Medial Displacement Osteotomy of the Hip for the Control of Valgus Instability in Children. *Proceedings of A.O.A. Meeting,* July, 1975.
56. Sonstegard, D. A., Kaufer, H., and Matthews, L. S. *Ortho. Clin. N. Am., 5:*551, 1974.
57. Sonstegard, D. A., Kaufer, H., and Matthews, L. S. *Ortho. Clin. N. Am., 5:*551, 1974.
58. Tronzo, R. G. *Surgery of the Hip Joint,* p. 559, Lea & Febiger, Philadelphia, 1973.
59. Dimon, J. H., and Hughston, J. C. *J. Bone and Jt. Surg., 49A:*440, 1967.
60. Müller, M. E., Allgöwer, M., and Willenegger, H. *Manual of Internal Fixation,* p. 158, Springer-Verlag, Berlin, 1970.
61. Sahlstrand, T. *Acta Ortho. Scand., 45:*213, 1974.
62. Fielding, J. W., Cochran, G. V. B., and Zickel, R. E. *Ortho. Clin. N. Am., 5:*629, 1974.
63. Ender, H. G. *Treatment of Per- and Sub-trochanteric Fractures with Ender's Flexible Intramedullary Pins,* p. 30, de Kostendrukkers, Schiedam, Holland, 1976.
64. Mooney, V. Fractures of the shaft of the femur. In *Fractures,* p. 1075, edited by C. A. Rockwood and D. P. Green, J. B. Lippincott Co., Philadelphia, 1975.
65. Clawson, D. K., Smith, R. F., and Hansen, S. T. *J. Bone Jt. Surg., 53A:*681, 1971.
66. Roscher, J. J., Nahigan, S. H., Macys, J. R., and Brown, J. E. *J. Bone Jt. Surg., 54A:*534, 1972.
67. Tachdjian, M. O. *Pediatric Orthopaedics,* p. 1681, W. B. Saunders Co., Philadelphia, 1972.
68. Tachdjian, M. O. *Pediatric Orthopaedics,* W. B. Saunders Co., Philadelphia, 1972.
69. Mooney, V., Nickel, V. L., Harvey, J. P., Jr., and Snelson, R. *J. Bone Jt. Surg., 52A:*1563, 1970.
70. Küntscher, G. *The Practice of Intra-medullary Nailing,* p. 2, Charles C Thomas, Springfield, Ill., 1967.
71. Böhler, J. *Trauma, 5:*150, 1965.
72. Clawson, D. K., Smith, R. F., and Hansen, S. T. *J. Bone Jt. Surg., 53A:*681, 1971.
73. Müller, M. E., Allgöwer, M., and Willenegger, H. *Manual of Internal Fixation,* p. 82, Springer-Verlag, Berlin, 1970.
74. Goldstein, L. A., and Dickerson, R. C. *Atlas of Orthopaedic Surgery,* p. 634, C. V. Mosby Co., St. Louis, 1974.
75. Hall, R. M. *Air Instrument Surgery,* vol. 2, Springer-Verlag, New York, 1972.
76. Stewart, M. J., Sisk, D., and Wallace, S. L. *J. Bone Jt. Surg., 48A:*784, 1966.
77. Crenshaw, A. H., editor. *Campbell's Operative Orthopaedics,* p. 542, C. V. Mosby Co., St. Louis, 1971.
78. Brown, P. W. *Clin. Ortho. Rel. Res., 105:*167, 1974.
79. Watson-Jones, R. *Fractures and Joint Injuries,* p. 435, Williams & Wilkins Co., Baltimore, 1955.
80. Sarmiento, A. *Clin. Ortho. Rel. Res., 105:*202, 1974.
81. Dehne, E. *Clin. Ortho. Rel. Res., 105:*192, 1974.
82. Leach, R. E. *Fractures of the tibia.* In *Fractures,* p. 1286, edited by C. A. Rockwood and D. P. Green, J. B. Lippincott Co., Philadelphia, 1975.
83. Hohl, M. *J. Bone Jt. Surg., 49A:*1455, 1967.
84. Courvoisier, E. *Fractures of the Tibial Tables,* p. 4, Swiss Association for The Study of Internal Fixation, Berne, 1973.
85. Hohl, M. Fractures about the knee. In *Fractures,* p. 1131, edited by C. A. Rockwood and D. P. Green, J. B. Lippincott Co., Philadelphia, 1975.
86. Herold, Z. H. *J. Bone Jt. Surg., 45B:*805, 1963.
87. Speed, K. *A Textbook of Fractures and Dislocations,* p. 252, Lea & Febiger, Philadelphia, 1928.
88. Weissman, S. L., and Herold, H. Z. *J. Bone Jt. Surg., 48A:*257, 1966.
89. Speed, K. *A Textbook of Fractures and Dislocations,* p. 254, Lea & Febiger, Philadelphia, 1928.
90. Brown, P. W., and Urban, J. G. *J. Bone Jt. Surg., 51A:*59, 1969.
91. Allgöwer, M., and Rüedi, T. In press, 1978.
92. Karlström, G., and Olerud, S. *J. Bone Jt. Surg., 57A:*915, 1975.
93. Mears, D. C. *Ortho. Survey, 1:*64, 1977.
94. Allgöwer, M., Matter, P., Perren, S. M., and Rüedi, T. *The Dynamic Compression Plate,* p. 34, Springer-Verlag, Berlin, 1973.
95. D'Aubigne, R. M., Mouer, P., Zucman, J., and Mosse, Y. *Clin. Ortho. Rel. Res., 105:*267, 1974.
96. Lottes, J. O. *Clin. Ortho. Rel. Res., 105:*253, 1974.
97. Jergesen, F. *Clin. Ortho. Rel. Res., 105:*240, 1974.
98. Müller, M. E., Allgöwer, M., and Willenegger, H. *Manual of Internal Fixation,* p. 193, Springer-Verlag, Berlin, 1970.
99. Watson-Jones, R. *Fractures and Joint Injuries,* p. 862, Williams & Wilkins Co., Baltimore, 1955.
100. Lauge-Hansen, N. *Amer. J. Roentgen, Radium Ther. Nucl. Med., 71:*456, 1954.
101. Wilson, F. C. Fractures and dislocations of the ankle. In *Fractures,* p. 1361, edited by C. A. Rockwood and D. P. Green, J. B. Lippincott Co., Philadelphia, 1975.
102. Scranton, P. E., McMaster, J. H., and Kelly, E. *Clin. Ortho. Rel. Res., 118:*76, 1976.
103. Giannestras, N. J., and Sammarco, G. J. Fractures and dislocations in the foot. In *Fractures,* p. 1400, edited by C. A. Rockwood and D. P. Green, J. B. Lippincott Co., Philadelphia, 1975.

104. Essex Lopresti, P. *J. Bone Jt. Surg., 39B:*395, 1972.
105. Soeut, R., and Remy, R. *J. Bone Jt. Surg., 57B:*413, 1975.
106. Dunne, L. R., Jacobs, B., and Campbell, R. D. *J. Trauma, 6:*443, 1966.
107. Dart, D. E., and Graham, W. D. *J. Trauma, 6:*363, 1966.
108. Parkes, J. C. *Clin. Ortho. Rel. Res., 122:*28, 1977.
109. Neer, C. S. Fractures and dislocations of the shoulder. In *Fractures,* p. 585, edited by C. A. Rockwood and D. P. Green, J. B. Lippincott Co., Philadelphia, 1975.
110. Neer, C. S. *J. Bone Jt. Surg., 37A:*215, 1955.
111. Rush, L. V. *Atlas of Rush Pins Techniques,* p. 15, Berivon Co., Meridian, Miss., 1955.
112. Crenshaw, A. H., editor. *Campbell's Operative Orthopaedics,* p. 644, C. V. Mosby Co., St. Louis, 1971.
113. Tachdjian, M. O. *Pediatric Orthopaedics,* p. 1567, W. B. Saunders Co., Philadelphia, 1972.
114. Eaton, R. G., and Green, W. T. *Clin Ortho. Rel. Res., 113:*58, 1975.
115. Müller, M. E., Allgöwer, M., and Willenegger, H. *Manual of Internal Fixation,* p. 122, Springer-Verlag, Berlin, 1970.
116. Eppright, R. H., and Wilkins, K. E. Fractures and dislocations of the elbow. In *Fractures,* p. 487, edited by C. A. Rockwood and D. P. Green, J. B. Lippincott Co., Philadelphia, 1975.
117. Crenshaw, A. H., editor. *Campbell's Operative Orthopaedics,* p. 667, C. V. Mosby Co., St. Louis, 1971.
118. Anderson, L. D. Fractures of the shafts of the radius and ulna. In *Fractures,* p. 441, edited by

C. A. Rockwood and D. P. Green, J. B. Lippincott Co., Philadelphia, 1975.
119. Smith, H., and Sage, F. P. *J. Bone Jt. Surg., 39A:*91, 1957.
120. Rush, L. V. *Atlas of Rush Pin Techniques,* p. 199, Berivon Co., Meridian, Miss., 1955.
121. Nordin, B. E. C. *Lancet, 1:*1011, 1961.
122. Rang, M. *Children's Fractures,* p. 124, J. B. Lippincott Co., Philadelphia, 1974.
123. Sarmiento, A., Cooper, J. S., and Sinclair, W. F. *J. Bone Jt. Surg., 57A:*297, 1975.
124. Chase, R. A. *Atlas of Hand Surgery,* p. 246, W. B. Saunders Co., Philadelphia, 1973.
125. Heim, U., and Pfeiffer, K. M. *Small Fragment Set Manual,* p. 85, Springer-Verlag, Berlin, 1974.
126. Maudsley, R. H., and Chen, S. C. *J. Bone Jt. Surg., 54B:*432, 1972.
127. Watson-Jones, R. *Fracture and Joint Injuries,* ed. 4, p. 632, Williams & Wilkins Co., Baltimore, 1960.
128. Milford, L. The Hand. In *Campbell's Operative Orthopaedics,* p. 234, edited by A. H. Crenshaw, C. V. Mosby Co., St. Louis, 1971.
129. Morrison, W. A., O'Brien, B. M., and MacLeod, A. M. *Ortho. Clin. N. Am., 8:*295, 1977.
130. Kleinert, H. E., Juhala, C. A., Tsai, T., and van Beek, A. *Ortho. Clin. N. Am., 8:*309, 1977.
131. Stark, H. H. *A.A.O.S. Instruct. Course Lect., 19:*130, 1970.
132. Crawford, G. P. *J. Bone Jt. Surg., 58A:*487, 1976.
133. Müller, M. E., Allgöwer, M., and Willenegger, H. *Manual of Internal Fixation,* p. 278, Springer-Verlag, Berlin, 1970.

11

Percutaneous Pin Fixation

A variety of methods of skeletal traction or of fracture immobilization have been developed independently by workers using percutaneous stainless steel pins. Frequently, as in the treatment of femoral shaft fractures or of comminuted supracondylar humeral fractures in children, a skeletal traction pin is used as a temporary means for immobilization until sufficient callus has been deposited so that a plaster cast can be applied without loss of alignment of the fracture. In such examples the pins are generally connected to a system of balanced suspension which, in turn, is attached to the patient's bed. Where the patients have extensive open wounds or other medical problems, such as head injuries with confusion, their management can be rendered much more difficult by the apparatus for balanced suspension. Also, in the past decade when hospital costs have soared, the application of balanced suspension has become less favorable when other methods might be applied that would enable the patient to be discharged from the hospital. For these and other reasons methods of treatment have been devised in which the percutaneous pins are attached to a rigid stainless steel framework that stabilizes the impaired extremity so that the patient is independent of his surroundings. In this chapter the development and clinical application of such external pin fixation devices are described.

From about 1900 Lambotte[1] and subsequently other workers[2-5] independently developed methods of stabilization of open fractures with the use of external transfixation. In the United States perhaps the best known examples of the use of external fixation were the techniques employed by Anderson,[3] primarily for the treatment of complex fractures or osteotomies in children, and the clamps devised by Charnley[6] for the arthrodesis of the ankle or knee joint. Figure 11-1 shows an example of the Anderson device employed on the humerus for correction and stabilization of an osteotomy to correct cubitus varus deformity secondary to a malunion of a distal humeral fracture. Figure 11-2 shows an example of the use of the Charnley external device for arthrodesis of the knee joint. In view of complications such as pin tract infections, instability, malalignment and soft tissue injuries, the methods failed to gain widespread popularity in North America. Nevertheless, many European workers continued to explore the possible applications of external fixation. The AO group* developed a simple system with Steinmann percutaneous pins and threaded external uprights for use on infected nonunions and arthrodeses of joints. Workers, such as Weber,† achieved remarkable degrees of success in certain instances of severe bone loss concomitant with infected nonunions. In a few cases the author has replicated these results, as seen in Figure 11-3. Frequently two separate systems of the AO external device were employed in parallel to augment the stability of the device. Nevertheless, it was difficult to erect the AO frame in such a way that truly stable fixation could be achieved. Elsewhere in Europe, several groups attempted to use external fixation for minimally to moderately displaced pelvic ring fractures and they reported favorable results in a few cases.[8-10] In the U.S.S.R., Ilisarov[11] developed an external fixation device which was employed for a variety of fracture problems primarily in the lower extremity. Excellent results were reported for a group of 912 patients with various bone and joint injuries and diseases. Figure 11-4 illustrates one of these cases. Meanwhile others such as D'Aubigne and Dubousset[12] attempted to perform leg lengthening by the use of a device similar to that of Anderson. Figure 11-5 shows one example of their method for lengthening of the tibia. Excellent results were reported for 3 cases with lengthening of 5 to 6 cm and union of

---

* Arbeitsgemeinschaft für Osteosynthesefragen or ASIF (Swiss) Association for the Study of Internal Fixation.

† B. Weber, personal communication, 1977.

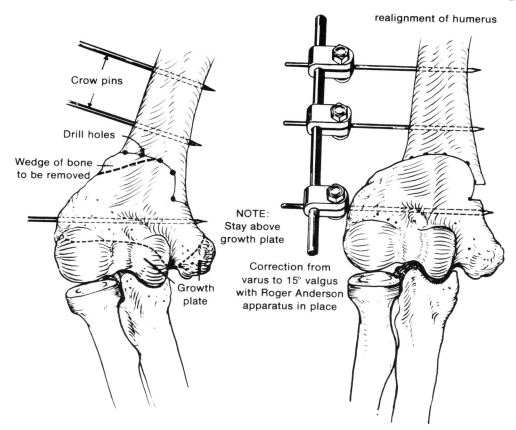

realignment of humerus

Crow pins

Drill holes

Wedge of bone
to be removed

NOTE:
Stay above
growth plate

Correction from
varus to 15° valgus
with Roger Anderson
apparatus in place

Growth
plate

Figure 11-1. A schematic illustration shows the application of the Anderson device for external fixation of a distal humeral osteotomy as treatment of a cubitus varus deformity. (Reproduced with permission of M. O. Tachdjian.[7]

bone was achieved within about 5 months after the osteotomy was performed.

One of the early embodiments of the "fixateur externe", as it is known in Europe, was developed by Hoffmann.[13, 14] At that time it was comparable to most other methods and without superiority. Subsequently the method was extensively modified by Vidal *et al.*[15, 16] and Adrey[17] so that an extraordinarily rigid double frame could be easily applied (Fig. 11-6).

About 10 years ago the author first used several types of external fixation device. While he was in England he saw numerous examples of arthrodesis of the knee or ankle with the use of the Charnley device. In many cases the device was unsatisfactory because it possessed insufficient stability and frequently culminated in persistent nonunion of bone. The pins were very difficult to insert with the appropriate alignment so that they could be attached to the external frame. The ability to make corrections in alignment of the extremity was limited. Subse-

quently, the author had the opportunity to work with Professor Willenegger, of Liestal, Switzerland, who achieved excellent results with the use of the AO external fixation device on infected nonunions of the lower extremity. While this apparatus was considerably easier to use in view of its enhanced versatility and aligning jigs for insertion of pins, nevertheless, it lacked adequate stability for many applications such as the arthrodesis of an infected total knee joint replacement. The author encountered similar limitations with the Anderson device. These and other experiences encouraged the author to design his own apparatus for the treatment of a grossly infected nonunion of a comminuted pelvic ring fracture (Figs. 11-7 to 11-9). The technique appeared to be very useful for pelvic trauma, especially for the extraordinarily difficult problem of wide abduction injuries with open wounds of the perineum. At about the same time, however, the author had the opportunity to see and use the Hoffmann device (Ets

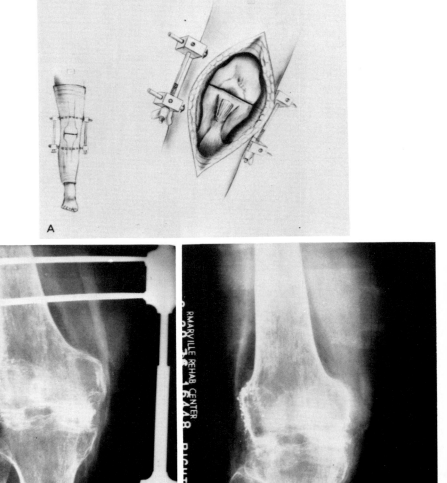

Figure 11-2. *A.* A schematic diagram shows the application of the Charnley external fixation device for fusion of a knee. *B.* An X-ray view shows fusion of the knee with the Charnley external fixation device. *C.* The same knee after fusion has occurred and the device has been removed.

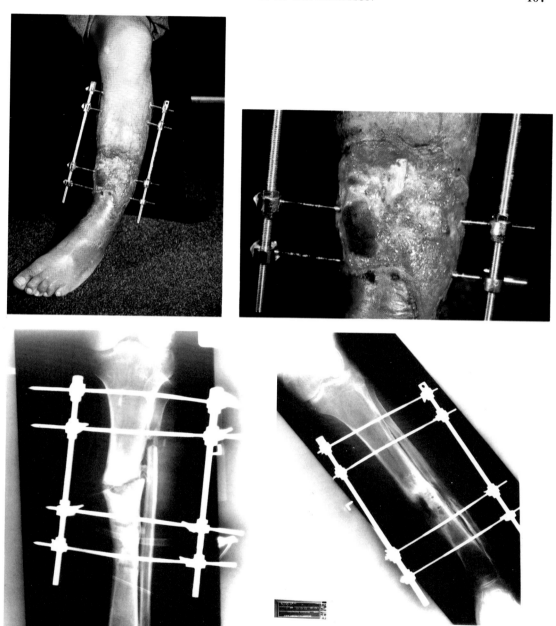

Figure 11-3. Photographs and radiological views of a midshaft tibial nonunion with absolute bone loss by the application of an AO threaded external fixation device. This man of 17 years had been treated 9 months earlier for a closed midshaft tibial fracture by the application of a screw. When loss of stability was observed in the postoperative period, eight subsequent operations were performed within 8 months which failed to provide stability but which provoked severe infection. *A* and *B*. The limb is shown with exposed tibia immediately after application of the device. *C*. An X-ray immediately after surgery. *D*. An X-ray shows the union of bone observed 6 months later.

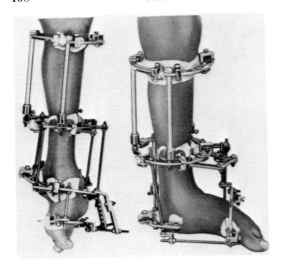

Figure 11-4. A photograph of a lower limb treated by the use of the Ilisarov device is shown in two stages of correction of the deformity.

Figure 11-5. Schematic diagrams reveal the application of the leg lengthening technique devised by D'Aubigne and Dubousset[12] by the use of a device similar to that of Anderson. (Reproduced with permission of M. O. Tachdjian.[7]

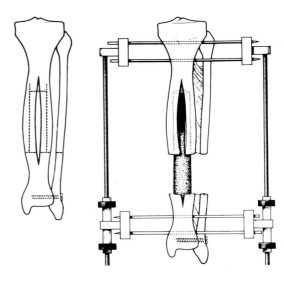

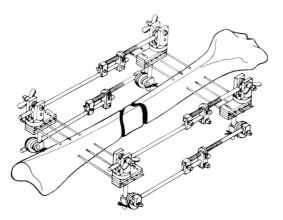

Figure 11-6. A schematic diagram of a Hoffmann device with the double upright frame developed by Vidal and Adrey.[16, 17] (Reproduced with permission of Ets. Jaquet Freres, Geneva, Switzerland.)

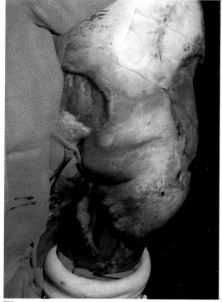

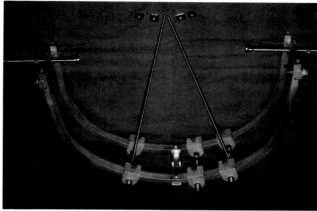

Figure 11.7A

Figure 11.7B

Figure 11-7. Photographs record the use of an external fixation device designed by the author for stabilization of a grossly infected nonunion of the pelvic ring in a woman of 21 years. (See also Figs. 11-8 and 11-9.) *A.* Preoperative photograph in which the large open wound extending from the posterior aspect of the lower leg and the perineum is visible. A large lateral sinus tract is evident which extends posterior to the hip joint and attaches to the perineal wound. Through the perineal wound, the bladder and bowel are visible. *B.* Photograph of the pelvic device designed by the author. An anterior hemihoop is attached to the ilium by large, threaded percutaneous pins. Supplementary posterior lateral pins impinge upon the superficial surfaces of the ilia. *C.* The patient is shown after application of the hemihoop and hip spica cast.

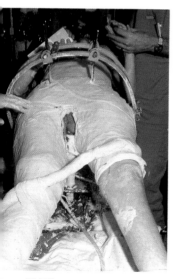

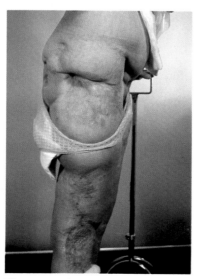

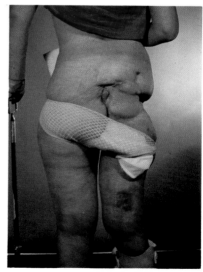

ʒure 11.7C

Figure 11.8A

Figure 11.8B

Figure 11-8. *A* and *B*. Photographs of the patient's wounds (seen in Fig. 11-7) 1 year after surgery when cutaneous coverage and union of fractures have been realized.

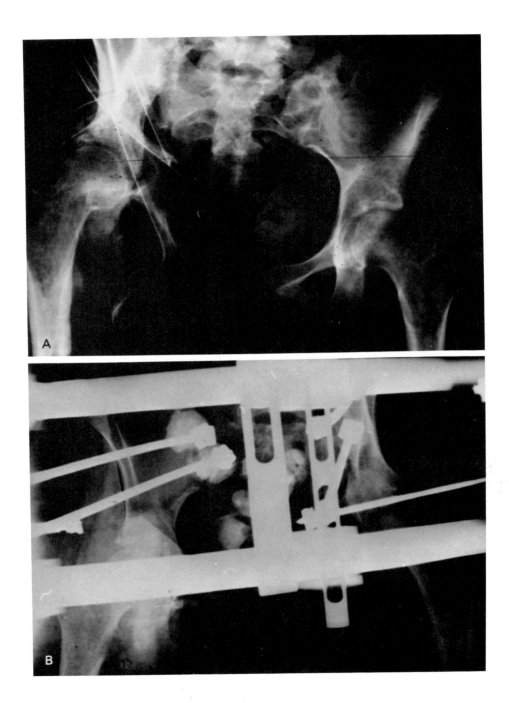

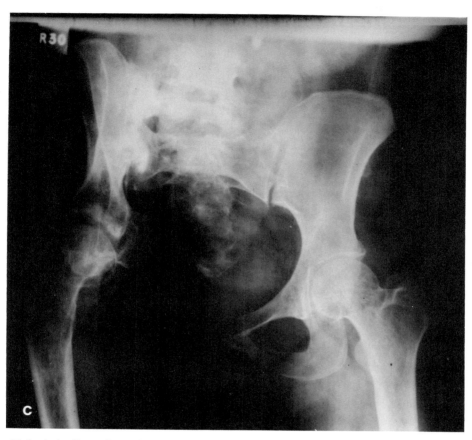

Figure 11-9. *A.* An X-ray shows the patient (seen in Figs. 11-7 and 11-8) 1 year after open pelvic fracture was sustained by which time she had an infected nonunion of the symphysis pubis, the right sacroiliac joint and osteomyelitis of the right hemipelvis. Drainage tubes are visible on the right side of the pelvis. *B.* An X-ray shows the pelvis after application of the hemihoop. *C.* An X-ray of the united pelvis 1 year after the osteotomy of the posterior ilium, beside the sacroiliac joint was performed and after external fixation was applied.

Jaquet Freres, 5 Route des Jeunes, 1211 Geneva 26, Switzerland). With the modifications of Vidal and Adrey, the Hoffmann apparatus was sufficiently versatile so that it could be employed for pelvic fractures and for many other applications. Subsequently the author has treated over 100 cases and assisted or reviewed an additional 200 cases where the Hoffmann device was applied to a great variety of complex fractures. The Hoffmann device appears to be the most satisfactory method of external fixation for most indications, other than leg lengthening, where the Wagner apparatus also is particularly useful. The remainder of this chapter is based heavily on the author's experience with the Hoffmann apparatus. It has become evident to him that external fixation is an extraordinarily valuable development in orthopaedic surgery for the treatment of complex fracture problems. It does not impinge upon the use of simpler techniques such as plaster casts for the treatment of closed, stable and simple fractures. It should not be used by itself to reduce and immobilize displaced interarticular fractures where the goal is restoration of joint function. Internal fixation remains the optimal method of treatment for such fractures, although combinations of external fixation with internal fixation may provide the optimal results for the treatment of many complex fractures.

Indications for Application of an External Fixation Device

The optimal indications for the use of the Hoffmann device are open, comminuted fractures or nonunions with extensive soft tissue loss or infection. The fractures amenable to such treatment include open, infected, comminuted and unstable fractures of the pelvic ring, central acetabular fractures and open fractures of the upper and lower extremity. The device is also a useful method for arthrodesis of joints, especially after infection of total joint replacements and after severe open injuries such as shotgun blasts. Where such fractures, nonunions or unstable joints are accompanied by loss of bone substance, external fixation is extremely valuable if it is followed by the application of autogenous bone graft. In a somewhat similar way such injuries can be treated by a combination of the use of the Hoffmann device with cutaneous and bone grafts on a vascular pedicle.

The method has certain indications in reconstructive surgery. Where complex 3-plane correction of an osteotomy site is necessary, the use of external fixation enables the surgeon to make multiple postoperative adjustments in alignment so that precise realignment is realized. The technique can be used for leg lengthening or, in exceptional cases, for lengthening of bones in the upper extremity.

Perhaps the most valuable attribute of the Hoffmann device over its rivals is its unique capability to permit the surgeon to reduce and immobilize all of the previously mentioned fracture problems, including pelvic stabilization by the use of a single apparatus.

In several European centers, the Hoffmann device is used as the routine method of treatment for tibial fractures in adults, including those closed injuries that show minor degrees of instability.[18] These workers argue that the method is so successful that it supplants the application of other methods. In the author's experience the application of a plaster cast is generally preferable for the treatment of such fractures, as was reviewed in Chapter 10. While the risk of pin tract infection is small, the sequelae of such infections can possess considerable morbidity. Nevertheless, there are certain relative indications for the use of the external fixation in acute closed tibial shaft fractures. In the presence of an unstable oblique fracture that cannot be controlled by the use of closed reductions and plaster casts, the Hoffmann device provides a suitable alternative to open reduction and internal fixation. With its provision of extremely rigid fixation, serial corrections and realignments of fractures and ready access to open wounds, the Hoffmann device is superior to percutaneous skeletal pins immobilized in a plaster cast. In such injuries, it is the only method of treatment that may enable the patient to rapidly resume a full weight-bearing gait. Another uncommon indication in closed tibial fractures is the presence of a dermatological disease, such as epidermolysis bullosa, in which chronic irritation from motion of the alternative of a plaster cast could aggravate the disease. In a somewhat similar way the use of plaster casts is greatly limited in hot tropical countries where severe fungal infections frequently develop under a cast. For this reason the use of the Hoffmann device has been widely employed in several African trauma centers.[19]

THE HOFFMANN DEVICE, ITS COMPONENTS AND METHODS OF APPLICATION

As a prerequisite to the satisfactory application of the Hoffmann device, the surgeon must familiarize himself with its numerous components and with the conventional ways in which

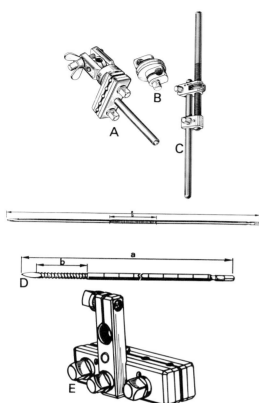

Figure 11-10. Schematic diagrams show the principal components necessary to construct a typical Hoffmann external fixation device: *A,* Universal ball joints; *B,* articulation couplings; *C,* adjustable connecting rods; *D,* threaded transfixing pins and half pins; *E,* complementary vise for parallel anchoring. (Reproduced with permission of Ets. Jaquet Freres, Geneva, Switzerland.)

they are combined to erect a stable extraskeletal frame. For the treatment of a fracture in an adult with a Hoffmann device, a surgeon requires the use of at least four components: universal ball joints, articulation couplings, adjustable connecting rods and threaded transfixing pins (Fig. 11-10). (Throughout this chapter the manufacturer's nomenclature for components of the Hoffmann device is used.) While nonthreaded pins have been available, their use has been abandoned by the author because they do not possess adequate fixation in bone. Of the several other components available, the complementary vise for parallel anchoring (Fig. 11-10*E*) is the most useful, especially for fixation in cancellous bone such as the metaphysis or in the os calcis. Prior to the application of the device, X-rays of the fracture are studied and the appropriate type of external frame is selected. The standard frames for treatment of most appendic-

ular fractures are discussed below. When the surgeon possesses no prior experience with the Hoffmann device he should build the appropriate external frame prior to the clinical application, so that he possesses both adequate numbers of components and the technique for its construction. For the most typical application, on a fresh open tibial shaft fracture, the patient is taken to the operating room and given a general or spinal anesthetic. The wound is cleaned and debrided by conventional techniques. Frequently a puncture wound or laceration must be extended so that adequate exploration is possible. Then the transfixing pins are inserted.

The author has found that three or four threaded transfixing pins should be inserted into each of the two major fracture fragments. The first pin is aligned in the midaxis of the medial or lateral surface of the tibia and aligned parallel to the knee joint (Fig. 11-11). A gap of at least 3 cm should be left between the limits of the fracture and the site on the undamaged bone where the pin is inserted. With a scalpel a stab wound is made at the appropriate site; the wound should be at least twice as long as the outside diameter of the pin. The first pin is mounted in a power drill for insertion up to its threaded portion. To minimize the pressure needed to insert the pin a power drill is preferred in place of a hand drill. Excessive pressure on the pin provokes unnecessary displacement of the fracture fragments which could complicate the subsequent reduction of the fracture. When the first pin has been inserted up to the threaded portion, the power drill is detached. While an assistant inserts a second pin into the power drill, the surgeon attaches the standard hand brace to the transfixing pin and completes its insertion. The surgeon must ensure that both cortices are secured by the threaded portion of the transfixing pin (Fig. 11-12).

In some young adults the resistance of the tibia to insertion of the transfixing pin by the use of a power drill is so great that slow progress is observed and considerable heat is produced. As soon as the surgeon detects this problem he should replace the transfixing pin with a 3-mm powered drill and a drill guide to make a hole through both cortices in the bone. Then the 4-mm transfixing pin is inserted with the hand brace.

After the first pin has been inserted, the aligning jig is placed on the pin (Fig. 11-11). The jig possesses holes through which four additional pins can be inserted into the bone to provide

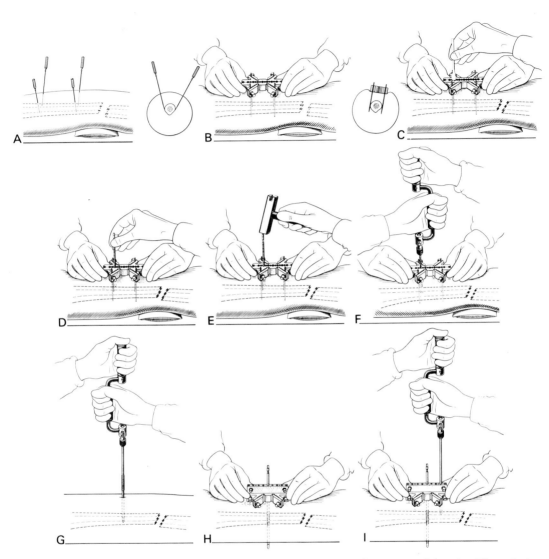

Figure 11-11. Schematic views reveal the stages in the insertion of Hoffmann transfixing pins. The technique is fully described in the text. *A.* Shown is a schematic view of locating the medial and lateral surfaces of a long bone by the insertion of specially designed percutaneous pins. In *B,* the specially designed percutaneous pin guide is used to facilitate the identification of the medial and lateral surface of the shaft of the bone. *C* shows the insertion of the special blade to make the incision in the skin at the pin site. *D* shows the insertion of the transfixing pin through the stab wound until it contacts the surface of the bone. In *E,* the pin is tapped gently to imbed the cutting edge into the proximal cortex. *F* shows the brace attached to the pin for additional insertion. Alternatively, in *G,* insertion of the pin by use of the brace without the pin guide is illustrated. In *H,* the pin guide is placed over the first pin to align the sites for insertion of additional pins. In *I,* the second pin is inserted through the appropriate hole in the pin guide. (Reproduced with permission of Ets. Jaquet Freres, Geneva, Switzerland.)

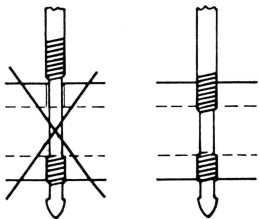

Figure 11-12. Schematic diagram illustrates the correct amount of insertion of a transfixing pin so that its threaded region contacts both cortices of bone. (Reproduced with permission of Ets. Jaquet Freres, Geneva, Switzerland.)

precise spacing between each pin. An assistant holds the aligning jig parallel to the long axis of the tibia. Next the pin most distal from the first pin is inserted in the same manner. Again the threaded portion of the pin is inserted by the hand brace while another assistant attaches a third transfixing pin to the power drill. After the insertion of the second pin the jig is maintained in satisfactory alignment by the two pins. One or two additional pins are now inserted through the appropriate holes in the jig. Since the threaded portion of the transfixing pin possesses a diameter that is larger than that of the hole in the jig, the two halves of the jig must be separated to enlarge the hole sufficiently to permit the passage of the threaded portion of the pin.

Subsequently three or four additional pins are inserted in a similar manner into the second major fracture fragment. An attempt is made to align the second row of pins with the first row of pins when the fracture fragments are held in anatomical alignment. While the Hoffmann device possesses sufficient intrinsic adjustments so that such exacting alignment of the pins is not essential, nevertheless, careful alignment of the pins within the fracture fragments greatly simplifies both the reduction of the fracture and the erection of the external frame. In the presence of a segmental fracture, additional transfixing pins are inserted into other fracture fragments of sufficient size (*e.g.*, greater than 3 cm in length).

The previous description of insertion of the pins refers to those fractures which permit insertion of all of the pins within the hard cortical bone of the diaphysis. When the pin approaches the peripheral portion of the diaphysis so that one set of pins must be inserted into the metaphysis, then the insertion of a second parallel row of metaphyseal pins with the use of a complementary vise should be considered. In young adults with strong cancellous bone a single row of pins may be adequate, but in older individuals and in those with osteoporosis of the metaphysis secondary to infection, disuse or through metabolic bone disease, two parallel rows of pins are essential.

All of the pins should be of sufficient length so that at least one transfixing pin separates the superficial surface of the skin and the universal ball joint with rod. This gap allows for the anticipated soft tissue swelling of the skin which otherwise might provoke cutaneous impingement upon the metal with subsequent ulceration and necrosis.

After the insertion of the pins a universal ball joint with rod is attached to both ends of the two rows of pins (Fig. 11-13). Each pin must fit into the cylindrical depression in the resilient material of the universal ball joint. An articulation coupling is attached to each of the rods on the universal ball joints. A spring-like "stop-clip" may be temporarily attached to the rod to prevent accidental removal of the articulation coupling. At this stage the nuts on the universal ball joints and the articulation couplings are tightened by hand. Next, adjustable connection rods of appropriate length are selected. The knurled wheel is turned to the midportion of the threaded segment on the adjustable connecting rod so that maximal adjustment in the alignment of the fracture is possible. Four adjustable con-

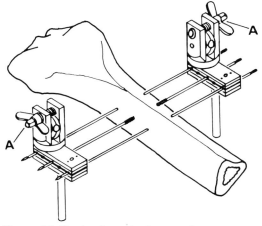

Figure 11-13. A schematic diagram shows two ball joint rods attached to a set of three transfixing pins. (See also Fig. 14, *A* to *E*.) (Reproduced with permission of Ets. Jaquet Freres, Geneva, Switzerland.)

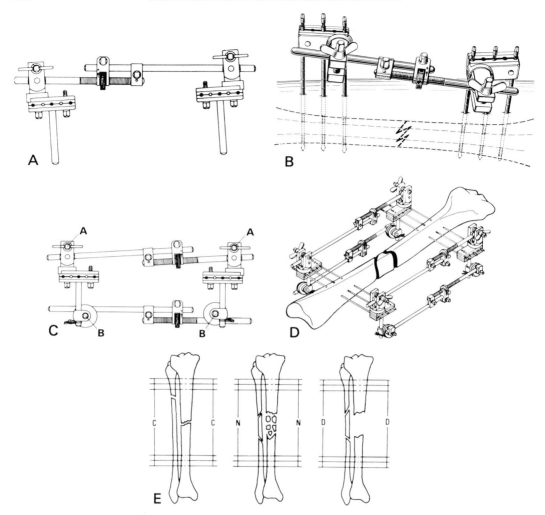

Figure 11-14. A series of schematic diagrams (Figs. 11-13 and 11-14 *A* to *E*) show the stages in the erection of a double upright frame. *A.* A schematic view shows an adjustable connecting rod is attached to two ball joint rods to form a simple frame. *B.* A schematic diagram of a ball joint with rod and slider bar attached to one side of bone. *C.* A schematic diagram shows one side of a double upright frame. *D.* A schematic view of a double upright frame. *E.* A schematic view of three tibial fractures with conventional sites for insertion of the transfixing pins. (Reproduced with permission of Ets. Jaquet Freres, Geneva, Switzerland.)

necting rods are attached between the proximal and distal fracture fragments (Fig. 11-14*A* to *E*). An assistant aligns the fracture with appropriate traction on the extremity and the surgeon tightens the square nuts with one of the two special wrenches. At this stage additional adjustments in the alignment of the fracture are frequently performed. The nuts may be loosened for manual corrections in the alignment. Alternatively, all of the nuts except the one on the distal end of the threaded portion of the adjustable connecting rod may be tightened. Then the knurled knob on the adjustable connecting rod

may be rotated by the use of the special rods which insert into the three equally-spaced depressions in the knurled knob. Angular deformities are corrected by lengthening the shorter side. Such angular correction must be made before the fracture surfaces are approximated. Otherwise impingement of the fracture fragments initiates large bending moments and, ultimately deformation of the transfixing pins, so that the desired alignment of the fracture is not realized. When a clinical appearance of the limb suggests that satisfactory alignment has been achieved, all of the nuts on the device are tightened. Subsequent adjustments in the alignment of the device are made after careful radiological views have been taken. The duration of anesthesia needed for the initial application of the Hoffman device is greatly foreshortened if such adjustments are made at a later time, such as the first or second postoperative day. Subsequently additional X-rays and minor adjustments in alignment may be repeated.

After the device has been tightened and the limb is stabilized, careful examination is made of the cutaneous sites of entry and exit of the percutaneous pins. If the skin is stretched over a pin, the stab wound is lengthened until relief of the pressure is achieved. Excessive pressure on the skin initiates local ischemia and may culminate in necrosis of the skin or even pin track infection. Where considerable correction of a deformity is made after insertion of the pins, a lengthy release of the skin may be necessary to prevent this complication. Small cotton roll dressings are applied to the pin sites for the first 24 hours after surgery. The wound at the fracture site is packed open or, in the presence of a smaller puncture wound, the cutaneous margins are loosely approximated without the use of sutures.

When a portion of the tibia is lost at the time of the fracture, the limb is aligned in anatomical configuration with 1 to 2 mm of excessive distraction. Stabilization of the extremity with the small amount of excessive distraction facilitates the secondary application of autogenous iliac crest cancellous bone which is described in Chapter 10.

When the patient is in bed the injured extremity is elevated by overhead traction to a position of 90° of flexion of the hip and knee. The suspension system can be attached to the Hoffmann device to facilitate the elevation.

On the day after surgery the dressings are removed and daily pin care is initiated. Each pin site is swabbed with hydrogen peroxide and a small amount of Betadine or bacitracin antibiotic ointment is applied. The patient or his relatives are taught to undertake this pin care. Most open wounds at the fracture site are treated with daily dressing changes of saline soaked cotton gauze. Where necessary sequential debridements of the wound are performed. All of the nuts on the Hoffmann device should be tightened on the first and third postoperative days, and subsequently, once a week. The nuts on the universal ball joint which secure the percutaneous pins are the most susceptible to loosening in view of the inelastic nature of the

resilient material that grips the pins. Loosening greatly enhances the likelihood of pin track infection, delayed union and mechanical pain experienced by the patient at the fracture site or the pin tracks.

Usually, serial X-rays of the fracture site are taken, one to three times in the first week after treatment and in the 4th, 8th and 16th weeks after injury. If the postoperative X-rays indicate malalignment, readjustment of the Hoffmann device is performed at the bedside on the first or second postoperative day, usually, with the use of mild analgesics and sedatives. Careful calculation from the postoperative X-rays enables the surgeon to quantify the desired correction. One revolution of the knurled knob on the adjustable connecting rod provides $\frac{1}{10}$ inch of axial correction. Deformities must be corrected by lengthening the appropriate side of the fracture so that bending moments on the percutaneous pins are minimized. After the fracture has been realigned it is impacted by simultaneous adjustment of all four knurled knobs on the adjustable connecting rods of the double frame.

When an open tibial fracture is accompanied by loss of bone substance then a second stage for the application of autogenous iliac crest cancellous bone to the fracture gap is planned. This procedure is performed when the open wound shows a clean granulation bed, usually 7 to 14 days after the application of the Hoffmann device. In most instances, the bone graft is taken from the posterior iliac crest. Only cancellous bone is used as the cortical bone possesses excessive liability to sequestrum formation and infection. Also, cortical bone graft shows less satisfactory stimulation of osteogenesis and healing at the fracture gap. The strips of cancellous bone are inserted into the gap at the fracture site through the open granulating wound. The volume of bone graft, ideally, should approximate that of the lost bone substance. The granulation tissue on the opposing ends of the fracture fragments should be carefully preserved as it provides a local available source of capillaries for rapid invasion and revascularization of the bone graft. After the graft has been inserted, the wound is gently packed as previously described. At this time the excessive distraction of the fracture that was deliberately provided at the time of application of the Hoffmann is corrected. This maneuver should provide a continuous column of bone graft across the fracture site.

The rigid fixation of the Hoffmann device encourages the ingrowth of granulation tissue and a secondary spontaneous epithelization of open wounds of diameters up to 8 or 10 cm. For larger wounds, secondary application of split thickness skin grafts may be applied to a clean granulation bed. Complex rotational flap grafts of full thickness skin are rarely required. Where an open fracture wound displays denuded bone, the osseous surface is kept moist with periodic application of physiological saline solutions until clean granulation tissue covers the bone, usually within 2 to 3 weeks. The spontaneous epithelization of smaller wounds or the application of split thickness skin grafts can be pursued.

Postoperative Management of the Patient with the Hoffmann Device

On the first postoperative day the patient is encouraged to undertake quadriceps exercises and active range of motion exercises for the knee and ankle joints even though remaining in the traction with 90° of flexion of hip and knee. When the soft tissue swelling has diminished the traction is discontinued and gait training is initiated. The patient is encouraged to undertake a partial weight-bearing gait. Within a few weeks after surgery the patient is encouraged to increase weight bearing on the extremity. Provided that the patient has minimal swelling of the leg the patient is permitted to undertake full weight bearing. The duration of hospitalization for a patient with an acute open tibial fracture with moderate skin loss usually varies between 1 and 3 weeks. As soon as the open wound shows complete coverage with granulation tissue, the patient is permitted to take showers at home. When the wounds have completely healed the patient is permitted to take baths or to swim in fresh water. Swimming in chlorinated or salt water, however, is not permitted in view of the likelihood of corrosion of the exposed portions of the device.

On follow-up visits the patient is questioned about the amount of pain, soft tissue swelling, and drainage. Usually pain and soft tissue swelling are indicative either of loosening of the device or of excessive activity by the patient. When the percutaneous pins penetrate muscles on either side of the fracture, pain may arise from motion of the muscles around the pins. During the insertion of the transfixing pins, therefore, minimal penetration of muscle should be undertaken. Serous drainage of the pin tracks may occur with excessive activity. Usually the drainage ceases within 24 hours after the patient has initiated bed rest with elevation of the extremity. Purulent drainage of the pins is discussed in the section on complications of the Hoffmann device.

On examination of the fractured extremity with a satisfactory rigid external fixation, the fracture site should show minimal tenderness on palpation. Tenderness is an indication of instability or of infection. If the surgeon grasps the Hoffmann device and shakes the limb, the patient should not experience any discomfort at the site of the fracture or at the site of percutaneous pins. Sequential X-rays reveal evidence of primary or of secondary bone healing. If the patient undertakes full weight bearing then follow-up X-rays are likely to show evidence of secondary bone healing with callus formation. In many instances, however, the fracture heals with primary bone healing and minimal radiological evidence of callus formation appears. For patients who have had cancellous bone grafts, incorporation of the graft should be observed before considering the removal of the Hoffmann device. Open transverse or oblique fractures of the tibial shaft generally require 4 to 5 months of external fixation before metal removal can be considered. In some cases, especially after the application of bone graft to a site of a segmental loss, the period may be prolonged for 8 to 12 months. The author's findings are comparable to those reported by Karlström and Olerud.[20]

On clinical follow-up if the patient shows evidence of loosening of the Hoffman device, the surgeon must ensure that weekly adjustments to tighten the device have been undertaken by the patient, his relatives or others. If the device begins to loosen despite a proper tightening regime, it is likely that inadequate numbers of the pins have been inserted. This is particularly true where the bone is moderately osteoporotic. In such cases the patient should be readmitted and additional clusters of percutaneous pins should be inserted which are more distal from the fracture site. Appropriate connections are attached to the transfixing pins so that longer adjustable connecting rods may be attached to incorporate all of the pins.

Metal removal is generally performed in a hospital under ketamine hydrochloride anesthesia. The adjustable connecting rods are detached from both the universal ball joints and the articulation couplings. Then a clinical test for motion at the fracture site is performed. If clinical and radiological evidence of fracture healing are present the transfixing pins are removed and a short-leg walking cast is applied to the extremity for prevention of a spiral fracture, which might initiate at the osseous pin tracks. If on clinical examination the fracture is wholly unstable, then the connecting rods are reattached to the articulations and ball joints. Alternatively, when clinical and radiological assessment indicates that partial healing of the fracture has transpired the surgeon may elect to remove the transfixing pins and initiate conventional treatment with a plaster cast.

Application of Autogenous Composite Osseous and Cutaneous Grafts

Recently, O'Brien[21] and Taylor[22] have successfully applied autogenous composite grafts of bone with superficial full thickness skin to sites of open fractures with segmental loss of bone and skin. The procedure also has been used to replace bone after the excision of primary osseous tumors. The procedures require considerable competence in the application of microsurgery to anastomose the vascular pedicle which supplies the graft. Generally the vessels are about 2 mm in diameter. For this graft O'Brien has used a portion of the anterior iliac crest with superficial skin while Weiland* has used a section of the midshaft fibula. Three examples are shown in Figures 11-15 to 11-20. While the successful results are spectacular, the considerable technical difficulties and the prolonged time required for the surgical procedure are likely to prevent widespread application of these techniques in the near future.

Nature of Fracture Healing Encountered with External Fixation

In Chapters 5 and 9, the nature and significance of primary and secondary bone healing were fully described. A few studies have been undertaken in the laboratory to fully categorize the nature of bone healing that occurs when external fixation is applied to a fresh fracture. In many clinical applications of the Hoffmann device the extensive loss of periosteum by the open injury or by infection greatly inhibits secondary bone healing by periosteal ossification. Certain relevant clinical observations, however, have been made. Radiological evidence of both primary and secondary bone healing is frequently encountered (Figs. 11-21 and 11-22). With adequate numbers of pins and anatomical reduction of the fracture, primary bone healing without periosteal new bone formation may be observed. In most cases where the patient undertakes full weight bearing, some evidence of periosteal new bone formation is present. Even in those patients

who have had extensive loss of periosteum at the site of a segmental bone loss, strips of autogenous cancellous bone placed adjacent to surrounding muscle will show rapid evidence of revascularization and osteogenesis, usually within 4 to 6 weeks after surgery. Where inadequate stability is realized with the Hoffmann device, little or no evidence of new bone formation will be observed at the fracture site. Jorgensen[23] has attempted to correlate the angular deformity at a tibial fracture site immobilized with the Hoffmann device. From his observations and from the studies of Rahn et al.,[24] it appears that the capillary ingrowth necessary for primary bone healing will not occur at the fracture site unless rigid fixation is achieved. It will be recalled from observations by Rahn et al. that less than 5 to 10 μm of dynamic motion must occur at a fracture site, if primary bone healing is to be realized.

Observations by Rahn et al.[24] may also explain another observation on the clinical application of the Hoffmann device. While the incidence of nonunion is extremely low the duration of time required for fracture healing seems to be remarkably prolonged, particularly in view of the degree of rigid immobilization that is achieved.[16] It seems not unlikely that the degree of immobilization conventionally achieved by the use of the Hoffmann device with a Vidal double upright frame is such that periosteal new bone formation is inhibited by the limited amount of cyclic motion at the fracture site while the absolutely rigid fixation of bone with anatomical reduction of the fracture fragments (e.g., the optimal conditions for primary bone healing) is not achieved.

Application of the Hoffmann Device to Multiple Fractures in the Lower Extremity

As a sequelae to industrial accidents such as mining incidents, motor vehicular accidents and injuries to pedestrians, many patients sustain multiple trauma including severe and usually comminuted open fractures at multiple levels in a single extremity, often in combination with injuries to other organ systems such as the abdominal viscera, chest injuries and head injuries. In the author's experience the management of these patients is greatly facilitated by the application of the Hoffmann device to their injured extremity. After external stabilization of the extremity the open wound can be managed in a way that was previously discussed. Furthermore, injuries to other organ systems can be treated

---

* A. Weiland, personal communication, 1978.

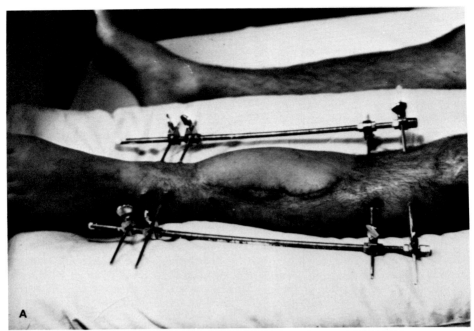

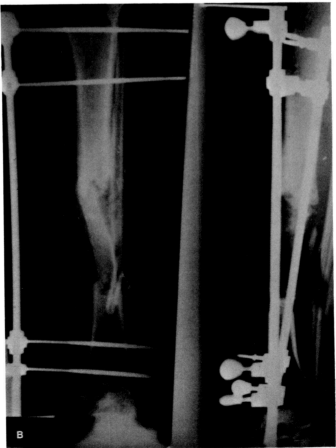

Figure 11-15. A photograph (*A*) and an X-ray (*B*) reveal evidence of the application of an autogenous composite graft of bone with superficial full thickness skin coverage on a vascular pedicle to an infected nonunion of the tibia. (Reproduced with permission of Dr. Bernard O'Brien.)

Figure 11-16. Shown schematically is the method of preparation of a vascularized fibular and cutaneous graft (B) to be inserted into the contralateral tibial defect (A), as shown in (C). (Reproduced with permission of Dr. G. Ian Taylor.)

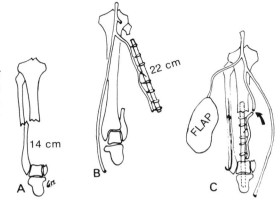

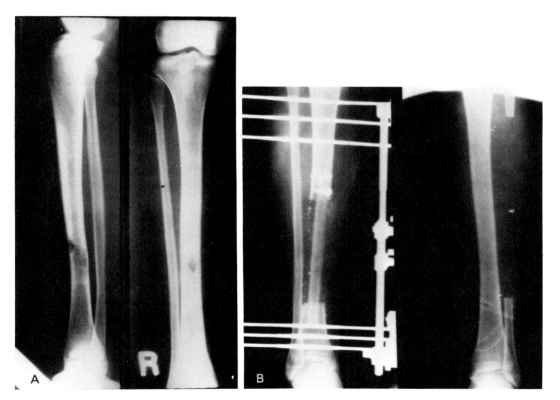

Figures 11-17. Two clinical examples of the application of autogenous bone grafts on a vascular pedicle for the treatment of massive resection of primary bone tumors are shown in Figures 11-17 to 11-20. A. An X-ray showing chondrosarcoma of the distal tibia seen in a lateral preoperative picture. B. Postoperative X-ray shows the free vascularized bone graft in place on the right and the donor site for the fibular graft on the left. (Reproduced with permission of Dr. Andrew Weiland.)

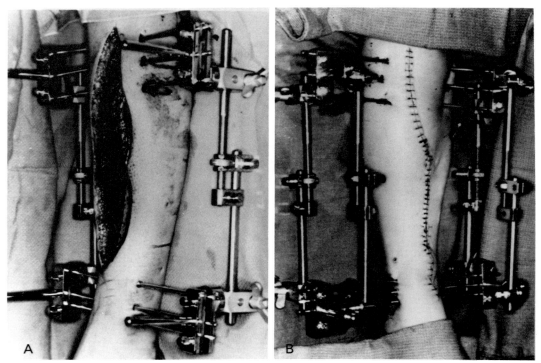

Figure 11-18. *A* and *B*. Intraoperative and postoperative photographs show the Hoffmann apparatus in place. (See also Figs. 11-17, 11-19 and 11-20. Reproduced with permission of Dr. Andrew Weiland.)

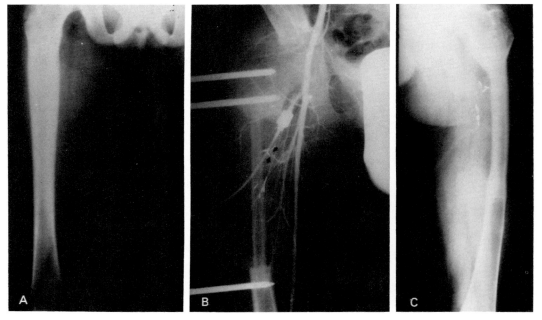

Figure 11-19. *A*. X-ray of an 11-year-old boy with chondrosarcoma of the right proximal femur. *B*. A postoperative arteriogram shows the patent anastomosis between the vascular graft and a branch of the femoral artery. *C*. An X-ray postoperative at 1 year. (See also Figs. 11-17, 11-18 and 11-20. Reproduced with permission of Dr. Andrew Weiland.)

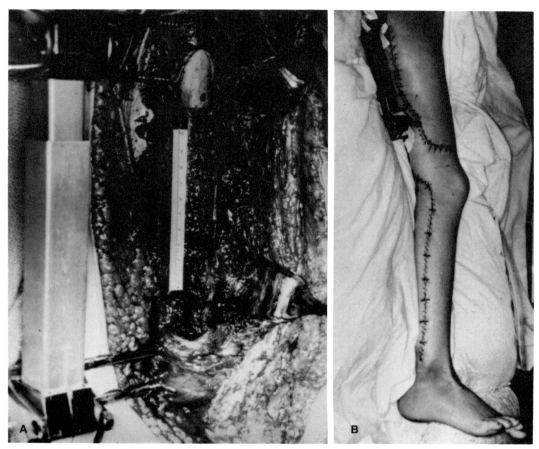

Figure 11-20. *A.* Intraoperative photograph. A ruler indicates the segment of excised femur. *B.* Postoperative photograph with the Wagner apparatus shown on the medial aspect of the thigh. (See also Figs. 11-17 to 11-19. Reproduced with permission of Dr. Andrew Weiland.)

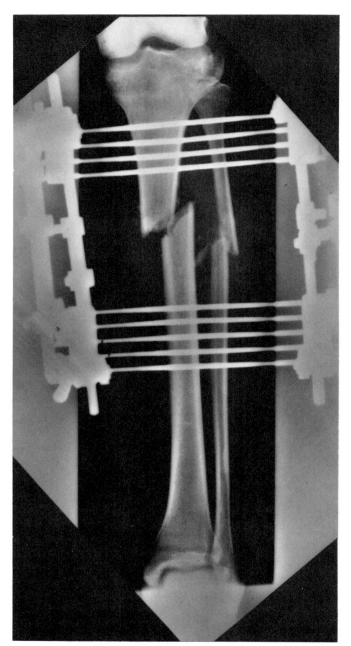

Figure 11-21. X-ray of bilateral open tibial fractures sustained by a pedestrian age 19, treated with bilateral Hoffmann devices. An oblique fracture with callus formation is shown. (See also Fig. 11-22.)

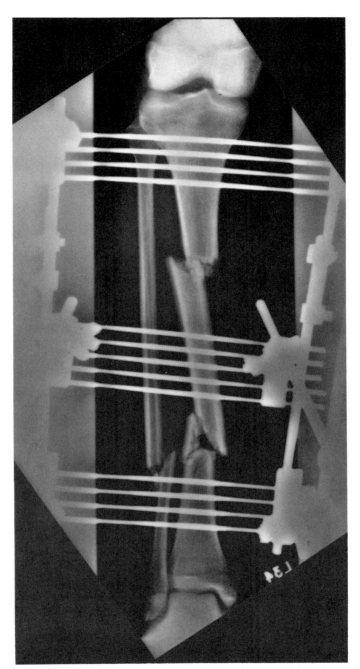

Figure 11-22. X-ray of same injury shown in Figure 11-21 reveals segmental fracture with minimal callus formation. Both tibiae were shortened by ½ inch. By 5 months both tibiae had healed without deformity and with equal leg lengths.

appropriately without the usual problems in transport and transfer of the patient who is suspended in balanced traction.

After X-rays of the injured extremity have been assessed, components for an appropriate Hoffmann device are selected which will permit rigid stabilization of the unstable portion of the extremity. For example, if the patient sustains open comminuted fractures of the midshaft tibia and the ipsilateral midshaft femur, then the device should extend from the distal diaphysis or metaphysis of the tibia to the proximal diaphysis or metaphysis of the femur. Depending upon the extent of the open wounds and the area of skin loss around the knee joint, the surgeon may elect to apply two separate Hoffmann devices to the tibia and femur respectively, or alternatively, he may elect to temporarily stabilize the entire extremity, including the knee joint, in a single Hoffmann device. At a later date, the single device can be reconstructed as two separate devices to enable the patient to perform active range of motion exercises of the knee joint. Where the fracture extends into the knee joint itself the surgeon must decide whether the knee joint can be salvaged as a useful articular joint or whether a primary arthrodesis should be performed. If the knee joint is to be salvaged then displaced interarticular fragments will require open reduction and internal fixation. The role of internal fixation in combination with the use of the Hoffmann device is discussed below.

For the application of the Hoffmann device to an extremity with multiple fractures, the general principles of application are similar to those described in the previous section. The open wounds are explored, debrided and irrigated. Then each of the major fracture fragments are impaled with three or four threaded transfixing pins. Where major fragments such as the tibial plateau or the proximal tibial metaphysis consist primarily of cancellous bone, two parallel rows of pins should be inserted by the application of the complementary vise for parallel anchoring (Fig. 11-10). For optimal stability the two parallel rows of metaphyseal pins should be inserted parallel to the knee joint so that they are mounted at right angles to the row of diaphyseal pins. Where the fracture extends into the proximal femur or into the distal tibia, supplementary pins in the ipsilateral ilium or the os calcis may be necessary. The reader is referred to the subsequent subsections that describe Hoffmann devices for various anatomical sites. Connes[10] and DuToit[25] have described a variety of exter-

nal frames for particular fractures. In the distal femur and in the entire length of the tibia, the pins may be inserted in the midaxis of the bone, from medial to lateral. Pins inserted in the proximal femoral shaft, however, should be directed more obliquely through the leg along the posterior border of the vastus medialis to exit on the posterior lateral aspect of the leg. This change in alignment of the pins avoids obstruction of the groin; also it minimizes the risk of penetration of the femoral artery or the sciatic nerve (Fig. 11-23). Additional half pins may be inserted to augment stability. The half pins with continuous threads are particularly useful in the greater trochanter. The stability engendered by the half pins is not comparable to that achieved by the use of transfixing pins so that they should only be applied in a supplementary role. Universal ball joints with rods are attached to the most proximal and distal sets of transfixing pins and long adjustable rods are attached to them to roughly stabilize the limb. Universal ball joints are attached to the additional groups of pins. Then connecting rods are attached between the ball joints and the long adjustable connecting rods by the use of articulation couplings (Fig. 11-10C). As previously described, a clinical assessment of alignment is used at the time of application and small amounts of excessive distraction at the fracture sites are achieved by adjustments on the connecting rods. Supplementary corrections of alignment are made at a later time after another careful radiological assessment. The adjustments can be time consuming; they should not compromise other urgent aspects of management of the acutely ill patient.

In many of these injuries large areas of skin loss are present. Frequently the transfixing pins have to be inserted at sites of full thickness skin loss and denuded bone (Fig. 11-24). Provided that absolute stability of the extremity is achieved, the absence of skin and other soft tissues around the pin sites does not appear to be deleterious.

Use of the Hoffmann Device in Patients with Multiple Trauma

Many of the patients with multiple trauma possess open fractures to several extremities as well as other injuries to their head, chest and abdomen. The Hoffmann device is a valuable tool for rapid stabilization of their open fractures. It provides ready access to the open wounds for appropriate management. It enables the patient to be transported with ease. It can be used as a definitive method for immobiliza-

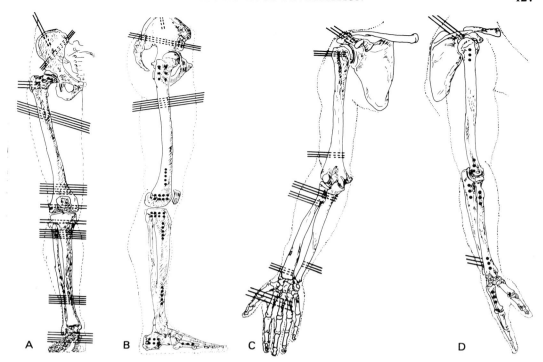

Figure 11-23. Schematic diagrams indicate the conventional sites for insertion of transfixing pins into the lower extremity (*A* and *B*) and the upper extremity (*C* and *D*). *A* and *C* are anterior views of the lower and upper extremity. *B* and *D* are lateral views of the lower and upper extremity.

tion of the fractures. Alternatively, after the open wounds have healed and the acute management of the injuries to other organ systems has been undertaken, one or more of the Hoffmann devices may be replaced by other forms of immobilization. Where the initial management of the patient's medical or surgical problems limits the time available for the application of external fixation, temporarily, simpler devices of lesser rigidity may be applied. A single external frame (Fig. 11-14C) is adequate for temporary stabilization. Otherwise the application of the devices is performed as previously described. For application of the device on the upper extremity, the relevant following subsections should be examined. In the upper extremity, the transfixing pins should not penetrate major muscle groups because the impaled muscles undergo scar formation around the pins so that joint contractures of adjacent joints ensue.

Combinations of Internal and External Skeletal Fixation

While the Hoffmann device is a satisfactory form of immobilization for the shafts of long bones or for joints where arthrodesis is desired,

its great limitation is its failure to provide satisfactory treatment for most interarticular fractures. When conventional methods of application are undertaken the Hoffmann device does not permit accurate anatomical alignment of an articular fracture nor does it permit early postoperative mobilization of the joint. As such it contravenes the methods necessary to achieve good results for interarticular fractures. If displaced interarticular fractures accompany extensive, open comminuted fractures, treatment by a combination of internal and external fixation should be considered. Initially, the badly contaminated wounds are debrided and the entire comminuted region is stabilized with external fixation. Usually within 1 to 3 weeks, when the soft tissue wounds show evidence of sufficient healing, such as clean granulation coverage, open reduction and internal fixation are undertaken. Ideally the joint is approached through undamaged skin, although when this is unfeasible it is approached through clean granulation tissue. Usually cancellous or malleolar screws are used to stabilize the interarticular fractures, as described in Chapter 10. In view of the supplementary external stabilization, the use of but-

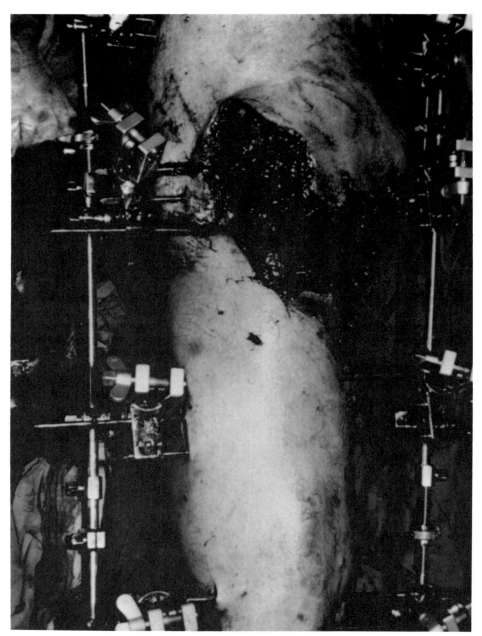

Figure 11-24. A photograph reveals evidence of extensive open fractures of the lower extremity where transfixing pins have been inserted directly into denuded bone. Absolute stability of the extremity could not have been achieved without this procedure. (Reproduced with permission of Dr. W. S. Nettrour.)

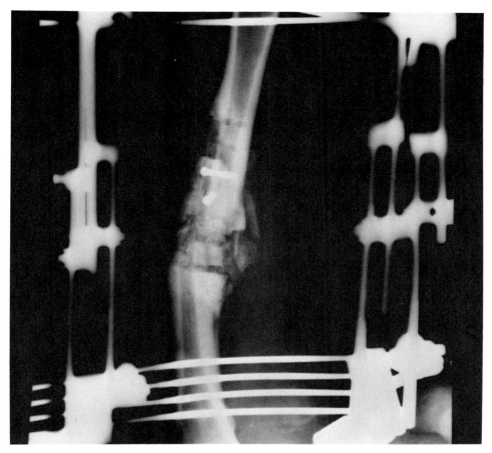

Figure 11-25. An X-ray of a leg lengthening procedure on a mature femur is shown. Previously this motorcyclist had sustained a midshaft femoral fracture which healed with 1½ inches of foreshortening and 30° of internal rotational deformity. At a secondary procedure the rotational and lengthening osteotomy was performed with the application of screw fixation. A Hoffmann device also was applied.

tress plates is rarely necessary. When extensive traumatic insult to the skin and underlying tissues has occurred, minimal exposure of the joint and the adjacent bone is advised.

Where the fractures violate open growth plates, primary or secondary open reduction of the displaced fracture is performed in a similar way as was previously described in Chapter 10.

In many of the patients who sustain violent trauma with metaphyseal fractures, cancellous bone of the region shows marked diminution in volume. In such instances, secondary application of autogenous iliac crest cancellous bone is necessary, as described in Chapter 10. Figure 11-25 shows the application of a Hoffmann device to a malunited femur for stabilization, at the time of leg lengthening and derotational osteotomy, where supplementary internal fixation was re-

quired. Also for fractures of the forearm in which extensive comminution of one bone precludes the use of internal fixation, the comminuted fracture may be stabilized with a Hoffmann device, while the simple fracture is treated by internal fixation (Fig. 11-26).

Application of the Hoffmann Device to Nonunions and Infected Nonunions

In the management of nonunions, either internal or external fixation may be applied. In many cases an equally good result can be achieved by the use of either method. There are certain relative indications, however, for either method. Where dense uninfected bone is present on either side of a nonunion that possesses good skin coverage the author generally prefers to use internal fixation, such as a compression plate or

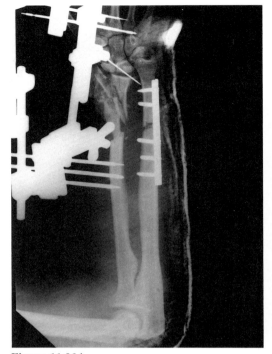

Figure 11.26A

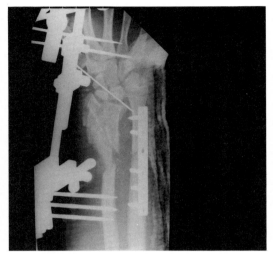

Figure 11.26B

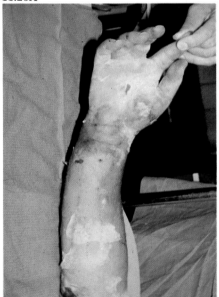

Figure 11.26C

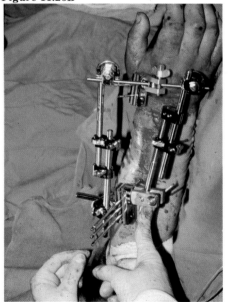

Figure 11.26D

an intramedullary rod. The advantages include compression of the nonunion site, and generally greater convenience and cosmesis for the patient. For the treatment of displaced interarticular nonunions, internal fixation is preferable so that accurate anatomical reduction can be achieved. Where the bone on either side of the fracture is markedly osteoporotic or where skin coverage at the nonunion is of poor quality, generally the use of external fixation is preferred. The Hoffmann device permits fixation of bone more distant from the fracture site where more dense bone stock may be encountered. Also tenuous skin coverage at the site of the fracture may be left intact.

When the Hoffmann device is applied to stabilize a pseudarthrosis, the technique of application is similar to that previously described. Adequate numbers of pins are essential if rigid stability is to be achieved. Where the opposing unstable bone ends are not in direct continuity and where the areas of contact of the bone fragments are significantly less than the diameter of the intact bone, autogenous cancellous bone graft should be added. The technique of bone graft was fully described in Chapter 10. After the addition of bone graft the fracture is compressed by adjustment of the connecting rods. No other form of immobilization is necessary. The patient is encouraged to undertake partial or full weight bearing and to exercise adjacent joints and muscle groups.

For the treatment of infected nonunions the application of the Hoffmann device is generally preferred to the use of techniques of internal fixation.[26] Admittedly, as Meyer et al.[27] have shown, rigid internal fixation can provide a satisfactory result for patients with infected nonunions. Frequently, however, the technical problems in the application of internal fixation to the osteoporotic infected bone is a formidable one. If the implant fails to provide rigid fixation then it serves as a sequestrum to aggravate the infection and to further compromise the likelihood for union. The one site where, in the author's experience, internal fixation may be generally preferable to external fixation of infected nonunions is in the forearm. For the treatment of most other infected nonunions, however, the

author prefers the use of the Hoffmann device.

The treatment of an infected nonunion of a long bone is undertaken in two stages. In the first stage the nonunion site and soft tissue extensions of the wound are thoroughly debrided. Next, three or four transfixing pins are inserted through the adjacent bone, preferably through nonosteoporotic areas. While insertion of the pins through intact skin is preferable, in many cases this is impossible. As previously mentioned, insertion of pins into denuded, viable bone does not preclude a satisfactory outcome provided that rigid stabilization is achieved. The external frame is attached to the transfixing pins and the limb is aligned with minor excessive distraction of the fracture site. If excessive foreshortening of the extremity has previously occurred at the nonunion site, especially in the lower limb, an attempt is made to distract the limb to its anatomical length.

When the entire length of the involved bone is markedly osteoporotic, double rows of metaphyseal pins are inserted. Occasionally, rigid stabilization of the nonunion can be achieved only by the insertion of additional pins into an adjacent bone (Fig. 11-27).

In many of these examples the use of the Hoffmann device represents the terminal salvage procedure prior to amputation of a limb that has undergone many previous operations. As such, extension of the Hoffmann device across adjacent joints, even with the likelihood of subsequent permanent limitation of joint motion frequently is preferable to amputation.

The wound is packed and daily dressing changes are undertaken. Usually within 1 to 2 weeks after the debridement and immobilization the second stage is undertaken when autogenous cancellous bone is added to the nonunion site. The bone is inserted through the open wound as previously described. Then the graft is compressed by adjustment of the connecting rods.

Where the whole extremity is substantially osteoporotic, postoperative limitation on weight bearing may be necessary. Whenever possible at least 25 pounds of weight bearing, measurable by bearing weight on the afflicted limb on a bathroom scale, is permitted on the limb so that further disuse osteoporosis is minimized. Fre-

Figure 11-26. X-rays reveal the application of the Hoffmann device and internal fixation to fractures of the forearm. The simple ulnar fracture was easily treated by the use of a plate while the comminuted distal radial fracture was more readily treated by the use of a single Hoffmann external frame. A. A preoperative X-ray of the described forearm fractures with dislocation of the elbow. B. Postoperative X-ray with Hoffmann device on comminuted distal radial fracture and the dynamic compression plate on the ulna. A technical error is inadequate reconstitution of the length of the radius. C and D. Pre- and postoperative views of the forearm to show the single frame applied to the radius. (Reproduced with permission of Dr. J. Imbriglia.)

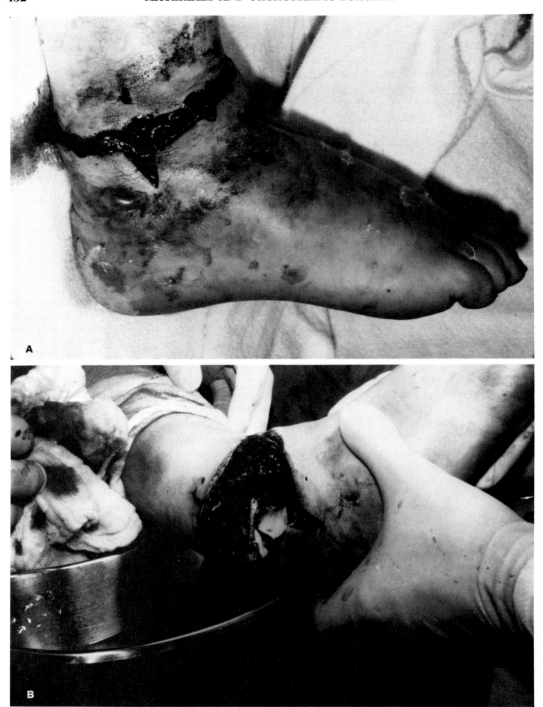

Figure 11-27. Photographs and X-rays show the application of two parallel rows of pins inserted into metaphyseal bone anchored to a complementary vise. *A* and *B*. Preoperative views of open fracture/dislocation of ankle and subtalar joints with traumatic loss of body of the talus in a girl of 20. *C*. Photograph of the Hoffmann device with a double row of pins emerging from the calcaneus. Betadine discolors the skin in this view although the open wound is clearly visible. *D*. Preoperative X-ray which shows loss of most of the talus. *E*. Postoperative X-ray to show the application of the Hoffmann device. Bone graft has been applied to the former site of the body of the talus.

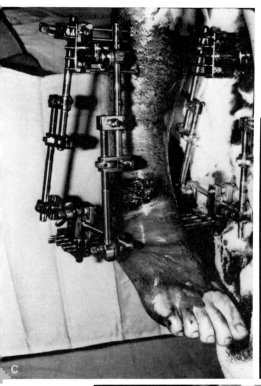

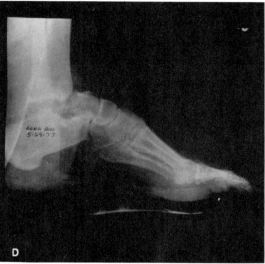

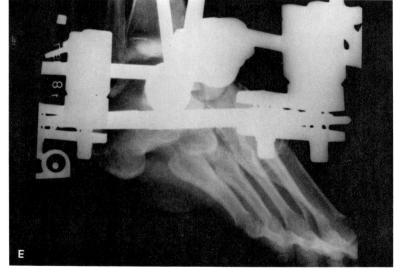

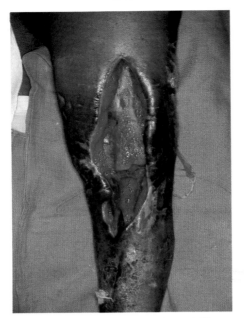

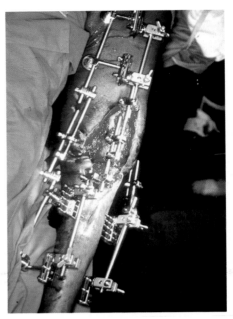

Figure 11-28. A series of photographs and X-rays, presented in Figures 11-28 to 11-31, show an infected total knee joint replacement with extensive loss of anterior skin coverage with evidence of granulation tissue that forms after the joint is stabilized with a Hoffmann device. Figure 11-28 shows the open wound after removal of a Guepar total knee joint replacement prior to definitive treatment.

Figure 11-29. The wound (seen in Fig. 11-28) is shown after granulation tissue covers the anterior defect. The extensive Hoffmann device is clearly evident. (See also Figs. 11-30 and 11-31.)

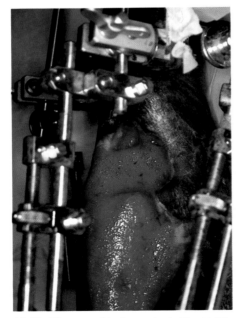

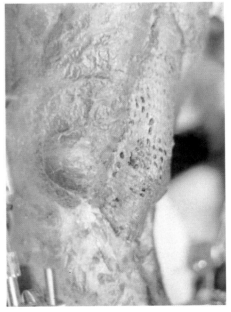

Figure 11-30. The wound is shown (as in Fig. 11-29) after granulation tissue covers the anterior defect. The extensive Hoffmann device is clearly evident. (See also Figs. 11-28 and 11-31.)

Figure 11-31. The anterior defect of the wound shown in Figure 11-28 is seen after coverage with split thickness skin graft. (See also Figs. 11-29 and 11-30.) (Figures 11-28–11-31 reproduced with permission of Dr. H. Phillips.)

quently the external fixation device remains in place for 6 to 12 months. If sequential X-rays show sites of sequestrum formation adjacent to sites of the incorporation of the bone graft further sequestrectomy is undertaken, often with simultaneous application of additional autogenous cancellous bone.

The management of open wounds accompanying infected nonunions is undertaken in the same way as was described for fresh open fractures. In brief, the denuded bone should be kept moist with periodic applications of physiological saline solution until granulation tissue covers the bone (Figs. 11-28 to 11-31). Subsequently, spontaneous epithelization may occur over the granulation tissue or, for large wounds, the application of split thickness skin grafts may be performed.

Arthrodesis by the Use of the Hoffmann Device

In Chapter 10 the role of internal fixation for arthrodesis of joints was described. For uninfected joints, and where nonosteoporotic bone is present, internal fixation is frequently the method of choice. Where an infected unstable joint is present, particularly after failed total joint replacement, the application of the Hoffmann device is frequently the preferred and, in some cases it may be the only method available to salvage the extremity. With the current popularity of total hip and knee joint replacements, the Hoffmann device provides a satisfactory method to salvage failures of both procedures. While it is generally applied with a goal of fusing the joints, it can be used as a method to stabilize the infected total hip so that a satisfactory pseudarthrosis is achieved, comparable to that described by Girdlestone[28] and Duthie and Ferguson.[29] With the application of the Hoffmann device, most of the postoperative convalescence may be continued at home as an inexpensive alternative to the prolonged course of skeletal traction necessary for a satisfactory Girdlestone procedure. At present it is unclear whether a Girdlestone procedure or a hip fusion is the optimal solution for the failed total hip. The recent observations of Hamblin[30] indicate that a pseudarthrosis of the failed total hip continues to improve in quality for at least a decade after the time of failure. Ultimately, the patient is likely to possess a pain-free, mobile and moderately stable hip. While the details of the application of the Hoffmann device to the hip joint and the knee joint are described below, the general principles are described here.

A 2-stage procedure is planned where the first stage represents removal of the implant and debridement of the joint. The joint is stabilized by the application of the Hoffmann device and the joint is distracted by a few millimeters to facilitate the subsequent addition of the bone graft. The systemic application of appropriate antibiotics is initiated and daily dressing changes on the open wound are performed. When a clean granular wound is present, the application of autogenous cancellous bone is undertaken. After removal of an infected total knee joint prosthesis, usually the residual adjacent ends of the femur and tibia consist of hollow cylinders of bone with thin osteoporotic cortices (Figs. 11-32 to 11-34). It is essential that the cavity is filled with bone graft if union of bone is to be achieved without excessive foreshortening of the limb. Figure 11-34 illustrates an example where arthrodesis of a failed Guepar total knee joint with a fulminant open infection was achieved although excessive foreshortening of the limb is clearly evident, with the proximal fibula adjacent to the distal femoral shaft.

After debridement and external fixation of an infected total hip joint, arthrodesis may be facilitated by a second procedure when autogenous bone graft is applied and a vertical osteotomy is performed through the acetabulum posterior to the sciatic notch. After the osteotomy, the segment of pelvis hinged at the symphysis can be distracted by 2 to 6 cm so that its lateral edge is depressed to the level of the femoral neck. The osteotomy prevents the marked foreshortening of the extremity that would otherwise result from fusion of the acetabulum to the proximal femoral neck. Bone graft is added between the exposed surfaces of the pelvic osteotomy and the femoral neck. The procedure is described in the subsequent subsection on the pelvis.

After the second stage of the procedures for fusion of the hip or the knee, the patient is permitted to undergo partial or full weight bearing. Usually 6 to 12 months are required before union is achieved.

Where a pseudarthrosis of the hip joint is desired, the hip joint is debrided and the Hoffmann device is applied. After 8 weeks it is removed and motion exercises of the established pseudarthrosis are initiated.

Limitations and Complications of the Hoffmann Device

The principal limitation of the Hoffmann device is its inability to satisfactorily immobilize displaced interarticular fractures or growth plate injuries where accurate reduction and internal

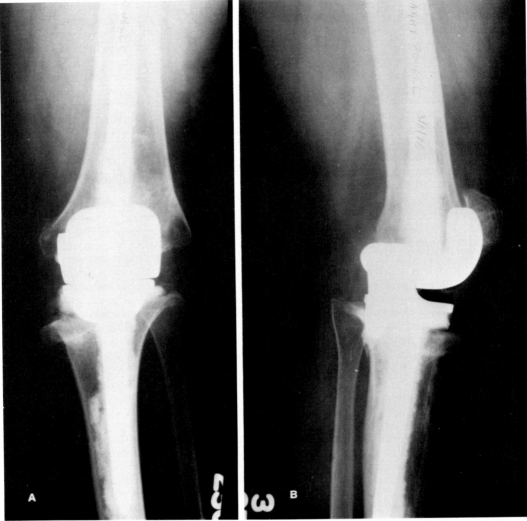

Figure 11-32. X-rays of the infected total knee joint from the patient previously shown in Figures 11-28 to 11-31. *A* and *B*. show the infected Guepar prosthesis in place. (See also Figs. 11-33 and 11-34.) (Reproduced with permission of Dr. H. Phillips.)

fixation are generally required. When displaced physeal or interarticular fractures accompany extensive open comminuted fractures of adjacent bones, external fixation may be used to stabilize the extremity and supplementary open reduction and internal fixation may be applied to the physeal or interarticular fractures. In certain cases of pathological fractures secondary to widespread disuse osteoporosis such as some cases of paraplegia or of metastatic bone disease, the osteoporotic bone may preclude satisfactory application of the Hoffmann device.

The complications of external fixation arise both during the application of the device and during its subsequent use. At the time of appli-

cation, impalement of neurovascular structures or of adjacent viscera is a considerable hazard. Also, the reader is referred to the detailed description of percutaneous pin insertion by Junkin.[31] Impalement of muscles may provoke contractures of adjacent joints. In the forearm, surgical exposure of the bone at the sites for pin insertion should be seriously considered so that the main flexor and extensor groups are avoided. When transfixing pins are inserted into the pelvis, open exposure of the bone is essential. A rigid and precise aligning jig also is necessary to carefully direct the pins during insertion.

The second group of complications associated with the use of external fixation results from

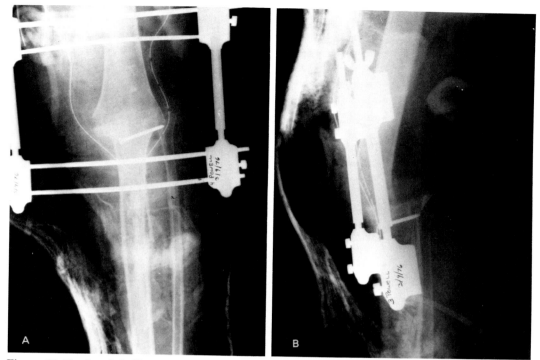

Figure 11-33. *A* and *B*. X-rays of patient seen in Figure 11-32 show a lateral view of the knee joint after removal of the implant and attempted stabilization with a Charnley external device and a cast. This procedure failed. (See also Fig. 11-34.) (Reproduced with permission of Dr. H. Phillips.)

inadequate stabilization of the fracture. The patient may experience pain or motion at the fracture site. He may experience pain, soft tissue swelling, and drainage of the pin sites secondary to instability. The instability may result from inadequate tightening of the Hoffmann device, insufficient numbers of pins, or from incorrect construction of the external frame. Drainage at a pin site may occur in the presence of stable fixation if insufficient release of a cutaneous wound is performed. This complication is prevented if large incisions at the entry and exit sites of pins are performed. Also the pin sites should be carefully examined in the first 24 hours after the application of the device. Frequently extension of the percutaneous wounds are necessary when redness, soft tissue swelling or pain are present. Drainage from pin sites also occurs when the patient undergoes exessive activity. If the patient undertakes 24 hours of bed rest with elevation of the extremity, cessation of the drainage usually follows.

Once a pin tract infection has developed with purulent drainage, often with X-ray confirmation by the presence of a radiolucent tract

around the pin, the pin must be removed. Usually the pin is loose and can be withdrawn by hand. Curettage of the pin tract is undertaken and the entry and exit sites are debrided. Insertion of additional transfixing pins may be necessary. In the presence of one or more pin tract infections, the surgeon may be tempted to prematurely remove the Hoffmann device. In the presence of an infected and unstable nonunion this temptation should be resisted. Generally it is quite unnecessary; upon removal of the device the recurrence of gross motion at the pseudarthrosis will stimulate the infection to spread. Alternatively a more rigid device should be applied to eliminate motion at the nonunion site. Admittedly, when the fracture site has begun to heal, the Hoffmann device may be removed and a plaster cast applied.

While not a complication, strictly speaking, a relative shortcoming of the Hoffmann device is the prolonged period necessary for union to occur. Frequently the addition of supplementary bone graft will shorten the anticipated healing period, especially in the presence of inadequate bone mass.

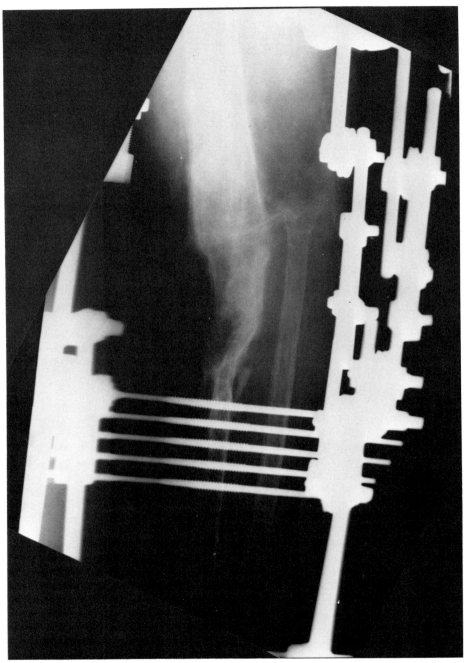

Figure 11-34. X-ray of patient seen in Figures 11-32 and 11-33 shows the knee after stabilization with Hoffmann external fixation. Without the application of cancellous bone graft, approximation of the opposing bone ends was achieved by excessive compression so that the proximal end of the fibula is visible along the lateral aspect of the distal femur. (Reproduced with permission of Dr. H. Phillips.)

Treatment of Leg Length Discrepancy by Application of External Fixation

In children the arrest of growth by epiphysiodesis and, in adults, the shortening of the longer limb have been the procedures of choice for equalizing leg length discrepancies.[32, 33] Surgical leg lengthening of the femur was first reported by Codivilla[34] in 1905. Subsequently, numerous other authors have described methods of treatment by lengthening, many of which have been condemned because of their numerous complications.[35-38] In the last decade there has been a resurgence of interest in leg lengthening, initiated by Anderson.[39] Prior to the contribution by Anderson, some workers had attempted to lengthen abruptly by performing a midshaft osteotomy with immediate distraction equivalent to 5 to 15% of the overall length of the bone followed by insertion of bone graft. Complications including irreversible nerve palsies, nonunion, dislocation of adjacent joints and dislodgement of the graft with loss of correction were not uncommon. Also the techniques of internal fixation of the graft were likely to provoke fracture of the adjacent segments of the bone. Other workers employed Steinmann pins for skeletal traction and distraction of the osteotomized bone. Such an unstable system of skeletal traction showed an unsatisfactory incidence of pin track infection, malunion and nonunion. In contrast for lengthening of the tibia, Anderson recommended fibular osteotomy with distal tibiofibular synostosis, subcutaneous division of the tibia into proximal and distal segments and daily distraction of the tibial segments by means of transfixing pins held in a screw distraction apparatus. Subsequently Kawamura et al.,[36] devised a simple, inexpensive apparatus in which four smooth Steinmann transfixing pins are inserted above and below the osteotomy site and an external frame is attached (Fig. 11-35). Osteotomy of the fibula and tibia are performed through separate incisions with minimal surgical trauma. If equinus deformity of the foot is anticipated or if it develops during the leg lengthening procedure, surgical lengthening of the Achilles' tendon is performed. In the early postoperative period daily incremental lengthening is undertaken until a total lengthening of 10% of the initial length of the tibia is achieved. When callus begins to consolidate at the osteotomy site the external frame is replaced by a plaster cast incorporating the transfixing pins. Weight bearing is limited by the use of crutches until x-rays of the osteotomy site indicate continuity of a structurally adequate amount of bone. The lengthening period is monitored by symptomatic indications from the patient such as complaint of pain, observation of the amount of active motion of adjacent joints, assays of enzymes including aldolase, creatine-phosphokinase, glutamic-oxaloacetic transaminase, measurement of action potentials of the electrical activity of the skeletal muscles and blood flow, estimated by venous occlusion plethysmography. From these and other observations on a canine model and from several hundred patients mostly with the diagnosis of old anterior poliomyelitis, Kawamura et al.[36] confirmed that leg lengthening of the tibia or femur can be performed safely if the lengthening is limited to a maximum of 10% of the initial length of the bone. The lengthening procedure can be repeated on an individual bone after an interval of 1 to 3 years. The method developed by Kawamura et al.,[36] however, lacks sufficient rigidity so that the patient is unable to be ambulatory while the lengthening is under-

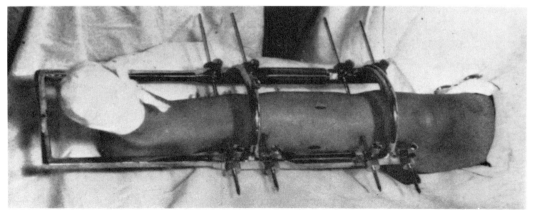

Figure 11-35. Photograph shows the application of the Kawamura device for leg lengthening of the tibia. (Reproduced with permission of Dr. B. Kawamura.)

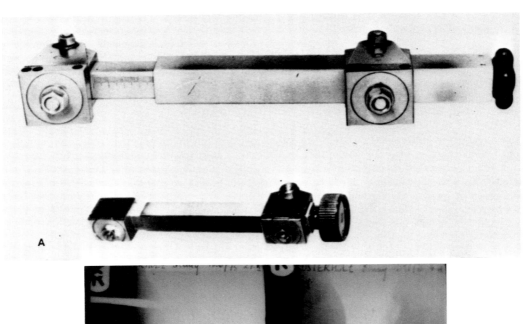

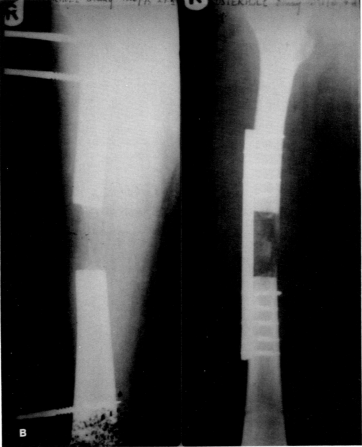

Figure 11-36. *A.* A photograph shows the larger and smaller models of Wagner apparatus for leg lengthening. *B.* The special AO plate developed by Wagner for stabilization of a bone after lengthening is shown. (Reproduced with permission of Dr. B. Rahn.)

way. Furthermore, the patient requires close supervision in a hospital for this period. The more elegant apparatus devised by Wagner[40] overcomes these liabilities.

The Wagner Apparatus

During the past decade, Wagner[40] and his colleagues have developed both a simple apparatus for leg lengthening and also an exacting clinical method for the procedure. Fastidious attention to clinical detail is essential if the numerous hazards and complications of leg lengthening are to be avoided.

The device consists of two concentric tubes, of square cross-section, one of which can be distracted with respect to the other by the rotation of a knob (Fig. 11-36A). An articulation is attached to each of the tubes. Two percutaneous pins insert into each of the articulations. With the aid of an aligning jig two pins are inserted into the proximal and distal ends of the shaft of the relevant long bone. The Wagner apparatus is attached to four or six Schanz pins or screws. The pins must be carefully aligned with respect to the axis of the knee joint. Otherwise, rotational malalignment of the bone will occur during the lengthening process. The bone is lengthened at the rate of 1.5 mm per day or 1.0 cm per week. The average femoral lengthening performed by Wagner has been 7.5 cm. During the lengthening the patient is requested to perform active flexion of the knee each day. If the flexion of the knee diminishes to less than 60° the lengthening is stopped. If the patient rapidly regains knee motion the lengthening schedule is resumed. If the knee motion does not improve further lengthening is abandoned for at least 1 to 2 years.

When the desired length of the bone is achieved, a unique AO plate with a thickened cross-section is applied to stabilize the osteotomy (Fig. 11-36B). The patient walks with the use of two canes and applies approximately 15 kg of force to the foot on the lengthened limb. Rahn and Perren[41] have recorded the rate of advancement of the mineralization front as 0.5 mm per week from each end of the osteotomy gap. Up to 22 cm of length have been achieved.

Healing of the bone is very slow over the age of 20 years, however, and prohibitively slow over the age of 40 years. The critical stages in the technique of application are now discussed.

A 3.6-mm drill is used to prepare the holes for the Schanz screws. The holes are made slightly anterior to the midaxis of the bone. The cutaneous incision is 2 cm in length for each screw.

At the proximal end of the bone the screws are inserted into the distal end of the wound. The distal screws are inserted into the proximal end of the cutaneous wound. This positioning minimizes the pressure exerted by the pin on the adjacent skin during the lengthening process. The self-tapping screws are inserted by the use of a hand chuck. The final turn of the chuck should align the screw so that its flat distal portion corresponds to the long axis of the bone. Such positioning provides maximal holding power for the screw. With the use of the drill guide, additional holes are made and the screws are inserted. The lengthening device is applied to the Schanz screws and then distracted by small amounts so that the device is stabilized.

After the device has been applied to the lateral aspect of the femur, a posterior lateral longitudinal incision is made and extended down to the lateral intermuscular septum. The vastus lateralis is released and a transverse midshaft femoral osteotomy is performed. The bone fragments should spring apart by about 3 or 4 mm. In children the periosteum is divided to minimize stretching and pain. In contrast, the periosteum is maintained intact in adults to provide maximal nutrition to the osteotomy site. A longitudinal incision in the periosteum minimizes disruption. Closed suction drainage is applied to the wound and motion of the knee is checked.

On the following day the lengthening is initiated at a rate of 1.5 mm per day. Usually 8 cm of lengthening is achieved within the first 8 weeks. If another 8 cm of lengthening were desired, an additional 12 weeks of time would be anticipated. The delay would be encountered usually because of temporary limitation of knee motion to less than 60° of active flexion. Lengthening is terminated when the desired goal has been achieved or when other clinical problems have intervened. In patients over the age of 16 years, cessation of lengthening is followed by the application of a special AO plate (Fig. 11-36B). For patients under age 16 years, provisional callus formation is visible on X-rays by about 8 weeks after full lengthening is achieved. At this time the osteotomy site is compressed by the adjustments in the device. After an additional 4-week period radiological formation of matured callus should appear.

For the application of the plate in individuals over age 16 years, the patient is placed on the operating table in a prone position. Through the previous posterolateral incision on the thigh the plate is applied to the posterior aspect of the femur. The plate is bent to correspond to the physiological bow of the femur. The plate has a special low modulus of elasticity to permit the bending maneuver. If a varus deformity of the femur is observed at the time of internal fixation, the deformity is corrected to minimize bending moments on the plate. To assist with such adjustments the Wagner apparatus is not removed until after interoperative adjustments of alignment of the bone have been made. Also, at the time of internal fixation a decision on whether to use autogenous posterior iliac crest bone graft is made. When applied the strips of graft are inserted into longitudinal slots made in the provisional callus. Also they are packed around the callus.

While the application of the plate permits early removal of the external fixation device, it is not without problems. The plate provides a considerable degree of "stress protection" to the bone with diminution in the stimulus for adequate callus formation. The callus is often atrophic, osteoporotic and of lesser diameter than that of the ends of the shaft. If at 1 year after internal fixation, inadequate callus formation is present the plate is replaced with a smaller one with a lower modulus of elasticity. Usually the smaller AO plate can be removed 1 year later. The patient is always informed that this change of the plate may be necessary. Similarly, before leg lengthening is undertaken he is informed that fatigue fracture of the plate is likely to occur. Subsequently, the origin of such potential *complications* is understood by the patient to have been *anticipated problems*.

Two groups of patients possess a particularly high risk to develop a marked flexion contracture of the knee. On patients who previously have sustained a fracture of the femur with substantial foreshortening, the scar formation associated with the fracture healing engenders their risk for flexion contracture of the knee. A similar risk is shared by patients with a congenital short femur. In the latter group the intramuscular septum and the fascia lata are released at the time of application of the Wagner apparatus. Where the patients possess a valgus knee or other congenital deformities, these problems are treated prior to lengthening of the congenital short femur.

Lengthening of the tibia has certain important differences from that of the femur. The external device is applied on the medial aspect of the tibia. At the time of osteotomy of the tibia, screws are inserted into 3.2-mm drill holes between the proximal tibia and proximal fibula and the distal tibia and distal fibula. The screws prevent subluxation of the proximal or distal tibiofibular joints. Both bones are osteotomized at the same level in the midshaft region. If the patient possesses an equinus foot, the heel cord is lengthened before tibial lengthening is initiated. Of the patients who do not have a preoperative heel cord release, 30% require subsequent open lengthening of the heel cord when active ankle motion diminishes to 20°. The external fixation device is applied and a midlateral longitudinal incision is made to expose the fibula and tibia. The deep fascia is split in a longitudinal axis to expose the fibula. Afterward, muscles attached to the interosseous membrane are released. The tibia is exposed through the same or a separate incision. A space of 11 mm is left at the osteotomy site for subsequent application of the plate. The osteotomy of the bones is performed with a reciprocating saw. Next an anterior longitudinal incision is made for release of the anterior fascia. The tibia is exposed and osteotomized. The use of two incisions provides a less hazardous exposure and wide release of the fascial compartments to prevent a compartmental syndrome.

On the following day lengthening is initiated at a rate of 1.5 mm per day. Wagner has averaged about 4.5 cm of tibial lengthening per case. A dearth of callus formation is anticipated so that application of the plate and a bone graft are generally employed. The graft consists of superficial strips of autogenous corticocancellous bone with deeper layers of cancellous strips.

Where lengthening is performed as treatment of a congenital short tibia, very tight bilateral soft tissue structures are anticipated. Usually, wide release procedures are necessary. Frequently the peroneal nerve itself must also be released.

After lengthening of a femur or a tibia Wagner usually maintains the patient in the hospital for a period of 6 weeks to 6 months. Bony consolidation generally requires 8 weeks to 8 months. Where a deformity of the lower extremity exists concurrently with a congenital short tibia the deformity is corrected prior to the lengthening procedure. Where the femur and tibia are short on the same side of the body simultaneous lengthening procedures can be undertaken. The rates of lengthening of each bone are the same as previously described for separate procedures.

In Wagner's experience the most common source of compromise of nerve function associated with lengthening is compression of the nerve, especially of the peroneal nerve. When clinical evidence of this problem arises, a release procedure of the proximal fibula is performed, often under local infiltration of a xylocaine hydrochloride local anesthetic. Similarly the sciatic nerve may be compromised by tension of the hamstrings, the posterior fascia or the iliotibial band. When it is recognized a release procedure is performed and lengthening of the bone is continued.

Wagner has applied similar lengthening techniques to the upper extremity. Such procedures should be limited to those clinicians who have considerable experience with the technique in the lower extremity. A particularly useful application is a discrepancy in the length of the radius and the ulna where the shorter bone may be lengthened. This application has an especially low risk associated with it. Wagner has, however, lengthened both bones of the forearm simultaneously by the application of two separate devices. Pronation and supination were maintained during the lengthening procedure.

Leg Lengthening by the Application of the Hoffmann Device

The author has applied the Hoffmann device to children with a congenitally short femur or short tibia and to adults with a traumatic foreshortening of the tibia or femur, with or without concomitant rotational deformities. The technique of lengthening has been similar to that previously described by Wagner, as in the last subsection. While the Hoffmann device is not as simple as the Wagner apparatus, it provides a more rigid fixation. Also, the extraordinary versatility of the Hoffmann device permits its use for all of the applications where external fixation is necessary. The use of a single device limits the necessary stock by the hospital and it enables orthopaedic residents to be trained to use one method of highly versatile external fixation.

APPLICATION OF THE HOFFMANN DEVICE IN THE LOWER EXTREMITY

Treatment of Pelvic Fractures

Fractures of the pelvis comprise a highly diverse group of skeletal injuries which are fully reviewed elsewhere.[42–44] In brief, they can be classified as minor avulsion fractures, isolated fractures of the rami, usually with minimal displacement, acetabular fractures and pelvic ring fractures. The acetabular fractures include minor fractures of the acetabular rim and central acetabular fractures. Disruption of the pelvic ring requires at least two sites of injury at the sacroiliac joint or the symphysis pubis and/or the rami, the ilium, or sacrum. Numerous combinations of these injuries have been described.

As mentioned in Chapter 10, numerically most pelvic fractures consist of avulsion injuries or undisplaced rami fractures which resolve with conservative management. The treatment of many acetabular lip fractures, with or without dislocation of the hip, requires accurate open reduction and internal fixation. Treatment of central acetabular fractures and of unstable pelvic ring fractures has remained a problem to the present time. With the very considerable impact forces necessary to provoke such injuries, adjacent soft tissues are likely to undergo disruption, especially with bleeding from the internal or external iliac arterial or venous systems. After the patient's general medical condition has stabilized, various methods of immobilization of the pelvis have been employed, including the use of a pelvic sling, skeletal traction and the application of a hip spica cast. None of these methods provides accurate or controlled reduction of the fractures. Apart from the use of the hip spica cast, the others require prolonged hospitalization, usually for about 3 months. Previously several workers, notably Judet[45] and Willenegger,* have employed internal fixation with accurate reduction of these fractures. Where gross displacement and comminution of the fractures has occurred, these methods are exceptionally difficult. Also, in view of the disruption of the iliac vessels, catastrophic intraoperative bleeding has been widely reported. In light of these hazards, most authors have discouraged the use of open reduction and internal fixation.

Several groups have favored the use of an external fixation device for certain unstable pelvic fractures. A trapezoidal compression frame has been attached to multiple pins inserted into the superior surfaces of the iliac crest. Favorable results have been described for pelvic ring fractures of minor displacement. In the author's opinion, however, the trapezoidal device lacks adequate rigidity to cope with grossly unstable pelvic ring fractures. Furthermore, the pins in the iliac crest are embedded in bone of moderate holding capacity. While this site is adequate for supplementary control in pelvic stabilization, it is wholly inadequate for stabilization of a grossly unstable pelvic ring.

In view of the limitations of previous methods of treatment the author has devised a technique whereby the Hoffmann device is used to reduce pelvic ring fractures and to rigidly stabilize them. The method has also been used satisfactorily for

---

* H. Willenegger, personal communication, 1977.

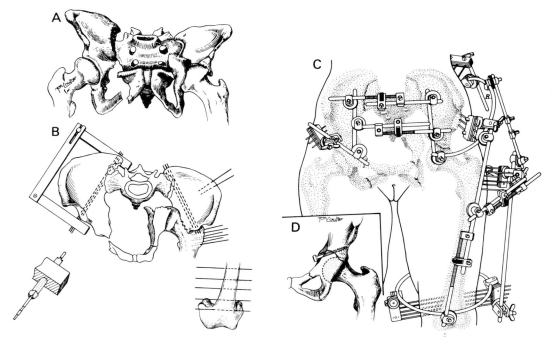

Figures 11-37. Schematic diagrams of the application of the Hoffmann device to two representative pelvic fractures on a single skeleton, a pelvic ring fracture and a central acetabular fracture. The fractures are illustrated in Figure 11-37A. In *B*, the insertion of the transfixing pins from the region of the anterior inferior iliac spine to the posterior inferior iliac spine is shown with the use of a jig to align the pins. *C* shows the external device attached to the pins. In the text the description of the construction of the device for either the treatment of a pelvic ring fracture or of a central acetabular fracture is given. Only those pertinent parts of the device would be applied for either fracture alone. *D* shows the reconstruction of the acetabulum after a central acetabular fracture by the use of cancellous lag screws.

the treatment of central acetabular fractures and for combinations of pelvic ring fractures with central acetabular fractures which are now described in turn.

Unstable Pelvic Ring Fractures

Generally the Hoffmann device is applied after the patient's cardiovascular status has been stabilized. There is one notable exception, where wide abduction injuries of the pelvic ring have occurred in which abduction of a leg beyond 100° occurs with open injuries of the perineum, either through, or adjacent to, the urogenital organs and bowel. In such injuries where fecal contamination of the perineal area and where concurrent laceration of the femoral vessels occur, the application of the Hoffmann device assists in the reduction of the fracture, the control of bleeding and in wound care. In the presence of an extensive perineal wound and especially with laceration to the large bowel or rectum, diversion colostomy should be performed as soon as possible.

For the application of a pelvic Hoffmann device the transfixing pins are inserted after direct exposure of the anterior and posterior surfaces of the ilium (Fig. 11-37). Open insertion minimizes the risk of damage to adjacent abdominal viscera or neurovascular structures. The patient is positioned on his left side for insertion of the pins through the right ilium. Subsequently he must be turned onto his right side for insertion of the pins into the left ilium. An incision is made from the region of the anterior superior iliac crest to the anterior inferior iliac crest. It is extended down to periosteum which is incised. The anterior rounded surface of the region between the superior and inferior crests is removed with a rongeur so that the pins will not slip from the optimal site of insertion. A similar approach is made to the region from the posterior superior iliac crest to the posterior inferior iliac crest. A jig is applied (see Fig. 11-37*B*) which permits accurate alignment of three parallel iliac transfixing pins. The jig possesses three series of parallel, cannulated screws which are embedded

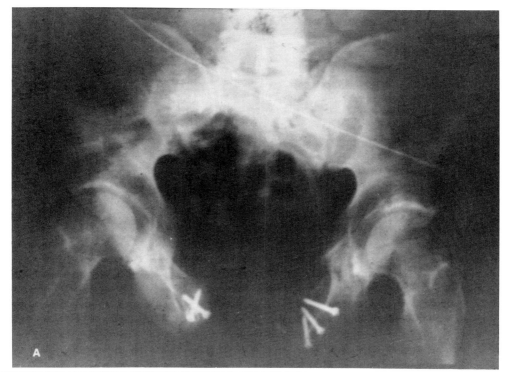

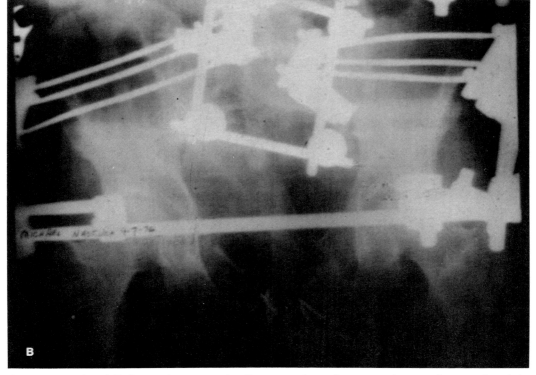

Figure 11-38. *A* and *B*. Pre- and postoperative X-rays are shown for a case of traumatic exstrophy of the bladder which was treated by the author 6 months after the initial injury when the complications, an infected nonunion of the pelvic ring with exposed bladder and symphysis, persisted.

into the surfaces of the anterior and posterior iliac crest. From the anterior approach, three 400-mm transfixing pins of 6.0 mm outside diameter with extended segments of thread are inserted. The wounds are closed loosely around the pins. The patient is turned onto his opposite side and the other ilium is transfixed with three similar pins. The patient is then placed in a supine position. The exposed ends of the pins are grasped to align the fracture fragments. Where superior migration of a hemipelvis has occurred, longitudinal traction is applied on the ipsilateral extremity to achieve a reduction. Ball joints with a series of two parallel adjustable connecting rods are attached to the exposed anterior and posterior segments of the pins respectively. Supplementary adjustments of the knurled knobs on the adjustable connecting rods permits further reduction and compression of the fractures. Pelvic inlet views are the most helpful radiological confirmation of accurate reduction of the fractures.

After surgery the patient may lie on either side without significant discomfort from the device. As soon as the patient's other soft tissue problems have healed he is permitted to sit and to walk with a partial weight-bearing gait. Six weeks after surgery the external fixation device is removed under general anesthesia. Subsequently the patient is allowed to resume full weight-bearing gait.

For wide diastasis of the symphysis pubis, often with traumatic exstrophy of the bladder, the device provides an excellent method for reduction of the fracture in view of the great mechanical advantage that the exposed ends of the transfixing pins provide for use by the surgeon. The mechanical advantage is further increased if a long tube is attached to the exposed parts of the percutaneous pins. Figure 11-38 shows the pre- and postoperative X-rays for a case of traumatic exstrophy of the bladder which was treated 6 months after a mining accident when the injury persisted as an infected nonunion with an exposed bladder. The excellent reduction of the fracture is readily visible. The reduction greatly facilitates urological reconstruction and cutaneous coverage of the bladder.

For wide abduction injuries of the pelvis with laceration of the femoral artery (Figs. 11-43 and 11-44), the application of the Hoffmann frame facilitates the vascular surgeons with their vascular repair. Also compression of the exposed fracture fragments diminishes the early post-traumatic bleeding.

Central Acetabular Fractures

For the treatment of a left central acetabular fracture the patient is placed on the operating table on his right side. Three iliac pins are inserted from the anterior to the posterior iliac crest in the same method that was described under the previous subsection (Fig. 11-39). Two additional half pins are inserted into the superior portion of the iliac crest. A hemihoop is attached to the three portions of exposed pelvic pins. Four to six half pins are inserted into the greater trochanter and three pins are inserted as a longitudinal row into the distal femur. A solid stainless steel ring is attached to the distal femoral

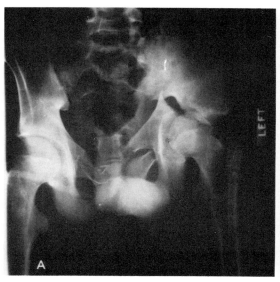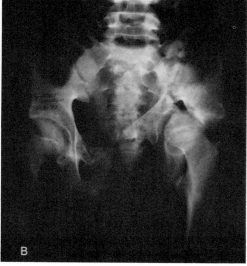

Figure 11-39. *A* and *B*. Two X-rays of a malunion of a central acetabular fracture of the pelvis.

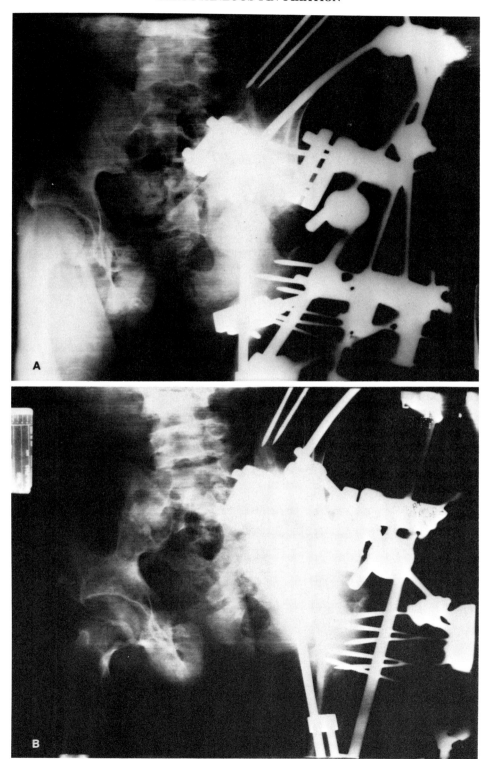

Figure 11-40. *A* and *B*. Two X-rays after open reduction and internal fixation of the acetabulum. Fixation has been achieved with 6.5-mm cancellous lag screws. The pubic fragment was osteotomized because its medial aspect had united with the ischial fragment so that the obturator artery was encased in bone.

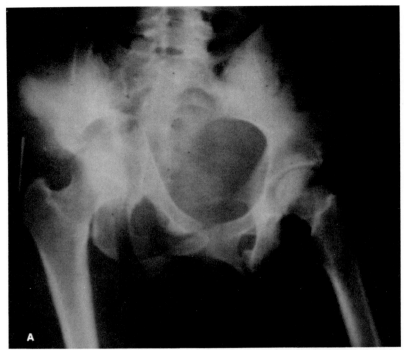

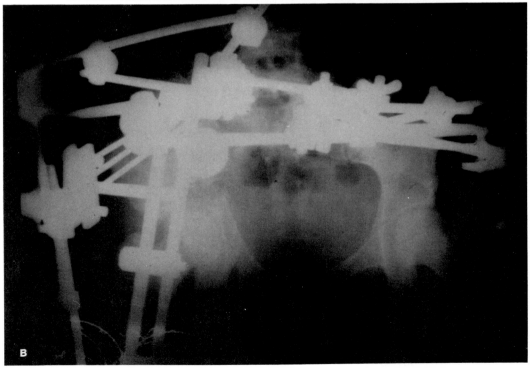

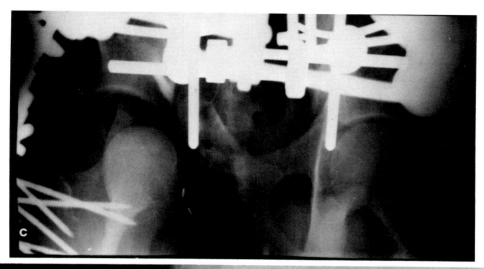

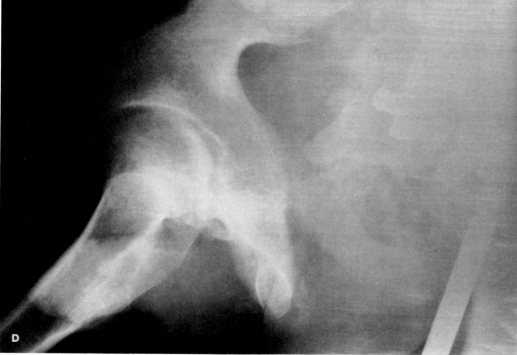

Figure 11-41. X-rays and photographs of a 35-year-old woman who fell from a 2-story window and sustained a central acetabular fracture and a pelvic ring disruption. A pelvic Hoffmann device is shown in place. *A.* Preoperative view to show disruption of the pelvic ring and the central acetabular fracture. *B.* Application of the Hoffmann device and reduction of the femoral head as well as pelvic ring. *C.* An oblique X-ray of the pelvis to show reduction of the femoral head with residual displacement of the acetabulum. *D.* Tomography of the acetabulum 6 months after the second operative procedure with open reduction internal fixation of the acetabulum was undertaken. Satisfactory alignment of the acetabulum is visible.

pins by the use of the universal ball joints or ball joint with rods. An anterior and a posterior long adjustable connecting rod connects the hemi-hoop to the distal femoral ring. Additional lateral long adjustable connecting rods connect the hemihoop to the greater trochanteric pins and the distal femoral ring (Fig. 11-40). By adjustment of the connecting rods the femoral head is distracted and moved in a lateral direction until anatomical location is achieved. Accurate radiological confirmation of the reduction is essential. Unfortunately the acetabulum remains in its displaced position. X-rays of a clinical example of a central acetabular fracture treated with external fixation device are shown in Figure 11-41.

At a second operation an anterior approach to the hip joint is made, by the use of a Smith-Petersen approach,[46] to undertake accurate reduction and internal fixation of the central acetabular fracture (Fig. 11-42). Both exposure of the articular surface of the acetabulum and the internal surface of the pelvis are necessary to achieve accurate reduction. The femoral head is used as a mold around which the acetabular fragments are positioned. The larger fragments are secured with 6.5-mm cancellous lag screws. Frequently ancillary autogenous cancellous bone graft is necessary to supplement the fixation.

After surgery the patient is permitted to sit and to walk with the use of crutches or a walker. The Hoffmann device provides such stable fixation that full weight bearing would be feasible although it is discouraged to prevent high shearing stresses on the skin around the pelvic pins. When the patient's general condition has stabilized he is discharged. From 6 to 8 weeks after surgery the patient is readmitted and the device is removed. Active range of motion exercises of the hip are initiated. The patient resumes walking but with a non-weight-bearing gait for an additional period of 4 to 6 weeks.

For treatment of a central acetabular fracture the use of the Hoffmann device has several advantages. It permits accurate anatomical reduction and fixation of the femoral head. It greatly facilitates surgical reconstruction of the acetabulum. In the postoperative period the fragile acetabular fragments are not subjected to weight-bearing forces that would be very likely to provoke substantial displacement. With the stable configuration of the external fixation device the patient is able to be discharged in the early postoperative period, as soon as he can undertake independent transfers from bed to chair and walk with aids. The pelvic Hoffmann technique has several potential complications including errors in insertion of the pins, pin tract infection and loss of correction of the fractures. The first complication is eliminated by the use of the previously described insertional technique. Loss of reduction of the fracture should not occur provided that the screws on the Hoffmann device are not permitted to loosen. Drainage from the pin tracts is not uncommon if the pins are maintained in place for more than about 8 weeks, especially if the patient is grossly obese. Daily care of the pin sites is essential.

Unstable Pelvis Ring Fractures Combined with Central Acetabular Fractures

In the presence of such grossly comminuted pelvic fractures, the author has found it very helpful to apply a Hoffmann device that embodies the features of the two separate devices described for use on pelvic ring fractures and on central acetabular fractures (Fig. 11-37). All of the pins required for the two separate fractures are inserted in the previously described manner. The external fixation device for stabilization of the pelvic ring fracture is applied and the pelvic ring is reduced on the operating table. An extension of the device from the pelvic hemihoop to a distal femoral ring is made as was described in the previous subsection. The femoral head on the side of the central acetabular fracture is reduced and the patient is transferred to a bed. On the following day X-rays are taken and serial adjustments in the position of the Hoffmann device are made until satisfactory reduction of the pelvic ring fracture and of the position of the femoral head are achieved. Subsequently open reduction and internal fixation of the central acetabular fracture are made as previously described. Afterward the patient is permitted to undertake transfers and to walk with a partial weight-bearing gait. Eight weeks after surgery the device is removed and active range of motion exercises of the involved hip are undertaken. A non-weight-bearing gait is maintained for an additional 4 weeks or until the central acetabular fracture has healed. Two clinical examples are shown in Figures 11-43 to 11-46.

The Hip Joint and the Femoral Neck

For the treatment of infected and failed total hip joint replacements and infected nonunions of the proximal femur, the Hoffmann device may provide stabilization of the relevant extremity with continuation of partial or full weight bearing for the patient. The same device is applied

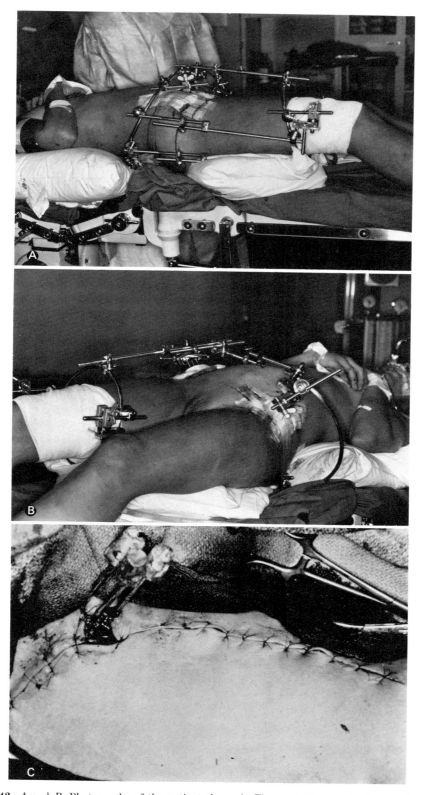

Figure 11-42. *A* and *B.* Photographs of the patient shown in Figure 11-41 *A* to *D* after application of the Hoffmann device. *C.* Line of cutaneous incision marks the approach to the hip and anterior acetabulum.

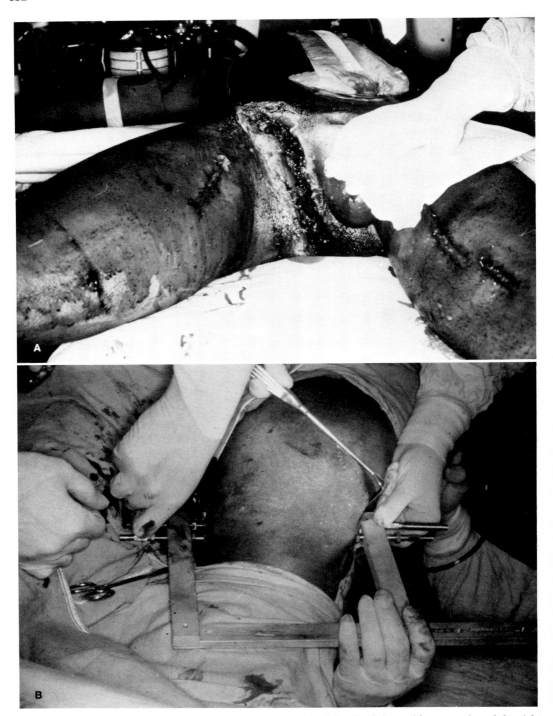

Figure 11-43. Photographs of a patient who sustained a wide abduction injury with transection of the right femoral artery, extensive peroneal wound, disruption of pelvic ring and right central acetabulum fracture. *A.* Peroneal wound is shown. *B.* Shown is the application of pelvic jig to insert transfixing pelvic pins. (See also Figs. 11-44 to 11-46.)

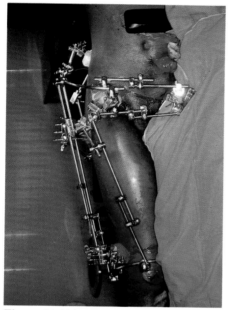

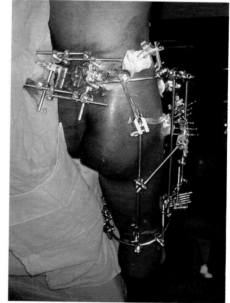

Figure 11.44A   Figure 11.44B

Figure 11-44. *A* and *B*. Postoperative views of the pelvis after application of the Hoffmann device for injury shown in Figure 11-43. The anterior view is seen in *A*. (See also Figs. 11-45 and 11-46.)

as was previously described for the treatment of central acetabular fractures (Fig. 11-37 *C* and *D*). The ipsilateral ilium is stabilized to the distal femur by the use of a hemi-iliac hoop, a solid femoral ring and multiple adjustable connecting rods. Transfixing pins are essential in both the proximal and distal osseous segments if adequate stability of the extremity is to be achieved. Supplementary half pins, inserted into the lateral iliac crest and into the greater trochanter or proximal femoral shaft greatly augment the rigidity of the device.

After failed total hip replacement the surgeon may elect to create a stable pseudarthrosis of the hip joint as Girdlestone[28] and Duthie and Ferguson[29] described or alternatively he may elect to fuse the hip joint. At the present time it is unclear which of these methods is generally preferable. From the observations of Campbell *et al.*[30] in Glasgow, it seems likely that hip fusion may provide superior early results but that the quality of the result of the pseudarthrosis may gradually improve for at least a decade after it is performed. If the surgeon elects to perform a pseudarthrosis, the hip joint is debrided and the unilateral pelvic Hoffmann device is applied as previously described for use in central acetabular fractures. Between 6 and 8 weeks after surgery the device is removed and physical therapy is initiated. If the surgeon elects to salvage an

infected total hip by a fusion procedure, a 2-stage operation is necessary. In the first stage the hip joint is debrided and packed in an open manner, or a closed, suction-drainage system is applied. At the same time the unilateral pelvic Hoffmann device is constructed. Within 1 to 2 weeks after surgery when the active cellulitis has subsided, a pelvic osteotomy with centralization of the femur and the application of bone graft is performed. At that time autogenous cancellous bone from the posterior iliac crest is first taken. Through a Smith-Petersen approach,[46] the acetabulum and the deep surface of the pelvis are exposed. An osteotomy is made through the acetabulum in the long axis of the body (Fig. 11-47). The osteotomy extends from the anterior inferior iliac crest to the sciatic notch. Afterward the medial portion of the acetabulum can be hinged at the symphysis pubis and distracted in a distal fashion so that its lateral border impinges upon the residual femoral neck. The proximal femur is centralized by appropriate adjustment in the Hoffmann device. The autogenous cancellous bone graft is placed in the vicinity of the centralized proximal femoral neck and the adjacent portion of pelvis.

After surgery the patient is maintained in the Hoffmann device preferably for 8 to 12 weeks. Afterward partial weight bearing may be necessary until the hip has fused.

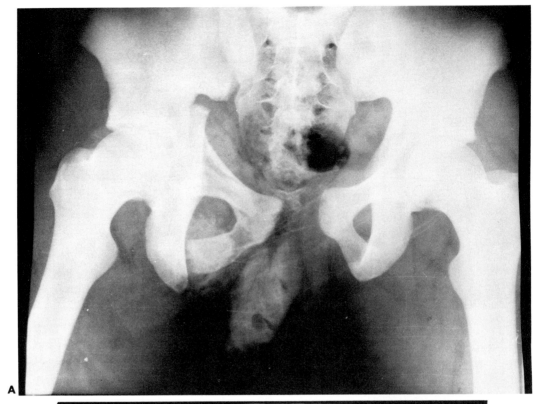

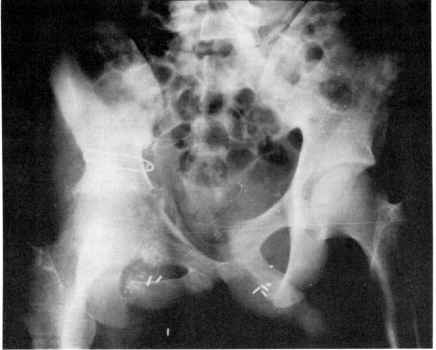

Figure 11-45. Preoperative X-rays of injury shown in Figure 11-43. *A.* X-ray prior to vascular repair of femoral artery. *B.* X-ray after vascular repair when further displacement of the right hemipelvis is evident. (See also Figs. 11-44 and 11-46.)

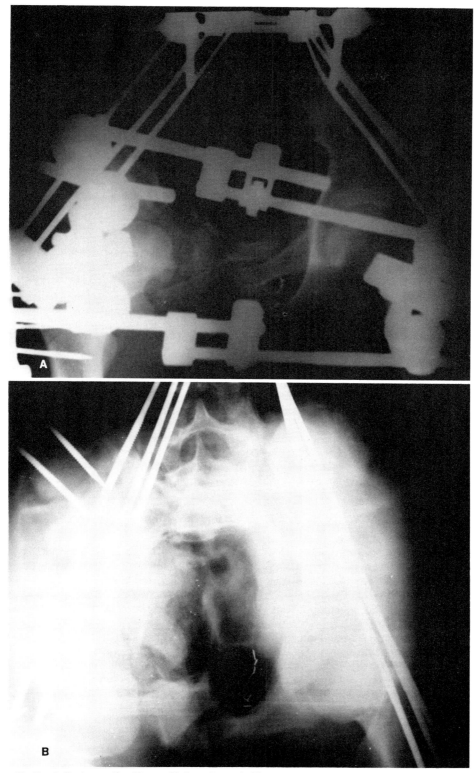

Figure 11-46. *A*. Postoperative X-ray of injury shown in Figure 11-43 after application of Hoffmann device. *B*. Oblique X-ray or pelvic inlet view to show reconstitution of pelvic ring and the position of the transfixing pins and the right half pins. (See also Figs. 11-44 and 11-45.)

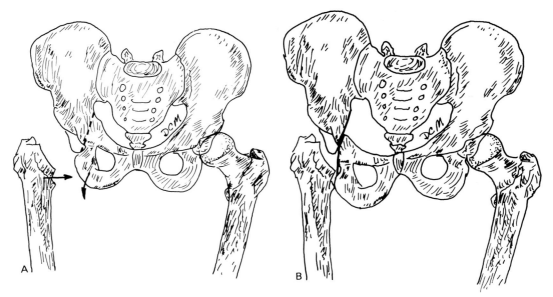

Figure 11-47. *A*. Schematic diagram to show the site for a pelvic osteotomy in an attempt to fuse a failed total hip joint replacement. *B*. The osteotomy has been displaced and the proximal femur has been centralized.

For unusual cases of infected nonunions of the femoral neck, a similar type of Hoffmann device is applied (Figs. 11-48 and 11-49). Again in many of these cases a 2-stage procedure is desirable where the first stage consists of debridement and application of the Hoffmann device and the second stage consists of the application of autogenous cancellous bone. After the application of the graft the fracture site can be compressed by adjustment of the Hoffmann device.

The Femoral Shaft

In the presence of badly contaminated, open, comminuted femoral shaft fractures the Hoffmann device may be the optimal method of treatment. It provides an alternative to skeletal traction and the application of a hip spica or internal fixation. The stable fixation may facilitate soft tissue management and eliminate the need for an internal fixation device at the site of denuded bone. Also, in cases of an infected nonunion of the femoral shaft, especially when accompanied by severe osteoporosis of the bone, the Hoffmann device may be one of the few methods of treatment available which enables the surgeon to stabilize the limb at more distant portions of normal bone with a lesser degree of osteoporosis. If a very lengthy segment of bone is of poor structural quality, the device may be extended in a proximal direction, to the ilium or in a distal direction, to the tibia. An example is shown in Figure 11-48 and 11-49. Proximal trans-

fixing pins are applied obliquely through the femur, from anterolateral to posteromedial. The distal pins are inserted parallel to the knee joint. Additional half pins may be inserted into the greater trochanter. Additional stability may be provided by the addition of short connecting rods between the adjacent adjustable connecting rods.

The optimal sites for insertion of percutaneous pins in the femur are shown in Figure 11-23.

The Knee Joint

The Hoffmann device is frequently suitable for fusion of the knee after failed total knee joint replacements as well as for other applications of arthrodesis of the knee (Figs. 11-50 and 11-51). After failed and infected total knee joint replacement, the femoral condyles and the tibial plateau are frequently markedly osteoporotic. Upon removal of the total knee joint prosthesis, a considerable gap exists between the adjacent bone ends, usually not less than 2 cm. After curettage of residual infected bone, a gap of up to 3 to 4 cm may exist. The central cancellous portion of the femoral condyles and the tibial plateau are usually absent as a result of the previous surgery and of the infection (Figs. 11-32 to 11-34). If an osseous union is to be achieved between the femur and the tibia, a column of bone must be restored across this site. The union may be achieved either by considerable fore-

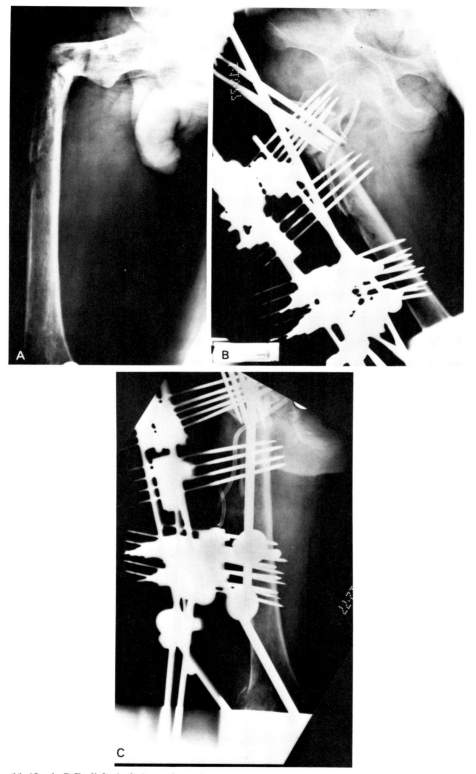

Figure 11-48. *A–C.* Radiological views of a patient before and after debridement and application of an external fixation device for an infected nonunion of the proximal femur with severe disuse osteoporosis of the entire extremity provoked a second pathological fracture of the distal femoral metaphysis. (See also Fig. 11-49.) (Reproduced with permission of Dr. W. S. Nettrour.)

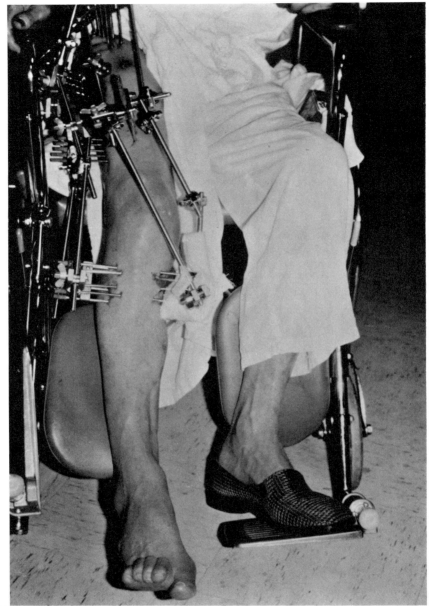

Figure 11-49. Photograph of the patient shown in Figure 11-48. (Reproduced with permission of Dr. W. S. Nettrour.)

shortening of the extremity with impaction of the adjacent bone ends or, alternatively, at a second stage the large cavity may be filled with autogenous cancellous bone. The latter method is generally preferable to minimize the otherwise anticipated extensive foreshortening of the limb.

To stabilize such an unstable site as the knee after failed total knee joint replacement, the Hoffmann device must be exceptionally rigid. Two separate sets of pins in the femur and the tibia are necessary. Optimal stability is achieved if one set of pins in the distal femur and the proximal tibia are inserted parallel to the knee joint. If the metaphyseal bone is markedly osteoporotic a second series of transfixing pins are inserted into the metaphyseal region by the use of the complementary vise for parallel anchoring (Fig. 11-10E). Universal ball joints with rods are attached to the most proximal and the most distal sets of pins. Long adjustable connecting

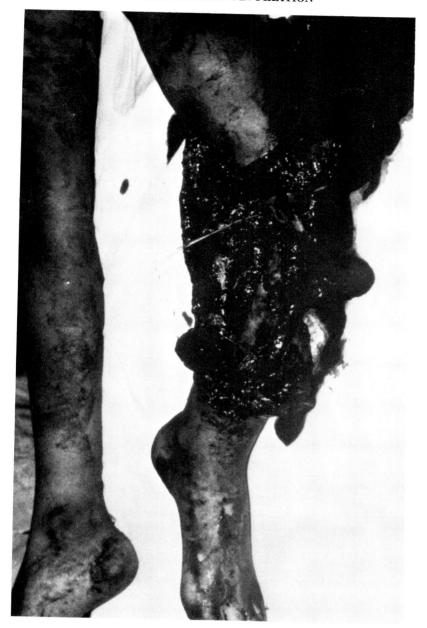

Figure 11-50. Photograph of a young motorcyclist who sustained an open traumatic dislocation of his knee joint which was debrided and treated with external fixation. (See also Fig. 11-51.) (Reproduced with permission of Dr. W. S. Nettrour.)

rods are attached between these ball joints to erect the conventional double frame. Universal ball joints are attached to the metaphyseal pins on either side of the knee joint. Short connecting rods are attached from the universal ball joints to articulation couplings mounted on the long adjustable connecting rods. The knee joint is debrided in the conventional manner and packed in open fashion. After the cellulitis has largely resolved, the application of autogenous cancellous bone graft is performed. Once the bone graft is in place the knurled knobs on the long adjustable connecting rods are manipulated to foreshorten somewhat the extremity and thereby to stabilize the graft.

In the postoperative period the patient is per-

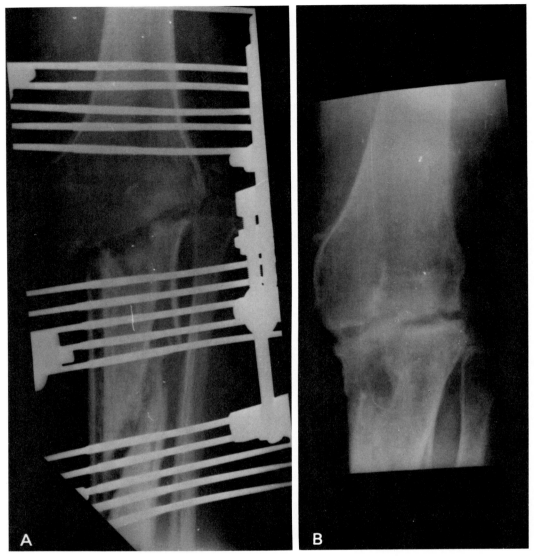

Figure 11-51. *A*. X-ray shows application of the Hoffmann device to injury sustained by the motorcyclist shown in Figure 11-50. *B*. X-ray after stable union is achieved shows spontaneous ingrowth of granulation tissue in the postoperative view. (Reproduced with permission of Dr. W. S. Nettrour.)

mitted to undertake partial or full weight-bearing gait. The fusion generally requires 4 to 8 months to unite. The period may be foreshortened somewhat if, at the time of monthly postoperative visits, secondary adjustments on the connecting rods are made to further compress the bone graft by about ¹⁄₁₀ inch per visit.

Tibial Shaft Fractures

The largest clinical experience in the use of the Hoffmann device has been accrued by its application to open tibial shaft fractures and to infected nonunions of the tibia. The method has achieved such a high level of success that some workers, such as Roy-Camille *et al.,*[18] have employed it for treatment of closed tibial shaft fractures. The advocates of such treatment for closed fractures suggest that comparable high levels of uncomplicated union are achieved. While the author has not employed the method for simple, stable tibial shaft fractures, he has used it for unstable fractures that were initially treated by the application of a cast without satisfactory maintenance of the reduction. Also,

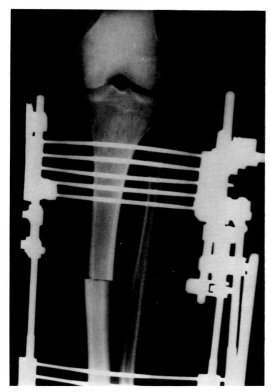

Figure 11-52. X-ray after application of the Hoffmann device of a patient who required a complex 3-planed corrective osteotomy of the tibia. Previously the patient had sustained a crush injury to his foot with a traumatic arthrodesis of his subtalar and ankle joints. The patient was referred with gross malalignment of the hind foot and the entire foot showed tenuous blood supply. After the osteotomy was made and the external fixation device was applied, the patient was permitted to walk. He made his own recommendations in the optimal position of his foot for walking and adjustments were made in the Hoffmann device to provide this position. (See also Fig. 11-53.)

he has employed it for complex osteotomies of the tibia that require 3-plane correction (Figs. 11-52 and 11-53). The treatment of metabolic bone diseases such as hypophosphatasia or vitamin D resistant rickets are two excellent indications. Multiple levels of osteotomies can be performed and the fragments can be easily stabilized. A somewhat similar indication is the treatment of fibrous dysplasia, where lengthy segments of involved bone can be curetted and grafted (Figs. 11-54 and 11-55).

As previously mentioned, the use of the Hoffmann device for the treatment of shaft fractures is a reliable method to achieve union although

the time required for such unions to transpire may be very lengthy. In an effort to enhance the rate of fracture healing, Roy-Camille et al.[18] have attempted to alter the rigidity of the device. By the use of a less rigid frame a closed and moderately stable tibial fracture, with largely intact periosteum, shows much more rapid evidence of callus formation and fracture healing than in a case where a rigid double frame is employed. In the latter case only primary healing of bone is observed. If the double frame is not absolutely stable or if the patient is exceptionally active, it seems likely that even the primary fracture healing is retarded somewhat. The potential hazard of deliberately lowering this rigidity of the frame is that motion of the pins may increase the likelihood of pin track infection. Also, where the periosteum has been severely compromised by the presence of severe

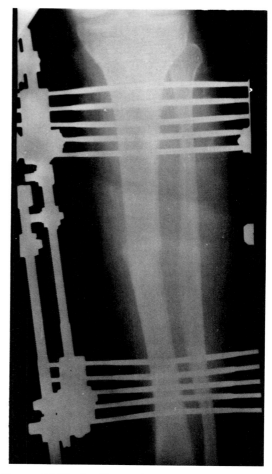

Figure 11-53. An X-ray of the patient shown in Figure 11-52 12 weeks after osteotomy.

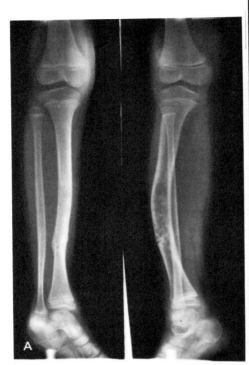
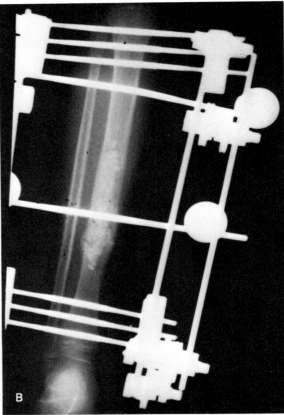

Figure 11-54. The use of the Hoffmann device for the correction of a pathological fracture secondary to fibrous dysplasia of the tibia is shown. *A* and *B* show the pre- and postoperative X-rays with subsequent bone healing. For bone graft "Bethesda bone", was kindly provided by Lt. Comdr. Gary Friedlaender, M.D., MC, USNR, Director, Tissue Bank Naval Medical Research Institute, Bethesda, Maryland. The freeze-dried allographic tissue is used in children in view of their limited resources of autogenous cancellous bone. (See also Fig. 11-55.)

open injuries with loss of soft tissue and bone substance, then the only method of fracture healing available to the body is the primary modality. In this case an absolutely rigid device becomes mandatory.

In light of the previous discussion, it is recommended that surgeons without previous experience with external fixation should initially employ the device only in those cases of open tibial fractures or of infected nonunions where its use cannot be questioned. As their experience grows they can extend the indications for its use and they can attempt to employ the device in those ways that would lead to secondary fracture healing.

Weber* and his colleagues have had considerable experience in the application of the AO external fixation device to nonunions of the tibia

* B. Weber, personal communication, 1978.

often with extensive bone loss. For comminuted fractures with extensive soft tissue injury they have employed lag screw fixation of fracture fragments after the initial external stabilization and soft tissue healing of the open wounds. The lag screws permit close approximation of adjacent fracture fragments to augment the rate of primary fracture healing. The screws prevent motion between adjacent fracture fragments so that the optimal rate of primary bone healing is observed.

For fractures with extensive bone loss, Weber and his colleagues emphasized the need for serial applications of autogenous cancellous bone. The first application of graft should span the entire length of the gap even though the diameter of the bone graft may be very small, in view of the limited amount of bone that is available (Figs. 11-56 and 11-57). Subsequently, at 6- to 12-week intervals, additional cancellous bone graft may

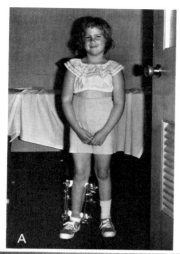

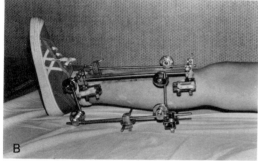

Figure 11-55. *A* and *B*. The child, seen in Figure 11-54, is shown with the external fixation device when she undertook full weight-bearing gait and participated in activities at school.

be inserted adjacent to the initial graft so that a larger column of bone accumulates at the fracture gap. While the several stages may occupy many months, nevertheless the patient is able to be out of the hospital during virtually all of the period. The method also may enable a clinician to salvage an extremity with an intact foot when otherwise amputation would be indicated.

Fractures of the Distal Tibia, Talus and Calcaneus

In the management of severe open injuries involving the distal tibia, the talus or certain calcaneal injuries as well as fracture dislocations of the ankle and subtalar joint or for the treatment of infected nonunions of these joints, the Hoffmann device provides its usual attributes of stable fixation with ready access for the treatment of soft tissue injuries. For this wide variety of fracture problems one standard Hoffmann frame is usually suitable. Figures 11-58 to 11-66 illustrate two clinical examples.

A longitudinal row of five transfixing pins are inserted into the tibia at least 1 inch proximal to a tibial fracture, if the latter is present. In the absence of a fracture of the distal tibia, the longitudinal row of pins is inserted into the distal third of the tibial shaft. One or two rows, each of at least three transfixing pins, is inserted into the os calcis parallel to the plantar surface of the foot (Fig. 11-23). The talus is not routinely employed for insertion of percutaneous pins because of its small size and because of the proximity of the posterior tibial artery. When two rows of pins are inserted into the os calcis, a universal ball joint with rod and a complementary vise for parallel anchoring are attached to each of the exposed rows of pins. The freely mobile clamp is removed from the universal ball joint and the rod portion is directed in a cephalad fashion. In this way the pins and the ancillary fixation are kept well away from the plantar surface so that the patient may walk on the sole of his foot. An articulation coupling is attached to the rod portion of the universal ball joint and a short connecting rod is inserted into the articulation coupling. A universal ball joint with rod is attached to either end of the row of pins in the tibia. Next the conventional double frame can be assembled by the use of four long adjustable connecting rods.

Where the os calcis is osteoporotic, or when its mechanical integrity is otherwise compromised, additional stability can be achieved by the use of a third row of transfixing pins inserted into the metatarsals. Then a triangular framework can be assembled with the use of adjustable connecting rods that attach the tibial pins to the os calcis, the tibial pins to the metatarsal pins and the os calcis pins to the metatarsal pins. This frame is described in the next subsection.

For severe open injuries of the distal tibia, the ankle, or subtalar joints, the open injuries are debrided, irrigated and packed in an open manner, and the external fixation device is applied. Subsequently, maximal elevation of the extremity is achieved by suspending the Hoffmann device from a system of overhead traction and suspension to achieve 90° of flexion of the hip and the knee. When the condition of the soft tissues has stabilized, consideration for bone grafting can be given. In many of these injuries either the ankle joint or the subtalar joint, or both, may not be subject to reconstructive procedures. Both the complexity of the joints' surfaces and the severe comminution of the subchondral bone may favor primary arthrodesis of one or both joints so that the optimal result for

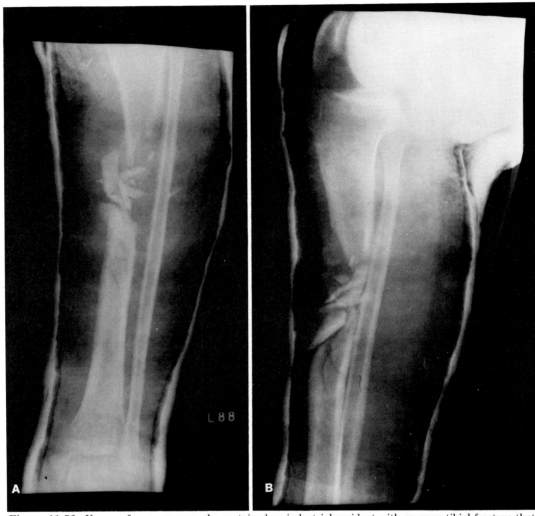

Figure 11-56. X-rays of a young man who sustained an industrial accident with an open tibial fracture that progressed to infected nonunion is shown at the time of primary debridement (*A*) and the application of an external fixation device, and a second procedure when autogenous cancellous bone graft was applied to the nonunion site (*B*). (See also Fig. 11-57.).

the patient is achieved as rapidly as possible. In such instances a second stage is undertaken in which residual articular cartilage is removed and autogenous cancellous bone is packed between the exposed subchondral surfaces. As previously described after the initial application of the Hoffmann device, the fracture site is deliberately distracted by a small amount so that the secondary grafting procedure may be accomplished with less intraoperative damage to the granulation tissue on the fracture surfaces. Postoperative immobilization for about 4 months is generally required. During this period the patient may wear a sandal in which the straps are al-

tered to fit around the external fixation device. A rocker bottom is applied to facilitate walking, in the absence of motion of the ankle and subtalar joints.

The Midfoot

While the application of the Hoffmann device to the foot is a fairly limited application, nevertheless, it can be very useful for extensive soft tissue loss with fractures of the foot, usually combined with injuries to the hindfoot or ankle joint. For isolated injuries to the midfoot region, the os calcis can be stabilized to the metatarsals

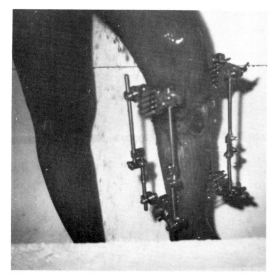

Figure 11-57. The patient, shown in Figure 11-56 is seen while taking a shower. His open wound with a clean granulating bed is visible.

by the insertion of rows of transfixing pins in both sites, parallel to the plantar surface. A single or double upright frame can be employed. For more extensive injuries, a device with triangular external frame is erected. Three distal tibial pins, one or two rows of three os calcis pins and three to five metatarsal transfixing pins are inserted (Figs. 11-61 to 11-66). Universal ball joints with rods are attached to each site of exposed pins. If a double row of pins is inserted into the os calcis a complementary vise for parallel anchoring is attached to the universal ball joint with rod on the os calcis pins. Long adjustable connecting rods are attached between the universal ball joints. The frame permits adjustment of eversion or inversion and dorsiflexion or plantar flexion of the foot, adjustment of the long and transverse arches of the foot and distraction or compression of the fracture sites. It may enable a patient to undertake partial or full weight bearing even in the presence of wholly unstable fractures. A sandal with a rocker bottom sole is prepared for use by the patient. Generally 6 to 12 weeks of immobilization is necessary for fracture healing to occur.

APPLICATION OF THE HOFFMANN DEVICE IN THE UPPER EXTREMITY

The Shoulder, The Proximal and Midshaft Humerus

In the author's experience the use of the Hoffmann device for somewhat uncommon problems

such as infected nonunions of the shoulder, or severe open injuries to the proximal humerus such as shotgun blasts, has been a useful method of treatment. As in all of its applications in the upper extremity, the insertion of the transfixing pins requires special care so that vital soft tissue organs are not impaled. The intrathoracic viscera, the numerous large vessels and nerves in the region of the shoulder joint and neck and not least of all, the main muscle groups risk impalement. Where the bone is not accessible by a subcutaneous route, consideration for open

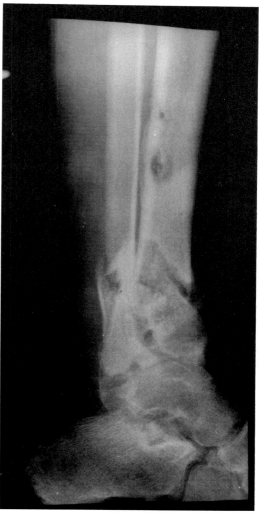

Figure 11-58. X-rays seen in Figures 11-58 to 11-60 illustrate the use of an external fixation device in a patient who had sustained an infected nonunion of a comminuted intra-articular distal tibial fracture with infective arthritis of the ankle joint. Two parallel rows of transfixing pins are visible in the os calcis. Figure 11-58 shows the preoperative X-rays.

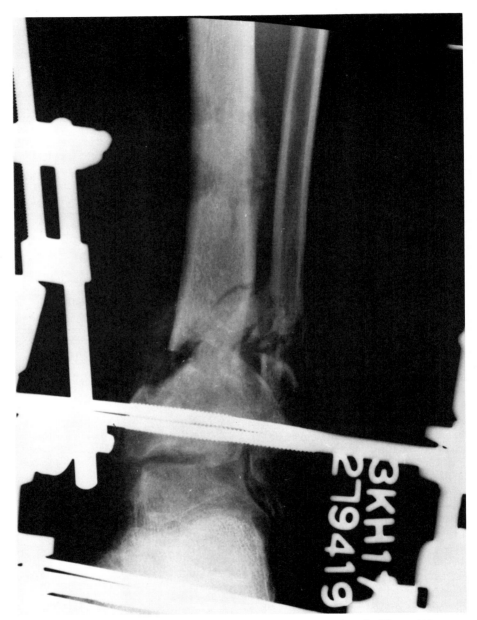

Figure 11-59. X-rays of the patient shown in Figure 11-58. (See also Fig. 11-60.)

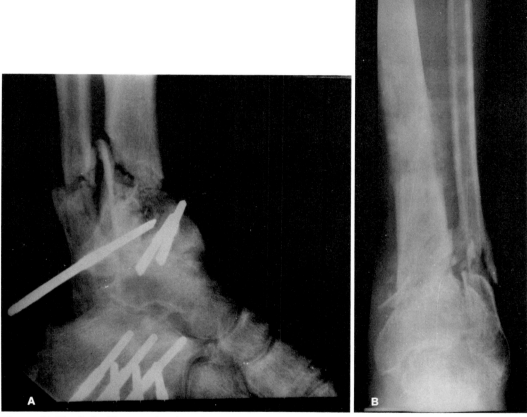

Figure 11-60. *A*. An X-ray at the time of removal of the Hoffmann device of patient shown in Figures 11-58 and 11-59. *B*. X-ray shows the healed fracture.

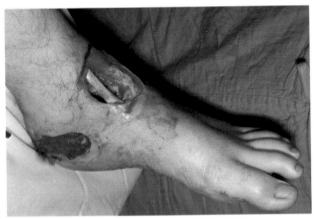

Figure 11-61. Photograph of a patient who sustained a shotgun blast through his foot is presented. The entry and exit wounds of the injury are clearly visible. (See also Figs. 11-62 to 11-66.)

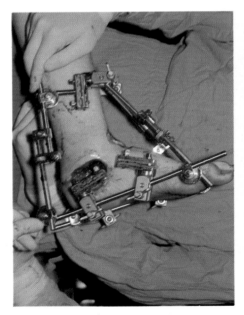

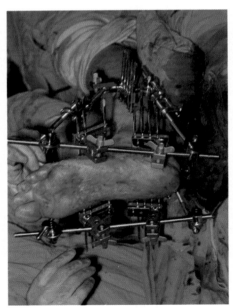

Figure 11-62. Photograph of the injury shown in Figure 11-61. (See also Figs. 11-63 to 11-66.)

Figure 11-63. Shown is the triangulation technique of external fixation of the injury seen in Figures 11-61 and 11-62. (See also Figs. 11-64 to 11-66.)

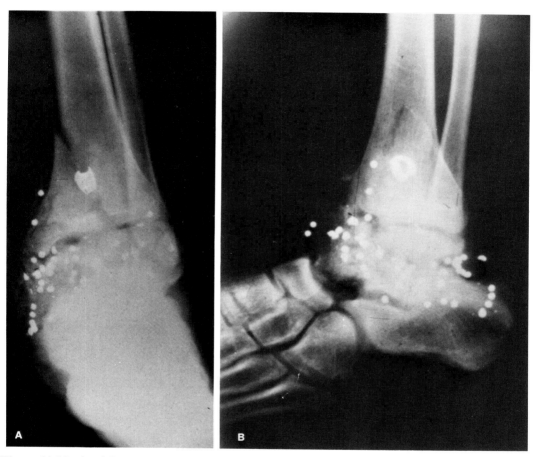

Figure 11-64. *A* and *B*. Preoperative radiological views are shown of the injury presented in Figures 11-61 and 11-62. (See also Figs. 11-63, 11-65 and 11-66.)

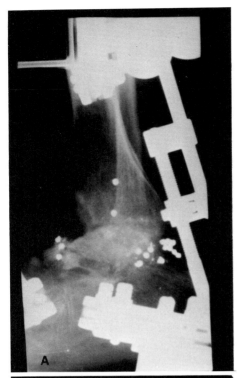

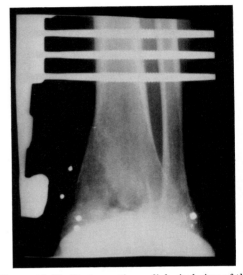

Figure 11-66. Postoperative radiological view of the injury shown in Figures 11-61 and 11-62. (See also Figs. 11-63 to 11-65.)

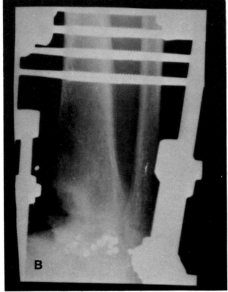

Figure 11-65. *A* and *B*. Postoperative radiological views are shown of the injury presented in Figures 11-61 and 11-62. (See also Figs. 11-63, 11-64 and 11-66.)

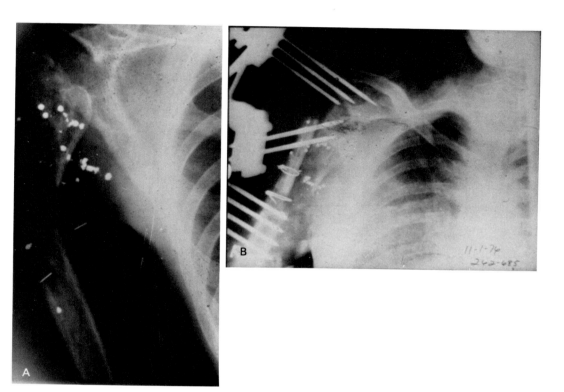

Figure 11-67. *A* and *B*. Pre- and postoperative X-rays of a patient who sustained a shotgun blast through his proximal humerus are shown. (See also Figs. 11-69 to 11-71.) (Reproduced with permission of Dr. S. Burton.)

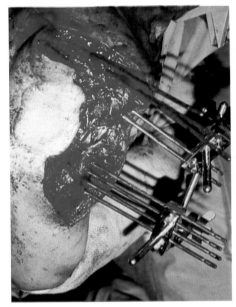

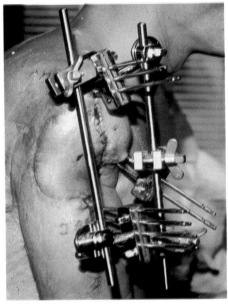

Figure 11-68. Photograph reveals the intraoperative view on the application of the Hoffmann device for the injury shown in Figure 11-67. (See also Figs. 11-69 to 11-74.)

Figure 11-69. Photograph reveals the postoperative view on the application of the Hoffmann device for the injury shown in Figure 11-67. (See also Figs. 11-68 and 11-70 to 11-71.)

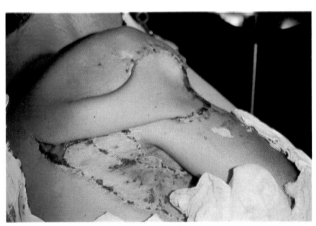

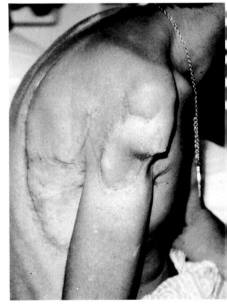

Figure 11-70. Photograph shows the application of a rotational tubular flap graft for the injury shown in Figure 11-67. (See also Figs. 11-68, 11-69, 11-71 and 11-71.)

Figure 11-71. Photograph of the wound shown in Figure 11-67 6 months later at which time cutaneous and osseus healing were completed. (See also Figs. 11-68 to 11-70.) (Figures 11-68–11-71 reproduced with permission of Dr. S. Burton.)

insertion of the pins through planes between adjacent muscle groups should be carefully considered. This becomes essential for use in the distal humerus and forearm where impalement of muscles provokes severe flexion contractures. The optimal sites for percutaneous pin insertion in the humerus have been described by Junkin[31] and are shown in Figure 11-23C and D. Fixation in the scapula is readily achieved by insertion of pins into the spine of the acromion. Transfixing pins can be inserted into the humerus both through the greater tuberosity and through the shaft of the bone. For most applications in the upper extremity a single frame is adequate. Three or four transfixing pins also provide sufficient stabilization in bone. A universal ball joint is attached to the pins so that an adjustable connecting rod can stabilize the relevant skeletal segment. Figures 11-67 to 11-71 show a typical application for immobilization of the shoulder joint and the midshaft humerus. For such shotgun blasts to the humerus and comparable open injuries with severe soft tissue damage, debridement of the wound is performed concurrently with the application of the Hoffmann device. Rotational flap grafts may be needed to provide skin coverage. Frequently an additional stage for the application of autogenous bone graft is necessary. The procedure is undertaken as previously described. In the humerus, however, moderate foreshortening of the limb is well tolerated, as an arm length discrepancy is not of such clinical significance as a leg length discrepancy. Nevertheless, certain of these injuries are accompanied by extensive loss of bone substance. In these situations the application of a large quantity of autogenous bone graft may prevent the otherwise anticipated gross foreshortening of the humerus.

The single frame device provides sufficient immobilization of the shoulder and proximal humerus so that the patient may continue most activity of the forearm and hand.

The Elbow

A single frame device can be readily employed to immobilize the elbow joint for arthrodesis in the presence of infected nonunions or severe open injuries. The insertion of three pins into the midshaft humerus and the midshaft ulna is undertaken. The single frame is applied to the lateral surface of the arm. Again it should be emphasized that the pins must be placed through subcutaneous margins of the bone, usually through open exposure of intramuscular planes. If the single frame lacks sufficient rigidity, a triangular device can be erected as was described for use in the midfoot. On exceptional cases where gross infection and osteoporosis of the distal humerus and proximal ulna are present, the pins can be inserted with the triangulation technique, including the use of a double upright frame, through the proximal and midshaft humerus and the midshaft or distal ulna.

The Midshaft Forearm and the Wrist Joint

For open fractures of the midshaft forearm with severe soft tissue compromise, the Hoffmann device can be applied to either the radius or the ulna or to both bones. Not infrequently a comminuted and/or open fracture of one bone such as the radius can be treated with the Hoffmann device while a concurrent closed fracture of the midshaft ulna can be treated with conventional internal fixation (Fig. 11-26). When the Hoffmann device is applied to one or both bones in the forearm, standard half pins are employed which penetrate but one bone (Figs. 11-72 to 11-74). For immobilization of a fractured ulna and radius, two separate Hoffmann devices are employed, one for each bone, so that pronation and supination are maintained during the period of immobilization. The use of two separate devices permits correction of alignment of each bone independent of the other. Great care must be taken during the insertion of the pins so that the flexor and extensor masses of muscle are not violated. Direct open exposure of the bone is virtually essential. After three transfixing pins have been inserted into the major proximal and distal fracture fragments, careful alignment must be performed. The rotational alignment is especially critical if pronation and supination are to be preserved. The rotational alignment can be checked by the residual amount of passive pronation and supination.

Comminuted fractures of the distal radius can be treated by the use of a single external frame that extends from the proximal or midshaft radius to transfixing pins inserted in the metacarpals (Fig. 11-72). Two or three transfixing pins are inserted into either site. Prior to attachment of the external frame, preservation of pronation and supination must be ascertained. The wrist joint is immobilized with about 10 to 15° of dorsiflexion. Such a frame is sufficiently rigid so that the patient can continue to use his hand both for active exercises and for light activities. In the presence of neuromuscular injury whereby the extensors or flexors of the hand are impaired, dynamic splints can be attached to the

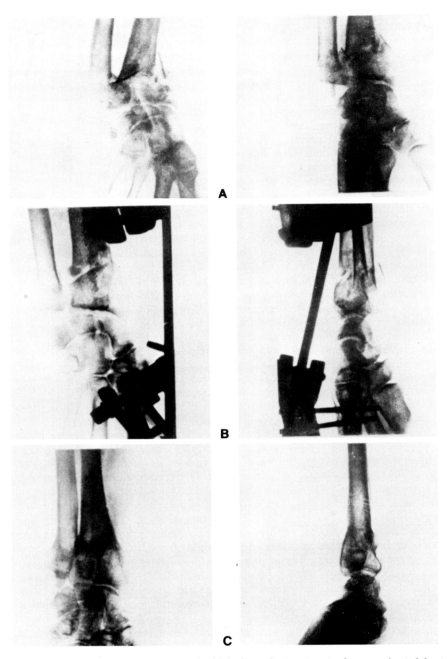

Figure 11-72. A series of X-rays are presented which show the treatment of a comminuted fracture of the distal radius and ulna by the application of a single frame external fixation device (*B*). Excellent correction of the fracture deformity has been achieved (*C*).

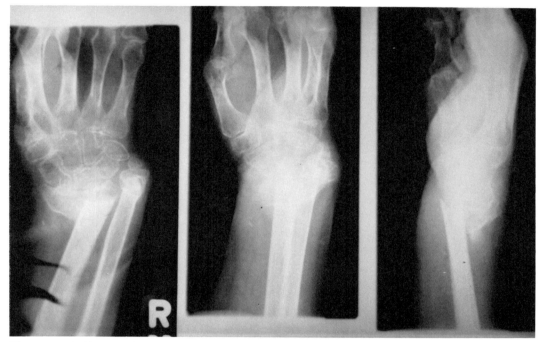

Figure 11-73. Preoperative X-rays of a severely open comminuted fracture of the distal radius treated with a single external frame. (See also Fig. 11-74.)

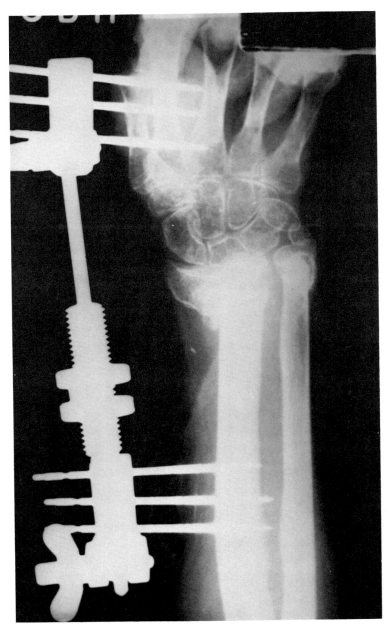

Figure 11-74. Postoperative X-ray of fracture shown in Figure 11-73.

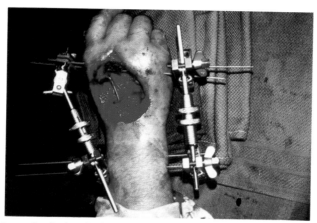

Figure 11-75. A photograph of a hand after treatment of multiple open metacarpal fractures by the use of external fixation is presented. The device consists of several 3-mm transfixing pins and two continuous compression rods all of which are smaller than the usual Hoffman device.

Hoffmann device which support the relevant digits.

For guillotine-type amputations of the upper extremity, at the level of the wrist joint or distal forearm, a single external frame can be employed as a rapid method for skeletal stabilization, prior to the vascular reanastomosis. A double frame is specifically contraindicated, at least prior to the vascular reanastomosis, as it occludes access for the operating microscope and microsurgical reconstruction of the vessels. In cases of more distal amputation, through the metacarpals or phalanges, endoskeletal stabilization with Kirschner wires is preferred as the most rapid method and one which does not block access to the extremity for vascular anastomosis.

Hoffmann External Minifixation for the Hand

Previously, for open fractures of the hand, where the author felt that external fixation was indicated, he applied 3-mm transfixing pins with two continuous compression rods (Fig. 11-75). This combination provided somewhat smaller instrumentation than the conventional Hoffmann apparatus. It also was useful for pediatric applications.

Recently a novel system of miniaturized external fixation has been introduced which consists of a series of external fixation devices for use on the hand, and in addition, for use on infants, and in maxillofacial surgery. The devices consist of a series of small but highly versatile frames which could be employed for a great variety of hand injuries. Usually 2-mm half pins are inserted into each major fracture fragment.

Single or double clamps are available to attach to the pins (Fig. 11-76). With the considerable variety of the available frames a wide variety of open injuries to the hand and the fingers should be amenable to their use, although the author has had limited experience in their application.

CONCLUSIONS

The development of sophisticated, stable and highly versatile systems for external fixation of fractures has greatly extended the ability of orthopaedic surgeons to salvage severely comminuted open fractures, infected nonunions and infected unstable joints. Of the numerous available devices, the Hoffmann device appears to be the most versatile and stable and the one which permits complex realignment of an extremity after the apparatus has been applied. For leg lengthening, the Wagner device is an elegant system which is cosmetically superior to the Hoffmann device. Other workers, however, have also achieved impressive results with the use of the AO system, the Kawamura leg lengthening instrumentation and others. It should be emphasized that external fixation is not perceived as the ultimate method in the stabilization of fractures but one additional modality of treatment which supplements skeletal traction, plaster casts and internal fixation and which is particularly valuable for those fractures which have severe soft tissue injuries. In many cases, such as in multiple trauma and in fractures of the forearm an external fixation device may be employed concurrently with a method of internal fixation such as a self-compression plate. For the treatment of open, comminuted interarticular

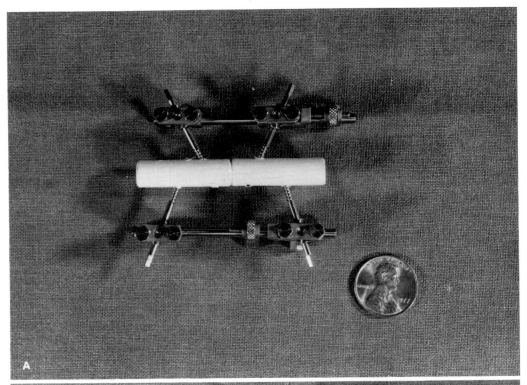

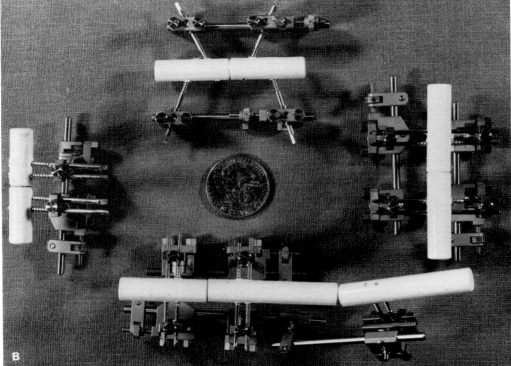

Figure 11-76. *A.* A photograph of one variant of the mini-Hoffman device is seen. *B.* Several types of mini-Hoffmann device are shown, also next to a quarter as a comparison for size.

fractures such as central acetabular fractures, both cancellous bone screws and a Hoffmann device may be used together to great advantage.

The liabilities of an external fixation device include the hazards of percutaneous pin insertion, pin track infection, and the slow rate of healing of bone which is generally encountered. An adequate explanation for the retardation of fracture healing observed in many cases of use of the Hoffmann device is not yet available. The relative roles of primary and secondary fracture healing associated with the use of external fixation have been described. For closed tibial fractures with largely intact periosteum, some workers have lowered the rigidity of the external frame, hopefully to encourage callus formation and more rapid healing. Alternatively, other workers, such as Weber, have provided supplementary lag screw fixation of tibial fractures that are immobilized with the Hoffmann device. The lag screw enhances the rigidity of the fracture site and decreases the fracture gap so that the demands on primary bone healing are minimized. Further work is clearly necessary to establish useful clinical methods for enhancing the rate of fracture healing when an external fixation device is used.

REFERENCES

1. Lambotte, A. L'intervention Operatoire dans les Fracteurs, p. 3, Lamartin, Brussels, 1907.
2. Müller, M. E., Allgöwer, M., and Willenegger, H. Manual of Internal Fixation, p. 170, Springer-Verlag, New York, 1970.
3. Anderson, R. Surg. Gyne. and Obst., 58:639, 1934.
4. Stader, O. N. Am. Vet., 18:37, 1937.
5. Haynes, H. H. A. Med. J., 32:720, 1939.
6. Charnley, J. Compression Arthrodeses, p. 7, E. & S. Livingstone, Edinburgh, 1953.
7. Tachdjian, M. O. Pediatric Orthopaedics, W. B. Saunders Co., Philadelphia, 1972.
8. Carabalona, P., Rabischong, P., Bonnel, F., Perruchan, E., and Peguret, F. Montpellier Chirurg., 19:61, 1973.
9. Slatis, P., and Karaharju, E. O. Injury, 7:53, 1974.
10. Connes, H. Hoffmann's Double Frame External Anchorage, p. 69, Gead, Paris, 1973.
11. Ilisarov, L. Results of Clinical Tests and Experience Obtained from the Clinical Use of the Set of Ilisarov Compression-Distraction Apparatus, p. 3, Med export., Moscow, 1976.
12. D'Aubigne, R. M., and Dubousset, J. J. Bone Jt. Surg., 53A:420, 1971.
13. Hoffmann, R. In Congres Francais de Chirurgie, p. 601, 1938.
14. Hoffmann, R. Acta Chir. Scand., 107:72, 1954.
15. Vidal, J. Montpellier Chirurg., 14:451, 1968.
16. Vidal, J., Rabischong, P., Bonnel, F., and Adrey, J. Montpellier Chirurg., 16:52, 1970.
17. Adrey, J. Le Fixateur Externe d'Hoffmann Couple' en Cadre, p. 11, Gead, Paris, 1970.
18. Roy-Camille, R., Reignier, B., Saillant, G., and Berteaux, D. Rev. Chirurg. Ortho., 62:347, 1976.
19. Fowles, J. In Press, 1978.
20. Karlström, G., and Olerud, S. J. Bone Jt. Surg., 57A:915, 1975.
21. O'Brien, B. M. Microvascular Reconstructive Surgery, p. 23, J. & A. Churchill, Edinburgh, 1976.
22. Taylor, G. I. Ortho. Clin. N. Am., 8:425, 1977.
23. Jorgensen, T. E. Acta Orthop. Scand., 43:264, 1972.
24. Rahn, B. A., Gallinaro, P., Baltensperger, A., and Perren, S. M. J. Bone Jt. Surg., 53A:783, 1971.
25. DuToit, G. T. Hoffmann's "Exoskeleton" for Fractures, Osteotomies and Arthrodesis, p. 2, Report No. 7: 76/77, Cripples Research Association of South Africa, Johannesburg, 1977.
26. Rittmann, W. W., and Perren, S. M. Cortical Bone Healing after Internal Fixation and Infection, p. 58, Springer-Verlag, Berlin, 1974.
27. Meyer, S., Weiland, A. J., and Willenegger, H. J. Bone Jt. Surg., 57A:836, 1975.
28. Girdlestone, G. R. J. Bone Jt. Surg., 6:519, 1924.
29. Duthie, R. B., and Ferguson, A. B., Jr. Mercer's Orthopaedics, p. 723, Williams & Wililkins Co., Baltimore, 1973.
30. Campbell, A., Fitzgerald B., Fisher. W. D. and Hamblem, D. L. S. Bone Jt. Surg. 60B:441, 1978.
31. Junkin, H. D. The Topography of Pins, Precision Pinning of Fractures, p. 2, American Fracture Association, Bloomington, Ill., 1971.
32. Tachdjian, M. O. Pediatric Orthopaedics, p. 1469, W. B. Saunders, Philadelphia, 1972.
33. Duthie, R. B. and Ferguson, A. B., Jr. Mercer's Orthopaedics, p. 344, Williams & Wilkins Co., Baltimore, 1973.
34. Codivilla, A. Am. J. Ortho. Surg., 2:353, 1905.
35. Compere, E. L. J. Bone Jt. Surg., 18:692, 1936.
36. Kawamura, B., Hosono, S., Takahashi, T., Yano, T., Kobayashi, Y., Shibata, N., and Shinoda, Y. J. Bone and Jt. Surg., 50A:851, 1968.
37. Bosworth, D. M. Surg. Gyne. and Obstet., 66:912, 1938.
38. Abbott, L. C., and Saunders, J. B. Ann. Surg., 110: 961, 1939.
39. Anderson, W. V. J. Bone Jt. Surg., 34B:150, 1952.
40. Wagner, H. Surgical lengthening or shortening of the femur and tibia. In Progress in Orthopaedic Surgery, Vol. 1, p. 7, edited by N. Gschwend et al., Springer-Verlag, New York, 1977.
41. Rahn, B. A., and Perren, S. M. Experientia, 26:519, 1970; Stain Technol., 46:125, 1971.
42. Kane, W. J. Fractures of the pelvis. In Fractures, p. 905, edited by C. A. Rockwood and D. P. Green, J. B. Lippincott Co., Philadelphia, 1975.
43. Hoaglund, F. T., and Duthie, R. B. Fracture and joint injuries, In Principles of Surgery, p. 1791, edited by S. I. Schwartz, McGraw-Hill Book Co., New York, 1969.
44. Watson-Jones, R. Fractures and Joint Injuries, p. 934, Williams & Wilkins Co., Baltimore, 1960.
45. Judet, R. Act. Chir. Ortho. L'Hospital Raymond-Poincaré, p. 25, Masson, Paris, 1964.
46. Crenshaw, A. H., editor. Campbell's Operative Orthopaedics, p. 90, C. V. Mosby, St. Louis, 1971.

12

Instrumentation in Spinal Surgery

Michael F. Schafer

The human spine tends to grow and to maintain the head and shoulders in a central position above the pelvis in both the frontal and sagittal planes. Both muscular activity and the sense of balance hold the spine in an erect position. Some degree of lumbar lordosis or dorsal kyphosis, however, is normal. As a result of congenital malformations, trauma, neuromuscular, inflammatory, metabolic and other diseases, deformity of the spine may transpire. Scoliosis, a lateral and rotatory deviation of the spine, is usually of idiopathic origin and is considerably more common than kyphotic or lordotic deformities. For a comprehensive description of spinal deformities the reader is referred elsewhere.[9, 80]

In the past two decades, tremendous progress has occurred in the methods of treatment for children with spinal deformity. External braces have been developed for use by certain children with mild scoliotic or kyphotic deformities which encourage subsequent normal growth of the spine. In many children with more severe spinal deformities, surgical correction of the deformity and fusion of the spine is necessary to prevent further progression of the deformity. In the present chapter the anatomy of the spine and the pathogenesis of the abnormal spine are discussed. Then the methods of correction of spinal deformity are reviewed. Subsequently the techniques of posterior and anterior spinal instrumentation and fusion are presented.

ANATOMY

The spinal column is composed of vertebrae, joints, ligaments, intervertebral discs and muscles. The basic components of the vertebrae include the body which bears most of the weight and is separated from an adjacent body by an intervertebral disc. The vertebral arch is composed of two pedicles attached to the vertebral body. These pedicles are united dorsally by paired laminae that have a spinous process projecting posteriorly from the union of the two

laminae. Near the junction of the laminae and pedicles are the transverse processes (Fig. 12-1A).

Each vertebra has two paired articular processes that form the articulations between the vertebral arches. The superior articular process is directed posteriorly to some extent, and the inferior articular process is directed somewhat anteriorly. These joints are surrounded by a thin, loose capsule that permits the necessary sliding motion between the adjacent processes (Fig. 12-1 A and B).

The ligaments which unite the vertebral bodies are the anterior and posterior longitudinal ligaments (Fig. 12-2 A and B. The anterior longitudinal ligament is strong and resists hyperextension of the spine. This ligament has a firm attachment to the ends of the vertebral bodies and a loose attachment in the middle. The posterior longitudinal ligament is attached primarily to the ends of the vertebrae and to the intervertebral disc. In both the thoracic and lumbar regions, the ligament is a narrow band over the middle part of the body with expansions laterally over the intervertebral discs.

The ligamentum flavum is a paired ligament that passes between the laminae of adjacent vertebral bodies from the second cervical vertebra to the lumbosacral joint (Fig. 12-2 A and B). The attachment is from the ventral surface of the upper laminae to the superior ventral portion of the lower laminae. The ligamentum flavum has a high elastic content which permits a wide range of interlaminar movement.

The supraspinous ligaments and intraspinous ligaments are attached to the spinous processes. These ligaments are well developed in the lumbar area, and help prevent hyperflexion of the spine (Fig. 12-2B).

The intervertebral disc consists of two main components—the nucleus pulposus and the annulus fibrosis. The nucleus is composed of a combination of water, collagen and mucopoly-

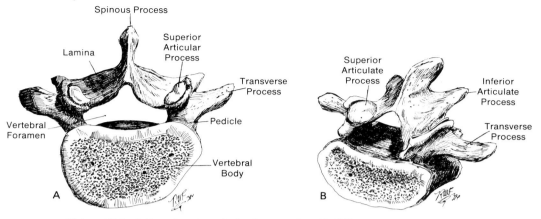

Figure 12-1. *A.* Superior view of a lumbar vertebra. *B.* Oblique view of a lumbar vertebra.

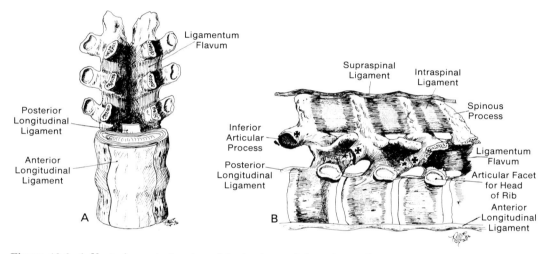

Figure 12-2. *A.* Ventral or anterior view of the lumbar and thoracic vertebrae. *B.* Lateral view of the lumbar and thoracic vertebrae: ⊣⊢ Inferior articular process; ★ a superior articular process.

saccharides. The principal mucopolysaccharides are chondroitin 4-sulfate, chondroitin 6-sulfate, and keratin sulfate. These are attached to a core of noncollagenous protein.[9] The annulus is composed of collagen fibers arranged in an X pattern. This enhances the strength of the annulus and provides for elasticity of the disc.

The muscles of the spine are more complex than the limb muscles.[40] The spinal muscles have mulitple origins and insertions, and the fiber bundles from any one origin diverge to several insertions. Each insertion is composed of fiber bundles converging from several origins.[40]

SCOLIOSIS

Scoliosis is a complex deformity of the spinal column that is characterized by lateral bend of the spinal column as well as rotation of the column on its longitudinal axis (Fig. 12-3). This causes alterations to occur in the vertebrae, joints, ligaments, intervertebral discs and muscles of the spinal column.

Pathology

For comprehension of the difficulties associated with the surgical correction of scoliosis, the structural changes in the spinal column have to be appreciated. As curvature of the spine progresses, the vertebral bodies in the major curve rotate so that the spinous processes rotate toward the concavity of the curve. With the rotation, the ribs on the convex side of the curve move posteriorly, and the ribs on the concave side move anteriorly. With the anterior rotation

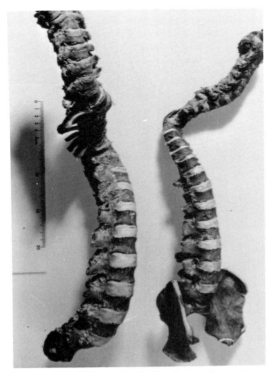

Figure 12-3. Dissected spinal column of a patient with scoliosis. This specimen demonstrates both the lateral spinal curvature and the rotation of the spine on its longitudinal axis. (Courtesy of G. M. Bedbrook, Perth, Western Australia.)

of the ribs on the concave side, the chest wall shows an anterior prominence.

With progression of the curvature, the convex surfaces of the laminae thicken and become widely separated while their concave surfaces decrease in breadth and approximate each other. The concave pedicles become shorter and stubbier. With these changes the neural canal becomes distorted.[41] In severe cases, the spinal cord may be angulated and stretched; but it is unusual for there to be any interference with the neural function, unless a diastematomyelia is present. In diastematomyelia, the spinal cord is usually split into two columns by a mass fixed anteriorly to the vertebral body and posteriorly to the dura. This mass can be osseous, cartilaginous, or a fibrous septum partially or completely dividing the neural canal.[9]

Adjacent soft tissues undergo changes with the progression of the spinal deformity. On the concave side of the curvature, the muscles and ligaments thicken and contract, while on the convex side they stretch and atrophy. In severe cases, ligamentous calcification may ensue, so

that adjacent arches and intervertebral articulations undergo spontaneous fusion.[41]

The compressive and distractive forces on the scoliotic spine provoke alteration of the intervertebral disc. On the concave side, the disc is compressed with a diminution of the vertical height. On the convex side, the intervertebral space appears widened because of the diminution on the concave side.

During the growth period, the vertebral shape is altered as a result of asymmetrical influences on the spine. The growth rate will be slower in the areas of excess pressure and will increase on the contralateral side.[6] Therefore, the vertebral body height will be decreased on the concave side and higher on the convex side.

Deformity of the thoracic spinal column provokes changes in the thoracic viscera. With an increasing curvature, the distance from the apex to the base of the lung on the concave side will become shorter. Both Makley et al.[51] and Bjure et al.[3] found that the lung volume and maximum voluntary ventilation are reduced in proportion to the degree of spinal angulation.

Riseborough and Shannon[71] report that in curves greater than 65° there is not only a decrease in the total lung capacity and vital capacity, but also an increase gradient between the alveolar oxygen content and the arterial oxygen content. This is defined as a shunt; that is, blood is being passed through the lung without being oxygenated. These factors are responsible for an arterial hypoxemia in curves greater than 65°. Bergofsky et al.[2] postulate that this eventually causes an increase in the pulmonary artery pressure which causes right heart failure.

Development of Techniques for Correction of Scoliosis

In 1911, Hibbs[37] described a posterior spinal fusion for the treatment of tuberculosis. In 1924, he described the use of this posterior arthrodesis for the treatment of scoliosis.[38] In 1948, Cobb[13] estimated that surgery is required in approximately 5% of patients with scoliosis secondary to poliomyelitis, and in most patients with scoliosis secondary to neurofibromatosis.

In 1945, Blount and Moe[6] and Schmidt[75, 80] developed the Milwaukee brace as a means of preventing the scoliotic deformity from increasing following surgery. The brace consists of a pelvic girdle which is molded to the lateral abdominal musculature above the iliac crest, the gluteal area below the crest, and the anterior abdomen. This is essential because the brace cannot be effective without a firm base. There

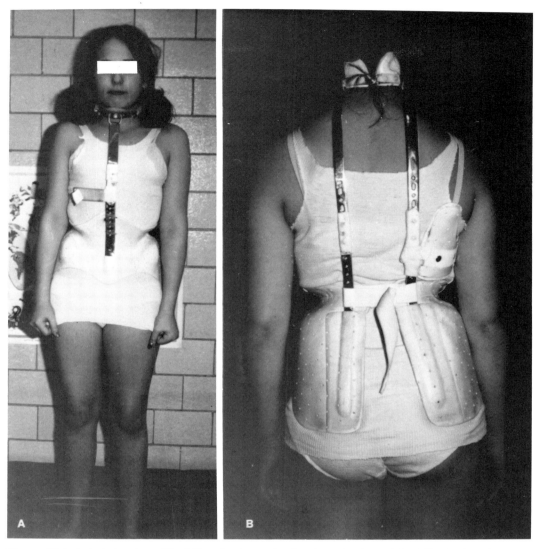

Figure 12-4. *A.* Anterior view of the Milwaukee brace showing the orthoplast pelvic girdle that is molded over the iliac crest and anterior abdominal wall. The anterior upright connects the pelvic girdle to the neck ring that contains the throat mold. *B.* Posterior view of the Milwaukee brace showing the two occipital pads, the right thoracic pad and the pelvic girdle which is molded over the iliac crest and the gluteal area below the crest.

are one anterior and two posterior uprights connecting the pelvic girdle to the neck ring and throat mold. Depending upon the type of curve, either thoracic or lumbar pads can be added to the posterior uprights. The neck ring consists of paired occipital pads in the throat mold (Fig. 12–4).

When the Milwaukee brace is worn, the spinal curvature is improved by a combination of distraction and a 3-point holding force. The 3-point force includes the pelvic girdle, neck pad and thoracic pad. For the moderate curves, the 3-point holding force of the pads is more efficient than distraction. However, as the magnitude of the curve increases, more distraction is desirable.[6]

The Milwaukee brace is an effective means for the nonoperative treatment of spinal curves of less than 40°. However, Blount and Moe[6] found that the mean total brace wearing time was 34.4 months. Therefore, in order to obtain the best results with the Milwaukee brace, the attending physician must depend upon rapport that he develops with the patient and family.

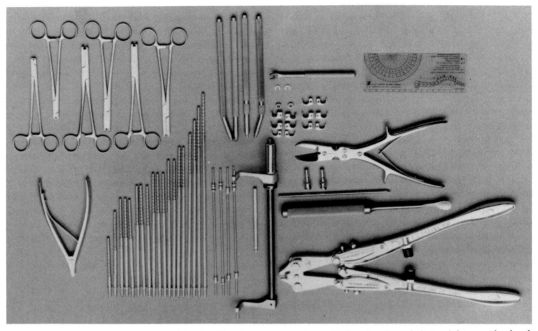

Figure 12-5. Instrumentation used in the Harrington procedure. At the *top* from left to right are the hook holders, hook drivers and flat wrench to turn the hex nuts on the compression rods. Immediately below the flat wrench are the C clamps to prevent the rod from slipping on the hook. Below the C clamps are the hex nuts of the compression assembly and the various Harrington hooks. In the *bottom row* are the Harrington spreader, various sized Harrington rods, the compression rod assembly and the outrigger distraction unit. Other equipment included in the picture on the *far right* from top to bottom include the Harrington goniometer, bone cutting forceps, sacral bar eyelet, sacral bar, Cobb periosteal elevator and double action pin cutter. (Photograph courtesy of Zimmer, U.S.A., Warsaw, Ind.)

During the past 30 years, there has been an evolution of the operative techniques in the treatment of scoliosis. Risser,[72] Risser and Norquist,[73] Cobb,[13–15] Blount et al.,[7, 8] Moe[53] and Goldstein[28, 29] have reported on the various casting and operative methods for obtaining and maintaining a correction of spinal deformity in scoliosis without instrumentation. Despite their efforts, there was a high incidence of pseudarthrosis or nonunion and loss of correction.

The epidemics of poliomyelitis in the late 1940s and the early 1950s produced numerous patients with paralytic spinal deformities. Their spinal deformities were frequently associated with cardiopulmonary compromise. The usual methods of casting and spinal fusion were hazardous for such patients. In the 1950s, Harrington attempted unsuccessfully to prevent progression of spinal deformity by internal fixation of the spine with the application of screws for immobilization of the facetal joint. Next, he attempted to develop a distraction and compression system using hooks and rods. Initially, he felt that this system would provide a means for dynamic stabilization of the spine without the need for an arthrodesis. Frequently, the rods underwent metal fatigue with failure, or the hooks disengaged. Thus, in addition to using internal fixation, he began to fuse the spine posteriorly.[32]

The instrumentation developed by Harrington must stabilize the spine for a minimum of 9 months before adequate fusion of the operative site will have transpired. The distraction rod is designed to withstand at least 3.5 million undulations of force, with up to 75 pounds of stress per undulation, before breaking. During normal activity, the human being will exert undulating forces in the instrumented spine between 7,000 and 10,000 times a day. Therefore, the instruments can survive as a distracting force for 12 to 18 months.[33]

In addition to the inherent strength needed in the instrumentation, material used in manufacturing the rods must be tolerated by the body tissues without corroding. This is accomplished by making the hooks and rods from 316 L stainless steel produced by consumable electrode vacuum melting. The hooks and rods are fabricated from this material which is cold-worked to a hardness of approximately 35 on the Rockwell C scale. This level of hardness will give a tensile strength from 130,000 to 140,000 psi.[34]

Instrumentation

The Harrington instrumentation (Fig. 12-5) consists of a distraction rod which is available in one of several sizes, is circular and ratcheted on one end to receive a hook. The hooks are designed to meet four basic requirements: (1) the design must accommodate the multicontoured posterior elements of the spine; (2) the area of contact of the hook with the spine must be amenable to varying amounts of force; (3) the hooks must have a common uniform aperture to allow the introduction of a common purpose adjustable rod and yet allow that rod to be as close as possible to the hook so as to reduce the undesirable mechanics that can be set up by movements of the force upon an eccentrically loaded system; and (4) the hooks must center themselves in an optimal mechanical position on the common rod, so that the ill effects of eccentric loading can be minimized. In this way, the correcting and holding qualities of the system will vary with changes in external forces.[34]

In order to meet all of these requirements, seven types of hooks are available. The hooks vary from blunt to sharp edged, depending upon the type of bone fixation that is desired. The hooks also vary in size to enable them to be placed either in the area of the small thoracic facetal joint and pedicle or in the upper lumbar laminae. In addition, an alar sacral hook is available for fusion that extends to the sacrum. This enables the sacral rod to be eliminated.

The compression rod, which is 3.2 mm or 4.8 in diameter, is threaded and contains hexagonal nuts to hold the hooks in place. This apparatus is applied on the convex side of the curve.

The outrigger distraction unit enables a distraction force to be applied prior to the insertion of the rod. The spreader enables a correcting force to be applied to the hooks of the distraction rod. Other equipment includes a hook clamp and driver.

Biomechanics

The actual force which may be applied to the spine is limited not so much by the strength of the device as by the strength of the bone into which the hooks are placed. When the distraction hooks are properly placed, a distraction force of greater than 300 pounds (136 kilograms) can be applied.[34] However, with the possibility of dislocation of the upper hooks, Waugh[85] and Nachemson and Elfstrom[57, 58] recommend that the force of distraction should not exceed 35 to 40 kiloponds. Nachemson and Elfstrom[58] also found that the flexible curve could be corrected between 55 and 70% when this force was used. In contrast to the considerable correction of flexible curves with the application of modest force, Schultz and Hirsch[77] showed that even immense forces would not provide much additional correction of a rigid curve. With simulation of spinal curvature in a computer, Schultz and Hirsch[77] observed that as the distraction increases, the distraction force would rise sharply with relatively less curve correction. Therefore, there is usually little advantage to increasing the distracting force above 35 to 40 kiloponds, because the additional correction could be relatively small and the risk of hook dislocation high. Although some bone absorption at the fixation site of the distracting hook has to be expected in spinal instrumentation, it is desirable to minimize the amount as much as possible. When the compression system is used, there is a decrease in the amount of bone absorption at the distraction purchase site[33] and a decreased likelihood of the hook cutting out. In support of this finding, Harrington performed a series of cases without the compression system. His average correction in this group was 51% while with the combined distraction and compression system his correction was 64%.[34]

TRACTION

In 1959, Perry and Nickel[68] described the use of the halo in the treatment of paralysis of the muscles of the cervical spine secondary to poliomyelitis. The halo was a modification of a device developed by Bloom for facial maxillary traction.[67] Since 1959, the halo has been used for the treatment of unstable cervical spines secondary to paralysis, trauma, rheumatoid arthritis or extensive laminectomies.

Winter et al.[87] reported on the use of the halo and bilateral femoral or tibial Steinmann pins for the preoperative correction of curvatures of the spine (Fig. 12-6). They stated that this technique provided better correction of the curve than could be obtained by plaster cast techniques or bracing. Pelvic obliquity could be controlled by the application of more weight on the lower extremity of the high side of the pelvis.

De Wald and Ray[18] developed a pelvic hoop which could be attached to the halo by four uprights that contain turnbuckles. The hoop was

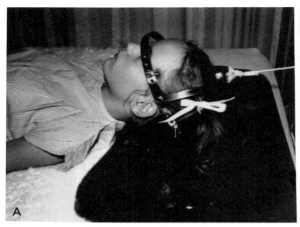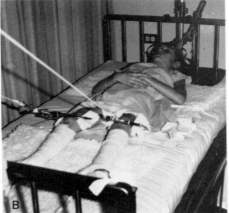

Figure 12-6. *A*. The halo is positioned so that it fits below the maximum diameter of the skull. *B*. This patient has bilateral Steinmann pins placed in the femur and bilateral traction bows for the attachment of the weights. Weight is also applied through the halo.

fixed to the pelvis by two threaded rods. With the halo hoop apparatus, longitudinal traction could be applied while the patient remained ambulatory (Fig. 12-7). In addition, it enabled both anterior and posterior surgical procedures to be performed without removing the apparatus.

Halo and Pelvic Apparatus

Application. The halo and the pins are sterilized. Although the pins are threaded, the end is smooth. This enables a sharp pin tip to catch in the outer surface of the skull. The threaded end of the pin fits into a halo channel which is also threaded. Therefore, the pin acts as an expanding wedge between the halo and the skull. Displacement is prevented by the simultaneous tightening of the diagonally opposite pin.

The halo is positioned on the head, so that it is below the maximum diameter of the skull. This will prevent progressive peripheral migration that can result from bone erosion. In order to ensure that the halo is below the maximum skull diameter, the anterior pins are centered in the groove at the upper margin of the eyebrows. The posterior pins should be positioned so that the halo is about ⅛ inch to ¼ inch above the ear. In addition, there should be more space posteriorly than anteriorly in order to allow for the edema that can develop in nonambulatory patients who are in the supine position more than the prone position.

After the pins have been tightened by finger pressure, a torque screwdriver is used to apply the final pressure. The maximum tension that should be used is 5 to 6 inch pounds.[67] After the

desired tension is obtained, the pins are locked by a nut that is placed tightly against the outside of the halo. This prevents an inadvertent skull penetration if a screw becomes loose.

After the halo has been applied, the pins should be cleansed each day with an antiseptic solution, such as hydrogen perioxide or Betadine. The pins should not be continually tightened, because necrosis of the outer table of the skull can occur. The only indications for tightening the pins are drainage or inflammation around a pin. If the inflammatory process continues despite tightening, the pins should be replaced.

The pelvic pins are positioned according to the technique of O'Brien.[62, 65, 66] In order to obtain precise pin placement, a drilling jig has been designed that is similar to the one developed by Cass and Dwyer.[10] The jig is applied so that the pins will enter just lateral to the anterior superior iliac spine and emerge at the posterior superior spine. A hand drill is used instead of a power drill to insert the pins in order to prevent necrosis of the bone which could lead to infection. In addition to daily cleansing with Betadine or hydrogen peroxide, a topical antibiotic is applied around the pins.

Biomechanics. The development of the halo-pelvic apparatus and halofemoral traction has been a useful adjunct in the treatment of spinal deformities. With both of these methods, greater longitudinal traction forces can be applied than with either braces or plaster techniques. The greatest difficulty with these methods is to determine the maximum amount of correction that can be obtained. The amount of correction that

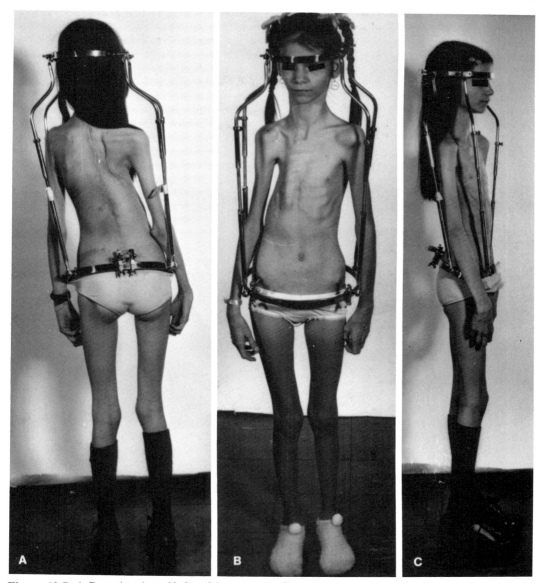

Figure 12-7. *A*. Posterior view of halo pelvic apparatus. *B*. Anterior view of halo pelvic apparatus. *C*. Lateral view of halo pelvic apparatus. (*A, B* and *C*, courtesy of William J. Kane.)

is obtained, and the load that is applied, depends upon the following factors: deformity, shape, length and level of the deformity, the stiffness or rigidity of the curve, the body weight of the patient, the etiology of the deformity, and the biomechanical properties of bone, intervertebral disc, ligaments, nerves and other soft tissues.[12]

Although the ligamentum flavum, annulus fibrosis and bone are known to be viscoelastic, the reaction of the spine as a whole to correction is impossible to predict. In addition, it is important to understand the relationship of stretching on nerve fibers to the development of neuropraxia. OBrien[65] states that a slow stretching of the nerve will give a greater increase in length without a disturbance of function.

Clark *et al.*[12] have shown, through the use of a compression spring in each of the vertical uprights, that the halopelvic distraction procedure can be divided into three phases: First, the initial short period required to overcome gravity in the form of the superincumbant body weight above the deformity; second, a creep phase where the load increase is comparatively small and most of the correction is obtained; and third, a nonlinear portion with the load rising quickly to maximum value without further correction of the deformity. They state that the maximum tolerated load is usually accompanied by neck pain and there is no further clinical or roentgenographic improvement.

Letts et al.[47] analyzed their results to determine the length of time that preoperative halofemoral traction was required. They found that the majority of the correction occurred within 7 days of the application of skeletal traction and little further correction was obtained by either increasing the amount of weight or by continuing traction for a longer period of time. If the traction was continued for longer than 3 weeks, the vertebrae became osteoporotic and were much less suitable for Harrington instrumentation due to weakening of the vertebral laminae.

Indications. The main use of either halofemoral or halopelvic traction is in older patients with curves that exceed 80° and are rigid. Other indications include patients with congenital curves, curves from neurofibromatosis and cervical thoracic curves. Since greater force can be applied for longer periods of time with halopelvic traction, it is mainly indicated in cases with severe rigid curves that need a longer period of preoperative traction.

Complications. The complications with the use of halopelvic traction include those involving either the halo or pelvic pins and neurological complications. The halo must be rigidly fixed to the skull to prevent loosening and potential pin track infection. This is usually accomplished by initially tightening the pins to 5 to 6 inch pounds of pressure with the torque screwdriver. At the end of 1 week, the pins are checked and tightened again to this pressure. If drainage occurs from the pin site, a culture should be taken for gram stain and for sensitivity. If this is positive, the skull pins should be replaced. If the culture is negative, local wound care should be given and the pins tightened. It is important that this approach be used whenever there is drainage, because there has been a reported case of a brain abscess following the use of the halo which eventually required a craniotomy and drainage of the abscess.[84]

Ransford and Manning[69] reported a case in which three pins penetrated the inner table of the skull despite the use of the torque screwdriver. The penetration was diagnosed by the failure of tightening of the pins after minimal screwing. The penetration was confirmed by a tangential roentgenogram of the skull.

O'Brien[62] studied the amount of force that was required to dislodge a halo from cadaver skulls. He found that a force equal to or greater than the body weight was required before the halo pins cut through the bone and slipped off. However, a large force can be applied to the halo pins during distraction, and any loosening of the pins would enable the halo to become dislodged.

As a result of the distraction, O'Brien et al.[65] reported that 50% of their patients showed some degenerative changes in the cervical spine. These changes usually occurred in the posterior joints and were more likely to occur in older patients with rigid spinal deformities. These patients were frequently treated for long periods of time and had higher corrective forces used. When force measurements of the spine were performed during distraction, it seemed that the critical level was 60% of the body weight.[62]

Tredwell and O'Brien[82] reported a 13.9% incidence of avascular necrosis of the proximal end of the dens in patients undergoing halopelvic traction. Roentgenographically, this was manifested by cystic areas in the dens, sclerosis and irregularity of contour. Force measurements were available in 10 of 14 patients with avascular necrosis of the dens, and the average distraction force was 78.1% of the body weight, as compared to 64.9% of the body weight in patients without avascular necrosis.

Schatzker et al.[74] reported that there are two major sources of blood supply to the dens. The central artery enters the dens anteriorly and goes to the center of the body of the dens. The second major source of the blood supply enters through the apical, alar and accessory ligaments. Tredwell and OBrien[82] feel that these ligaments are either stretched or ruptured with the resultant decrease in blood supply to the dens leading to avascular necrosis. At the present time, the clinical significance of this avascular necrosis is unknown.

The atlanto-occipital and atlanto-axial joints are the most mobile in the skeleton due to the absence of an intervertebral disc between the vertebral bodies. O'Brien et al.[65] noted an atlanto-axial subluxation in three patients after treatment with halopelvic traction. This subluxation was not present 6 months after cessation of traction. Therefore, lateral cervical spine films should be obtained during distraction with halopelvic traction.

Ransford and Manning[69] reported two cases of paraplegia secondary to halopelvic distraction. Although O'Brien et al.[65] do not report any paraplegia, they do report that three patients had episodes of temporary spasticity and lower limb weakness during the course of their treatment. Although the exact etiology of the paraplegia is unknown, it is felt that it may result because of damage to the anterior spinal artery. When distraction forces are applied slowly over a long period of time, the nerve trunks can be stretched well beyond their normal range of elasticity without disturbance of function. When the trunks are distracted rapidly, the elastic limits of the nerve are rapidly exceeded and lesions in the nerves occur.[65] Therefore, to minimize the risk of paraplegia, the distraction should be carried out slowly.

O'Brien[62] has reported temporary cranial nerve palsies in patients undergoing halopelvic distraction. Nerves most frequently injured are the 6th, 10th and 12th. These nerves run a vertical or obliquely vertical course which makes them more susceptible to injury during distraction.

Although it is possible to perforate the bowel with the insertion of the pelvic pins, O'Brien[62] states that he knows of only four instances of damage to either the peritoneum or bowel with pelvic pin insertion. When the patient has abdominal pain, elevated temperature and a rising pulse rate, the possibility of bowel damage should be considered. If it is felt that a perforation has occurred, the pelvic pins should be left in place and a laparotomy performed. If a perforation of the small intestine, cecum or sigmoid colon has occurred, it should be overlapped and sewn and the surrounding area drained. If there is an extensive injury to either the cecum or sigmoid colon, a right or left hemicolectomy should be performed.

The incidence of perforation of the bowel is higher in cases of pelvic obliquity. Therefore, an initial period of halofemoral traction may be indicated prior to the insertion of the pelvic pins. This distraction would tend to level the pelvis and facilitate the insertion of the pelvic pins.[62]

Loosening of the pelvic pins is common due to the constant reciprocal action of the pins against the cancellous bone. In addition, there is a resorption osteoporosis that occurs around the pelvic pins with resulting resorption of the bone trabeculae.[62] Ransford and Manning[69] reported that in nine patients, one pin hole required attention for a chronic discharge and one developed a small abscess. However, all of them had healed by 3 months, and there was no evidence of long term osteomyelitis.

Cotrel Traction

In 1971, Cotrel[17] discussed the use of the E.D.F. technique for the preoperative management of spinal deformities. This method combines three corrective forces: elongation, derotation and lateral flexion of the spine toward the convexity of the curve. There are two stages involved in this technique. The first stage consists of continuous spinal traction to stretch the trunk and make the curve supple. The second stage consists of a plaster cast that is made to correct the thoracic asymmetry, strengthen the trunk musculature and reduce the scoliotic rib hump.

The traction is composed of a head halter which has an occipital piece and a chin strap. This is attached by standard spreader bar to a rope that drops over one pulley. Weights of between 5 and 8 pounds are attached to the rope (Fig. 12-8A). It is essential that a 45° angle of pull between the horizontal plane and the rope be maintained, so that the pull is on the occiput instead of the chin.[44]

The second part of the traction is the counterbalancing force (Fig. 12-8B). This consists of two separate systems of straps for each side of the pelvis. The pelvic portion consists of a triangular shaped trochanteric pad that is placed directly over the greater trochanter. Each pad has an attached buckle and two straps. One strap goes under the patient's back, around the iliac crest to the contralateral side and crosses anteriorly over the abdomen to fasten onto the buckle on the trochanteric pad. The straps, which are encased by foam over the area where they rest above the iliac crest and anterior-superior iliac spine, cross anteriorly above the symphysis and posteriorly over the sacrum. The second strap passes distally and fastens around the foot of the bed. This strap, plus elevation of the foot of the bed 10 cm provides the counter traction.[44]

The third component is dynamic because the patient elongates the spine against resistance (Fig. 12-8C). This is accomplished by extending the hips and knees down on two foot plates. These foot plates are connected to the occipital chin strap by an intermediary pulley. This permits the patient to stretch the spine while lying supine.

The actual place of the Cotrel traction in scoliosis is debatable at present. Rigid curves are best treated by halofemoral or halopelvic traction while more flexible curves of lesser magnitude may be treated by Cotrel traction. Nachemson and Nordwall[59] studied a group of patients that were treated with Cotrel traction followed by Harrington instrumentation, and compared them with a similar group treated by Harrington instrumentation alone. He concluded that there was no advantage to using preoperative Cotrel traction.

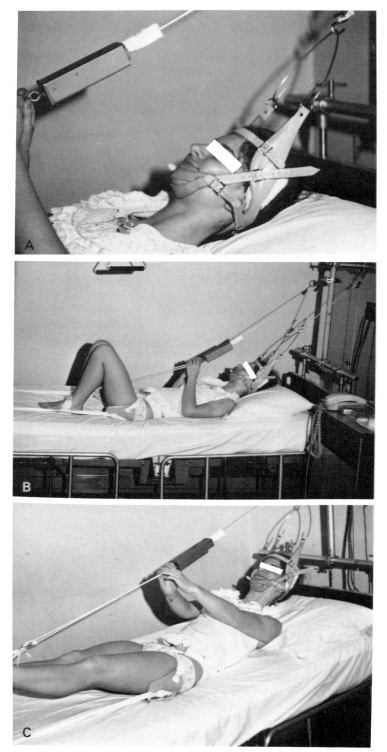

Figure 12-8. *A.* The head halter, which contains a chin strap and occipital portion, is attached to a spreader bar. Weights between 5 and 8 pounds are attached to the head halter. *B.* The counter-balancing system consists of the trochanteric pad and associated straps. *C.* The dynamic portion of the Cotrel traction consists of the patient extending the hips and knees against foot straps that are connected to the chin piece by an intermediary pulley.

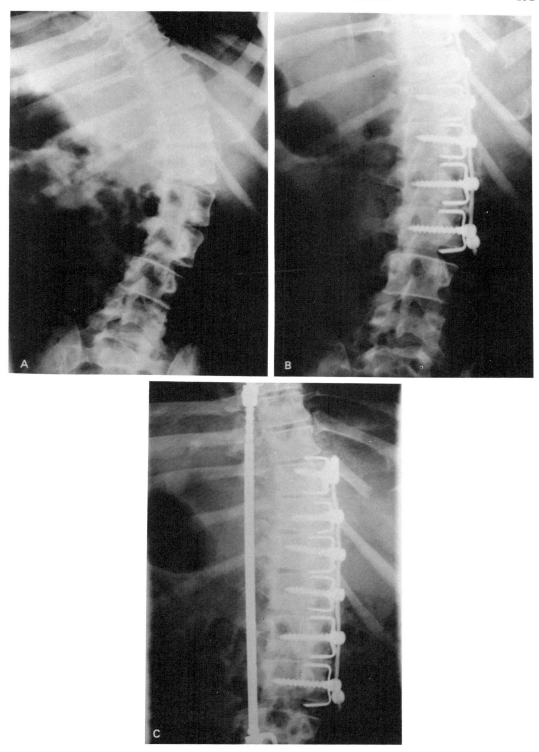

Figure 12-9. *A.* Long paralytic C curve caused by poliomyelitis. *B.* Dwyer fusion has been performed from T10–L3. *C.* Two weeks after the Dwyer fusion, a posterior fusion using Harrington instrumentation was performed from T7–L4.

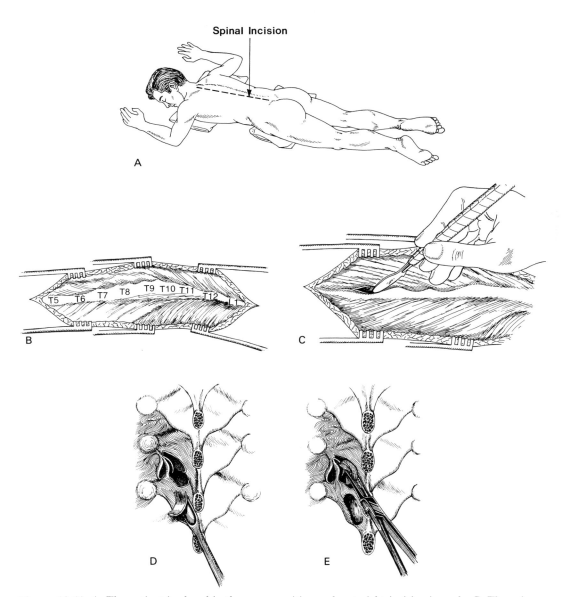

Figure 12-10. A. The patient is placed in the prone position and a straight incision is made. B. The spinous processes are exposed from T5–L1. C. After the exposure of the spinous processes, the cartilaginous cap on the process is split. This incision extends to the bony tip of the process. (B and C, reproduced with permission of M. O. Tachdjian.[81]) D. Two hinged fragments of bone have been raised from the cephalad articular process and the adjacent transverse process and overlapped in the intertransverse process space. E. The spinous process is removed, rotated and placed into the denuded joint area. (D and E, reproduced with permission of J. H. Moe.[55])

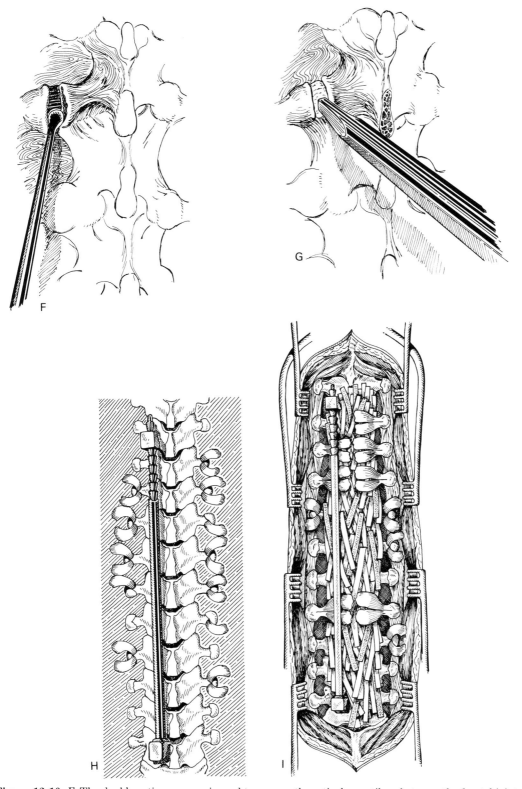

Figure 12-10. *F.* The double action rongeur is used to remove the articular cartilage between the facetal joints in the lumbar area. *G.* A block of cancellous bone is driven into the defect created by the removal of the articular cartilage. (*F* and *G,* reproduced with permission of J. H. Moe.[55]) *H.* After the decortication is completed, the Harrington rod is inserted. *I.* After the rod has been inserted, strips of cancellous and cortical bone are laid along the spine. (*H* and *I,* reproduced with permission of H. A. Keim.[43])

FUSION

Selection of the Fusion Area

The area of the fusion depends upon many factors: age of the patient, etiology of the curve, the type of curve and the length of vertebral rotation. In a younger child, a longer fusion is usually required to maintain correction. If a short fusion is performed, the curve may lengthen or the graft may bend. On the other hand, a shorter fusion can be performed if the Milwaukee brace is used during the period of growth.

The etiology of the curve determines the extent of the fusion. In general, the paralytic curves tend to be long C curves that frequently extend into the sacrum and require an extensive posterior fusion. In fact, O'Brien and Yau[63] prefer to treat these curves with a Dwyer anterior fusion followed by a posterior fusion with Harrington instrumentation (Fig. 12-9). The paralytic curves associated with pelvic obliquity have been handled by preliminary traction and require anterior spinal fusion by the Dwyer technique to the level of L5 and posterior spinal fusion to the sacrum with Harrington rods.[64]

The pattern of the curves is important in the determination of the extent of the fusion. A double major curve requires that both curves be fused, especially in a double major thoracic curve. If only the lower thoracic curve is fused, the upper curve will be exaggerated with a resultant asymmetry of the neck. The single major curve with a flexible compensatory curve requires only the major curve to be fused.

In the right thoracic left lumbar curvature, Moe[55] has emphasized the need to take lateral side bending roentgenograms of the spine. These roentgenograms are taken by having the patient first bend to the right side and then to the left side while lying in the supine position. The right thoracic curve nearly always has a large structural component to it and is fairly rigid. Frequently, the left lumbar curve is flexible so that only the thoracic curve needs fusion and correction. The flexible lumbar curve will balance and compensate the thoracic curve.[55]

Moe[55] has demonstrated that vertebral rotation of the scoliotic segment is important in the selection of the fusion area. His rule is to fuse from neutral vertebrae to neutral vertebrae. This must be considered in the thoracic curve with vertebral rotation of the upper lumbar vertebrae. If the upper vertebrae are not included in the fusion, the curve will lengthen when the cast is removed. The only exception to this rule

is the rotation that may disappear with traction or casting correction. The fusion may be shortened, but usually by only one segment.

In lumbar curves, fusion to the sacrum is rarely indicated.[55] The presence of spondylolisthesis, which is the slipping of a superior vertebral body forward on an inferior vertebral body, is an exception to this rule.

Technique for Posterior Fusion and Insertion of a Harrington Rod in Idiopathic Scoliosis

In the treatment of scoliosis, the primary operative goals are correction of the curve and a solid fusion. The technique of Harrington instrumentation of the spine has been described by many authors, and only the major steps will be reiterated.[29, 30, 34, 35, 55]

After induction by endotracheal anesthesia, the patient is placed in the prone position. A straight incision over the operative site gives a much better cosmetic appearance than an incision which follows the curve (Fig. 12-10A). Sharp dissection is continued through the subcutaneous fascial planes until the tips of the spinous processes are exposed (Fig. 12-10B). During this stage, meticulous hemostasis must be achieved.

With the exposure of the tips of the spinous processes, a straight incision bisects the cartilaginous cap on the spinous process. This incision is extended to the bony tip of the process (Fig. 12-10C). After exposure of several tips of the spinous processes, the soft tissues are stripped from the spinous processes with a Cobb elevator. This is performed in a plane deep to the periosteum. The stripping is continued until all of the bone on either side of the spinous processes is exposed. In the thoracic spine, the dissection is extended to the tips of the transverse processes and in the lumbar spine until the facetal joints are exposed.

At this time identification of the vertebrae is performed by intraoperative roentgenograms. It is important to remember that the thoracic spinous processes project caudally and their identification by roentgenograms may be difficult. On the other hand, the 12th thoracic and lumbar spinous processes project directly posteriorly. A towel clip, therefore, should be placed on the superior portion of the spinous processes of either the 12th thoracic or the 1st lumbar vertebrae and be accurately identified by a roentgenogram.

After the vertebrae have been properly identified, the ligamentous tissue, which covers all of the joints, must be removed with a sharp curet.

Then the level for insertion of the upper hook is identified. In order to facilitate the placement of the upper hook, a small portion of the inferior articular process is removed. This increases exposure of the facetal joints. The sharp-edged 1251 hook is placed between the facetal joint surfaces to the center of the cephalad pedicle. This is tapped into place to indent the pedicle. After tapping the 1251 sharp hook, it is removed and a dull 1252 hook is inserted.

The lower hook is placed in the cephalad portion of the lumbar laminae. The ligamentum flavum is detached from its attachment on the laminae. The laminae edge is removed either with a Kerrison rongeur or with a sharp osteotome and curet.[55] After the dura is visualized, the 1254 dull hook is inserted under the full thickness of the laminae. This hook has been found to fit the best in this area.

After firm fixation of the hooks has been obtained, the correcting outrigger is attached. The outrigger may be gradually lengthened during the remainder of the procedure as the soft tissues on the concave side stretch. Moe[55] prefers to obtain his correction with a cast or some form of distraction prior to surgery. He feels that the outrigger provides less control of the forces of distraction.

As previously noted, Harrington applies a compression system to the convex side of the curve.[32-36] He states that the correction obtained using the combination of distraction and compression was 64% in 1,000 cases. In the 100 cases without compression, the correction was 51%.[34] On the other hand, Moe states that the compression system increases the amount of lordosis in a curve area. Therefore, he advises that this system be used only in spines that are kyphotic in the area of the curve.[9, 55] Elfstrom and Nachemson[26] evaluated the effect of the compression system using telemetry. They felt that in curves exceeding 50°, there was no improvement with the compression system as compared to the distraction rod alone. At present, it appears that the compression system should be used in cases of scoliosis with a kyphotic component to the curve (Fig. 12-11).

When the hooks and the distraction outrigger are in place, the fusion is performed. With the Moe fusion, two hinged fragments of bone are

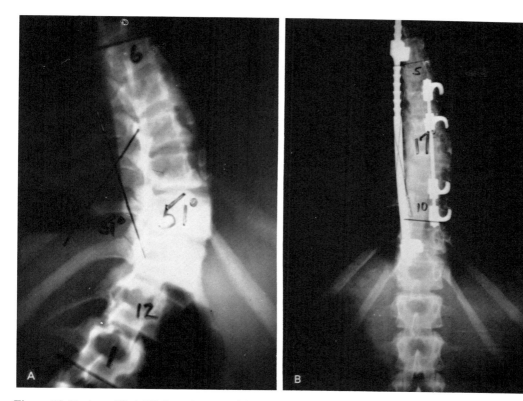

Figure 12-11. *A. and B.* A 51° thoracic curve with associated kyphosis was corrected to 17° using a combination of the distraction and compression system.

raised from the cephalad articular processes and from adjacent transverse processes in the thoracic area. This creates two flaps of bone which overlap across the intertransverse process space (Fig. 12-10D). The superior flap involves only the superficial part of the inferior articular process. The remaining portion of this articular process is removed separately. The superior articular process is removed with a curet.[55] The spinous process is removed, rotated and placed into the joint area (Fig. 12-10E). This is gently impacted in place. In the transitional T11 and T12 area, the superior articular process is removed by means of a gouge. When this is removed, a trough is formed with the floor of the trough being the outer half of the articulation. This half, which still contains articular cartilage, is removed with a curet. The defect is filled with cancellous iliac bone. In the lumbar region the double action rongeur is used to remove the articular cartilage (Fig. 12-10F). A block of either cancellous or cortical cancellous bone is driven into the defect (Fig. 12-10G).

On the convex side, the facetal joints are decorticated. A meticulous facetal block fusion is not performed on this side but all the remaining exposed bone on the convex side is decorticated. In addition, the remainder of the bone on the concave side is also decorticated, but care is used so that the facetal block fusions do not become dislodged. With the completion of decortication, the outrigger is removed and the Harrington rod is inserted (Fig. 12-10H). After the insertion of the Harrington rod, either a small C washer or wire is placed immediately beneath the superior hook, in order to prevent the hook from slipping on the rod.

Although experimental studies have shown that the distracting force on the rod declines rapidly from the viscoelastic deformation of the paraspinous soft tissues,[58] it provides enough internal fixation to allow the patient to be ambulatory in a snug cast until the fusion has matured (Fig. 12-12).

After the rod has been inserted, cancellous bone which has been taken from the iliac crest is laid along the spine. Cortical bone is laid over this cancellous bone (Fig. 12-10I). The highest

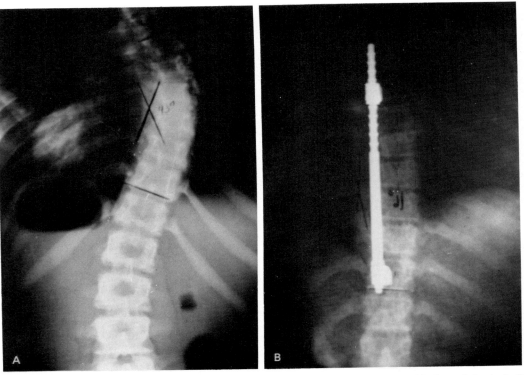

Figure 12-12. *A.* Shown is a patient with a right thoracic curve of 43° associated with thoracic lordosis. In addition, the patient refused to wear her brace and the curve had increased 10° in a 6-month period. *B.* After Harrington instrumentation and fusion, the curve measured 16°.

rate of pseudarthrosis occurs in the thoracolumbar spine; abundant bone graft should therefore be placed in this area.

Postoperative

Prior to the development of Harrington instrumentation, a Risser cast was applied to obtain correction of the curve, the fusion was performed and the patient was continued in the cast with bed rest for 6 months. Following the development of Harrington instrumentation, the patients were still continued at bed rest for 6 months in a cast following their fusion.

Since the majority of the patients with idiopathic scoliosis were teenagers, there were numerous problems with keeping them in bed for 6 months. Therefore, during the 1960s, both Harrington[32, 36] and Leider et al.[46] began shortening the period of time that a child spends in bed. When the results were analyzed, it became apparent that the use of early ambulation did not have an adverse effect upon the final results. Leider et al.[46] reported an average loss of only 5° in 106 patients treated by spinal fusion, Harrington instrumentation and a Risser-Cotrel cast with early ambulation. Harrington feels that the use of early ambulation stimulates the development of the fusion mass.[32, 34]

Complications

Because of the complexity of the problem, the surgical treatment of scoliosis is associated with a variety of intraoperative and/or postoperative complications.

The major intraoperative complications include cardiac arrest and damage to the spinal cord. The cardiac arrest can be the result of hypovolemia. When the operation is performed meticulously, the blood loss can be minimized. However, in a number of cases, the blood loss can be high. Therefore, a careful record should be kept of the blood loss by weighing the sponges and recording the drainage in the suction bottles. Then accurate blood replacement can be given. In an attempt to decrease the amount of blood loss at the time of surgery, hypotensive anesthesia has been used. A ganglionic blocking agent, pentolinium tartrate, is used to induce the hypotension. Because of the possibility of decreased perfusion to the central nervous system, heart and kidney, the pressure should not fall below 60 mmHg. In addition, the arterial pO_2 should be kept higher than normal in order to increase the amount of oxygen to the vital organs. The development of hypopoxemia in a hypotensive patient could result in damage to the vital organs.[52] Alternatively, an attempt to decrease blood loss has been made by injecting epinephrine, 1 to 5 hundred thousand solution, into the skin, subcutaneous tissue and paraspinous muscles.

Spinal cord injury can be caused directly by instrumentation or indirectly by excessive traction. The direct injury should be preventable with careful operative technique. However, caution should be exercised in the surgical treatment of patients with spina bifida, that is, partial or complete absence of the vertebral laminae. If any doubt exists preoperatively concerning whether the posterior elements of the spine are intact, an anteroposterior tomogram of the spine can be performed.

The morbidity and mortality committee of the Scoliosis Research Society collected and studied the cases of neurological damage to the spinal cord. One of the factors that they found associated with the development of neurological complications included severe kyphosis in patients with a pre-existing neural deficit. Also, 32% of the neurological complications reported occurred in cases of congenital scoliosis. In this group, there were nine patients who developed neurological complications secondary to their Harrington instrumentation without preoperative traction. When preoperative traction followed by Harrington instrumentation was used in this group of patients, there was only one case of neurological damage to the spinal cord. They concluded that the Harrington rod should only be used in congenital scoliosis to maintain the correction that was obtained by preliminary traction.[50]

If Harrington instrumentation is used in patients with diastematomyelia, damage to the spinal cord is likely. Winter et al.[88] report a 4.9% incidence of diastematomyelia in patients with congenital scoliosis. Therefore, roentgenograms of all patients with scoliosis should be examined for widening of the interpedicular distance and for a midline bone spur. These signs are compatible with diastematomyelia, although the condition may be present when the roentgenograms are normal. If there is any question regarding the presence or absence of diastematomyelia, a myelogram is mandatory prior to surgery. In patients with a negative myelogram who have congenital scoliosis with a widened interpedicular distance and a neurological deficit or foot deformity, Winter et al.[88] advocate that the spinal cord be explored prior to the surgical correction of the spinal deformity.

The use of preoperative skeletal traction was

also studied by the committee. They felt that the patient had to be closely followed during traction for the development of either cranial nerve palsy or long tract signs. The presence of either of these findings necessitated an immediate reduction of the traction. Since the traction is such a powerful correcting force, Harrington instrumentation to obtain further correction after traction is not warranted because of the increased risk.[50]

In order to minimize the use of excessive traction on a spinal cord with possible neurological damage, Stagnara et al.[78] partially awakens the patient after insertion of the Harrington rod and distraction. The patients are instructed to move their toes in order to assess their neurological condition. If they are unable to move their toes, the distraction on the rod is decreased until they can.

If a neurological complication arises after instrumentation, the rod should be removed promptly. The prognosis for recovery from incomplete lesions of the spinal cord is better than from complete lesions, especially if the rod is removed.[50]

Following scoliosis surgery, atelectasis and pneumonia are the major respiratory complications, especially in patients with compromised preoperative respiratory function. The postoperative application of blow bottles, respiratory exercises and intermittent positive pressure ventilation tends to diminish the incidence of atelectasis and pneumonia.

If the patient is found to have poor preoperative respiratory function, the use of a nasal endothracheal tube postoperatively will enable effective suctioning procedures to be carried out and permit efficient mechanical ventilation. Usually the tube can be removed within 2 or 3 days, and the patient will be able to ventilate spontaneously on his own.

The use of Harrington instrumentation has increased the incidence of infection in scoliosis surgery from 2 to 7%.[54] Because of the increase in incidence of infection, Bradford et al.[9] recommend the use of prophylactic antibiotics. With prophylactic antibiotics, the incidence of infection is then reduced to 1%.

When an infection does occur, prompt recognition and treatment is mandatory. If the wound becomes red and swollen with increased warmth or if drainage occurs, aspiration is performed. After careful preparation of the skin, a needle for aspiration is introduced lateral to the incision to prevent the possibility of contamination by insertion directly through the incision.[42] The aspirate is examined grossly for evidence of pus, after which it is sent to the laboratory for gram stain and culture.

After the culture has been obtained, the patient is taken to surgery and the wound is opened widely down to the fusion mass. Repeated cultures are obtained and all necrotic tissue is debrided. Only the bone graft material that appears to be floating in purulent exudate is removed. The wound is irrigated thoroughly and suction tubes are inserted for the installation of suction irrigation. Since the majority of infections are caused by Staphylococcus aureus, both semisynthetic penicillins (e.g., oxacillin) and cephalosporin (e.g., Keflin) have been used in the suction irrigation and by intravenous administration.[42]

Keller and Pappas[42] reported a series of cases treated with removal of the rods, and although the infection was resolved, the spinal curve increased. This supports the work of other authors, who agree with leaving the rod in place.[9] The suction irrigation system is usually discontinued after 7 days or when the irrigating solution is clear. At this time both the prior input and output tubes are placed on suction for several days, after which they are removed.

In addition to the suction irrigation, the patient is placed on intravenous antibiotics. The choice of the antibiotics depends upon the sensitivity of the organism. The intravenous antibiotics are maintained for 2 weeks. When the 2 weeks of intravenous antibiotics are finished, the patient is placed on oral antibiotics for another 6 weeks.

The use of Harrington instrumentation, facet block fusion and supplemental autogenous cancellous bone has decreased the incidence of pseudarthrosis from levels as high as 50%[9] to 4.7%.[46] Although the incidence of pseudarthrosis has decreased, early recognition and treatment are important.

When the cast is removed at 9 months, oblique roentgenograms are taken of the fusion area. If there is evidence of a pseudarthrosis, the fusion is re-explored.

The most common sites of pseudarthrosis are the thoracolumbar junction and the lumbar spine. It is more common in patients with paralytic curves and curves associated with neurofibromatosis than in idiopathic or congenital curves.

A loss of correction usually signifies the presence of a pseudarthrosis. When this loss of correction occurs, oblique roentgenograms are used to evaluate the fusion. In addition, tomography

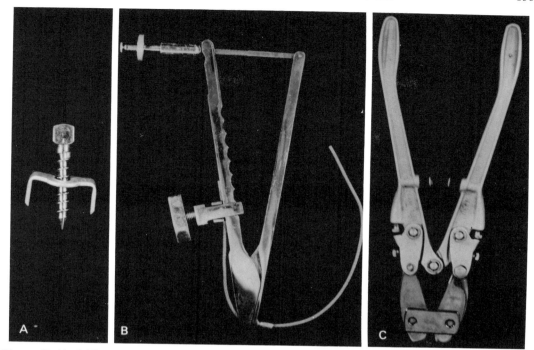

Figure 12-13. *A.* The cannulated screws with deep threads are placed through the hole in the vertebral plates and are screwed into the vertebral body. The vertebral plates come in graded sizes to provide a snug fit to the vertebral bodies. *B.* The tension device with the cable threaded through it has a spring gauge which records the tension in 20-pound increments. The maximum tension that can be applied is 100 pounds. *C.* The mechanical swage produces a force of around 4,000 to 5,000 pounds on the screw head and prevents the cable from slipping.

has been useful in certain cases. If there is any doubt concerning an adequate fusion, re-exploration is essential. In some cases, the entire fusion mass may need to be decorticated before the pseudarthrosis is found.

Fracture of the distraction rod is the most common metal failure of the instrumentation. This usually occurs between the 18th and 36th postoperative month, and occurs at the first ratchet junction. The usual cause of the fracture of the rod is the failure to include the upper hook in the fusion mass.[34] Therefore, even though a solid fusion may occur, with repetitive loads the rod undergoes fatigue failure with fracture.

When the distraction rod does break, it is not necessary to remove it unless it is associated with a loss of correction and progressive overlap of the rod. Therefore, roentgenograms should be taken periodically to determine whether there is a loss of correction or overlap of the rod. If these signs are positive, re-exploration of the spine with removal of the rod, repair of the pseudarthrosis, and insertion of a new rod is recommended.

DWYER INSTRUMENTATION

During the past decade the development of the Dwyer instrumentation has provided a powerful tool for the correction of scoliosis and/or lordosis. This operation utilizes an anterolateral approach to the convex side of the spinal column. The intervertebral discs are removed; special instrumentation is applied to correct the curvature, and an intervertebral body fusion is performed.

Instrumentation

To perform this procedure, special equipment is needed. The equipment is made of titanium, selected for its inertness and strength, and includes cannulated screws, vertebral plates, tension apparatus and a swaging clamp (Fig. 12-13). The screws have deep threads for rigid fixation in the vertebral body and cannulated heads for the passage of the cable. The vertebral plates come in graduated sizes to provide a snug fit with the vertebral bodies. The design of the plate impedes the distraction of the screws from the vertebral body by the tension apparatus. The cable is composed of multiple strands to increase its tensile strength. It has an end button on its superior end, and another end button is placed on the cable after the last screw head has been swaged. The end button enhances a grip on the cable and is necessary because motion of the spine increases the amount of stress on the end screws. The tension device is a spring gauge which records the tension in increments of 20 pounds. The maximum tension which can be applied is 100 pounds. The tension device enables the surgeon to estimate the force applied during the correction. Although Dwyer initially used a hydraulic clamp to provide a strong swage between the screw heads and cable, most surgeons use a mechanical swage because it is less cumbersome. Swaging produces a force of about 4,000 to 5,000 pounds between the screw heads and the cable.[24]

Biomechanics

From mechanical tests, the force required to break the cable is 350 pounds. The force required for removal of the end button exceeds 350 pounds. After swaging the cable to the screw head, the minimum force required for slippage of the cable through the screw head is 150 pounds.[23]

Waugh[85] and Nachemson and Elfstrom[58] have demonstrated that the distracting force of the Harrington rod declines rapidly in the operative and in the postoperative period. Diminution of the distraction force represents a time-dependent relaxation of the spinal ligaments and the intervertebral disc in response to stress.

Although such studies have not been completed after Dwyer instrumentation, clinical experience suggests a similar stress relaxation. After the tension apparatus has been applied, the vertebral bodies are approximated by gradual elevation of the tension. If the tension is increased slowly, the surgeon will observe that the amount of force required to approximate the vertebral bodies will gradually decline. The decline may be due to the stress relaxation of the soft tissues on the concave side of the curve. To obtain the maximum correction of the curve, therefore, the tension should be applied slowly at each intervertebral level. Another application of the concept of stress relaxation of the soft tissues on the concave side of the curve is when direct pressure is applied to the screw heads of two adjacent vertebrae as they are being approximated. This pressure provokes elongation of the tissue on the concave side of the curve

with subsequent decline in the amount of tension needed to approximate the vertebral bodies.

Indications

Although Dwyer invented this approach for the treatment of scoliosis in 1964, indications for its application are still debated. The only absolute indications appear to be idiopathic thoracolumbar and lumbar curves and scoliotic curves associated with deficient posterior elements and lumbar lordosis, such as myelomeningocele (Fig. 12-14). Patients with idiopathic thoracolumbar and lumbar curves are ideal candidates because of the large size of the vertebral bodies; this permits the application of greater force to the vertebral bodies without crushing them. In addition, excision of their larger intervertebral disc provides greater mobility and correction of the curve.

Prior to the development of the Dwyer instrumentation, the management of scoliosis in patients with myelomeningocele was disappointing because of deficient posterior elements and a high incidence of pseudarthrosis. Since the application of the Dwyer instrumentation requires an anterior approach, it has met with greater success in these patients. In curves that extend into the sacrum, a supplemental posterior fusion with Harrington instrumentation is recommended.[64]

Idiopathic thoracic curves and paralytic curves appear to be relative indications. There has not been a definite advantage in treating the routine thoracic curve with Dwyer instrumentation. On the other hand, paralytic curves are often associated with a high incidence of pseudarthrosis. Winter has stated it to be as high as 20%.[88] Although the Dwyer instrumentation provides an excellent means for obtaining and maintaining correction, O'Brien and Yau[63] have reported that the application of the Dwyer procedure alone is inadequate for patients with paralytic scoliosis. They advocate the use of Dwyer instrumentation for correction of the scoliosis at the apex of the curve. Subsequently, a more extensive posterior fusion with the use of Harrington instrumentation is performed. This combination provides better correction of the curve, and it decreases the incidence of pseudarthrosis at the level of the deformity.[64]

Lordotic deformities of the spine are best handled by the use of Dwyer instrumentation. In patients who are paraplegic, the instrumentation can be applied to the front of the vertebral bodies with subsequent correction of the lordosis.

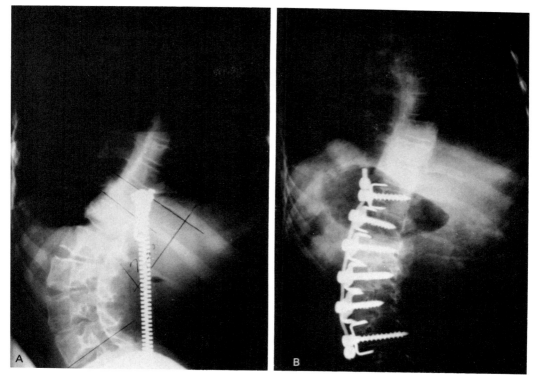

Figure 12-14. *A and B.* A 13-year-old myelomeningocele patient, who has an associated 78° thoracolumbar curve, was treated by means of Dwyer instrumentation. The postoperative curve measured 30°.

A major contraindication to this procedure is the presence of a kyphotic deformity. After the intervertebral discs have been removed, application of anterior instrumentation will increase the kyphosis. Curves which originate higher than T5 should be treated by another method. The exposure is difficult for the insertion of the upper screws in these curves; also, it is difficult to swage the upper screws. The vertebral bodies are small so that less force can be applied to them by the tension apparatus. With excision of the smaller intervertebral discs, there is less mobility and correction of a high thoracic curve.

Preoperative Management

In patients with supple idiopathic thoracolumbar or lumbar curves of less than 75°, preoperative traction is not needed. In patients with rigid curves, Cotrel traction, halofemoral or halopelvic traction should be utilized. Before anterior spinal surgery is performed, pulmonary function studies are mandatory. They should include an assessment of arterial blood gases, vital capacities and maximum breathing capacities. These studies permit estimation of the magnitude of intraoperative and postoperative

risk to the patients with impairment of pulmonary function. Furthermore, they allow planning for appropriate postoperative pulmonary care. Where the studies indicate that the patient may require respiratory assistance for longer than 48 hours after surgery, preoperative tracheostomy is indicated.

Operative Technique

After the administration of a general anesthetic, the patient is placed in the lateral decubitus position, so that the convex side of the curve is uppermost (Fig. 12-15). The upper arm is brought forward so that the scapula rotates away from the vertebral column. This enables exposure of higher vertebrae if necessary. For accentuation of the intervertebral discs, a kidney rest is elevated at the apex of the curve. This allows an easier removal of the intervertebral discs. After excision of the disc tissue, the rest is lowered to increase the mobility of the curve.

Adequate exposure requires removal of the correct rib. In general, the removal of the 5th rib will allow an exposure from T5 to T11. The removal of the 6th rib will allow an exposure from T6 to T12. On the other hand, in patients

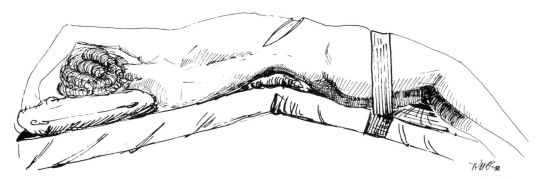

Figure 12-15. The patient has been placed in the lateral decubitus position with the right arm positioned forward. This rotates the scapula away from the vertebral column. The incision is placed directly over the rib that is to be removed. It starts lateral to the midline of the back, follows the rib around the lateral portion of the thorax, and extends down in the abdomen.

with a sloping rib cage, the removal of the 5th rib may limit access from T6 to T11. In a thoracolumbar curve, the removal of the 10th rib with a dissection to the retroperitoneal plane can provide access from T10 to the sacrum.

In thoracolumbar curves, division of the diaphragm is necessary to obtain a complete exposure of the entire curve. The posterior wall of the diaphragm is divided about ½ inch from its peripheral attachment. Prior to division of the diaphragm, stay sutures are placed on each side of the proposed incision. This facilitates the subsequent closure of the diaphragm.

For curves in the thoracic spine, the exposure of the vertebral bodies and intervertebral discs is completed by incision of the pleura and ligation of the intercostal segmental arteries. The ligation of these vessels at the midportion of the vertebral body enables the surgeon to avoid the vascular anastomosis located at the intervertebral foramen. Alternatively, for curves of the thoracolumbar spine, detachment of the crura of the diaphragm and origin of the psoas muscle from the vertebral bodies and ligation of the lumbar segmental vessels are necessary.

After exposure of the vertebral column has been completed, the intervertebral discs are removed. To maximize mobility of the curve, all the disc material must be excised. This stage demands fastidious technique so that the thin, fragile posterior longitudinal ligament is not broached with the inevitable penetration of the dura or even the spinal cord. After removal of the disc, the cartilaginous vertebral end plates are excised by the use of either a fine chisel or ring curet. Only the cartilaginous end plate is removed so that the vertebral body is not weakened.

The vertebral plates are available in graded

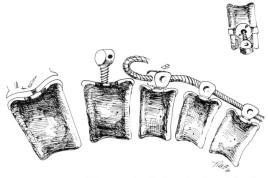

Figure 12-16. The vertebral plate is placed in the center of the vertebral body. A spike driver is used to start the hole in the vertebral body for the passage of the self-tapping screw. This diagram also illustrates the passage of the cable through the eye hole in the screw.

sizes. The plate is selected which fits snugly over the vertebral body (Fig. 12-16). After the plate is positioned, small starter holes for the screws are scored on the bone with a spike driver (Fig. 12-16). The deep threaded screw is secured to the vertebral body. The position of the screw should be aligned carefully, so that inadvertent penetration of the spinal canal does not occur. The screw should be long enough so that it engages the opposite cortex of the vertebral body. Then the cable is threaded through the cannulated screw head.

At this stage, bone graft is prepared from the resected rib. The rib is cut into small pieces which are placed between the vertebral bodies. Now the tension apparatus is applied; tension is gradually increased until the vertebral bodies are approximated (Fig. 12-17). Then the cannulated screw heads are swaged before the removal

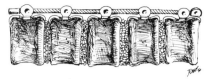

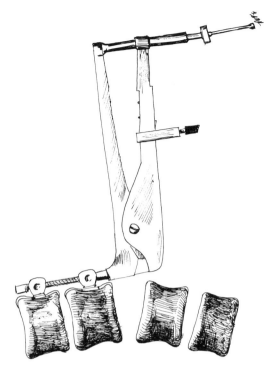

Figure 12-18. At the completion of the technique, the vertebral bodies are approximated, and the rib graft is placed in the intervertebral disc space. All screw heads and the end button are swaged to prevent cable slippage.

Figure 12-17. The cable has been threaded through the eye holes of the first two screws. After passing through the eye holes, it is threaded through the tension apparatus and fastened by the clamp to the handle. The spring gauge on the tensioner is gradually tightened until the vertebral bodies are approximated. Before the cable is released from the tensioner, the screw heads are swaged to prevent the cable from slipping.

Complications

The major potential operative complications include fracture of the vertebral body, pulling out of the vertebral screws, vascular insult to the spinal cord, damage to the aorta or vena cava and mechanical damage to the spinal cord. In the thoracic spine, the maximum compressive force that can be applied between adjacent vertebrae during the approximation stage of the operation is between 30 and 40 pounds. As the curve progresses caudally, greater force can be applied. When the vertebral screw is inserted, it must contact the opposite cortex of the vertebrae to minimize the likelihood of the screw pulling out. When the segmental vessels are ligated opposite the midportion of the vertebral body, the vascular anastomosis near the intervertebral foramen is avoided so that vascular insult to the spinal cord becomes less likely. The aorta and vena cava are located on the concave side of the curve. When the rim of the annulus is removed, care must be exercised so that these vessels are not damaged. Upon removal of the intervertebral disc or insertion of screws into the vertebral bodies, mechanical damage to the spinal cord is possible unless these procedures are undertaken with great care. Prior to insertion of a screw, appropriate alignment of the screw with the posterior longitudinal ligament is necessary to avoid penetration of the spinal canal.

of the tension apparatus. Swaging prevents slippage of the cable in the screws. Placement of additional plates and screws, with approximation of vertebral bodies and swaging, is repeated at each level of the curve (Fig. 12-18).

Postoperative Care

When the pleural cavity is entered, a large chest tube should be inserted and connected to closed under water seal drainage prior to closure of the chest. The tube can be removed when roentgenograms show re-expansion of the lungs and when pleural drainage is less than 30 ml per 24 hours. This usually requires approximately 72 hours.

When the incision is healed and the sutures are removed, the patient is placed in a plaster of Paris body jacket that is carefully molded over the iliac crests. Plaster immobilization continues for 5 to 6 months, or until it is felt that union of the spinal fusion has occurred.

The immediate postoperative complications include atelectasis and superficial wound infection. With the magnitude and location of the operative incision, patients tend to hypoventilate during the early postoperative period. Vigorous intraoperative and postoperative intermittent positive pressure ventilation lessens the incidence of atelectasis. With the prolonged and extensive tissue dissection, prophylactic antibiotics should be administered prior to surgery and continued for approximately 5 days after surgery.

Because the overall length of the spinal column is shortened with the excision of the disc, paraplegia secondary to traction is unlikely to occur. If the patient wakes up paraplegic postoperatively, biplane roentgenograms or a C.A.T. scan should be obtained to rule out screw penetration of the spinal canal. If the screw has penetrated the canal, the patient should undergo surgical exploration with repositioning of the screw. Another potential cause of paraplegia is a vascular insult to the spinal cord. In a series of cases reported by Dwyer and Schafer,[24] this complication did not occur. However, if biplane roentgenograms or a C.A.T. scan were normal, one could assume that the cause of paraplegia was vascular and not reoperate to remove or replace the Dwyer apparatus. In either case, the author feels that steroids should be administered as soon as possible after the diagnosis of paraplegia has been made. Dexamethasone (Decadron), beginning with 10 mg intravenously at 12 hourly intervals with a gradual reduction over the next 5 days, is the drug of choice. The steroids help reduce the cellular edema, maintain cellular membrane integrity and stabilize the membranes of the intercellular lysosomes. This prevents the hydrolytic lysosomal enzymes from digesting the cells and extending the inflammatory tissue damage.[79]

Dwyer did not report any deep infections in his first series.[24] A recent report from Hong Kong discusses the management of three cases of deep infection, paravertebral abscesses, secondary to Dwyer instrumentation. It was the conclusion of Dwyer and Shafer[24] that early recognition and debridement of the paravertebral abscess should be performed. In addition, the patients were treated with intravenous antibiotics. If possible, the Dwyer apparatus should be left in place until the fusion has occurred. If the infection cannot be controlled with the instrumentation in place, the Dwyer apparatus should be removed and a posterior fusion with Harrington rod instrumentation performed so that the curve does not progress.[25]

Late Complications

Dwyer reported a 96% fusion rate in his series.[24] In the two cases that failed to fuse, neither patient had been placed in plaster of Paris jackets after surgery.

In his original series, Dwyer had two cases of mechanical failure. The screw broke at the junction of the head and shaft in the superior vertebrae. Neither of these cases had been immobilized in a plaster jacket postoperatively.[24]

Comparison

Although Dwyer's initial fusion rate was 96%, he states that there has not been a case of pseudarthrosis since the use of the plaster of Paris body jacket. This compares favorably with the incidence of pseudarthrosis recorded in the series of Goldstein,[30] Harrington[36] and Leider et al.,[46] with the application of posterior spinal fusion and Harrington rod fixation. A majority of the Dwyer patients showed radiological evidence of fusion by 6 months after instrumentation. Therefore, the duration of time required for plaster immobilization is less than that required for patients with Harrington instrumentation.

Advantages

With the application of Dwyer instrumentation, there is firm mechanical fixation at each segment of the curve; alternatively after Harrington instrumentation, the load is concentrated at the top and bottom of the curve. Anterior instrumentation maintains the correction achieved at surgery until fusion has occurred. In contrast, Goldstein[30] reported a 2.8° loss in correction, and Leider et al.[46] reported a 5° loss of correction following posterior instrumentation and fusion. With anterior instrumentation, the majority of cases show radiographic evidence of fusion between the 5th and 6th month, whereas with Harrington instrumentation, radiographic union is usually not present until the 9th month. Dwyer instrumentation requires fusion only of the primary curve. However, when posterior instrumentation is used, it is usually necessary to fuse two or three segments beyond the primary curve.

CONCLUSIONS

Treatment of scoliosis by either Harrington rod instrumentation or Dwyer instrumentation has provided a better understanding of the use and limitations of instrumentation in spinal surgery. Thoracic curves are best handled by Harrington instrumentation whereas thoracolumbar curves are best handled by Dwyer instrumentation. Curves that are caused by paralysis or are associated with pelvic obliquity are handled by a combination of Dwyer anterior fusion and Harrington posterior fusion.

Although such instrumentation has improved the ability of orthopaedic surgeons to treat difficult spinal problems, neurological complications occur in spinal surgery. Further research efforts are needed to improve spinal cord monitoring in order to prevent neurological complications during surgery. The principles that have been learned by instrumentation of scoliotic spines are beginning to be applied in spinal cord injuries and in kyphotic deformities of the spine. Further research in these areas is needed before the place of instrumentation in spinal cord injuries and kyphosis is known.

REFERENCES

1. Bake, B., Bjure, J., Kasalecky, J., and Nachemson, A. *Thorax, 27:*703–712, 1972.
2. Bergofsky, E. H., Turino, G. M., and Fishman, A. P. *Medicine, 38:*263, 1959.
3. Bjure, J., Grumby, G., Kasalecky, J., Lindh, M., and Nachemson, A. *Thorax, 25:*451–456, 1970.
4. Block, A. J., Wexler, J., and McDonnell, E. V. *J. Am. Med. Assn., 212:*1520–1522, 1970.
5. Blount, W. P. *Bull. Hosp. Joint Dis., 19:*152–165, 1958.
6. Blount, W. P., and Moe, J. H. *The Milwaukee Brace,* Williams & Wilkins Co., Baltimore, 1973.
7. Blount, W. P., Schmidt, A. C., and Bidwell, R. G. *J. Bone and Joint Surg., 40A:*526–528, 1958.
8. Blount, W. P., Schmidt, A. C., Keever, B. D., and Leonard, E. T. *J. Bone and Joint Surg., 40A:*511–525, 1958.
9. Bradford, D. S., Moe, J. H., and Winter, R. B. Scoliosis. In *The Spine,* edited by R. H. Rothman and F. A. Simeone W. B. Saunders, Philadelphia, 1975.
10. Cass, C. A., Dwyer, A. F. *J. Bone and Joint Surg., 53B:*135–139, 1969.
11. Clark, J. A., and Kesterton, L. *J. Biomechanics, 4:*589, 1971.
12. Clark, J. A., Hsu, L. C. S., and Yau, A. C. M. C. *Clin. Orthop., 110:*90–111, 1975.
13. Cobb, J. R. *AAOS Instructional Course Lectures, 5:*261–275, 1948.
14. Cobb, J. R. *Bull. Hosp. Joint Dis., 19:*187–209, 1958.
15. Cobb, J. R. *AAOS Instructional Course Lectures, 9:*65–70, 1952.
16. Compere, E. L., Metzger, W. I., and Mitra, R. N. *J. Bone and Joint Surg., 49A:*614–624, 1967.
17. Cotrel, Y. The "E.D.F." technique. In *Postgraduate Course on the Management and Care of the Scoliosis, Patient 22–31,* edited by H. A. Keim, New York Orthopaedic Hospital, 1971.
18. De Wald, R. L., and Ray, R. D. *J. Bone and Joint Surg., 52A:*233, 1970.
19. Dickson, J. H., and Harrington, P. R. *J. Bone and Joint Surg., 55A:*993–1002, 1973.
20. Dwyer, A. F. *J. Western Pacific Orthop. Assn., 6:*63–96, 1969.
21. Dwyer, A. F. *Israel J. Med. Sci. 9:*805–812, 1973.
22. Dwyer, A. F. *Clin. Orthop., 93:*191–206, 1973.
23. Dwyer, A. F., Newton, N. C., and Sherwood, A. A. *Clin. Orthop., 62:*192–202, 1969.
24. Dwyer, A. F., and Schafer, M. F. *J. Bone and Joint Surg., 56B:*218–224, 1974.
25. Dwyer, A. P., O'Brien, J. P., Seal, P. V., Hsu, L., Yau, A., and Hodgson, A. R. *Deep Para-Vertebral Infection Following Dwyer's Anterior Spinal Instrumentation,* Scoliosis Research Society, 1975.
26. Elfstrom, G., and Nachemson, A. *Clin. Orthop., 93:*158–172, 1973.
27. Gazioglu, K., Goldstein, L. A., Femi-Pearse, D., and Yu, P. N. *J. Bone and Joint Surg., 50A:*1391–1399, 1968.
28. Goldstein, L. A. *J. Bone and Joint Surg., 41A:*321–335, 1959.
29. Goldstein, L. A. *Clin. Orthop., 35:*95–115, 1964.
30. Goldstein, L. A. *Clin. Orthop., 93:*131–157, 1973.
31. Hall, J. E. *Orthop. Clin. N. America, 3:*81–98, 1972.
32. Harrington, P. R. *Clin. Orthop., 93:*110–112, 1973.
33. Harrington, P. R. Instrumentation in Structural Scoliosis. In *Modern Trends in Orthopaedics,* pp. 93–123, edited by D. Graham, Butterworths, London, 1967.
34. Harrington, P. R. *Orthop. Clin. N. America, 3:*49–67, 1972.
35. Harrington, P. R. *J. Bone and Joint Surg., 44A:*591–610, 1962.
36. Harrington, P. R., and Dickson, J. H. *Clin. Orthop., 93:*113–130, 1973.
37. Hibbs, R. A. *New York Med. J., 93:*1013, 1911.
38. Hibbs, R. A. *J. Bone and Joint Surg., 6:*3–37, 1924.
39. Hirsch, C., and Waugh, T. *Acta Orthop. Scand., 39:*136–144, 1968.
40. Hollinshead, W. H. *Instructional Course Lectures, 18:*120–125, 1962–1969.
41. James, J. I. P. *Scoliosis,* E. & S. Livingstone, Edinburgh, 1967.
42. Keller, R. B., and Pappas, A. M. *Orthop. Clin. N. America, 3:*99–111, 1972.
43. Keim, H. A. *Clinical Symposia, 24* No. 1, 1972.
44. La Breche, B. G., Levangie, P. K., and Sharby, N. H. *Physical Therapy, 54:*837–842, 1974.
45. Larson, A. G. *Anesthesiology, 25:*682–706, 1964.
46. Leider, L. L., Moe, J. H., and Winter, R. B. *Bone and Joint Surg., 55A:*1003–1015, 1973.
47. Letts, R. M., Palakar, G., and Bobechko, W. P. *J. Bone and Joint Surg., 57A:*616–619, 1975.
48. Levine, D. B., Wilson, R. L., and Doherty, J. H. *J. Bone and Joint Surg., 52A:*408, 1970.
49. Lonstein, J., Winter, R. B., Moe, J. H., and Gaines, D. *Clin. Orthop., 96:*222–233, 1973.
50. MacEwen, G. D., Bunnell, W. P., and Sriram, K. *J. Bone and Joint Surg., 57A:*404–408, 1975.
51. Makley, J. T., Herndon, C. H., Inkley, S., Doershuk, C., Matthews, L. W., Post, R. H., Littell, A. S. *J. Bone and Joint Surg., 50A:* 1379–1389, 1968.
52. McNeill, T. W., De Wald, R. L., Kuo, R. N., and Bennett, E. V. *J. Bone and Joint Surg., 56A:*1167–1172, 1974.
53. Moe, J. H. *J. Bone and Joint Surg., 40A:*529–554, 1958.
54. Moe, J. H. *Clin. Orthop., 53:*21–30, 1967.
55. Moe, J. H. *Orthop. Clin. N. America, 3:*17–48, 1972.
56. Moe, J. H., and Gustilo, R. B. *J. Bone and Joint Surg., 46A:*293–312, 1964.
57. Nachemson, A., and Elfstrom, G. *J. Bone and Joint Surg., 51A:*1660–1662, 1969.
58. Nachemson, A., and Elfstrom, G. *J. Bone and Joint Surg., 53A:*445–465, 1971.
59. Nachemson, A., and Nordwall, A. *The Cotrel Dynamic Spine Traction—An Ineffective Method for Pre-Operative Correction of Scoliosis,* Scoliosis Research Society, 1975.
60. Nickel, V. L., Perry, J., Garrett, A., and Heppenstall, M. *J. Bone and Joint Surg., 50A:*1400–1409, 1968.

61. Nickel, V. L., Perry, J., Garrett, A., and Heppenstall, M. *J. Bone and Joint Surg.*, *50A*:1400–1409, 1968.
62. O'Brien, J. P. *Acta Orthop. Scand., Suppl. 163*, 11, 1975.
63. O'Brien, J. P., and Yau, A. *Clin. Orthop.*, *86*:151–153, 1972.
64. O'Brien, J. P., Dwyer, A. P., and Hodgson, A. R. *J. Bone and Joint Surg.*, *57A*:626–631, 1975.
65. O'Brien, J. P., Yau, A. C. M. C., and Hodgson, A. R. *Clin. Orthop.*, *93*:179–190, 1973.
66. O'Brien, J. P., Yau, A. C. M. C., Smith, T. K., and Hodgson, A. R. *J. Bone and Joint Surg.*, *53B*:217–229, 1971.
67. Perry, J. *Orthop. Clin. N. America, 3*:69–80, 1972.
68. Perry, J., and Nickel, J. L. *J. Bone and Joint Surg., 41A*:37–60, 1959.
69. Ransford, A. O., and Manning, C. W. S. F. *J. Bone and Joint Surg., 57B*:131–137, 1975.
70. Riseborough, E. J. *Israel J. Med. Sci. 9*:787–790, 1973.
71. Riseborough, E. J., and Shannon, D. C. The effects of scoliosis on pulmonary function and the changes occurring in the lungs following surgical correction of idiopathic scoliosis. In *Postgraduate Course on the Management and Care of the Scoliosis Patient, 10–17*, edited by H. A. Keim, New York Orthopaedic Hospital, 1970.
72. Risser, J. C. *AAOS Instructional Course Lectures, 5*:248–260, 1948.
73. Risser, J. C., and Norquist, D. M. *J. Bone and Joint Surg., 40A*:555–569, 1958.
74. Schatzker, J., Rorabeck, C. H., and Waddell, J. P. *J. Bone and Joint Surg., 53B*:392–405, 1971.
75. Schmidt, A. C. *Clin. Orthop., 77*:73–83, 1971.
76. Schultz, A. B. *Clin. Orthop., 100*:66–73, 1974.
77. Schultz, A. B., and Hirsch, C. *J. Bone and Joint Surg., 55A*:983–992, 1973.
78. Stagnara, P., Vauzelle, C., and Jauvinraux, P. *Functional Monitoring of Spinal Cord Activity during Spinal Surgery,* Presentation at Scoliosis Research Society, Wilmington, Delaware, September, 1972.
79. Streeten, D. H. P. *J. Am. Med. Assn., 232*:944–977, 1975.
80. Tachdjian, M. O. *Pediatric Orthopaedics,* p. 1190, W. B. Saunders Co. Philadelphia, 1972.
81. Tachdjian, M. O. *Pediatric Orthopaedics,* W. B. Saunders Co., Philadelphia, 1972.
82. Tredwell, S. J., and O'Brien, J. P. *J. Bone and Joint Surg., 57A*:332–336, 1975.
83. Vauzelle, C., Stagnara, P., and Jauvinraux, P. *Clin. Orthop., 93*:173–178, 1973.
84. Victor, D. I., and Keller, R. B. *J. Bone and Joint Surg., 55A*:635–639, 1973.
85. Waugh, T. R. *Acta Orthop. Scand. Suppl. 93,* 1966.
86. Winter, R. B. The effect of early fusion on spine growth. In *Scoliosis and Growth,* edited by P. A. Zorab, Proceedings of a Third Symposium held at the Institute for Diseases of the Chest, Brompton Hospital, London, England, November 13, 1970, Churchill, Livingstone, London, p. 98, 1971.
87. Winter, R. B., Moe, J. H., and Eilers, V. E. *J. Bone and Joint Surg., 50A*:15–47, 1968.
88. Winter, R. B., Haven, J. J., Moe, J. H., and LaGaard, S. M. *J. Bone and Joint Surg., 56A*:27–39, 1974.

13

Reconstruction of
Articular Joints

During the past century, many surgeons have questioned how they might reconstruct impaired articular joints. In view of the enormous number of patients who possess painful, stiff, deformed or unstable joints, the widespread interest in arthroplastic techniques is not surprising. While restoration of an arthritic joint to its inherent, painfree, functional state was the obvious goal, the slow rate of improvement in arthroplastic techniques encouraged many surgeons to attempt alternative solutions to those arthritic joints where nonoperative methods of treatment had failed. Where a single joint was involved, arthrodesis, or fusion, was often the best solution. It eliminated painful motion and instability, and permitted the surgeon to correct a previous deformity. Arthrodesis remains an excellent and even preferred method of treatment for many reconstructive problems, particularly for patients with infected or neuropathic joints, but also where available arthroplastic techniques might be excessively fragile or unavailable. Techniques of arthrodesis were reviewed in Chapters 9 and 10 and are described in detail elsewhere.[1, 2] Alternatively, for patients with multiple arthritic joints, fusions frequently are contraindicated because motion cannot be sacrificed at several joints without a stringent functional compromise. For example, in the rheumatoid hand, while the distal interphalangeal joints can be fused without excessive loss of function, supplementary fusions of more proximal finger joints create a claw-like hand with excessively poor grasp. Excision of the proximal joints, especially the metacarpophalangeal joints, was devised whereby the opposing ends of the two bones were resected. Fibrous tissue is regenerated in the interval with the elimination of pain. Motion of the joint can be restored, although stability is compromised by foreshortening, elimination of joint congruity and the presence of other pathological alterations. In certain cases, the postoperative stability gradually improves to a surprising degree. Hurri *et al.*[3] and Vainio *et al.*[4] have documented the results

of excisional arthroplasty in the elbow and the metacarpophalangeal joints. Within 2 to 3 years after surgery, the joint stability is restored to a highly functional degree.

The Keller arthroplasty of the great toe, with excision of the proximal end of the proximal phalanx, is widely employed to restore a painfree functional great toe as the treatment of painful hallux valgus or hallux rigidus.[5] After excisional arthroplasty of many weight-bearing joints such as the knee, however, an unacceptable degree of instability, sometimes accompanied by pain, is created. Surgical techniques of pseudarthrosis and excisional arthroplasty are described elsewhere.[2, 6]

In the present chapter, the evolution of presently available arthroplastic techniques is described. The methods rest on a solid foundation of biomechanics, the knowledge required by the bioengineer for the selection of appropriate materials and the optimal design parameters. The chapter is organized by anatomical regions. In each subsection, the biomechanics of the joint is discussed, after which the available arthroplastic methods are reviewed. Clinical applications of the procedures are described in Chapter 14. Miscellaneous arthroplastic techniques such as the reconstruction of the proximal joint in the great toe and the intercarpal joints are presented in Chapter 15.

ARTHROPLASTIC RECONSTRUCTION OF THE HIP

Biomechanics of the Hip

The biomechanics of the hip joint has been described in great detail by several workers.[7–12] In the following brief review, and in the comparable ones that follow on other joints, the biomechanics of the region is divided into four domains. The first, the mechanical properties of the tissues in question, was described in Chapter 5. Likewise, the anatomical form of the unit substructures also was presented in Chapter 5. Kinematics, the third domain, describes the mo-

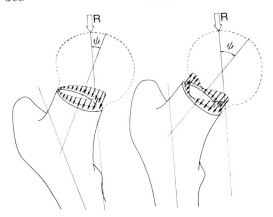

Figure 13-1. *Left.* Schematic distribution of compressive and tensile strains in the cortical shell of the femoral neck. When the femur is loaded in a physiological fashion, there is a distribution of compressive stresses in the cortical shell of the neck. No stresses or strains are found in the superior cortex of the neck and there is increasing compressive stress and strain as the inferior cortex is approached. The femoral neck is under a bending load of such a character that no tensile strains are recorded. *Right.* Distribution of compressive and tensile strain when the shaft is loaded more vertically in a nonphysiological manner. Large tensile strains are presented in the superior cortex and higher compressive strain levels are found in the inferior cortex. (Reproduced with permission of V. H. Frankel.[15])

tion of the whole joint or the motion on and about the articular surfaces. The fourth domain dwells with the loading of the structure during use. The last two domains are now described in turn.

The collagenous tissues display viscoelastic, time-dependent, anisotropic behavior. Accurate mechanical tests must include the appropriate rate of load or strain, the orientation of the sample relative to the axis of the structure under test and the method of procurement, storage and preparation of the specimen. With the considerable variation in the local variations of mechanical properties, the correct anatomical orientation of the specimen under test is essential.

Determination of the substructural mechanical properties of the hip joint requires a preliminary assessment of the direction of the reactionary load against the femur.[7] Available methods include static[13] and dynamic studies,[12] cadaveric preparations[14] and telemetry from instrumented prostheses *in vivo.*[15] From these and ancillary techniques, the distribution of compressive and tensile strains in the cortical shell of the femoral neck and the femoral head can be described. The former are shown diagrammatically in Figure 13-1. Previous workers described a medial trabecular and so-called compressive system, and a lateral trabecular and so-called tensile system. Large tensile strains were described in the superior cortex with compressive strains in the inferior cortex. This configuration of loading applies only when the shaft is loaded more vertically in a nonphysiological manner. From the studies of Rydell,[16] it is now evident that under physiological load there is a distribution of compressive stresses in the cortical shell of the neck. No stresses or strains are found in the superior cortex of the neck and there is increasing compressive stress and strain as the inferior cortex is approached. The femoral neck is under a bending load of such a character that no tensile strains are recorded. Torsional loading of the femoral neck appears to be insignificant.

The kinematics of the hip joint is best perceived as the motion of a spherical joint around the center of rotation of the femoral head to produce sliding at the joint surfaces.[7] Numerous methods have been employed to determine the displacement, velocities and acceleration of the femur in relation to the pelvis. Such data has also been correlated with the phasic muscular activity around the hip joint to determine the function of muscles in gait.[17] From the acceleration data, calculations of forces and moments acting on the hip joint and on various arthroplastic joints can be determined.

Local variations of forces imposed on the femoral head have been determined by many workers. Pauwels[18] and Blount[19] have emphasized that the force in the head of the femur is about 2½ times that of body weight in static, single leg stance. Small changes in the relationship of the muscle arm to the gravitational arm will alter this relationship considerably. For example, when lying on the back and raising the leg 2 inches off the ground, approximately 2½ times body weight is imposed upon the femoral head. Similar calculations can be performed for other static activities. The large joint loads attributable to muscular force have been confirmed by Rydell[16] through the use of an instrumented prosthesis. During dynamic activity, considerably larger loads on the femoral head will be encountered. They have been measured directly and indirectly through the use of kinematic data and a force plate which gives the ground reaction. The force on the head of the femur during gait can attain levels of 5 to 6 times body weight during stance phase, and at least that of body

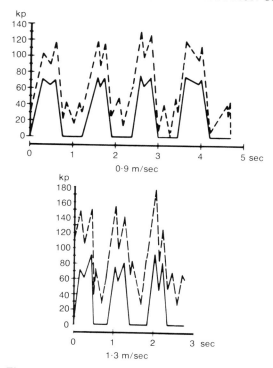

Figure 13-2. Force on a femoral head prosthesis during gait. The *dashed line* indicates the force on the prosthesis. The *solid line* indicates the force of the foot against the foot plate. During swing phase, when the force of the foot against the foot plate is zero, large forces are still measured in the prosthesis due to the action of muscles about the hip joint. When the gait velocity is increased, a corresponding increase is found in the load on the femoral head during both swing and stance phases. (Reproduced with permission of N. W. Rydell.[16])

weight during swing phase. Shown in Figure 13-2 are the dynamic forces imposed upon a femoral head prosthesis, as reported by Rydell.[16] The forces are perhaps somewhat smaller than anticipated because of slower gait and tilting of the trunk over the prosthesis. It is of note that increase in the force occurred when the speed of gait was increased from 0.9 m/sec to 1.3 m/sec. During stance phase, the reaction against the head of the femur depends in part upon the ground reaction, although this is not true during swing phase. Forces on the femoral head are found from the relationships: Force = mass times accleration for linear motion; torque = mass moment of inertia times angular acceleration for angular motions. These relationships can be used to calculate the forces acting on the head of the femur during any part of swing phase. A more detailed account of the dynamics

of the lower extremity has been provided by Kummer[20] to which the interested reader is referred.

Kummer also has described the stress distribution in the articular surfaces of the hip joint. In such a spherical joint, the area of support need not be identical with the area of contact, nor with the anatomical articular surface. As seen in Figure 13-3A, the supporting area is delineated either by the borders of the anatomical articular surface or by the principal circle on the sphere, comparable to the equator on the globe if the point of penetration of the stressing force, R (the hip resultant), is considered as the "pole." With this assumption, no normal forces can be transmitted from the socket to the articular head below the equator. Also, where the border of the socket lies above the equator, it delineates the area of force transmission. It should be self-evident that the pole cannot extend beyond the borders of the area of contact. For theoretical calculation of the stresses, the hip resultant, R, is divided into partial forces, p_i, and distributed in such a way that the sums of rotational moments of opposite sides are equal to zero (Fig. 13-3B). This discussion is extended by Kummer, who shows that the principal stresses in the articular surface are proportional to the normal components of p_i (Fig. 13-3C). If

$$p_i = \text{the partial forces}$$
then
$$R = \sum p_i$$

and, assuming an elastic but not visibly deformable material, the principal stresses in the articular surface are proportional to the normal components of p_i:

$$\sigma_i = -p_i \sin \alpha_i$$

where α_i is the angle between p_i and the equator (angle of latitude). If the principal circle through the pole and the apex of the border of the socket is taken as the "zero meridian" and the angle of inclination of the acetabular border to the equatorial plane is ρ, the smallest angle α on the zero meridian will be (Fig. 13-3C):

$$\alpha_0 = \rho$$

This angle increases as the resultant, R, approaches the acetabular border. Since the sum of all moments equals zero, the stresses must increase in the area between R and the border of the surface of contact. Consequently, an increased angle, ρ, is associated with enlarged stresses at the articular border (Fig. 13-3C).

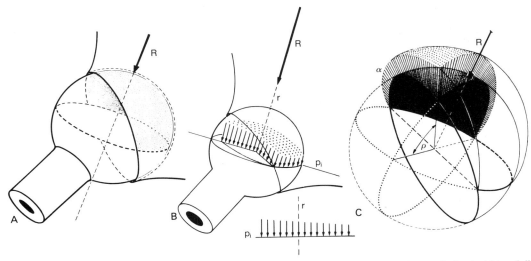

Figure 13-3. *A.* The supporting area of a spherical joint is represented schematically as a "spherical biangle". The spherical head may be covered by cartilage. The area of contact on the anatomical surface of the femoral head with the socket comprises the supportive area of contact or shadowed biangle. *R,* the hip resultant, penetrates the joint at the "pole". *B.* A schematic diagram shows the division of the hip resultant, *R,* into partial forces p_i. The distribution of the p_i takes place in a plane perpendicular to the line of action *r* of *R*. *C.* The stress distribution in a spherical joint is represented where *R* is the hip resultant and ρ is the angle between the plane of the border of the socket and the equatorial plane. (*A, B* and *C,* reproduced with permission of B. Kummer.[21])

Since the magnitudes of the transmitted normal forces and, consequently, the normal stresses, depend upon the angle α, the stresses will be greatest and equal to the partial force p_i at the pole and will decrease to zero at the equator.

The hypothesis developed by Kummer assumes that the opposing layers of articular cartilage possess slightly different radii of curvature in the unloaded state, but wholly congruent surfaces under the imposition of anatomical load. As Greenwald[22] and others[23, 24] have pointed out, anatomical joints do not appear to be strictly congruent; the unloaded surfaces of the joint are, in fact, not perfectly spherical. Since the joint is multiaxial, the degree of congruency must vary throughout the range of movement. At least for light loads, there must be contact and noncontact zones within the joint. The incongruity of such spherical joints appears to contribute to their efficient mechanisms for lubrication. At least in the early stages of osteoarthritis, the joints become progressively more congruent.

In a somewhat similar way, Dietschi *et al.*[25] have investigated the biomechanics of the acetabulum. These workers have provided a distribution diagram of the compressive stresses around the acetabulum and on the opposing surface of the pelvis. Compressive stresses ranging between 0.051 and 0.082 kp/mm² have been

recorded for a hypothetical individual of body weight 60 kg in weight-bearing configuration. At the upper limit, this value is about 3 times the magnitude of the ultimate static strength of cancellous bone.

While at first glance the articular surface of the joint appears to be absolutely smooth and regular, closer scrutiny reveals local undulations and depressions. Several workers have attempted to characterize both the degree of irregularity of the surfaces and the local variations in their mechanical properties.[24-27] The studies are hampered by the changes in the surface that accompany fixation and other aspects of preparation of the specimen.

Previous Arthroplastic Methods for Reconstruction of the Hip

The first great milestone in surgical reconstruction of the diseased hip joint was the cup, or "mold" arthroplasty devised by Smith-Petersen.[28] In principle, the diseased acetabulum and femoral head were reamed to provide opposing concentric surfaces. A smooth interpositional material was positioned between the reamed surfaces. Of the various materials employed, cobalt-chromium (Co-Cr) alloy has been used most recently. In the postoperative period, the raw bony surfaces adjacent to the cup are enveloped by fibrocartilage which, in certain instances, may show hyaline cartilage similar to articular cartilage.[29] A bursa-like sac develops around the arthroplastic joint which produces synovial fluid and simulates the lining of an anatomical joint. A pain-free, mobile arthroplastic joint may result if the patient follows an elaborate regime of exercises for many months. Once a cup arthroplasty has become functional and painless it may remain so for many decades.[30] Unfortunately, the success rate has not been particularly high apart from the encouraging figures of the inventor. The principal problems include avascular necrosis of the femoral head and neck with late collapse of bone. Migration of the cup, also, is not uncommon. Many patients have prolonged mechanical pain despite an apparently satisfactory result as assessed by active motion of the hip and by X-rays.

Prior to the development of total hip joint replacement, cup arthroplasty was the method of choice for treatment of degenerative and rheumatoid hips, infected hips and many other infections. With its superior reliability, total hip joint replacement has succeeded cup arthroplasty for most of these indications. The best indication for cup arthroplasty remains the reconstruction of an infected hip joint or infected cup arthroplasty. Cup arthroplasty can be used to retain joint mobility despite the presence of old, healed infections and active infections of pyogenic or tuberculous nature. Prior to primary or revision cup arthroplasty, however, the infection must be brought under control by debridement of infected tissue and aggressive antibiotic therapy. While cup arthroplasty can provide gratifying results, it is a most demanding procedure for the surgeon and subsequently for the physical therapist. The technical details of the surgical reconstruction and the rehabilitation are described by Harris[31] and Leddy et al.[32]

Cup arthroplasty has also been recommended for treatment of juvenile rheumatoid arthritis of the hip with minimal joint destruction, traumatic arthritis in young adults with painful mobile hips, and selected adolescent hip disorders such as slipped capital femoral epiphysis, avascular necrosis and Perthes' disease.[30] Many surgeons, however, would argue that even in such young adults, total hip joint replacement provides a much greater likelihood for a clinically satisfactory result despite the fact that presently available implants are likely to fail during the patient's lifetime.

Other complications of cup arthroplasty are ectopic bone formation in about 30%, stiffness and even ankylosis and infection which in some

series is about 4%. The exacting regime of physical therapy has been described by Tronzo et al.[30] It requires 6 months of patient and diligent effort by the patient with close assistance from the therapist.

In certain uncommon infections of the hip joint where the femoral head and neck are largely destroyed, trochanteric arthroplasty has been performed whereby a cup is positioned on the greater trochanter which is then inserted into the acetabulum. This and other uncommon reconstructive procedures are reviewed elsewhere.[30, 33]

Within a historical perspective, the lessons learned from cup arthroplasty are the value of a carefully planned and well documented attempt to develop a new arthroplastic procedure and the insight into ways that man-made materials may be employed in reconstructive procedures to encourage the regeneration of useful biological tissues.

Endoprosthetic Arthroplasty

While hemiarthroplasty might seem appropriate to describe an arthroplasty of the femoral head, this term could also apply to reconstruction of the acetabulum. By tradition, "endoprosthetic arthroplasty" implies isolated femoral head replacement which was first popularized by the Judet brothers.[34] In 1950, Moore[35] and Thompson[36] independently conceived of the femoral head replacement with anchorage of the prosthesis within the proximal femur. The Thompson prosthesis possesses a short, solid curve stem with the head in slight valgus position (Chapter 1, Fig. 1-14). The Moore prosthesis (Chapter 1, Fig. 1-14) has unique fenestrations for ingrowth of bone. Despite the appearance of numerous competing designs, these two, with slight modifications, have withstood the test of time. At present, a straight-stemmed version of the Moore prosthesis is most widely employed in the United States. The Thompson prosthesis is used frequently in conjunction with methylmethacrylate cement for rigid fixation.[37]

Initially, endoprostheses were used to treat femoral nonunions, although they rapidly gained favor for primary replacement of acute femoral neck fractures. As the limitations of cup arthroplasty became evident, the use of the endoprosthesis was extended to some types of the arthritides. Anderson et al.[38] however, showed that the results of femoral head replacement were most successful where the primary disease affected only the femoral head with minimal involvement of the acetabulum. More recently,

Salvati and Wilson[39] have reported their results of the long-term expectations of endoprosthetic arthroplasties for various disorders of the hip. They used 5 years as a minimum follow-up period with a maximum of 20 years and an average of 5.6 years: (A) 70% showed excellent to good results in fresh fractures and nonunions of the femoral neck; (B) 86% gave excellent to good results for avascular necrosis; (C) 60% gave excellent to good results for degenerative joint disease; (D) 63% gave good to excellent results for a failed prosthesis undergoing revision.

Despite this favorable impression, it is clear the endoprosthetic replacement of the femoral head frequently culminates in a painful hip joint with erosion of the opposing acetabular surface. Such mechanical hip pain usually arises about 10 years after implantation. Rheumatoid arthritic patients and others with osteoporosis of the pelvis are likely to show marked erosion of the acetabulum within a much shorter period of time.[40] While the clearest indication for endoprosthetic replacement of the femoral head remains treatment of acute femoral neck fractures, most surgeons agree that the procedure should not be undertaken in patients younger than 65 years because a healed femoral neck will provide a more durable result than an artificial femoral head.[37] Furthermore, only displaced femoral neck fractures should be treated with endoprosthetic replacement because basicervical and undisplaced neck fractures are easily nailed and show better prognoses. Other uncommon indications for femoral head replacement are grossly comminuted pertrochanteric fractures in elderly

patients with limited ambulation and life expectancy, nonunions of the femoral neck, pathological fractures of the proximal femur secondary to metastatic bone disease, and occasionally, primary tumors of the proximal femur and avascular necrosis of the femoral head. These indications are discussed elsewhere.[37] The contraindications for proximal femoral replacement include rheumatoid arthritis or advanced degenerative arthritis with distortion or destruction of the acetabular articular cartilage, neuropathic joints, previous infections of the hip joint or inadequate bone stock. The specific complications of endoprosthetic procedures include protrusion of the stem, malposition, fracture of the femoral shaft, dislocation and rarely, neurovascular problems. Late failures may include infection, myositis ossificans, protrusio acetabulum, sciatic or femoral nerve damage, broken prostheses, mechanical hip pain secondary to loosening or to acetabular erosion, and bony fractures around the distal prosthetic stem.

Biomechanics of the Reconstructed Hip

Biomechanical abnormalities of the hip arise from a physiological imbalance between the mechanical stresses that occur in the joint and the ability of the involved tissues to sustain them. The imbalance may result from the presence of congenital deformities or the presence of arthritis which may disrupt the normal distribution of forces in the joint to provoke further disintegration and pain. As part of the reconstructive procedure, the compressive force acting across the articular surfaces may be decreased either

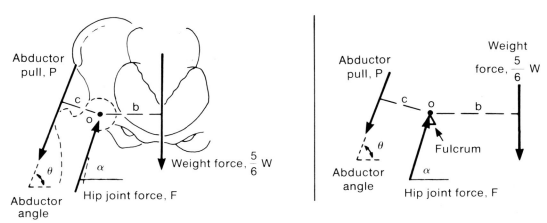

Figure 13-4. The schematic diagram shows the determination of the force acting on the hip joint in unilateral stance. The figures show the lever arm system present in the frontal plane. (Reproduced with permission of A. S. Greenwald and C. L. Nelson.[41])

by increasing the weight-bearing surface of the joint or by decreasing the load that acts across these areas.

When the hip is perceived as a system of levers, as shown in Figure 13-4, it is apparent that the reduction of force on the hip can be undertaken in several ways. The most obvious is a reduction of the patient's weight. For each pound of weight loss, the force on the hip is reduced by approximately 3 pounds. Force reduction also may be accomplished by the patient leaning toward the involved hip. Concurrently, the center of gravity shifts toward the center of the affected femoral head to reduce its lever arm about this fulcrum. In turn, the magnitude of abductor muscle force necessary to achieve rotational stability in the frontal plane decreases and the net force that acts across the articular surface is reduced. Other methods to diminish the force on the hip joint include the use of a cane in the opposite hand and a reduction in walking speed.[16] Alternatively, proximal femoral

varus or valgus osteotomies described by Pauwels[18] increase the articular weight-bearing area to reduce and redistribute the interarticular force. In this way, osteotomy may increase the surface area of contact between the opposing joint surfaces.

More recently, total hip joint replacement has provided several ways in which the forces across the hip joint may be diminished. As Charnley[42] emphasizes, diminution of the forces across the arthroplastic hip may prolong the anticipated duration of function of the man-made device. Charnley attempted to diminish the load that acts across the arthroplastic hip by medial displacement of the acetabular cup and lateral displacement of the greater trochanter with the attached abductor muscles (Fig. 13-5). Medial displacement was enhanced by diminution in the size of the arthroplastic femoral head. The mechanics of these alterations are indicated by a static force analysis shown in Figure 13-4. They represent the hip in the frontal plane during one-legged stance. The hip is represented as a fulcrum in which the abductor and body weight lever arms may be determined by measurements from X-ray films. With the knowledge of the weight force and the abductor angle estimated from X-ray films, three simple equations described the equilibrium of the skeletal system and permit an estimate of the force generated at the hip.

For rotational stability in the frontal plane $\swarrow = \searrow$:

$$\tfrac{5}{6}\, Wb = Pc \tag{1}$$

For horizontal equilibrium $\rightarrow = \leftarrow$:

$$F_{\text{horz.}} = P \cos \theta \tag{2}$$

For vertical equilibrium $\uparrow = \downarrow$:

$$F_{\text{vent.}} = P \sin \theta + \tfrac{5}{6}\, W \tag{3}$$

By use of Pythagoras' theorem:

$$F^2 = F^2_{\text{horiz.}} + F^2_{\text{vert.}} \tag{4}$$

Substitution provides the following expression for the force on the hip joint:

$$F = W(\tfrac{5}{6})[(b/c^2) + 2bc \sin \theta + 1]^{1/2} \tag{5}$$

The angle of the hip joint force with respect to the horizontal is obtained from:

$$\text{Tan } \alpha = F_{\text{vent.}}/F_{\text{horz.}} = \frac{b/c \sin \theta + 1}{b/c} \tag{6}$$

By the use of these equations and several clinical examples, Greenwald and Nelson[44] have

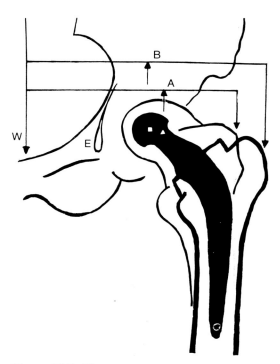

Figure 13-5. The moment arms about the hip joint are shown before operation, A, and after reconstruction, with a small diameter femoral head replacement, B (22 mm). The arthroplastic hip shows medial displacement of the center of rotation and lateral projection of the greater trochanter. (Reproduced with permission of J. Charnley.[43])

shown how total hip joint replacement frequently lowers the force of the hip joint to one-half of the preoperative values. The principal goal of the surgeon, to lower the force of the hip joint, is achieved by displacement of the fulcrum of the hip in a medial direction. While transferring the greater trochanter in a lateral direction provides a similar benefit, distal migration of the greater trochanter down the shaft of the femur or changing the abductor angle is of little benefit. Distal displacement restores physiological tension in the abductor musculature, but does little to influence the lever arm system.

During the development of his low friction arthroplasty, Charnley[42] was well aware of the previous considerations and of several others. Charnley defined the principal mechanical considerations for the arthroplastic hip joint as follows:

A hemispherical bearing was expected to function for at least 20 years in the human hip. The range of diameters of the femoral head replacement that could be considered was 20 to 40 mm (⅞ to 1⅝ inches) which should function under the following physical conditions: (1) Oscillation through approximately 20° in the loaded half-cycle followed by a similar unloaded half-cycle; (2) sliding speeds of 0.75 to 1.5 feet per minute; (3) stresses on the projected area of the hemispherical bearing from 330 to 120 psi; (4) estimates of the viscosity of synovial fluid range from 5.7 to 1160 poise (1 poise $= 0.1$ $Ns/m^2)^{45}$; (5) operating temperature constant at 37°C; (6) maximum angular range of motion required 100 to 120°; (7) maximum available external diameter of 50 mm, although 40 mm would be advantageous in many applications. The direction of main load is approximately vertical.

Arthroplastic Fixation with Methylmethacrylate Cement

The early attempts of total hip joint replacement employed either intramedullary stems or screws to attach the implants to bone. After surgery, the implants were observed to undergo loosening with migration, pain, or destruction of adjacent bone.

A few early workers had attempted to use methylmethacrylate cement to secure orthopaedic implants.[46] In 1941, Kiaer used the cement to attach the Judet prosthesis. With the short stem of the prosthesis, mechanical failures arose for which the cement was incorrectly implicated as the source of the problem. In 1953, Haboush reported the use of cement to attach a femoral prosthesis with a long stem. He applied the cement only to the cut surface of the neck of the femur to improve the seating of the metal on the bone and avoid local sites of high pressure. The technique failed in view of the use of insufficient cement in the incorrect location. The subsequent contribution of Charnley[42, 46] was attributable to the insertion of cement deeply into the medullary canal to provide transference of load from the distal two-thirds of the stem of the prosthesis to the endosteal surface of the femoral cortex.

Polymethylmethacrylate cement possesses no intrinsic adhesive property against wet bone. A bond between cement and bone represents an intimate mechanical interlocking of superficial irregularities. The irregularities can be natural features at the bone surface such as the interstices of cancellous bone or they may comprise man-made slots, drill holes or other undulations of the surface. In clinical applications under conditions of load bearing the cement-bone interface tolerates compressive forces much more satisfactorily than shearing forces. Where shearing forces are imposed upon the surface, the quality of the bond is enhanced if the design combines shearing and compressive forces. If the union fails with even a microscopic degree of looseness, histological and radiological changes in the adjacent bone occur which augment the degree of looseness.

Methylmethacrylate, the monomer from which polymethylmethacrylate is formed, has the general structure $CH_2:C(CH_3)\cdot COO:CH_3$

Methylmethacrylate is a volatile liquid with a boiling point of 100°C. Upon exposure to light it polymerizes into a solid resin. Spontaneous polymerization can be prevented by the addition of an inhibitor such as 0.1% hydroquinone. In contrast, rapid and controlled polymerization is realized by the addition of a chemical initiator such as 2% benzoyl peroxide. Even after the addition of an initiator, polymerization does not start immediately unless the reaction is activated by heat or the addition of a chemical activator. In bone cement the activator is about 2% dimethyl-p-toluidine. Self-curing acrylic bone cement consists of liquid and solid constituents. Upon mixture of the ingredients a dough or paste is formed which ultimately hardens spontaneously as an exothermic reaction. A typical formulation of the liquid constituent is: Methylmethacrylate, 97.8%; tertiary amine (dimethyl-p-toluidine), 2% (initiator); and hydroquinone, 0.1% (inhibitor). The powder constituent of the typical formulation consists of: Polymethylmethacrylate, 97%; benzoyl peroxide, 2%

(activator); and pigmented fillers, 1%. On microscopic inspection the amorphous white powder consists of minute spherical balls. In production liquid monomer is polymerized and dispersed as a suspension. The suspension is ground in a ball mill to yield spherical granular polymer. The polymeric powder contains benzoyl peroxide so that admixture with the liquid monomer provokes dissolution of some of the powder. In the presence of the tertiary amine activator in the liquid, the monomer then polymerizes and combines the spherical granules and powder into a solid aggregate.

The rate of polymerization following admixture of the liquid and powder in a bone cement depends upon several factors controlled by methods of manufacture. The molecular weight of the polymer and the textures of the powders can be altered. Both the proportions of the activator and initiator, as well as the proportions of liquid and powder, can be adjusted. At the time of application, the ambient temperature influences the time for solidification.

In orthopaedic surgery, the proportion of liquid to powder should be the smallest volume of liquid that will render the mass sufficiently plastic for application. A minimum amount of liquid and a maximum amount of powder generates the minimum amount of heat. The usual proportion of powder to liquid is in the region of 40 g of powder to 20 ml of liquid. Very small variations in the volume of liquid can affect the viscosity of the mixture.

As an example of the effect of room temperature on the setting time of a typical mixture, a prolongation of setting time of about 2 minutes follows ambient cooling from 67 to 58°F (20 to 15°C), and an acceleration of 1 minute by warming from 67 to 76°F (20 to 25°C). The temperature generated as the cement solidifies depends greatly upon the volume of polymerizing cement. A mass of cement about the size of a golf ball reaches an exterior temperature of about 80°C. In contrast, a 1-cm cube of cement shows a superficial temperature of about 70°C. When the cement is employed with a metal prosthesis in the intramedullary canal of a femur the layer of cement rarely exceeds a thickness of about 5 mm and it is more typically from 1 to 2 mm in thickness. Both the implant within the cement and the wet bone surrounding the cement serve to remove heat. In a test with thermal measurements on a cadaveric specimen, Charnley and Smith[46] observed a maximal rise in temperature of 12°C above the starting temperature which persisted for 30 seconds and decreased abruptly.

Recently Reckling and Dillon[47] have reported the bone-cement interface temperature recorded during total hip joint replacement. Thermoprobe measurements were recorded during 20 total hip joint replacement procedures. A range of elevation in temperature between 3 and 17°C was recorded. The highest temperature, 48°C, was well below the denaturation point (56°C) of protein. These workers felt that the presence of blood and other liquid at the interface, the large surface area, the poor heat conductivity of methylmethacrylate and the relatively thin layers of cement generally employed for total joint replacement prevented further elevation in the superficial temperature of the cement. Lundskog[48] and Feith[49] have studied the influence of a temperature of 50°C applied to living bone for 30 seconds. These workers observed no demonstrable death of osteocytes or changes in the regenerative process. From these observations it seems unlikely that routine application of cement provokes thermal damage to adjacent tissues. Where a large bolus of cement is employed, however, there seems to be little doubt that thermal damage can provoke substantial changes to adjacent tissues. In separate experiments, Linder[50] has studied the reaction of bone to the acute chemical trauma of bone cement in conditions of minimal thermal elevation. He concludes that the local release of monomer and possibly of other constituents of cement has no deleterious effect on adjacent bone.

During polymerization the volumetric change in the cement as recorded by Haas et al.[51] is a shrinkage of about 5% by volume. This magnitude of volumetric shrinkage could seriously impair the ability of the cement to bond the prosthesis to bone. In clinical use, however, the shrinkage of cement has not been a problem. It is conceivable that expansion of the cement during the mixture of liquid and powder occurs by the admixture of minute air bubbles. During the injection process, further expansion of the air bubbles could help to inject the plastic into the investment. Porosities ranging from 1% to 10% of the volume of the cement have been recorded by Haas et al.[51]

Charnley[52] and others[51] have measured the monomeric constituents of solidified surgical cement. Shortly after solidification, the amount of retained monomer ranges from 3.5% to 1.9%. Over the following year approximately 0.3% reduction in the concentration of free monomer is noted. One specimen removed from a patient after 2 years implantation in the femur showed residual monomer of 0.85%. Residual peroxide

Table 13-1
Mechanical Properties of Bone Cement[a]

	Radiopaque cement	Radiolucent cement
Tensile strength, psi[b]	4,190.00 (230)[c]	4,730.0 (170)
Compressive strength psi	13,300.00 (360)	13,500.0 (570)
Transverse breaking load lb force[d]	9.43 (0.70)	10.8 (0.29)
Modulus of rupture psi	7,410.00 (450)	8,250.0 (230)
Young's modulus:		
From transverse loading data psi	0.30×10^6 (0.013×10^6)	0.32×10^6 (0.011×10^6)
From compressive loading data psi	0.32×10^6 (0.009×10^6)	0.33×10^6 (0.007×10^6)

[a] Reproduced with permission of S. S. Haas, G. M. Brauer and G. Dickson.[51]
[b] To convert psi to MP_a, divide by 145.
[c] Standard deviations are shown in parentheses.
[d] To convert lb force to N, divide by 0.225.

contents of approximately 0.35% have been measured soon after solidification. Over the following year the concentrations drop to a final value of about 0.05%.

Haas et al.[51] have provided a detailed characterization of polymethylmethacrylate bone cement. The data is presented similarly to that reported by Charnley and Smith,[46] although with greater detail. Their methods of standardization, such as the molecular weight of the constituents, are presented. The porosity of the material was observed to increase greatly with rapid mixing so that figures of 10% might be reached. In Table 13-1, their mechanical characterization of radiopaque and radiolucent cement is shown. All of the strengths are about 25% lower than the upper limits of normal cortical bone, and its stiffness is about 5 to 10 times lower. Usually, the cement is employed in juxtaposition to the cancellous bone which probably shows a compressive strength of about 1000 psi, although osteoporotic bone may be in the order of a magnitude less than this figure.

Freitag and Cannon[53] have studied the fracture characteristics of presently available orthopaedic bone cements including Simplex-P (Howmedica, Inc., Rutherford, N. J.) and Zimmer, (Zimmer U.S.A., Warsaw, Ind.). The Zimmer acrylic bone cement shows superior fracture toughness and longer fatigue life than the Simplex-P material.

Recently, Taitsman and Saha[54] have studied the tensile strength of a bone cement reinforced with a stainless steel wire, as well as comparable specimens in which Vitallium wires were embedded. The results show that the tensile strength of bone cement can be substantially increased by reinforcement with metal wires. Increase in strength is proportional to the number of wires used. Even after mechanical failure of cement,

the reinforcing wires may carry an appreciable amount of load. The minimum cross-sectional area of reinforcing wires necessary for a highly significant improvement of stress is 1.5% to 2% of the cross-sectional area of the specimen. This study and others employing reinforcement of cement with carbon fibers indicate a method for future improvements in the mechanical properties of bone cement.

Barium sulfate frequently is admixed to the bone cement to provide radiopacity. The optimal radiographic densities for the acetabulum is provided by the addition of 2.5 g of barium sulfate to 40 g of powder and 5 g of barium sulfate for the shaft of the femur.[46] Rae[55] has studied the influence of sterile barium sulfate particles on mouse peritoneal macrophages grown in tissue culture. The macrophages show phagocytosis of the particulate barium sulfate with vacuolization of the cytoplasm. Barium sulfate, however, did not cause a release of lactic dehydrogenase from the macrophages and phagocytosis could not be implicated as a precipitant of intracellular damage. While barium sulfate is relatively insoluble, it has a solubility in water of about 2.5 μg/ml. It is conceivable that soluble moieties of barium sulfate could influence cells, although this seems unlikely in view of the small amount of material present and the slow rate of solubilization of barium sulfate.

Surface Finish of Articular Surfaces in Total Joint Replacements

For over a decade, Charnley[42] has argued that the surface finish of total joint replacements should be as smooth and regular as possible. Various workers have questioned the relationship between surface finish and the rate of erosion of surfaces. The more recent studies by Scott et al.[56] and Scott and Westcott[57] strongly suggest that a superior surface finish is consistent with a minimal rate of erosion. The degree of irregularity of a hemispherical surface is characterized by two criteria. Center line average (CLA) represents the average deviation of a surface profile from a line which makes the sum of the areas contained between itself and those parts of the profile which lie on either side of it. Whereas, CLA represents sphericity at the equator of a sphere, the total indicator reading (TIR) is a similar index of sphericity that represents sphericity of sagittal sections through the sphere as well as the sphericity of the equators. Root mean square (RMS) is an index of out-of-roundness that indicates both the width and depth of surface irregularities. The typical TIR of the best femoral head prostheses is about 2.5 μm. Out-of-roundness of a Stanmore total hip prosthesis is less than 10 μm RMS. These values suggest that a fluid-film thickness greater than 0.3 μm could be maintained. Ungethüm et al.[58] have measured the out-of-roundness of the McKee-Farrar metal-on-metal total hip and the Weber-Huggler metal-on-polymer model. The out-of-roundness figures varied greatly between comparable McKee-Farrar implants provided by different manufacturers, although the Weber-Huggler type prostheses exhibited relatively small roundness deviations. The standard deviations calculated for the femoral head prostheses ranged from 0.1 μm to 40 μm; the figures for the sockets ranged from 0.1 μm to 21 μm. The implants provided by two manufacturers consistently showed roundness deviations of the articular surfaces of less than 3 μm. These workers suggest that the maximum tolerable standard deviation of sphericity of the articulating surfaces should be 3.0 μm.

The friction in a total joint replacement is dependent upon the mode of lubrication, the nature of the materials, the geometry of the joint and the load imposed upon the joint. The measurements of the coefficient of friction between Co-Cr metal-on-metal prostheses are 0.4 to 1.5 in the dry state while similar measurements for Co-Cr on high density polyethylene (HDP) are 0.15 to 0.40. For stainless steel and HDP with synovial fluid lubricant in vitro, Walker and Bullough[59] report a coefficient friction of about 0.1. For artificial joints in vivo they estimate a coefficient of friction of about 0.8 for metal-on-metal joints and 0.02 for metal-on-plastic. The last results indicate a considerable degree of fluid film lubrication for artificial joints in man. They compare favorably with the figures obtained for cartilage-on-cartilage of 0.008. The coefficients of friction of various sliding materials are given in Table 13-2. After the initial postoperative healing period, the joint lubricant in vivo is likely to be highly similar to normal synovial fluid. The latter is a complex lubricant with non-Newtonian characteristics.[60] At low shear rates its viscosity is about 1 to 10 Ns/m^2 and at high shear rates its viscosity falls to 10^{-3} to 10^{-2} Ns/m^2. The static friction or "stiction-friction" in McKee-Farrar and Charnley-Müller prostheses has been compared with dynamic friction, recorded under oscillating conditions, by Simon et al.[61] Under physiological conditions, stiction-friction differs little from dynamic friction in both metal-on-metal and metal-on-plastic prostheses and is little affected by the lubricant as long as some fluid is present. Somewhat similar results have been reported by Chen et al.[62] Amstutz,[63] Gold et al.[64] and Walker and Salvati[65] have reported the coefficients of fric-

Table 13-2
Coefficients of Friction of Sliding Materials

Materials	Lubricant	Coefficient of friction
Cast cobalt-chromium alloy (metal-on-metal)	Dry	0.80
	Distilled H$_2$O	0.38
	Synovial fluid	0.16
	Globulin solution	0.16
	Albumin solution	0.18
	In vivo	0.04
Cast cobalt-chromium alloy against high density polyethylene	Synovial fluid	
	In vitro	0.04
	In vivo	0.02
AISI 316 alloy against high density polyethylene	Synovial fluid	
	In vitro	0.10
	In vivo	0.02
Cartilage-on-cartilage	In vivo	0.008

tion and wear analysis for a variety of polymeric materials articulating against Co-Cr or stainless steel alloys. None of the materials under test show superiority to HDP when various attributes of wear, coefficient of friction and potential toxicity of wear products are considered. Walker and Erkman[66] have studied the wear characteristics of HDP reinforced with carbon fibers, a material also discussed in Chapter 16. The reinforced material appears to have about a 30% superiority in wear rate. After wear tests with the carbon fiber reinforcement shell, however, slight scratching of the metal surface was observed which was not seen after comparable tests in which unreinforced HDP was studied. These workers also studied the effect of polymeric wear when the opposing metal surface was smooth or previously roughened with scratches up to 20 μinch (0.5 μm) in depth. No difference in polymeric wear was noted between the smooth and roughened metal surfaces. Perhaps the best explanation for this observation is the nature of the adhesive wear process of a polymer on a metal surface, whereby the initial erosion of polymer provokes transfer of the wear particles to the opposing metal surface. For the metal implants in their study, the degree of smoothness was between 2 μinch and 0.35 μinch CLA. On the basis of their study they questioned whether the expense needed to provide a greater degree of smoothness was justified. They provided some reassurance that minor scratches that arise accidentally during surgery should not

substantially affect the rate of wear of the polyethylene component. These findings have been confirmed by Buchholz and Strickle.[67]

Polyethylene acetabular cups have been fabricated in various ways. Hoechst, a West German supplier of ultra high molecular weight polyethylene in powder form, compresses some of the powder into a block, designated RCH-1000. Some manufacturers of orthopaedic products purchase RCH-1000 polyethylene blocks from which they prepare acetabular cups with a machine finish. Other manufacturers, such as Zimmer, mold acetabular cups directly from ultra high molecular weight polyethylene powder.[68] The latter process does not require the addition of releasing agents or other similar impurities to the polyethylene. The molded cups show a superior degree of surface finish without presence of machining grooves or other irregularities. Ainsworth[68] suggests that the superior surface finish may contribute to a lower degree of erosion in service.

Assessment of Wear in Total Hip Replacements

Prior to clinical application, all of the materials for use as bearing surfaces in total joint replacements have required examination in laboratory conditions which attempt to accurately simulate conditions of wear *in vivo*. Many workers have developed somewhat different types of laboratory screening tests, shown schematically in Figure 13-6*A*, for which the interested reader

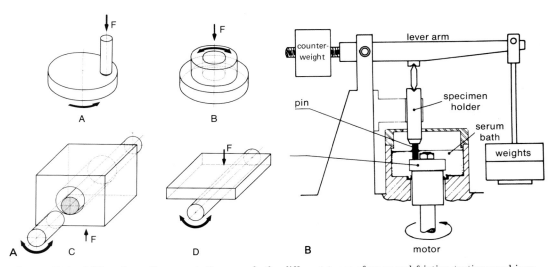

Figure 13-6. *A.* The schematic presentation reveals the different types of wear and friction testing machines: *A*, Pin-on-disc; *B*, ring-on-disc; *C*, journal-on-bush; *D*, block-on-journal. (Reproduced with permission of M. Ungethüm.[69]) *B*. The schematic diagram shows a pin-on-disc machine to assess wear rates for bearing surfaces for total joint replacements. (Reproduced with permission of J. T. Scales and K. W. J. Wright.[70])

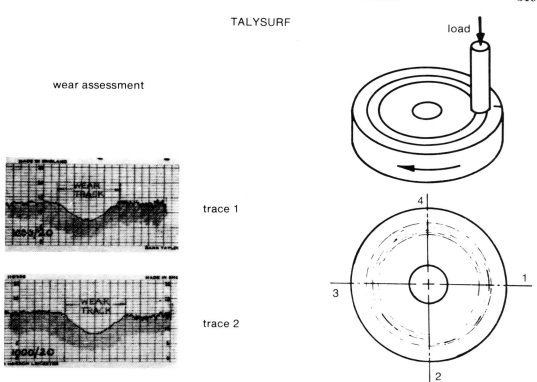

TALYSURF

load

wear assessment

trace 1

trace 2

Figure 13-7. The method and documentation of Talysurf assessment of wear track on disc is shown. (Reproduced with permission of J. T. Scales and K. W. J. Wright.[70])

is referred to the original reports.[63–65, 71, 72] At Stanmore a simple and reproducible study of wear characteristics of materials has employed a pin-on-disc machine (Fig 13-6B). The method employs a pin with a spherical radius at one end loaded vertically against the surface of a thick disc rotating about a vertical axis in a bath of bovine serum. An annular wear track is produced. Although tests can be performed for varying periods of time, measurable tracks are usually produced within 48 hours of study. The volume of eroded material is calculated from magnified profiles of the wear track using a Talysurf machine (Fig. 13-7). The attributes of the technique include much greater accuracy than assessment of weight loss from an eroded specimen and the inaccuracies of weight loss assessment of polymeric materials which can absorb water from the serum bath to show a spurious weight gain after test. While the pin-on-disc technique is notable for its simplicity it suffers from certain limitations.[73, 74] Unlike natural joints the relative motion of the rubbing surfaces is continuous rather than oscillatory to produce different lubrication regimes. The technique alters the wear areas of two bearing sur-

faces from those observed in hip prostheses. The effective radius of the contacting surfaces cannot readily be adjusted to give similar values to those of prostheses. Particularly for metal-on-metal combinations the surface stresses differ widely from those that would be observed in total hip joint replacements. With the pin-on-disc technique, wear debris is not necessarily trapped between the surfaces to augment wear in the way which may occur with total joint replacements. Scales and Wright[71] have employed a journal or bush test rig to overcome these limitations. The journal, mounted on a horizontal spindle, is oscillated at physiological rates comparable to relative loss of these bearing surfaces. The bush slides on the journal while immersed in a serum bath. The bush-housing is loaded with weights which are monitored by a strain gauge transducer to replicate the frictional torque developed across the bearing surfaces of total joint replacements *in vivo*. At Stanmore a hip joint simulator also is available which replicates a prosthetic ball and socket. In Figure 13-8, two comparable hip joint simulators to test the rate of wear of a ball-and-socket or cup are shown schematically. By the use of these and

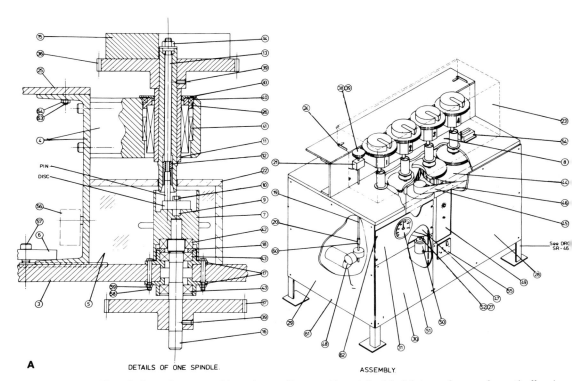

A   DETAILS OF ONE SPINDLE.   ASSEMBLY.

Figure 13-8. Two designs of wear machines that replicate motion at the hip joint are shown schematically. *A*, Stanmore MK 2 pin-on-disc machine (both pins and discs can be rotated). In *B* (p. 522), a ball-and-socket design used at Stanmore is seen, while in *C*, a hip joint simulator of the München type is revealed. (*A* and *B* reproduced with permission of J. T. Scales and K. S. J. Wright[70]; *C* reproduced with permission of M. Ungethüm.[73])

PIN on DISC MACHINE.(Mk.2.)

Part NO.	DRG NO.	Description	NO. off	Comments	Part NO.	DRG NO.	Description	NO. off	Comments
—	SR-18	GENERAL ASSEMBLY	—		24	SR-40	HINGE	2	
—	SR-46	Sub Assembly of STAND & MOTOR MOUNTING BRACKET	—		25	SR-45	TOP PLATE	1	
1	SR-19	STAND	1		26	SR-44	BEARING SPACER	4	
2	SR-31	MOTOR MOUNTING BRACKET	1		27	SR-51	MOTOR SHAFT EXTENSION	1	If required
3	SR-20	BASE PLATE	1		28	SR-48	PANEL (Front Right)	1	
4	SR-21	SPINDLE MOUNTING - 4a & BACK SUPPORT - 4b	4, 1		29	SR-49	PANEL (Side)	2	
5	SR-42	KEY (To mate part 3 with 4b)	2		30	SR-47	PANEL (Front Lower Left)	1	
6	SR-28	CLAMP	3		31	SR-50	STD INSTRUMENT PANEL	1	
7	SR-25	DISC CARRIER	4		32	SR-54	COVER HANDLE	1	
8	SR-43	TRIP PIN	1		33	SR-55	PROTECTIVE COVER	4	
9	SR-26	DISC SPIGOT	4						
10	SR-26	DISC NUT	4						
11	SR-29	COLLET HOLDER (Complete)	4		36	COMMERCIAL	GEAR (Pin Drive)	4	12 D.P × 100 teeth ¾ Face Width (Bore to suit SR-29)
12	SR-27	COLLET	4		37	"	GEAR (Disc Drive)	4	12 D.P × 100 teeth ¾ Face Width (Bore to suit SR-24)
13	SR-30	DRAW BAR	4		38	"	GEAR (Pin Drive)	1	12 D.P × 20 teeth ¾ Face Width (Bore to suit SR-35)
14	SR-30	NUT	4		39	"	M6 × 12LG Grub Screw	17	For securing gears to drive shafts
15	SR-41	WEIGHT	4		40	"	SUPPORT BEARING	4	T 37 (Hoffman)
16	SR-24	DRIVE SHAFT	4	Cut to appropriate length	41	"	LINEAR ROTATING BEARING	4	BIMO 4060 (Sterox)
17	SR-22	RADIAL BEARING HOUSING	8		42	"	THRUST BEARING	4	8205 (Claude Rye Ltd.)
18	SR-23	THRUST BEARING SUPPORT DISC	4		43	"	RADIAL BEARING	8	204 (Claude Rye Ltd.)
19	SR-35	LOW SPEED DRIVE SHAFT	1		44	"	PULLEY (Driven)	1	120 H 150 Taper Lock Bush to suit
20	SR-35	CONNECTOR	1		45	"	PULLEY (Driver)	1	20H 150 Taper Lock Bush to suit
21	SR-34	BEARING BLOCK	1		46	"	BELT	1	700 H 150
22	SR-39	SHEILD	1		47	"	MOTOR (Disc drive)	1	Morse Motor NO. MD 90130L (Borg Warner)
23	SR-53	HINGED COVER	1		48	"	MOTOR (Pin drive)	1	SD 13 MM (Parvalux Electric Motor Co.Ltd)

PIN on DISC MACHINE.(Mk.2.)

Part NO	DRG NO.	Description	NO. off	Comments	Part NO.	DRG NO.	Desciption	NO. off	Comments
49	COMMERCIAL	MOTOR SPEED CONTROL	1	Morse Cadet 75L (Borg Warner)	74	COMMERCIAL	M5 × 20LG Pan HD Self Tapping Screw	8	See DRG NO SR-40
50	"	TACHOMETER	1	ACA2/R3P Circscale Alternator (Record Electrical Co.Ltd.)	75	"	M4 × 20LG Cheese HD Screw	1	For securing MOTOR SPEED CONTROL to STAND
51	"	REV COUNTER DIAL	1	0/60 rpm. 6PA Circscale round indicator (Record Electrical Co.Ltd)	76	"	M4 Hex Nut	1	
52	"	COUPLING	1	Flexible Coupling DRG NO 900147 (Record Electrical Co.Ltd)	77	"	M3 × 10LG Csk HD Screw	2	For securing 3 PIN SWITCH SOCKET to PANEL (Front Right)
53	"	000 TAPER PIN	2	To suit COUPLING	78	"	M3 Hex Nut	2	
54	"	COUNTER	1	Type NO.032001 Lever NO 500005 Ratchet Counter (Hengstler)	79	"	M5 × 16LG Pan HD Self Tapping Screw	8	See DRG NO SR-53
55	"	3 PIN SWITCH SOCKET	1	STD 13 amp	80	"	M6 × 20LG Hex HD Screw	4	See DRG NO SR-54
56	"	MICRO SWITCH	1	4 CRQ (Burgess)	81	"	M5 × 30LG Hex HD Screw	4	For securing MOTOR (Pin drive) to STAND
57	"	M10 × 40LG Socket HD Bolt	3	See G.A.	82	"	M5 Hex Nut	4	
58	"	M6 × 45LG Titanium Hex HD Bolt	16	"	83	"	M4 × 40LG Hex HD Bolt	4	For securing COUNTER to BASE PLATE
59	"	M6 Hex Nut	16	"	84	"	M4 Hex Nut	4	
60	"	M6 × 8LG Grub Screw	2	"					
61	"	M4 × 10LG Pan HD Self Tapping Screw	28	"					
62	"	M6 × 12LG Pan HD Screw	4	"					
63	"	M6 × 25LG Csk HD Screw	3	"					
64	"	M6 Hex Nut	3	"					
65	"	M10 × 45LG Socket HD Bolt	12	See DRG NO SR-21					
66	"	Ø8 × 45LG Steel Dowel	8						
67	"	M10 × 25LG Socket HD Screw	4	For securing MOTOR (Disc drive) to MOTOR MOUNTING BRACKET					
68	"	M8 × 50LG Hex HD Bolt	4	For securing MOTOR MOUNTING BRACKET to BASE PLATE					
69	"	M8 Hex Nut	4						
70	"	M6 × 15LG Hex HD Screw	2	See DRG NO SR-31					
71	"	M6 Hex Nut	2						
72	"	M6 × 30LG Hex HD Screw	4	For securing BEARING BLOCK to BACK SUPPORT					
73	"	M5 × 16LG Pan HD Self Tapping Screw	11	See DRG NO SR-39					

Figure 13-8 Part A Cont.

Figure 13-8—cont.

1. Motor
2. Moving cam
3. Load cam
4. Spring assembly
5. Ball and cup

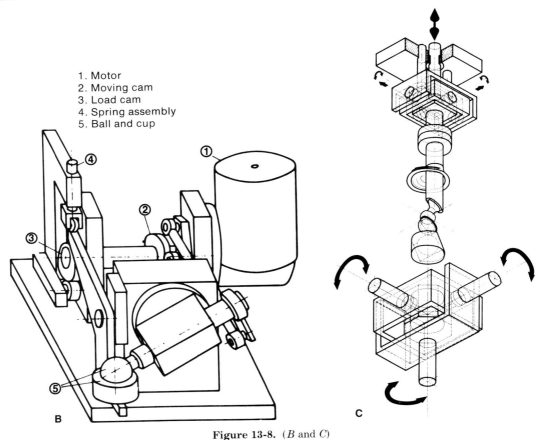

Figure 13-8. (*B* and *C*)

ancillary techniques the wear rates for a variety of materials currently in use and for potentially superior materials have been assessed. The tests provide a valuable qualitative assessment of the relative rates of erosion of various combinations of materials. As an accurate assessment of the absolute rate of wear predicted for total joints *in vivo* the methods are of limited accuracy. Charnley and Cupic[75] estimate the rate of wear of HDP components as 1.3 mm in 10 years (0.13 mm per year), but the method used to measure wear was criticized on the grounds that it could be influenced by the direction of wear of the prosthetic head into the socket. Estimates from the clinical impressions between 5 and 6 years after surgery suggested that the wear rates *in vivo* were from 0.1 to 0.2 mm per year. Charnley and Halley[76] employed a radiographic technique for patients with stainless steel on polyethylene joint replacements over a period of 9 to 10 years after surgery. For the group of patients the average age was 73.3 years at the end of the period of study. The average rate of wear was 0.15 mm per year and 68% of the patients followed this

pattern. Wear of more than 2.5 mm per decade occurred in 15%. There was a diminution in the rate of wear with the passage of time so that the rate of wear was approximately 40% less in the second 5-year period than in the first 5 years. Body weight and physical activity did not appear to have any relationship to the final amount of wear. In another report Halley and Charnley[77] evaluated a group of 39 patients under 30 years of age with diagnoses including rheumatoid arthritis, ankylosing spondylitis, congenital dislocation of the hip and various others. The wear did not seem to be any greater in this younger age group as compared to the previous study in older patients. The built-in restraints, however, of this group of patients largely with multiple joint disease may have influenced the rate of wear of the joints. Clarke *et al.*[78] have criticized the radiographic assessment of wear and cited its limited accuracy in view of the very low rate of erosion. In a limited study, Charnley* has recovered total hip joint replacements from pa-

---

* J. Charnley, personal communication, 1976.

tients who previously underwent total hip joint replacement and subsequently died from some unrelated cause such as myocardial infarction or cerebrovascular disease. He observed that the laboratory assessments of wear are about 100% overly optimistic compared with the observations for total hip joint replacements *in vivo.* Gold and Walker[64] reported the rates of wear for a variety of commercially available total hip joint replacements. The wear of Charnley joints made from stainless steel and Co-Cr alloy, was about the same. The 28-mm diameter joints showed less wear than the 22-mm diameter joints; whereas, the 32-mm models were no better than the 28-mm and were probably a little more inferior. There was no difference in wear between joints with about 100 μm clearance and 500 μm clearance. Lack of sphericity up to 10 μm in the femoral component did not appreciably alter wear. A surface finish of 0.05 to μm probably provoked less wear than a surface roughness greater than 1 μm. In the study of the rates of wear of a variety of polymeric materials, Amstutz,[63] failed to observe any material which showed superior rates of wear to those recorded from HDP. Walker *et al.*[72] studied the wear on removed McKee-Ferrar total hip prostheses that had remained *in vivo* for nearly 4 years. The articular surfaces showed multidirectional scratches with evidence of a secondary process of more generalized adhesive wear. A wear-depth of about 1 μm was observed on the specimens with an estimate of volumetric wear at about 5 mm^3. This can be compared with volumetric wear from metal-on-polymer joints, using the average annual wear depth of 130 μm quoted by Charnley and Cupic[75] which gives a volume of 50 mm^3. While the volume of metallic wear is much less than that of the polymer other considerations which determine the extent of tissue reaction to wear products include the sizes and number of particles and the ways in which the particles interact with body tissues.

Design Features in Total Hip Replacements

In addition to the characteristics of the articular surfaces, many other features of the design of a total hip replacement may contribute to its stability, range of motion and strength. These are discussed in turn for the femoral and the acetabular components.

Femoral Component

Stability and Range of Motion. One of the principal goals of total joint replacement is the

return of the joint to approximately normal function. Within the constraint previously described by Charnley[42] whereby excessive range of motion of the prosthetic joint might compromise long term fixation, nevertheless, the clinical goal is a range of motion that is not significantly less than that of a normal hip joint. The postoperative range of hip motion is related to many factors including the etiology of the disease, the quality of capsuloligamentous supports and features of design of the implant. Restricted motion of the implant secondary to neck-socket impingement of the component may contribute to subluxation and dislocation. Early postoperative dislocations may occur when the components forcibly exceed the permitted range of motion and overcome the passive capsular or active muscular retaining forces. Either the ball can climb the socket wall and ride over the socket rim without neck-socket impingement or, alternatively, the neck can contact the acetabular rim and lever the ball up and out of the recess. Rarely, a third mode of dislocation, impingement of bony prominences such as the greater trochanter against the lateral pelvic wall, may occur. In the first situation the diameter of the prosthetic femoral head is the main factor. With a larger ball a greater vertical distance must be transgressed before the ball reaches the rim so that a large ball will not dislocate as readily as a smaller one (Fig. 13-9). In the second mode, the ball-neck diameter ratio and the neck-socket

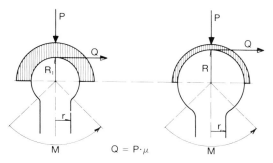

Figure 13-9. A schematic diagram shows two total hip joint replacements of smaller, R_1, and larger, R, radii of curvature of articulating surfaces. With a larger ball a greater vertical distance, Q, must be transgressed before the ball reaches the rim so that a large ball will not dislocate as readily as a smaller one. The large ball is also preferable because it will permit a greater arc of motion prior to impingement of the neck, r, on the socket. For a given sized space in the acetabulum, however, the wall of the socket can possess a greater thickness for the smaller ball than for the larger one.

Table 13-3
Simulated Ranges of Motion of Total Hip Protheses[a]

	Charnley	Bechtol	Harris	Trapezoidal-28	Aufranc-Turner	Müller
Flexion[b]	80	93	93	114	101	96
Internal rotation in flexion	0[c]	2	3	36	14	6
Abduction in extension	42	45	57	60	56	57
External rotation in extension	42	52	66	74	69	68

[a] Reproduced with permission of H. Amstutz and K. Markolf.[79]

[b] The flexion reported here is measured at 0° abduction and 0° external rotation; increases in either abduction or external rotation will increase the given angles.

[c] At 90° of flexion and 0° of abduction the femur was in external rotation.

rim shape are important factors. Early neck-socket impingement favors subluxation or dislocation. If the acetabular cavity is deepened either as a result of design or with prosthetic wear, the stability is enhanced but the range of motion is diminished. For example, the Charnley socket which accepts an 11-mm radius ball is intentionally deepened to 13 mm. Preservation of the capsular attachments at surgery and increasing passive muscular tension by trochanteric advancement also help to prevent dislocation.

Clinical dislocations occur most frequently during internal rotation with flexion and external rotation with extension. Various laboratory tests to record the degree of stability of total hip joint replacements have been discussed by Amstutz and Markolf.[79] The simulated ranges of motion of several currently available total hip prostheses are described in Table 13-3. The Trapezoidal-28 (T-28) design (Zimmer U.S.A., Warsaw, Ind.) shows the greatest degree of flexion, internal rotation, abduction with extension and external rotation with extension. The acetabular position for all prostheses tested was arbitrarily chosen for reference at 42° lateral opening and 22° anterior opening (anteversion). The femoral component was placed in a neutral position with 0° anteversion. While an increase in anteversion of either the socket or femoral neck will increase the arc of flexion and internal rotation with flexion, it will provide a corresponding decrease in external rotation and extension. Conversely, a decrease in anteversion of either component will result in increased external rotation and extension but a loss of both flexion and internal rotation and pure flexion. An increase in lateral opening will result in increased internal rotation and flexion as well as increased abduction but a loss of external rotation and extension will occur. The converse is likewise true. The T-28 prosthesis has a neck

with a noncircular cross-section. This feature of design is largely responsible for the enhanced motion of the prosthesis compared to the original Charnley design (Thackray, Ltd., Leeds, U.K.). It will be observed that flexion is increased by 34° or 42% while internal rotation with flexion is increased from 0 to 36° and external rotation with extension is increased from 42 to 74°.

In their electrogoniometric study Johnson and Smidt[80] observed that an average of 140° of hip flexion was required for sitting, 172° to rise from sitting to standing, 114° to squat, and 125° to stoop to pick up an object from the floor. While most total hip reconstructions would not permit these functions without subluxation, flexion can be increased by supplementary flexion of the pelvis on the lumbosacral spine. Greater arcs of flexion are also possible as some abduction and external rotation of the hip is permitted. In general 1° of flexion is gained for each degree of external rotation when abduction angles are near zero. This effect is enhanced as abduction increases and is diminished as external rotation increases. For all of the post-Charnley designs the increased range of motion has been accomplished by reduction in the socket depth, increased ball-neck diameter ratios and changes in neck and socket rim shape. Enhanced stability has been achieved by increasing the ball-neck diameter ratio to prevent a greater range of movement without neck-socket contact. Other clinical factors involved in dislocation, however, should be emphasized. The principal concern is an excessive angle of inclination of the acetabular cup although excessive anteversion of the acetabular cup or femoral component or insufficient muscular tension with improper reconstruction of the abductor muscles are contributing factors.

The safety factor in necks of many design appears to be adequate since no mechanical

Table 13-4

Head/Neck Diameter Ratios for Various Total Hip Replacement Prostheses[a]

Prosthesis	Head diameter	Head-neck diameter ratio
	mm	
Charnley	22.0	1.74
Bechtol	25.4	2.00
Harris	26.0	2.03
Trapezoidal-28	28.0	
Long axis of neck		1.72–2.01
Short axis of neck		2.97–3.24
Aufranc-Turner	32.0	
Long axis of neck		2.00
Short axis of neck		2.32
Müller	32.0	1.98

[a] Reproduced with permission of H. Amstutz and K. Markolf.[79]

failures have been recorded.[79] For the smaller diameters, between 22 and 28 mm, the neck cross-sectional area has been reduced with apparent safety. The T-28 total hip replacement has the lowest cross-sectional area of any available unit although the strength is augmented by the trapezoidal shape of the cross-section. The Aufranc-Turner prosthesis (Howmedica, Inc., Rutherford, N.J.) has an elliptical cross-section for a similar reason, to selectively improve the range of motion in flexion and in flexion with internal rotation. The head-neck diameter ratios for all hip units tested by Amstutz and Markolf[79] are shown in Table 13-4. Increased thickness in the vertical dimension of the neck theoretically should reduce abduction. This potential loss has been recovered in the T-28 unit by chamfer of the socket rim to provide an actual increase in the range of abduction. The socket chamfer has the additional advantage of guiding the prosthesis back into the socket should subluxation occur. Admittedly the long term stability of any of the prostheses may be altered by the degree of wear on the prosthetic components.

Strength of the Femoral Stem. The strengths of femoral stems have been reported by Markolf and Amstutz[79] and Weightman.[81] In 1973 Charnley[82] reported six femoral stem fractures from his early implants. Subsequently, Galante *et al.*,[83] and others[81] have reported mechanical failures of stems. Whereas one of the principal concerns by early workers was the optimal shape of stem to interdigitate with cement, more recently, workers have studied the attributes of strength of the femoral component to lessen the

likelihood of late fatigue fractures. Amstutz and Markolf[79] compared the features of the T-28, the Charnley and Müller prostheses (Protek, Ltd., Berne, Switzerland). Strain gauge instrumentation was applied to the femoral stems at the sites seen in Figure 13-10. Records were made while compressive forces were applied to the femoral heads in the frontal plane at nine different angles of inclination to simulate loading situations that might occur *in vivo*. The stresses at 12 locations on the stem and neck were calculated from the strain gauge readings and compiled as a function of loading angle. All strains were measured within the elastic limits. Two critical locations of interest, the neck and the stem were tested as simple cantilever beams (Fig. 13-11). The test results show the relative strengths of the various stem and neck configurations and indicated various potential sites of weakness. The cantilever beam mode of testing is the most severe in terms of tensile stress produced on the lateral surface of the stem. At the critical middle to distal stem locations where clinical failures have been observed, the higher stresses were recorded for the Müller prosthesis. The T-28 prosthesis showed relatively high stresses at the upper neck-flange junction (Fig 13-11A). Design modification of the neck reduced these stress values to the level for the Charnley and Müller prostheses while sacrificing only 1 or 2° from the range of motion previously described.

Loading tests on prostheses embedded in polymethylmethacrylate showed that the re-

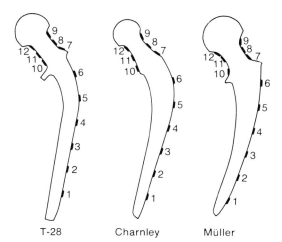

Figure 13-10. A schematic diagram shows the locations of strain gauges on the lateral aspect of the stems and on the superior and inferior aspects of the necks of three prostheses under test. (Reproduced with permission of H. C. Amstutz and K. L. Markolf.[84])

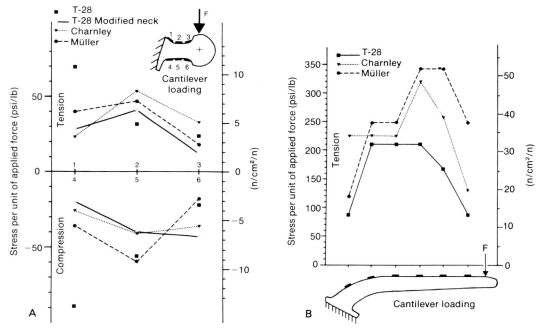

Figure 13-11. *A.* The results of cantilever loading of the femoral neck are shown. The highest stresses were measured at the upper neck-flange junction of long-necked Trapezoidal-28 (T-28) prostheses. *B.* The results of cantilever loading of the femoral stem are shown. The highest stresses in the distal half of the stem are recorded on Charnley and Müller prostheses. (*A* and *B*, reproduced with permission of H. C. Amstutz and K. L. Markolf.[84])

corded stress in the lateral surfaces of the stems are quite similar for all three prostheses despite substantial differences in stem geometries.

In Weightman's study,[81] the Charnley, Charnley extra-heavy duty, the Imperial College and the computer-aided design stem (CAD) standard curved and standard straight prostheses (Howmedica, Inc., Rutherford, N.J.) were compared (Fig. 13-12). The study was designed to extend the observations of Amstutz and Markolf.[79] Former workers[83] had shown that the stress levels and the stems were much higher when they were loose or supported only distally than when they were rigidly fixed over their entire length. While these results supported the conclusion of Charnley,[82] that the fatigue failure occurs because of a lack of proximal support, they did not answer the question of whether the stresses developed in properly cemented prostheses were dangerous and likely to provoke stem fractures. Weightman emphasized that the stress levels measured in stems rigidly fixed in acrylic cement are influenced by the thickness of the cement mass and may not be relevant to the *in vivo* situation. Alternatively, Amstutz and Markolf[79] concluded that inadequate stem de-

sign, varus placement, low strength metal and lack of adequate proximal medial support secondary to osteoporotic bone or inadequate supportive cement could contribute to dangerously high stress levels in femoral stems. Galante *et al.*[83] considered the question of stress levels in properly oriented and cemented stems. Although these workers found that the locations of fractures corresponded to the sites of maximal surface tensile stress predicted by the stress analysis of stems in a varus position, or loosened cement, they possessed insufficient knowledge about the fatigue properties of implant materials to predict whether current designs of femoral stems that were correctly positioned in the femur, would function indefinitely without undergoing fracture. In his study on the strength of femoral stems, Weightman observed that the optimal fatigue life for any given material will be found when the tensile stress on the convex lateral surface of the femoral stem is minimized. In any given situation of good or bad cement fixation, high or low strength bone, valgus or varus positioning of the stem, the value of the maximum tensile stress produced in a stem is a function of a design of the stem. Recently, two

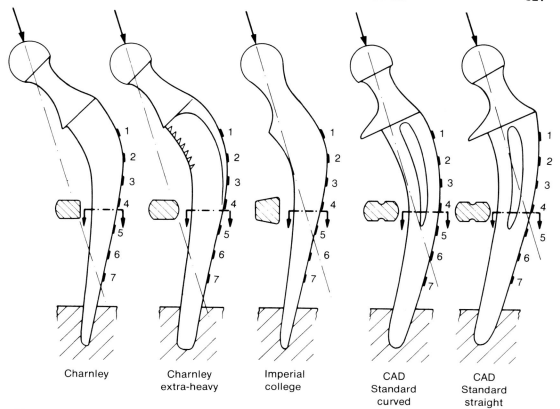

Charnley Charnley extra-heavy Imperial college CAD Standard curved CAD Standard straight

Figure 13-12. The schematic diagram indicates the details of five femoral stems under test. Both the stem profiles and the cross-sections of the midstem are revealed. The positions of the strain gauges are indicated along with the line of load action and the position of the clamp in the distal fixation test. (CAD, computer-aided design stem.) (Reproduced with permission of B. Weightman.[85])

new designs of stems have been introduced in an effort to thwart fatigue fractures. Howmedica has provided the CAD and Thackray has marketed the Charnley heavy and extra-heavy duty "cobra" design. The Howmedica design has been produced with the aid of a finite element computer program while the Charnley design attempts to reduce the stress in the stem by transferring an increased proportion of the supply load directly to the cement. Weightman employed strain gauge instrumentation to determine stress values in various regions of the femoral stems when implants were loaded in one of two configurations seen in Figure 13-12. In one case the stem was clamped at the tip in an especially designed fixture with the stem at an angle of 24° to the vertical and loaded to 2 KN in a material's testing machine. The angle of 24° was chosen so that the vertically applied load would simulate the average angle at which the resultant force is imposed upon on the hip *in vivo* in normal walking. In a second series of

tests designed to simulate the ideal clinical situation of cement fixation of the implant in bone along the entire length of stem, comparable loading conditions were repeated.

From the fatigue failure point of view the maximum tensile stress produced in each stem is the critical factor. The results for tests in which the stems were clamped at the tip indicate in decreasing order of merit the maximum tensile stresses shown in parentheses:

CAD standard straight	(20 MN/m^2)
Imperial College	(40 MN/m^2)
CAD standard curved	(50 MN/m^2)
Charnley extra-heavy duty	(95 MN/m^2)
Charnley	(145 MN/m^2)

At any given load the maximum tensile stress produced in the CAD standard straight stem, under conditions of zero proximal support will be a factor of 7.25 less than that produced in the

Charnley stem; in the Imperial College stem a factor of 3.6 less; in the CAD standard curved stem a factor of 2.9 less; and in the Charnley extra-heavy duty a factor of 1.5 less. Tensile stresses are produced on the lateral surface of the stems by the bending action of the applied load. For a given load the magnitude of the tensile stresses depends upon the moment arm of the load about the stem and the resistance to bending offered by the shape of the stem cross-section. Three factors contribute to the substantial difference in the results for the CAD standard straight stem and those observed for the Charnley stem. The moment arm of the applied load about the proximal stem is reduced by the increased neck angle of the CAD standard straight stem. Second, a moment arm is further reduced by the decreased curvature of the stem itself. Third, the cross-sectional area, or more accurately the second moment of area, of the CAD standard straight stem is greater to provide an enhanced resistance to bending. The explanation also applies to the other configurations of femoral stems.

The high compressive stresses produced at the distal end of the CAD standard straight and the Imperial College stems are the direct result of reducing the moment arm of the applied load about the proximal stem. As shown in Figure 13-12, the design features which reduced the moment arm about the proximal arm increase the moment arm about the distal stem.

Where the stems were totally embedded in cement the results in decreasing order of merit were as follows:

CAD standard straight	(22 MN/m^2)
CAD standard curved	(45 MN/m^2)
Imperial College	(55 MN/m^2)
Charnley	(68 MN/m^2)
Charnley extra-heavy duty	(72 MN/m))

For various experimental reasons including the position of the femoral stem, varying amounts of varus alignment, the diameters of the femoral shaft, the differences in the results should not be considered to reflect merely the design of the implants. Nevertheless, it is still evident that the maximal tensile stress in the Charnley and the Charnley extra-heavy duty stems are significantly lower when they are fully cemented in bone than when they are distally clamped. When a weak stem is reinforced by adequate amounts of cement and the presence of sound bone, the combined structure including

the cement and bone may carry a substantial portion of the applied load. For a strong stem the addition of cement and bone shows less effect. The maximum tensile stress in the distally clamped Charnley stem was over 100% greater than when it was cemented. In the Charnley extra-heavy duty the maximum tensile stress was 30% greater without cement and bone support and in the CAD standard curved about 10% greater. With the Imperial College stem and the CAD standard straight stem the maximum tensile stress actually increased when cemented in bone although this probably represented variable amounts of varus alignment of the stem.

The results of the tests suggest that the large neck collars on the CAD stems, the T-28 stem or the cobra-like flange on the Charnley extra-heavy duty stem have little or no effect on the stresses produced in the stems. Although the collars are designed to reduce the load and the stress on the stems by transferring part of the applied load directly to the cortical bone, they do not function as anticipated.

The results indicate that on the commercially available femoral stems under scrutiny the Howmedica CAD stems are the least likely to experience fatigue failure *in vivo*. Unfortunately, the observation that the peak stresses in these stems and in the Imperial College stem were not significantly reduced when they were cemented in bone, suggests another liability of these designs. The stems are so stiff that most of the applied load is carried directly by the stem and little by the adjacent cortical bone of the proximal femur. Stress protection, therefore, with secondary osteoporosis of the protected bone, may be anticipated. Wilson and Scales[86] and Charnley[82] have all observed clinical evidence of such stress protection. Further work on the optimal configuration of femoral stem design is clearly indicated. The design should possess excellent resistance to fatigue failure without excessive stiffness (*e.g.*, less than a magnitude greater than that possessed by the bone itself). Alternatively, at least for many applications, future implants may attempt to eliminate the need for the stem altogether, as described below.

Firm statistical data on fatigue fracture femoral stems are not readily available. Charnley[82] reported on his 10-year experience with 6500 prostheses followed for at least 3½ years. Fractures of the femoral component were observed between 1½ and 6 years after surgery. The overall rate of incidence of fractures was 0.23% with an incidence of 6% in patients weighing more than 88 kg. Andriacchi *et al.*[87] published an investigation of 6 cases involving failed femoral components. The literature was reviewed and incidence of fractures between 0 and 1% were reported. Ducheyne *et al.* reported two fractured femoral components by 2½ years postsurgery out of a total of 90 Charnley total hip prostheses. For 56 Charnley-Müller total hip prostheses the incidence of fracture was 11%, 6 prostheses failing out of a total of 56. It seems likely that substantially larger numbers of fractures will emerge unless substantial changes are made in the design of presently available implants.[87]

Acetabular Design Component

A variety of minor alterations of the acetabular component has been undertaken by several workers in an attempt to provide greater motion and stability. From the early experience of Charnley, the general configuration of the acetabulum has been a polyethylene cup with a metal wire to serve as a radiological marker of alignment of the acetabulum. Charnley and others have attempted to employ the metallic marker as an index of the amount of erosion of the socket. The distance between the most superior and medial portion of the femoral head and the plane of a wire marker was measured on X-rays taken at various times after surgery. The rate of wear of presently available sockets is of such a small magnitude that the radiological measurements are of limited value. As an index of alignment of the acetabulum, likewise the wire provides an inaccurate assessment. Clarke *et al.*[78] have undertaken radiological studies *in vitro* which confirm the difficulty in assessment of the position of acetabular wires *in vivo*. To enhance the range of motion of the socket and to limit the likelihood for posterior dislocation, Charnley extended the posterior rim with favorable results. On the T-28 design a chamfer was provided to encourage spontaneous reduction of a subluxed femoral head. The nonarticular surface of the implant has been altered with a variety of grooves and ridges to augment interdigitation of cement into the implant. To the author's knowledge, no studies are available which reveal the superiority of any available design.

During the early years of clinical implantation of polyethylene sockets, many workers anticipated a moderately rapid rate of erosion of polyethylene with a need for replacement of the articular surface after 5 to 10 years.[88] As mentioned previously, this problem has not arisen in practice. Nevertheless, the concern stimulated workers such as Harris[89] to develop acetabular

components in which the articular surface could be replaced without disturbing the cement interface with bone. Harris designed a Vitallium socket which cemented into the pelvis. The socket was lined with a polyethylene component that could be unscrewed for rapid replacement upon surgical revision. With the anatomical limitations on the outer diameter of a socket, the polyethylene liner was necessarily of diminished thickness compared to a solid polyethylene socket. At present there appear to be no indications for the use of such a multicomponent socket.

Harris[89] and others have also attempted to use polyethylene sockets in which the principal weight-bearing portion subjected to erosion was of substantially greater thickness than the nonweight-bearing portion of the socket. This technique appears to have considerable merit.

Variations in the Design of Total Hip Joint Replacements

Since the introduction of total hip arthroplasty by Charnley, numerous workers have introduced unique designs with various attributes. Most of these have not withstood the test of time. The interested reader can study these designs elsewhere.[90] Nevertheless, four design parameters are of particular interest and are mentioned briefly.

Within the inherent liability of separate acetabular and femoral components to sublux or dislocate, Sivash[91] was encouraged to design a mechanically articulating prosthesis. The articulation was accomplished by the prosthetic socket encompassing more than 50% of the ball. The fixed articulation of the ball-and-socket simplified insertional techniques and reduced the usual requirement for careful positioning. A range of flexion of 88° was provided. As initially designed, the implant did not require the use of cement, although it could be employed if the surgeon so desired. The design was brought to the United States by Russin,[92] who observed similar good results in a series of animal experiments. The implant was constructed in a somewhat unusual fashion. The stem and acetabular components are made of 6-Al 4-V titanium alloy. The ball of the prosthesis is composed of HS-21 cast Co-Cr alloy. The Co-Cr ball is controlled to a tolerance of sphericity of 50-millionths of an inch with a smoothness tolerance of 4-millionths of an inch. The plastic socket liner is made of RCH-1000C ultra high molecular weight polyethylene. The surgical indications for the implant were listed as degenerative arthritis (pro-

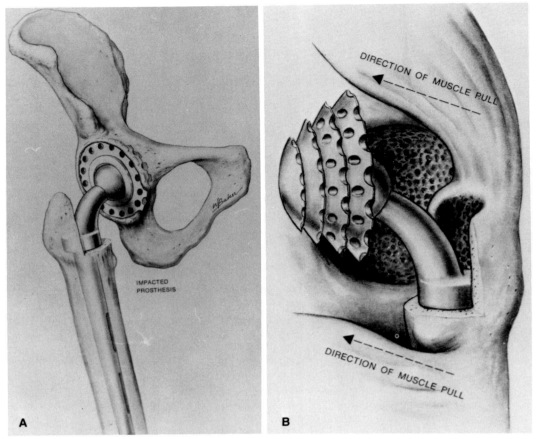

Figure 13-13. *A* and *B.* Schematic diagrams show the Sivash total hip joint prosthesis. (Reproduced with permission of L. A. Russin.[92])

vided that the bone is not osteoporotic), congenital dysplasia of the hip where the acetabulum will accommodate the prosthetic component, acetabular fractures where total hip joint replacement is indicated and replacement of failed prostheses. The device is shown in typical application in Figure 13-13.

The Sivash prosthesis is shown as an example of conflicts that arise in the mechanical criteria and design of total joint replacement. Most attempts to provide marked increase in the stability of a prosthesis provoke the transfer of dynamic loads to undesirable sites such as the interface between the implant and the bone. The articulating surfaces also share in these excessive loads and are thereby rendered more likely to undergo mechanical failure. Where the implant is used to augment the apparently deficient biological stability, mechanical failure of the implant or loosening is even more likely to occur. Therefore, the author would not recommend the Sivash device for any application.

Several workers have studied metal-to-plastic trunnion-bearing prostheses. In these implants the femoral component ends abruptly in a short cylindrical shaft with a flange at the level of the anatomical femoral neck. A polymeric ball is free to rotate on this shaft and articulates with the hemispherical bearing surface of the acetabular component, as indicated in Figure 13-14. Christiansen and Weber,[93] two proponents of this system, recommend that the wear is distributed between pairs of bearing surfaces and that the ball can be replaced, if necessary, without disturbing the attachment of either the femoral or the acetabular component to bone. Antagonists argue that the heaviest loads in the ball act nearly through its center but at an angle of about 35° to the axis of the shaft, so that high stresses are concentrated at the lower part of the flange and at the upper end of the shaft to provide rapid eccentric wear of the plastic ball. Somewhat similar implants have been employed for endoprosthetic replacement when the ball

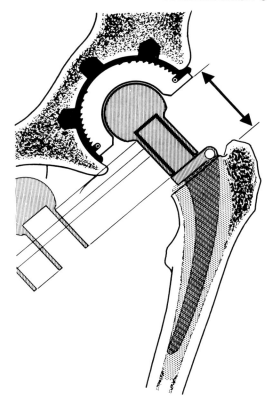

Figure 13-14. A schematic diagram shows the Weber trunnion-bearing prosthesis (Reproduced with permission of Allo Pro Ag, Baar/Zug, Switzerland.)

articulates against the cartilaginous surface of the acetabulum and rotates on a trunnion.[94, 95]

The shortcomings of the trunnion-bearing systems have been reported by several workers.[42] Perhaps the most serious flaw in the design is that dislocation of the ball on the trunnion is virtually inevitable if the ball dislocates from its opposing acetabular surface. Open reduction becomes the only method of treatment with its likelihood for deleterious side-effects such as a deep wound infection. Charnley and others have observed that when the polyethylene component is the ball instead of the socket, progressive erosion of polyethylene is accompanied by eccentricity of the ball. In contrast, the eroded polyethylene socket is observed to be a highly regular surface. Even with the 11-mm Charnley device, the central cylindrical erosion in polyethylene shows a regular hemispherical surface. With the eccentricity of wear observed in the trunnion-bearing system, the rate of wear of the ball is likely to increase with time.

For at least a decade the surface replacement of the hip joint has been studied by several workers, including Freeman,[96] Walker, Wagner[97] and Amstutz et al.[98] All of these workers have employed a polyethylene socket to line the acetabulum and a stainless steel or Co-Cr hemisphere to cover the articular surface of the proximal femur. The opposing hemispheres or shells have been attached to bone by methylmethacrylate cement. The early observations in experimental animals indicated several problems including avascular necrosis of the femoral head with late collapse and loss of alignment of the implants, fractures of the femoral neck, loosening of the components, and difficulties in the surgical alignment of the femoral component. Most of these problems have been solved by the various workers in this field. Reaming of the femoral head requires careful alignment and the use of jigs since the osteoarthritic femoral head may be markedly irregular. Careful selection of the cases is necessary so that femoral heads with marked destruction secondary to avascular necrosis or other pathological entities are treated with conventional prostheses. Until further clinical evaluation is available, the role of these implants remains unclear. Intrinsic advantages should include the minimal removal of bone stock and a provision for fusion of a failed total hip. It is not unlikely that the infection rates observed for the resurfacing procedures will be less than those documented for patients in which the implants possess intramedullary stems.

One other type of implant under assessment is the coated porous prosthesis in which anchorage is achieved by ingrowth of bone into a highly irregular surface. Sintered Co-Cr implants, a variety of ceramics and others are under scrutiny at the present time. For at least 2 years the ceramic devices[99, 100] (Fig. 13-15) have been employed while the author has utilized the sinter-coated Co-Cr implants for approximately 1½ year. The preliminary observations suggest that

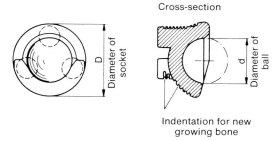

Figure 13-15. A schematic diagram shows a ceramic socket for replacement of the acetabulum. The device consists of a spherical cup with three anchoring pins. (Reproduced with permission of M. Salzer et al.[101])

ingrowth of bone provides a rapid, secure attachment of the prostheses which is maintained for the limited period of observation currently available. The excessively brittle ceramics are liable to brittle fracture, which would appear to be a substantial liability. Further observations are clearly needed. The ideal combination would appear to be porous coated resurfacing prostheses so that two hemispheres are employed without the need for methylmethacrylate cement. This concept is discussed in Chapter 16.

Complications of Total Hip Joint Replacements

After total hip joint replacement, a number of complications may arise which can be classified into those of a strictly mechanical nature, biological problems related to the presence of the implant or to the operation itself, and still others that are of general medical implication such as thromboembolic disease. In the following discussion the local problems are described while those that are primarily of clinical implication, such as thromboembolic disease, are presented in Chapter 14.

Subluxation and Dislocation of Implants. With the presently available implants, most dislocations arise as the result of a surgical error. The problem is prevented if the surgeon undertakes a trial range of motion prior to and after cement fixation of the components. Since the hip can be located by positioning the hip in internal rotation with flexion or external rotation with extension, dislocation in the early postoperative period may occur if the hip assumes a similar position. In the immediate postoperative period when the patient may be drowsy, the position of the lower extremity should be controlled by traction or an abduction splint or pillow so that undesirable positions cannot occur. For about 6 weeks after surgery, the patient must avoid excessive flexion of the hip or extension with external rotation while the capsule heals around the prosthesis. After that period of time, spontaneous dislocation of a correctly aligned implant is unlikely to occur. Nevertheless, Charnley[42] has documented a series of patients who undergo apparently spontaneous dislocation of the implant with minimal trauma many years after surgical implantation. The explanation for this problem remains obscure. Another group of patients may show traumatic dislocation of their prosthetic hip such as might also be observed for patients with anatomical hips. Usually, closed reduction is successful.

For those patients who show early postoperative and atraumatic dislocation of their prosthetic hip, malalignment is the likely cause. Even if a closed reduction is successful, subsequent surgical correction of the malalignment is usually necessary to prevent the otherwise anticipated recurrent dislocation.

Loosening of Implants. Loosening of implants is an uncommon problem that is generally accompanied by mechanical hip pain. It is likely that many implants that ultimately are found to be loose show micromotion immediately after solidification of cement. Close scrutiny of the interface between the cement and the bone may reveal the presence of bubbles or of a transmitted fluid wave when a compressive force is applied to it. When these diagnostic signs of loosening are present, the implant and cement should be removed immediately and a new implant should be inserted. Loosening is of particular concern in patients who undergo recurrent falls, such as alcoholics or certain competitive athletes. Loosening also may be indicative of infection with resorption of bone. A slightly higher incidence of loosening has been observed with the McKee-Ferrar metal-on-metal prosthesis than with the metal-on-polymeric implants. Charnley[42] attributes this difference to the discrepancy in the coefficient friction of the dissimilar implants. At the time of surgery, close approximation of the cement to the bone substantially lessens the likelihood for a poor bond. An intervening layer of blood is likely to hinder such a close approximation. The bony surfaces should be rendered dry and free of blood immediately prior to the insertion of cement.

Wound Infection after Total Hip Replacement. Perhaps the single greatest complication of total hip joint replacement remains postoperative infection. In his early studies, Charnley[42] noted an incidence of infection of up to 8%. Rigorous aseptic measures were developed, as described in Chapter 8, which greatly diminished the concentration of bacteria in the intraoperative environment and was associated with diminution of the infection rate. At present, acceptable rates of infection are less than 1%. In addition to a rigorous aseptic technique, many workers have questioned the role of antibiotics in the immediate preoperative period as well as during and after the procedure. Interested readers should see several other reviews.[102-104] Kolczun and Nelson[105] and others have shown that within 2 hours after intravenous administration of various antibiotics, a concentration is realized in bone that approximates the level recorded in the blood stream. There seems no need, therefore, to provide antibiotic coverage for more than 2 hours prior to surgery. Antibiotics administered for a longer duration provide enhanced opportunity for resistant organisms to multiply. Several workers[106] have reported that upon the application of routine, so-called prophylactic antibiotics, the incidence of infection may assume the same low level as those series in which clean air environment and other more elaborate measures are used. At this time, the relative merits of routine antibiotics and of other methods remain unclear. The protagonists of routine antibiotics suggests that a single agent such as an antistaphylococcal antibiotic may be employed to prevent spread through the blood or from the wound to the site of the implant at a time prior to multiplication of the organisms. The antagonists of this method argue that there is no statistical data to support the routine administration of antibiotics and that drug resistance is much more likely to develop with such widespread application. In the author's practice, a cephalosporin is given by intravenous administration from about 2 hours prior to surgery until about 2 days after surgery.

Another concept in the use of antibiotics with total joint replacement has been the incorporation of an antibiotic into methylmethacrylate cement. Levin,[107] Hill et al.[108] Elson et al.[109] and many others have reported on the incorporation of fusidic acid, gentamicin and clindamycin into acrylic cement. The results have been somewhat conflicting. There seems little doubt that the antibiotics may be slowly released from the cement into the surrounding tissues at the site of minimal host resistance to infection for periods of up to a few months. The precise durations of clinically effective antibiotics in useful concentrations have been highly variable. Some workers, such as Buchholz and Engelbrecht[110] have recommended highly this practice, while others such as Hill et al.[108] discourage it from several points of view. The need for prolonged antibiotic activity depends upon the unproven role of blood-borne infection and the causation of periarticular infection. The presence of a small concentration of antibiotics over a prolonged time provides the optimal environment for the development of resistant organisms. Antibiotics can provoke hypersensitivity to adjacent or distant tissues. When an antibiotic is released slowly from cement, it provides an excellent opportunity for initiation of hypersensitivity which could necessitate removal of the implant and the adjacent cement. Further observations in this field are clearly needed.

Other Biological Complications of Total Hip Joint Replacement. Hypersensitivity of Co-Cr wear particles in McKee-Farrar total hip joint replacements has been described by several workers and is fully discussed in Chapter 7. Cutaneous hypersensitivity to methylmethacrylate cement also has been reported by surgeons and is discussed in Chapter 7. The latter is prevented by avoidance of cutaneous exposure to cement. Deep vein thrombosis, occasionally with pulmonary embolus, is a well recognized complication of all types of hip surgery, including total hip joint replacement. It is discussed in Chapter 14. Intra-abdominal complications of total hip joint replacement have included paralytic ileus secondary to the evolution of heat from solidifying cement, direct trauma to major vessels and intra-abdominal organs and aneurysms of the common iliac artery and its branches, secondary to the solidification of cement and to infections in the prosthetic joint. All of these are discussed in Chapter 14.

Tools for Use with Total Hip Joint Replacement

Several of the surgeons who have developed total hip joint replacement have provided a complete set of instruments to facilitate the operation. Interested readers should consult the original authors.[42, 111] Nevertheless, a few salient features of their designs merit comment here. Charnley[42] developed a unique series of instruments, including retractors and acetabular reamers, which have been widely employed by other workers. The acetabular reamer has a similar appearance to a conventional brace and bit. The diameter of the cutting head can be altered during use by rotation of an attached wheel. The reamer requires a central pilot hole for anchorage. Many other types of reamers have been provided by other workers, of which the author favors the MIRA power reamer with disposable blades. This device provides exceptionally rapid cutting of bone and an inexpensive method for replacement of the cutting edges. Whereas Charnley employs a Gigli wire saw, other workers have developed oscillating blades to facilitate transection of the femoral neck. The author prefers one of the latter designs of air-powered instruments with reciprocal motion of the cutting edge. Similarly, power drills are available to prepare the anchoring holes in the acetabulum. Injection of cement into the intramedullary cavity of the femur is facilitated by the use of an injection gun.[112] With such an instrument, the proximal femur can be completely filled with methylmethacrylate. Concern has arisen, however, that fat emboli may be disseminated into the systemic circulation when cement is injected with such force. The clinical significance of such emboli remains unclear. For insertion of the acetabular and femoral components a variety of jigs have been employed to assist in alignment of the implant. The use of an acetabular jig is essential if correct alignment is to be realized.

ARTHROPLASTIC RECONSTRUCTION OF THE KNEE

Biomechanics of the Knee

The development of arthroplastic techniques for use in the knee joint has been greatly hampered by the complexities and limited knowledge of the biomechanics of the knee joint.

A mobile knee joint is needed for efficient human walking and sitting. In walking, the knee permits the lower extremity to become a multisegmental pendulum to ease the energy required for swing and deceleration. Acting in concert with the hip and ankle, the bendable knee shortens the leg during swing and allows for movement without unnecessary vertical motion of the center of gravity as would be required if the pelvis had to be elevated to clear the swinging limb. In sitting, flexion of the knee permits comfortable hyperflexion of the hips so that the gluteal fat pads approximate the sitting surface. While knee motion is not employed in standing and lying, the fully extended knee locks spontaneously so that standing on straight knees can be accomplished without muscular activity. The knee locks by a screwing-home mechanism so that active muscular activity is needed to unlock it. As the knee approximates full extension, the femur rotates internally on the tibia. Rotation of the knee permits the tibiofemoral angle to be slightly valgus and still permits the tibia to flex in alignment with the femur. Tibiofemoral angulation, combined with adduction of the hip, diminishes excessive lateral displacement of the center of gravity and gait by enabling the feet to be positioned much closer together than they would be if the limbs were parallel (Fig. 13-16). With the feet close together, walking can be accomplished without marked shift in the center of gravity across the lateral plane which would require much greater expenditure of energy for gait.

As Radin[114] has emphasized, the knee is a hinge joint with gliding surfaces and no fixed articulation. The articular surfaces are curved in

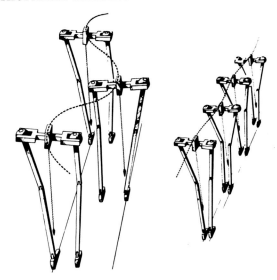

Figure 13-16. Through the influence of the tibiofemoral angle and adduction of the hip, excessive lateral displacement of the center of gravity in gait is prevented and the energy requirement for walking is diminished. (Reproduced with permission of J. B. Dec et al.[113])

three planes so that rotation may occur. The spaces created by the rounding of the corners are filled with washers made of fibrocartilage, the menisci, which provide additional stability.

Stability in the knee is realized both by the intricate design of the articular surfaces and by the presence of dense ligaments. The central aspects of the femoral condyles articulate against the periphery of the tibial spines. The unequal size of the femoral condyles (Fig. 13-17) directs rotational motion of the tibia on the femur.[116] The medial condyle is larger than the lateral so that the tibia is encouraged to rotate externally during extension. In flexion, the tibia rotates internally. The rotation of the tibia on the medial condyle is readily perceived as the tibia forming an arc about the lateral condyle during knee motion.

Motion of the knee is largely governed by the cruciate ligaments. As Huson[117] has pointed out, the cruciate ligaments function as a closed kinematic chain between the femur and the tibia (Fig. 13-18). The two chains or cruciate ligaments remain in tension throughout the range of motion and the axis of motion shifts during rotation. During extension, the tibia glides in an anterior direction on the femur while the opposite occurs with flexion. As Goodfellow* has

---

* J. Goodfellow, personal communication, 1976.

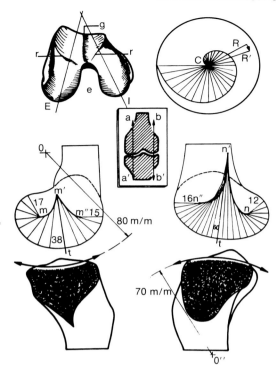

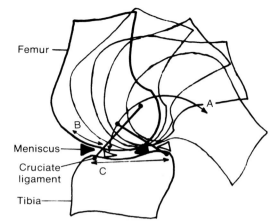

Figure 13-18. With flexion and extension of the knee, anteriolposterior gliding movement occurs between the inferior surface of the menisci and the tibial plateaus. (See also Fig. 13-19.) (Reproduced with permission of F. B. Smith and J. Blair.[118])

Figure 13-17. The marked asymmetry of the medial and lateral compartments of the knee joint is shown. The medial compartment is on the *right* and the lateral compartment is on the *left*. (Reproduced with permission of N. Gschwend.[115])

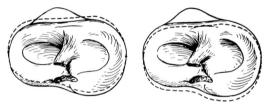

Figure 13-19. The menisci move anteriorly in full extension (*left*). The menisci move posteriorly in flexion (*right*). (See also Fig. 13-18.) (Reproduced with permission of F. B. Smith and J. Blair.[118])

shown, the rolling motion of the knee occurs between the femoral condyles and the superior surfaces of the menisci. The anteroposterior gliding motion occurs between the inferior surface of the menisci and the tibial plateaus (Figs. 13-18 and 13-19). The medial and to a lesser extent, the lateral collateral ligament remains taut in all degrees of flexion.[119] The posterior and posteromedial capsules augment stability of the knee. The medial ligament is the main strut of the capsular tissues of the knee. The deep portion is a thickened part of the capsule itself and is adherent to the meniscus. The superficial part forms a strong broad strap of triangular shape. It takes origin immediately distal to the adductor tubercle and inserts broadly into the medial surface of the tibia at least 1½ inches distal to the joint line. Its posterior border has continuity with the strong posterior capsule of the knee joint. Anteriorly, it has fibrous connections with the quadriceps expansion and the patellar ligament. Inevitably, such a broad and firm structure participates in all movements of the knee both by its structure and its intimate connec-

tions with the anterior and posterior muscles of the thigh. The lateral ligament extends in two layers from the lateral epicondyle of the femur to the head of the fibula and plays a minor role in the stability of the knee joint.

A prerequisite for successful tibiofemoral motion is alignment in the frontal plane. The body weight is exerted along the vertical line from the center of gravity and normally passes medially to the knee of a human standing on one foot. This vector tends to make the femur tilt on the tibia. It is counterbalanced by a lateral dynamic stay comprised of the iliotibial band, the tensor fascia lata and the gluteus maximus. The summation of these frontal forces represents the total load supported by the knee in this plane. The resultant force crosses the knee in the area of the tibial spine (Fig. 13-20). The surface area of the knee joint under physiological load has

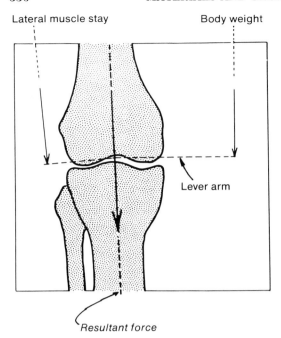

Figure 13-20. Both body weight and the lateral dynamic stay act on the knee through a lever arm. The resultant force passes through the tibial spines. (Reproduced with permission of E. L. Radin.[120])

been estimated at about 23 cm², which is larger than the contact area of the hip joint.

The dynamics of knee motion has been studied in great detail by many workers for which the interested reader is referred to the studies by Paul,[121] Frankel[122] and Maquet.[123] During a normal walking cycle, maximal flexion and swing-phase is about 75°. Rotation of the knee joint in the horizontal plane ranges from about 4 to 13° with a mean of 8.7°. Other workers, such as Kettelkamp and Nasca,[124] have observed a larger range of rotation with a mean of about 13°. Normal sitting requires better than 110° of flexion. There remains a considerable controversy in the literature as to the role of the so-called "instant centers" of knee motion as viewed laterally (Fig. 13-21A).[114, 125] It is likely that there are individual variations in the locations of these instant centers even in normal individuals. An analysis of forces transmitted through the knee is well described by Paul.[121]

The patella functions as a sesamoid bone to augment the mechanical advantage of the quadriceps tendon (Fig. 13-21B). The articular surface of the patella is divided into three principal facets, a large lateral, a smaller medial and an odd facet. None of these areas is truly congruous

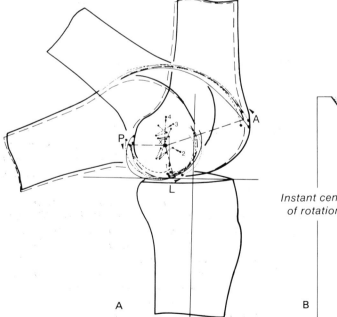

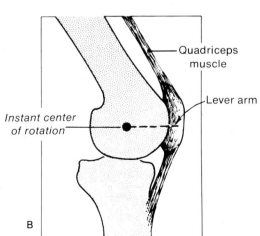

Figure 13-21. A. The flexion of four normal knees is described by tracing points P, A and L on the femur relative to the tibia. The loci of the instant centers of rotation are plotted for each knee and the differences are apparent. X is the "average instant center" and if the paths of P, A and L are traced about the fixed point X, the result is close to the normal. (Reproduced with permission of P. S. Walker.[125]) B. The patella serves to increase the lever arm of the quadriceps force as it acts upon the knee. (Reproduced with permission of E. L. Radin.[126])

with the patellar groove of the femur. The medial and lateral facets are separated by a vertical rounded ridge which fits into the trochlear surface of the femur. When the knee is flexed, the patella migrates to the under aspect of the femoral condyles, where the trochlear surface is prolonged onto the inner condyle. In flexion, the patella tilts away from the lateral condyle so that only the inner part of its articular surface rests against the medial condyle. As Bullough *et al.*[23] have shown, physiological incongruity is a feature of healthy joints such as the patellofemoral articulation. With early degenerative change, the joints become progressively more congruent. The physiological significance of the incongruity appears to be related to the lubrication of joints.

Biomechanical Changes in the Arthritic Knee. The pattern of knee motion during walking is substantially altered in both degenerative and rheumatoid arthritis. It is useful to compare and contrast these changes with the events that occur in the normal knee. As mentioned previously, the normal knee shows about 75° of flexion in walking, 85° while climbing stairs, 100° while sitting and 120° when picking up an object from the floor. During normal walking, over 3 times body weight is imposed upon the tibial plateaus, while over 4 times body weight is imposed when climbing stairs. Degenerative arthritis is usually accompanied by varus deformity of the knee. With genu varum there is a decrease or loss of stance phase flexion-extension. The pattern of abduction-adduction and rotation also is abnormal, although without an absolute diminution in the range of motion. In severe rheumatoid arthritis, often with concomitant valgus deformity, there is virtually no flexion-extension throughout gait. Abduction-adduction and rotation persist in mostly abnormal patterns. Other changes have been discussed by Kettelkamp and Nasca.[124] With severe degenerative or rheumatoid change, fixed flexion deformity is a constant finding which compromises gait and other activities.

Walker[125] has provided a concise outline of the mechanical principles of the knee which are shown schematically in Figures 13-22 to 13-24. As a reference to describe the motion and forces, orthogonal axes, X, Y and Z, are drawn. Abduction and adduction occur about the X-axis, rotation about the Y-axis and flexion-extension about the Z-axis. Anteroposterior glide is a linear movement along the X-axis. If the femur flexes through a small angular range in the lateral XY plane, then a point can be located about which the femur rotates relative to the tibia. This point is termed the "instant center" of rotation. Since the instant center changes continuously as the knee moves, the locus of its path can be used to describe the motion.

The forces and moments acting at the knee joint produce stresses of various structures. As seen in Figure 13-22, force, T, in the extensor tendon of an area, A, creates a tensile stress, TA. The load on the condyle compresses the cartilage to form areas of contact A_m and A_l in the medial and lateral compartments, with compressive stresses of W_m/A_m and W_l/A_l. When there is sliding between the condyles, shear stresses are developed due to friction. Their magnitude is given by the friction force, F, divided by area, A. The force, F, itself is related to the vertical (normal) force by the coefficient of friction, μ: $F = \mu : W$. In human joints, μ is minute, usually about 0.01, although it can be 0.05 to 0.15 in artificial joints.

Passive rotation of the femur on the tibia about the Y-axis (transverse rotation) increases as the flexion angle is increased, and although only a few degrees at full extension, it usually reaches 30° at midflexion. Walking is characterized by phasic internal and external rotation of about 13°. The highest vertical forces on the joint occur immediately after heel-strike of 2 to 3 times body weight and just before toe-off of 3 to 4 times body weight. The forces in ascending or descending stairs are 12% to 25% higher than those for level walking. In walking, the peak force at 10% and 50% of the cycle occurs at about 25° of flexion, whereas in ascending or descending stairs there are force peaks at flexion angles of up to 80°. In Figure 13-23, the contact areas on the articular cartilaginous surfaces are seen. At twice body weight, areas measured *in vitro* on the medial and lateral condyles are 1.8 cm² and 1.4 cm² respectively. Walker[125] estimates that at peak loads, areas of about 2.5 cm² are in contact. In Figure 13-21A, the instant centers of rotation of four normal knees are shown. The differences between the values of apparent normal knees are evident.

Laxity and flexibility of the allied soft tissues around the knee also influence the mechanics of the knee. If a force is gradually applied to the knee, there is a large initial displacement with little resistance, after which progressively higher forces are needed for further displacement. The initial displacement is static laxity and the further displacement in response to a defined maximum force is dynamic laxity. These concepts are shown in Figure 13-24.

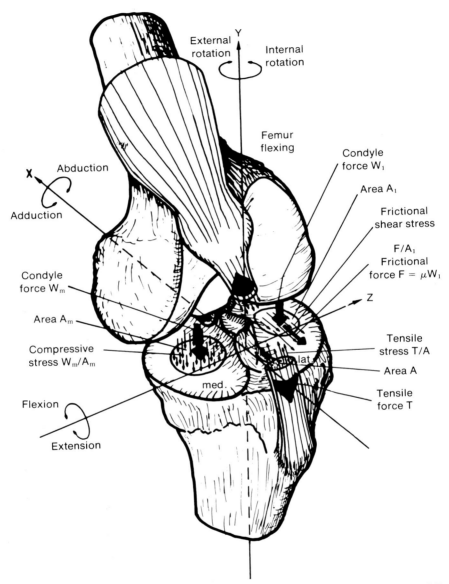

Figure 13-22. Some mechanical principles of the knee joint are shown. Orthogonal axes X, Y and Z are drawn with respect to the tibia and forces in motion are described relative to the axes. Tensile, compressive and shear stresses are illustrated. (Reproduced with permission of P. S. Walker.[127])

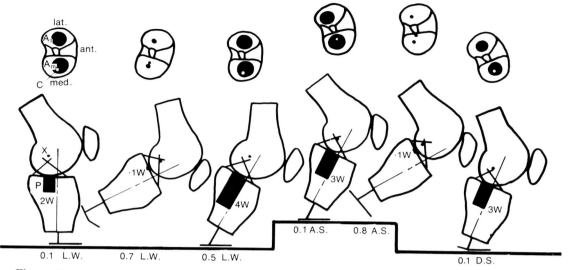

Figure 13-23. The knee is shown schematically at various phases of level walking, *L. W.,* ascending stairs, *A. S.,* and descending stairs, *D. S.* The stance phase is 0.0 to 0.6 of the full cycle and the swing phase is 0.6 to 1.0. The instant center of rotation in the lateral plane, *X,* and in the transverse plane, *C;* internal and external rotation; joint force, *P,* as a factor of body weight, *W;* and contact areas on the condyles (A_1A_m) are shown. (Reproduced with permission of P. S. Walker.[127])

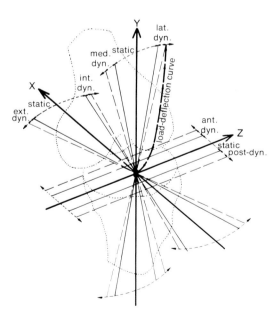

Figure 13-24. Laxity and flexibility of the knee are expressed as static laxity and dynamic laxity. Lateral laxity, vertical transverse rotation and anteroposterior glide are illustrated. The shape of the load deflection graph shows the tightening of the joint in extension. (Reproduced with permission of P. S. Walker.[127])

Mechanical Principles of Total Knee Joints. From the previous discussion, the varieties of motion and forces and the complex kinematic and elastic response of the knee should be apparent. If an arthroplastic device only partially replaces the structures of the knee, such as the unicompartmental replacement, then the device should function in harmony with the existing biological structures. If the prosthesis is a radical alteration in biomechanical concept, such as a hinge with a single axis of rotation, it should permit the ligaments and muscles to function correctly and provide appropriate range of motion. The mechanical factors that define prosthetic design are now described. Figure 13-25 reveals the principal anatomical dimensions of the knee, as recorded by Walker[125] from X-rays and cadavers. The average dimensions obtained from a number of specimens were $w_f = 8.0$ cm and $f_m = f_l = 7.1$ cm. Other comparable measurements of the femoral condyles have provided average dimensions of about 10% smaller figures than these. Despite the range of sizes, the knees show considerable symmetry so that pairs of dimensions are closely equal: f_{lat} and f_{med}, f_m and f_l, h_m and h_l. Also, t_{lat} and b_m are only about 10% greater than t_{med} and b_l respectively. In a design for surface replacement prostheses, the normal lateral outline of the femoral condyles should be closely replicated to permit

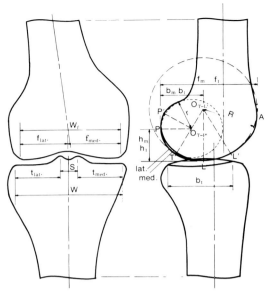

Figure 13-25. The principal dimensions of the adult knee recorded from a radiograph are shown. The dimensions made from the anteroposterior view are self-explanatory. On the lateral view, P, A and L are at the posterior, anterior and lower aspects respectively; $f_m f_l$ denote the anteroposterior widths from P to A for the medial and lateral condyles respectively; $b_m b_l$ denote the anteroposterior distance from P to L of the medial and lateral condyles respectively; $h_m h_l$ are the vertical heights between L and P of the medial and lateral condyles. The lateral outline of the femoral condyles can be closely described by the arcs of two circles as shown. The two arcs sweep L' to T from $0°$ to $30°$ flexion and T to P' from $30°$ to $120°$ flexion. (Reproduced with permission of P. S. Walker.[127])

a full range of motion and to preserve the correct lengths of the cruciate and collateral ligaments. Two circular arcs describe the shape of the femoral condyles almost exactly (Fig. 13-25), although a portion of an ellipse is also accurate (Fig. 13-17). The curvature of the tibial spines with which the inner femoral condyles conform is another important parameter. The spines control rotational laxity of the joint by distracting the joint as rotation occurs and by tightening the ligaments. Lateral subluxation also is inhibited by a similar mechanism.

In normal human subjects there is a wide variation in the patterns that describe the lateral instant centers of the knee during flexion (Fig. 13-21A). For surface replacement prostheses, the knee may retain its anatomical rotational axis. In a prosthesis that is designed to provide partial or complete stability, however, some stable axis

of rotation must be inherent in the prosthesis itself. Whenever possible, the passive soft tissue structures and the musculature should guide the motion. When a simple hinge is employed, the axis cannot replicate normal rotational axis of the knee even when the hinge is positioned in the most advantageous site. As the soft tissues impose forces upon the hinge in an attempt to define the anatomical arc of motion, the constraint in the hinge engenders forces in the mechanical components that will tend to loosen the implant or to initiate fatigue failure. Four types of abnormality of motion result: impingement of the posterior femoral condyle on the tibia; distraction of the femur from the tibia; anterior displacement of the femur; and posterior displacement of the femur. Whenever the knee joint shows a compromise of stability which must be replaced at least in part by the design of the implant, the guided motion must be a compromise. On the one hand the knee should be able to choose its own position without excessive instability and subluxation; on the other hand, high torsional forces will be imposed on a prosthesis with excessive restraint which in the long run could adversely affect fixation between the prosthesis and the bone or the mechanical integrity of the device itself.

Previously, the magnitude of the forces imposed during normal activities was described. Ideally, the prosthesis should transmit these forces to the bone to restore stresses that would occur normally, both to limit the forces imposed upon the implant and to provide physiological stresses on the bone that prevent osteoporosis. Surface replacement implants satisfy this criterion to a large degree, particularly if the components are located against the condylar surfaces. In certain pathological conditions, however, the ability of the bone to withstand normal stresses is compromised. Osteoporosis is a common feature of rheumatoid arthritis or diseased states where disuse has been a chronic problem. Osteoporosis also may accompany many other diseases including iatrogenic states such as chronic systemic administration of steroids. In normal joints at 3 times body weight with a contact area of 2 cm^2 on each condyle, the stresses in the bone will be about 50 kg/cm^2. The force is transmitted by the underlying trabecular bone to the cortical walls. Normal trabecular bone has a compressive strength of about 140 kg/cm^2 while osteoporotic trabecular structures may show strengths of between 19 and 45 kg/cm^2. If a surface replacement prosthesis is employed in a joint with osteoporotic bone, the implant should distribute the load over a larger surface area than normal to prevent localized compressive failure of the bone. After surgical joint replacement, at least in some instances, bone remodeling may occur so that osteoporotic bone is strengthened. Unfortunately, this does not always occur.

Whenever possible, physiological force transferred from the implant to bone should be transmitted in a nearly normal way to reduce the stresses on the prosthesis and on the fixation. For example, when the tibial component is supported flat on the underlying bone it transmits mainly compressive stresses. In a hinge prosthesis, however, stabilization is realized largely by the presence of intramedullary stems. Under weight-bearing conditions at large flexion angles, considerable bending moments are imposed upon the femoral stem.

Methods to Test Novel Designs. The preliminary mechanical tests needed to study novel designs of total knee joint replacements are difficult to undertake.[125] Initially, a new design can be subjected to force analysis on a computer to provide a rapid screening technique. Ultimately, a suitable model of a prosthetic-bone system must be studied in laboratory tests. Either the prosthesis can be attached to a cadaveric knee under simulated anatomical conditions or, alternatively, a mechanical knee simulator can be employed. The tests should employ strain gauges to measure stresses at strategic points on the prosthesis during the application of dynamic loads and motion of the joint. Rotational forces must be incorporated into the tests. In view of the complex arc of motion described by the human knee, accurate simulation is difficult to replicate and requires expensive instrumentation.[128] The test environment should be a physiological solution at body temperature. The results should indicate the strength of the device, the strength of the fixation, and the wear of the components. Shaw and Murray[128] have described their knee joint simulator which is representative of various testing devices that are currently employed.

Currently Available Total Knee Joint Replacements

During the past 20 years, two early concepts in arthroplasty of the knee were femoral moulds[129] and interpositional metallic plates.[130, 131] The femoral moulds consisted of femoral condylar surfaces of Co-Cr alloy attached to the femur by the use of an intramedullary stem (Fig. 13-26). The device provided a

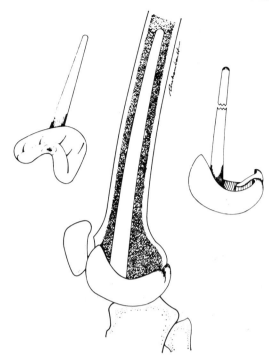

Figure 13-26. An implant for femoral mould arthroplasty is shown. The device consists of a large condylar replacement with an intramedullary stem. (Reproduced with permission of T. A. Potter.[132])

smooth gliding surface to articulate with the tibia. The results were highly variable, probably in view of the difficulty of realizing geometric compatibility within the joint. Alternatively, MacIntosh[130] developed plates for insertion on the tibial plateau. The plates had a knurled surface to oppose the tibia, although they were not routinely cemented in place. Rotation occurred between the femur and the superior surface of the plates while anteroposterior gliding of the plates on the tibial plateau was confirmed by radiological studies. Moderate success was realized by MacIntosh and others although the postoperative convalescent period was prolonged and arduous. The plates provided a smooth tibial bearing surface and increased the stability of the joint by the return of physiological tension on the collateral and cruciate ligaments after the arthritic process had provoked destruction and collapse of the tibial plateaus.

Apart from some of the earlier designs of hinges, virtually all of the presently available total knee joint replacements consist of a femoral component of stainless steel or Co-Cr alloy and a plastic tibial component of ultra high molecular weight polyethylene. Some of the designs permit independent resurfacing of the medial or lateral or patellofemoral compartments. In other designs, the femoral condyles and the tibial plateaus are joined by anterior ridges. While the separate pieces provide greater versatility, they necessitate considerable surgical skill to accurately position the medial and lateral prosthetic joints and thereby provide concentric motion of the knee. Other differences in the prostheses are the degree of conformity between the femoral and tibial articular surfaces and the amount of inherent stability provided by the contour of the implant. High conformity will decrease contact stress but may increase abrasive wear by retention of wear particles. Low conformity will increase contact stresses and may induce fatigue wear, although abrasive wear will be diminished. A few generic types of presently available models are reviewed briefly.

Unicompartmental Replacements. One of the first resurfacing prostheses employed metallic half-discs fitted into slots cut into the posterior femoral condyles and plastic runners fitted into slots in the upper tibia.[133] Only the surfaces over the load-bearing arcs of the femur and the tibia were replaced with a design that permitted "polycentric" motion (Fig. 13-27). With its narrow articular surfaces, stresses on the implant were high and stability was reduced. Furthermore, the device necessitated the use of complex jigs to permit accurate alignment of the implants. All of the more recent designs have tended to increase the articular surface area. The unicondylar system (Chapter 14, Fig. 14-7C to F) from the Hospital for Special Surgery in New York,[134] the Marmor modular system (Fig. 13-28)[135], the Buchholz SLED system[136] and the Charnley system[137] are representative examples. All of these prostheses permit resurfacing of either one or both compartments where the patient shows good bone stock, muscle strength and normal ligaments with less than 10° of angular deformity. In the SLED system the femoral component possesses a lateral outline identical to that of the femoral condyles. The tibial plateaus are flat to provide freedom of motion without any stability. In the unicondylar design, the shape of the femoral condyles is replicated but tibial spines are provided that match the inner curve on the femoral component to increase rotational stability.

Bicompartmental Resurfacing Implants. For knees that show bicompartmental disease but with good supporting tissues, as in the previous group, the UCI[138, 139] and the duocondylar sys-

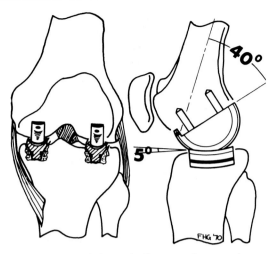

Figure 13-27. Schematic diagrams show a polycentric knee prosthesis in anteroposterior and lateral views.

tems[140-142] attempt to provide resurfacing with retention of anatomical geometry of the femoral condylar and tibial surfaces. These systems allow near-normal rotation as well as flexion and limited gliding. Minimal bone need be removed and angular flexion deformities of up to 15 to 20° can be corrected. These systems permit surgeons to treat moderately to severely involved arthritic knees and still obtain good results with 90 to 110° of knee flexion. The system requires, however, good bone stock, muscle tone and ligaments to realize optimal results. The UCI prosthesis (Figs. 13-29 and 13-30) was one of the first systems available that attempted to replicate the configuration of the femoral condyles. The tibial component is of crescentic shape and of much simpler configuration than the anatomical tibial plateaus. While this combination permits rotation, it substantially decreases the weight-bearing surface area of contact between the articulating surfaces. The force per unit area on the weight-bearing portion of the polymeric tibial prosthesis is sufficiently high so that cold-flow or creep of the plastic is observed. The articular surface of the tibial component of the duocondylar implant more closely approximates the anatomical configuration. The reasonable accuracy of the prosthetic motion and the instant center of rotation is apparent and probably contributes heavily to the better than 100° of flexion that is realized in most patients. It should be consistent with a greater functional life-expectancy of the polymeric prosthesis. The prosthetic devices provide an accurate replication of

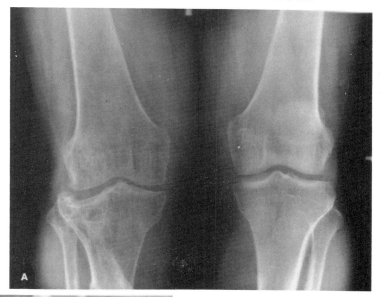

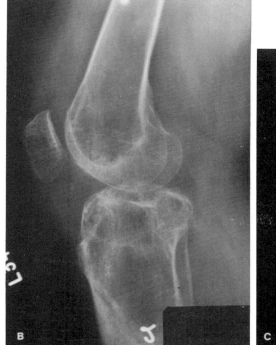

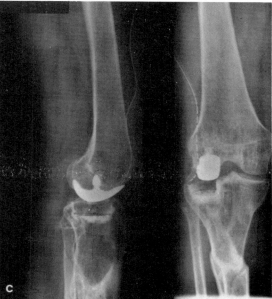

Figure 13-28. *A, B and C.* Pre- and postoperative X-rays reveal the treatment of traumatic arthritis of a lateral compartment of the knee secondary to a tibial plateau fracture with the use of a Marmor modular system. The wavy line along the anterior and lateral femoral surface represents a suction drain employed at the time of surgery.

anatomical motion. The radius of curvature of the femoral condylar component is adjusted to provide stability in full extension but some rotational freedom in flexion. Excessive rotation is restrained by impingement of the inner aspects of the femoral condyles on spines incorporated into the plastic tibial plateaus.

For attachment to bone, the femoral components of the UCI and the duocondylar systems are highly similar. Both implants show a large

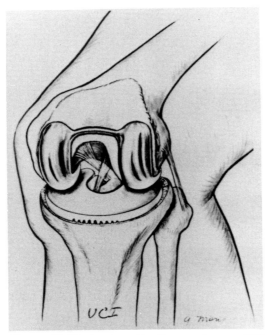

Figure 13-29. A schematic diagram shows a UCI prosthesis after surgery. The flexed view of the knee shows the position of the prostheses with respect to the collateral and cruciate ligaments. The potential for rotation of the femoral prosthesis on the tibial plateau is evident. (Reproduced with permission of T. R. Waugh et al.[138])

surface area of contact with the underlying bone, and both devices have small antirotational pegs which insert into slots in the femoral condyles. For the tibial components, both devices have comparable large areas of contact with the underlying bone. In both implants the surface impinging on the tibial plateau shows irregularities for interdigitation of cement. Drill holes are made in the bone to provide rotational stability of the cement. With the provision in both designs of implant for rotational laxity in flexion and for anteroposterior sliding with flexion and extension, the dominant forces on the components will be compressive rather than rotational or angular moments, which in the long term, could provoke deterioration of the cement fixation.

For the knee with more marked flexion, angular and rotational deformities with loss of bone substance, attenuated ligaments, subluxation and poor muscle control, a system which provides more stability than that provided by the anatomical surfaces is required. As the prosthetic stability is increased beyond that normally provided by the articular surfaces, the ultimate motion of the knee is likely to be limited, especially in rotation. Appropriate systems include the geometric,[143, 144] the Freeman-Swanson[145–147] and the total condylar prostheses.[148] While good collateral ligaments are required the cruciates are not necessary. Angular deformities of up to 45° and flexion deformities of up to 60° can be corrected.

One of the first implants which was designed to satisfy these criteria was the geometric (Fig. 13-31). The outline of the femoral condyles is a circular arc which restricts the range of flexion to about 90°. It provides some rotational stability and some anteroposterior stability although anteroposterior stability is reduced with flexion, as in the normal knee. For several years this implant has been widely employed for the reconstruction of degenerative joints with intact ligamentous structures. With its substantial limitation of anteroposterior glide the implant is subjected to rigorous shearing and impulsive loads. As shown in Figure 13-32, the anterior ends of the tibial articular surfaces are liable to creep or fracture from these excessive forces. For a knee with an intact cruciate system, premature mechanical failure of the tibial component could be predicted from the current biomechanical concept of the knee. Mechanical failure is much less likely to occur, however, if the implant is employed in a rheumatoid knee with compromised cruciate function.

The Freeman-Swanson prosthesis was designed for use in rheumatoid patients with moderate to marked osteoporosis and compromised cruciate function. In an effort to enlarge the surface area between the implant and the bone, the entire condylar region of the distal femur and the superior surface of the tibia are resurfaced to lower the force per unit area on the osteoporotic bone. While this feature lessens the likelihood of subsidence or settling of the tibial component, it necessitates excision of the cruciate ligaments, although frequently in rheumatoid patients they are absent or of little strength. To augment the stability of the knee, the tibial component was shaped like a trough into which a roller-like component on the lower end of the femur was restricted (Fig. 13-33).

In a recent follow-up on 116 knees operated by Freeman et al.[147] at the London Hospital, the Freeman-Swanson design, now known as the ICLH (Imperial College London Hospital) prosthesis, has shown surprisingly good results in a group of patients who showed moderate to severe deformities prior to surgery. Two of the implants underwent progressive loosening with

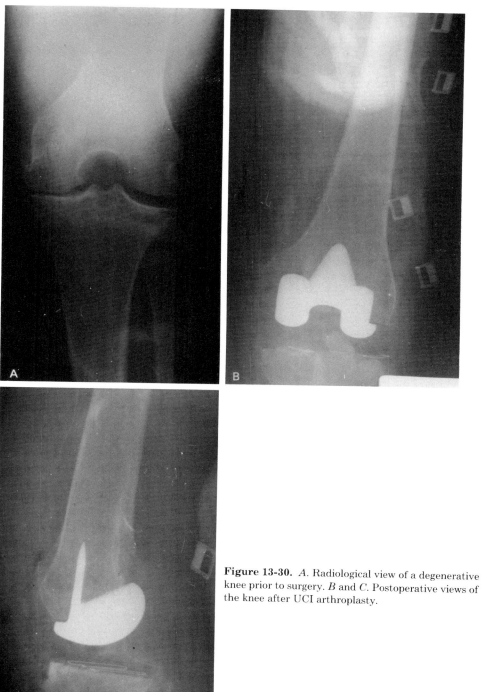

Figure 13-30. *A.* Radiological view of a degenerative knee prior to surgery. *B* and *C.* Postoperative views of the knee after UCI arthroplasty.

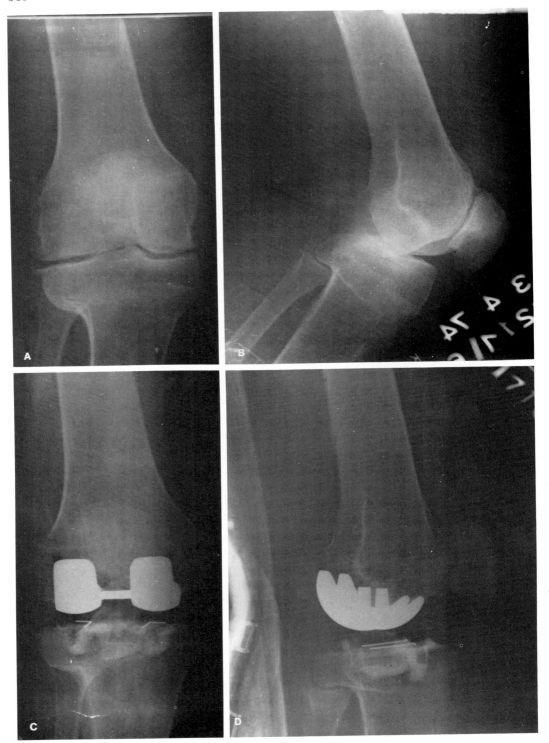

Figure 13-31. *A to D.* A series of X-rays show pre- and postoperative radiological views of a rheumatoid knee treated with a geometric knee replacement.

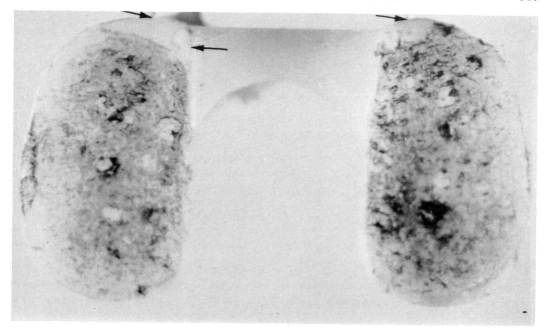

Figure 13-32. A photograph shows the articular surface of a geometric knee replacement which was removed 3 years after implantation when the patient complained of mechanical knee pain. The anterior end of the articular surface (*arrows*) shows fracture of the leading edges. The surfaces have undergone deformation with creep. The lightest areas on the articular surfaces represent inclusions of polymethylmethacrylate cement which serve as abrasive bodies to increase the rate of erosion of high density polyethylene. The darkest discoloration represents small amounts of metallic debris that is eroded by the presence of the cement particles.

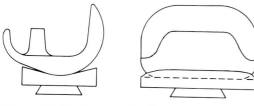

Figure 13-33. A schematic diagram shows antero-posterior and lateral views of the Freeman-Swanson or Imperial College London Hospital (ICLH) prosthesis. (Reproduced with permission M. A. R. Freeman, S. A. B. Swanson and R. C. Todd.[145])

sinkage of the tibial component into the cancellous bone of the tibia. The range of motion realized depended upon a number of factors including the state of the quadriceps muscle and is not subject to a simple interpretation. The implant can be used in combination with a patellofemoral replacement which is discussed below.

Surface Replacements with Enhanced Stability. A variety of systems has been developed for use in severely compromised knees where stability is substantially compromised in addi-

tion to a painful limited arc of motion with moderate to severe deformities. As a group, the implants possess broad condylar bearing surfaces with some type of intercondylar stabilizing mechanism for mediolateral and anteroposterior stabilization. Although clinical experience with these systems is limited, the preliminary results suggest that they offer the best hope for reconstruction of a severely compromised and unstable knee. While Deane's prosthesis[149] achieves fixation solely by a metaphyseal extension of the femoral component and small tibial anchoring rails that embed in the tibial plateau, most of the other devices possess short intramedullary stems on both the femoral and tibial components. Representative examples of the latter group include the spherocentric[150, 151] the Attenborough[152] and the stabilocondylar devices.[153, 154] The examples are described briefly in turn.

The Deane prosthesis is notable for its elegant simplicity and its preservation of the integrity of the intramedullary cavities. The latter feature might lessen the higher infection rate and the incidence of prosthetic loosening that is generally associated with the presence of intramedullary stems. Also, the fracture of bone around

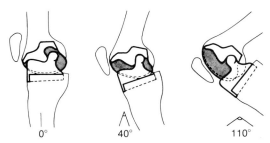

Figure 13-34. A schematic diagram illustrates the mechanism of the Deane prosthesis from a stable position at full extension. Sliding occurs for 40° when a smooth transition to a ball-and-socket load permits further flexion with axial rotation up to 110°. (Reproduced with permission of G. Deane.[149])

intramedullary stems with less than the anticipated breaking force should not arise. The implant is unusual in that the femoral component consists of HDP while the tibial component is made of Co-Cr alloy. To accommodate the stabilizing mechanism the femoral component requires extensive osseous resection within the intercondylar space. With the retention of the peripheral portions of the femoral condyle, however, fusion of a knee after a failed prosthesis should be possible without excessive foreshortening of the extremity. Stabilization of the implant is realized by the presence of an intercondylar sphere on the posterior portion of the superior surface of the tibial component which fits into a recess in the femoral component (Fig. 13-34). The complex shape of the implant permits anatomical variation of the center of prosthetic rotation throughout flexion. At full extension a subtle configuration provides stability without rotation. Beyond 40° of flexion the intercondylar mechanism provides a ball-and-socket design so that multiaxial movement with rotation occurs between the femoral and tibial components.

The spherocentric knee is a nonhinged, intrinsically stable knee joint prosthesis which permits controlled triaxial rotation and was designed specifically for use in severely deformed and grossly unstable knees. The principal femoral and tibial components are made of Co-Cr alloy. HDP inserts rest on the articular surface of the tibia and a comparable polyethylene socket fits over a ball on the tibial unit (Fig. 13-35). Short intramedullary stems augment fixation in bone. Two runner-and-track articulations occur between the femoral and tibial condyles. A ball-and-socket joint is situated in the intercondylar portion of the implant. The tibial component possesses a central sphere above a cylindrical

shaft. The sphere is contained within a polyethylene socket which is housed within the femoral component. The ball-and-socket joint permits triaxial rotation although dislocation is not possible in any direction. The center of the sphere approximates the average flexion axis of the normal knee. The location, dimensions and contour of the femoral runners and their mating tibial polyethylene tracks direct and control flexion, varus-valgus movement and rotation. The contours (Fig. 13-35B to D) of the femoral condylar surfaces of the prosthesis in the sagittal plane include an anterior part with a larger radius of curvature which is not concentric with the surface of the sphere, and a posterior part with a smaller radius of curvature which is concentric with the surface of the sphere. As the knee approaches full extension, the anterior surface of the femoral condylar runners, with their larger radius of a curvature, bear increasingly on the plastic tibial tracks thereby to unload the top of the sphere and force the underside of the sphere against the surrounding plastic socket. The central pillar is placed in tension and hyperextension is arrested by a gradual deceleration without a rigid extension stop. Impact loading during extension is minimized. At full extension the prosthesis is fully stabilized in all directions except flexion.

As the prosthesis is flexed from its fully extended position (Fig 13-35B to D), the femoral condylar surfaces slowly lift off the plastic tibial tracks and transfer weight-bearing load to the dome of the sphere. As the condylar runners lift further and further off the tracks, triaxial rotation of increasing amplitude is permitted. At maximum flexion of 120°, the prosthesis permits up to 30° of tibial rotation and up to 5° of varus and valgus motion. The polymeric articular surfaces are readily replaceable if they undergo excessive wear.

Sonstegard *et al.*[150, 151] have reported extensive laboratory tests on the spherocentric knee. One of the tests was the insertion of the prosthesis into cadaveric bones and the application of an Instron testing machine for evaluation of deflection under load and energy absorption in a position of hyperextension. The tests were repeated on a hinge prosthesis and anatomical preparations as well as the spherocentric implant. The mode of failure for all of the cemented prostheses was separation at the cement-bone interface but at load levels far above the tolerance of the intact control knee. Although the hinge specimens were strongest they were extremely rigid and therefore transmitted high

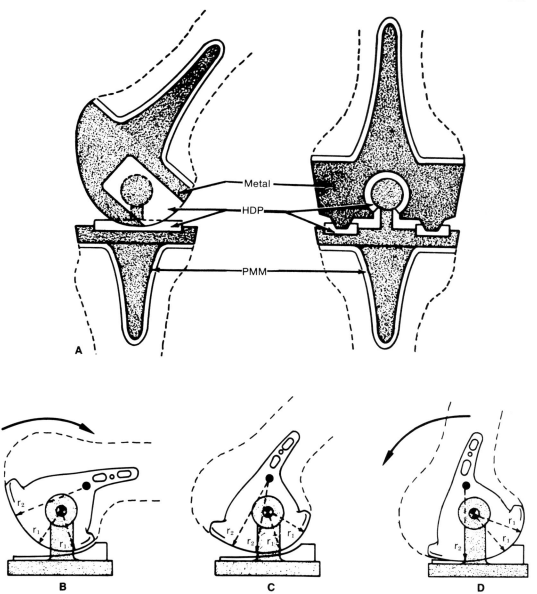

Figure 13-35. *A.* The schematic diagram shows the frontal and lateral views of the spherocentric knee. The bearing surfaces consist of high density polyethylene (HDP) on metal to diminish friction and wear. The interface between bone and implant consists of polymethylmethacrylate (PMM) cement to diminish shear effects. (Reproduced with permission of L. S. Matthews, D. A. Sonstegard and H. Kaufer.[155]) *B* to *D.* Schematic lateral views of the articular portions of a spherocentric knee are shown. *B.* Moderate flexion is shown. The posterior part of each femoral condyle or runner has a small radius of curvature, r_1, and is concentric with a sphere. Its surface is not in close contact with the tibial track in this position thus permitting triaxial motion centered about the sphere. *C.* As the prosthesis moves toward extension, the surface of the anterior part of each femoral condyle or runner, which has a larger radius of curvature, r_2, and is not concentric with this sphere, approaches the tibial track. As the prosthesis moves toward complete extension, triaxial motion is progressively diminished. In any flexed position, virtually all of the load on the prosthesis is born by this sphere; the runners and tracks serve primarily to modulate the excursion of triaxial motion. *D.* Nearly complete extension is shown. The anterior part of each femoral condylar runner with its largest radius of curvature, r_2, is now in close contact with the tibial track. Further extension is arrested in a graduated fashion by the cam-like action. With the considerable load transmitted by the tracks and the runners in the fully extended position, triaxial motion is eliminated and the prosthesis is completely stable. (Reproduced with permission of D. A. Sonstegard, H. Kaufer and L. S. Matthews.[156])

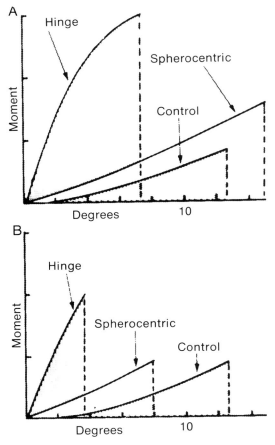

Figure 13-36. *A.* Plots of the average moments in angular deflection of control, spherocentric and hinge specimens tested in extension are shown. The slope of the load-deflection curve for spherocentric knees is quite similar to that of the control knees but shows a capacity for greater strain without permanent deformation, greater load and greater energy absorption prior to ultimate failure. *B.* Plots of the average moments in angular deflections of control, spherocentric and hinge specimens tested in extension and loaded up to the energy level that caused failure of the average control knee are shown. At this energy level, a hinged-knee subjects the supporting bone to more than twice the moment of a similarly loaded spherocentric knee. (Reproduced with permission of D. A. Sonstegard, H. Kaufer and L. S. Matthews.[157])

loads to the implant-cement-bone junction. The loads would be expected to contribute to loosening of the implant. The spherocentric specimens were stronger than the intact knees but were much less rigid than those with a hinge. The capacity of the spherocentric knee to deflect reversibly under load would diminish the force at the implant-cement-bone junction in compar-

ison with a hinge-prosthesis subjected to similar load (Fig. 13-36) and should lessen the risk of late separation of the implant-bone interface around a spherocentric prosthesis. *In vivo,* triaxial motion of a spherocentric knee may permit surrounding muscle and supporting soft tissues to share in the dissipation of energy resulting from torsional or valgus-varus stresses. In contrast the uniaxial hinge must transmit all of the energy derived from varus-valgus or torsional stresses directly to the implant-bone interface. With the rigidity of the hinge, the absorbed energy will be manifested as a large load and a small deflection, or impact.

Sonstegard *et al.*[150] have reported the results of the application of the spherocentric knee in a small group of patients with severe deformities and instability. Typically after surgery the patient shows about 90° of flexion, an increase of about 20° compared to the preoperative average arc, and a stable knee with minimal pain. While their 2-year period of follow-up is too brief to provide an indication of prolonged function, nevertheless, additional reports of their results are eagerly awaited.

Attenborough[152] has designed the stabilizing gliding prosthesis which functions along a similar concept. The device consists of a Co-Cr femoral component with two femoral condyles attached to a tapered intramedullary stem 75 mm in length. The tibial component of HDP has a broad tibial plateau and a hollow intramedullary stem 70 mm in length. A cylindrical metal stabilizing stem inserts into the tibial component. The upper end of the stem has a sphere which articulates with the intercondylar region of the femoral component (Fig. 13-37). In flexion the stabilizing rod articulates with a widened portion of the intercondylar region of the femoral unit so that some rotation and lateral mobility is permitted. As the unit is brought into full extension the sphere articulates with a femoral surface of a smaller radius of curvature so that stability is increased. In view of the polycentric nature of the principal articulating surfaces, engendered by the variation in the radius of curvature of the femoral condyles, the stabilizing rod must move vertically with flexion and extension. The inventor has employed this feature to provide a unique mechanism for lubrication of the joint. The stabilizing rod has one flattened surface so that synovial fluid can run into the bottom of the central hole when the knee is flexed. With extension of the knee the rod functions as a piston to drive synovial fluid through two small lateral holes close to the main weight-bearing

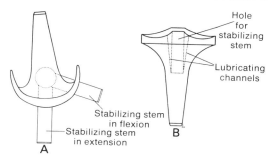

Figure 13-37. A schematic diagram shows the Attenborough total knee joint replacement. *A*. The diagram shows the femoral component with its stabilizing stem in extension and in flexion. *B*. The diagram reveals the tibial component with its cylindrical cavity for the stabilizing stem and two parallel lubricating channels. (Reproduced with permission of C. G. Attenborough.)[152]

surfaces and around the shaft of the stabilizing rod. Laboratory tests have confirmed the efficiency of this small pump.

One liability of the design would appear to be the metal-on-metal articulation of the stem on the femoral component. With a minor alteration in the design these surfaces could be separated by a polyethylene cap such as is the one in the spherocentric design. Nevertheless, Attenborough has reported favorable results on his initial series of 53 operations performed on degenerative and rheumatoid knees with a follow-up period of up to 2½ years. A detailed assessment of his results is published elsewhere.[152]

Hinge-type Prostheses. The first types of total knee joint available were rigid uniaxial hinges. Representative examples were the Waldius[158, 159] followed by the Shiers[160] in Great Britain, Buchholz[161, 162] in Germany and more recently the Guepar[163, 164] in France. As the surface replacements became available, the indications for the use of hinge-type implants receded progressively to the present time. At present if they have any indication it is the severely deformed and painful knee with minimal intrinsic stability. The hinge-type prostheses have major disadvantages.[165] With their large intramedullary stems and broad articular surfaces, extensive bone resection is necessary at the time of implantation. If the procedure fails so that arthrodesis is needed, the latter exercise is extremely difficult to undertake and has been accompanied by high rates of failure with pseudarthrosis. The extremity is markedly foreshortened in view of the extensive bone resection. Several of the hinges have been

devised which fit almost entirely within the central portion of the bone to leave a peripheral rim up to the level of the tibial plateau and the distal femoral condyle. One example of such an implant is the Herbert.[166] While arthrodesis of such a failed knee might appear to be more easily undertaken in practice this is not the case. When such an arthroplastic joint becomes infected with osteomyelitis and accompanying osteoporosis of bone the residual thin walled cylinders of bone are difficult to stabilize, and the bone is liable to subside with substantial late foreshortening of the extremity. With poor bony contact of the adjacent femoral and tibial surfaces, fusion is difficult to realize.

The early hinges such as the Waldius and Shiers had other substantial disadvantages. Fractures of bone around the long intramedullary stems were not uncommon. Loosening of the implant was almost a constant finding after 8 to 10 years of function. With loosening, the stems were likely to erode through adjacent bone and the patient was likely to complain of mechanical pain. Also the axes of the hinges were not positioned to be consistent with a full range of motion and with a sufficient lever arm of the quadriceps muscle. More recently the introduction of the Guepar model lessened the undesirable features of the hinge-type implants. Less than 2 cm of bone are removed from the articular surfaces. The axis of rotation is placed close to the ideal axis position to provide a greater range of motion. Left- and right-hand models are available for provision of physiological valgus, the lateral angulation of 8 to 16° in the normal distal femur. The high forces imposed at large flexion angles are not transmitted entirely to the stem since a substantial portion of the femoral component is contained within the distal femur.

Trillat and Bousquet[125] have devised an ingenious hinge-type prosthesis that uses a cam-like arrangement to provide internal and external rotation. As in the normal joint, rotation increases progressively with flexion angle. The prosthesis is preassembled to simplify surgical implantation. Unfortunately a large amount of bone must be resected before its insertion. To diminish bone resection several workers have attempted to develop intercondylar hinges. The design by Herbert[166] was one of the first of these which unfortunately has been associated with many mechanical failures. Biomechanical tests have indicated that the forces on the stem-bearing junction in the intercondylar region are excessive. Lagrange and Letournel[167] employ a plastic box about 4 cm wide embedded in the femoral condyles. Stability is achieved by the use of intramedullary stems. All of the devices that remove forces from the femoral and tibial condyles and transmit them to the cortical wall through intramedullary stems appear to be fundamentally unsound. With the unnatural stress pattern at the bone ends in the diaphysis, remodeling of bone is likely to result in osteoporosis with failure of fixation and late settling of the implants.

Patellofemoral Arthroplasty. Early studies on arthroplastic techniques in the knee joint focused primary attention on the tibiofemoral articulations. Certain patients, however, have isolated patellofemoral arthritis. Also it has become apparent that unsatisfactory pain relief following knee arthroplasty is often attributable to deterioration of the patellofemoral articulation. About 15% of the patients with tibiofemoral arthroplasty have severe and disabling pain from this source and many others have minor intermittent symptoms. The problem is greater in osteoarthritic than in rheumatoid arthritic patients. Where conservative measures have failed the principal solution has been patellectomy. With its biomechanical compromise to the quadriceps mechanism, residual weakness with buckling of the knee has been a major problem. After patellectomy many adults continue to have minor or moderate mechanical patellofemoral pain. In recent years considerable attention has been focused on attempts to provide comparable arthroplastic solutions for the patellofemoral joint. Bechtol[168] and Ewald* have developed techniques for arthroplasty of the patellofemoral articulation that can be used alone or in conjunction with other total knee joint replacements. The implants consist of a stainless steel or Co-Cr alloy insertion for the intercondylar region of the femur and a HDP patellar component. The femoral component replicates the natural contour of the patellofemoral facet of the femur. The under surface is irregular with antirotational pegs to provide firm stability in bone cement. The patellar component shows medial and lateral articular facets and a central peg on the nonarticular surface to provide stabilization in bone cement.

Where patellofemoral arthroplasty is undertaken as the sole operative procedure, somewhat conflicting results have been reported by different workers and no long term follow-up studies

are yet available. While some workers have indicated favorable results, others such as Ewald have been dissatisfied with the stability of the implants or of the relief of pain. Clearly further studies are indicated.

In the past 5 years many workers have attempted to incorporate patellofemoral articulations into the designs of femoral-patellar arthroplasties. Most workers are now agreed that in the presence of triple compartment arthritis resurfacing of all three joints provides a far superior result to isolated femorotibial replacement. Many implants are now available wherein the femoral component shows a large anterior flange which covers the patellofemoral facet of the femur and is employed with a polyethylene patellar component. Of the numerous implants of this type currently available the duopatella,[125] the total condylar,[141] and the modified ICLH design of Freeman and Swanson[145] are representative examples. The duocondylar design is similar to the duocondylar prosthesis previously described but with a patellar flange and a plastic patellar button. The principal components possess substantial grooves to permit retention of the cruciate ligaments. Alternatively, where the cruciate ligaments are ineffective or absent or where the bone is markedly osteoporotic so that a larger area of contact between the implant and the underlying bone is desired, the total condylar design can be employed (Chapter 14, Fig. 14-11A and B). Its articular surfaces are highly similar to those of the duocondylar or duopatellar design.[169] The implants fill the intercondylar region and the polymeric tibial unit shows a metaphyseal stem. Severe flexion contractures and varus or valgus deformities can be corrected. For degenerative knees with triple compartment arthritis and intact cruciate ligaments, some workers favor the use of the total condylar design with the deliberate excision of the cruciate ligaments. They argue that retention of the cruciates and the use of the duopatellar design might restore a knee in which the center of rotation preserved by the cruciates is not concentric with that provided by the arthroplastic surfaces. This situation would arise if the surgeon fails to align the implants with the anatomical axis of motion. If the cruciate ligaments are deliberately sacrificed and the total condylar implant is employed, then the arthroplastic surface defines the center of rotation of the knee so that this problem does not arise. Long term follow-up studies will be necessary to determine which argument is correct.

---

* F. C. Ewald, personal communication, 1977.

For those severely arthritic knees with triple compartment disease and substantial instability and deformity a stabilocondylar prosthesis is available.[153] The implant provides an intercondylar stabilizing unit in which a polymeric extension of the tibial component articulates with the intercondylar region of the femoral unit. The prosthesis permits a −5 to 115° arc of flexion with 10° of internal-external rotation and adduction when the unit is fully flexed. With the unit positioned in extension supplementary motion is inhibited. An intramedullary tibial stem augments anchorage in bones.

The follow-up periods for available clinical studies in all of these designs are fairly limited. Insall et al.[170] have reported the results on 116 total condylar prostheses implanted for periods of up to 2½ years. In 81 of these patients the patellar implant was employed. Sixty-eight patients were osteoarthritics, 40 were rheumatoid arthritics, 3 showed post-traumatic knees, 4 had failure of other prostheses and 1 had osteonecrosis. In the postoperative follow-up the pain relief has been more uniformly predictable than after the use of other implants which these workers attribute to replacement of the patellofemoral articulation. Loosening has not been observed although incomplete radiolucent lines at the cement-bone interface of the tibial component has been observed in 18% of the immediate postoperative films and an additional 17% in subsequent X-rays. The lucent line has not exceeded 1 mm in thickness. In the former case it is felt to represent a thin film of blood between the cement and bone. Initial radiolucencies were observed around 3.5% of patellar components. Tibial radiolucencies were present after a similar follow-up period in 55% of the duocondylar, 65% of the unicondylar and 85% of the geometric prostheses.

Many of the patients with degenerative arthritis show instability in extension in which asymmetry of the collateral ligamentous lengths develops from the stress of walking on a deformed knee. In the more common varus deformity the medial ligament shortens and the lateral ligament stretches. Unless corrected, this imbalance persists after knee replacement. Fifteen degrees of fixed deformity can be corrected by asymmetric bone resection without fear of postoperative instability. The greater deformities require tightening of the lateral ligament or lengthening of the medial ligament by its release from the tibia. The "medial release" has provided more satisfactory results for Insall et al.[170]

It is achieved by elevation of a flap consisting of the deep portion of the medial ligament, the periosteum with the insertion of the pes tendons and the superficial medial ligament. These structures are divided at their distal insertion on the tibia. When traction is subsequently applied to the tibia, the medial "flap" slides proximally and rapidly adheres in the postoperative period despite the absence of postoperative immobilization. A similar release of the lateral soft tissue structures for correction of fixed valgus deformities is not recommended because of the risk of peroneal nerve palsy.

Accurate realignment of the deformed knee is a critical stage in total knee joint replacement. The deformities are sufficiently complex that attempts to correct them by visual appraisal is most unlikely to succeed. Insall,[134, 148] Freeman[145] and other workers[135-164] have devised complex jigs which assist in the realignment of the knee by proper determination of each of the tibial and femoral resections of bone. Prior to surgery the surgeon must be familiar with the appropriate set of jigs for many of them have certain details of insertion that are not readily appreciated at the time of surgery. Some of the designs require the use of reciprocating or oscillating power saws of which the Insall design is an example. Others permit the use of osteotomes. Power saws are preferred for these procedures since they permit the resection of precise amounts of bone of uniform thickness and straight transected surfaces. Some of the presently available power saws possess inadequate power for the resection of dense sclerotic degenerative bone. The saws show excessive evolution of heat during prolonged application. Nevertheless, osteotomes are much more difficult to employ. In view of thickness of many osteotome blades the relevant jigs are used to insert Steinmann pins at the limits of the osteotomy. Then the jig is removed and the osteotome is applied between two pins. A few jigs, such as that devised by Kenna,* permit the application of either an oscillating blade or an osteotome.

To anchor a knee prosthesis the insertion of methylmethacrylate cement requires even greater attention to detail than the comparable stage of total hip joint replacement. Excessive cement is likely to fracture and free bodies of cement are likely to settle and become trapped between the principal articulating surfaces. The loose bodies of methylmethacrylate provoke

---

* R. Kenna, personal communication, 1977.

rapid abrasive wear of HDP. Alternatively, in the hip joint under the influence of gravity, particles of cement settle into the inferior recesses of synovium where they are usually embedded.

Recent Concepts in Total Knee Joint Replacement

Two concepts in total knee joint replacement have emerged in recent years which merit comment. Goodfellow* has designed an arthroplastic knee that embodies two separate femoral components and two tibial components, all constructed of polyethylene, and two metallic "meniscal" units. The advantage of this system is its precise replication of the anatomical motion of the knee without excessive constraint. Rotation of the knee occurs between the femoral units and the superior surfaces of the meniscal implants. Anteroposterior glide occurs between the inferior surfaces of the meniscal units and the polymeric components on the tibial plateaus. This system is currently under clinical evaluation in Oxford. The principal liability of Goodfellow's design is the surgical complication associated with the insertion of six independent parts. Accurate alignment of the femoral and tibial components both with respect to the medial and lateral compartments and between both compartments would be difficult. Unless precise realignment was realized, late subluxation of the meniscal units would be likely to occur. Nevertheless, future embodiments of the design might show a common femoral component and a single tibial unit.

Another concept under study by Kenna† is a femorotibial arthroplasty which replicates anatomical knee motion and is attached to bone by the use of a sinter coated Co-Cr alloy for the ingrowth of bone. Antirotational pegs are inserted into the distal femur and the proximal tibia to control rotation during the critical period of early ingrowth of bone. In view of the primary compressive forces to which the knee is subjected and the limitation of rotation shearing forces, the mechanical environment is ideal for the satisfactory function of a porous coated implant. The design is of particular value in the knee where loose bodies of methylmethacrylate cement are particularly deleterious. The results of a clinical trial are awaited with interest.

---

* J. Goodfellow, personal communication, 1976.

† R. Kenna, personal communication, 1977.

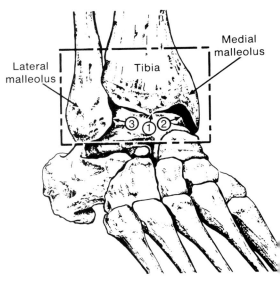

Figure 13-38. The anatomical features of the ankle joint are shown in a schematic mortise view. The numbers refer to the three sets of articular surfaces that comprise the ankle joint: *1*, The distal tibia and the superior surface of the talus; *2*, the medial malleolus and the medial side of the talus; and *3*, the lateral malleolus or fibula and the lateral side of the talus. (Reproduced with permission of Zimmer U.S.A., Warsaw, Ind.)

ARTHROPLASTIC RECONSTRUCTION OF THE ANKLE JOINT

The ankle joint and subtalar complex (Figs. 13-38 to 13-40) permit flexion of the foot on the leg with supplementary inversion or eversion of the foot so that gait may be undertaken on both level and irregular terrain. Historically, the ankle joint has been construed as a simple hinge with a single axis of motion.[172] The axis of motion is felt to pass transversely through the body of the talus.[173] In one of the early comprehensive studies on ankle motion, Hicks[174] observed two axes of ankle motion, one in dorsiflexion and another in plantar flexion. In one of the early biomechanical evaluations Wright *et al.*[175] concluded that the subtalar and ankle joints function in harmony as a universal joint. During normal walking these workers recorded 6° of subtalar motion and 14° of ankle rotation. They attempted to correlate the motion of the joints with the contraction of adjacent muscles and the weight-bearing forces imposed upon the joints for walking on level and irregular terrain. Isman and Inman[176] studied the axis of ankle motion with respect to the plane of the leg. They showed that the ankle axis is directed laterally and pos-

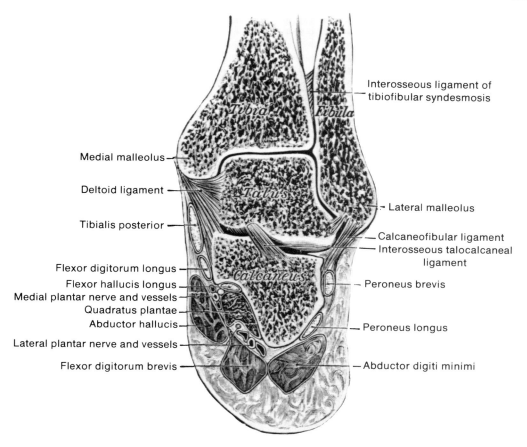

Figure 13-39. A detailed cross-section of the tibiotalar (ankle) joint and the talocalcanceal (subtalar) joint. (Reproduced with permission of C. M. Goss.)[171]

teriorly as projected on the transverse plane of the leg but it is also directed laterally and downward as seen in the coronal plane (Fig. 13-41). In their anthropometric studies they found that in the coronal plane the functional axis of the ankle may deviate from 88° to 68° in the vertical axis of the leg. An examiner may obtain a reasonably accurate estimate of the position of the axis by placing the end of his index fingers at the most distal bony prominences of the malleoli. With the oblique orientation of the ankle joint axis, horizontal rotations in the foot or the leg must accompany movements of the ankle. The rotations of ankle motion are clearly depicted in Figures 13-42 and 13-43. With the foot free and the leg fixed the oblique ankle joint axis causes the foot to deviate outward on dorsiflexion and inward on plantar flexion. The projection of the foot under the transverse plane, shown by the shadows in the sketches, reveals the extent of this external and internal rotation of the foot (Fig. 13-42). The amount of the rotation varies

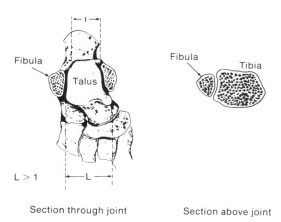

Figure 13-40. Two sectional views through and above the ankle joint. (Reproduced with permission of Zimmer U.S.A., Warsaw, Ind.)

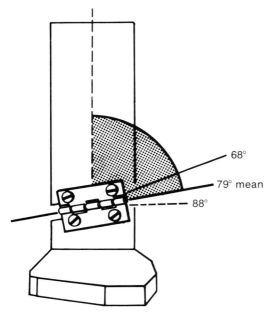

68°

79° mean

88°

Figure 13-41. The schematic diagram shows the physiological variation in the inclination of axis of the ankle joint. (Reproduced with permission of V. T. Inman and R. A. Mann.)[172]

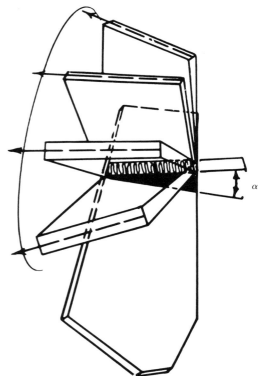

α

Figure 13-43. With the foot planted on the floor, plantar flexion and dorsiflexion of the ankle produce horizontal rotation of the leg because of the obliquity of the ankle axis. (Reproduced with permission of V. T. Inman and R. A. Mann.)[177]

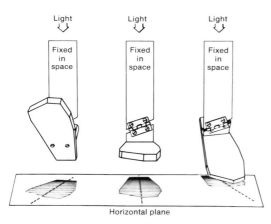

Horizontal plane

Figure 13-42. The effect of the obliquely positioned ankle axis upon the rotation of the foot in a horizontal plane is shown during plantar flexion and dorsiflexion. The foot is in a non-weight-bearing position and displacement is reflected in the shadows of the foot. (Reproduced with permission of V. T. Inman and R. A. Mann.)[177]

with the obliquity of the ankle axis and the amount of dorsiflexion and plantar flexion. Alternatively with the foot fixed on the ground during midstance, the body passing over the foot produces dorsiflexion of the foot relative to the

leg. Again the degree of internal rotation of the leg and the foot depends upon the amount of dorsiflexion and the obliquity of the ankle axis. With conventional walking the average amount of this rotation is 19° with a range of 13 to 25°. More recently Sammarco *et al.*[178] have provided a detailed kinematic study of the ankle joint. By use of X-rays they observed the range of motion, centers of rotation and the surface motion of the articular cartilage during weight bearing and non-weight-bearing. Abnormal ankle joints of patients with various orthopaedic disorders also were examined. Their techniques are described fully elsewhere.[178] Twenty-four normal ankles were studied which showed a variation in the total range of motion from 24 to 75° with an average of 43 ± 12.4° (mean ± standard deviation). The average ankle dorsiflexion was 21 ± 7.21° and the average ankle plantar flexion was 23 ± 8°. In a series of 10 abnormal weight-bearing ankles afflicted with rheumatoid, degenerative or traumatic arthritis, a range of motion

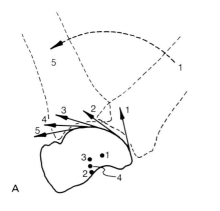

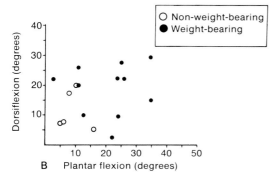

Figure 13-44. *A.* In the schematic view of the lateral ankle joint in a normal non-weight-bearing male, all of the instant centers are located within the talar body. Surface velocity shows joint distraction at the beginning of motion but sliding thereafter. (Reproduced with permission of G. J. Sammarco, A. H. Burstein and E. H. Frankel.)[179] *B.* Ranges of motion for a series of abnormal ankles in weight-bearing and non-weight-bearing conditions are shown. (Reproduced with permission of G. J. Sammarco, A. H. Burstein and E. H. Frankel.)[180]

from 21 to 61° with an average 37 ± 6° was recorded. The average angle of dorsiflexion was 18 ± 9.4° (mean ± standard deviation) and the average angle of plantar flexion was 21 ± 9.3°. There was a significant decrease in the range of motion while non-weight-bearing when compared with a weight-bearing study.

The instant centers of rotations and surface velocities at the points of contact were constructed for 22 normal ankles. In only 12 ankles did the instant centers fall within the body of the talus. In Figure 13-44A, the surface velocities along with the instant centers are shown for a normal non-weight-bearing male. Surface velocity indicates distraction of the joint at the begin-

ning of motion but sliding thereafter. The same techniques were applied to a variety of patients who had sustained bi- or trimalleolar fractures with the subsequent onset of traumatic arthritis, or patients with rheumatoid arthritis or other diseases. The results vary considerably with the stage of any particular disease process.

From these studies it is clear that a normal ankle shows a series of instant centers of rotation that occur from the time motion begins as plantar flexion until its termination at the limit of dorsiflexion. The centers occur anatomically both within and without the body of the talus. The normal ankle shows a tendency toward distraction early in motion followed by sliding throughout the midportion and terminating in compression at the end of dorsiflexion. The process reverses itself when the joint is moved in the opposite direction. The diseased ankle shows a different pattern in the placement of instant centers and in the ranges of motion (Fig. 13-44B) from that observed in a normal ankle. The surface velocities for abnormal ankles did not follow a specific pattern as noted in normal ankles. During weight-bearing most velocities were directed parallel to the joint surface. Abnormal, somewhat unpredictable changes in surface velocity were noted in the pathological ankles. These workers suggest that the abnormal instant centers noted in arthritic joints may lead to altered surface velocities which in turn may provoke more rapid deterioration of the articular surfaces.

Techniques of Total Ankle Joint Replacement

The previous methods of treatment for the arthritic ankle joint have been limited to conservative procedures such as limited weight bearing or analgesics, or alternatively, arthrodesis.[181-183] The numerous available methods of arthrodesis are a reflection of the limitations and complications of current procedures, particularly delayed or nonunion, but also neurovascular complications. In view of the unusual blood supply of the talus,[184, 185] avascular necrosis of its body has been reported after various surgical procedures such as triple arthrodesis, as well as after fractures of the bone. The major part of the blood supply to the talus enters anteriorly and inferiorly through the neck of the talus. There is also a rich blood supply entering from the medial surface below the articular facet of the tibial malleolus.

For about 7 years, several workers have attempted to develop a total ankle joint replacement. In 1970, Lord and Marotte[186] in Paris, implanted a ball-and-socket ankle prosthesis which was comparable to a small inverted hip prosthesis. The stem of the metallic ball component was situated in the medullary cavity of the tibia and the plastic socket was housed in the talus. From 1972, the St. Georg group[187] in Hamburg and the ICLH in London[188] independently implanted prostheses consisting of part cylindrical, convex metallic talar components and matching concave plastic tibial components. In the St. Georg design (Fig. 13-45) the tibial component is a large polyethylene block with fenestrations on a superior surface and a concave articular surface with a radius of 32 mm, which approximates the physiological curve of the articular surface of the tibia in a large individual. The metallic talar component has a convex articular surface with a radius of curvature of 25 mm. It has a maximum height of 7 mm with 6 studs on its inferior surface for anchorage into cement. The opposing articular surfaces provide an almost linear contact zone which facilitates lubrication with synovial fluid. Unlike most of the other total joint replacement techniques, the St. Georg system employs osteotomy of the lateral malleolus for dislocation of the ankle joint. This extensive surgical procedure facilitates resection of the opposing articular

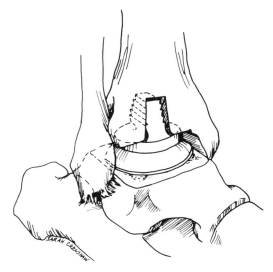

Figure 13-46. Schematic diagram shows a Smith total ankle joint replacement *in vivo*. (Reproduced with permission of Wright Manufacturing Co.)

surfaces in a highly precise manner. Appropriate depressions are made in the distal tibia and the talus for anchorage of cement to secure the implants. Subsequently, the ankle joint is reduced and the lateral malleolus is immobilized with a cancellous bone screw. The alternative types of total ankle joint replacement are performed through an anterior approach which is relatively atraumatic provided that the dorsalis pedis artery and the deep peroneal nerve are carefully retracted. Through the anterior approach, total ankle joint replacement is a much more benign procedure to soft tissues than arthrodesis of the ankle. One of the first American designs of ankle joint replacement was by Smith,[189] who developed a simple design with a stainless steel tibial component, and a HDP talar unit (Fig. 13-46). The articular surfaces were of hemispherical configuration so that minimal forces on the bone cement interface would be imposed even if the alignment of the prosthesis was not concentric with the anatomical axis. The cross-sectional area of the articular surfaces was of the order of 1 inch^2 so that the force per unit area in the weight-bearing extremity was high. The operative procedure is quite simple, although radiological control is advisable so that the implants are positioned close to the center of rotation of the anatomical ankle joint. In the author's experience, the range of dorsal or plantar flexion achieved after surgery is rarely more than 10° to 15°. Nevertheless, the procedure can provide a relatively benign form of "instant"

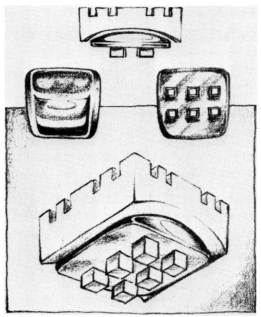

Figure 13-45. A schematic diagram of the St. Georg total ankle joint replacement. (Reproduced with permission of Richards Manufacturing Co.)

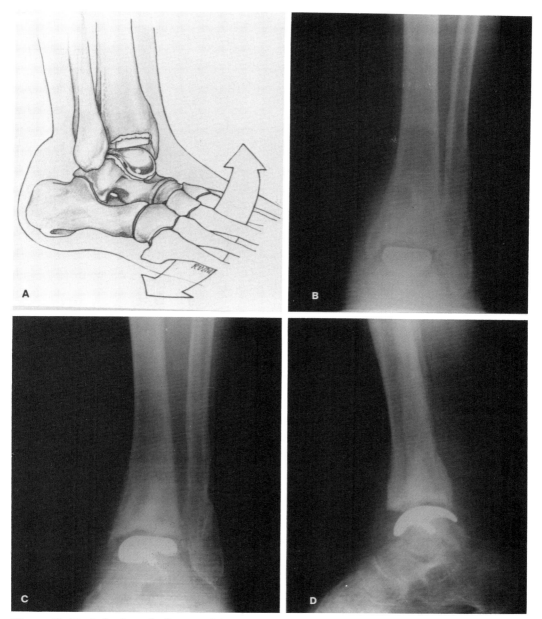

Figure 13-47. *A.* A schematic diagram of the Thompson-Parkridge-Richards (TPR) total ankle joint replacement. (Reproduced with permission of Richards Manufacturing Co.) *B* to *D.* X-rays show anteroposterior, oblique and lateral views of a TPR total ankle joint replacement undertaken for traumatic arthritis in an adult male. (Reproduced with permission of C. Stanitski).

ankle arthrodesis with a modest range of motion as a fringe benefit. Unfortunately, many patients have complained of mechanical pain after the surgery. The rival design by Thompson,[190] the TPR system, (Thompson-Parkridge-Richards, Richards Manufacturing Co., Memphis, Tenn.) also provides arthroplasty of the ankle with min-

imal bony resection. The articular surfaces approximate a cylindrical configuration with beveled edges to permit modest abduction and adduction (Fig. 13-47). The implant is available in two sizes and two thicknesses to allow for variations in patient size and joint laxity. The polymeric tibial unit has recesses for anchorage in

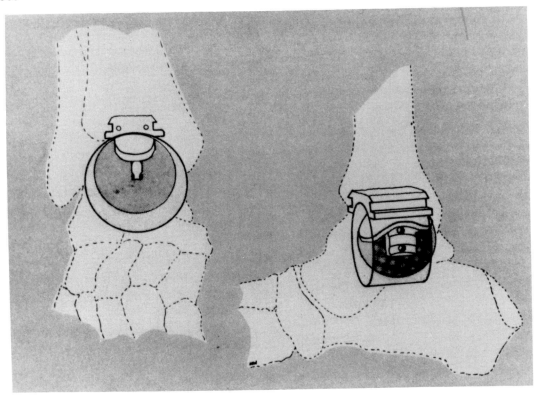

Figure 13-48. Schematic diagram shows the Newton total ankle joint replacement. (Reproduced with permission of S. E. Newton.)[191]

the cement while the stainless steel talar component has a short stem for attachment to the bone. Another design by Newton,[191] consists of a HDP tibial prosthesis and a Co-Cr unit for the talus (Fig. 13-48). The tibial implant possesses an articular surface with a cylindrical configuration while the talar unit is a section of a sphere with a slightly smaller radius. The arthroplasty permits both gliding as well as inversion and eversion and rotation. The talar implant rests on the articular surface of the talus so that no bone needs to be resected. As with the other units, methylmethacrylate cement is employed for fixation.

Recently, Pappas et al.[192] have classified the available types of total ankle joint replacements into two configurations, seen in Figures 13-49 to 13-51. While all of the implants consist of a polymeric and a metallic unit for the articular surfaces, certain of the designs show incongruent surface types, while others show congruent surfaces. The incongruent types have been classified as trochlear surfaces, concave/convex (sledge) and convex/convex surfaces. All of the designs show normal axial rotation, in addition

to flexion-extension. These designs, however, will show relatively poor wear and deformation resistance due to high local stress from the incongruent surface contact and the relatively poor inherent stability (Fig. 13-51). The high local stresses and pressures associated with normal walking loads would be likely to provoke permanent deformation of the ultra high molecular weight polyethylene. Also, the kinematic properties of such joints will be markedly different from the anatomical joint surface. For the Newton ankle design, using values of 2.4 cm for the radius of the cylindrical section, and 1.9 cm for the radius of the spherical section, a Young's modulus of 69,000 N/cm^2 (100,000 psi) and a Poisson's ratio of 0.33, the value of K is approximately 430 (1028) where P is in Newtons (lb). If yielding is to be avoided in a material with a yield strength of 2750 N/cm^2 (4000 psi), typical for ultra high molecular weight polyethylene at 37°C, the maximum load that can be applied to the prosthesis is only 262 N (59 lb). In contrast, during level walking, a man weighing 700 N (157 lb) would produce a joint load of about 1050 N (236 lb) and as much as 2800 N (629 lb) in

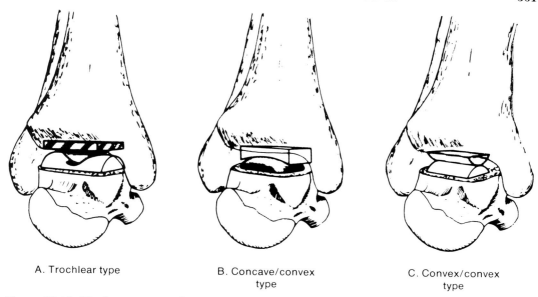

A. Trochlear type   B. Concave/convex   C. Convex/convex
                                    type   type

Figure 13-49. The incongruent surface types of total ankle joint replacements are shown. (Reproduced with permission of M. Pappas, S. S. Buechel, and A. F. DePalma.)[193]

climbing stairs. Pappas concludes that the New-ton prosthesis would suffer substantial local de-formation, fatigue and wear as a result of normal activity. In contrast, these workers argue that a congruent-type ankle with a typical contact area of about 5.2 cm^2 could support a load of 14,300 newtons (3200 lb) on UHMWPE (ultrahigh mo-lecular weight polyethylene) without substantial yielding. This value is much greater than the anticipated physiological loads.

Four basic variations of congruent surface types have been identified, as shown in Figure 13-50. The types are spherical (ball-and-socket), spheroidal (barrel-shaped), conical and cylindri-cal arrangements. Congruent surfaces permit good pressure distribution and offer superior wear and surface deformation resistance when compared to incongruent types. In addition, they provide some enhanced stability (Fig. 13-51).

The spherical type permits three independent axes of rotation. It allows actual rotation and inversion-eversion, which is especially important where a degenerative subtalar joint accompanies arthritis of the ankle joint. The liabilities of this consideration include the need for proper loca-tion of the center of rotation. This consideration, coupled with the geometry of the talus and the space available in the joint, favor a surface ge-ometry with a relatively shallow spherical seg-ment. The shallowness tends to limit the flexion-extension excursion and the shear resistance,

increasing the possibility of dislocation. The sur-face configuration is also less resistant to inver-sion-eversion injuries. As in the incongruent sledge-type, the pivot center during extreme in-version or eversion is at the center, rather than at the end of the talus, resulting in substantially greater than normal loading of the ligaments.

The spheroidal type provides two independ-ent rotations: plantar and dorsiflexion and in-version-eversion. Since it fails to provide axial rotation, the spheroidal type does not appear to be useful where subtalar motion is absent. Otherwise, it possesses the same disadvantages as the spherical type, without other desirable features of the cylindrical or conical configura-tions for patients with good subtalar joints.

The conical type prosthesis employs dual cones with a single horizontal axis. It provides some mediolateral thrust resistance, although this resistance is less than that offered by some cylindrical designs. The design has an ample range of motion which is obtained by a greater than normal rotational axis. Greater resection of bone is necessary with it than with other designs.

With this review in mind, Pappas et al.[192] designed a total ankle joint with a cylindrical shape because of its simplicity and inherently greater range of motion for a given axis location and bearing-contact area. It provides essentially normal stability and resistance to inversion-ev-ersion injuries. The talar component approxi-

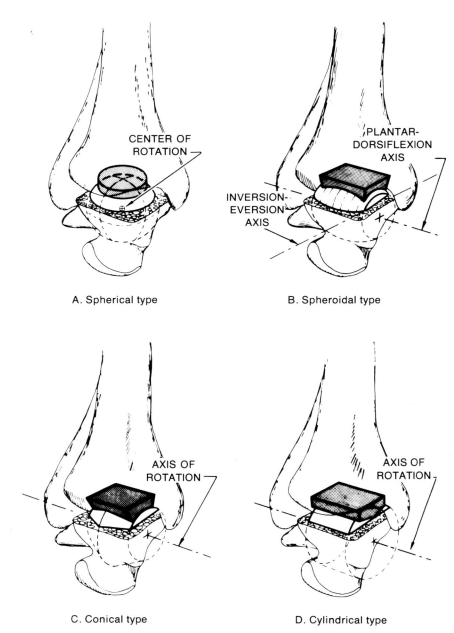

Figure 13-50. The congruent surface types of total ankle joint replacements are shown. (Reproduced with permission of M. Pappas, S. S. Buechel, and A. F. DePalma.)[194]

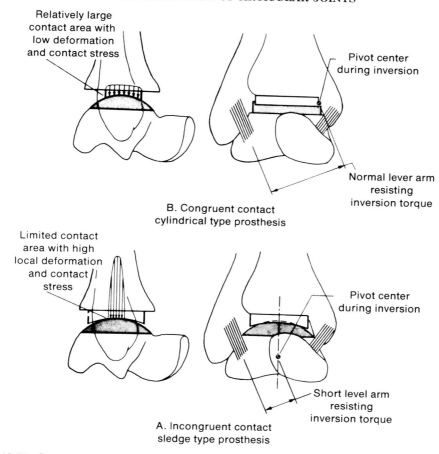

Relatively large contact area with low deformation and contact stress

Pivot center during inversion

Normal lever arm resisting inversion torque

B. Congruent contact cylindrical type prosthesis

Limited contact area with high local deformation and contact stress

Pivot center during inversion

Short level arm resisting inversion torque

A. Incongruent contact sledge type prosthesis

Figure 13-51. Contact stress in and stability of congruent and incongruent ankle prostheses are revealed. (Reproduced with permission of M. Pappas, S. S. Buechel, and A. F. DePalma.)[195]

mates the main diameter of the dome it replaces to minimize bone resection. A posterior extension is employed to permit an increase of flexion-extension range with a total of 65° of motion, realized as 20° of dorsiflexion and 45° of plantar flexion. Conical bearing surfaces in the sides of the talar component engage and interact with the mortise surfaces of the tibial component. The mortise sides improve stability and permit a maximum of 10° of talar tilt without dislocation of the prosthesis. The area of cylindrical surface contact is 5.2 mm², in comparison with 1.9 cm² for the Charnley 22-mm total hip replacement, and 3.5 cm² for the Müller 30-mm total hip prosthesis. Again, the results of prolonged clinical assessment will be necessary to determine the efficacy of the design.

Most recently, the Oregon total ankle joint replacement has emerged, which provides mediolateral stability and a unique carbon fiber reinforced UHMWPE component to articulate with a cast Co-Cr-Mo alloy. Most of the previous designs consisted of two sliding surfaces. For the Oregon model, like the design by Pappas *et al.*, the ankle joint is perceived as a series of three sets of articular surfaces: the distal tibia and the superior surface of the talus; the medial malleolus and the medial side of the talus; and the lateral malleolus or fibula and the lateral side of the talus. This perception of an ankle is shown schematically in Figures 13-38 to 13-40. The lateral profile of the talar dome can be approximated by a single circle, whereas the medial profile requires two circles, although the centers of the two circles are in close proximity. They record a range of motion of the anatomical ankle during walking af about 30° with a peak load of about 5 times body weight.

The Oregon total ankle possesses three sets of congruent articular surfaces. The central portion

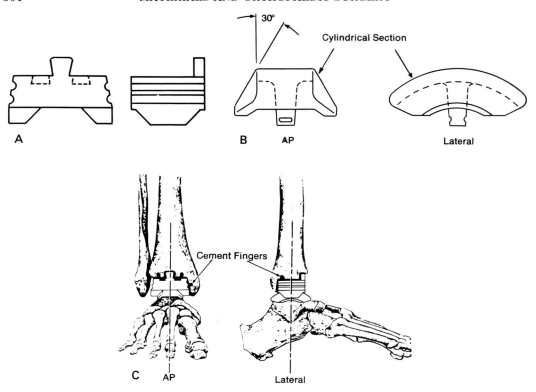

Figure 13-52. *A.* Anterior and lateral views of the Oregon tibial prosthesis are shown. *B.* Anteroposterior and lateral view of the Oregon talar prosthesis are shown. The Oregon total ankle prosthesis *in situ* is shown schematically. (*A, B* and *C*, reproduced with permission of Zimmer U.S.A.)

is a horizontal cylinder with a diameter slightly smaller than the average measurement of the talar profile. It provides a total range of flexion and extension of 40°. The lateral and medial surfaces are oriented at 30° in the vertical and provide transverse stability with a provision for 10° of rotation. The unit is shown schematically in Figure 13-52. For insertion of the talar unit, only the medial and lateral borders of the talus are resected while the superior surface of the talus is retained. The subchondral cortical bone provides a good buttress for the prosthesis. A small fixation post provides cement fixation along with two shallow recesses. The tibial component decreases posteriorly to fit into the wedge-shaped recess of the distal tibia. The posterior cortex of the distal tibia is left intact to provide good support for the implant and minimize the potential for loosening from sharing forces. Also, the retention of the posterior cortex prevents extrusion of bone cement into the posterior joint capsule. Such cement might damage posterior vessels and ligamentous structures and

impede motion of the arthroplastic joint. Only the anterior margin of the distal tibia and a small area of the medial malleolus are resected for insertion of the tibial unit. A few biomechanical observations on the Oregon total ankle are available.[196] The calculated maximum stress at the prosthetic interface during walking is estimated at a maximum of 1067 to 1443 psi over a surface area of 0.61 to 0.78 inch^2. Comparable figures for the geometric total knee replacement are 425 to 888 psi with a calculated contact area of 1.28 inch^2 and for the Charnley total hip replacement 1076 to 763 psi with a calculated contact area of 0.49 to 0.58 inch^2. For the Oregon ankle, the loosening torque measured at 200 lb of vertical compression force is 300 inches per pound, whereas that for the Freeman-Kempson ankle joint replacement is 192 inches per pound.

To date, the clinical observations on total ankle joint replacements are limited to a few cases studied over a few years. The principal problems have been prosthetic loosening, limited motion of the arthroplastic joints and me-

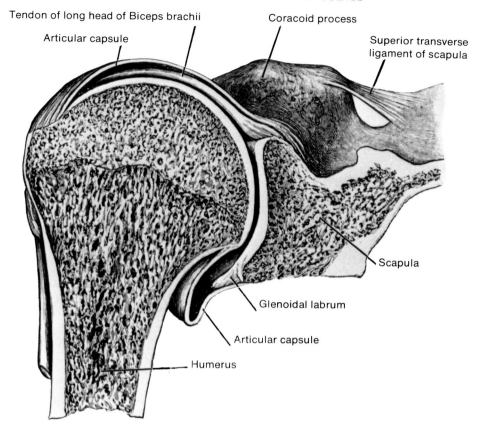

Tendon of long head of Biceps brachii

Articular capsule

Coracoid process

Superior transverse ligament of scapula

Scapula

Glenoidal labrum

Articular capsule

Humerus

Figure 13-53. The anatomy of the glenohumeral joint is revealed. (Reproduced with permission of C. M. Goss.)[200]

chanical pain at the ankle joint. Clearly, much further work remains to be undertaken in this field.

ARTHROPLASTIC RECONSTRUCTION OF THE SHOULDER JOINT

The shoulder consists of several joints which act in concert to provide motion of the upper extremity on the thorax.[197-199] The relevant joints include the articulation of the scapula on the rib cage, the sternoclavicular joint, the coracoacromial articulation and the glenohumeral joint (Fig. 13-53). The last mentioned is a ball-and-socket articulation, which may be afflicted by a variety of pathological conditions, including traumatic insults, rheumatoid arthritis, avascular necrosis and occasionally, degenerative arthritis, as well as others. In recent years a few attempts have been undertaken to develop arthroplastic reconstructions of the glenohumeral joint. Previously, painful arthritic afflictions with limited range of motion have been treated

by fusion of the joint.[201] Inevitably, fusion of such a highly mobile joint must compromise substantially the function of the upper extemity. Three radically different approaches have been undertaken in an effort to reconstruct a mobile glenohumeral articulation. Before these are reviewed, the biomechanics of the shoulder is discussed.

Anatomical Considerations of the Shoulder Joint

Numerous anatomical features of the shoulder joint function in unison to provide the most mobile joint in the body. The radius of the articular surface of the glenoid is relatively large, so that the glenoid articular surface is almost flat. The radius of the articular surface of the humerus is relatively small to provide a hemispherical configuration.[202] The incongruent surfaces provide an inherently unstable joint, with an extraordinary degree of motion. The capsule of the glenohumeral joint is relatively thin, with

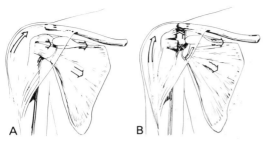

Figure 13-54. *A.* The function of the supraspinatus is to depress the greater tuberosity while compressing the humeral head against the glenoid articular surface. The more inferior muscles on the scapula, the subscapularis, infraspinatus and teres minor, are more powerful depressors of the humeral head. They function simultaneously and synergistically with the deltoid muscle throughout the range of elevation. *B.* A complete tear of the rotator cuff sacrifices the ability to fix the glenohumeral fulcrum. The deltoid is unable to elevate the humerus and dislocates the humeral head under the acromion. (*A* and *B*, reproduced with permission of J. M. Fenlin, Jr.[204])

many folds and pouches. To permit the greatest degree of mobility of the joint, the capsule is so lax that it provides little stability. The musculotendinous rotator cuff surrounding the joint provides stability with freedom of motion.[203] Furthermore, it fixes the fulcrum against which the deltoid can contract and elevate the humerus with power. As seen in Figure 13-54A, the supraspinatus tendon depresses the greater tuberosity, while compressing the humeral head against the glenoid articular surface. The more inferior muscles on the scapula, the subscapularis, infraspinatus and teres minor, are more powerful depressors of the humeral head. They function simultaneously and synergistically with the deltoid muscle throughout the range of elevation. They serve primarily to fix the fulcrum while permitting mobility, and to a lesser degree they assist with the power of elevation. Complete paralysis, or rupture of the rotator cuff sacrifices the ability to fix the glenohumeral fulcrum (Fig. 13-54B). The deltoid then is unable to elevate the humerus, and merely shrugs the shoulder. If the derangement is partial paralysis, or partial avulsion of the rotator cuff, the resulting disability is usually weakness in elevation.

The musculotendinous cuff, along with the greater and lesser tuberosities must glide freely under the coracoacromial arch for optimal function. The narrow subacromial space is occupied by a bursa. Minor anatomical derangement in this area can provide substantial disability of the shoulder. For example, degeneration of the rotator cuff, exostoses of the acromion or of the greater tuberosity, all may interfere with the smooth gliding mechanism.

Biomechanics of the Shoulder

Recently, Poppen and Walker[205] have reviewed the center of the rotation and motion of the glenohumeral joint. In a series of normal patients, a radiographic method revealed that up to 30° of abduction occurred chiefly at the glenohumeral joint. From 30° to the maximum abduction, the ratio of glenohumeral to scapulothoracic motion was 5:4. This observation agreed with that of Freedman and Munro,[206] but differed somewhat from Inman *et al.*[203] The centers of rotation are mostly within 6 mm of the center of the humeral ball, which was correlated to an average excursion of the ball up or down the face of the scapula of only 1 mm. The average glenoid encompasses an angle of 80° and the humeral head conforms closely with it at all angles of abduction. With this provision, the instant center of rotation is close to the center of the ball.

These workers also correlated the electromyographic records of muscle activity with shoulder motion. In abduction in the plane of the scapula and neutral rotation, the compressive component increases steadily to 1 times body weight at 90° abduction, and then diminishes to 0.95 times body weight at 150°. The upward shearing force reaches its maximum of 0.65 body weight at 60° and then diminishes to close to zero at 120° to 150° of abduction. At 90° of abduction the resultant force peaked at just over 1 times body weight. Comparable measurements were undertaken in abduction with internal rotation and abduction with external rotation. The measurements also show that the humeral head is inherently more stable in a superior-inferior plane in external rotation.

Biomechanics of Shoulder Joint Replacement

In recent years at least eight different medical centers have studied the design or implantation of glenohumeral joint prostheses. Several different designs have been studied for which Fenlin[202] has provided an excellent conceptual review. The following discussion is based on his observations.

Historically, the first satisfactory arthroplastic technique was that devised by Neer[207] for replacement of the humeral head. This hemiarthroplasty was designed for use after four-part

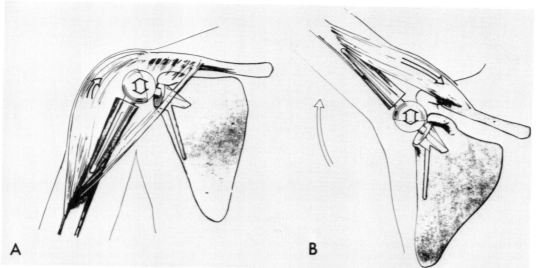

Figure 13-55. A prosthesis with an inherently stable fulcrum allows the deltoid bone to elevate the humerus. (Reproduced with permission of J. M. Fenlin, Jr.[208])

fracture/dislocations of the shoulder where avascular necrosis of the principal articular component is almost inevitable, and for use in rheumatoid and degenerative arthritis (Chapter 14, Fig. 14-14G). For success, the shoulder requires a normal rotator cuff function, with a smooth subacromial gliding mechanism. The glenoid articular surface also must be relatively normal. By the application of meticulous surgical reconstruction and postoperative rehabilitation, Neer reported excellent results after the use of this arthroplasty. In view of its success, he extended the system to applications for patients with glenoid destruction as well as deterioration of the humeral head. The glenoid articular surface was reconstructed by the use of a cylindrical plug of HDP (Chapter 14, Fig. 14-14H). The glenoid replacement provided a smooth articular surface and enhanced the stability of the glenohumeral joint. Nevertheless, the system still required a normally functioning rotator cuff. With this criteria satisfied, Neer has reported highly satisfactory results. At present, the glenohumeral arthroplasty of Neer is the optimal form of treatment for the patients who satisfy the appropriate criteria.

As Fenlin[202] has emphasized, unfortunately many patients with deterioration of the glenohumeral joint possess compromised function of the rotator cuff. The other designs of glenohumeral joint replacement have been directed toward a satisfactory solution to this complex problem. If the prosthesis were designed with an inherently stable fulcrum, the deltoid alone could elevate the humerus without the assistance of the rotator cuff (Fig. 13-55). In this instance, the incompetent rotator cuff could be resected along with the greater and lesser tuberosities to provide substantial flexibility in the design of the prosthesis, such as a stable ball-and-socket configuration. Fenlin favors a large ball from several points of view. To stabilize a small ball, the appropriate socket must extend more degrees beyond the equator than is true for a large ball (Fig. 13-56A). From this parameter, more degrees of range of motion are lost to the socket with a small ball. With a large ball, the range of motion of the prosthesis can be in excess of the active range of motion of the patient. If the end stages of motion are not reached, then the bump at the extremes of motion which might provoke prosthetic loosening does not occur. Another advantage of a large ball, is that its larger radius represents the lever arm across which the deltoid contracts to initiate elevation (Fig. 13-56B). The force initiating elevation, therefore, is greater, and is proportional to the radius of the ball. This advantage is particularly important where the only force initiating elevation is the deltoid muscle. If the rotator cuff is resected, a considerable soft tissue void arises between the deltoid muscle and the prosthesis. By the use of a larger prosthesis, the void is filled to provide a cosmetic contour to the shoulder.

As with other total joint replacements, HDP

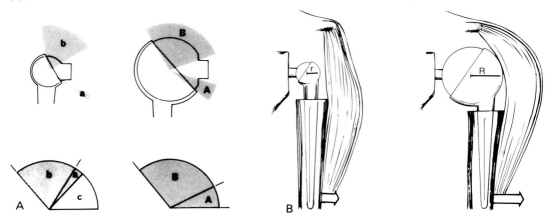

Figure 13-56. *A.* The axle attached to the ball subtends a greater number of degrees on the circumference of a small ball than that of a large ball. In addition, to gain the same degree of stability, it is necessary for the cup to extend more degrees beyond the equator of a small ball than of a large ball. The total loss of motion is depicted by arc *C*.(Reproduced with permission of J. M. Fenlin, Jr.[209]) *B.* The radius of the ball represents a lever arm across which the deltoid contracts to initiate elevation. The elevation force with the large ball is, therefore, greater and is proportional to the length of the radius. The larger prosthesis offers a better cosmetic contour for the shoulder. (Reproduced with permission of J. M. Fenlin, Jr.[210])

articulating with a metallic alloy has been common practice. Fenlin uses the 6Al-4V titanium alloy in view of its resistance to fatigue and corrosion. In view of the greater strength and structural rigidity of the metal, this material is employed for the cup so that it may have a relatively thin wall. In this way, the polyethylene ball may have the largest possible diameter for any given anatomical space available.

While the anatomical joint shows the ball attached to the humeral side with the cup on the scapular side, the arthroplastic device of Fenlin reverses this arrangement. In the anatomical arrangement, the potential to dislocate is always greatest when the alignment of the humerus is perpendicular to the open mouth of the cup. In this position a longitudinal pull on the humerus can provoke dislocation. With the cup attached to the humerus, however, its open face is aligned at 45° to the shaft of the humerus, so that the potential to dislocate is greatly diminished.

One of the most difficult features of total glenohumeral joint replacement is the limited bone stock available in the scapula for the fixation of the relevant prosthesis. Apart from the glenoid, the scapular wing is a thin, flat sheet of bone. Other prostheses, such as the Stanmore design (Fig. 13-57A), possess a glenoid replacement with three stems for cement fixation. Preparation of the scapula for anchorage of the stems

is excessively difficult. Loosening of the glenoid component complicates most applications of the Stanmore design. The design by Fenlin shows a unique scapular anchor which seats well in bone. Alteration from the anatomical design, with the ball attached to the scapula, lessens the potential loosening forces on the anchor. In Figures 13-57A and B, the Stanmore design with a medium size ball prosthesis and a small ball prosthesis are shown. With the smaller ball, the fulcrum of the joint can technically be placed within the cavity of the glenoid. Forces radiating from the fulcrum are distributed to the cortical walls of the cavity and are mostly compressive forces which the cement tolerates quite well. The intermediate size ball prosthesis displaces the center of the fulcrum beyond the confines of the cancellous cavity by the distance X. In turn, the shearing forces imposed upon the scapular fixation device are augmented to jeopardize the cement fixation. With a large diameter ball prosthesis, the distance X from the center of the fulcrum to the cancellous cavity of the scapula is even greater, so that the shearing forces would be proportionally greater and even less desirable. As previously mentioned, a large diameter ball shows a number of other marked advantages. The potential disadvantages of the large ball are obviated if the ball is attached to the scapula instead of the humerus. With the Fenlin design (Fig. 13-57C), the scapular anchor may fill the

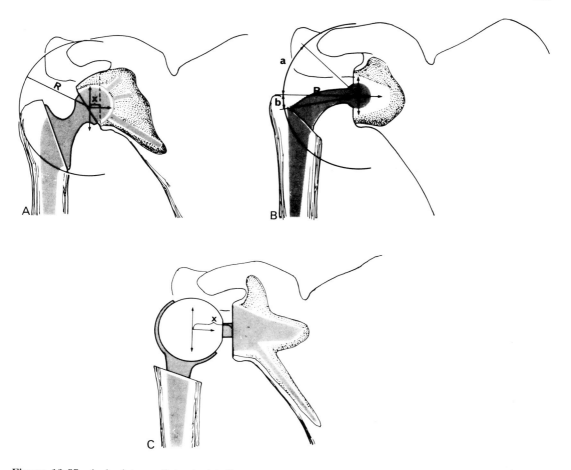

Figure 13-57. *A.* An intermediate sized ball prosthesis of the Stanmore design is shown. The center of the fulcrum is displaced beyond the confines of the cancellous cavity by the distance *X*. This adds more shear stress to the scapular fixation device. The spike extends partly into the medullary canal of the axillary border of the scapula. The scapular wing, however, is a particularly thin and fragile bone. (Reproduced with permission of J. M. Fenlin, Jr.[211]) *B.* A composite of a small ball prosthesis shows that the fulcrum can be placed within the confines of the cancellous cavity. The forces radiating from the fulcrum are distributed to the cortical walls of the cavity and are mostly compressive forces. The long radius, *R*, does not permit the greater tuberosity to clear the acromion and limits motion. Some motion can be gained by resection of the tuberosity or shortening the radius. (Reproduced with permission of J. M. Fenlin, Jr.[212]) *C.* A schematic view shows the Fenlin design for a total joint replacement with a large ball prosthesis. The ball is attached to the scapula and the socket is anchored to the proximal humerus. The distance, *X*, from the center of the fulcrum to the cancellous cavity of the scapula is great so that the shear effect is enlarged. The scapular anchor fills the medullary cavity as much as possible with a metallic device and utilizes a relatively thin wall and cement as a filler. A long spike inserts into the medullary canal of the axillary border of the scapula. (Reproduced with permission of J. M. Fenlin, Jr.[211])

entire glenoid portion of the scapula so that the fixation is substantially augmented.

One other prosthesis has been devised in an attempt to restore pain-free function and stability to the glenohumeral joint. A design by Macnab and English[213] shows anchorage surfaces for fixation in bone which are sinter-coated Co-Cr alloy, to permit fixation by ingrowth of bone. The humeral component shows a highly polished hemispherical articular surface, comparable to the anatomical design. The glenoid articular surface is made of HDP attached to a Co-

Cr base. The base has a sinter-coated surface for fixation to the scapula. It also shows an outrigger stabilizer that is secured in the acromion to resist rotational forces and prevent loosening of the glenoid component. The polymeric glenoid component shows a large superior lip which establishes a stable point of leverage to prevent superior migration of the humeral head prosthesis. This feature will compensate in part for loss of leverage due to degenerative changes or traumatic tear in the rotator cuff. The implant is shown in Chapter 14, Figure 14-13A.

Few clinical results have been reported for any of the previous systems. The best documentation is that provided by Neer[207] in those patients with an intact rotator cuff. Fenlin[202] has reported the results of a few patients in which his device was employed. While these are highly promising, larger numbers of cases observed over longer periods of time will be needed to make a useful assessment of his or other devices. Similar reports by Letten and Scales,[214, 215] present encouraging results with the Stanmore design, although other workers have not replicated their favorable results. Much further work remains to be undertaken on the development of glenohumeral joint replacements.

ARTHROPLASTIC RECONSTRUCTION OF THE ELBOW JOINT

The elbow joint is a hinge or ginglymus joint (Fig. 13-58), which primarily permits flexion and extension.[199, 217-219] In fact, it also participates in pronation and supination of the forearm at the humeroradial articulation. Detailed biomechanical analysis of the elbow joint has lagged behind comparable evaluation of other joints. As such, previous workers have considered the elbow to be purely a uniaxial hinge. Many of the early attempts at elbow joint replacement employed metallic uniaxial hinges which showed a surprisingly high incidence of loosening.[219] The explanation for this complication is the previously unrecognized axial rotation of the elbow on the humerus. The newer biomechanical studies on the elbow have clearly shown that the elbow, like the knee, is a polycentric hinge with a complex arc of motion, which shall be described shortly.

For over 100 years, various workers have attempted to reconstruct the elbow joint with a variety of arthroplastic techniques.[220, 221] In the past century, when tuberculosis was a frequent affliction of joints, interpositional arthroplasties of the elbow, with the application of various biological tissues such as fascia lata, were widely

undertaken. To the present time, various workers including Vainio, recommend biological interpositional arthroplasties of the elbow.[222, 223] The convalescence period is prolonged in view of the early postoperative instability which gradually resolves over a 2- to 3-year period. Other surgeons have employed hemiarthroplastic techniques with resurfacing of the trochlea on the distal humerus[224, 225] or of the trochlear notch in the proximal ulna.[226, 227] Street and Stevens[224] reported 7-year follow-ups on their trochlear and capitellar replacement of stainless steel or titanium alloy, which was employed on patients with rheumatoid arthritis, hemophilia and posttraumatic lesions. Patients with post-traumatic insults showed a stable, pain-free elbow, with a functional range of motion while those with inflammatory arthritis or hemophilia had a poor result. The operation was difficult to undertake and did not gain widespread popularity. The attempts to resurface the trochlear fossa with a saddle-shaped implant of Co-Cr alloy, also have not achieved favorable results. Where the arthritic process involves opposing joint surfaces, it is unlikely that such hemiarthroplastic techniques would be successful.

The Biomechanics of the Elbow

In a recent report, Morrey and Chao[228] have provided an elegant description of the 3-dimensional motion of the elbow joint, which is a marked improvement on previous knowledge. They studied normal upper extremities in fresh cadaveric specimens. Metallic markers were inserted into the bones, along the axes of the humerus, radius and ulna. By the use of these and other markers, X-rays were taken throughout ranges of motion, with elbows positioned in flexion and rotation. A fixed system of coordinates, based on the humerus was employed. The elbow flexion and rotation were studied both separately and in combination. Biplane X-rays were employed to record the joint motion, at various increments of elbow flexion. Flexion-extension changes in carrying angle and actual rotation were calculated using a 3 by 3 transformation matrix and expressed as Eulerian angles. The accuracy of the calculations of the Eulerian angles is within ± 2.5°. The details of their analytic technique deserve scrutiny in their original paper.

During elbow flexion, the carrying angle (Θ) formed by the long axis of the forearm and by the long axis of the humerus in the frontal plane, shows a linear change (Fig. 13-59A). The pattern of change is independent of forearm position in

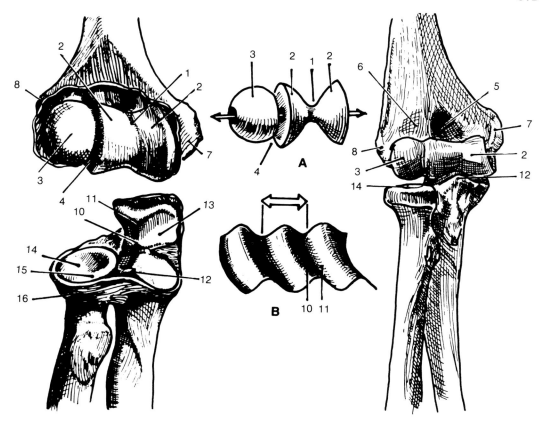

Figure 13-58. A detailed anatomical drawing of the elbow joint is shown. The numbers refer to the same portions of the articular surfaces in all of the drawings. The distal end of the humerus has two articular surfaces: the trochlea, *2*, a pulley-shaped structure with a central groove, *1*, lying in a sagittal plane and embodied by two convex lips, *2*; and a capitulum, a spherical surface, *3*, positioned lateral to the trochlea. The capitulum is an anteriorly placed hemisphere which, unlike the trochlea, does not extend posteriorly. The proximal ends of the forearm bones show articular surfaces corresponding to those in the distal ends of the humerus. The trochlear notch of the ulna articulates with the trochlea. It consists of a longitudinal rounded ridge, *10*, extending from the olecranon process, *11*, superiorly to the coronoid process, *12*, anteriorly and inferiorly. On either side of the ridge which corresponds to the trochlear groove is a concave surface, *13*, corresponding to the lips of the trochlea. The articular surface is shaped like a segment of a corrugated iron sheet formed by a ridge, *10*, and two gutters, *11* (*B*). The cylindrical surface of the head of the radius possesses a central concavity on its proximal end which corresponds to the convexity of the capitellum humeri. It is bound by a rim which articulates with the capitellotrochlear groove. The figure on the *right* shows apposition of the articular surfaces with the olecranon fossa, *5*, above the trochlea and the radial fossa, *6*, the medial epicondyle, *7*, and the lateral epicondyle, *8*. (Reproduced with permission of I. A. Kapandji.[216])

neutral, supination or pronation. Morrey and Chao[228] observed a valgus carrying angle of 10° in full extension, and a varus angle ranging between 6 and 10° in full flexion. While the magnitude of carrying angle varies with sex, height and body habitus, nevertheless, these figures are indicative of the changes in carrying angle that occur during elbow flexion. During elbow flexion, the forearm was also observed to rotate about its long axis. The rotation was observed while the forearm was in fixed supination, neutral and pronation, and hence represented axial rotation resulting from the configuration of the humeroulnar articular surfaces and ligamentous constraints. The long axis of the forearm was calculated to rotate about 5° internally during early elbow flexion and about 5° externally during terminal flexion (Fig. 13-59B).

In the assessment of changes accompanying supination-pronation (Fig. 13-60A), for the ex-

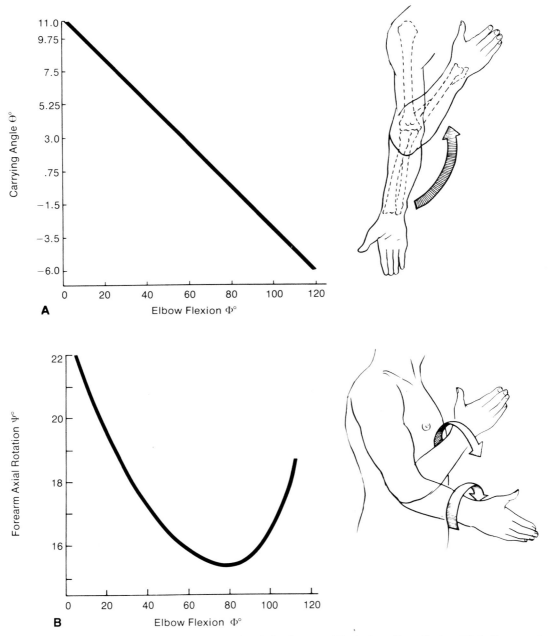

Figure 13-59. *A.* The change in carrying angle of the forearm (Θ) during elbow flexion (Φ) is linear and progresses from a valgus (+) to a varus (−) angle. *B.* Axial rotation about the long axis of the forearm taken as a unit (Ψ) during elbow flexion (Φ) is internal for 0° to about 80° of flexion and external thereafter. (*A* and *B*, reproduced with permission of B. F. Morrey and E. Y. S. Chao.[229])

tended elbow the ulna shows virtually no valgus deviation with respect to the humerus during forearm rotation from supination to pronation. The long axis of the radius deviates medially during this motion because rotation of the forearm is accomplished by a rotation of this bone.

The long axis of the radius is deviated medially 6 to 10° with respect to the long axis of the humerus during pronation. There is no significant axial rotation of the ulna during pronation and supination with the elbow fully extended.

The instant centers of rotation during elbow

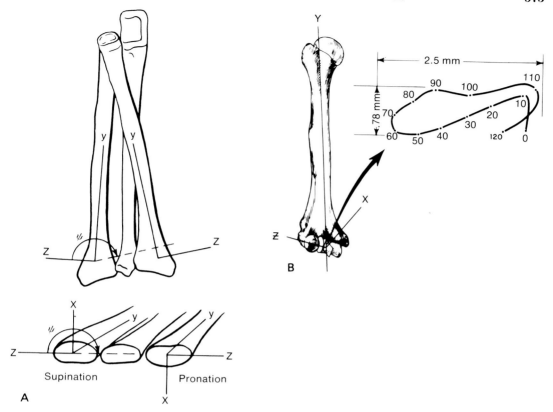

Figure 13-60. *A.* The changes accompanying supination and pronation of the extended elbow are shown. *B.* Configurations and dimensions of the locus of the instant centers of rotation of the elbow are seen. (Reproduced with permission of B. F. Morrey and E. Y. S. Chao.[229])

flexion were determined to verify the approximate location of the axis of flexion-extension. In a previous study Fischer[231] described the locus of the instant centers of rotation of the elbow in flexion and extension at the center of the trochlea with an area 2 to 3 mm in diameter (Fig. 13-60B). Fischer employed the Reuleaux technique[232] with a 2-dimensional analysis. Morrey and Chao[228] were able to verify the results of Fischer, namely, that the axis of elbow flexion is fixed and passes through the center of the trochlea. The axis must be oriented obliquely, however, with respect to the forearm axis since the carrying angle changes during elbow flexion and extension. (The axes of rotation of the elbow passing through the center of the trochlea are located in the plane of the anterior border of the humerus as seen on a lateral X-ray.)

Elbow Joint Arthroplasties

During the past decade several workers have attempted to employ uniaxial hinges for replacement of the humeroulnar articulation, usually in combination with excision of the radial head. Since most of the weight-bearing forces at the elbow joint are transmitted through the humeroulnar joint, resection of the radial head does not substantially effect stability in the mature elbow and it obviates the need for more complex implants that would resurface the radiohumeral articulation. The earliest designs were minor modifications of the hinge prostheses, such as the Schiers device employed for reconstruction of the knee.[233] The implants were reduced in size and secured with methylmethacrylate cement. In view of the rapid onset of loosening other designs altered the alignment of the two intramedullary stems to conform to the "carrying angle" between the natural axes of the humerus and ulna. The surgical alignment of the altered prostheses, such as that designed by Dee[234] (Fig. 13-61), was even more difficult than the previous types of implants. Schlein[235] has designed an implant with an inherent 7° carrying

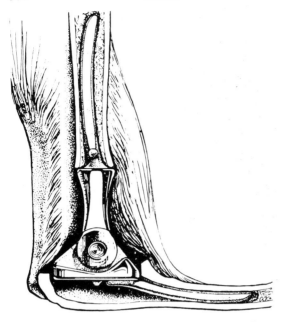

Figure 13-61. A schematic lateral view of a Dee elbow prosthesis. Apart from a portion of the humeral intramedullary stem the remainder of the implant is buried within bone. (Reproduced with permission of R. Dee.[230])

angle that shows an intrinsic degree of freedom of 4 to 6° in all three planes. The cobalt-chromium prosthesis possesses an ultra high density polyethylene bearing surface by press-poppet fit. The polymeric unit is machined into a commercial snap fit and a bearing surface. The ulnar component is joined to the bearing surface by the snap fit. Over 400 of the Schlein constrained elbow prostheses have been inserted over the past 3 years. Eleven cases of prosthetic loosenings were reported in which 3 cases occurred after major trauma. Seven of the prostheses were reinserted with longer humeral stems; subsequently they appeared to function satisfactorily. Two cases of prosthetic subluxation were reported. In 5 cases fracture of the humeral condyles occurred during insertion of the prosthesis. Apart from retardation of the rehabilitation program the ultimate outcome was not influenced by this complication. Transient neurapraxias were noted although only one permanent ulnar nerve palsy was reported. Perhaps the outstanding improvement in the Schlein design was the loosening rate of about 3% which is approximately 1/10 of the loosening of the conventional hinge-type arthroplasties. Nevertheless, it seems likely that more prolonged follow-up periods will reveal a higher incidence of prosthetic loosening.

Another problem with elbow-joint arthroplasty is related to the limited soft tissue coverage of the implant. The dorsal portions of the humeroulnar articulation are largely subcutaneous. Whenever implants are not surrounded by an envelope of muscle postoperative wound infections are more likely to occur.[234] Portions of the early hinge-type prostheses were deep to the skin and subcutaneous tissues. More recent designs have attempted to diminish the size of the hinge so that it would fit entirely within the confines of the distal humerus or the proximal ulna. Most of the articular portion of the Dee prosthesis fits entirely within the proximal ulna. A short section of the humeral component, connecting the intramedullary stem to the hinge, does not reside within bone although it is surrounded by the brachialis and brachioradialis on the anterior surface and by the triceps muscle on the posterior aspect. In another clinical report Ewald[219] has reported on a group of traumatic rheumatoid and degenerative patients who underwent hinge arthroplasty of the elbow and were followed for periods of up to 2½ years. Of the patients, 75% showed satisfactory results with 110° to 120° of flexion. In other patients loosening of the implant often with marked erosion or fracture of bone was observed. Some of the patients also showed infections which were difficult to manage. In an effort to lessen these complications, Ewald* has devised a nonconstrained system with metal-on-polyethylene surface replacements of the humeroulnar joint. His preliminary clinical observations have been encouraging.

One other constrained design, the Swanson flexible silicone rubber hinge has been used extensively.[236] The implant is an enlargement of the similar prostheses used by the inventor for treatment of metacarpophalangeal arthritis. Both in the hands of the inventor and in other workers the implant has shown excessive liability to undergo fatigue fracture of the hinge. In view of its fixed center of rotation and inability to accommodate the change in carrying angle of the elbow with flexion, the fractures are not surprising.

ARTHROPLASTIC RECONSTRUCTION OF THE WRIST

Experience with replacement arthroplasty of the wrist joint has been very limited. Especially

---

* F. C. Ewald, personal communication, 1977.

in patients with rheumatoid arthritis but also in others with traumatic lesions, fusion of the wrist has been a moderately successful form of treatment provided that the patient possesses adequate motion of adjacent joints.[237, 238] As the quality of results of other total joint replacements has improved interest in the development of a similar device for the wrist joint has rekindled. All of the presently available systems have been designed without access to a detailed biomechanical analysis of the wrist joint. The surgical techniques of implantation have been further hampered by the absence of clinical techniques to determine the center of rotation of the wrist joint. Without this knowledge the surgeon was likely to implant the hinge with incorrect inclination and orientation. In the postoperative period, fracture of the hinge or loosening of the anchorage site would be anticipated. These problems have been encountered frequently in the limited clinical trials. Recently Hamas* has studied the center of rotation of the wrist and defined relevant clinical techniques which can be used at the time or total wrist arthroplasty. His elegant method is described shortly.

Biomechanics of the Wrist

From an anatomical view point the wrist represents a complex joint with remarkable flexibility and stability.[239, 240] The wrist joint or radiocarpal joint permits flexion, extension, adduction and abduction. A combination of these movements represents circumduction of this ellipsoidal articulation. The socket is formed by the lower articular surface of the radius with the articular disc (Fig. 13-62). The convex ellipsoidal surface is formed by the proximal articular surfaces of the scaphoid, lunate and triquetrum plus the interosseous ligaments binding the three bones together. The proximal bearing surfaces of the scaphoid and lunate are approximately equal in area while that of the lunate is extremely small. The carpal bones do not articulate with the ulna but with the disc which excludes the ulna from the wrist joint (Fig. 13-62B). Stability of the wrist is achieved mainly by the dorsal and volar ligamentous and capsular structures with additional support provided by the close proximity of the wrist flexors and extensors to the carpus. The configuration of the proximal carpal row in the anteroposterior plane is one of an arc of much greater diameter than the second smaller arc, composed of the lesser multangular, capitate and hamate (Fig. 13-62A).

The kinesthesiology of the wrist comprises motion of the radiocarpal articulation and of the intracarpal motion. The instant center, or axis of motion of the radiocarpal complex, is located within the head of the capitate. Although the configuration of the head of the capitate, as it articulates within the concavity formed by the navicular and lunate, would suggest that some rotatory motion occurs at the wrist, rotational movement about a single axis does not occur at the radiocarpal complex. Rotational movement at the wrist occurs through the proximal and distal radioulnar joints and is expressed as supination and pronation.

The normal arc of flexion occurring at the wrist approximates 85° to 90° with 50° or 65% occurring at the radiocarpal articulation. The residual 35% arises from the midcarpal articulation. Values for extension usually approach 80 to 85° with about 35° arising from the radiocarpal articulation while 50° occurs at the midcarpal joint. The contribution of the radiocarpal and midcarpal joints to radial and ulnar deviation is nearly equal. The radioulnar motion occurs between the proximal and distal carpal row in a somewhat paradoxical way. With ulnar deviation the proximal carpal row moves toward the radial side of the wrist, while the distal carpal row shifts toward the ulnar side of the carpus. The opposite prevails with radial deviation. The reciprocal motion facilitates radial and ulnar deviation without an appreciable change in the linear alignment of the hand with reference to the forearm. It should be noted that the triquetrum only articulates with the distal radius at the extremes of radioulnar motion.

The Designs of Total Wrist Joint Replacements

Whereas the goal of arthroplastic reconstruction of many joints is strictly to resurface the opposing articular surfaces, this is not the case in a substantial number of patients with defective interfaces between the radius and the proximal carpal row. Many disease processes create diffuse mechanical problems at the wrist with subluxation or dislocation and destruction of musculotendinous structures. An implant for a wrist joint arthroplasty, therefore, should replace the articular surfaces and restore motion in the anatomical axes of the radiocarpal complex. The design of the implant also must reflect the variable amount of space available for implantation of the prosthetic interface.

Wrists that exhibit substantial degenerative change following trauma usually show principal

* R. S. Hamas, personal communication, 1978.

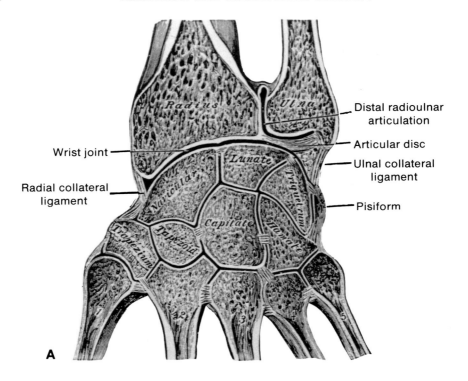

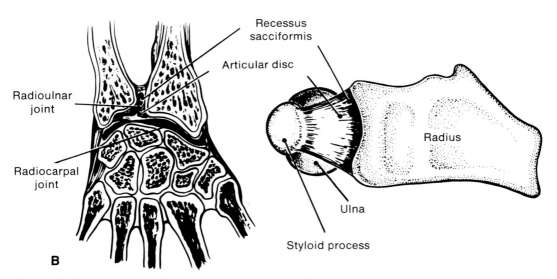

Figure 13-62. *A.* Anatomical features of the wrist joint are shown. *B.* The joint space itself is highlighted and the appearance of the distal end of the radius with the articular disc and the styloid process of the ulna is presented. (*A*, reproduced with permission of C. M. Goss.[241])

destruction at the level of the proximal carpal row. Nonunion of the scaphoid and aseptic necrosis of the scaphoid and lunate are not infrequent sequelae of such trauma. The resection of the scaphoid and lunate is a logical part of the total wrist joint replacement. Resection of the head of the capitate at the level of the lesser multangular provides a space 6.5 cm^2 (1 in.^{2}) in an anteroposterior plane to augment the space available for the implant and to facilitate its fixation in the metacarpals.[242] Attachment to the radius is readily achieved by the use of a prosthetic stem in the radial medullary canal.

The site of principal concern for prosthetic loosening is attachment to the second and third metacarpals where intramedullary stems are cemented in place. Jobbins *et al.*[243] report that about 250 kg is required to disrupt a metallic-cement interface around a pin 9.5 mm in diameter and 22 mm in length. From this observation Volz[242] estimates that the failing point of the metacarpal attachment is about 99 kg. With knurled segments in the prosthetic stems he estimates that the force of failure could be elevated to about 150 kg. In contrast the ultimate tensile strength of a metacarpal with the cortical thickness of about 0.5 mm is approximately 153 kg while the ultimate tensile strength of a Co-Cr alloy stem of appropriate diameter to fit in the metacarpal is approximately 840 kg.

Other desirable features of prosthetic design should include an adequate range of motion in the two axes observed at the wrist joint, adequate stability and location of the moving surfaces so that they restore the instant center of motion observed in a normal wrist. Three prosthetic designs are currently available which satisfy these criteria to a variable degree. Each is discussed briefly in turn.

The most widely employed total wrist arthroplasty is the silicone rubber design by Swanson.[244] This model is fully described by its inventor in Chapter 14. In brief it represents a flexible hinge arthroplasty comparable to that more extensively used at the metacarpophalangeal joint. It permits flexion and extension without other motion. The implant is inserted loosely into the intramedullary cavity of the radius and into the third metacarpal. Comparable to other silastic arthroplasties the implant can "piston" in a proximal or distal direction to center itself near the center of rotation of the joint. This capability should lessen bending moments and shear stresses on the implant and on the interface between the implant and bone. The unnatural constraint imposed by the implant, without pro-

vision for adduction or abduction provokes excessive bending moments on the implant.

Meuli[245] has devised a ball-and-socket system in which a polyethylene ball is mounted on a cylindrical metallic trunnion of Co-Cr alloy (Fig. 13-63). The socket is made of the same alloy. Both of the metallic elements possess two prongs that are secured to the intramedullary cavities of the radius and to the second and third metacarpals, respectively, with methylmethacrylate cement. The arthroplasty permits flexion and extension, abduction and adduction and circumduction comparable to that in the anatomical wrist. Loosening of the implant has been a considerable problem. Many cases of loosening arise because the implant is not centered in the anatomical axis of motion. Alleviation of this problem is discussed shortly.

A recent design by Volz[242] employs a toroidal sector in which the articular surfaces possess radii of different dimensions (Fig. 13-64). Motion can occur in two planes without appreciable circumduction. The distal component consists of Co-Cr alloy and shows a convex surface that fits into a concave, recessed radial articular surface. The latter implant possesses a polyethylene articular surface with a Co-Cr alloy stem. The articular interface possesses sufficient stability so that physiological forces of distraction of up to 40 lb are not likely to provoke subluxation or dislocation. The implant permits 90° of flexion and extension and 50° of radioulnar deviation.

In a series of 17 total wrist joint replacements undertaken in 14 patients with severe deformities secondary to trauma or rheumatoid arthritis, Volz has documented results for up to 13 months after surgery. The range of postoperative motion has averaged about 50° of flexion and extension and 25° of radioulnar deviation. The pain relief has been good. Postoperative ulnar deviation has been observed in some patients. This tendency is diminished if tenotomy of the flexor carpi ulnaris and palmaris longus are performed at the time of total wrist replacement. Nevertheless, two patients failed to develop significant motion after surgery. Restoration of motion and prolonged fixation of the implants in bone demands that the prosthetic joint is centered coaxial with the anatomical axis of motion. Previously no clinical technique has been available to assist the surgeon in this crucial stage of the reconstructive procedure. Recently Hamas* has devised a simple and elegant technique which is presented here.

_____
* R. S. Hamas, personal communication, 1978.

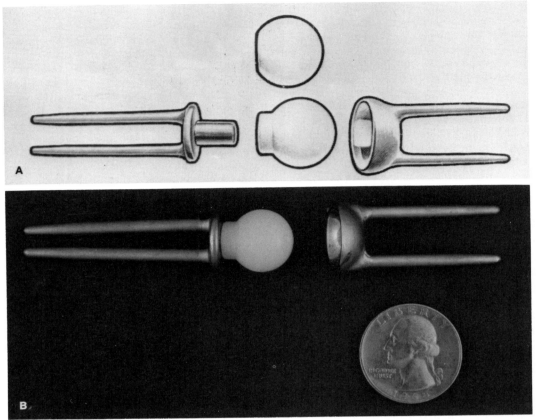

Figure 13-63. *A* and *B*. The schematic diagram and photograph reveal the Meuli total wrist joint prosthesis.

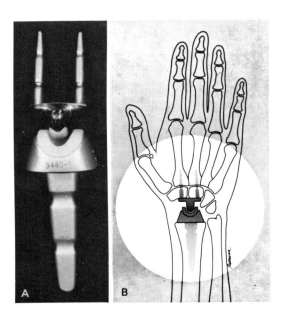

Figure 13-64. *A* and *B*. A Volz total wrist joint prosthesis is shown in an anteroposterior view. The larger component represents the radial implant with a polyethylene concave interface. The distal component possesses a polished hemisphere with radii of two different dimensions. The pair of metallic prongs insert into the medullary cavities of the second and third metacarpals (Reproduced with permission of R. G. Volz.[246])

Biomechanical Considerations in Total Wrist Arthroplasty*

Total wrist arthroplasty provides an alternative to arthrodesis and Silastic arthroplasty for patients with degenerative, traumatic or rheumatoid arthritis. The procedure is indicated for relief of pain, correction of deformity and restoration of motion. Two designs of prosthesis are now available: the Meuli[245] and Volz.[242] Both procedures require resection of the distal radius, the scaphoid, lunate, triquetrum, proximal one-half of the capitate and proximal one-half of the hamate (Fig. 13-65A). The proximal component of the prosthesis is implanted in the radius and the distal component in one or two metacarpal shafts.

The wrist has axes of radioulnar deviation and an axis of flexion-extension which do not intersect; there is no coaxial rotation of the hand on the radius. In reconstructive arthroplasty, the objective is to position the prosthesis by bending or tilting so that its axes of motion lie concentric with the axes of motion of a normal wrist.[242, 247, 248] (In certain wrists with severe soft tissue deformities, it also may be necessary to release contractures and restore soft tissue balance relative to the repositioned axes of motion.) It can then be expected that the reconstructed wrist will be balanced and have optimal mechanics with relation to the motor units moving the wrist. If this is not done, it can be expected that the wrist will be imbalanced to some degree and that the abnormal stresses applied may eventually loosen the prosthesis, as has been found with malpositions of other joint prostheses.

A major problem at the time of surgery is the location of the site for the axes of prosthetic motion after performing the resection shown in Figure 13-65A. Although normally the axes of motion of the wrist pass through the head of the capitate, this structure is excised along with most of the radiocarpal joint and precludes the use of these anatomical landmarks. Preoperative radiographs also are of little use in the rheumatoid patient since the carpus is often collapsed proximally, subluxed volarly, and translocated ulnarly (Fig. 13-65B) with distortion of the normal relationship of the head of the capitate to the distal radius.[249, 250] No carpal or hand structure, therefore, can serve as a reference to position the proximal component of the prosthesis in the radius. Without objective guidelines, surgeons subjectively position the axes of motion of the prosthesis where they think the axes of motion normally would lie until they achieve a balanced "feel" of the arthroplastic wrist.[248,*] This technique lacks reproducibility and predictability and it does not assure *optimal* positioning of the axes of motion of the prosthesis. Because of this, imbalance of the wrist has been reported as a major complication of total wrist arthroplasty.[242, 247, 248] The imbalance presents clinically as a limitation and an asymmetry of motion and an abnormal resting posture of the hand. The usual deformity is ulnar drift and flexion because of excessive radial and dorsal placement of the prosthesis.

It is possible to have the axis of radioulnar deviation excessively radial and yet observe a balanced appearance of the wrist rather than the expected ulnar drift deformity. This situation can occur in one of four ways: (1) By tenotomy of the flexor carpi ulnaris which removes an ulnar deviating force[242, 247, 248]; (2) by transfer of the extensor carpi ulnaris to the base of the third or fourth metacarpal to decrease its ulnar deviating force[248]; (3) by use of a cast to prohibit radioulnar deviation for 6 to 12 weeks. With immobilization a restrictive capsular scar forms which resists ulnar drift[248]; and (4) by preservation of the triquetrum (Fig. 13-65C). The bone impinges upon the distal radius or ulna and acts as a mechanical bone block to prevent excessive ulnar drift.[248]

To optimally position a total wrist prosthesis, it is necessary to locate the anatomical site of the axes of motion. The site may be obscured if the radiocarpal joint is distorted by disease or if the joint previously has been excised. Previous studies of the wrist have failed to provide a suitable method to identify this site. Recently a quantitative radiographic method has been developed which identifies the anatomical axes of motion of the wrist in relation to radiographic references in the hand and forearm.

Normal Location of Axes of Motion. In a study of the biomechanics of the normal wrist, Youm *et al.*[251] (Fig. 13-66A) showed that the perpendicular distance, u, from the longitudinal axis of the ulna to the axis of radioulnar deviation had a constant ratio to the length of the third metacarpal, MC_3, as measured on a posteroanterior radiograph:

$$\frac{u}{MC_3} = 0.3$$

---

* R. S. Hamas, personal communication, 1978.

* R. G. Volz, personal communication, 1978.

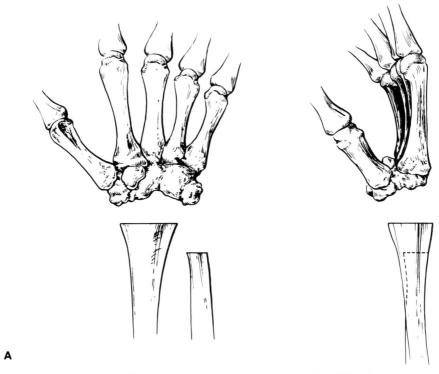

A

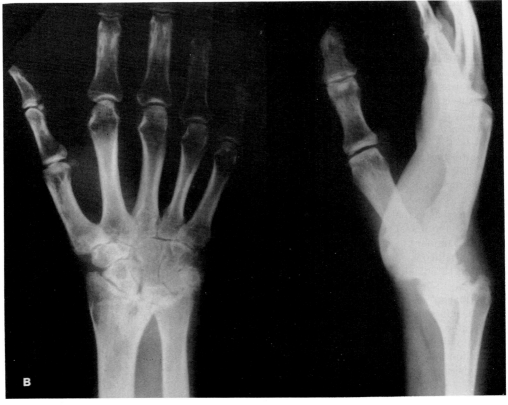

B

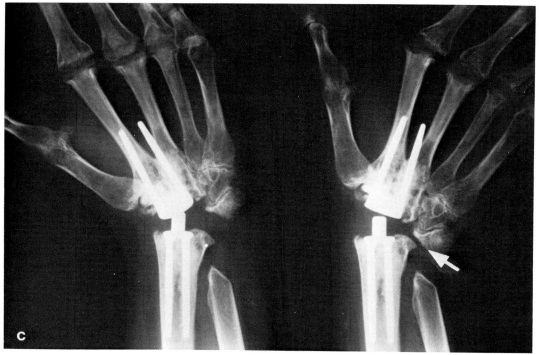

Figure 13-65. *A.* Bone resection needed for a total wrist prosthesis is seen. *B.* Radiographs show the typical deformities of the rheumatoid wrist. *C.* Although this wrist has balanced radioulnar deviation, the axis of motion of the prosthesis is too radialward. The expected ulnar drift deformity is prevented by a mechanical bone block (*arrow*). (*A, B* and *C* reproduced with permission of R. S. Hamas.)

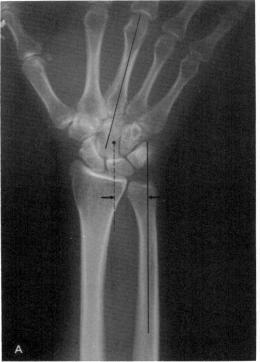
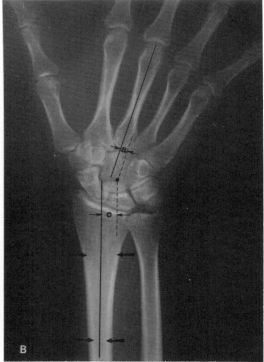
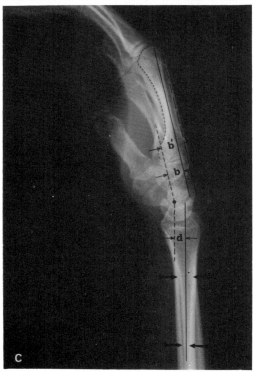

Figure 13-66. *A.* A posteroanterior radiograph shows the axis of radioulnar deviation (*dot*), the axes of the third metacarpal and ulna (*solid lines*), and a *dashed line* parallel to the ulnar axis. The *arrows* indicate the distance, *u*, from the ulnar axis to the axis of radioulnar deviation. *B.* A posteroanterior radiograph shows the axis of radioulnar deviation (*dot*), the third metacarpal and distal radius reference axes (*solid lines*), and *dashed lines* parallel to the reference axes. The *light arrows* indicate the distances *a* and *c* from each reference axis to the axis of radioulnar deviation. The *heavy arrows* indicate where the medullary canal is bisected to define the distal radial axis. *C.* A lateral radiograph shows the axis of flexion-extension motion (*dot*), the third metacarpal and the distal radius reference axes (*solid lines*), an alternate reference line through the dorsal cortex of the third metacarpal, and *dashed lines* parallel to the reference axes. The *light arrows* indicate the distances *b*, *b'* and *d* from each reference axis to the axis of flexion-extension motion. The *heavy arrows* indicate where the medullary canal is bisected to define the distal radial axis. (*A, B* and *C* reproduced with permission of R. S. Hamas.)

The axis of radioulnar deviation was noted to lie ulnad to the axis of the third metacarpal but the distance between them was not quantified. The axis of flexion-extension was not described relative to references in the hand and forearm. The method of Youm established a location of the axis of motion relative to a radiographic reference axis. An expression defines the site as a ratio of the distance between the reference points and the length of the third metacarpal. The expression, thereby, accounts for changes in the site of the axes of motion that arise from variations in wrist size.

For use in positioning a total wrist prosthesis, the normal location of each axis of motion must be described relative to a reference in the hand, for the distal component, and a reference in the forearm, for the proximal component. The references allow each component to be positioned independently so that its axis of motion lies in normal relationships to its reference axis. When the components are joined, anatomical alignment of the hand and forearm will be assured. The longitudinal axis of the third metacarpal and the longitudinal axis of the distal radius are chosen for the hand and forearm references because these bones articulate directly with the carpus and are used for implantation of the prosthesis. The axis of the ulna does not meet these criteria and, therefore, is not used. The forearm and hand radiographic reference axes are defined as follows: *the axis of the distal radius* is the line bisecting the medullary canal of the straight portion of the distal radius (for about 5 cm proximal to the start of the distal flair); the *axis of the third metacarpal* is the line bisecting the medullary canal of the third metacarpal shaft.

The axis of the radioulnar deviation can be located on the posteroanterior radiograph (Fig. 13-66B) using the distance, a, from the axis of the third metacarpal and the distance, c, from the axis of the distal radius. To adjust for differences in wrist size, each distance is expressed as a ratio in respect to the length of the patient's third metacarpal, MC_3:

$$\frac{a}{MC_3} = A$$

$$\frac{c}{MC_3} = C$$

Similarly, the axis of flexion-extension motion can be located on the lateral radiograph (Fig. 13-66C) using the distance, b, from the axis of the third metacarpal and the distance, d, from the axis of the distal radius. To adjust for differences in wrist size, each distance can be expressed as a ratio with respect to the length of the patient's third metacarpal, MC_3:

$$\frac{b}{MC_3} = B$$

$$\frac{d}{MC_3} = D$$

The ratios A, B, C and D are constants.

To provide reproducible and comparable distances on the radiographs for each patient, standardized posteroanterior and lateral radiographic views were established. For the *standardized posteroanterior view* (Fig. 13-67A), the palm is placed flat against the X-ray plate with contact of the second and third metacarpal heads. This maneuver elevates the volar aspect of the wrist from the plate by a small distance. Care is taken to prevent rotation of the metacarpals. The *length of the third metacarpal,* determined from this view, is used in the calculation of all ratios. For the *standardized lateral view* (Fig. 13-67B), the ulnar aspect of the hand, wrist and forearm is placed flat against the X-ray plate. The metacarpals are positioned so that the third metacarpal is slightly more dorsal than the other metacarpals. In each view, the X-ray tube is positioned 40 inches from the plate. The X-ray beam is perpendicular to the plate and is centered on the wrist joint. Since there is no coaxial rotation of the hand on the radius, positioning the third metacarpal as previously described simultaneously provides true posteroanterior and lateral views of the radius. The standardized views are unaffected by the rotatory position of the ulna relative to the radius.

Occasionally, it may be difficult for the surgeon to locate precisely the axis of the third metacarpal on the standardized lateral view because of the overlap of the other metacarpals. An alternate reference line was established parallel to the axis of the third metacarpal and through the dorsal cortex of the bone (Fig. 13-66c). The axis of flexion-extension is located by the distance, b' from this alternate reference line. The distance is expressed as a constant ratio, B', with respect to the length of the third metacarpal, MC_3:

$$\frac{b'}{MC_3} = B'$$

To determine normal values for the five ratios, 25 wrists were studied in patients between the ages of 20 and 30 years and without a history of previous injury. For each wrist, standardized

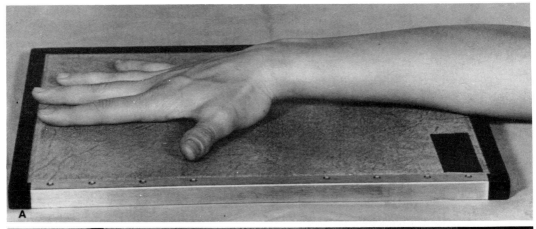

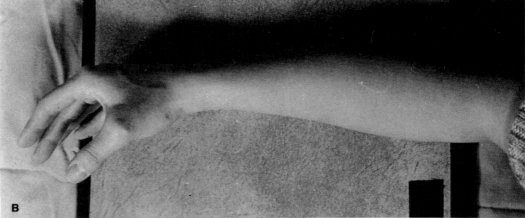

Figure 13-67. The positions of the upper extremity for the standardized radiographs are seen: *A.* Posteroanterior view; *B.* lateral view. The degree of pronation-supination is not important. (*A* and *B*, reproduced with permission of R. S. Hamas.)

posteroanterior radiographs were taken in 10° of radial deviation and 20° of ulnar deviation. By trial and error, a point was found around which these two X-ray films could be rotated to exactly superimpose the radii or third metacarpals (Fig. 13-68). The point represents the axis of radioulnar deviation for that wrist. The distances from the axis of the third metacarpal, a, and from the axis of the distal radius, c, to the axis of radioulnar deviation were measured and expressed as the ratios A and C with respect to the length of that patient's third metacarpal. Similarly, standardized lateral radiographs were taken in 25° of flexion and 25° of extension. By trial and error, a point was found around which these two X-ray films could be rotated to exactly superimpose the radii or third metacarpals. The point represents the axis of flexion-extension motion

for that wrist. The distances from the axis of the third metacarpal, b, from the alternate reference line, b', and from the axis of the distal radius, d, to the axis of flexion-extension were measured and expressed as the ratios B, B' and D with respect to the length of that patient's third metacarpal.

The axis of radioulnar deviation was always ulnar and the axis of flexion-extension was always volar to the reference axes. The mean values and standard deviations for the ratios found from 25 normal wrists are shown in Table 13-5.

To locate the anatomical axes of motion in a wrist, standardized posteroanterior and lateral radiographs are obtained and the reference axes are drawn on them. The length of the patient's third metacarpal, MC_3, is measured on the pos-

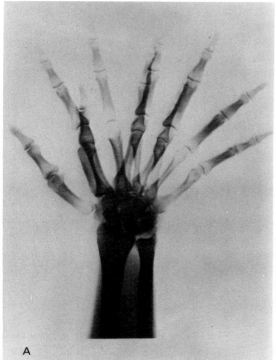 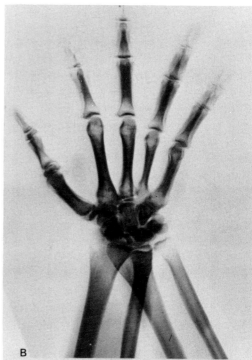

Figure 13-68. A technique for locating the axis of radioulnar deviation in normal wrists uses one standardized posteroanterior radiograph taken in radial deviation and one taken in ulnar deviation. *A*, radii superimposed; *B*, third metacarpals superimposed. The *dot* identifies the point around which the two radiographs were rotated. (*A* and *B*, reproduced with permission of R. S. Hamas.)

Table 13-5
25 Normal Wrists

Ratio	Mean	Standard deviation
A	0.052	± 0.004
B	0.15	± 0.02
B′	0.20	± 0.02
C	0.12	± 0.01
D	0.095	± 0.01

teroanterior view and multiplied by the mean value for each ratio from Table 13-5:

$MC_3 \times A = a$ = normal distance from third metacarpal axis;

$MC_3 \times C = c$ = normal distance from distal radial axis;

$MC_3 \times B = b$ = normal distance from third metacarpal axis;

$MC_3 \times B' = b'$ = normal distance from dorsal cortex of third metacarpal;

$MC_3 \times D = d$ = normal distance from distal radial axis.

These normal distances from the reference axes to the normal locations of the axes of motion are best demonstrated by drawing parallel lines on the posteroanterior radiograph at the distances, *a* and *c*, ulnar to the reference axes and on the lateral radiograph at the distances, *b* or *b′* and *d*, volar to the reference axes as shown by the dashed lines in Figure 13-66 *B* and *C*.

The normal locations for the axes of motion of that patient's wrist lie on the parallel lines.

Clinical Assessment. To utilize this method, it is first necessary to place a large Kirschner wire transversely through the midshaft of the radius parallel to the plane of the table when the hand is positioned as shown in Figure 13-67A. After the radiocarpal joint is resected, small metal clips are placed on the cortex of the distal radius and the carpal remnant (Fig. 13-69). A Kirschner wire is used instead of the metacarpals to show the rotatory orientation of the radius. The optimal location for the axes of motion is determined relative to the radiographic reference axes as previously described.

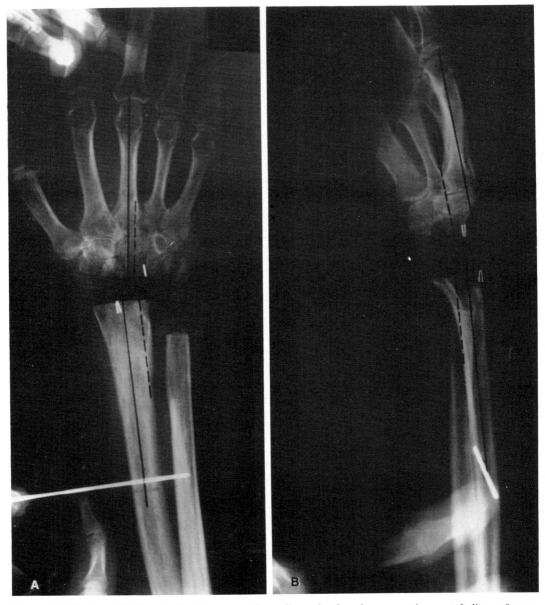

Figure 13-69. *A* and *B.* Standardized intraoperative radiographs show bone resection, metal clips, reference axes (*solid lines*), and *dashed lines* parallel to the reference axes. (*A* and *B*, reproduced with permission of R. S. Hamas.)

The distance from each metal clip to each axis of motion is measured and used to position the axes of motion of the prosthesis in the patient's wrist. The Meuli prosthesis is either bent or a stem is removed from each component. The implant is tilted to achieve the desired position (Fig. 13-70). Active exercises are begun on the third postoperative day with the forearm verti-

cally positioned with the elbow resting on a table. A small volar splint is worn continuously for 2 weeks, and at night for another week.

The quantitative data accrued from 10 arthroplastic wrists is shown in Table 13-6. After follow-up periods from 3 to 18 months, all of the patients showed good relief of pain and improved grip strength. As shown by the ratios, it was

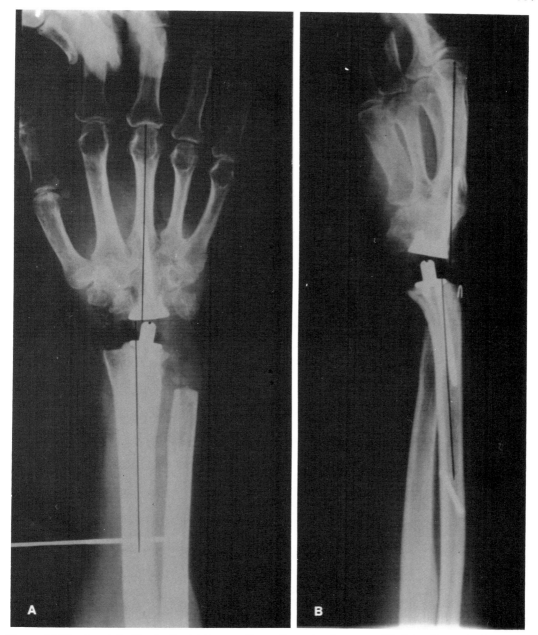

Figure 13-70. *A* and *B*. Standardized intraoperative radiographs show a modified Meuli prosthesis with its axes of motion (*dot*) at the optimal location. The reference axes are shown by the *solid lines*. (*A* and *B*, reproduced with the permission of R. S. Hamas.)

usually possible to position the axes of motion of the prostheses within 2 mm of the optimal locations determined from the radiographs. No patients underwent a tenotomy, tendon transfer, mechanical bone block or cast immobilization to prevent radioulnar deviation or ulnar drift. These early results strongly suggest that quantitative positioning of the axes of motion of wrist prostheses results in balanced wrists with excellent ranges of motion.

ARTHROPLASTIC RECONSTRUCTION IN THE HAND

Where severe arthritic change in the hand necessitates surgical treatment a variety of potential solutions are available. Particularly for

Table 13-6
Ten Meuli Wrist Prostheses *in vivo*

Patients	Flexion	Extension	Radial	Ulnar	Ratios			
					A	B	C	D
1	55	55	20	35	0.052	0.16	0.12	0.103
2	45	55	5	50	0.033	0.13	0.11	0.100
3	35	55	0	50	0.083	0.15	0.10	0.108
4	25	55	45	15	0.054	0.15	0.14	0.092
5	50	40	20	35	0.054	0.15	0.11	0.100
6	35	50	25	30	0.060	0.11	0.16	0.127
7	35	35	20	40	0.046	0.16	0.13	0.092
8	60	45	30	30	0.052	0.16	0.11	0.097
9	15	35	25	25	0.065	0.20	0.11	0.101
10	45	60	20	35	0.015	0.14	0.12	0.110
Average	40	48.5	21	34.5	0.051	0.15	0.12	0.103

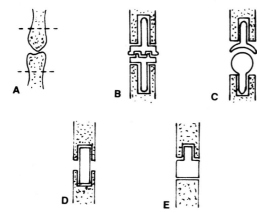

Figure 13-71. Schematic diagrams indicate the various types of resectional and implant arthroplasties available for treatment of joints in the hand. (Reproduced with permission of R. I. Burton.[252])

the distal joints in the fingers, fusion irradicates pain and restores stability although motion is sacrificed. Where more proximal joints are afflicted, the loss of motion consistent with arthrodesis of a joint is less desirable, particularly if multiple joints are involved. As seen in Figure 13-71, several types of joint arthroplasties have been developed for use in the hand.[252] One of the earliest solutions was the excision of a joint, comparable to the Girdlestone hip procedure or the Keller great toe arthroplasty (Fig. 13-71A). Pain is usually relieved and deformity may be corrected, although stability and strength may be lacking. Alternatively, a hinge-type prosthesis may be inserted (Fig. 13-71B), although its axis of motion may not duplicate that of the normal joint. Flatt[253] developed one of the first hinge prostheses for use in the hand. The metallic joints were difficult to align correctly. Particularly where they were malaligned, they were liable to undergo loosening, excessive wear and breakage. Subsidence of implants secondary to bone resorption also was encountered. The Niebauer-Cutter silicone rubber-Dacron prosthesis is secured by ingrowth of tissue into the Dacron weave on the stems.[254] It flexes and extends much like a hinge. Alternatively, articulated prostheses such as the Steffee prosthesis (Steffee Finger Prosthesis, DePuy, Warsaw, Ind.) have been developed which provide polycentric motion similar to the metacarpophalangeal joint. Ultimately, polycentric hinges (Fig. 13-71C) may be the design of choice in view of their combination of stability, durability and anatomical motion. Another design in widespread application is the malleable, dynamic spacer which stimulates the formation of a pseudocapsule around the implant (Fig. 13-71D). The Swanson prosthesis[255] is a representative example in which a flexible silicone rubber rod bridges the resected joint. In view of the reciprocal motion of the implant, it seeks the site of lowest stress. Alternatively for certain sites, hemiresectional arthroplasty can be undertaken in which a "space filler" with a medullary stem is inserted into an adjacent bone (Fig. 13-71E). The implant provides temporary stability until the pseudocapsule has formed. Examples include the trapezium, scaphoid, lunate, ulnar head or radial head arthroplasties, discussed in Chapter 15. Where the implant serves as a dynamic spacer, the collagen and fibrous tissue of the pseudocapsule which develops around the implant is an integral part of the arthroplasty. The postoperative exercise program is directed to form the optimal shape and consistency of pseudocapsule. In general, implant arthroplasty can be considered for the rheumatoid or osteoarthritic joint that is substantially deformed, stiff, unstable or painful. Contraindications include a history of regional sepsis, neuropathic joints, mutilans rheumatoid arthritis and juvenile patients with open epiphyses. Implant arthroplasty should not be employed if there are inadequate musculotendinous units to power the reconstructed joint. Alternative procedures including arthrodesis, excisional arthroplasty, ligamentous reconstruction and tendon rebalancing procedures are discussed elsewhere.[253, 256] Where the preoperative joint shows deformity with imbalance of adja-adjacent musculotendinous structures, the arthroplastic procedure must include a reconstruction of the soft tissues to release the deformities and balance the musculotendinous units. The general principles of the biological reconstructions are described in Chapter 14.

Biomechanical Assessment of Finger Joints and Prosthetic Joint Design

Napier[257] and Landsmeer[258] have divided the activities of the normal hand into power grasp and precision handling. Power grasp is a forceful act performed with the fingers flexed at all three joints so that the object is grasped between the fingers and the palm. It is usually performed with the wrist deviated ulnad and dorsiflexed to augment the tension in the flexor tendons. The thumb is positioned on the palmar side of the grasped object to force it securely into the palm. Precision handling involves manipulation of small objects in a finely controlled manner. The object is gripped between the opposed thumb and the index and long fingers. The wrist position may be variable to increase the manipulative range. The fingers are generally held in a semiflexed position with the thumb extended and opposed. There are numerous variations and combinations of these activities.

Landsmeer and Long,[259] Flatt[253] and Smith[260] have described the anatomy of the hand from an analysis of structure and function of the components. A finger consists of a multilinked structure provided with adequate controls so that the structure does not collapse into a zigzag or accordian fashion under compressive force (Fig. 13-72A). The interphalangeal joints act in a synchronous fashion in both flexion and extension.[262] Angular displacement in a ratio of approximately 2:1 occurs between the proximal and distal interphalangeal joints. At the distal interphalangeal joint, extension is provided by a conjoint tendon of the lateral bands and flexion is supplied by the flexor profundus tendon. Flexion at this joint would normally increase exten-

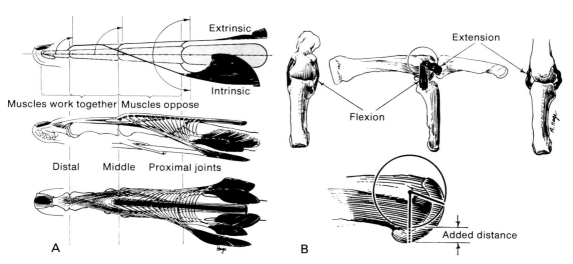

Figure 13-72. *A.* A schematic diagram of a finger indicates the principal musculotendinous structures. The intrinsic muscles approach the metacarpophalangeal joints from the depth of the palm and lie on the palmar aspect of the axis of the joint. Subsequently the tendons pass dorsal to the axis of the interphalangeal joints so that the intrinsic muscles flex the metacarpophalangeal joints and extend the interphalangeal joints. *B.* A schematic diagram shows the metacarpophalangeal joint. When the joint is in extension, the collateral ligaments are slack to permit abduction and adduction. The joint is stabilized in flexion because the ligaments are tightened in both longitudinal and transverse planes. (*A* and *B*, reproduced with permission of A. E. Flatt.[261])

sor tension at the proximal interphalangeal joint if tension were supplied directly over the top of the joint. The lateral bands, however, diverge over the top of the proximal interphalangeal joint. With increasing distal joint flexion, the lateral bands displace further toward the center of rotation of the proximal interphalangeal joint so that the moment contributed by the lateral bands is decreased. In addition, the oblique retinacular ligament originating on the volar aspect of the flexor tendon sheath of the proximal interphalangeal joint and inserting into the conjoint tendon on the dorsum of the distal interphalangeal joint, may act as a static structure to encourage synchronous motion of the two joints.

The extraordinarily dextrous hand undergoes reciprocal angular displacement between the interphalangeal joints and the metacarpophalangeal joints. This combined motion is directed by the extensor hood mechanism which consists of the extensor tendon applied over the dorsum of the metacarpophalangeal joint with its insertion into the dorsal lip of the middle phalanx. It directs extension of the metacarpophalangeal joint through a sling mechanism which inserts in a common ligamentous area at the palmar base of the proximal phalanx. These insertions form a common meeting of the transverse intermetacarpal ligament, the volar plate and the proximal pulley of the flexor sheaths and the metacarpal glenoidal ligaments. This unique arrangement of the extensor hood enables it to slip proximally and distally on the proximal phalanx to accommodate interphalangeal joint motion while concurrently allowing either synchronous or reciprocal motion at the metacarpophalangeal joint (Fig. 13-72A).

The metacarpophalangeal joints are positioned by the relative moments between the extensor tendons, the finger flexors and the interosseous tendons. Through both their phalangeal and their extensor retinacular insertions, the interosseous tendons exert forces for flexion, adduction, abduction, supination and pronation of the proximal phalanx on the metacarpal. The mobility of the ulnar side of the hand is increased by the additional flexion and extension possible through the fourth and fifth metacarpal joints.

Pinch requires a radially directed force on the index and long fingers to oppose the action of the thumb. This force is supplied by the first and second dorsal interosseous muscles and is aided by the asymmetrical contour in the frontal plane of the index and long finger metacarpals. The metacarpal heads show enhanced width on the volar surface which has a marked effect on the mobility of the joints owing to the disposition of the collateral ligaments (Fig. 13-72B). These become more taut with increasing flexion of the metacarpophalangeal joint as a result both of accommodating to the width of the volar aspect of the metacarpal head and, in the case of the radiocollateral ligament, of its position dorsal to the axis of rotation in the extended position. The ligament shows increase in tension during flexion as it crosses the center of rotation in the metacarpal head (Fig. 13-73). Collateral ligaments, the thickened portions of the metacarpophalangeal joint capsules, provide the main constraints to motion at these joints. The radial collateral ligaments tend to be stronger and run a course that is more perpendicular to the longitudinal axis of the metacarpal than the ulnar collateral ligaments. This orientation toward the perpendicular diminishes with progression from the index to the little fingers. The ulnar collateral ligament is more parallel to the longitudinal axis of the metacarpal and this feature becomes more striking as the little finger is approached. The strong and perpendicular displacement of the radial collateral ligament in the index finger aids in resisting the pronatory torque produced by pinching the end of the thumb. It also produces a supinatory torque on the fingers when they undergo ulnar deviation. In pathological states such as rheumatoid arthritis the disposition of the collateral ligament has a distinct bearing on the alterations of motion observed in the metacarpophalangeal joints.

The eccentric nature of the metacarpophalangeal joints produces a rolling motion in addition to the more obvious sliding motion. Pagowski et al.[263] have shown that the rolling motion tends to pump synovial fluid through the joint space. These workers provide a detailed assessment of the fluid flow through the joint, the coefficient of friction and an estimate of joint spacing.

Biomechanical Aspects of Prosthetic Design

Projected prosthetic designs for finger joint should consider the vectors of the forces about the joint, the relative displacements of the tendons with their effects on the adjacent joints and the type of motion in the joint. One approach is to prepare free-body diagrams of the finger elements during pinch as seen in Figure 13-74A. The forces involved are the pinch force, F, the deep flexor muscles, P, the superficial flexor muscles, S, and the average of the interosseous muscles, I. This analysis assumes a value for the

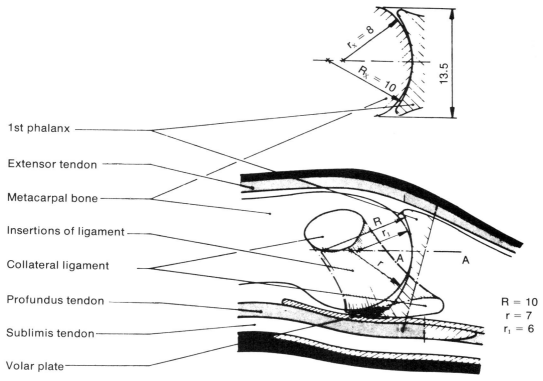

1st phalanx

Extensor tendon

Metacarpal bone

Insertions of ligament

Collateral ligament

Profundus tendon

Sublimis tendon

Volar plate

R = 10
r = 7
r₁ = 6

Figure 13-73. In the metacarpophalangeal joint the attachments of the collateral ligaments are positioned eccentrically to produce a rolling motion in addition to the more obvious sliding joint motion. (Reproduced with permission of F. Pagowski, M. Munro and K. Piekarski.[263])

forces produced by the interosseous and lumbrical muscles. Moment equations at the three joints are solved by insertion of measurements of the lengths of the articulated segments and the moment arms of the tendons of each articulation obtained from cadaveric studies. With this method, Smith *et al.*[266] conclude that a flexor force of 6 units is necessary to produce 1 unit of pulp force. A vector summation of the moment forces supplied by the superficial and deep flexor muscles and the combined interosseous and lumbrical muscles with the pulp force provides a value for the compressive force of the joint 7.5 units. The limitations of this technique have been described by Linscheid and Chao.[262] They point out that the magnitudes of the interosseous forces and the lumbrical forces at the metacarpophalangeal joints usually are unknown. Also, the joint compressive force calculated here is a complex assessment of the lateral and dorsal constraint forces at the joint provided by the collateral ligaments and the volar plate as well as the actual joint contact force normal to the joint surface. Furthermore, the pinch

action is believed to be 3-dimensional in nature so that the present planar analysis is inappropriate.

Flatt and Fischer[267,268] modified the moment equations for the finger joints in the sagittal plane and subjected these to analysis in fresh fingers for verification in a sophisticated electromechanical test system. The force diagram in their moments with respect to finger joint centers are shown in Figure 13-74B. The moment equations are obtained from free-body diagrams for the distal phalanx, middle phalanx and proximal phalanx. These equations are:

$$T(HE_3) - P(HP_3) = 0 \tag{1}$$

$$T(HE_{12}) + M(HE_2) - P(HP_2) = 0 \tag{2}$$

$$E(HE_1) - P(HP_1) - I(HI_1) = 0 \tag{3}$$

These equations assume that frictional, inertial and viscoelastic effects on soft tissues are negligible; joint surfaces are cylindric; that the bearing force in each joint is directed toward the axis of rotation; and that the link system is rigid and tendons are inextensible and lined by frictionless

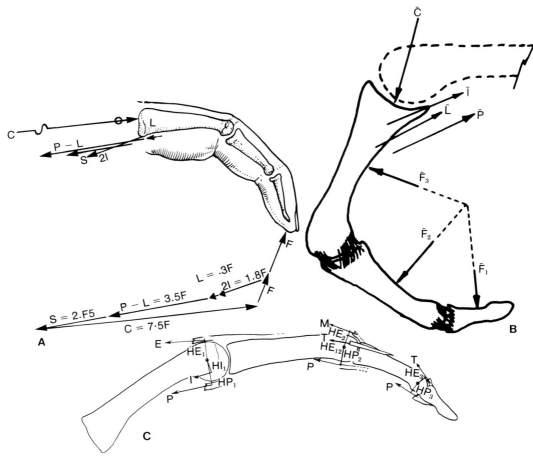

Figure 13-74. *A.* A free-body diagram shows the force equilibrium for a finger during pinch. *C*, bone compressive force; *F*, load force; *L*, lumbrical force; *I*, interosseous force; *P*, flexor digitorium profundus force; *S*, flexor digitorium sublimus force. (Reproduced with permission of R. L. Lindscheid and E. Y. S. Chao.[264]) *B.* A tendon force diagram at the finger joints are revealed. Vectors indicates forces of: *T*, terminal tendon; *M* (central slip), medial bend; *E*, extensor tendon; *P*, profundus; *S*, sublimus; *I*, interosseous. *H* describes the height of moment arm. *C.* A free-body diagram of a finger during grasp action is shown. $\bar{F}_1$, $\bar{F}_2$ and $\bar{F}_3$ are distributed forces on each phalanx. $\bar{C}$ is a joint reactive force. (*B* and *C*, reproduced with permission of R. L. Lindscheid and E. H. S. Chao.[265])

pulleys. The equation for the proximal interphalangeal joint has two extensor moments. The value of the moment arm, HE_{12}, is variable and decreases with increasing flexion of the joint. Landmeer[269] emphasizes that this decrease in moment arm at the proximal interphalangeal joint is necessary for synchronous motion to occur in the distal and proximal interphalangeal joints. With the proper substitution of values, these equations may be solved simultaneously so that a mathematical model that predicts the relationship among the three joints at given positions may be obtained.

Analysis of forces on the finger during grasp is more complex and is not known in detail. The force is exerted against the grasped object over the variable surface of each of the three phalanges. Resolution of the forces at the interphalangeal and metacarpophalangeal joints into a joint compressive force and a tangential subluxing force is helpful for prosthetic design (Fig. 13-74C). The range of compressive forces within the joint permits the selection of materials with adequate strength and appropriate bearing surfaces. The force of subluxation determines the strength necessary to insure adequate joint constraints and the optimal configuration of anchorage of the device. The range of these forces, particularly the upper limits, is as yet not adequately determined.

Recently Swanson et al.[270] measured an average maximum index pinch of 5.05 kg and 3.45 kg for normal men and women, respectively. In view of the observation by Lindscheid and Chao,[262] that the compressive force is about 7.5 times pinch force, the maximum forces for normal men and women will be 37.8 kg and 25.9 kg respectively. Walker and Erkman[271] reported the maximum likely lateral moment on the index finger at 0° flexion. For 20 male and 20 female patients, the average moments were 23.6 kg/cm (± 7.05 S.D.) and 12.3 kg/cm (± 3.8 S.D.) respectively. These workers also determined the average lateral force with the finger in flexion for the index finger of male and female patients. The figures were 7.5 kg and 4.8 kg respectively. Hence, the torque on prosthetic joint components are: male metacarpals, 52.5 kg/cm; female metacarpals, 24.0 kg/cm; male phalanges, 37.5 kg/cm; female phalanges, 16.8 kg/cm. Much of these torques would be carried by ligaments, capsule and muscles, although the proportion is difficult to estimate.

The mathematical analysis involved in obtaining the moment equations assumes that the center of rotation of the joint remains constant and that the motion described by the joints is circular. This has been confirmed for the distal and proximal interphalangeal joints. Flatt and Fisher[268] suggested that the motion of the metacarpophalangeal joint is circular within an arc of 25°. The arc of adduction-abduction about the metacarpophalangeal joints also approximates a circular motion.

Prosthetic Joint Constraints

The uniaxial motion at the distal and proximal interphalangeal joints markedly simplifies prosthetic design because the constraints for motion, other than in the flexion-extension plane, may be incorporated into the prosthetic components. Alternatively, the metacarpophalangeal joint presents complex problems in design and joint constraint. If motion in three planes is to be preserved, the design must incorporate constraints within the prosthetic system or the reconstruction must include repair or preservation of the normal ligamentous restraints.

The average range of flexion-extension at the metacarpophalangeal joint is 110 to 120°, of which 10° is for flexion and 10 to 20° for hyperextension. This range of motion decreases from the index to the little finger joints. When the joints are in extension, radial-ulnar deviation of 60° for the index, 50° for the little, and 45° for the middle and ring fingers are recorded. There are no radial-ulnar movements when the metacarpophalangeal joints are in a flexed position. The interphalangeal joints show 110 to 130° of flexion without other motion.

The force analysis of the restraints about the metacarpophalangeal joint was performed with trigonometric analysis by Flatt.[272] Linscheid and Chao[262] provide an abbreviated discussion of this technique. The results from the mathematical analysis indicate that the forces encountered in the metacarpoglenoidal ligament and volar plate of the joint increase with increasing flexion. Pagowski et al.[263] estimate a physiological joint load between 10 and 1000 Newtons. Other observations indicate that the metacarpophalangeal ligaments are the primary restraint to palmar subluxation of the proximal phalanges and that the metacarpoglenoidal ligaments provide restraint to subluxation of the flexor mechanism. Sectioning the metacarpoglenoidal ligaments of the index and longer finger allows the flexor tendons to bowstring in an ulnar direction and induces an ulnad deviating force on the digits. Attenuation of these ligaments and the difficulties in their reconstruction have proved to be a problem in presently available prosthetic joint replacements. Correction of the ulnar translation of the proximal phalanx on the metacarpal tends to decrease the ulnar moment that the flexors may exert.

Presently Available Finger Joint Arthroplasties

Of the presently available finger joint prostheses, the standard against which the others are judged is the Swanson silicone rubber implant (Fig. 13-75A).[255] Over 25,000 patients have been treated with this technique. The dynamic joint spacers provide sufficient internal stability to maintain anatomical alignment and space between the bone ends while early motion of the joint is resumed. The implant glides about 1 to 2 mm in the intermedullary canals on flexion-extension movements. The mobile implant seeks the axis of rotation of the joint and thereby limits stress on adjacent tissues and itself. The implant has been used successfully for both metacarpophalangeal joints[273] and proximal interphalangeal joint resectional arthroplasties.[255] The principal liabilities of the system have been fractures of the implant which occur primarily when inadequate soft tissue reconstruction of the joint is undertaken.[274] With severe joint deformities, particularly in rheumatoid arthritis,

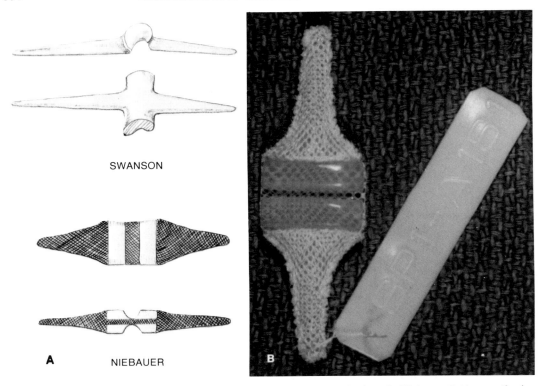

SWANSON

A   NIEBAUER

B

Figure 13-75. *A*. Schematic views show a Swanson silicone rubber prosthesis and a Niebauer-Cutter prosthesis. *B*. A photograph reveals a Niebauer-Cutter finger joint prosthesis.

reconstruction of the soft tissues to rebalance the principal motor units around the joints is difficult. With its limited capacity for stabilization, the Swanson technique may show postoperative recurrence of ulnar deviation and other deformities, even in the hands of experienced surgeons.

The Niebauer-Cutter prosthesis (Fig. 13-75) was developed concurrently with the somewhat similar Swanson silicone rubber hinge. The intermedullary stems of the former implant are covered with coarse-woven Dacron.[254] After an initial period when its inherent mobility permits the implant to seek the optimal center of rotation of the joint, it is immobilized by ingrowth of tissue into the Dacron. The hinge is a biconcave design (Fig. 13-75*B*). The silicone is molded over a core of Dacron mesh to augment strength and stability. Urbaniak[254] has compared the clinical results of the application of Niebauer-Cutter and Swanson-type finger joint prostheses over a 5-year period of clinical application. Despite the differences in design and the theoretical arguments in favor of or against each implant, the clinical trial appears to show remarkably similar results of surgery. Assessment by postoperative

range of motion, residual pain, stability and late fracture of the prosthesis are highly comparable. For metacarpophalangeal joints, the average range of motion is about 50° with an increased range of active motion of about 20°. Swanson[255] has reported on the results of his technique, employed in the proximal phalangeal joints. Again, he emphasizes the need for reconstruction of the soft tissues and a postoperative goal of 0 to 70° of active flexion.

Recently Beckenbaugh *et al.*[275] reported a series of 530 consecutive metacarpophalangeal joint arthroplasties using Swanson or Niebauer prostheses. After surgery, the patients were followed for up to 2½ years. For joints treated with Swanson prostheses, the ultimate average motion was 38°, the fracture rate was 26.2% and the recurrence of clinical deformity was 11.3%. For joints treated with Niebauer prostheses, the ultimate average motion was 35°, the fracture rate was 38.2% and the recurrence of clinical deformity was 44.1%. The patient population, with 116 rheumatoid patients, may have contributed heavily to the high incidences of implant failure and recurrent deformity. The surgeons favored the Swanson design although improvements are

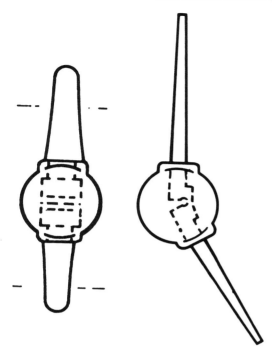

Figure 13-76. Schematic diagrams show anteroposterior and lateral views of the Calnan-Nicolle encapsulated finger joint replacement.

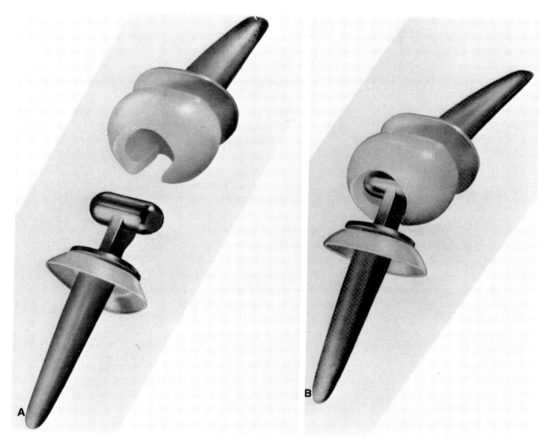

Figure 13-77. *A* and *B*. Two views of the Steffee finger joint prosthesis are shown.

recommended for the designs of both prostheses. Despite the high rates of complications, Beckenbaugh et al.[275] stress that most of the patients were clinically improved and pleased with the surgical results.

Another design of mobile spacer, is that provided by Calnan.[276] Calnan and Reis[276] initially designed a polypropylene integral hinge. Subsequently, the prosthesis was modified to present a silicone integral hinge enclosed in a polypropylene capsule which maintains circulating joint fluid (Fig. 13-76). Apart from its encapsulation, the unit functions in the same way as the Swanson prosthesis. The spherical housing provides a useful spacer and prevents the ingrowth of fibrous tissue around the hinge, thereby to limit the resistance of the hinge to deformation. While the design may appear attractive in principle, from practical considerations it appears to be a needless complication of the Swanson prosthesis.

A recent design, the Steffee prosthesis, provides a polycentric hinge with inherent stability.[271] The articulating surfaces are a Co-Cr alloy cylinder, against a HDP socket (Fig. 13-77). Each component possesses a metallic intramedullary stem which is cemented into the intramedullary cavity of the metacarpal and proximal phalanx respectively. The unit provides superior stabilization of the joint with retention of roughly anatomical motion. At present, a detailed biomechanical assessment is not available, although preliminary clinical experience has been satisfactory. A mechanical characterization of a somewhat similar polycentric hinge has been reported by Walker and Erkman.[271] These workers are concerned that permanent deformation of the polyethylene may occur in clinical use. The conformity between the ball and the collar is desirable to absorb shearing forces, which occur in most normal actions of the hand, in combination with compressive forces. The location of the axis of rotation may be critical to obtain the correct balance of forces between the various tendons which cross the joint. The insertion technique must permit the correct placement of the device to achieve consistent results. Degenerative conditions of tendons and supporting structures may require modification of this location. The pull-out strength between cement and bone in cadaver bones was about 100 kg; metal stems in cement pulled out at about 50 kg and plastic stems at 10 to 20 kg. Slippery stems pulled out at much lower values. Hopefully, future studies on polycentric hinges will yield improvements in implant design and function.

REFERENCES

1. Crenshaw, A. H. Arthrodesis. In *Campbell's Operative Orthopaedics*, edited by A. H. Crenshaw, p. 1125, C. V. Mosby Co., St. Louis, 1971.
2. Müller, M. E., Allgöwer, M., and Willengger, H. *Manual of Internal Fixation*, p. 278, Springer-Verlag, Berlin, 1970.
3. Hurri, L., Pulkki, T., and Vainio, K. J. *Acta Chir. Scand., 127*:459, 1964.
4. Vainio, K. J., Reiman, I., and Pulkki, T. *Reconstr. Surg. Traum., 9*:1, 1967.
5. Edmonson, A. S. Postural deformities. In *Campbell's Operative Orthopaedics*, edited by A. H. Crenshaw, p. 1815, C. V. Mosby Co., St. Louis, 1971.
6. Duthie, R. B., and Ferguson, A. B., Jr. *Mercer's Orthopaedic Surgery*, p. 723, Williams & Wilkins Co., Baltimore, 1973.
7. Frankel, V. H. Biomechanics of the hip. In *Surgery of the Hip Joint*, edited by R. G. Tronzo, p. 105, Lea & Febiger, Philadelphia, 1973.
8. Greenwald, A. S., and Nelson, C. L. *Ortho. Clin. N. Am., 4*:435, 1973.
9. Brekelmans, W. A. M., and Poort, H. W. *Acta Orthop. Belg., 39*, Suppl. 1, 3, 1973.
10. Walker, P. S. *Acta Orthop. Belg., 39*, Suppl. 1, 43, 1973.
11. Dietschi, C., Schreiber, A., Huggler, A. H., and Jacob, H. *Acta Orthop. Belg., 41*, Suppl. 1, 153, 1975.
12. Paul, J. Magnitude of forces transmitted at the hip and knee. In *Lubrication and Wear in Joints*, edited by V. Wright, p. 77, J. B. Lippincott, Philadelphia, 1969.
13. Inman, V. T. *J. Bone Jt. Surg., 29*:607, 1947.
14. Frankel, V. H. *The Femoral Neck. Function, Fracture Mechanisms, Internal Fixation*, p. 13, Charles C Thomas, Springfield, Ill., 1960.
15. Frankel, V. H. Biomechanics of the hip. In *Surgery of the Hip Joint*, p. 109, edited by R. G. Tronzo, Lea & Febiger, Philadelphia, 1973.
16. Rydell, N. W. *Acta Orthop. Scand., Suppl. 88*, 10, 1966.
17. Murray, M. P. *Am. J. Phys. Med., 46*:290, 1967.
18. Pauwels, F. *Der Schenkelhalsbruch Mechanisches Problem*, p. 127, Ferdinand Enke, Stuttgart, 1936.
19. Blount, W. P. *J. Bone Jt. Surg., 38A*:695, 1956.
20. Kummer, B. Biomechanics of the hip and knee joint. In *Advances in Artificial Hip and Knee Joint Technology*, p. 24, edited by M. Schaldach and D. Hohmann, Springer-Verlag, Berlin, 1976.
21. Kummer, B. Biomechanics of the hip and knee joint. In *Advances in Artificial Hip and Knee Joint Technology*, p. 33, edited by M. Schaldach and D. Hohmann, Springer-Verlag, Berlin, 1976.
22. Greenwald, A. S. Joint congruence, a dynamic concept. In *The Hip*, edited by W. H. Harris, p. 3, C. V. Mosby, St. Louis, 1974.

23. Bullough, P., Goodfellow, J., Greenwald, A. S., and O'Connor, J. J. *Nature, 217*:1290, 1968.

24. Oonishi, H., Shikita, T., and Hamoguchi, T. *Acta Orthop. Belge., 42*, Suppl. 1., 153, 1976.

25. Dietschi, C., Schreiber, A., Huggler, A. H., and Jacob, H. *Acta Orthop. Belge., 41:* Suppl. 1, 153, 1975.

26. Redler, I., and Mow, V. C. Biomechanical theories of ultrastructural alterations of articular surfaces of femoral heads. In *The Hip*, p. 23, edited by W. H. Harris, C. V. Mosby, St. Louis, 1974.

27. Kempson, G. E. Mechanical properties of articular cartilage. In *Adult Articular Cartilage*, p. 171, edited by M. A. R. Freeman, Grune & Stratton, New York, 1973.

28. Smith-Petersen, M. N. *J. Bone Jt. Surg., 30B*:59, 1948.

29. Aufranc, O. E. *Constructive Surgery of the Hip*, p. 125, C. V. Mosby, St. Louis, 1962.

30. Tronzo, R. G., Lowell, J. D., and Sbarbaro, J. L. Cup arthroplasty of the hip joint. In *Surgery of the Hip Joint*, edited by R. G. Tronzo, p. 725 Lea & Febiger, Philadelphia, 1973.

31. Harris, W. H., and Aufranc, O. E. *J. Bone Jt. Surg., 47A*:31, 1965.

32. Leddy, J., Grantham, S. A., and Stinchfield, F. E. *J. Bone Jt. Surg., 53A*:37, 1971.

33. Wilson, P. D. *J. Bone Jt. Surg., 29*:313, 1947.

34. Judet, J., and Judet, R. *J. Bone Jt. Surg., 32B*:166, 1950.

35. Moore, A. T. *J. Bone Jt. Surg., 39A*:811, 1957.

36. Thompson, F. R. *Clin. Orthop., 44*:73, 1966.

37. Tronzo, R. G., and Whittaker, R. Endoprosthetic Arthroplasties. In *Surgery of the Hip Joint*, p. 698, edited by R. G. Tronzo, Lea & Febiger, Philadelphia, 1973.

38. Anderson, L., Hansa, W. R. and Waring, T. L. *J. Bone Jt. Surg., 46A*:1049, 1964.

39. Salvati, E. A., and Wilson, P. D. Long-term results of femoral head replacements. AAOS, Washington, 1972.

40. Lowe, L. W. Rheumatoid arthritis of the hip joint, clinical aspects and their management. In *Surgery of the Hip Joint*, p. 597, edited by R. G. Tronzo, Lea & Febiger, Philadelphia, 1973.

41. Greenwald, A. S., and Nelson, C. L. *Ortho. Clin. N. Am., 4*:438, 1973.

42. Charnley, J. *Clin. Orthop., 72*:39, 1970.

43. Charnley, J. *Clin Orthop., 72*:16, 1970.

44. Greenwald, A. S., and Nelson, C. L. *Clin. Orthop. N. Am., 4*:435, 1973.

45. Ropes, M. W., and Bauer, W. *Synovial Fluid Changes in Joint Disease*, p. 59, Harvard University Press, Cambridge, Mass., 1953.

46. Charnley, J., and Smith, D. C. *The Physical and Chemical Properties of Self-curing Acrylic Cement for Use in Orthopaedic Surgery*, Wrightington, Int. Publ. No. 16, Leeds (Thackray), 1968.

47. Reckling, F. W., and Dillon, W. L. *J. Bone Jt. Surg., 59A*:80, 1977.

48. Lundskog, J. *J. Plast. Reconstr. Surg., Suppl. 9*, 35, 1972.

49. Feith, R. *Acta Orthop. Scand., Suppl. 161*, 16, 1975.

50. Linder, L. *J. Bone Jt. Surg., 59A*:82, 1977.

51. Haas, S. S., Brauer, G. M., and Dickson, G. *J. Bone Jt. Surg., 57A*:380, 1975.

52. Charnley, J. *Acrylic Cement in Orthopaedic Surgery*, p. 23, E. & S. Livingstone, Edinburgh, 1970.

53. Freitag, T. A., and Cannon, S. L. *J. Biomed. Mater. Res., 11*:609, 1977.

54. Taitsman, J. P., and Saha, S. *J. Bone Jt. Surg., 59A*:419, 1977.

55. Rae, T. *J. Biomed. Mater. Res., 11*:839, 1977.

56. Scott, D., Seifert, W. W., and Westcott, V. C. *Sci. Am., 230*:88, 1974.

57. Scott, D., and Westcott, V. C. *Wear, 44*:173, 1977.

58. Ungethüm, M., Jäger, M., Witt, A. N., and Hildebrandt, H. J. *Acta Orthop. Scand., 45*:421, 1974.

59. Walker, P. S., and Bullough, P. G. *Ortho. Clin. N. Am., 4*:275, 1973.

60. Walker, P. S., and Salvati, E. *J. Biomed. Mater. Res., 4*:327, 1973.

61. Simon, S. R., Paul, I. L., Rose, R. M., and Radin, E. L. *J. Bone Jt. Surg., 57A*:226, 1975.

62. Chen, S. C., Lowe, S. A., Scales, J. T., and Ansell, R. H. *Acta Orthop. Scand., 45*:429, 1974.

63. Amstutz, H. *J. Biomed. Mater. Res., 3*:547, 1968.

64. Gold, B. L., and Walker, P. S. *Clin. Orthop., 100*:270, 1974.

65. Walker, P. S., and Salvati, E. *J. Biomed. Mater. Res., 4*:327, 1973.

66. Walker, P. S., and Erkman, M. J. *Wear, 21*:377, 1972.

67. Buchholz, H. W., and Strickle, E. *Is the Congruence of the Components of the Total Hip and Fine Polish of the Metallic Head Really an Advantage?*, p. 12, Richards Manufacturing Co., Memphis, Tenn., 1973.

68. Ainsworth, R. D. *Molded Polyethylene Acetabular Cups*, p. 3, Zimmer USA, Warsaw, Ind., 1976.

69. Ungethüm, M. Requirements of operational tests and test results in total hip and knee arthroplasty. In *Advances in Artificial Hip and Knee Joint Technology*, p. 495, Springer-Verlag, Berlin, 1976.

70. Scales, J. T., and Wright, K. W. J. *Acta Orthop. Belge., 41*, Suppl. 1, 163, 1975.

71. Scales, J. T., and Wright, K. W. J. *Acta Orthop. Belge., 41*, Suppl. 1, 160, 1975.

72. Walker, P. S., Salvati, E., and Hotzler, R. K. *J. Bone Jt. Surg., 56A*: 92, 1974.

73. Ungethüm, M. Requirements of operational tests and test results in total hip and knee arthroplasty. In *Advances in Artificial Hip and Knee Joint Technology*, p. 498, edited by M. Schaldach and D. Hohmann, Springer-Verlag, Berlin, 1976.

74. Walker, P., Dowson, D., Longfield, M., and Wright, V. A joint simulator. In *Lubrication and Wear in Joints*, p. 104, J. B. Lippincott, Philadelphia, 1969.

75. Charnley, J., and Cupic, Z. *Clin. Orthop., 95*:9, 1973.

76. Charnley, J., and Halley, D. K. *Clin. Orthop., 112*: 170, 1975.

77. Halley, D. K., and Charnley, J. *Clin. Orthop., 112*:180, 1975.

78. Clarke, I., Black, K., Rennie, C., and Amstutz, H. C. *Clin. Orthop., 121:*126, 1976.
79. Amstutz, H. C., and Markolf, K. L. Design features in total hip replacements. In *The Hip,* p. 111, edited by W. H. Harris, C. V. Mosby, St. Louis, 1974.
80. Johnson, R. C., and Smidt, G. L. *Clin. Orthop., 72:*205, 1970.
81. Weightman, B. The stress in total hip prosthesis femoral stems. In *Advances in Artificial Hip and Knee Joint Technology,* p. 138, edited by M. Schaldach and D. Hohmann, Springer-Verlag, Berlin, 1976.
82. Charnley, J. A. *Clin. Orthop., 111:*105, 1975.
83. Galante, J. O., Rostoker, W., and Doyle, J. M. *J. Bone Jt. Surg., 57A:*230, 1975.
84. Amstutz, H. C., and Markolf, K. S. Design features in total hip replacement. In *The Hip,* p. 117, edited by W. H. Harris, C. V. Mosby, St. Louis, 1974.
85. Weightman, B. The stress in total hip prosthesis femoral stems. In *Advances in Artificial Hip and Knee Joint Technology,* p. 140, edited by M. Schaldach and D. Hohmann, Springer-Verlag, Berlin, 1976.
86. Wilson, J. N., and Scales, J. T. *Clin. Orthop., 72:*145, 1970.
87. Andriacchi, T. P., Galante, J. O., Belytschko, T. B., and Hampton, S. *J. Bone Jt. Surg., 58A:*618, 1976.
88. Charnley, J., and Kamangar, A. *Med. Biol. Eng., 7:*31, 1969.
89. Harris, W. H. *Clin. Orthop., 95:*168, 1973.
90. Charnley, J. *Clin. Orthop., 72:*2, 1970.
91. Sivash, K. M. *Alloplasty of the Hip Joint,* p. 1, Medical Press, Moscow, 1967.
92. Russin, L. A. *The Sivash Total Hip Prosthesis,* p. 3, U. S. Surgical Corp., New York, 1974.
93. Weber, B. G. *Clin. Orthop., 72:*79, 1970.
94. Bateman, J. E. *Orthop. Digest, 3:*15, 1974.
95. Giliberty, R. P. *Orthop. Rev., 3:*40, 1974.
96. Freeman, M. A. R. Some disadvantages of cemented intramedullary stem fixation and their remedies. In *Advances in Artificial Hip and Knee Joint Technology,* edited by M. Schaldach and D. Hohmann, Springer-Verlag, Berlin, 1976.
97. Wagner, H. *Arch. Orthop. Unfallchir., 82:*101, 1975.
98. Amstutz, H. R., Clarke, I. C., Christie, J., and Graff-Radford, A. *Clin. Orthop., 128:*261, 1977.
99. Hulbert, S. F., and Klawitter, J. J. Ceramics as a new approach to the improvement of artificial hip and knee joint technology, In *Advances in Artificial Hip and Knee Joint Technology,* p. 287, edited by M. Schaldach and D. Hohmann, Springer-Verlag, Berlin, 1976.
100. Griss, P., Heimke, G., Krempien, B., and Jentschura, G. Ceramic hip joint replacement—experimental results and early clinical experience. In *Advances in Artificial Hip and Knee Joint Technology,* p. 446, edited by M. Schaldach and D. Hohmann, Springer-Verlag, Berlin, 1976.
101. Salzer, M., Locke, H., Plenk, H., Jr., Ponzet, G., Stark, N., and Zweymuller, K. Experience with bioceramic endoprostheses of the hip and knee joint. In *Advances in Hip and Knee Joint Technology,* p. 463, edited by M. Schaldach and D. Hohmann, Springer-Verlag, Berlin, 1976.
102. Eftekhar, N. S. Controversy of clean air and total hip replacement. In *The Hip,* p. 266, edited by W. H. Harris, C. V. Mosby, St. Louis, 1974.
103. Charnley, J. *Cleveland Clin. Quartr., 40:*99, 1973.
104. Dixon, R. E. *Cleveland Clin. Quartr., 40:*115, 1973.
105. Kolczun, M. C., and Nelson, C. L. Antibiotic concentration in human bone. In *The Hip,* p. 206, edited by W. H. Harris, C. V. Mosby, St. Louis, 1974.
106. Amstutz, H. C. *Cleveland Clin. Quartr., 40:*125, 1973.
107. Levin, P. D. *J. Bone Jt. Surg., 57B:*234, 1975.
108. Hill, J., Klenerman, L., Trustey, S., and Blowers, R. *J. Bone Jt. Surg., 59B:*197, 1977.
109. Elson, R. A., Jehcott, A. E., McGechie, D. B., and Verettas, D. *J. Bone Jt. Surg., 59B:*200, 1977.
110. Buchholz, H. W., and Engelbrecht, H. *Chirurg., 41:*511, 1970.
111. Müller, M. E. *Clin. Orthop., 72:*46, 1970.
112. Markolf, K. L., and Amstutz, H. C. *Clin. Orthop., 121:*99, 1976.
113. Dec, J. B., Saunders, M. D., Inman, V. T., and Eberhart, H. D. *J. Bone Jt. Surg., 35A:*543, 1953.
114. Radin, E. L. *Orthop. Clin. N. Am., 4:*539, 1973.
115. Gschwend, N. Design criteria present indication and implantation techniques for artificial knee joints. In *Advances in Artificial Hip and Knee Joint Technology,* p. 91, edited by M. Schaldach and D. Hohmann, Springer-Verlag, Berlin, 1976.
116. Gschwend, N. Design criteria, present indication and implantation techniques for artificial knee joints. In *Advances in Artificial Hip and Knee Joint Technology,* p. 90, edited by M. Schaldach and D. Hohmann, Springer-Verlag, Berlin, 1976.
117. Huson, A. *The Knee Joint—Int. Congress, Rotterdam 1973,* p. 163, Excerpta Medica, Amsterdam, 1974.
118. Smith, F. B. and Blair, J. *J. Bone Jt. Surg., 36A:* 88, 1954.
119. Helfet, A. J. *Disorders of the Knee,* p. 11, J. B. Lippincott, Philadelphia, 1974.
120. Radin, D. L. *Orthop. Clin. N. Am., 4:*543, 1973.
121. Paul, J. P. Loading on normal hip and knee joints and on joint replacements. In *Advances in Artificial Hip and Knee Joint Technology,* p. 53, edited by M. Schaldach and D. Hohmann, Springer-Verlag, Berlin, 1976.
122. Frankel, V. H. *Orthop. Clin. N. Am., 2:*175, 1971.
123. Maquet, P. *Acta Orthop Belg., 38,* Suppl. 1, 33, 1971.
124. Kettelkamp, D. B. and Nasca, R. *Clin. Orthop., 94:*8, 1973.
125. Walker, P. S. Engineering principles of knee prostheses. In *Disorders of the Knee,* p. 261, edited by A. S. Helfet, J. B. Lippincott, Philadelphia, 1974.
126. Radin, E. L. *Orthop. Clin. N. Am., 4:*544, 1973.
127. Walker, P. S. Engineering principles of knee prostheses. In *Disorders of the Knee,* p. 262, edited by A. J. Helfet, J. B. Lippincott, Philadelphia, 1974.

128. Shaw, J. A., and Murray, D. G. *Clin. Orthop.,* *94:*15, 1973.
129. Jones, W. N. Mold replacement in the rheumatoid knee. In *Surgery of Rheumatoid Arthritis,* p. 35, edited by R. L. Cruess and N. Mitchell, J. B. Lippincott, Philadelphia, 1971.
130. MacIntosh, D. L. Arthroplasty of the knee in rheumatoid arthritis using the hemiarthroplasty prosthesis. In *Surgery of Rheumatoid Arthritis,* p. 29, edited by R. L. Cruess and N. Mitchell, J. B. Lippincott, Philadelphia, 1971.
131. Campbell, W. C. *Clin. Orthop.,* *120:*4, 1976.
132. Potter, T. A. Correction of arthritic deformities. In *Arthritis and Allied Conditions,* p. 651, edited by J. L. Hollander and D. J. McCarty, Lea & Febiger, Philadelphia, 1972.
133. Ilstrup, D. M., Combs, J. J., Bryan, R. S., Peterson, L. F. A., and Skolnick, M. D. *Clin. Orthop.,* *120:*18, 1976.
134. Insall, J., and Walker, P. *Clin. Orthop.,* *120:*83, 1976.
135. Marmor, L. *Clin. Orthop.,* *120:*86, 1976.
136. Engelbrecht, E. *Der. Chirurg.,* *11:*510, 1971.
137. Charnley, J. *The Charnley Load-Angle Inlay Arthroplasty of the Knee,* p. 2, Leeds (Thackray), 1975.
138. Waugh, T. R., Smith, R. C., Orofino, C. F., and Anzel, S. M. *Clin. Orthop.,* *94:*196, 1973.
139. Evanski, P. M., Waugh, T. R., Orofino, C. F., and Anzel, S. H. *Clin. Orthop.,* *120:*33, 1976.
140. Ranawat, C. S., and Shine, J. J. *Clin. Orthop.,* *94:*185, 1973.
141. Ranawat, C. S., Insall, J., and Sine, J. *Clin. Orthop.,* *120:*76, 1976.
142. Walker, P. S., and Masse, Y. *Acta Orthop. Belge.,* *39:*151, 1973.
143. Coventry, M. B., Upshaw, J. E., Riley, L. H., Finerman, G. A. M., and Turner, R. H. *Clin. Orthop.,* *94:*177, 1973.
144. Ilstrup, D. M., Coventry, M. B., and Skolnick, M. D. *Clin. Orthop.,* *120:*27, 1976.
145. Freeman, M. A. R., Swanson, S. A. V., and Todd, R. C. *Clin. Orthop., 94:* 153, 1973.
146. Bargren, J. H., Freeman, M. A. R., and Swanson, S. A. V., and Todd, R. C. *Clin. Orthop.,* *120:*65, 1976.
147. Freeman, M. A. R., Scales, T., and Todd, R. C. *J. Bone Jt. Surg.,* *59B:*64, 1977.
148. Insall, J. N., Ranawat, C. S., Scott, U. N., and Walker, P. S. *Clin. Orthop.,* *120:*49, 1976.
149. Deane, G. *The Deane Knee,* p. 1, Instn. Mechn. Engr., London, 1975.
150. Sonstegard, D. A., Kaufer, H., and Matthews, L. S. *J. Bone Jt. Surg.,* *59A:*602, 1977.
151. Sonstegard, D. A., Kaufer, H., and Matthews, L. S. *Sci. Am.,* *238:*44, 1978.
152. Attenborough, C. G. *Ann. Roy. Col. Surg. (E),* *58:*4, 1976.
153. Walker, P. S., and Shoji, H. *Clin. Orthop.,* *94:*222, 1973.
154. Ghelman, B., Walker, P. S., Shoji, H., and Erkman, M. J. *Clin. Orthop.,* *108:*149, 1975.
155. Matthews, L. S., Sonstegard, D. A., and Kaufer, H. *Clin. Orthop.,* *94:*238, 1973.
156. Sonstegard, D. A., Kaufer, H., and Matthews, L. S. *J. Bone Jt. Surg.,* *59A:*604, 1977.
157. Sonstegard, D. A., Kaufer, H., and Matthews, L. S. *J. Bone Jt. Surg.,* *59A:*606, 1977.
158. Jones, G. B. *Clin. Orthop., 94:*50, 1973.
159. Wilson, F. C., and Venters, G. C. *Clin. Orthop.,* *120:*39, 1976.
160. Arden, G. P. *Clin. Orthop.,* *94:*92, 1973.
161. Engelbrecht, E., Siegel, A., Röttger, J., and Buchholz, H. W. *Clin. Orthop.,* *120:*54, 1976.
162. Engelbrecht, E. *Mater. Med. Nordmark, 27:*117, 1975.
163. Mazas, F. B., and the Guepar. *Clin. Orthop.,* *94:*211, 1973.
164. Deburge, A., and the Guepar. *Clin. Orthop.,* *120:*47, 1976.
165. Blouth, W., Skripitz, W., and Bontemps, G. Problematics of current hinge-type artificial knee joints. In *Advances in Artificial Hip and Knee Joint Technology,* p. 374, edited by M. Schaldach and D. Hohmann, Springer-Verlag, Berlin, 1976.
166. Herbert, J. J., and Herbert, A. *Clin. Orthop.,* *94:*202, 1973.
167. Letournel, E., and Lagrange, J. *Clin. Orthop.,* *94:*249, 1973.
168. Bechtol, C. O. *Bechtol Patello-femoral Joint Replacement System,* p. 3, Richards Manufacturing Co., Memphis, Tenn., 1974.
169. Walker, P. S., and Hsieh, H-H. *J. Bone Jt. Surg.,* *59B:*222, 1977.
170. Insall, J. N., Ranawat, C. S., Aglietti, P., and Shine, J. *J. Bone Jt. Surg., 58A:*754, 1976.
171. Goss, C. M., editor. *Gray's Anatomy,* p. 361, Lea & Febiger, Philadelphia, 1975.
172. Inman, V. T., and Mann, R. A. Biomechanics of the foot and ankle. In *DuVries' Surgery of the Foot,* p. 3, edited by V. T. Inman, C. V. Mosby, St. Louis, 1973.
173. Morris, J. M. *Clin. Orthop., 122:*10, 1977.
174. Hicks, J. H. *J. Anat.,* *87:*345, 1953.
175. Wright, D. G., Desai, S. M., and Henderson, W. H. *J. Bone Jt. Surg., 46A:*361, 1964.
176. Isman, R. E., and Inman, V. T. *Bull. Pros. Res., 97:*10, 1969.
177. Inman, V. T., and Mann, R. A. Biomechanics of the foot and ankle. In *DuVries' Surgery of the Foot,* p. 16, edited by V. T. Inman, C. V. Mosby, St. Louis, 1973.
178. Sammarco, G. J., Burstein, A. H., and Frankel, V. H. *Orthop. Clin. N. Am., 4:*75, 1973.
179. Sammarco, G. J., Burstein, A. H., and Frankel, E. H. *Orthop. Clin. N. Am., 4:*85, 1973.
180. Sammarco, G. J., Burstein, A. H., and Frankel, E. H. *Orthop. Clin. N. Am., 4:*84, 1973.
181. Laurin, C. A. The surgical management of degenerative lesions of the foot and ankle. In *Surgical Management of Degenerative Arthritis of the Lower Limb,* p. 215, edited by R. L. Cruess and N. S. Mitchell, Lea & Febiger, Philadelphia, 1975.
182. Jones, W. N. Treatment of rheumatoid arthritis of the foot and ankle. In *Surgery of Rheumatoid Arthritis,* p. 87, edited by R. L. Cruess and N. S. Mitchell, J. B. Lippincott, Philadelphia, 1971.
183. Crenshaw, A. H. Arthrodesis. In *Campbell's Operative Orthopaedics,* p. 1125, edited by A. H. Crenshaw, St. Louis, (C. V. Mosby), 1971.
184. Haliburton, R. A., Sullivan, C. R., Kelly, P. J., and Peterson, L. F. A., *J. Bone Jt. Surg., 40A:*1125, 1958.

185. Crock, H. V. *The Blood Supply of the Lower Limb Bones in Man*, p. 76, E. & S. Livingstone, Edinburgh, 1967.
186. Lord, G., and Marotte, J. H. *Rev. Chirurg. Orthop. Repar. l'Appar. Moteur, 59:* 139, 1973.
187. Buchholz, H. W. *Der Chirurg., 44:*5, 1973.
188. Freeman, M. A. R. Some disadvantages of cemented intramedullary stem fixation and their remedies. In *Advances in Artificial Hip and Knee Joint Technology*, p. 127, edited by M. Schaldach and D. Hohmann, Springer-Verlag, Berlin, 1976.
189. Smith, R. C. *Smith Total Ankle Surgical Procedure*, p. 2, Wright Manufacturing Co., Memphis, Tenn., 1973.
190. Thompson, P. C. *TPR Total Ankle*, p. 1, Richards Manufacturing Co., Memphis, Tenn., 1976.
191. Newton, S. E. *Surg. Update, 2:*6, 1975.
192. Pappas, M., Buechel, F. F., and DePalma, A. F. *Clin. Orthop., 118:*82, 1976.
193. Pappas, M., Buechel, S. S., and DePalma, A. F. *Clin. Orthop., 118:*83, 1976.
194. Pappas, M., Buechel, S. S., and DePalma, A. F. *Clin. Orthop., 118:*84, 1976.
195. Pappas, M., Buechel, S. S., and DePalma, A. F. *Clin. Orthop., 118:*85, 1976.
196. Groth, H., Fagan, P., and Shen, G. *The Oregon Total Ankle System*, p. 3, Zimmer U.S.A., Warsaw, Ind., 1977.
197. Kopandji, I. A. *The Physiology of the Joints*, p. 10, E. & S. Livingstone, Edinburgh, 1970.
198. Goss, C. M., editor. *Gray's Anatomy*, p. 317, Lea & Febiger, Philadelphia, 1975.
199. Grant, J. C. B. *A Method of Anatomy*, p. 176, Williams & Wilkins, Baltimore, 1958.
200. Goss, C. M., editor. *Gray's Anatomy*, p. 317, Lea & Febiger, Philadelphia, 1975.
201. Neer, C. S. The rheumatoid shoulder. In *Surgery of Rheumatoid Arthritis*, p. 117, edited by R. L. Cruess and N. Mitchell, J. B. Lippincott, Philadelphia, 1971.
202. Fenlin, J. M., Jr., *Orthop. Clin. N. Am., 6:*565, 1975.
203. Inman, V. T., Saunders, J. B., and Abbott, L. C. *J. Bone Jt. Surg., 26:*1, 1944.
204. Fenlin, J. M., Jr. *Orthop. Clin. N. Am., 6:*567, 1975.
205. Poppen, N. K., and Walker, P. S. The mechanics of the shoulder (glenohumeral) joint. In *Transactions of the 22nd Ann Meeting, Orthop. Res. Soc., 1:*65, 1976.
206. Freedman, L., and Munro, R. R. *J. Bone Jt. Surg., 48A:*1503, 1966.
207. Neer, C. S. *J. Bone Jt. Surg., 56A:*1, 1974.
208. Fenlin, J. M., Jr. *Orthop. Clin. N. Am., 6:*568, 1975.
209. Fenlin, J. M., Jr. *Orthop. Clin. N. Am., 6:*569, 1975.
210. Fenlin, J. M., Jr. *Orthop. Clin. N. Am., 6:*570, 1975.
211. Fenlin, J. M., Jr. *Orthop. Clin. N. Am., 6:*575, 1975.
212. Fenlin, J. M., Jr. *Orthop. Clin. N. Am., 6:*574, 1975.
213. Macnab, I., and English, T. *Glenohumeral Prosthesis*, p. E 1, Medishield Inc., Paramus, N. J., 1976.
214. Letten, A. W. F., and Scales, J. T. *Proc. R. Soc. Med., 65:*373, 1972.
215. Letten, A. W. F., and Scales, J. T. *J. Bone Jt. Surg., 55B:*217, 1973.
216. Kapandji, I. A. *Physiology of the Joints*, p. 81, E. & S. Livingstone, Edinburgh, 1970.
217. Goss, C. M., editor. *Grays Anatomy*, p. 326, Lea & Febiger, Philadelphia, 1975.
218. Kapandji, I. A. *The Physiology of the Joints*, p. 78, E. & S. Livingstone, Edinburgh, 1970.
219. Ewald, F. C. *Orthop. Clin. N. Am., 6:*685, 1975.
220. Campbell, W. C. *Ann. Surg., 76:*615, 1922.
221. MacAnsland, W. R. *N. Eng. J. Med., 236:*97, 1947.
222. Hurri, L., Pulkki, T., and Vainio, K. *Acta. Chir. Scand., 127:*459, 1964.
223. Vainio, K. Arthroplasty of the elbow and hand in rheumatoid arthritis. In *Synovectomy and Arthroplasty in Rheumatoid Arthritis*, p. 66, edited by G. Chapchal, G. Thieme Verlag, 1967.
224. Street, D. M., and Stevens, P. S. *J. Bone Jt. Surg., 56A:*1147, 1974.
225. Mellen, R. H., and Phalen, G. S. *J. Bone Jt. Surg., 29:*348, 1947.
226. Johnson, E. W., and Schlein, A. P. *J. Bone Jt. Surg., 52A:*721, 1970.
227. Peterson, L. F. A., and Jones, J. M. *Orthop. Clin. N. Am., 2:*667, 1971.
228. Morrey, B. F., and Chao, E. Y. S. *J. Bone Jt. Surg., 58A:*501, 1976.
229. Morrey, B. F., and Chao, E. Y. S. *J. Bone Jt. Surg., 58A:*503, 1976.
230. Dee, R. *J. Bone Jt. Surg., 54B:*91, 1972.
231. Fick, R. *Handbuch der Anatomie and Mechanik der Gelenke, unter Berucksichtigung der Bewegenden Muskeln*, p. 299, vol. 2, Jena, 1911.
232. Reuleaux, F. *Kinematics of Machinery: Outlines of a Theory of Machines*, p. 56, translated and edited by A. B. Kennedy, Dover, New York, 1963.
233. Souter, W. A. *Orthop. Clin. N. Am., 4:*395, 1973.
234. Dee, R. *J. Bone Jt. Surg., 54B:*88, 1972.
235. Schlein, A. P. *Clin. Orthop., 121:*22, 1976.
236. Swanson, A. B. *Flexible Implant Resection Arthroplasty in the Hand and Extremities*, p. 276, C. V. Mosby, St. Louis, 1973.
237. Clawson, D. K., and Convery, F. R. Surgery in rheumatoid arthritis of the wrist. In *Surgery of Rheumatoid Arthritis*, p. 135, edited by R. L. Cruess and N. Mitchell, J. B. Lippincott, Philadelphia, 1971.
238. Chase, R. A. *Atlas of Hand Surgery*, p. 288, W. B. Saunders, Philadelphia, 1973.
239. Kaplan, E. B. *Functional and Surgical Anatomy of the Hand*, p. 216, J. B. Lippincott, Philadelphia, 1953.
240. Kapandji, I. A. *The Physiology of the Joints*, p. 122, E. & S. Livingston, Edinburgh, 1970.
241. Goss, C. M., editor. *Gray's Anatomy*, p. 333, Lea & Febiger, Philadelphia, 1975.
242. Volz, R. G. *Clin. Orthop., 128:*180, 1977.
243. Jobbins, B., Flowers, M., and Reeves, B. F. *Biomed. Eng., 8:*380, 1973.
244. Swanson, A. B. *Flexible Implant Resection Arthroplasty in the Hand and Extremities*, p. 291, C. V. Mosby, St. Louis, 1973.
245. Meuli, H. C. *Z. Orthop., 113:*476, 1975.
246. Volz, R. G. *Clin. Orthop., 128:*181, 1977.

247. Linscheid, R. L., and Beckenbaugh, R. D. *Geriatrics, 31:*48, 1976.

248. Beckenbaugh, R. D., and Linscheid, R. L. *J. Hand Surg., 2:*337, 1977.

249. Hastings, D. E., and Evans, J. A. *J. Bone Jt. Surg., 57A:*930, 1975.

250. McMurtry, R. Y., Flatt, A. E., and Gillespie, T. E. *J. Bone Jt. Surg.*, in press, 1978.

251. Youm, Y., McMurtry, R. Y., Flatt, A. E., and Gillespie, T. E. *J. Bone Jt. Surg.*, in press, 1978.

252. Burton, R. I. *Orthop. Clin. N. Am., 4:*313, 1973.

253. Flatt, A. E. *The Care of the Rheumatoid Hand*, p. 220, C. V. Mosby, St. Louis, 1974.

254. Urbaniak, J. R. *Clin. Orthop., 204:*9, 1974.

255. Swanson, A. B. *Orthop. Clin. N. Am., 4:*1007, 1973.

256. Chase, R. A. *Atlas of Hand Surgery*, p. 321, W. B. Saunders, Philadelphia, 1973.

257. Napier, J. R. *J. Bone Jt. Surg., 38B:*902, 1956.

258. Landsmeer, J. M. F. *Ann. Rheum. Dis., 21:*164, 1962.

259. Landsmeer, J. M. F., and Long, C. *Acta Anat. (Basel), 60:*330, 1965.

260. Smith, R. J. *Clin. Orthop., 104:* 92, 1974.

261. Flatt, A. E. *The Care of Minor Hand Injuries*, ed. 3, C. V. Mosby, St. Louis, 1972.

262. Linscheid, R. L., and Chao, E. Y. S. *Orthop. Clin. N. Am., 4:*317, 1973.

263. Pagowski, S., Munro, M., and Piekarski, *J. Appl. Phys., 47:*2156, 1976.

264. Lindscheid, R. L., and Chao, E. Y. S. *Orthop. Clin. N. Am., 4:*321, 1973.

265. Lindscheid, R. L., and Chao, E. Y. S. *Orthop. Clin. N. Am., 4:*322, 1973.

266. Smith, E. M., Juvinall, R. C., Bender, L. F., and Pearson, J. R. *Arth. Rheu., 7:*467, 1964.

267. Flatt, A. E., and Fischer, G. W. *Surg. Forum, 19:*459, 1968.

268. Flatt, A. E., and Fischer, G. W. *Ann. Rheum. Dis., Suppl.* 28, 36, 1969.

269. Landsmeer, J. M. F. *Acta Morphol. Neerl. Scand., 2:*59, 1958.

270. Swanson, A. B., Matev, I. B., and deGroot, G. *Bull. Prosth. Res., 13:*1, 1974.

271. Walker, P. S., and Erkman, M. J. *Clin. Orthop., 112:*349, 1975.

272. Flatt, A. E. The pathomechanics of ulnar drift: a biomechanical and clinical study. Final report, Social and Rehabilitation Services, grant no. RD 2226M, 1971.

273. Swanson, A. B., and Mater, I. B. *J. Bone Jt. Surg., 52A:*1265, 1970.

274. Swanson, A. B., Meester, W. D., Swanson, G. deG., Rangaswamy, L., and Schut, G. E. D. *Orthop. Clin. N. Am., 4:*1097, 1973.

275. Beckenbaugh, R. D., Dobyns, J. H., Linscheid, R. L., and Bryan, R. S. *J. Bone Jt. Surg., 58A:*483, 1976.

276. Calnan, J. S. *Br. J. Hosp. Med., 5:*240, 1971.

14

Clinical Methods of
Total Joint Replacements

There is a need for engineers, as well as surgeons, to appreciate the clinical aspects of total joint replacement so that they can incorporate clinical considerations into the designs of superior methods of joint reconstruction. This chapter provides specific guidelines on some accepted and successful methods of total joint replacement with principal discussion on the hip where most clinical experience has been obtained. Operative indications, surgical techniques, postoperative care and the management of common postoperative complications are reviewed.

The classic interpositional arthroplasties and hemiarthroplasties that still find clinical application are viewed in Chapter 13. Other recently devised arthroplastic procedures such as the reconstruction of metatarsophalangeal joints, and replacement of carpal bones, tendons and ligaments are discussed in Chapter 15. Most techniques of total joint reconstruction of finger joints are, perhaps, best classified as interpositional arthroplasties. Nevertheless, the methods are discussed in this chapter. The length of the subsections on the several total joint replacements varies considerably and reflects the present state of knowledge and clinical experience on each technique.

TOTAL HIP JOINT REPLACEMENT

Total hip joint replacement is experiencing its second decade of extraordinary clinical success which rarely has been rivaled by any other major reconstructive procedure.

For 10-year follow-up on 379 primary operations, Charnley[1] reported a mortality of 2.1% of which two out of three deaths were from pulmonary embolism. Early evidence of infection occurred in 1.6% but in a further 2.2%, infection became apparent months or years later. Late mechanical failure occurred at a rate of 1.3%. Of the remaining patients, 90% obtained complete relief of pain and restoration of normal ability to walk. The other 10% had slight or intermittent pain and walked with a limp without the use of walking aids. Restoration of motion was not quite so spectacular, although in all cases the range of motion was improved, as outlined in Chapter 13.

The results reported by Müller,[2] Eftekhar[3] and others[4, 5] are comparable to those reported by Charnley. Over 90% of the patients routinely show excellent relief of pain and improved mobility and function. About 1% to 1.5% of the patients have to undergo reoperation for early or late complications each year. This figure represents 10% to 15% of the patients in the first decade.

Since the early clinical studies on total hip replacements by Charnley,[6, 7] McKee[8] and others[9–11] the author has had the privilege to visit the Wrightington Hip Centre on several occasions, to observe Maurice Müller in Berne, and to visit numerous other experienced hip surgeons on both sides of the Atlantic. From these observations, from the voluminous literature and from his clinical practice in Pittsburgh, the author has evolved the following rationale for the management of patients with severe arthritis of the hip before, during and after total hip replacement.

A subsection on the intra-abdominal complications of total hip replacement is included for which the author is grateful to Dr. Daniel H. Brooks, head of the Division of General Surgery at Allegheny General Hospital in Pittsburgh, Pennsylvania.

Indications for Total Hip Joint Replacement

The primary indication for total hip joint replacement, and similarly for comparable arthroplastic procedures of other joints is intolerable joint pain provoked by: (1) degenerative, traumatic, rheumatoid or other inflammatory arthritis; (2) arthritis secondary to various congenital or idiopathic conditions such as congenital dislocation of the hip, Perthes' disease, slipped capital femoral epiphysis or Paget's disease; and (3) other less frequently encountered conditions.[12, 13] The one main type of end-stage arthritis where total joint replacement is contraindicated is septic arthritis where the surgical procedure is likely to provoke an exacerbation of the infection with clinical failure. The other notable exception is a neuropathic or Charcot joint where the loss of sensation of pain and position-sense in the joint renders the arthroplastic procedure unduly susceptible to subluxation, dislocation and infection. Where pain is the indication for surgery, other modalities of treatment such as diminished activity, the use of walking aids, and simple analgesics should be employed prior to a precipitous decision to undertake surgery. Where a degenerative hip is painful but mobile, with better than 90° of flexion, a medial, varus displacement osteotomy through the intertrochanteric region may be preferred, especially in patients under the age of 50 years.[14] While the osteotomy does not provide relief of pain in all patients, when successful it provides a biological solution without the inherent liabilities of an artificial joint, including an indefinite predilection for septic arthritis that results from a transient hematogenous dissemination of organisms to an arthroplastic joint. Other hip surgeons, such as Charnley,[7] argue that osteotomy as a treatment for degenerative arthritis is never indicated because of its high incidence of failure to provide prolonged relief of pain and because the osteotomy and the subsequent surgery to remove the fixation device provide two procedures with the associated risk of a deep wound infection that could jeopardize the subsequent execution of a total hip joint replacement with its greater likelihood for relief of arthritic pain.

Another indication for total hip joint replacement is severe limitation of motion, especially where the patient has other stiff joints. Patients with ankylosing spondylitis frequently have involvement of both hips and the spine with progressive flexion deformities at both sites.[9] Rheumatoid arthritic patients may have numerous stiff or painful appendicular and axial joints. In certain instances the inflammatory disease abates after a prolonged course so that the patient possesses numerous stiff joints or grossly deformed joints which subsequently undergo secondary degenerative changes.

Another uncommon indication for total hip joint replacement is relocation of a dislocated hip of congenital origin, where, in addition to relief of pain from secondary degenerative change, the surgical procedure provides an opportunity for the surgeon to reconstruct the acetabulum at the anatomical site.[15] The surgery provides a substantial improvement of the patient's apparent and true leg length discrepancy and a marked improvement in the patient's gait, both from cosmetic and functional aspects. Such a formidable operation, however, should not be performed by a surgeon unless he has considerable experience with similar arthroplastic problems and unless the patient has been informed of the possible complications of surgery.

Other reconstructive procedures of the hip such as fusion and cup arthroplasty have limited applications which are discussed elsewhere.[16–19]

An accurate documentation of the preoperative condition of the patient should be prepared using a standard format such as that devised by d'Aubigne and Postel,[20] Harris[21] or Wilson,[22] so that follow-up data may be correlated. The Charnley adaptation[23] of the scheme by d'Aubigne and Postel is presented in Table 14-1 with minor modifications by Amstutz.[24]

Preoperative Preparation for Total Hip Joint Replacement

Prior to surgery, medical assessment should be performed with scrutiny for possible septic foci such as the urinary tract and the ears, nose and throat.[25] Particularly in the adult males over the age of 50 years, the urinary tract should be assessed for possible causes of postoperative obstruction which could require treatment by the insertion of a urinary catheter. Such instrumentation is accompanied by a likelihood of transient septicemia and migration of organisms to the arthroplastic joint. Especially when an adult male shows historical and clinical evidence of prostatic enlargement which affects micturition, surgical correction of the urological obstruction prior to total hip joint replacement should be carefully considered.

The role of prophylactic antibiotics has been questioned by many workers[1, 26, 27] as discussed in Chapter 13. The author prefers to use a cephalosporin administered by the intravenous route. If the surgeon elects to use systemic chemotherapy, he should select an antibiotic, such as a variety of cephalosporins, that is effective against Staphylococcus and common commensal organisms in the urinary tract. The drug should first be given between 2 and 6 hours prior to surgery so that the patient's flora do not have a prolonged period of exposure to the drug be-

Table 14-1
Evaluation Scheme for the Arthritic Hip

Pain	*Walking*
0. Continuous. Intolerable. Strong medication frequently.	0 Bedridden.
2. Continuous but tolerable. Salicylates frequently.	2. Wheelchair activities. Independent transfers.
4. Little or none at rest but pain with activities. Salicylates frequently.	4. Walks with crutches or walker but less than 2 blocks.
6. Pain with certain activities and morning pain which abates spontaneously. Salicylates occasionally.	6. Walks with one support and more than 5 blocks.
8. Occasional, slight pain.	8. Walks without support at home, outside with one support or without, with a mild limp.
10. No pain.	10. Normal walking.
Muscle Power (MP) and Motion	*Function*
0. Ankylosis with deformity.	0. Completely dependent and confined.
2. Ankylosis with good functional position.	2. Partially dependent.
4. MP, poor or fair. Flexion less than 90°. Restricted lateral and rotary movement.	4. Independent. Limited housework and shopping.
6. MP, fair or good. Flexion up to 90°. Fair lateral and rotary movement.	6. Undertakes most housework, desk-type work and shops freely.
8. MP, good or normal. Flexion more than 90°. Good lateral and rotary movement.	8. Minimal restriction. Can undertake jobs with prolonged standing or walking.
10. MP-normal. Motion-normal or near normal.	10. Normal activities.

fore surgery.[28] Two hours of intravenous exposure to common antibiotics provides adequate concentrations of the agent in articular joints.

For the optimal brief exposure of the patient to the potentially hazardous hospital flora, such as resistant strains of *Staphylococcus aureus,* the patient should be admitted to hospital on the day prior to surgery. Where more extensive tests for medical screening are necessary, they should be undertaken on a preliminary admission, or as an outpatient. The patient should not share a room with another patient who has open or infected wounds.

Preoperative instructions to the patient should include a brief format of postoperative traction, physical therapy and the temporary postoperative restriction on certain positions of the lower extremities.[25]

The Surgical Technique of Total Hip Joint Replacement

Irrespective of the operative exposure of the implant which is employed, certain general principles of surgery are highly recommended. As with other arthroplastic procedures the goal remains the optimal, realistic reconstruction of the hip rather than hip replacement. A knowledge of the anatomical landmarks is a prerequisite for the surgeon, including topographical features such as the anterior superior iliac spine, the greater trochanter, as well as intimate features of the hip joint, such as the angle and inclination of the acetabulum. Frequently, the anatomy of the severely arthritic hip is grossly abnormal and appropriate operative adjustments are necessary.

The surgical team should consist of the operator, the first and second assistants and the scrub and circulating nurses. Optimal conditions for sterility of the operating field are essential. The technique of the surgical team, including attention to details such as the method of application of surgical gowns and gloves, minimal movement around the operating room and minimal realistic duration of the operation is more important than the provision for clean air rooms.[29] The significance of clean air facilities is reviewed in Chapter 8.

Operative gowns and gloves are of moderately standardized form apart from the ancillary apparatus necessary for clean air technique. The most useful supplementary technique is the application of double gloves by the team, as advised by Charnley.[30] The outer pair should be a half or whole size larger than the regular size employed by the team member. The looser gloves lessen the likelihood of perforation of a glove which otherwise is extremely likely, in view of the numerous pointed cutting tools and bone. Alternatively, an outer pair of protective nylon gloves, as designed by Müller* is helpful.

The patient is positioned carefully so that the surgical team is aware of the orientation of the acetabulum. The three operative exposures described below require different positioning of the patient. Whichever exposure and appropriate position are employed, the team must ensure that the position will not shift during surgery so that their orientation of the acetabulum is lost prior to insertion of the acetabular component. The patient's skin on the relevant extremity, the groin and the hip proximal to the umbilicus and/or the equivalent region in the back are prepared in routine fashion, with 2% iodine or Betadine scrub solution. The limb is draped free with sheets and a stockinet is rolled to midthigh. A medium sized Vi-Drape is applied to the exposed thigh, the inguinal region and the perineum with retention of abduction and flexion of the hip. On large or obese patients a second Vi-Drape may be required to provide complete coverage of the operative field.

The Operative Exposure for Total Hip Joint Replacement

Three operative exposures to the hip have been widely employed for arthroplastic procedures.[31] Each has staunch advocates and opponents. Each approach is used by a variety of centers where excellent results are obtained in vast numbers of patients. In capable hands, the duration of surgery is about the same irrespective of the approach. For the inexperienced hip surgeon, however, some recommendations may be helpful. For a routine total hip joint replacement in an uncomplicated case, the author prefers the posterolateral, or Gibson approach,[24] with the patient firmly supported on his nonoperative side in a well defined position. The surgeon should be aware of the tendency, particularly of the obese patient, to gradually list toward his ventral surface. The posterolateral approach is the simplest approach, without excision of the greater trochanter, which shows excellent exposure of the acetabulum and the proximal femur with minimal bleeding. Its principal liabilities are a tendency for the surgeon to position the acetabular component in excessive retroversion, especially if the patient lists toward his ventral surface. Also, the surgeon must deliberately avoid the tendency to insert the femoral stem with excessive varus deformity by its inser-

tion in the lateral aspect of the superior extent of the proximal femur. The use of a box chisel, which is routinely employed for the preparation of the femur prior to insertion of a Moore straight-stemmed femoral prosthesis,[32] is recommended.

Where the patient presents with one of several complicating factors such as protrusio-acetabulum, previous reconstructive procedures such as cup arthroplasty, femoral osteotomy with retained metal, or femoral head replacement, congenital dislocation of the hip or rarely, gross obesity, the author prefers a lateral approach with the technique described by Harris.[33] With the patient positioned on his nonoperative side, and through a curved incision, the surgeon possesses excellent visualization of the depth of the wound. Alternatively, the straight lateral incision described by Charnley,[6] with the patient positioned on his back, can be used. Admittedly, the latter approach provides optimal knowledge by the surgeon of the orientation of the acetabulum. Yet, as Coventry[34] has emphasized, a lateral approach to the hip, with the patient on his side, provides superior exposure. With the patient supine, only the surgeon and the first assistant can observe the surgical procedure while the second assistant, who is across the table from the operative hip, contributes little to the surgery and does not learn the exacting details of the surgery. In the teaching hospital, where many hip arthroplasties are performed, all of the surgical assistants who are in training should participate intimately in operations. With the patient positioned on his side all of the assistants can observe the surgical field.

The anterolateral approach of Watson-Jones has been preferred by many surgeons including Müller[35] and Evarts et al.[36] because of the greater distance between the incision and the perirectal region. The approach is more difficult than the posterolateral one and visualization of the acetabulum and proximal femur is less satisfactory. The author is unaware of a difference in the incidence of infection when any of the surgical approaches are used by knowledgable surgeons with otherwise similar techniques.

The relative merits of a variety of available total hip joint prostheses are described in Chapter 13. The author prefers to use the Trapezoidal-28 (T-28) system which provides a wide variety of implants of different sizes and configurations, one of which is suitable for most reconstructive problems.[24] With two exceptions the subsequent discussion refers to the application of the T-28 prosthesis. For the straight lateral

---

* M. E. Müller, personal communication, 1969.

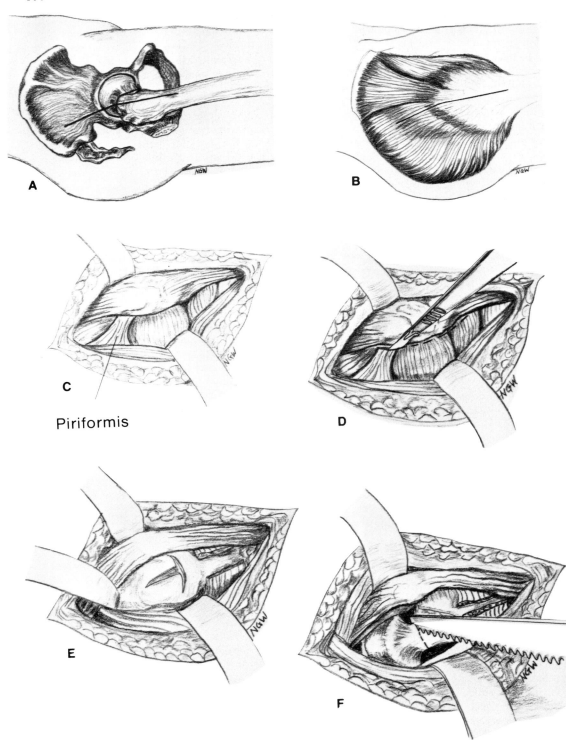

Piriformis

Figure 14-1. *A* to *K*. Technique for total hip joint replacement through a posterolateral approach.

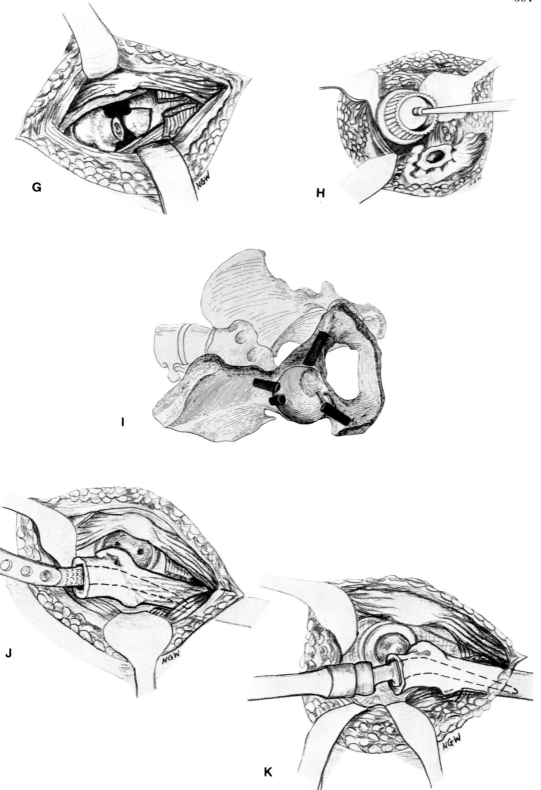

and the anterolateral approaches, the instrumentation systems of Charnley and Müller, respectively, are described.

A Posterolateral Approach. The patient is placed in a lateral position and secured firmly with anterior and posterior supports. The involved leg is draped to permit free movement during the procedure. With the hip flexed, a longitudinal incision is extended from the posterosuperior iliac spine over the greater trochanter and distally along the lateral aspect of the leg (Fig. 14-1*A*). The fascia lata is opened longitudinally, beginning in the distal portion of the wound, and extended proximally (Fig. 14-1*B*). The gluteus maximus is divided in line with its fibers to a level above the acetabulum. The gluteus maximus muscle and the fascia lata are retracted posteriorly to visualize the short external rotators (namely, the piriformis, obturator internus, gemelli and the upper part of the quadratus femoris) (Fig. 14-1*C*). The short external rotator muscles are divided close to their attachments into the femur as in Figure 14-1*D*. The surgeon should be aware of the proximity of the sciatic nerve to the posterior portion of the wound although direct visualization of the nerve is unnecessary.

The capsule of the hip joint is opened along the posterolateral aspect of the femoral neck from its insertion on the femoral neck to its origin on the rim of the acetabulum (Fig. 14-1*E*). For wider exposure of the hip joint the capsular incision can be converted into a "T". The femoral head is dislocated posteriorly. Dislodgement is facilitated by the insertion of a uterine skid or periosteal elevator into the hip joint to pry the femoral head away from the acetabulum. If there is mild protrusio acetabuli or ankylosis of the hip joint, it will be preferable to first divide the femoral neck and subsequently to remove the femoral head with a corkscrew or by fragmentation. Excessive force should not be applied to the femur during dislocation of the femoral head or the risk of fracture of the femur becomes substantial. An oscillating saw is useful to section the femoral neck (Fig. 14-1*F*). The optimal plane for division of the femoral neck is about 1.5 cm (1 fingerbreadth) above the lesser trochanter medially to the base of the greater trochanter laterally (Fig. 14-1*G*). This cut is 45° to the long axis of the femur with 0 to 5° of anteversion. The trial femoral component may be used as a template.

The acetabulum is curetted to remove residual articular cartilage. Marginal osteophytes at the edge of the acetabulum may be excised to facilitate proper placement of the acetabular component. In most instances, further resection of capsule is unnecessary unless a segment of capsule obstructs the insertion of the reamers or the implants. The acetabulum is reamed with a series of graduated reamers until the optimal size is achieved (Fig. 14-1*H*). Of the many types of reamers available, the air-powered instruments with a disposable bladed MIRA system appear to be optimal for rapid enlargement or redirection of the acetabulum. In a simple degenerative joint, reaming is terminated when a hemispherical surface of subchondral bone is reached. The dense subchondral bone should not be removed because the acetabular component is likely to undergo gradual central migration if it is surrounded by cancellous bone. An acetabular thickness of at least 0.5 cm should remain intact. A trial acetabular cup is placed into the acetabulum to determine bone coverage. The cup should be covered with bone, especially at its superior and posterior borders. A ⅜-inch drill is used to prepare cement holes in the ilium, ischium and pubis (Fig. 14-1*I*). The depth of the holes should be 1 to 2 cm although it should not penetrate the pelvis. Each hole is undercut slightly with a curet. The hip joint is irrigated periodically with triple antibiotic solution, such as a mixture of 50,000 units of bacitracin, 0.5 g of neomycin and 50 mg of polymyxin B per 0.5 liter of normal saline.

The medullary space of the proximal femur is prepared with a rasp (Fig. 14-1*J*) so that the femoral component, subsequently, will be inserted in a position of 5 to 10° anteversion. Progressively larger femoral rasps are used to permit the use of the largest stem that can be safely inserted into the femur.

The methylmethacrylate is mixed to a doughy consistency and packed firmly into the acetabular cementing holes. Further cement is placed in the acetabulum and the acetabular component is guided into place with the use of an acetabular guide. The cup is placed at a 45° angle to the long axis of the body and 5 to 10° of anteversion. Firm pressure is applied to the cup, by means of the acetabular guide. Excessive pressure, however, is deleterious because the cement is extruded. While the cement is pliable, peripheral excrescences are trimmed. Ten minutes after the cement is first mixed, the acetabular guide is removed and the cup is inspected. Excessive cement is carefully removed. Pressure is applied to the cup and the interfaces between the bone and cement and the cement and cup are inspected. If microscopic motion is detected at an interface, the cup and cement are removed and another attempt is made to cement the cup.

A trial femoral component is selected and inserted into the proximal femur. A trial reduction of the hip joint is undertaken and the stability of the joint is ascertained. An attempt is made to use the femoral component with the longest length of neck so that the risk of impingement of the greater trochanter or the prosthetic femoral neck on the lateral aspect of the pelvis or the acetabular component is minimized. Such impingement is a common cause of subsequent loosening of an implant. Attention also is focused on the flange of the femoral component where it seats on the proximal femur. If the flange fails to seat correctly, the bone is trimmed appropriately. The medulla is carefully aspirated of residual blood. A clean sponge is placed in the cup to prevent subsequent contamination of the socket with cement. A second batch of methylmethacrylate is mixed until it acquires a dough-like consistency. It is rolled into a cylinder which can be packed into the proximal femur. Impactors or injection apparatus may facilitate the insertion so that cement wholly fills the cavity in bone beyond the tip of the femoral component. Prior to insertion of cement, a polyethylene tube may be inserted into the femur to allow air and blood to escape. The femoral component is introduced into the proximal femur with great care in a position of slight valgus of the stem (Fig. 14-1K). The valgus alignment provides optimal transfer of load between the implant and the bone. While the cement hardens, the implant is immobilized with an impactor as in Figure 14-1K. Afterward, the hip joint is reduced and a trial range of motion is performed. The positions in which spontaneous dislocation occur are recorded, with particular attention to the positions of flexion with internal rotation and extension with external rotation. If the arthroplasty lacks adequate stability, revision of the malpositioned component should be undertaken.

The hip should be stable in 90° of flexion with 30° of internal rotation and 0° of flexion with 30° of external rotation. A final irrigation of the wound is performed and a suction drainage tube is placed in the hip joint. A second tube may be placed along the subcutaneous layer. The short external rotator muscles and the fascia lata are repaired with interrupted 0-0 vicryl polyglactin 910 (Ethicon, Inc., Somerville, N. J.) sutures. The subcutaneous tissue is closed with interrupted 3-0 polyglactin 910 sutures and the skin is closed with interrupted Vicryl polyglactin 910 or nylon sutures. Dry dressings and an abduction splint are applied prior to the transfer of the patient to his bed.

If the patient has severe bilateral arthritis of the hips so that bilateral total hip replacements are indicated, the experienced team of hip surgeons may elect to undertake bilateral arthroplastic surgery under one anesthetic. After the first procedure is completed, the patient is repositioned on his opposite side and reprepared and draped for the second procedure. Particular caution is necessary so that dislocation of the arthroplastic hip does not occur during the repositioning. For hip surgeons with less experience, sequential procedures undertaken with an interval of 6 weeks to 6 months are preferred.

A Lateral Exposure. For more difficult reconstructive problems in total hip joint replacement, a lateral approach with excision of the greater trochanter is preferred. At least three slightly different lateral exposures have been widely employed. Charnley[23] uses a straight lateral approach with the patient positioned on his back. Figure 14-2A to I illustrate total hip replacement through this exposure. Coventry[34] uses a similar incision with the patient positioned on his nonoperative side. Harris[33] modified the lateral approach with a curved incision that provides more extensive visualization. The patient is carefully placed on his side with adequate anterior and posterior supports so that his position cannot shift during the operation. Perhaps the most useful application of the Harris technique is for reconstruction of a painful congenital dislocation of the hip,[37] as shown in Figures 14-3 A to J and 14-4 A to C. Excellent visualization of the false acetabulum is essential.[15, 38] The skin incision parallels the posterior border of the muscle belly of the tensor fascia lata and courses to the posterosuperior corner of the greater trochanter. It then passes straight down the femur about 3 inches and curves anteriorly as in Figure 14-3A. After incision of the subcutaneous tissues, the fascia lata is divided from the distal end of the wound (Fig. 14-3B). The index finger is passed through the division in the fascia lata to palpate the tendon of gluteus maximus. The fascia lata incision is placed 1 fingerbreadth in front of the maximus tendon. The fascial incision is continued proximally in this way so that the substance of the gluteus maximus is not violated. The bursa over the greater trochanter is dissected away so that the proximal origin of the vastus lateralis can be clearly seen. If the posterior iliotibial band is excessively tight it is incised proximal to the attachment of the gluteus maximus to the femur

Figure 14-2. *A* to *I.* Technique for total hip joint replacement through a straight lateral approach of Charnley. The patient is prepared in the careful fashion previously described by the innovator and positioned on the operating table in the supine position under general anesthesia. A longitudinal skin incision (Fig. 14-2*A*) is centered over the middle of the trochanter and extends at least 3 inches (7.5 cm) proximal to the tip of the trochanter and distally to the level of midfemur. The hip is flexed to 30° and adducted until the buttock is elevated from the table. This maneuver facilitates exposure especially in obese patients. The deep fascia is incised parallel to the shaft of the femur and in its midaxis. A transverse relaxing incision in the fascia lata proximal to the trochanter may relieve excessive tension. The gluteus maximus is split in line with the muscle fibers. With the hip externally rotated the cleft between gluteus medius and tensor fascia lata is developed to expose the anterior surface of the capsule of the hip joint. The capsule is incised at the long axis of the neck of the femur. A curved bone retractor is positioned on the inferior femoral neck while cholecystectomy forceps are passed on the superior neck of the femur until they protrude through the posterior capsule. With the forceps a Gigli saw (Fig. 14-2*B*) is passed through the interior of the joint cavity for division of the greater trochanter. Periosteum is incised on the lateral surface of the greater trochanter and periosteal flaps are developed. The greater trochanter is detached and retracted in a superior direction (Fig. 14-2*C*). The short external rotators of the hip are incised close to their insertion on the greater trochanter. The acetabular labrum is incised posterosuperiorly to facilitate dislocation.

With the hip positioned in adduction and external rotation dislocation is accomplished. The femoral neck is divided with a Gigli saw to leave about 5 mm of superior cortex in the femoral neck. The centering drill with its centering guide is inserted into the acetabulum and the preliminary hole is made at 20 to 30° from a transverse axis. The centering drill is replaced with a pilot drill which enlarges the preliminary hole. Next the expanding reamers are used to enlarge and deepen the acetabulum (Fig. 14-2*D*). Deepening continues until ⅛ inch (3 mm) of bone remains in the pilot hole. A trial fit of the socket is performed and appropriate adjustments are made. A ½-inch diameter cement hole is made in the ilium. Cement is mixed and inserted after which the socket is positioned with the socket guide holder. The socket is aligned with an axis of 45° to the long axis of the body and 0 to 5° of anteversion. Afterward, excessive cement is removed. Figure 14-2*E* shows the socket cemented in place.

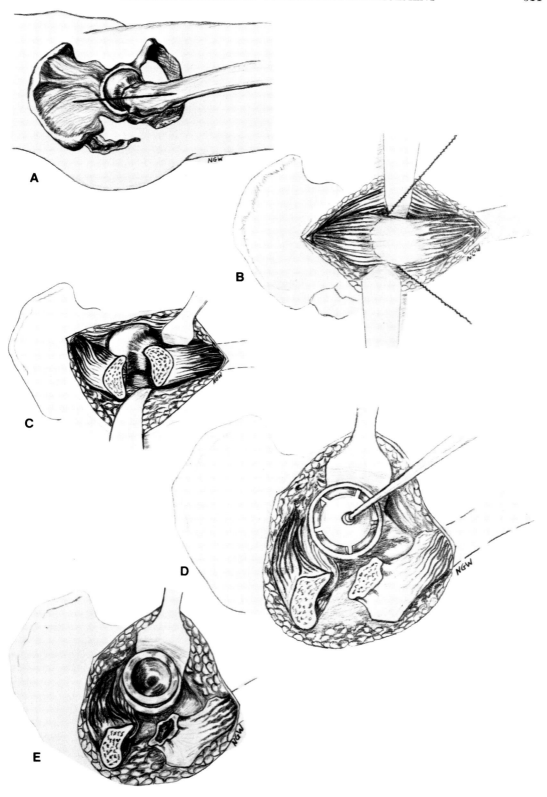

With the hip externally rotated and the knee flexed to 90° the exposed surface of femoral neck is delivered to the wound. The "taper-pin" reamer is used to prepare the proximal femur and to prevent subsequent reamers from piercing the lateral femoral cortex. The femoral broaches (Fig. 14-2F) are used to prepare the intramedullary cavity in a neutral position of version. A trial femoral prosthesis is inserted and the hip joint is reduced for a test of stability and motion.

With the special male and female reamers the osteotomized surfaces of the greater trochanter are prepared. The reamers permit adjustment in the site of attachment of the greater trochanter to optimize the tension in the abductor muscles. Appropriate drill holes are made for insertion of the wires to reattach the greater trochanter. When the wires have been positioned cement is mixed and inserted into the proximal femur. The implant is inserted with an attempt to achieve valgus alignment of the stem (Fig. 14-2G). The hip joint is reduced (Fig. 14-2H) and the greater trochanter is reattached (Fig. 14-2I) by the use of a Kirschner wire-tightener. Excessive wire (20 s.w.g. (standard wire gauge)) is removed and the exposed wire is covered by a flap of vastus lateralis aponeurosis. Suction drains are inserted and the wound is closed in layers. Charnley recommends the use of pull-out fat sutures of novel design.

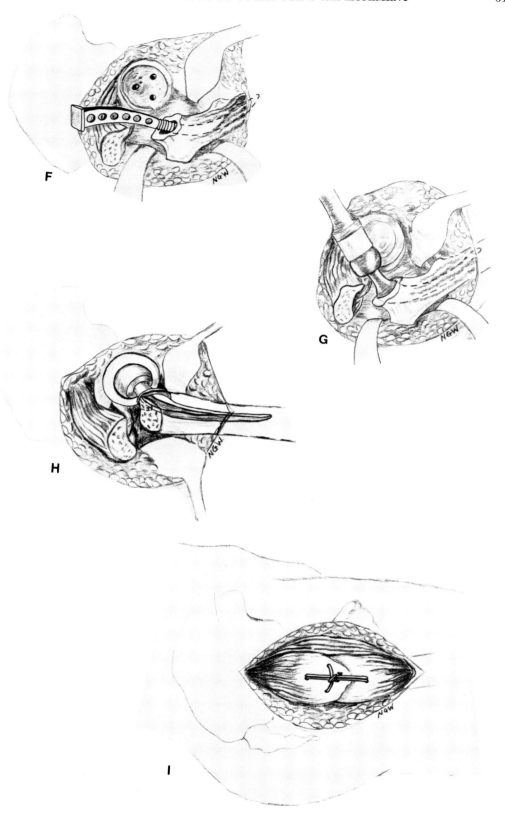

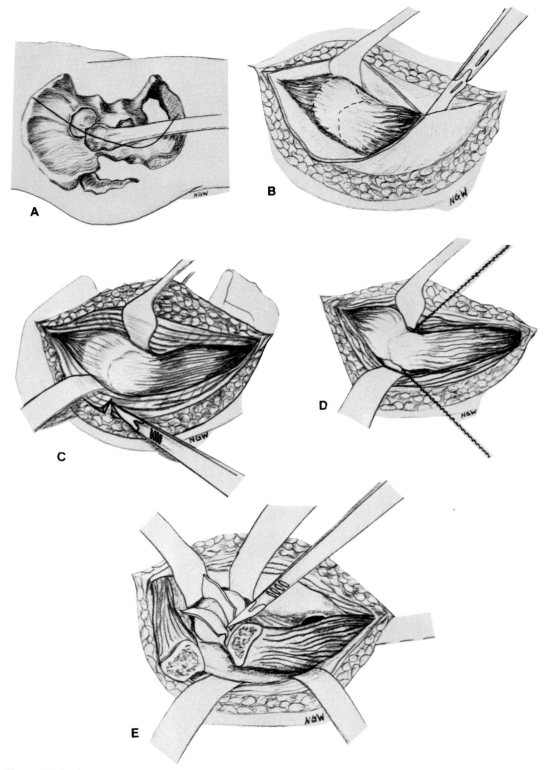

Figure 14-3. *A* to *J.* Technique for total hip joint replacement through a lateral exposure of Harris for reconstruction of a congenital dislocation of the hip.

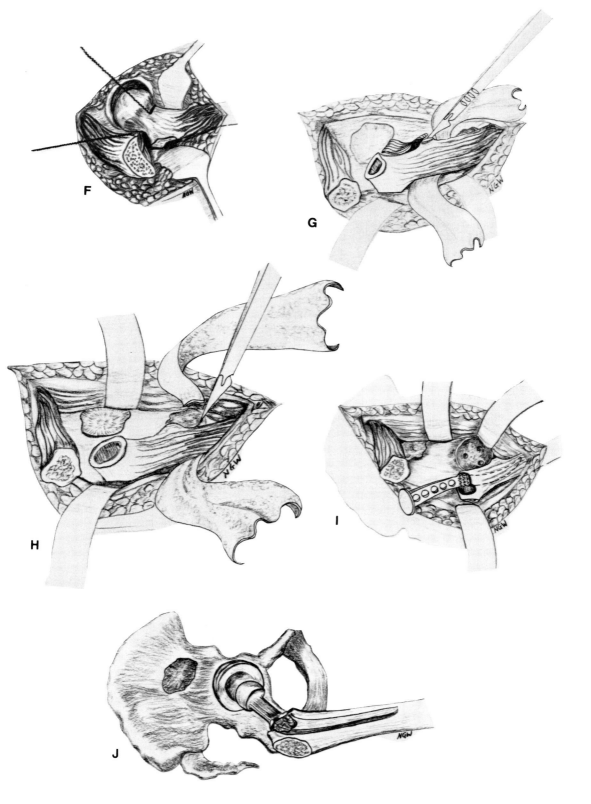

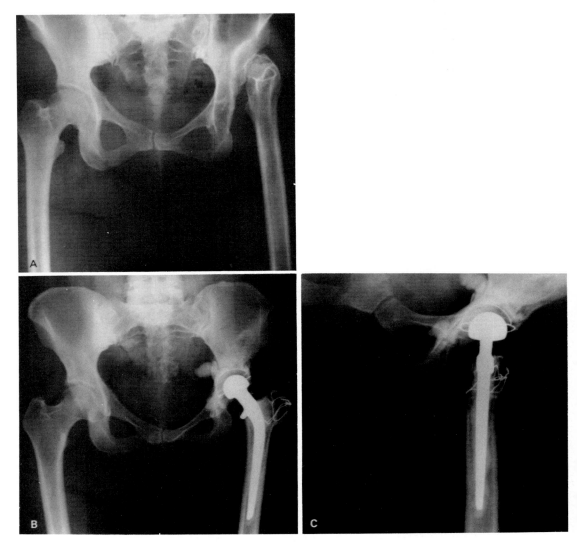

Figure 14-4. *A* to *C*. Figure 14-4*A* is a preoperative X-ray of a painful dislocated hip of congenital origin in a woman of 35 years. The dysplasia of the entire hemipelvis on the involved side is evident. Figure 14-4 *B* and *C*, postoperative X-rays of the same patient taken 3 years after surgery reveal the location of the socket in the true acetabulum.

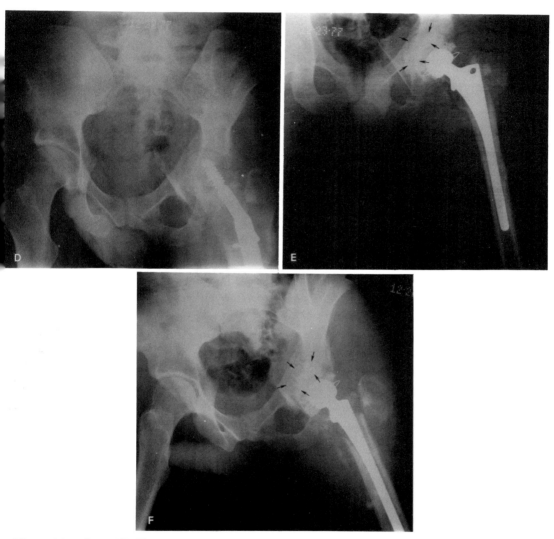

Figure 14-4. *D* to *F*. In Figure 14-4*D* an X-ray reveals the painful stiff hip of a man of 22 years who, 1 year earlier, had sustained a left pertrochanteric femoral fracture with a displaced central acetabular fracture. The former progressed to a nonunion while the latter healed with substantial displacement and severe traumatic arthritis of the hip joint. In Figure 14-4 *E* and *F*, postoperative X-rays reveal the use of the femoral head as a bone graft (*arrows*) to fill and strengthen the acetabulum. The femoral component possesses a porous sinter coated surface for ingrowth of bone so that methylmethacrylate is not employed.

(Fig. 14-3C). By blunt dissection the anterior border of gluteus medius is identified and retracted cephalad with a right-angle retractor. The limb is externally rotated and the anterior portion of the capsule of the hip joint is visualized. A Gigli saw is passed between the proximal femur and the capsule as in Figure 14-3D. Alternatively, if this cannot be undertaken, the saw can be passed through a curved trocar. The saw is positioned posterior and distal to the styloid of the greater trochanter, where the tendon of gluteus medius attaches to the femur. The bone is divided and the greater trochanter is retracted cephalad. The dissection is continued to the lateral iliac wall. In the presence of a dislocated hip, the gluteus medius is elevated until the entire false acetabulum is visualized. The capsule, now exposed, is incised longitudinally from the superior rim of the false acetabulum to its superior attachment on the proximal femoral neck (Fig. 14-3E). Each anterior and posterior portion of capsule is removed as a separate intact layer. The femoral neck is divided with a Gigli saw (Fig. 14-3F). For exposure of the posterior capsule that extends distal to the true acetabulum, incision of the short external rotator muscles and the iliopsoas tendon from their insertions on the posterior femoral neck is essential (Fig. 14-3G). Removal of the largely redundant capsule in two large pieces enables the surgeon to retain his orientation amidst the confusing distortions in anatomy that are present in such patients. The confusion is compounded by the presence of capsular folds that extend from the femoral neck to both the false acetabulum and to the true acetabulum. The origin of the capsular folds has been elegantly described by Ferguson.[39] Ultimately, the entire capsule is excised to permit visualization of the hypotrophic true acetabulum (Fig. 14-3H) which is filled with fibrous and fatty tissue.

The whole ipsilateral pelvis of patients with congenital dislocation of the hip is poorly developed and of inferior bone stock to the contralateral hemipelvis. While the true acetabulum is exceptionally small, it provides the sole location with adequate bone stock where the cup may be situated.[15, 37, 38] Starting with small reamers, the true acetabulum is carefully enlarged. Special small cups are necessary in view of the limited available space. For a grossly deficient pelvic wall, Harris[40] has devised a unique method for stabilization of the acetabular component. The dysplastic femoral head is trimmed appropriately and anchored to the superior aspect of the true acetabulum. Cancellous bone screws are used to attach the bone graft. Subsequently, the acetabulum is reamed. The true acetabulum serves as the medial pelvic wall while the femoral head functions as a superior bony buttress for the cup.

Pelvic cement holes are prepared, with particular caution while drilling the pubic hole, in view of the proximity of the femoral vessels.

The proximal femur is prepared after assessment of the rotational deformity. In many cases a deformity of up to 90° of anteversion may be present. In such instances a new site on the proximal femur is required for the arthroplastic femoral neck. The site is made by the use of a rongeur and a small femoral rasp is carefully inserted into the medullary cavity (Fig. 14-3 I and J). Special small femoral components with a straight stem are necessary because the maldevelopment of the proximal femur may prevent the insertion of a standard curve stem.

The acetabular component is cemented in place and excess cement is removed. Anterior encroachment of molten cement to the femoral vessels must be avoided. A trial femoral component is inserted and the hip is reduced (Fig. 14-4J). A trial range of motion is undertaken to ensure adequate stability of the implant. The trial prosthesis is removed and the wires for reattachment of the greater trochanter are inserted into the femur. The cement is mixed and introduced into the proximal femur after which the femoral component is inserted. The hip joint is reduced and a trial range of motion is repeated. Provided that the trial is satisfactory, the greater trochanter is reattached with the wires. The position of the greater trochanter can be altered to provide optimal tension in the gluteus medius and minimus. If the rim of bone at the false acetabulum impedes the optimal positioning of the glutei and, thereby the desired distal reattachment of the greater trochanter, the rim can be removed. Suction drainage tubes are inserted into the hip joint and subcutaneous regions respectively. The tensor fascia lata with its extension along the aponeurosis of the gluteus maximus is carefully sutured and the subcutaneous tissue and skin are closed. Prior to location of the prosthetic joint, the hip and knee are flexed about 30 to 50° to avoid tension on the sciatic nerve. Radiographs of a typical painful congenital dislocation of the hip before and after arthroplastic surgery are seen in Figure 14-4 A to C.

In view of the dysplasia of the ipsilateral hemipelvis and proximal femur in patients with congenital dislocation of the hip, several surgical aspects should be emphasized. Adequate mobilization of the proximal femur is essential so that the femur can be shifted to a distal position for insertion of the prosthetic femoral head into the true acetabulum. The distal migration provides excellent correction of the apparent leg length discrepancy. It can be accompanied, however, by traction injuries to the sciatic nerve. Prior to location of the femoral head in the true acetabulum, the hip joint and knee joint should be flexed to at least 30° to lessen the likelihood of nerve palsy. The new acetabulum must be reconstructed in its normal physiological site because it is the only region in the dysplastic hemipelvis where adequate bone stock is potentially available. In view of the pelvic dysplasia, neurovascular injuries especially to the femoral nerve, artery and vein are more likely to occur than during reconstruction of a conventional osteoarthritic hip, especially during the reaming of the acetabulum. Usually, the anterior wall of the acetabulum is the most defective site. No attempt is made to ream the acetabulum to the conventional diameter. Alternatively, smaller sized reamers and smaller acetabular cups are necessary. In view of the lack of thickness of the inner wall of the pelvis, special preparation of the true acetabulum may be necessary. The use of the femoral head as a bone graft was described. Alternatively, a titanium mesh liner may be inserted which has extensions onto the lateral aspect of the pelvis.[41] By the preparation of supplementary drill holes in the lateral pelvis superior to the acetabulum, the metal may be anchored to augment the support of the acetabular component. Occasionally, the cup may have to be inserted in a somewhat more vertical position (less than 45°) although this position compromises the stability of the hip joint. When cement is applied to the acetabulum, caution is necessary so that cement does not flow anterior to the acetabulum with damage to the femoral nerve.

While full correction of the apparent leg length discrepancy is possible, no attempt should be made to correct a true discrepancy of femoral length by the application of a special long neck prosthesis.[15, 37, 38, 42] Excessive correction of the leg length discrepancy may render location of the femoral head and the acetabulum excessively difficult so that fracture of the bone ensues. It is safer to restore leg length by the application of a lift on the shoe.

When a lateral approach is undertaken for the treatment of a degenerative hip secondary to other conditions a few other technical details should be noted. Patients with rheumatoid arthritis or certain other inflammatory diseases are likely to have excessive osteoporosis secondary to long-term steroid therapy and the disease itself.[9] Manipulation of a limb should be performed with extreme care to avoid spiral fracture of the femur. In a patient with severe protrusio acetabuli, posterior capsular release and removal of osteophytes as well as marked adduction of the femur may facilitate dislocation of the femoral head. Alternatively, preliminary osteotomy of the femoral neck may be helpful. The floor of the acetabulum in severe protrusio acetabuli may be thin or defective so that fracture is likely to occur during the reaming procedure. If the acetabular component is inserted into such an acetabulum, late fracture and central migration of the bone is likely to occur. The acetabulum can be reinforced by one of two methods. The femoral head can be shaped to provide a hemispherical plug of bone which fills the cavity. In Figure 14-4 D to F, X-rays reveal the use of such a bone graft in a traumatic protrusio. Alternatively, titanium and stainless steel mesh is available as a reinforcing agent.

Where previous reconstructive procedures have failed, the lateral approach may be helpful from several points of view.[43] After proximal femoral osteotomy, metal removal may be accomplished without difficulty. The bony block in the intramedullary cavity secondary to the osteotomy may be reamed without difficulty. When a rotational deformity is created by the femoral osteotomy, accurate realignment of the femoral component is necessary. Removal of the greater trochanter simplifies this effort.

During the removal of a failed Austin-Moore prosthesis, considerable force may be necessary to loosen the stem. Prostheses with multiple large fenestrations or bony ingrowth can be especially difficult to distract. Bone may be osteotomized from a large proximal fenestration. Removal of the greater trochanter permits the surgeon to apply longitudinal blows with a mallet to the extraction device. Curettage of the fibrous track around a prosthesis is essential so that the methylmethacrylate cement may bond to the underlying cancellous bone. Where a prosthesis is cemented in place, tightly adherent cement may be left in situ rather than risk the fracture of adjacent bone. Conversion of a cup arthroplasty usually is easier than the conversion of a femoral head prosthesis. If such a hip is excessively stiff, osteotomy of the femoral neck should be performed prior to dislocation. Other unusual problems, such as total hip replacement in Paget's disease and failed hip fusion or pseudarthrosis are described elsewhere.[44, 45]

An Anterolateral Approach.[35] Where the surgeon prefers this approach, the patient is placed in the supine position with a small roll measuring about 14 by 4 inches beneath the ipsilateral buttock. The roll serves to accentuate the hip joint structures anteriorly and is removed at the time of acetabular cup insertion. A Watson-Jones incision[31, 35] is used to expose the hip (Fig. 14-5A). The incision starts about 2 inches distal and lateral to the anterosuperior iliac spine and curves slightly distally and posteriorly over the anterolateral aspect of the greater trochanter and lateral surface of the femoral shaft. After the skin and subcutaneous tissues are divided the fascia lata overlying the vastus lateralis is incised distally. The interval between the gluteus medius and tensor fascia lata muscles is identified as in Figure 14-5B. This step is simplified by proceeding proximally from the origin of the vastus lateralis. After the interval is identified, the gluteus medius and other abductors are retracted by a smooth Hohmann retractor placed behind the femoral neck and in front of the greater trochanter.

In obese patients and in others where visualization is difficult, the interval between the insertion of gluteus medius and the origin of vastus lateralis may be partly, or rarely, completely incised (Fig. 14-5C). The anterior attachment of gluteus medius is reflected in a lateral direction. Where visualization is particularly troublesome, excision of the greater trochanter is recommended. A second Hohmann retractor is placed along the medial aspect of the neck and directed toward the lesser trochanter to allow retraction of the tensor fascia lata muscle and exposure of the precapsular fat. The precapsular fat is removed with a periosteal elevator and the third Hohmann retractor, with a broad blade and a sharp point, is placed over the anterior medial rim of the acetabulum to allow full exposure of the hip joint. The capsule is debrided of fat and soft tissue both medially and laterally as far as possible with a periosteal elevator. The capsule of the hip joint is incised to permit exposure of the femoral head and neck. With an oscillating saw the femoral neck is osteotomized at 45° to the long axis and 5° of anteversion (Fig. 14-5D). The cut is made 1 fingerbreadth proximal to the lesser trochanter. Next, the femur is prepared to accept the femoral prosthesis. Temporary retention of the femoral head facilitates exposure of the distal osteotomized surface as the lesser

trochanter rests on the proximal osteotomized surface and displaces the opposing cut surface from the wound (Fig. 14-5E). A few fibers of the abductor musculature, at their insertion, may be divided to improve the exposure. The table may be flexed to shift the legs downward and augment exposure of the proximal femoral shaft. If there is marked contracture of the short external rotator muscles they can be divided at their insertion on the femur.

The leg is properly positioned in adduction and external rotation. A Hohmann retractor is placed beneath the greater trochanter and the proximal femur is supported anteriorly on the proximal femoral neck. Afterward the rasp may be readily inserted into the shaft of the femur. Initial introduction of the rasp is undertaken by hand to lessen the likelihood of penetration of the shaft with the tip of the rasp. The final 1 to 2 cm of penetration can be achieved with a mallet.

Attention now shifts to the acetabulum. A large periosteal elevator is inserted into the acetabulum behind the femoral head to expedite the dislocation. A corkscrew can be inserted into the periphery of the femoral head to facilitate its removal. Subsequently, the Hohmann retractors are repositioned inside the capsule to augment exposure of the acetabulum. Residual cartilage in the acetabulum is removed with a curet. The acetabulum is reamed with graduated reamers positioned at approximately 45° with the long axis of the body and 10° of anteversion (Fig. 14-5F). Where the surgeon desires to undertake substantial medial displacement of the cup, the acetabulum may be enlarged with Smith-Petersen curved gouges. Cement holes are made in the ilium, ischium and pubis as in Figure 14-5G and a trial acetabular component is inserted.

At this time the pillow is removed from beneath the hip prior to insertion of the cement. The methylmethacrylate is mixed to a doughy consistency and packed firmly into the cement holes. The proper cup is inserted into the acetabulum and held until the cement has solidified (Fig. 14-5 H to J). The cup should be placed in a 45° angle to the long axis of the body and 10° of anteversion. Excessive cement is trimmed. A trial femoral component is inserted and the hip is reduced. Selection of a femoral component with the appropriate length of neck permits the surgeon to achieve optimal tension in the abductor muscles. After reduction of the hip, tension should be moderate and the hip should not dislocate throughout a normal range of motion. If dislocation occurs, attention should be directed toward the muscle tension in the neck size, and a search should be made for impingement of the greater trochanter on the pelvis or acetabular component.

After the appropriate femoral component is selected, the shaft of the femur is irrigated with antibiotic solution and a polyethylene catheter is introduced 8 to 10 cm into the shaft of the femur (Fig. 14-5K). The prepared methylmethacrylate is packed vigorously into the femoral shaft allowing air and blood to escape through the polyethylene vent tube. The femoral prosthesis is inserted into the shaft of the femur with slight valgus alignment of the prosthetic stem (Fig. 14-5 L and M). Afterward, the femoral head is reduced and moved through a range of motion. Drainage tubes are inserted and the wound is closed as previously described for other approaches to the hip.

In the presence of moderate to marked protrusio acetabuli, a "spacer" is necessary to fill and strengthen the capacious acetabulum. As mentioned previously either a portion of the femoral head (Fig. 14-5I) or metallic mesh and methylmethacrylate may be used. Exposure of the acetabulum may be greatly facilitated by excision of the greater trochanter. When the femoral head is used as a spacer, it is carefully reamed with a Smith-Petersen cup reamer *prior* to its removal. It can be anchored into the acetabulum with cancellous bone screws, provided that they are deeply countersunk, to permit subsequent reaming of the acetabulum.

Postoperative Care

Numerous hospitals have designed their own elaborate system for the postoperative management of a patient undergoing a total hip replacement. The reader is referred elsewhere for scrutiny of some detailed accounts that may have particular application.[30, 34-36] The brief following discussion provides the main theme of management as observed by the author.

After completion of the surgery, dry dressings are applied to the wound. Elastic stockings may be applied to the extremity to limit venostasis. An abduction splint is applied to the patient to ensure safe transfer to a postoperative bed. X-rays are taken in the postoperative recovery room to ensure location of the arthroplasty. Split Russell's traction is applied to both lower extremities. The early postoperative period when the patient lacks total awareness of his surroundings and the ability to fully co-operate with instructions provides a particular risk for dislocation of the arthroplasty. By the application of traction or the abduction brace, the risk of dislocation is greatly lessened.

On the first postoperative day the patient is encouraged to undertake gentle active flexion of his hip and knee. On the second postoperative day he is stood on a tilt table at physical therapy and encouraged to walk between parallel bars. Gradually the patient progresses to the use of a walker or crutches with a partial weight-bearing gait. Toward the end of the first postoperative week the patient is instructed in a method of transfer from the bed to an erect position that avoids flexion of the hip beyond 60°. Also, he is taught a method to sit on an elevated toilet seat. The elevated segment fits on a standard toilet and is used postoperatively by the patient in his home for the first 6 weeks. Usually he is discharged within 6 to 8 days after surgery, when he is able to transfer and to walk independently with crutches. The patient is discharged home in an ambulance or a comparable vehicle in which excessive hip flexion is avoided. During the first 6 weeks at home he is encouraged to spend most of his time in bed with two pillows between his legs or walking. To sit he assumes semiupright position by the use of pillows or uses an elevated seat. The initial postoperative visit is undertaken 6 weeks after surgery when transfers in a car are first permitted.

As previous studies have shown many adults with arthritis of the hip have considerable frustrations with sexual relationships in view of their hip pain and stiffness.[46] Counseling by the medical team is greatly appreciated. After total hip joint replacement, the patient should be advised to restrain from sexual activities for the first 6 to 8 weeks in view of the considerable risk of dislocation of the prosthetic joint. Subsequently, no limitations are necessary.

Two therapeutic aspects of the postoperative management have remained controversial to the present time. For a full discussion on the role of prophylactic antibiotics after hip arthroplasty, the reader is advised to consult elsewhere.[26, 30, 47-50] The author prefers to employ a cephalosporin by intravenous administration which is first given 2 hours prior to surgery and continued for 5 days after surgery. Afterward, antibiotics are terminated. The high incidence of thromboembolic complications following hip surgery have stimulated numerous studies into the role of prophylactic anticoagulation.[51-56] Therapeutic regimens which employ heparin, coumadin, dextran or aspirin have been widely used. Unfortunately, the more effective the an-

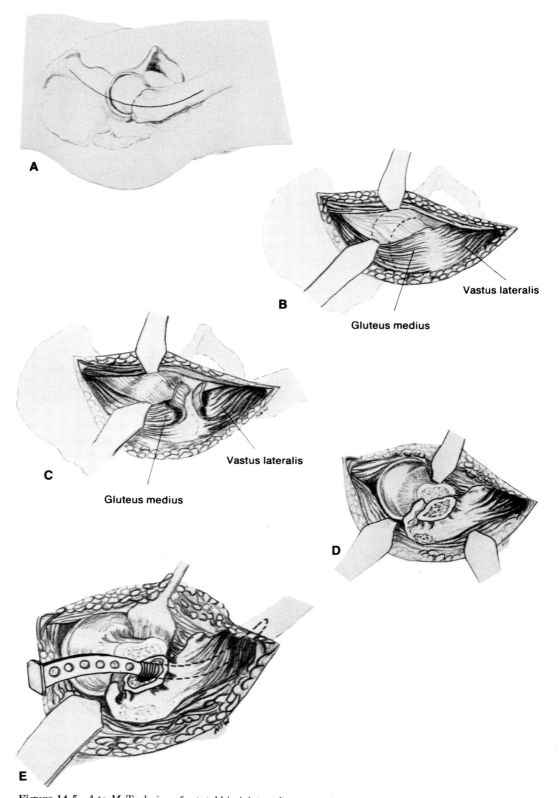

A

B

Vastus lateralis

Gluteus medius

C

Vastus lateralis

Gluteus medius

D

E

Figure 14-5. *A* to *M*. Technique for total hip joint replacement showing the anterolateral approach to the hip.

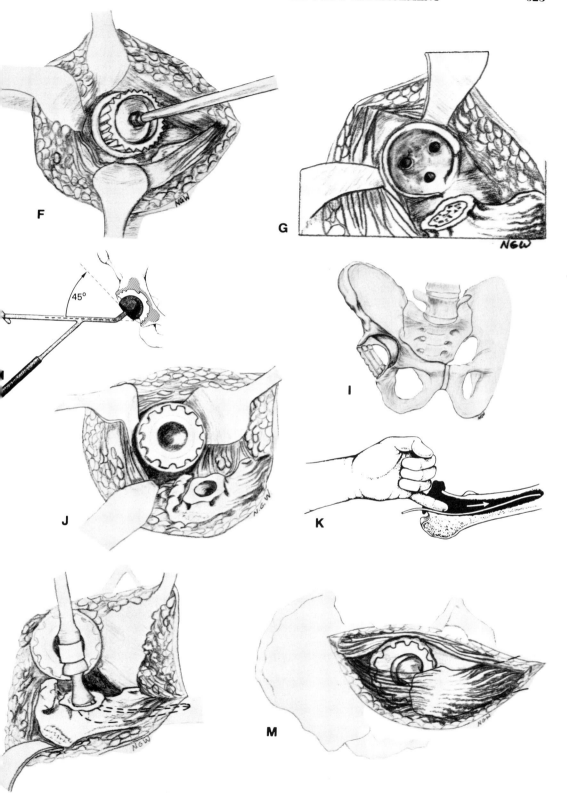

ticoagulant, the greater its tendency to initiate excessive bleeding at the operative site or excessive bleeding tendency elsewhere in the body. Certain patients possess specific contraindications to a program of prophylactic anticoagulation such as those with hypertension above 110 mmHg diastolic blood pressure, active peptic ulcer disease, a previous bleeding tendency or excessive bleeding at the operative site. Other patients with a past history of thromboembolic complications possess a definite indication for prophylactic anticoagulation. It is for the large residual population where controversy remains. For routine prophylactic anticoagulation the author prefers to employ low dose, subcutaneous injections of heparin.[55] The anticoagulant is terminated when the patient is discharged from the hospital.

Most aspects of routine postoperative management have been fully discussed elsewhere.[11, 23, 30, 34–36] One infrequently discussed aspect is after total hip arthroplasty in the patient with congenital dislocation of the hip. Usually, reduction of the prosthetic hip into the site of the anatomical acetabulum is accompanied by significant apparent lengthening of the extremity. After reduction of the hip the limb should be maintained in 30 to 50° of flexion of the hip and knee, to relieve potential longitudinal traction on the sciatic nerve. Particular caution is necessary until the patient is fully aroused from the general anesthetic. Subsequently, the patient is positioned in split Russell's traction with progressive extension of the hip and knee, as tolerated by the patient.

Complications of Total Hip Replacement

Previously Amstutz[57] has usefully classified the principal complications of total hip joint replacement by the time period after surgery when they occur (Table 14-2).

In a somewhat arbitrary way the postoperative period is deemed to extend up to 3 months. The interim period persists for 3 years and the long-term period refers to the time course over 3 years. The major systemic complication, thromboembolic disease, has not been greater for patients with total hip joint replacement than for those who have had other major hip surgery. Nevertheless, the incidence of recognized phlebitis, depending upon the method of diagnosis, ranges between 5% and 15% with an incidence of 2% pulmonary embolus. Useful general accounts of complications after total hip joint replacement are available elsewhere.[28, 58–60] A brief conspectus is now given.

Table 14-2
Complications after Total Hip Joint Replacement

Immediate postoperative period
  Systemic
  Local
    Sepsis
    Dislocation
    Periarticular calcification and/or ossification
    Complications due to trochanteric osteotomy migration.
    nonunion, wire breakage
Interim period
  Sepsis
  Prosthetic loosening
Long-term
  Wear debris accumulation and bearing failure
    Local effects
    Systemic effects
  Sepsis
  Prosthetic loosening

Infection

Following total hip joint replacement, infection has remained a disastrous complication, since the irradication of the infection usually cannot be achieved without removal of the implant. A full discussion on infection after total hip joint replacement is presented in Chapter 13 and is described in detail elsewhere.[61] Usually the diagnosis is recognized by the persistence or recurrence of drainage from the wound or a sinus tract with appropriate bacteriological confirmatory techniques. Alternatively, the patient may present with persistent or recurrent hip pain, whereupon needle aspiration of the hip joint performed with the use of X-ray image intensification may permit confirmation of the diagnosis. Less frequently the patient may present with evidence of systemic upset such as fever, weakness, malaise or with other sites of infection. The last presentation is most frequently encountered in patients with compromised immune mechanisms such as rheumatoid arthritic patients, especially those who are on large doses of systemic steroids or immunosuppressive chemotherapy.

Inevitably the best treatment of sepsis is prevention, which was fully emphasized in the previous chapter. Once an infection is recognized, consideration for immediate debridement of the wound with or without replacement of the implant should be given.

Salvati[62] and others have emphasized that immediate surgical treatment of the infection may permit a way to salvage the arthroplasty whereas a more conservative approach including the application of systemic antibiotics is very likely to fail. Once the patient has persistent drainage from the total hip joint replacement, Charnley prefers to continue conservative management as long as possible. Provided that the patient has minimal pain and no systemic signs of infection, he may continue his activities. In patients with poor medical history or who refuse removal of the implant, this course may be advisable or essential. As the infection persists, however, in many patients the proximal femur and ipsilateral hemipelvis become markedly osteoporotic, often with considerable destruction. Pathological fractures may occur or the implant may erode its way through the bone. A traumatic dislocation of the hip joint is likely to follow a shift in position of the implant.

The conventional procedure for treatment of a chronic infection of a total hip joint replacement is removal of the implant with debridement of the infected or necrotic tissue.[63, 64] Either at the first procedure or as a secondary effort, the hip joint may be converted into a formal Girdlestone arthroplasty whereby the surgeon attempts to prepare two flat congruous surfaces on the femoral neck and the opposing pelvic wall. The excellent results reported by Girdlestone were, for the most part, achieved in aseptic but arthritic hips and by the application of a prolonged course of hospital traction and therapy.[65, 66] The Girdlestone procedure currently employed for the treatment of septic total hip joint replacement differs greatly from the previous attempts, both by the presence of the infection and by the excessively expensive course of hospital management, with therapy needed to undertake a classic Girdlestone procedure. Two modern variations, therefore, are generally employed. After debridement of the hip joint and conversion to the pseudarthrosis, a provisional period of skeletal traction with the use of a tibial traction pin may be undertaken. When the wound shows evidence of satisfactory healing, the patient may be placed in a hip spica cast. Alternatively, many surgeons apply the hip spica cast at the time of the surgical debridement. A window is cut in the cast to permit dressing changes on the wound. Alternatively, closed suction drainage may be coupled with the skeletal traction or with the application of the cast. For the management of late infections with gross obstruction of the proximal femur and/or the opposing pelvis, the application of external fixation (see Chapter 11) may permit the surgeon to achieve a superior alignment of the pseudarthrosis, may simplify the management of the

wound by open or closed suction drainage techniques and may permit early ambulation of the patient.

Where the patient with the failed septic total hip joint replacement possesses normal knees, a normal contralateral hip and lumbosacral spine, consideration for conversion to a fusion of the hip can be given. The author has undertaken the fusion as a 2-stage procedure. First, the hip joint is debrided and a Hoffmann external fixation device is applied from the ipsilateral pelvis to the distal femoral shaft. By adjustments of the device, the proximal femur is displaced into a medial location. When control of the soft tissue infection is achieved, a transverse pelvic osteotomy is performed through the site of the previous acetabulum and the pelvic fragment with the rami is displaced in a distal direction until the osteotomized surface approaches the opposing femoral neck. Autogenous strips of cancellous bone are added to the fusion site. The procedure is elaborated in Chapter 11.

A question remains on the relative merits of permanent pseudarthrosis *versus* a fusion as the optimal treatment for a failed total hip joint replacement. Recently, Hamblin* and Hamblin *et al.*[67] have reported a 12-year follow-up on a series of patients in Glasgow on whom a conversion to pseudarthrosis had been undertaken for their infected total hip joint replacements. These workers report progressive improvement in the function of the pseudarthrosis observed over several years after surgery. Gradually the hip becomes more stable and the patient remains relatively pain-free so that a progressive functional improvement is documented. Nevertheless, further observations on the relative merits of Girdlestone arthroplasty and hip fusion are clearly necessary in the failed total hip.

Loosening

It is the author's impression that many loose implants were probably loose at the time of surgery. Unless the surgeon carefully scrutinizes the interfaces between bone, cement and the implant, he may fail to observe evidence of micromotion. Subsequent loosening of the implant is recognized when the patient presents with a complaint of mechanical hip pain. Loosening also may arise by impingement of the femoral neck or greater trochanter on the acetabular component or the lateral pelvis.[2] It is more likely to arise if the surgeon fails to achieve adequate interdigitation of cement between the available

* D. Hamblin, personal communication, 1977.

surfaces of the implant and the bone.[68, 69] Excessive bleeding at the time of insertion of the implant may preclude satisfactory mechanical interdigitation of cement into the bone in view of an interface of blood. Similarly, the surgeon must achieve adequate distal insertion of cement into the femoral shaft.[70] The application of a polyethylene vent tube and of a cement injector has been described.[2] Loosening appears to be more likely to occur after the use of all metal prostheses in view of the higher frictional torque at the articular surfaces. Loosening also can be observed after traumatic insults to the hip.

Patients with a minor degree of prosthetic loosening initially complain of mechanical hip pain. Loosening of the socket is generally associated with local tenderness over the posterior ilium. Alternatively, loosening of a femoral stem may be associated with a complaint of thigh pain. A variety of clinical tests have been described to confirm the site of the loose component although the author has not found them to be reliable.[68] With a grossly loose implant, a palpable or audible crepitus may be encountered. The gross loosening can be confirmed by image intensification or by arthrography. When the loose component exhibits micromotion, the diagnosis may be confirmed only by operative exposure. Prior to surgical intervention, appropriate diagnostic tests, including needle aspiration to eliminate the possibility of sepsis, should be performed. At surgery, the loose component is removed. For a loose acetabular cup, all of the methylmethacrylate cement should be removed prior to insertion of the replacement. When the femoral stem is loose, metal removal may be followed by the debridement of loose fragments of cement. Excessive enthusiasm for total removal of the cement should be dampened in view of the great risk of penetration or fracture of the bone.

Dislocation

The stability of the total hip arthroplastic reconstruction depends upon; (1) the inherent design of the arthroplastic components; (2) the orientation of the components in the acetabulum and the proximal femur; and (3) the tightness of the capsule and the muscles about the hip joint.[71] The features of design of the components and the orientation of the components have been discussed previously (see also Chapter 13). When the greater trochanter is osteotomized, its reattachment should be achieved while the hip is held in 20 to 30° of abduction so that the abductor muscles are tight. As previously emphasized, great caution is required in the early postoperative period to avoid excessive flexion or rotation of the arthroplastic hip. Minor limitations are maintained for the first 6 weeks after surgery.

If the arthroplastic hip dislocates spontaneously in the early postoperative period, an immediate attempt should be made to achieve a reduction. The dislocated hip is painful from capsular distention and the rapid onset of muscle spasm. For reduction of the hip adequate relaxation of the patient, usually under general anesthesia, is essential. After reduction the patient is maintained in 20 to 30° of abduction with extension of the lower extremities for a period of 1 to 3 weeks. Some surgeons prefer to immobilize the patient in a hip spica cast to permit regeneration of the capsule and tightening of other adjacent soft tissues. Alternatively, an abduction brace or bilateral split Russell's traction with abduction of the hips may be applied. The surgeon should examine carefully postreduction X-rays for evidence of gross errors in orientation of the components. If such an error is detected, consideration for surgical revision should be given as subsequent dislocations are almost inevitable.

Periarticular Calcification and Ossification

The incidence of periarticular ossification following total hip joint replacement approximates that observed after other major hip reconstructive procedures such as cup arthroplasty.[72] Most authors[73-75] have reported an incidence of between 15% and 30%, although Lazansky[76] reported a figure of 8%. The precise etiology and pathogenesis are unclear. Excessive intraoperative bleeding is one possible factor. Excessive stripping of periosteum or osteophytes from the ilium or the proximal femur is another possible cause. Throughout surgery, recurrent irrigation of the wound may facilitate removal of loose bone fragments and debris from the wound. Osseous particles provide another source for nucleation of mineral.

Usually the diagnosis of ectopic bone is made by radiological studies or when a limited range of motion of the arthroplastic hip is observed. In most cases, the myositis ossificans is not painful, and frequently it has surprisingly little influence on the functional result. The treatment, however, of symptomatic ectopic bone has remained unsatisfactory. Parenteral administration of diphosphonates[77] has been studied and some preliminary favorable results with diminished hip pain and increased hip motion have been reported.[78] At the present time, however, their role remains unclear. Surgical excision of the periarticular deposits should be discouraged in view of the high likelihood of recurrence often on an even greater magnitude.

Problems with a Trochanteric Osteotomy. In view of the theoretical inefficiency of reattachment of the greater trochanter by the use of wire loops and the technical problems that many surgeons observe when reattaching the greater trochanter by the use of wire, the complications of trochanteric osteotomy, have been surprisingly uncommon and of minor degree. Nonunion of the greater trochanter was observed in 1.8% of 501 hips by Lazansky,[79] 3.2% of cases by Nicholson[80] and in 2.7% of cases by Charnley.[81] Most of the cases reported by Charnley culminated in spontaneous osseous union. In the other cases remarkably little disability occurs after nonunion and symptoms are generally absent. Painful broken wires were removed by Lazansky in three patients with relief of symptoms. Late asymptomatic wire breakage is seen in about 5% of cases. The technical details for excision of the greater trochanter and its reattachment with wire must be carefully followed to maintain a low rate of nonunion. When the trochanter is osteoporotic or when bony contact after wiring is reduced by distorted anatomy, 2 or 3 weeks of bed rest in abduction may be indicated, rather than the usual 1 to 3 days. A case of fracture and migration of a trochanteric wire into the hip joint, after total hip joint replacement has been reported by Bronson,[82] although such cases of serious failure of trochanteric wires appear to be exceedingly uncommon.

Nevertheless, trochanteric osteotomy does present certain problems which, although minor, may thwart enthusiasm for routine application. The duration of surgery and operative blood loss are both increased. Wound hematomas and trochanteric bursitis after surgery are more common.[83] Mild trochanteric tenderness is more likely to occur if the wires break and penetrate superficial soft tissues. Breakage of the wires is not surprising in view of the cyclic bending moments to which they are exposed and the cold working of the wires, especially at the sites where they are twisted together. Premature breakage of the wire increases the incidence of nonunion or malunion of the greater trochanter.

Charnley[81] has emphasized, that breakage of the wires even in the early postoperative period does not preclude satisfactory active abduction by the patient provided that the fascia lata is carefully repaired by the surgeon. The Y-shaped

abductor mechanism that includes the gluteus maximus for the posterior superior limb, the tensor fascia lata for the anterior superior limb, and the fascia lata for a common distal limb substantially augments hip abduction by the gluteus medius and gluteus minimus.

Other workers have attempted to develop superior methods for reattachment of the greater trochanter. Müller[2] employs supplementary cancellous bone screws. Some attempts have been made to screw the osteotomized trochanter into a threaded receptacle that is welded to the prosthetic femoral stem. To date no alternative method has jeopardized the popularity of reattachment by the use of wire.

Intra-abdominal Complications of Total Hip Replacement*

Several intra-abdominal complications of total hip replacement have been well documented. Although unusual, such complications may be life-threatening so that their prevention and recognition are important in the overall management of the patient who undergoes total hip replacement. These complications are secondary to primary operative events or to unique characteristics of the cement utilized in the procedure. An awareness of such complications should allow the orthopaedist to avoid events which lead to intra-abdominal problems. Paralytic ileus is the most common postoperative intra-abdominal complication of total hip replacement. It occurs as a result of the local operative trauma in the pelvic region and is often aggravated by insufflation or swallowing of air by the patient in the early postoperative period. It has been suggested that heat generated by the cement may account for the ileus. Retroperitoneal hemorrhage and regional trauma, however, will also lead to the development of ileus; since ileus is observed in other hip procedures, it is likely to be of multifactoral origin.

Ileus has been reported in about 1% to 4% of total hip operations. Coventry et al.[84] reported 19 cases of ileus among 2012 total hips and noted the contribution of methylmethacrylate in the peritoneal cavity. Upon clinical recognition of the paralytic ileus, oral alimentation should be terminated until effective peristalsis resumes. Concurrently, intravenous fluids are administered by a conventional regime.[85] Second, in the patient with an ileus, the use of IPPB (intermittent positive pressure breathing) should be avoided because it increases swallowed intestinal

* This section was provided by Daniel H. Brooks.

gas. Alternatively, a nasogastric tube should be employed for decompression of the alimentary tract until peristalsis resumes.

The development of abdominal tenderness and distention, fever and leukocytosis after a total hip replacement may indicate an intestinal perforation. Such a perforation occurs from two possible mechanisms. First, the bowel, usually the cecum, may be perforated when pointed retractors are inserted, when the acetabulum is reamed, or when the acetabular cement holes are drilled. Second, and more commonly, during its insertion, cement may cause herniation through a hole in the acetabulum and contact an adjacent segment of bowel. Since the cement may reach a temperature of 80 to 100°C and protein coagulates at 56°C, any tissue which contacts the solidifying methylmethacrylate may be injured.[86, 87] Immediate perforation of the bowel may occur, or the local heat may create a small area of damage to the wall of the bowel with ischemia, whereupon delayed perforation is noted 36 to 48 hours after the operation.

Intestinal perforation should be considered in any patient who has abdominal tenderness, fever, leukocytosis and an X-ray which shows acetabular perforation with extravasation of cement. Prompt surgical intervention with closure, exteriorization or resection of the perforated segment of bowel and drainage of the abscess, combined with administration of intravenous antibiotics is essential.

A bladder fistula after total hip replacement also has been reported by Lowell.[59, 88] This complication may accompany perforation of the ischium or pubis in the preparation of a cement hole. Immediately prior to his departure to the operating room for total hip joint replacement, a patient should void to decompress his bladder. When a bladder perforation occurs it can be successfully managed by prolonged bladder decompression. Early recognition of the complication facilitates the prevention of a vesicoacetabulo-cutaneous fistula which may lead to infection and failure of the total hip joint replacement.

Intra-abdominal vascular complications probably represent the most life-threatening complication of total hip replacement. Occlusion of the external iliac artery has been reported as a result of extravasation of the cement.[89] Also perforation, hemorrhage and false aneurysm formation of the femoral or internal iliac artery and the common iliac vein have been reported.[89-94] Salama et al.[90] and Mallory[91] reported laceration of the femoral artery and the common iliac vein that accompanied reaming of the acetabulum. Tkaczuk[92] and Kroese[93] reported the late onset of false aneurysm formation of the internal iliac artery. In each case, during the preparation of pelvic cement holes the pelvic wall was wholly breached. Subsequently, during its insertion, the molten cement exuded through the cement hole to contact the vessel. The exothermic solidification of cement provoked thermal injury to adjacent tissues and culminated in deterioration of the arterial wall with hemorrhage or the formation of a false aneurysm. Alternatively, the thermal insult may provoke progressive fibrosis and vascular occlusion. Another, uncommon cause of false aneurysm formation of the internal iliac artery has been reported by Scullin et al.[94] Again, at surgery, cement holes breached the pelvic wall. Subsequently, the total hip joint replacement became infected and the infection tracked through the cement hole to the vicinity of the internal iliac artery. A false aneurysm in the vessel ensued as a result of the infection.

Vascular insult should be obviated if the surgeon exercises appropriate caution during the insertion of pointed (Hohmann) retractors around the pelvic wall and during the reaming process. If a large cement hole breaches the pelvis, subsequent herniation of the molten cement into the true pelvis can be prevented by the partial occlusion of the bony defect with a wire mesh plug. Once a vascular insult is recognized, urgent consultation with vascular surgeons is indicated. The general principles of management have been described by Scullin.[94]

Early recognition of intestinal perforation, bladder perforation or injury to the femoral or iliac vessels is essential so that prompt operative intervention can be performed to minimize the morbidity that otherwise follows these uncommon but serious complications of total hip joint replacement.

Accumulation of Debris and Failure of the Bearing Surfaces

In view of Charnley's initial difficulties when polytetrafluoroethylene was employed as a bearing surface in the early total hip joint replacements, comparable mechanical erosion of high density polyethylene was predictable.[6] Over the past decade the long-term rates of wear of polyethylene have been much lower than most earlier predictions. In most cases where excessive wear transpires, particulate polymethylmethacrylate cement is present as an abrasive agent to greatly accelerate the rate of wear of polyethylene.

Since 1963, Charnley[23] has incorporated a radiographic marker in the plastic socket of his prosthesis. Annual radiographs of patients have been undertaken to enable an estimate on the rate of wear. Considerable variations occur, ranging from a maximum of more than 1 mm in 5 years to nil at 7 years. A number of post mortem specimens have been recovered which permit direct measurement of polyethylene erosion. An average wear figure of about 0.13 mm per year has been documented although the rate appears to decrease after an initial "wearing-in" period. Actually, where no debris of methylmethacrylate is present, the wear rate of polyethylene may be as low as 0.01 mm per year.[1, 7] Many hip cups show no recordable wear after 10 years of service. As Clarke et al.[95] have shown, in view of the remarkable wear resistance displayed by polyethylene, radiographic methods to document the wear rate are unlikely to possess sufficient accuracy to be clinically applicable.

While the particulate and soluble moieties of erosion conceivably may be of some as yet unrecognized systemic importance, the erosion processes occur so slowly that mechanical failure from erosion would be most unlikely. To the present time there has been remarkably little evidence that wear debris from metal on high density polyethylene joints provokes the formation of particulate matter in such a concentration that deleterious biological side-effects occur. This topic is fully reviewed in Chapters 7 and 16. The erosion of metal-on-metal total joint replacements is discussed in Chapter 13.

Breakage of Femoral Stems

The highly significant incidence of mechanical failure of femoral prostheses is reviewed in Chapter 13. It seems likely that an ever increasing incidence of this failure will be reported over the next decade. Prophylactic measures are clearly indicated. The surgeon should use an adequate quantity of methylmethacrylate cement to totally surround the stem distal to its tip. During the insertion of the femoral component, a slight valgus position should be achieved. Where the surgeon elects not to remove the greater trochanter, particular care is necessary during the insertion if a varus malalignment of the stem is to be avoided. Once a fractured femoral stem is recognized, surgical replacement is generally indicated.

Hypersensitivity after Total Hip Joint Replacement

As described in Chapter 13 a few workers[96] have reported cases of cutaneous rashes that follow the insertion of metal-on-metal total hip joint replacements. Other workers[97] have postulated the possible hypersensitivity induced by metal wear particles as a cause for loosening of the implants although confirmation of such a mechanism for loosening remains unconfirmed. For the treatment of cutaneous hypersensitivity or other potentially allergic manifestations secondary to total hip joint replacement the reader is referred elsewhere.[96, 97]

Fractures of Acrylic Cement around the Femoral Stem

Much of the methylmethacrylate employed in orthopaedic surgery is rendered radiopaque by the addition of barium sulfate. When follow-up X-rays after total hip replacement are examined, fractures of acrylic cement related to the stem of the femoral head prosthesis have been observed. Weber and Charnley[98] observed these fractures in 1.5% of the radiographs of 6649 patients. Fracture of the cement was usually evident at the 6-month postoperative review and was sometimes associated with subsidence of the prosthesis. In most cases this radiological complication is devoid of symptoms. A few patients who complain of thigh pain in the first 6 months after surgery may have symptoms related to the cement fracture. Slight subsidence of the femoral prosthesis in the cement bed appears to result in a new position of superior stability. In a few cases where the separation of cement exceeds 4 mm the prognosis for stable positioning is poor but consideration for a diagnosis of chronic deep infection should be given. The mechanical causes producing fracture of cement remain speculative. Perhaps the most likely explanation is inadequate or eccentric introduction of cement at surgery so that the poorly supported stem becomes loose in the cement track. Under load bearing the prosthesis becomes "end bearing" on the distal part of the cement. Whereas the cement usually is exposed to compressive loads which it tolerates well, the distal part of the eccentrically positioned cement is subjected to tensile forces which it resists poorly. Ultimately the distal part fractures and the prosthesis subsides to assume a new, lower position in the tapered cavity. Again, a moderately uniform distribution of compressive load is imposed upon the cement. From the prognostic point, radiographic evidence of subsidence, even when accompanied by mild hip pain in the first 6 months after surgery, is not an indication for surgical revision of the prosthesis.

Radiological Demarcation of Cemented Sockets in Total Hip Replacement

Radiological evidence of demarcation between the cement of a total hip socket and the bone of the acetabulum has been observed by several workers.[99-102] Salvati et al.[100] reported on a subtraction technique of contrast radiography. They stated that the presence of a radiolucent line on a standard X-ray did not confirm the presence of loosening. Bergstrom et al.[101] observed a "radiolucent zone" less than 1 mm thick around some part of the acetabular socket in all 15 cases studied. They concluded that demarcation of nonprogressive nature and appearing in the first 6 months after operation was of no clinical significance. Recently DeLee and Charnley[102] reported on 141 Charnley low-friction arthroplasties followed for an average of 10 years in which 69% showed acetabular demarcation and 9% showed evidence of progressive migration of the socket. Most patients with acetabular demarcation were asymptomatic. Review of the operative report or the X-rays of the patients with acetabular migration generally provides evidence for a technical error which rendered the socket susceptible to migration. While present knowledge does not permit a satisfactory explanation of the radiographic changes in bone adjacent to cemented prostheses, a narrow demineralized demarcation zone without other change does not appear to be detrimental.

The Management of Osseous Fractures Adjacent to Total Hip Joint Replacement

A particularly difficult problem for a fracture surgeon is the management of a femoral fracture adjacent to the femoral stem or central acetabular fracture after total hip joint replacement. The insults may occur by conventional traumatic episodes such as automobile accidents. Alternatively many patients possess residual osteoporosis secondary to prolonged disuse or to other diseases or to medications such as steroids. Once the fracture has occurred the surgeon must review the quality of the bone stock and the relative merits of conservative and operative techniques. When fractures of the proximal femur occur, the fracture is usually observed at the tip of the femoral stem. In many instances satisfactory closed reduction is readily achieved. In the author's experience closed treatment by the use of traction and subsequently a hip spica cast is generally recommended. Usually the femoral shaft heals well with the implant in a satisfactory alignment. Perhaps more remarkably, the bone regenerated at the fracture site frequently provides adequate stabilization of the traumatically loosened implant and adjacent cement. If the implant is loose after the bone has healed, replacement of the implant does not provide a particularly challenging technical exercise. Alternatively if the surgeon elects to undertake open reduction and internal fixation of the fracture considerable technical difficulties may arise. The application of an onlay plate with screws may be exceptionally difficult because of the limited site for insertion of screws which may impinge upon the stem of the femoral component. The application of an intramedullary rod may be impossible unless the implant is replaced by a special model which possesses an exceptionally long femoral stem. If the fracture is comminuted even the insertion of such an implant may be challenging. Central acetabular fractures at the site of an acetabular cup, also, may occur as the result of pure traumatic insults or as pathological fractures in osteoporotic bone. Where there is minimal displacement of the implant, closed treatment with bed rest or the application of a hip spica cast is preferred. Where there is gross displacement of the acetabular component, formidable technical difficulties arise no matter what method the surgeon employs. The foremost problem is the restoration of a stable bony platform into which the acetabular cup can be stabilized. In many instances the reconstruction is simplified if primary conservative treatment is undertaken until union of the acetabular bone has occurred. At that time a grossly displaced acetabular component can be removed. The cavity can be filled by the insertion of bone graft. Alternatively, titanium or stainless steel wire mesh and supplementary methylmethacrylate cement may be used to restore a stable shelf. Where the central acetabulum is grossly displaced union of the bone may be impossible. In these cases surgical reconstruction of the acetabulum is necessary. The patient should be referred to major centers for total hip joint replacement in view of the complexities of the surgery.

Nerve Palsies Complicating Total Hip Joint Replacement

Another uncommon complication of total hip joint replacement is nerve injury. Most of the cases should be preventable. Patterson and

Brown[103] report 13 nerve palsies in 368 cases of which 6 involved the femoral nerve, 5 the peroneal nerve, 1 the sciatic nerve and 1 lateral femoral cutaneous nerve. The mechanisms of injury included hematomas secondary to anticoagulation, excessive retraction at surgery and scar formation around the lateral femoral cutaneous nerve. The peroneal injuries were secondary to misapplication of cutaneous traction or to abduction splints. Delayed sciatic nerve injuries secondary to heat necrosis from acrylic cement have also been reported. Virtually all of these injuries should be preventable by careful surgery and postoperative management. Peroneal nerve palsies may follow excessive intraoperative pressure on the nerve at the proximal fibula. Alternatively improper application of a hip abduction brace so that it provokes excessive pressure at the same site is another readily preventable complication. Once foot drop secondary to sciatic or peroneal nerve palsy is recognized the foot should be supported in a neutral position of the ankle until the motor imbalance resolves.

The Management of General Medical Problems that Accompany Total Hip Joint Replacement

In common with other major surgical procedures, numerous problems with potential complications may arise. There are many excellent reviews available which provide detailed discussions to which the interested reader is referred.[85, 104, 105] A few general problems with particular relevance to total hip surgery are reviewed briefly.

Intraoperative hemorrhage is a problem primarily for complicated cases, such as secondary reconstructive hip surgery or arthroplasty for congenital dislocation of the hip. For routine total hip replacement through a posterior approach we find that one or two units of blood are adequate transfusion. Frequently no replacement of red cells are necessary during the surgical procedure but they become necessary within a few days after surgery. For such cases, self-transfusion is ideal. During the 3-week period prior to surgery the patient donates one unit of blood on two occasions. The blood is frozen and stored for subsequent use. Alternatively, other centers employ hypotensive anesthesia as a technique to achieve decreased blood loss and thereby a decrease in the demand for blood replacement.[106, 107]

Where evidence of substantial early postoperative hemorrhage continues, consideration of the possibility of intraoperative damage of a major blood vessel around the hip should be given. In such cases, in addition to blood replacement, confirmation with arteriography and the need for surgical intervention may arise.

The problem of postoperative retention of urine secondary to obstructive problems such as benign prostatic hypertrophy was mentioned previously. The principal method of management should be prevention by appropriate clinical evaluation prior to hip surgery. Once total hip replacement has been performed, subsequent urogenital procedures such as urinary catheterization should be performed under optimal sterile conditions and under antibiotic coverage to prevent the likelihood of bacteriological "seeding" of urinary tract contaminants that otherwise might spread *via* the blood stream to the arthroplastic hip.

Postoperative prophylactic anticoagulation to prevent thrombophlebitis and pulmonary embolus was discussed previously. Certainly all patients with a predilection for thromboembolic disease should receive some sort of prophylactic anticoagulation such as low dose subcutaneous injections of heparin or oral anticoagulants such as Plaquenil (hydroxychloroquine sulfate).[108]

The Treatment of Pulmonary Embolus. Once the diagnosis of pulmonary embolus has been made by clinical assessment, chest X-rays, electrocardiograms or by lung scanning techniques, urgent medical management is essential, as other workers have outlined.[108-111] As a general rule, large continuous doses of intravenous heparin are recommended. Ideally the heparin is infused by a continuous pump so that the concentration of the agent in the peripheral blood shows minimal variation. Between 50,000 and 100,000 units of heparin can be given during the first 24 hours. Over the second 24 hours the dose must be diminished or excessive bleeding becomes extremely likely. Usually the dose can be stabilized at about 40,000 units per 24-hour period. The most hazardous period for recurrent embolus occurs when the patient is switched from intravenous to oral medications such as Coumadin. Usually oral anticoagulation is recommended for several months after surgery.

Occasionally patients have recurrent embolus despite the administration of otherwise adequate doses of anticoagulant. In this situation the insertion of a partial occluding device or "umbrella" into the inferior vena cava through a peripheral vein and the use of image intensification is recommended. Alternatively, if facilities are not available for the application of this technique, a partial occluding device can be applied to the inferior vena cava through an open surgical approach. The details of these procedures are described elsewhere.[110, 111]

Fat Embolism, Methylmethacrylate and Monomeric Toxicity following Total Hip Replacement. During the insertion of the femoral component in total hip replacement, intravascular dissemination of fat and marrow emboli have been documented by several workers.[112–114] Similarly, Dandy[115] reported four fatal fat embolic complications following methylmethacrylate stabilized prosthetic femoral head replacements for intracapsular hip fractures. In all of these patients a precipitous drop in blood pressure was documented during the operative procedure. Admittedly, the hypotension and pulmonary damage could have been provoked by a concurrent absorption in the lung of volatile monomer from the solidifying methylmethacrylate.[116] Salvati* has documented widespread dissemination of fat in the femoral vein during high pressure injection of methylmethacrylate into the femoral intramedullary cavity. The medullary pressure during the injection procedure is greatly diminished if a polyethylene vent tube is introduced prior to the insertion of cement. At the time of insertion of cement, the anesthesiologist should be alerted so that he may examine the patient for a clinical picture of tachypnea, hypoxemia, cyanosis and dimished $PaCO_2$, features of a physiological alveolar block consistent with fat emboli or pulmonary toxicity provoked by monomer. Both insults may cause pulmonary parenchymal damage with resultant interstitial fluid accumulation and a diffusion defect. Monomeric toxicity is heralded by a precipitous drop in blood pressure which the anesthesiologist should recognize immediately and treat with increased oxygen by inhalation. A concomitant drop in blood pressure is treated by appropriate adjustments in the intravenous fluids.

Fat embolism has been documented in the early postoperative period by Spengler *et al.*[117] After the patient became hypotensive and hypoxic these workers confirmed the diagnosis by the use of a xenon ventilation lung scan and the findings of a transient thrombocytopenia. Admittedly other factors such as pulmonary parenchymal damage resulting from blood transfusions could have contributed to the patient's condition although this seems unlikely. The patient responded to treatment with supplemental oxygen by mask and large doses of intravenous corticosteroids (1.5 g/24 hr).

* E. A. Salvati, personal communication, 1977.

In view of the increasing application of injection apparatus to ensure adequate penetration of methylmethacrylate around the femoral component, it seems likely that many more cases of fat embolus will be reported in the future. Orthopaedic surgeons and their anesthesiologists should be aware of this possibility as well as acute hypotension and pulmonary damage from volatile monomer in the solidifying cement. The volatile moieties can be largely eliminated by working the molten cement manually to increase superficial evaporation. Also the molten cement should not be introduced into bone until it "transforms" in the advanced state of solidiiication.[118] The "transformation" is evident when the cement shows greater cohesive properties than adhesive properties so that it tends to stick to itself rather than to the surgeon's gloves or to other foreign surfaces. Unless the cement is housed within a confined injection apparatus, the "transformation" point heralds the first moment that the surgeon can readily handle the cement.

TOTAL KNEE JOINT REPLACEMENT

A discussion of total knee joint replacement is necessarily much more involved than that of total hip joint replacement in view of the multiple joints which comprise the knee and of the varying degrees of stability that must be restored at the time of surgery. Total knee joint replacement is, therefore, a whole series of operations which have been designed for particular clinical problems around the knee. Unfortunately none of them is as satisfactory as total hip joint replacement. In view of their current limitations, numerous attempts are underway in an attempt to improve the arthroplastic procedures. The present discussion describes the use of a variety of implants that have been widely employed but which, no doubt, will be superceded in the near future. The description of the various surgical procedures is meant as a general guideline rather than a specific recommendation for the use of the articular implants mentioned in the present account.

The biomechanics of the knee joint is fully described in Chapter 13 and elsewherre.[119–121] The surgeon requires detailed knowledge of the function of the anatomical knee joint if his reconstructive procedures are to be selected appropriately. A series of reconstruction problems are described which start with the simplest problems and progress to the most difficult. The procedures are divided by the site and number of compartments of the knee joint that are involved in the arthritic process and upon the degree of residual stability of the knee at the time of surgery.

The reader should recognize that in the present state of the art, total knee joint replacement has considerable shortcomings. Other types of nonoperative management and surgical procedures such as proximal tibial valgus osteotomy,[122] MacIntosh plates[123, 124] for tibial arthroplasty and arthrodesis[125] continue to possess substantial therapeutic roles. A combination of quadriceps exercises, simple analgesics and diminution in activity may enable many patients to defer or avoid surgical reconstruction. Tibial osteotomy as a treatment for medial compartment arthritis provides a wholly biological solution which enables many patients to return to vigorous activity, a goal which is rarely achieved after arthroplastic procedures are performed on the knee. Similarly, for patients with severe triple compartment arthritis, arthrodesis may provide a realistic solution which enables a young man to return indefinitely to heavy laboring when he would fail to do so after total knee replacement. After a severe chronic intra-articular infection or in the presence of neuropathic, unstable joints, arthroplasty should not be performed. Either nonoperative treatment with external bracing or, arthrodesis should be undertaken.[126, 127] In the presence of a neuropathic joint, the surgeon should be aware of the high incidence of failure of all surgical procedures, including arthrodesis, and of the morbidity associated with operative intervention.

The Management of Unicompartmental Arthritis of the Femorotibial Articulation

Where the medial or lateral compartments of the knee joint show severe arthritic change secondary to traumatic or other secondary arthritides, a resurfacing procedure may be undertaken by the application of one of several implants which include: the Gunston or polycentric; the unicondylar system[128]; the Marmor modular system[129]; the Buchholz SLED system[130] and the Charnley system. The author's experience has been primarily with the Marmor modular system.[131] The prerequisites for the application of these components is a patient who shows good bone stock and muscle strength with normal ligaments and less than a 10° angular deformity of the knee joint with a near normal range of motion. Perhaps the ideal application is a patient who has traumatic arthritis secondary to a displaced fracture of a tibial plateau

usually in the lateral compartment. Where a patient presents with painful degenerative arthritis of the medial compartment, the author prefers proximal tibial valgus osteotomy to an arthroplastic procedure. The realigning procedure shifts the primary weight-bearing forces from the medial to the lateral compartment. As other workers have documented, excellent results may be obtained whereby the patient possesses a knee with the normal biological attributes and frequently has an ability to resume all employments including heavy manual labor.[122] The procedure also has merit where the medial compartment and the patellar-femoral articulation are compromised by degenerative arthritis. Despite the recommendations of a few workers, the treatment of lateral compartment arthritis by tibial osteotomy to shift weight-bearing forces to the medial compartment has not been generally satisfactory. In these instances the arthroplastic procedures appear to be the optimal form of treatment. A few workers still prefer to use a hemiarthroplasty such as the MacIntosh plate.[123, 124]

Prior to the introduction of any therapeutic measure, careful documentation of the symptomatic, anatomical and functional status of the knee is essential. The documentation helps to clarify the optimal modality of treatment. Subsequently, serial documentations enable the surgeon to ascertain the results of treatment and the possible need for changes in management. Table 14-3 presents a modified version of the Larson evaluation scheme. Of the numerous methods available, this system appears to be a reasonable compromise between an unwieldy detailed tabulation and a deficient evaluation. The Larson knee score is based on a 100 point system which allows 40 points for function, 40 points for pain, 10 points for anatomy and 10 points for range of motion.

Operative Technique for the Marmor Unicompartmental Arthroplasty of the Knee

The operative technique devised by Marmor[131] differs slightly for reconstruction of the lateral or medial compartments. A tourniquet is applied to the thigh and exsanguination is achieved by elevation or the use of an Esmarch's bandage. The extremity is draped and prepared in the conventional fashion. For reconstruction of the lateral compartment a lateral parapatellar incision is made of about 5 inches in length and 2 fingerbreadths lateral to the patellar border to expose the lateral compartment (Fig. 14-6A).

Table 14-3
Modified Larson Knee Score[a],[135]

Function (40 points)		Anatomy (10 points)	
Limp		Genu valgum or varum	
None	12	0–10	4
Slight	8	10–25	2
Moderate	6	over 25	0
Severe	2	Recurvatum	
Unable to walk	0	None	1
Support		Over 5	0
None	12	Flexion contracture	
Cane, long walks	8	None	1
Cane, full time	6	Over 10	0
Crutch	4	Patellar abnormality	
2 canes	2	None	1
2 crutches	1	Lateral position	0
Unable to walk	0	High riding	0
Distance walked		Increased mobility	0
Unlimited	12	Swelling	
6 blocks	8	None	3
2–3 blocks	6	Slight or occasional	2
Indoors only	2	Moderate or frequent	1
Bed and chair	0	Marked or persistent	0
Stairs		Pain (40 points)	
Normally	4	None	40
Normally with banister	2	Slight	35
Any method	1	Mild	25
Not able	0	Moderate	20
Range of motion (10 points)		Severe	10
0 to 45		Disabled	0
Deduct 1 for each 10 of loss. Max. 5 points		Subtotal	
45 to 90		Function	_____
Deduct 1 for each 15 of loss. Max. 3 points		Range of motion	_____
90 to 130		Anatomy	_____
Deduct 1 for each 20 of loss. Max. 2 points		Pain	_____
		Total rating	_____

[a] From D. B. Kettlekamp and M. S. Thompson.[132]

The knee joint is examined (Fig. 14-6B) to ensure adequate visibility of the opposing articular surfaces. If the entire tibial plateau cannot be visualized the distal ¼ inch of femoral condyle is osteotomized to achieve the exposure (Fig. 14-6 C and D). The tibial template is inserted and placed on the top of the tibial plateau. If the plateau possesses substantial irregularities secondary to the arthritic process the surface may be flattened by the application of an osteotome. The template is coated with methylene blue and inserted onto the tibial plateau to delineate an outline for the tibial component (Fig. 14-6E). With an air drill, bone is removed from inside the outline to a depth of 2 mm (Fig. 14-6F). The smallest tibial component, 6 mm in thickness, is impacted into place (Fig. 14-6G). Minor revisions in the depression may be necessary until satisfactory fit is achieved. At this time no attempt is made to determine the proper thickness of the tibial component. The knee is extended and the site where the anterior edge of the tibial plateau impinges upon the femoral condyle is marked with methylene blue as an indication of the anterior edge of the femoral component. The knee is flexed to 90° and a trial femoral template is selected (Fig. 14-6H). The template is screwed into the femoral driver and impacted into the femoral condyle that is congruent with the normal joint surface. The anterior edge of the femoral template coincides with the methylene blue line that was drawn previously in the femoral condyle. After the impaction a ⅜-inch drill hole is prepared in the bone at the appropriate site in the template to a depth of 1 to 1½ inches. The hole will accept the stem of the femoral component. Methylene blue is used to outline the slot in the template and the outer border of the entire template (Fig. 14-6*I*). The femoral template is removed and the air drill is used to cut a slot in the femoral condyle for acceptance of the fin of the femoral condylar component (Fig. 14-6*J*). A series of shallow cement anchoring holes are made in the cortical bone within the perimeter of the femoral template. A femoral trial component of appropriate size is selected and impacted into the condyle. A tibial plateau prosthesis of correct height is inserted and the knee is tested for range of motion and stability. In the presence of varus or valgus deformity either the depression in the tibial plateau can be deepened or the thickness of the tibial component can be altered by the selection of another implant. Excessive deepening is undesirable because of the osteoporotic nature of the bone deep to the subchondral plate which provides unsatisfactory support for the implant. When satisfactory realignment of the joint is realized, the trial components are removed and the joint is irrigated with antibiotic solution. Afterward the joint is dried and methylmethacrylate cement is mixed. Drill holes are prepared in the tibial depression to accept the cement. The cement is packed into the depressions and is applied as a coating on the underside of the implants. The implants are inserted and carefully seated in the proper position as in Figure 14-6 *K* and *L*. The tibial plateau should be horizontal when the knee is fully extended. Excessive cement is carefully removed. This is a critical stage in the procedure and particularly difficult to satisfactorily achieve in the posterior portion of the compartment.

When the cement has solidified, the joint is explored and excessive cement or free fragments of bone and cement are removed. A trial range of motion and a check for stability are repeated. Subsequently the wound is closed in layers with interrupted 0 polyglactin 910 sutures for the capsule, 3-0 polyglactin 910 for the subcutaneous tissue and 3-0 nylon, Prolene (polypropylene) or Vycril (polyglactin 910, Ethicon) for the skin. The use of closed suction drainage for the first 48 hours is helpful. A large compression dressing with a posterior splint is applied.

The operative technique for the insertion of a rival system, the unicondylar knee prothesis, is shown in Figure 14-7 *A* to *F*. The diagrams highlight the relationships of the implants to bony landmarks and ligaments.

Physical therapy is initiated on the day after unicompartmental arthroplasty. In fact the patient should be taught quadriceps exercises prior to the surgical procedure so that he compre- hends the technique from the first postoperative day. Satisfactory restitution of quadriceps strength is essential if a good result is to be achieved. Two days after surgery the posterior splint is removed and active range of motion exercises are encouraged. On the postoperative day the patient is stood out of bed, and on the following day he initiates walking training with the use of crutches or a walking aid. Partial weight-bearing gait is advised for 6 weeks after which the patient uses a cane for a supplementary period of 6 weeks. An attempt is made to regain 90° of active flexion within the first postoperative week. If the patient fails to achieve greater than 60° of flexion a manipulation of the knee under general anesthesia should be considered. The one contraindication for rapid restitution of knee motion is the presence of compromised skin. Especially in rheumatoid patients with cutaneous vasculitis or in those who have had chronic administration of large doses of systemic steroids, mobilization of the arthroplastic knee joint should be delayed until the skin has healed. Otherwise breakdown of the partly healed skin with dehiscence and infection of the wound are likely to occur.

The implants designed for unicompartmental application can, of course, be used for bicompartmental reconstruction of a knee. The author discourages this technique because the surgeon is presented with the difficulty of satisfactory alignment of the medial compartment with the lateral compartment as well as the other considerable difficulties of alignment of both knee components with the tibia and the femur and the patella. At least the former problem is obviated if a bicompartmental prosthesis is employed.

Bicompartmental Reconstruction in the Stable Knee

Where the patient presents with bicompartmental arthritis a variety of appropriate implants can be employed.[133, 134] The arthroplasties attempt to restore the anatomical motion of the knee, including rotation, although admittedly in a somewhat simplistic fashion.[120] The features of the implants are described in Chapter 13. Reconstruction with a UCI (University of California at Irvine) Wright Manufacturing Co., Memphis, Tenn., knee replacement is presented as a representative example.[134, 135] With the use of such implants angular and flexion deformities of up to 15 to 20° can be corrected. Prerequisites for their use, however, include satisfactory bone stock, muscle tone and ligamentous stability.

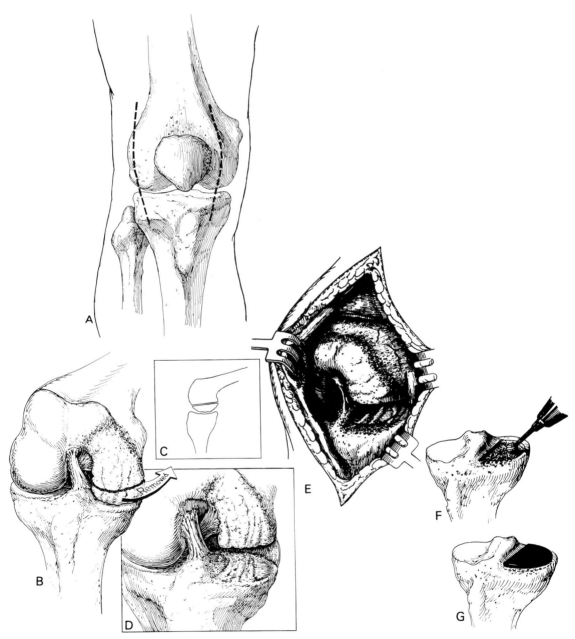

Figure 14-6. *A* to *L*. Technique for the Marmor unicompartmental knee arthroplasty. (Reproduced with permission of L. Marmor and The Richards Manufacturing Co.)

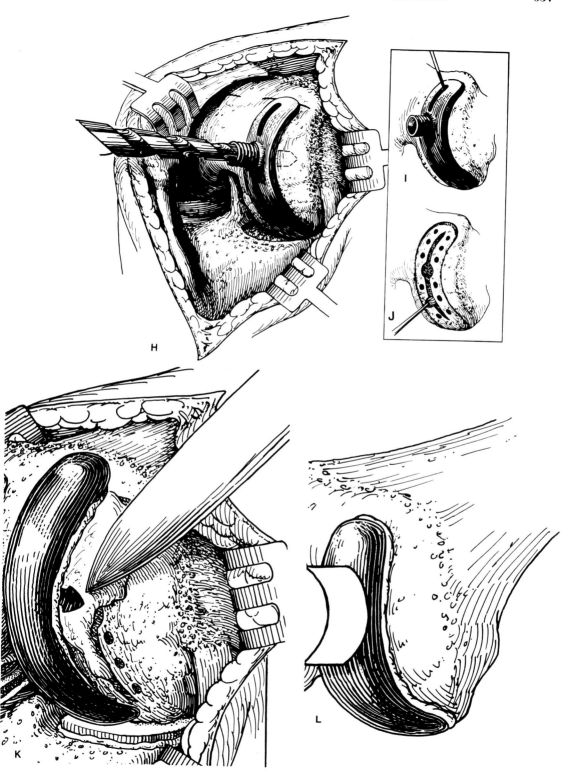

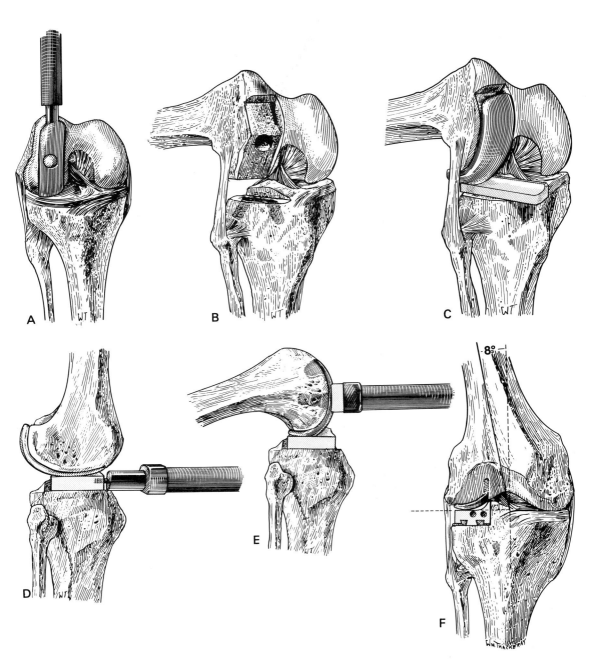

Figure 14-7. *A* to *F*. Technique for insertion of the unicondylar knee prosthesis for lateral compartment arthritis. A lateral parapatellar incision is made as shown in Figure 14-6*A*. The articular surfaces are exposed and the position of the femoral component is marked on the femoral condyle with the femoral jig (Fig. 14-7*A*). A fixation hole is drilled through the femoral jig. With an oscillating blade the femoral condyle is decorticated and the posterior portion of the condyle is removed (Fig. 14-7*B*). In a similar way part of the tibial plateau is excised to provide a surface transverse to the long axis of the tibia. The residual portion of meniscus is removed and cement holes of 1 cm in diameter and 2 cm in depth are prepared in the tibial plateau (Fig. 14-7*B*). Tibial and femoral trial prostheses are inserted (Fig. 14-7*C*) and a trial reduction is made. The knee should show 0 to 135° of stable motion with good alignment. With the tibial trial prosthesis (Fig. 14-7*D*), the correct thickness of tibial plateau is selected. Cement is applied to the tibial plateau and the tibial prosthesis is positioned with a tibial jig. Excessive cement is removed. The femoral trial prosthesis is inserted and the knee is extended until the cement solidifies. The knee is flexed to 100° and the femoral component is cemented with the use of a femoral pusher (Fig. 14-7*E*). Excessive cement is removed. The final alignment of the components is shown in Figure 14-7*F*. The components are aligned in the sagittal plane of the knee joint and the physiological 8° of valgus of the distal femur is maintained. (Fig. 14-7 *A* to *F*, reproduced with permission of Codman and Shurtleff, Inc., Randolph, Mass.)

Operative Procedure. A pneumatic tourniquet is applied to the thigh and the limb is exsanguinated. Prophylactic antibiotics are usually employed as described under total hip joint replacement. A long curved medial parapatellar incision is made which extends from the quadriceps tendon to the anterior tibial tubercle (Fig. 14-8*A*). Abrupt angulations along the incision are potentially disastrous, especially in rheumatoid patients who have cutaneous vasculitis, and may precipitate necrosis of skin superficial to the patella with a great likelihood for deep infection. Gentle retraction of the skin is essential for the same reason. An incision is made in the quadriceps tendon with a border of ½ inch of tendon attached to the vastus medialis (Fig. 14-8*B*). This incision is continued distally through the medial parapatellar retinaculum to the insertion of the patellar tendon. The superior, medial portion of the insertion of the patellar tendon may be incised to assist in the reflection of the patella. The patella is inverted and reflected in a lateral direction to expose the femoral condyles and tibial plateaus (Fig. 14-8*C*). The knee joint is explored to reveal the extent of synovitis and the condition of the cruciate ligaments. Synovectomy, particularly in the rheumatoid knee may be indicated. The anterior portions of the menisci are sharply excised. The more posterior portions can be removed subsequently when their visualization is improved by excision of bone. With the use of the femoral and tibial jigs and a power oscillating saw the femoral condyles and tibial plateaus are trimmed to receive the implants (Fig. 14-8*D*). The tibial plateaus are trimmed with the knee positioned in extension. Great care is necessary to ensure that the tibial cut is parallel to the horizontal in the anteroposterior and mediolateral planes. A total thickness of 1.7 cm of proximal tibial and distal femur is excised. If the knee shows a varus deformity with a lax medial collateral ligament the assistant distracts the leg prior to the excisional osteotomy to ensure correct orientation of the cuts. If the knee shows a flexion deformity, the excisional osteotomy of the distal femur is still performed transverse to the long axis of the bone. The knee is flexed to 90° for excisional osteotomy of the posterior femoral condyles (Fig. 14-8*E*). Even in the moderately deformed knee, 1.7 cm of bone is excised from the combined osteotomies of the tibial plateaus and the posterior femoral condyles. The "corner" of the bone on the distal femur between the posterior and the distal osteotomies is trimmed to an angle of 45° with respect to the posterior and the distal cuts. The first femoral aligning template assists in the preparation of the posterior osteotomy. The second femoral template is impacted into the distal femur as in Figure 14-8*F*. The template possesses a slot to delineate the site for slots that receive the fins of the prosthesis (Fig. 14-8*F*). The slots are cut with an air drill or an oscillating saw. With a curet, cement holes are prepared in the proximal tibia (Fig. 14-8*F*). Trial prosthesis are inserted and the knee is examined in extension, flexion, and through its arc of motion to ascertain the stability, axis of rotation of motion and the absolute range of motion of the knee. Adjustments should be undertaken as necessary.

Where a tibial plateau shows substantial erosion a special component may be employed to supplement the reconstruction. Minimal excessive bone stock should be removed from the cancellous portion of the tibial plateau, however, to lessen the likelihood of late settling of the tibial component. Once the subchondral bone on the proximal tibia is breached the underlying cancellous bone provides much less support.

The wound is irrigated to remove fragments of bone and other debris. Cement is mixed and inserted into the femoral slots. A small amount of cement is placed on the fins of the femoral component. The implant is carefully aligned and inserted with the use of an impactor and a mallet. During its solidification excessive cement is removed. Particular care is necessary to remove extraneous cement from the posterior portions of the knee. A second batch of cement is mixed and impacted into the appropriate depressions of the tibial plateau. Supplementary cement is applied to the tibial plateau and to the deep surface of the implant. The implant is carefully aligned and impacted with the knee joint held in full extension during the solidification process. Figure 14-8*G* reveals the implant after insertion. Again rigorous attention is necessary to ensure removal of all excessive cement.

The joint is irrigated and a large suction drainage tube is inserted. As previously described the wound is closed in layers and a compression dressing with a posterior splint is added. The postoperative exercise program is similar to that previously described for unicompartmental arthroplasties.

Two technical complications of bicompartmental arthroplasty are fracture of the central portion of the distal femur or of the tibial plateau with the attachments of the cruciate ligaments. The fragments can be reattached prior to insertion of the implants by the use of cancellous lag screws. In other cases after the insertion of the trial tibial and femoral components, impingement of the medial eminence of the tibia on the

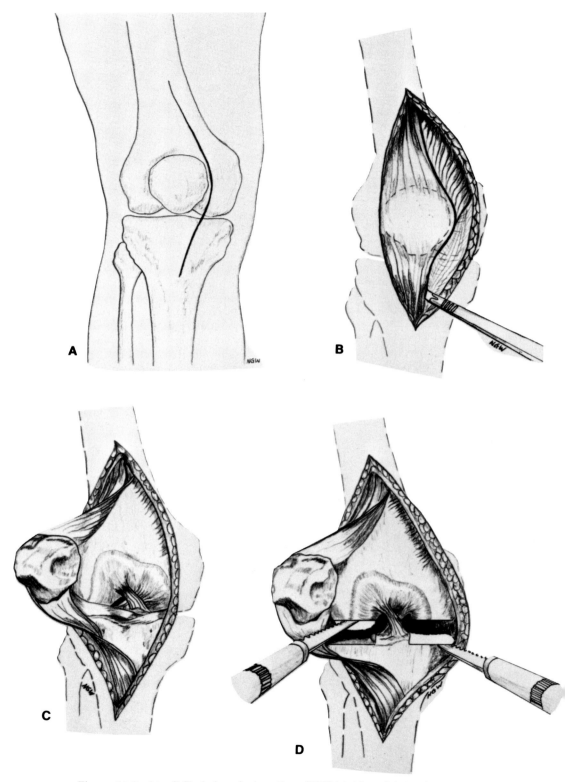

Figure 14-8. *A* to *G.* Technique for insertion of UCI total knee joint replacement.

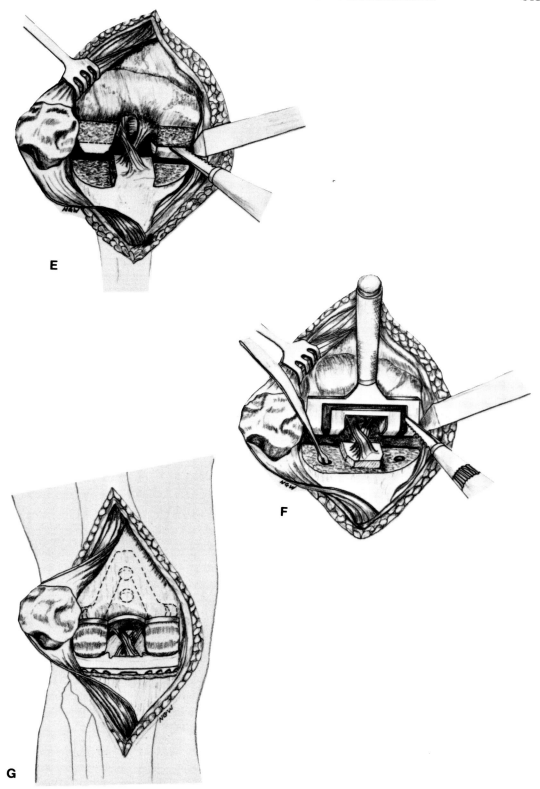

E

F

G

distal femur is noted. The eminence should be trimmed with a rongeur until the impingement is eliminated.

Other patients with bicompartmental disease show more marked flexion, angular and rotational deformities with loss of bone substance and attenuation of ligaments particularly the anterior cruciate ligaments. Patients with rheumatoid arthritis are particularly likely to present with these formidable reconstructive problems. Osteoporosis of bone is usually substantial so that settling of the implants is likely. Angular deformities of at least 40° of varus or valgus, and 60% of flexion are not uncommon. The surgical team should possess considerable experience with simpler arthroplastic reconstructions before they attempt to solve such problems. A variety of implants, described in Chapter 13 and elsewhere,[136-142] has been employed by different surgeons. A representative example, the Freeman-Swanson prosthesis,[141] is described which deliberately sacrifices the cruciate ligaments so that enhanced surface areas of contact between the implants and the underlying bone are possible. Freeman, Swanson *et al.*[142] report full correction of flexion deformities up to 90° and varus-valgus deformities up to 45°.

ICLH (Imperial College London Hospital) Arthroplasty of the Knee*

The Principles

In this operation approximately 1 cm of bone is resected from the distal end of the femur and the proximal end of the tibia. The bones are then resurfaced so as to provide movement and stability regardless of the initial deformity.

For the arthroplasty to be successful: (1) The distal end of the femur and the proximal end of the tibia must be cut in such a way that the prosthesis is horizontal and that the hip, knee and ankle lie in the same straight line; (2) the prosthesis must be inserted in such a way that the soft tissues are *tense* in the extended knee and only slightly lax in the flexed knee; and (3) the patella must lie in the midline of the knee throughout the range of movement.

The Instruments

Four straight cuts are made in the bones (three in the femur and one in the tibia). Each must be correctly placed. To ensure that this can be carried out in a repeatable fashion, three special instruments, the guide, spacer and tenser, are available.

The guide is used to determine the positions of those bone sections made in the flexed knee (*i.e.*, those in the posterior femur and proximal tibia) (Fig. 14-9*A*). The tenser is used to determine the position of section of the distal femur, to correct the varus/valgus alignment, and to regulate the tension in the soft tissues in the extended knee (Fig. 14-9*B*). The spacer is used in both the flexed (Fig. 14-9*A*) and the extended (Fig. 14-9*B*) knee to check that the bones have been correctly sectioned, that the appropriate soft tissue tension has been achieved, and that the knee has been correctly aligned. Additional instruments, including phantom prostheses, are used to implant the prosthesis.

The Stages of the Procedure

The arthroplasty is carried out in four stages: (1) Exposure; (2) tibiofemoral reconstruction: (a) soft tissue release and bone section at 90° flexion; (b) soft tissue release and bone section in full extension; (c) preparation of the bones to fit the prosthesis; (d) implantation of the prosthesis; (3) patellofemoral reconstruction: (a) soft tissue release; (b) preparation of the patella; (c) implantation of the prosthesis; (4) closure.

Pre-Operative Preparation

Under general anesthesia the patient is placed supine on a standard operating table and toweled so that the knee and tibia are visible. The skin is protected by a Steri-drape. When the limb is toweled, it is exsanguinated.

Operative Technique

Exposure. A straight midline incision is made, extending upward onto the thigh and downward onto the shin for a sufficient distance to ensure that when the knee is flexed the skin edges are not under tension. The incision is deepened to the quadriceps muscle, the patella, the ligamentum patellae and the tibia. The fascia covering the patella and the ligamentum patellae is dissected medially from the extensor mechanism. The incision is deepened through the medial patellar retinaculum and the rectus femoris tendon to expose the proximal tibia and the distal femur. A leash of vessels deep to the patellar retinaculum at the level of the ligamentum patellae requires coagulation.

The medial patellar retinaculum is elevated subperiosteally from the anteromedial aspect of the medial tibial condyle. Similarly, the retropatellar fat pad and the lateral patellar retinaculum are elevated in the midline and laterally.

* This section was provided by M. A. R. Freeman.

The patella is then dislocated laterally and the knee flexed, any anterior tibiofemoral adhesions being divided in the process. The operation is facilitated if a bandage is looped around the thigh at this stage so that an assistant can hold the knee in a flexed position.

Tibiofemoral Reconstruction. *Soft Tissue Release and Bone Section at 90° Flexion (Fig. 14-9A).* The soft tissues (including the cruciate ligaments) and marginal osteophytes in the intercondylar notch are removed so as to define its true margin. The supracondylar cortex of the femur is exposed.

A channel is cut in the midline of the anterior projection of the femoral condyles for the combined femoral template and drill *guide* (Fig. 14-9C). This instrument is placed on the front of the femur in such a way that its flat proximal portion rests accurately against the flat supracondylar region of the femoral cortex (Fig. 14-9D). (If bone is not resected to form a channel before the femoral drill guide is offered to the femur, the drill guide may be lifted forward by the femoral condyles.) When the drill guide has been appropriately placed, the surgeon notes which of the two holes in the drill guide lies opposite the apex of the arch of the intercondylar notch. A drill is passed through this hole (Fig. 14-9D). The choice of hole defines which of the two sizes of femoral component are to be used: the appropriate size is marked opposite the hole on the drill guide (Fig. 14-9C).

The intramedullary stem of the guide is passed through this hole into the medullary canal of the femur. The guide is pressed home until the plate on the guide touches the femur, and is rotated until it lies in the anteroposterior plane of the femur (Fig. 14-9E). Two marks are then made in the two femoral condyles opposite the posterior edge of the plate on the guide and the guide is removed. The posterior portions of both femoral condyles are then resected at the level of these marks in a plane which departs from the femoral shaft as it extends proximally (Fig. 14-9F). The extraction of the fragments from the knee is facilitated by levering them out with an osteotome. (It should be noted that this portion of the femur overhangs the back of the tibia in extension so that its removal would not prejudice the mechanical strength of the knee were it to undergo arthrodesis.)

Any adhesions that may be present between the capsule and the back and sides of the femoral condyles are separated from the bone with a periosteal elevator and complete division of the cruciate ligaments is confirmed. The guide, *pin*

carrier and *cuffed bar* are assembled and placed in the femur. The tibia in then placed parallel with the bar both in the anteroposterior and lateral views (Fig. 14-9G). It is *essential* that the gap between the femur and the tibia is now *opened as far as possible* by lifting the femur (*via* the bandage encircling the femur) against counter-traction through the tibia. When this position has been obtained, two Steinmann pins are driven through the tubes in the pin carrier into the tibia. The cuffed bar is then removed, the Steinmann pin carrier is moved out of the guide and the knee is further flexed to separate the guide from the pins. The guide is then removed.

The cuffed bar is now replaced in the Steinmann pin carrier so as to ensure that the pins are at right-angles to the top of the tibia both as viewed from the side and the front: if they are, the bar will be parallel to the shin in both views (Fig. 14-9H).

The tibia is now divided in the plane of the pins (Fig. 14-9I). Removal of the proximal tibia is facilitated by dividing the bone into medial and lateral halves and removing these separately: they may be elevated from the tibia itself with an osteotome, grasped in a bone-holding forceps and rotated out of the knee. In this way the fragments may be drawn forward so that the soft tissues can be cut at their bony attachment vertically downward against the cut surface of the tibia to protect the vital posterior soft tissues.

The knee is now fully flexed and any remaining adhesions between the posterior aspect of the femur and the posterior capsule are divided by sharp dissection and subperiosteal elevation. The posterior capsule should be sufficiently elevated from the femur to ensure that it will not interfere with the posterior flange of the femoral prosthesis and that it does not restrict the correction of a fixed preoperative deformity, especially a flexion deformity.

It should now be possible to place the spacer in the gap in the flexed knee. If this is possible, the surgeon knows that the prosthesis can be implanted in the flexed knee and that 90° of flexion can be obtained. If this is not possible, the bone preventing introduction of the spacer is removed. The spacer should fit firmly in the gap. If it is loose, too much bone has been removed and the replaced knee may be unstable in flexion. The cuffed bar is added to the spacer. The bar will be parallel with the shaft of the tibia if the tibia has been divided at right-angles to its long axis in both planes. If the bar is not

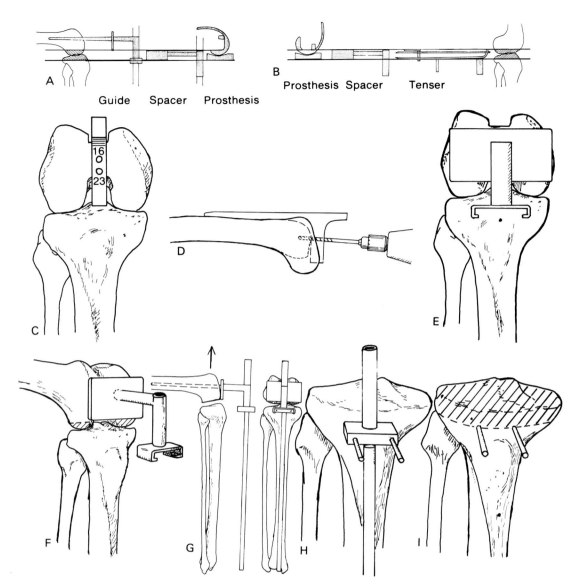

Figure 14-9. *A* to *S*. A series of schematic diagrams reveal the stages during the insertion of the Imperial College London Hospital (ICLH) arthroplasty of the knee. Figure 14-9 *A* and *B*. The special instruments, the guide, spacer and tensor, used to determine the positions of the bone resections in flexion (Fig. 14-9*A*) and an extension bracket (Fig. 14-9*B*) are shown. Figure 14-9 *C* to *F* shows the stages in the preparation of the flexed femoral condyles. In Figure 14-9*C*, the intercondylar channel in the femoral condyles with the combined femoral template and drill guide are seen. As shown in Figure 14-9*D*, a drill is passed through a hole in the drill guide which lies opposite the apex of the arch of the intercondylar notch. Figure 14-9*E* shows the intramedullary stem of the guide inserted through the drill hole into the intramedullary canal of the femur. The guide touches the femur and defines the anteroposterior plane of the bone. Figure 14-9*F*, the posterior portions of the femoral condyles are resected as shown. Figure 14-9*G*, the guide, pin carrier and cuff bar are shown in an assembled position after insertion into the femur. With the tibia aligned parallel to the bar in both the anteroposterior and lateral views two Steinmann pins are inserted through the tubes and the pin carrier into the tibia. Figure 14-9*H*, Steinmann pins are shown in position with the cuff bar replaced in the Steinmann pin carrier. The proximal tibia is resected in the plane of the pins as shown in Figure 14-9*I*. Figure 14-9*J*, the tenser is positioned in the extended knee. Figure 14-9*K* the bar is inserted through the tenser to ascertain the alignment of the knee. Figure 14-9*L*, by use of the tenser two marks are made on the femoral condyles opposite the proximal face of the marker. Figure 14-9*M* with the guide replaced in the flexed knee, the distal femoral condyles are resected through the marks made on the femur with a tenser. In Figure 14-9*N*, the knee is extended and the spacer is interpositioned between the femur and tibia. The bar is reattached to the spacer and correct alignment of the knee is confirmed. Minor adjustments may be made. Figure 14-9 *O* to *S* the final stages in preparation of the femoral condyles are shown. See text for detailed description. (Reproduced with permission of M. A. R. Freeman and S. A. V. Swanson and Deloro Stellite Co., Lancaster, N.Y.)

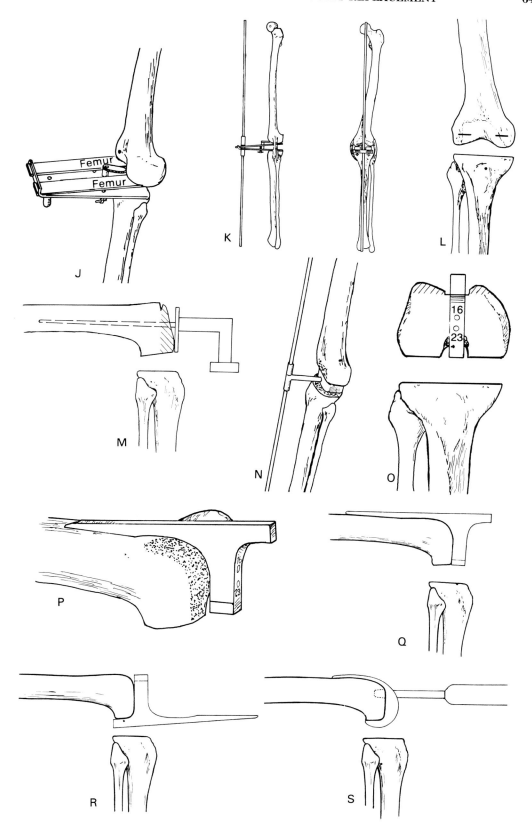

parallel to the shaft of the tibia, the cut surface of the tibia must be trimmed until the bar and the tibia are parallel.

Soft Tissue Release and Bone Resection in Full Extension (Fig. 14-9B). Unless a substantial fixed deformity has been present preoperatively, the removal of the upper tibia will have created a gap in the extended knee such that the tibia and femur can be placed in full extension. If the residue of a preoperative fixed flexion deformity prevents this, (1) the posterior capsule may be further relaxed by subperiosteal elevation from the femur, and (2) the distal end of the femoral condyle(s) may be removed progressively until full extension can be obtained.

With its blades closed, the tenser is introduced into the gap between the transected surface of the tibia distally and the femoral condyles proximally (Fig. 14-9J). The uninterrupted plate on the tenser (marked "tibia") should lie against the tibia and the two separate blades (marked "femur") should lie against the femoral condyles. The screws on the tenser are then turned in a clockwise direction, so as to separate the femoral blades from the tibial plate. In doing this, the ligaments on the medial and lateral sides of the knee can be tightened in turn. When the ligaments are tight a definite sense of resistance will be encountered as the screw is turned further. During this step in the procedure, care should be taken to keep the knee in full extension, since there is a tendency for it to flex as the soft tissues are tightened.

When the soft tissues on the medial and lateral side of the knee are tight, it should be possible to pick up the heel and to move the leg as a whole. Stressing the tibia in a medial or lateral direction should not produce opening of either compartment of the knee.

Both halves of the bar are then passed through the tenser, to check the alignment of the knee. The distal end of the bar should lie over the middle of the angle and the proximal end just medial to the anterior superior iliac spine (Fig. 14-9K). Viewed from the side the thigh and the shin should be parallel to the bar (*i.e.,* the leg should be straight). Small adjustments in the separation of the blades may be needed to achieve the required alignment and stability.

Soft Tissue Release to Correct Severe Fixed Varus or Valgus Deformity. If preoperatively the knee was in *severe fixed* varus or valgus, it may be found that the deformity persists at this stage, in spite of the small adjustments referred to above.

If fixed *varus* persists, all osteophytes should be removed from the medial femoral and tibial condyles. A medial soft tissue release may then have to be performed by releasing subperiosteally the tibial or the femoral attachments of the medial collateral ligament. (The deep portion of the tibial attachment is effectively released when the proximal tibia is resected but some further relaxation may be obtained by subperiosteal dissection of all the medial soft tissues from the remaining proximal tibia.) At its femoral attachment, the medial collateral ligament can be elevated by sharp dissection close to the bone. The soft tissues are then elevated from the medial aspect of the medial femoral condyle in both a proximal and posterior direction so as to expose the whole of the medial aspect of the medial femoral condyle. When the soft tissues have been released, the tenser will become loose in the medial compartment and should be tightened. Rarely, the medial hamstrings and the pes anserinus may also have to be released. In this way, the tibiofemoral angle can be adjusted until the correct valgus/varus alignment has been obtained (*i.e.,* until the proximal end of the bar lies over the hip).

If fixed *valgus* persists, a lateral soft tissue release should be carried out. Adhesions between the lateral femoral condyle and the posterior and lateral parts of the capsule are divided. A separate 2-cm incision is then made 6 cm proximal to the joint line of the knee in the transverse axis of the limb over the iliotibial tract which can be felt as a taut structure if the knee is stressed in a varus direction. Through this incision, the iliotibial tract, the tendinous portion of the biceps and the lateral intermuscular septum are divided. When this is done, the cut surfaces of the iliotibial tract will be found to spring apart, leaving a gap between them. Only the skin should be sutured. The femoral attachment of the lateral collateral ligament may have to be released in the same way as the femoral attachment of the medial collateral ligament. Little useful elongation can be obtained by tibial dissection. As with the correction of a fixed varus deformity the tenser is now adjusted until the correct tibiofemoral alignment has been obtained.

If a large valgus deformity is corrected, the lateral popliteal nerve should be exposed to ensure that it is neither under tension nor compressed against the neck of the fibula.

Bone Section. When the desired soft tissue tension and bony alignment have been obtained, the marker on the tenser is brought down to touch the two condyles of the femur (Fig. 14-9K). Two marks are made in the femur (one in each condyle) (Fig. 14-9L) opposite the *proximal face* of the marker.

The knee is now flexed to 90°, the guide is replaced, and the distal femoral condyles are resected through the marks made on the femur with the tenser (Fig. 14-9M). The plane of section as viewed from the side is given by the plate on the guide: the resected surface should be parallel with the plate.

The knee is extended and the spacer is placed in the gap between the femur and the tibia. The spacer should fit tightly in this gap so that, with the spacer in place, the knee is sufficiently stable to enable the surgeon to lift the ankle and to move the leg medially and laterally without causing angulation of the femur on the tibia. Both halves of the bar are now attached to the spacer. If the knee is in the correct alignment, the proximal end of the bar should lie over the hip (Fig. 14-9N). If the knee is not in the correct alignment, any residual valgus, varus or flexion deformity will be obvious and should be corrected by a further soft tissue release. (If a further soft tissue release is necessary at this stage, it implies that an inadequate soft tissue release was carried out when the tenser was in place and by this stage too much bone will have been removed.)

When the spacer has been satisfactorily positioned, the surgeon knows that it will be possible to achieve full extension, that the prosthesis can be inserted in this position, that the knee will be stable and that any preoperative malalignment has been eliminated.

It will be found that approximately 2 cm of bone will have been removed from the long axis of the limb. If instability or fixed deformity were present preoperatively, the planes of section will involve the removal of less bone on the collapsed side so that (1) the resected bone will be wedge-shaped, and (2) the plane of section may pass above, in the case of the tibia, or below, in the case of the femur, the collapsed surface so that no bone is actually removed from one or both of the condyles on the concave side of the deformity. If disease has produced severe bone destruction in this way or if excess bone has been removed in error, the resultant defect in the femur or tibia can be built up with cement.

Preparation of the Bones to Receive the Prosthesis. *The Femur.* The distal end of the femur is trimmed for a precise fit of the femoral component. The combined femoral drill guide and template is placed in the midline channel already cut in the femur (Fig. 14-9O) and the forward projection of the femoral condyles is resected (Fig. 14-9P) until the curvature of the template matches the curvature of the bone (Fig. 14-9Q). The line on the vertical limb of the template shows the length of the flat, distal surface of the small (*i.e.*, size 16) femoral prosthesis. The vertical limb itself is the same length as the corresponding surface on the large (*i.e.*, size 23) femoral prosthesis.

The template is removed and repositioned in the knee with its short arm lying opposite the cut surface of the posterior femoral condyles and the arm containing the two holes lying opposite the distal femoral surface. The curvature on the template between these two arms is now used to guide resection of the corner of the femur between its posterior and its distal surfaces until the curvature on the femur matches that on the template (Fig. 14-9R).

Finally a phantom femoral prosthesis of appropriate size, on its introducing handle, is offered to the femur and tapped onto the bone to ensure that it is a tight fit (Fig. 14-9S). (A spare femoral prosthesis should *never* be used for this and the subsequent stages of the operation, since bone fat will grease the inner surface of the prosthesis and thereafter cement will not bond to it. Attempts to cement a prosthesis which has been used for the trial stages of the operation may provoke premature prosthetic loosening.

The Tibia. The phantom femoral prosthesis is removed. The tibial template is inserted into the knee and positioned anteroposteriorly so that the stud on the under surface of the template hooks over the posterior tibial cortex. In the medial/lateral plane the template is centered in the knee. For rotational alignment, the template is positioned so that the bar overlies the tibial tubercle. When this position has been obtained, the phantom femoral prosthesis is inserted and the knee is extended. Full extension should be obtainable. The knee should be stable and the two components should match each other rotationally (Fig. 14-10A). If fixed external tibial rotation was present preoperatively, its correction may require the elevation of all the soft tissues attached to the proximal 1 cm of the whole of the circumference of the tibia. The correct alignment (in valgus, varus, extension and rotation) is confirmed by adding the bar (Fig. 14-10A). The surgeon should be able to push upward on the heel (as if the patient was standing on his leg) without causing the two elements of the prosthesis to buckle open. Should the prosthesis buckle open, the implica-

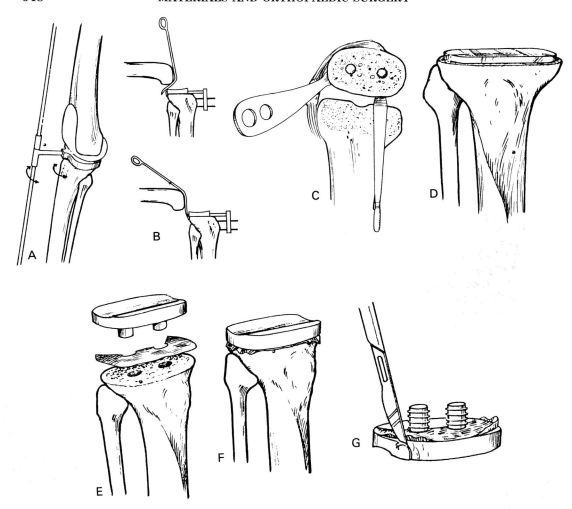

Figure 14-10. *A* to *O*. A series of schematic diagrams reveal the stages during the insertion of the Imperial College London Hospital (ICLH) arthroplasty of the knee (continued from Fig. 14-9 *A* to *S*). Figure 14-10*A*, with the phantom femoral prosthesis in place correct alignment is confirmed by addition of the bar. In Figure 14-10*B*, with the knee in a flexed position the template is fixed to the tibia with the two Steinmann pins. To expose the superficial surface of the tibial template a bone spike may be positioned posterior to the tibia, to lever the bone anterior of the distal end of the femur. Figure 14-10 *C* to *G* shows supplementary stages in the preparation of the proximal tibia. In Figure 14-10*C*, two pointed retractors are positioned in the posterior and the posterolateral surfaces of the tibia to expose the superior surface. Figure 14-10*D* shows a flat glass sheet positioned on the superior surface of the tibia to ensure that the surface is flat. In Figure 14-10*E*, a piece of foil and a large area of phantom tibial prosthesis are positioned on the exposed surface of the tibia. In Figure 14-10*F*, the sheet of foil is folded over the top of the tibia to define the maximal permissable size of the tibial prosthesis. In Figure 14-10*G*, the foil is removed from the knee and transferred to an actual tibial component. Extensions of polyethylene beyond the folds in the foil are removed. Figure 14-10*H* shows the insertion of the tibial component (*1*), and the femoral component (*2*). Figure 14-10*I* shows that after the knee is flexed, excessive cement is removed with a curet. In Figure 14-10 *J* to *O*, the stages in the preparation of the patellar polyethylene prosthesis are shown. Figure 14-10*J* shows a central drill hole in the patella. In Figure 14-10*K*, peripheral osteophytes on the patella are excised with a rongeur. Figure 14-10*L*, shows a special trephine with a central cylindrical shaft inserted into the patellar drill hole to prepare a suitable recess. In Figure 14-10*M*, the central drill hole is enlarged with a special bit or tap. Figure 14-10*N* shows the polyethylene patellar prosthesis inserted into the hole with or without the use of methylmethacrylate cement. In Figure 14-10*O*, posterior projections of the surrounding patellar articular surface are excised with the rongeur. (Reproduced with permission of M. A. R. Freeman and S. A. V. Swanson and Deloro Stellite Co., Lancaster, N.Y.)

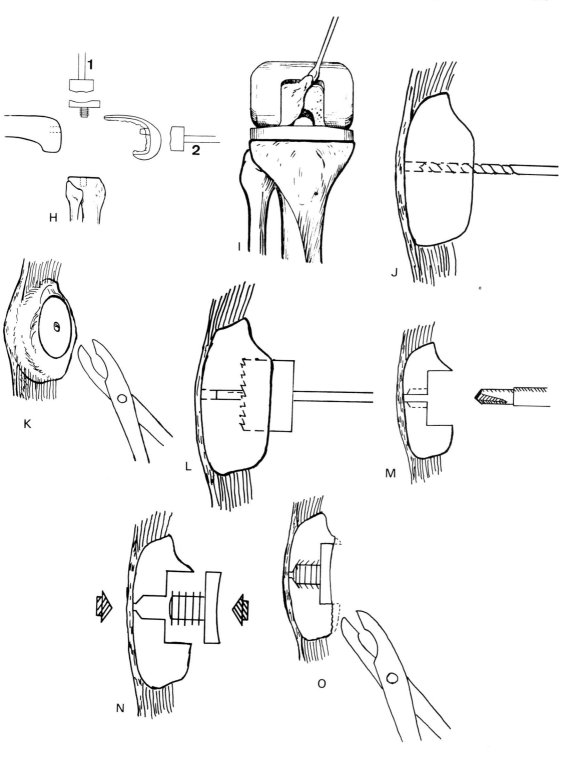

tion is that the knee is not in the correct valgus/varus alignment (which cannot be the case if the tenser and spacer have been used correctly).

When this situation has been achieved, the bar is removed and the template is fixed to the tibia by passing two Steinmann pins through the holes in the tube on the template into the tibia. The knee is fully flexed taking care not to move the tibial template relative to the tibia. The phantom femoral prosthesis is removed. To expose the tibial template sufficiently to allow the drill to be passed through it, it may be necessary to place a bone spike posterior to the tibia and to lever the bone forward relative to the femur (Fig. 14-10B). This should be done with great care so as not to disturb the tibial template. The drill guide is added to the template and the guarded drill is passed through one of the two holes in the tibial template to drill the tibia. When one hole has been drilled in the tibia, the plug is inserted into the hole to locate the tibial template. A second hole is then drilled. While these two holes are being drilled, the surgeon should check that the drill is not penetrating the tibial cortex; if it is, drilling should cease. (The stud on the tibial component will then have to be shortened sufficiently to match the depth of the hole that has been made.)

Implantation of the Tibial and Femoral Prostheses. The knee is fully flexed and the phantom prostheses are removed. The cut surface of the tibia is exposed by placing the angled retractor behind the tibia and levering the tibia forward relative to the femur. A second retractor is placed posterolaterally to retract the extensor mechanism away from the tibia (Fig. 14-10C). The surface of the bone is irrigated and residual soft tissue is removed.

The flat sheet of glass is placed on the top of the tibia and moved over the cut surface of the bone to ensure that this is flat (Fig. 14-10D). Any high points are trimmed away with a reciprocating saw. If a significant bone defect is present, cement will be required to fill it. If the whole cross-section of the tibia is flat and sound bone is available for contact with the tibial component no cement is required (but see "The Tibial Prosthesis").

The Tibial Prosthesis (inserted with or without Cement). A tibial prosthesis must be chosen of sufficient size to ensure that it rests upon all aspects of the tibial cortex. This usually requires the use of the large area tibial component. If, from inspection of the fit of the large area phantom tibial prosthesis, this component is

seen to be too large in certain directions, a piece of foil is placed under the phantom prosthesis (Fig. 14-10E) and folded down across the edge of the top of the tibia (Fig. 14-10F).

The phantom femoral component is inserted and a final check is made of stability and alignment in flexion and extension.

The knee is flexed and the phantom prosthesis is removed. The foil is then removed from the knee and transferred to the actual tibial component (Fig. 14-10G). Any polyethylene extending beyond the folds in the foil is removed with a knife or preferably with the ICLH polyethylene trimmer.

Care must be taken to ensure that the holes in the top of the tibia are the correct depth for the studs (if they are not, because the drill encountered the tibial cortex, the studs must be trimmed) and that the profile of the tibial component itself has been trimmed to match that of the tibia. Insertion of the tibial component then proceeds as follows:

The two flanged pegs on the prosthesis are inserted into their drill holes and impacted by hand. It will be found that about the first two flanges can be inserted in this way so as to steady the prosthesis. The prosthesis is then tapped down onto the tibia using the tibial impactor and a mallet (Fig. 14-10H). In its final placement the entire under surface of the tibial component should rest upon the cut surface of the tibia and the two studs should be fully engaged in their holes. If this is the case, the tibial component will have been absolutely immobilized on the tibia. The prosthesis should be horizontal, a placement which can be confirmed by placing the spacer plus the cuffed bar on the top of the tibia.

The Femoral Prosthesis. For the insertion of the femoral prosthesis, cement is placed on the surfaces of the femoral prosthesis and the prosthesis is driven lightly on to the femur with the impactor (Fig. 14-10H). Excess cement is removed and the knee is extended for impaction of the femoral prosthesis into the cement. Alignment may be checked by laying the two halves of the assembled bar along the leg. While the femoral prosthesis is steadied but *not impacted* with the impactor, the knee is again flexed and excess cement is removed (Fig. 14-10I). Excessive cement extrudes medially, laterally and into the intercondylar notch. Little or no cement extrudes past the proximal margins of the posterior flanges of the prosthesis and even if it is it can be reached through the intercondylar notch.

No cement is left in the posterior compartment of the knee.

The Femur. One femoral condyle may be so destroyed that the level of section of the distal femur indicated by the tenser passes distal to the bone end. In this event all soft tissue should be curetted from the condyle. Two screws are inserted into the condyle that protrude so that their heads lie at what would have been the desired level of bone section. The phantom femoral prosthesis is inserted and the screws are adjusted, if necessary, until the correct alignment of the extended knee is obtained. When the actual prosthesis is inserted, cement separates the prosthesis from the sectioned condyle. The screws pass through the cement and touch the prosthesis. Thus the screws may need to be backed out a little to offset the thickness of any cement on the other condyle. The cement sets to incorporate the screws which then become mechanically redundant.

If excess bone has been removed from both femoral condyles in error (so that the spacer and phantom prosthesis are loose in the *extended* knee), four screws should be inserted (two into each condyle) protruding sufficiently to tighten the knee when the actual prosthesis is in place.

Patellofemoral Reconstruction. *Soft-Tissue Release.* Whether the patellar surface is replaced or not, it is essential that the patella lies in the midline of the prosthesis both in full extension and throughout the range of flexion. Especially in knees with a preoperative valgus or external rotation deformity (in which there is usually a contracture of the lateral patellar retinaculum), there may be a tendency for the patella to sublux laterally. If this is found to be the case: (1) The patella should be released laterally by dividing the lateral patellar retinaculum (from its deep surface rather than through a separate skin incision); and (2) care should be taken to ensure that any fixed tibial rotation has been released and corrected by the division of the soft tissues attached to the proximal tibia.

Preparation of the Patella by Resection of Its Posterior Surface. If the patella is not to be replaced, the patella is everted, the synovium around its margin is excised and its posterior surface is resected flush with the posterior aspect of the ligamentum patellae distally, the patellar retinaculae medially and laterally, and the insertion of the quadriceps muscle proximally.

Patellar Resurfacing. When severe patellofemoral arthritis is present, the patellar articular surface is reconstructed with a polyethylene component, as seen in Figure 14-10 *J* to *O*.

A central drill hole is made in the patella (Fig. 14-10*J*) and the marginal osteophytes are resected (Fig. 14-10*K*). The hole is enlarged with a trephine (Fig. 14-10*L*) and the central drill hole is tapped (Fig. 14-10*M*).

A patellar implant is inserted with or without the use of supplementary cement (Fig. 14-10*N*). Posterior osteophytes or prominent projections of bone are removed with a rongeur (Fig. 14-10*O*).

Closure. The posterior layer of the suprapatellar pouch is closed with Dexon sutures over the proximal end of the anterior flange of the femoral prosthesis. Two 6.5 mm suction drains are placed in the synovial cavity of the knee and the wound is closed in three layers. The capsule and synovial membrane are closed with braided nylon and the edges of the incision are overlapped if necessary in order to draw the patella into the midline in both extension and in flexion. The superficial fascia is closed as a second layer with Dexon sutures to obliterate the dead space between the skin and the extensor mechanism. The skin is closed as a third layer with interrupted sutures. Tension sutures are employed if delayed healing is anticipated.

Postoperative Management. The knee is immobilized in a split plaster of Paris cylinder. Suction drainage is maintained for 2 days, and plaster of Paris for 5 days. During this time quadriceps exercises are commenced. If the wound is healthy in 5 days, active flexion is commenced and the patient may bear weight. It may be desirable (especially if the quadriceps muscles are weak) to support the knee in a splint when weight bearing begins and at night.

When the patient is able to stand unsupported on one leg, an anteroposterior and lateral weight-bearing X-ray of the knee should be taken. The anteroposterior X-ray should show that the two elements of the prosthesis are parallel with each other when under load (rather than buckling open), that they are accurately placed on the bone ends, that the prosthesis is horizontal, and that the leg is in the correct alignment. The lateral X-rays should show that there is no cement in the posterior compartment of the knee, that the prosthesis is accurately placed on the bone ends and that any pre-existing flexion deformity has been corrected.

If delayed wound healing necessitates the continued use of plaster of Paris, or if, in spite of early active flexion, 90° or the preoperative range plus 30° has not been obtained by the end of the third week, the knee should then be flexed under anesthesia with muscle relaxation.

Management of the Grossly Unstable Knee

Where the knee joint shows greater degrees of instability the surgeon must consider seriously whether reconstructive arthroplastic procedures are indicated. The question of a possible diagnosis of a neuropathic joint should be considered seriously and such joints should be treated in other ways, usually with external supports. The great variety of implants designed for treatments of grossly unstable knees are described in Chapter 13. The objectives of such surgery are to salvage the knee with the provision of stability, relief of pain and correction of deformities. The provision for an outstanding range of motion is a secondary consideration. Careful assessment of the patient may reveal that the instability is primarily secondary to loss of bone stock. In the author's experience most of the patients with unstable rheumatoid knees and indeed those with instabilities secondary to many other causes have potentially excellent stabilization by the collateral ligaments provided that prosthetic replacement of bone substance across the knee joint restores the physiological tension in the collateral ligaments. Such patients are suitable candidates for nonarticulated implants such as the Freeman-Swanson design. Restrained implants such as the hinge designs should be employed only where they are absolutely necessary. Their likelihood of loosening in the postoperative period is extremely great and probably approaches 100% within the first postoperative decade. The risk of severe infection possibly culminating in amputation of the limb is much greater than with the use of smaller implants that do not violate adjacent intramedullary cavities. Stress protection of the bone around the intramedullary stem of the implant provokes osteoporosis with a great likelihood for traumatic or pathological fracture of bone. It is the author's impression that far more constrained implants are being inserted at present than is necessary or advisable. The operative techniques required for the insertion of a variety of hinge-type constrained implants is fully reviewed elsewhere.[143–146] One uncommon indication for a hinge-type arthroplasty is after extensive resection of certain malignant tumors of bone such as giant cell tumors and fibrosarcomas. In most other situations a nonhinged intrinsically stable knee joint prosthesis such as the spherocentric design is preferred.[147, 148] While the general principles of the operative technique are similar to other total knee joint replacements, the interested reader should study the recommended method which is available elsewhere.[148]

Reconstruction of the Patellofemoral Articulation

In the past decade extensive experimental work has been undertaken in an attempt to provide satisfactory methods for the reconstruction of the patellofemoral articulation in the presence of unicompartmental or multicompartmental arthritis[149, 150]. A variety of implants is available in which the articular surface of the patella is replaced with high density polyethylene and the opposing intercondylar region on the distal femur is resurfaced with a stainless steel or Vitallium component.[151] In the present state of knowledge, these procedures are rarely indicated. Their use should be restricted to elderly patients and mainly those who have involvement of other compartments of the knee. Young patients with patellofemoral arthritis or chondromalacia patella refractory to conservative management should be treated with patellectomy rather than a resurfacing procedure until much greater experience is available. The early results of Ewald and Sledge,[152] and Mankin and Sledge* with the McKeever prosthesis and subsequently with a cemented polyethylene and Vitallium prosthesis should be noted. In 9 out of 10 rheumatoid patients in whom the McKeever prosthesis was applied the procedure failed with loosening of the components. With the limited patellar bone stock available for attachment of the patellar prosthesis, it is not surprising that loosening has been a problem. With the cemented polyethylene and Vitallium arthroplasty, mechanical erosion of the polyethylene initiated clinical failure. In view of the rigorous mechanical environment of the patellofemoral joint, the failure of polyethylene is not unanticipated. For the reconstruction of knees with triple compartmental arthritis, a variety of metallic femoral components are available that resurface both the femoral condyles and the intercondylar region.[153] The tibial plateaus and the patella are resurfaced with polyethylene. At present no clinical trials of adequate duration have been completed to allow useful evaluation. In most of these patients, however, the func-

---

* H. Mankin and C. B. Sledge, personal communication.

tional demands imposed upon their prosthetic joints are likely to be less than is observed in patients who require only patellofemoral arthroplasty.[154] If this is the case, the patients with triple compartmental arthroplasty may show more satisfactory performance of their patellofemoral articulation than the patients who undergo isolated patellofemoral arthroplasty.

Representative descriptions of isolated patellofemoral resurfacing and triple compartmental arthroplasty follow.

Isolated Patellofemoral Joint Replacement. A curvilinear medial parapatellar incision is made which extends from the insertion of the vastus medialis to the anterior tibial tubercle. The joint capsule is incised and the infrapatellar fat pad is excised. The under surface of the patellar tendon is freed from adherent fascia and the patella is retracted in a lateral direction to expose the patellar facet of the femur. The knee is flexed to 90° and the femoral marking template is positioned over the patellofemoral facet of the femur. The knee is extended to ensure that the femoral component does not interfere with joint motion. When the template is correctly positioned the knee is flexed to 90° and the outline of the template is marked on the femur with methylene blue. The femoral template is removed and the delineated region is contoured to the outline of the femoral drill jig. When the femoral facet is appropriately contoured the femoral jig is positioned and three ¼-inch drill holes are prepared through the guide holes in the jig to a depth of ½ inch. Each hole is undercut by the use of a curet. The trial femoral component is positioned and minor adjustments are made. After removal of the trial component the knee is extended and the patella is retracted in a lateral direction to expose its undersurface. The appropriate size for the patellar component is estimated by the use of a trial patellar component. The periphery of the correct component is delineated with methylene blue and the central, marked area is trimmed with an oscillating blade. The patellar drill jig is centered on the osteotomized patellar surface so that its long axis coincides with that of the patella. Prior to osteotomy of the patella two marking sutures may be secured to the adjacent deep surface of the patellar tendon and quadriceps tendon to indicate the central axis of the patella. After placement of the patellar drill jig, two ¼-inch drill holes are prepared through the guide holes in the jig. The guide is removed and the holes are deepened until they reach the cortical bone which should not be breached. The

femoral and patellar trial components are inserted and the joint is tested for stability and motion. Minor adjustments may be necessary. Subsequently additional small cement holes may be prepared in the opposing bony surfaces. Cement is mixed and the components are inserted. The general principles for closure of the wound and postoperative management follow those previously described for other arthroplastic procedures of the knee.

Arthroplastic Reconstruction of the Patellofemoral and Both Tibial Femoral Joints. For triple compartment arthroplasty the total condylar knee prosthesis is a representative example of current designs.[136] In fact this implant represents one of a series of devices that are available in different embodiments. One of the models is suitable for unicompartmental arthroplasty while others are designed for bicompartmental or triple compartmental resurfacing. Implants are available that restore varying degrees of constraint or stability. This system probably represents the most sophisticated one of total knee joint replacements that is currently available. The total condylar arthroplasty is indicated for rheumatoid or osteoarthritic knees with flexion deformities of up to 70° and fixed varus or valgus deformities of 15 to 40°.

Technique. The general principles of the bicompartmental arthroplastic part of the procedure are similar to those previously described. Through a long medial parapatellar incision the distal end of the femur and tibial plateaus are trimmed to appropriate configuration by the use of a series of special jigs (Fig. 14-11 *A* and *B*). The femoral components cover the entire anterior surface of the distal femur including the intercondylar region. The articular surface of the patella is osteotomized and a central cement hole is prepared with a patellar reamer of 12 mm (½ inch) in diameter and 13 mm in depth. In turn the tibial, femoral and patellar components are cemented in place. Otherwise the techniques of surgery are similar to those previously described. For comparable knee with triple compartment arthritis but with greater instability the Stabilo-condylar prosthesis in the same graduated series of implants designed by Walker and Shoji[155] may be employed. The implant is a lax hinge which permits −5° to 115° of flexion and 10° of internal-external rotation with supplementary abduction-adduction. The general principles for its insertion are similar to those described for the total condylar prosthesis and are described elsewhere.[155] An alternative, nonhinged intrinsically stable knee-joint prosthesis,

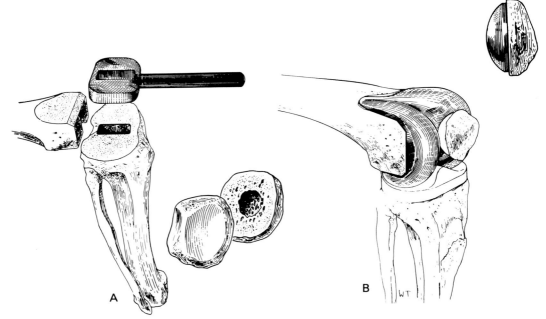

Figure 14-11. *A* and *B*. The final stages in the insertion of a total condylar knee prosthesis are shown. Figure 14-11*A* reveals the distal femur and tibial plateaus after the surfaces have been prepared by the use of special jigs and a reciprocating saw. Similarly the articular surface of the patella has been osteotomized and a central cement hole of 12 mm in diameter and 13 mm in depth has been prepared. A spacer is about to be placed on the exposed surface of the tibia. A rectangular slot is prepared in the center of the tibia as defined by the spacer. Previously the spacer has served to indicate the total thickness of bone removed through the extended knee joint. Figure 14-11*B* reveals the appearance of the flexed knee after insertion of the components. (Reproduced with permission of Codman, Randolph, Mass.)

the spherocentric system,[148] is described in Chapter 13.

The Limitations and Complications of Total Knee Joint Replacement

The limitations and complications of total knee joint replacement follow a similar pattern to those described for total hip joint replacement. The main difference between total hip joint replacement and total knee joint replacement is the markedly inferior clinical result which the patient with an arthroplastic knee of optimal surgical and postoperative management achieves. Many patients with total hip joint replacement possess a nearly normal functional result so that they may undertake most activities including their employment with virtually no limitations. In the author's experience this is rarely ever achieved after total knee joint replacement. The patient may be able to function around his house or to participate in a sedentary occupation. If his early postoperative result is particularly good and he undertakes more vig-

orous activity such as recreational sports including tennis or if he attempts to resume employment that requires considerable walking or climbing, within 1 to 3 years he usually experiences resumption of mechanical pain, swelling and stiffness so that the activities have to be terminated. As discussed in Chapters 7 and 13, the symptoms appear to result from excessive wear of high density polyethylene probably with a chemical synovitis secondary to the polyethylene wear particles. The erosion of polyethylene may be accentuated by creep or frequently by frank mechanical fracture of the polymeric material. The complications of total knee arthroplasty and the general principles of management are now reviewed.

Infection. As with all total joint replacement, sepsis is the most difficult frequently encountered complication. The incidence of infection appears to range between 2% and 10% depending upon the type of implant and the experience of the surgical team.[156-158] If the infection is recognized at an early state particularly in the preliminary postoperative period an attempt may be made to salvage the arthroplasty by immediate debridement following the insertion of closed suction and irrigation tubes and the administration of large doses of appropriate systemic antibiotics. Unfortunately, in many if not most cases, ultimately removal of the implant is necessary. For the treatment of a failed total knee joint the author prefers a 2-stage procedure with an initial debridement of the joint and application of the Hoffman external fixation device, as described in Chapter 11. The wound is packed in open fashion until the cellulitis resolves. At a second procedure, autogenous iliac crest cancellous bone is inserted into the joint space and the external fixation device is adjusted to provide compression between the femur and tibia. Fusion requires a minimum of 4 months of immobilization and frequently a much more extended period. The morbidity of the fusion in terms of compromise on the patient's activities is much greater than is encountered after a patient with a failed total hip joint undergoes conversion to a pseudarthrosis.

When infection presents in a patient with a large hinge-type prosthesis, removal of the implant is almost inevitable. Previous workers have presented a high incidence of major complications after infection associated with the use of constrained hinge-type devices including nonunion of the arthrodesis and above knee amputation.[156] In the author's experience, the 2-stage method of debridement and fusion with the use of the Hoffmann external fixation device has been particularly satisfactory. At the time of compression of the joint, bone graft should be applied to prevent the excessive shortening of the limb that is otherwise likely to occur. Usually, the distal femur and proximal tibia represent two hollow cavities which readily collapse with compression, so that a leg length discrepancy of 5 to 20 cm is not uncommon. The application of the bone graft combined with the rigid external stabilization permits fusion of the joint with an acceptable degree of foreshortening.

Thromboembolism. The incidence of thromboembolic phenomenon appears to be encountered less frequently after total knee joint replacement than after total hip arthroplasty. The general methods of treatment are similar and can be studied elsewhere.[109-111] Some workers have recommended routine prophylactic anticoagulation treatment. In the author's experience the deleterious side-effects of the medications, particularly excessive bleeding tendency are prohibitively common. Only patients with a history of thromboembolism or who present as particularly high risks should have prophylactic anticoagulation treatment by one of the accepted regimes.

Prophylactic Antibiotics. The author and numerous other workers[159] prefer to use routine prophylactic antibiotics as described under the section on total hip joint replacement. The course persists from 6 hours prior to surgery through the fifth postoperative day.

Loosening of Implants. The total knee components may be inadequately attached to the adjacent bone at surgery or they may loosen secondarily. Loosening presents as mechanical pain, which is relieved by immobilization. Where the magnitude of motion is small, confirmation may require arthrography or cine-studies with X-ray image intensification. Surgical treatment with replacement of the loose component is necessary. Implants are predisposed to loosen, or to wear excessively if the opposing femoral and tibial prostheses are malaligned to present incongruous surfaces or surfaces that do not move along the arc of motion defined by residual anatomical stabilizing structures, especially the collateral and cruciate ligaments.[160] During surgery the use of appropriate jigs to define the correct orientation for insertion of the implants is strongly advised.

Instability and Subluxation. These complications are, unfortunately, not uncommon, especially in very active patients, those with rheumatoid arthritis and grossly obese individuals. Prevention is the mainstay of treatment. The axis of the reconstructed knee must be horizontal.[160] If the axis is oblique, the femoral components are particularly likely to sublux on the tibial components. Surgical reconstruction is essential and should be undertaken at an early stage prior to severe subluxation or dislocation with possible damage to the collateral ligaments. Collapse of the osteoporotic bone, especially in rheumatoid patients and others on steroids is a formidable problem. Again, prevention is the most satisfactory form of treatment. Where possible, the subchrondral plate of more resilient bone should not be breached. In patients with osteoporotic bone, a broad implant such as the Freeman-Swanson or the total condylar design should be employed where a very large surface area of implant rests on adjacent bone. Furthermore, the large implants provide weight bearing through the stronger peripheral cortex. Once the implant has begun to drift, reconstruction should be undertaken as soon as possible before the technical problems grow to immense proportions. The tibial component is removed and the subchondral bone is curetted. The cavity thereby created is filled with a combination of a special tibial component that possesses a unilateral extension to occupy the cavity and with methylmethacrylate cement. When surgical reconstruction is contraindicated by the patient's general medical condition or by other factors, an external brace may enable the patient to walk.

Erosion of Implants. As previously described, erosion of an otherwise satisfactory total knee joint replacement remains an unsolved problem. Frequently the patient presents with symptoms of mechanical pain and swelling of progressive nature. Aspiration of synovial specimens under sterile conditions confirms the diagnosis (see Chapters 7 and 16). X-rays may indicate substantial erosion of the tibial polyethylene component. Ultimately, replacement of the polyethylene component is necessary. Excessive wear is provoked by malaligned components.[160] At the time of surgery the alignment should be carefully checked. If the femoral component, also, is malaligned it should be replaced. Many of the newer designs of implant possess more complex contoured surfaces which approximate those of the anatomical knee. It is not unlikely that these implants may show lower rates of erosion of the polymeric material. When the surgeon replaces a worn tibial implant, he should consider replacement of both components with such a newer design.

Breakage of Implants. The only type of fractures that have been reported are those of the constrained hinge-style implants.[154] Both the intramedullary stems and the metal axis of the hinge may undergo fatigue failure. Replacement of the hinge is necessary. Previous designs of hinges did not incorporate the physiological valgus of the distal femur. More recent designs, such as the Guepar, may show a somewhat lower breakage rate and are preferable for the replacement arthroplasty.

Osseous Fractures Adjacent to Total Knee Joint Replacements

The principal fractures have been observed in patients who have constrained hinge-type total knee joint replacements.[161] Spiral fractures may occur after conventional traumatic accidents; alternatively osteoporotic bone especially in rheumatoid patients is more likely to undergo pathological fractures. In most cases nonoperative methods with closed reduction of the fracture and immobilization in a cast are advisable. After the fracture has healed a loose implant may be replaced. Open reduction with internal fixation may present a formidable technical problem in view of the limited bone stock available for stabilization and the osteoporotic nature of the bone. As described previously, in fractures of the proximal femur adjacent to total hip joint replacement screws that anchor an onlay plate are difficult to apply and intramedullary rods are impossible to use. Alternatively, a special total knee joint replacement may be purchased which possesses an exceptionally long intramedullary stem to anchor the fractured long bone. The implants are difficult to insert. If postoperative infection occurs, it complicates both the arthroplastic joint and the union of the fracture.

TOTAL ANKLE JOINT REPLACEMENT

Until recently, arthrodesis of the ankle joint with severe arthritis has been recognized and accepted as the only reconstructive procedure.[162] The clinical results of ankle fusion have not been entirely satisfactory. Johnson and Bosekar[163] reviewed 140 ankle fusions performed at the Mayo Clinic. They observed that 17% of the patients had a persistent limp and inability to return to their former jobs; 12% had pseudarthrosis and 5.4% of the patients ultimately came to amputation. Lance *et al.*[164] reported the end result of 190 ankle fusions in which five different methods of arthrodesis were employed. The overall rate of nonunion was 22% with a 31% incidence of clinically unsatisfactory results. Inevitably, many workers have studied possible methods for total ankle joint replacement. The clinical role for arthroplasty of the ankle remains unclear. Nevertheless, some provisional results reported by Evanski and Waugh[165] and by Manes *et al.*[166] have been encouraging. The principal indications have included disability from traumatic arthritis, rheumatoid arthritis or rarely, avascular necrosis of the talus secondary to steroid ingestion that otherwise would warrant ankle fusion. An additional indication has been pseudarthrosis after a previous attempt at fusion or previous talectomy. The patient should realize that a secondary procedure with arthrodesis may be necessary if the replacement fails and that such failures are not unexpected in the current state of knowledge. Contraindications include previous infection in the ankle region, ligamentous instability and neuropathic arthropathy of the ankle. In the author's experience, total ankle arthroplasty has been followed by a limited range of motion of the ankle joint. Nevertheless, it has provided a technique for "fusion" of the ankle with much lesser morbidity than formal surgical attempts at ankle fusion. The limited ankle motion observed after arthroplasty has several explanations. Inadequate debridement of the posterior region of the ankle joint approached through an anterior incision is not unlikely. The surgeon may fail to position the implants concentric with the anatomical axis of the joint motion. Physiological positioning of the ankle joint prostheses is rendered much more difficult by the changes in ankle joint congruity that accompany degenerative or rheumatoid arthritis. The biomechanical studies by Sammarco et al.,[167] and others[168] have documented the alterations in the kinematics of ankle motion that accompany deterioration of the joint. For anatomical restoration of an arthritic joint by the insertion of prosthetic components, the surgeon has to restore accurately the anatomical joint surfaces and joint congruity or provide another complex pair of matching joint surfaces that behave similarly when constrained by the ligaments around the ankle. At present, either method seems an unduly overoptimistic attempt to restore ankle joint motion. Other workers,[164] however, have reported superior ranges of motion after surgery. The technique for insertion is described for a "Smith" total ankle joint although more recently the author has employed the Oregon ankle system (Zimmer USA, Warsaw, Ind.) by the use of a similar method.

Technique

With the patient supine under general or spinal anesthesia a pneumatic tourniquet is applied to the proximal thigh and the limb is exsanguinated. A small pad is placed under the greater trochanter to reduce excessive external rotation of the limb. The lower extremity is prepared and draped in conventional manner and an anterolateral approach is made to the talotibial joint parallel to the peroneus tertius muscle and approximately 4 ½ inches long (Fig. 14-12A). The common toe extensors and the neurovascular bundle are retracted medially. The anterolateral malleolar and the lateral tarsal arteries are sacrificed. The force of retraction should be carefully restricted to avoid excessive tissue trauma. The entire width of the joint space is exposed in the subperiosteal plane. The anterior talofibular ligament is carefully preserved.

With the spool-like template the proposed osteotomy sites in the talus and tibia are delineated (Fig. 14-12B). Two coronal osteotomies are made in the two bones with an oscillating blade. Excessive removal of the talus may predispose the residual portion of the bone to avascular necrosis in view of the tenuous and tortuous nature of its blood supply.[169] Particular care is necessary to avoid penetration of the posteromedial neurovascular bundle. A rongeur may be necessary to complete the posterior osteotomy. The cuts must be made parallel to the sole of the foot. As shown in Figure 14-12C, the template is inserted into the space to define its adequacy and alignment. The upper and lower diameters of the template are comparable to the diameters of the tibular and talar components. A slot in the template faces directly anterior. With an oscillating blade a slot of similar width and height is extended into the distal end of the anterior tibia. With a curet, the slot in the tibia is extended in a posterior plane to remove cancellous bone superior to the distal subchondral plate. The distal lip of cortical bone is carefully preserved in the posterior tibia (Fig. 14-12D) to interlock with a notch in the tibial component. Trial prostheses are inserted to allow proper seating of the tibial component. With a curet, four cement holes are prepared in the superior surface of the osteotomized talus (Fig. 14-12D). Both trial components are temporarily inserted and a trial range of motion is attempted. Great care should be taken to center the components concentric with the arc of motion of the anatomical talotibial articulation; otherwise inadequate range of motion is inevitable. X-rays in a mediolateral and anteroposterior plane should be considered to confirm proper positioning of the implants. Minor supplementary trimming and contouring may be necessary. When the range of motion is satisfactory, the trial components are removed and the wound is irrigated and dried. Cement is mixed and packed into the appropriate surface of the tibia. The tibial component is inserted and correctly situated in the midaxis of the joint. Excessive cement is removed while the cement solidifies. The use of excessive cement should be avoided because removal of solidified cement from the posterior ankle joint is extremely difficult after the insertion of the talar component. A second batch of cement is prepared and placed on the denuded surface of the talus. The talar component is centered under the tibial prosthesis and stabilized until solidification of cement. Further attempts are made to remove all excessive cement. Figure 14-12E reveals the ankle joint after insertion of both prostheses.

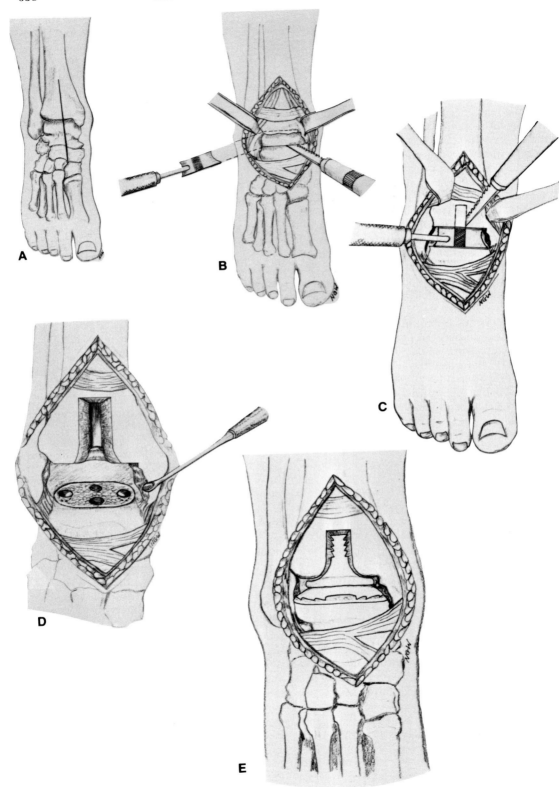

Figure 14-12. *A* to *E*. Technique for insertion of the Smith total ankle joint replacement.

The wound is closed in layers and a large bulky pressure-type dressing is applied with a posterior splint. A closed suction drain may be employed for the first 24 hours. The foot is elevated for about 3 days after which time, partial weight bearing with the use of crutches and active range of motion exercises are initiated. The regime of prophylactic antibiotics with intravenous cephalosporins is begun in the immediate preoperative period and continued after surgery 3 to 5 days. Rheumatoid patients may require 2 or 3 weeks of immobilization to ensure uncomplicated wound healing.

Postoperative Complications of Total Ankle Joint Replacement

The principle complications of total ankle joint replacement are wound infection, mechanical pain and loosening or migration of the components. Particularly in rheumatoid patients with cutaneous involvement deep wound infection, necrosis and sloughing of skin are likely to follow excessive intraoperative retraction. Most complications of ankle joint replacements culminate in subsequent arthrodesis. Usually the implants are removed, the wound is debrided and an external fixation device is applied. In the presence of active infection, the wound may be packed open until the cellulitis is brought under control. Alternatively, primary closure with the application of continuous irrigation through closed suction, irrigation tubes is undertaken. Subsequently, the external fixation device is adjusted to provide compression of the talotibial surfaces. At least 4 months of immobilization are required for fusion, although considerably more prolonged immobilization may be necessary. The details of the fusion procedure are described in Chapter 11.

TOTAL SHOULDER JOINT REPLACEMENT

Historically, attempts to surgically reconstruct the glenohumeral joint after significant derangement of the anatomy have produced unreliable and poor results. The milestone in arthroplastic procedures of the shoulder was achieved by Neer[170] in 1955 when he reported his earlier results with a humeral head prosthesis. Initially, the indication was comminuted fractures of the humeral head in which avascular necrosis was anticipated. The prosthesis replaces the articular surface of the humerus and it is anchored with an intramedullary stem. Success with the prosthesis requires precise anatomical reconstruction of the tuberosities of the humerus and an intact rotator cuff. An exacting procedure of physical therapy is essential to re-establish the subacromial gliding mechanism. In 1974, Neer[171, 172] extended the indications for his proximal humeral articular surface prosthesis in a series of patients with rheumatoid or degenerative arthritis. A high degree of success was encountered with patients who had a relatively normal rotator cuff function and minimal derangement of the glenoid articular surface. Marmor[173] has confirmed the favorable results of hemiarthroplasty in patients with rheumatoid arthritis involving the shoulder. More recently, Neer[171] has described a polyethylene cylindrical component for resurfacing the glenoid to accompany humeral head replacement.

Subsequently, several workers have turned to the more difficult reconstructive problem in the severely arthritic shoulder where the rotator cuff, also, is severely damaged. One attempt by Macnab and English[174] embodies a humeral component with an articular surface and an intramedullary stem combined with a glenoid prosthesis (Fig. 14-13A). The latter has an acromial outrigger which partly compensates for the compromised rotator cuff. The humeral stem and the glenoid base components are porous coated with a sintered powder of cobalt chromium alloy to provide a living bond between the bone and the implant. Provisional stabilization of the glenoid is achieved by the use of cancellous bone screws. Another novel approach has been described by Fenlin[175] in which the spherical surface for replacement of the humeral head is attached to the glenoid and the socket is secured to the humerus (Fig. 14-13B). As described in Chapter 13, Fenlin's reconstructive technique substantially alters the biomechanics of the shoulder in an attempt to lessen the considerable loosening forces imposed upon the implant-bone interface. A few satisfactory results have been reported by the inventor. A few other designs of glenohumeral replacement have been described, of which the Stanmore total shoulder replacement is the most widely employed.[176, 177] It is a ball-and-socket replica of the anatomical shoulder with components of cobalt chromium and a narrow polyethylene rim on the glenoid component. Most surgeons have experienced considerable technical difficulty in the insertion of the device. Anchorage of the glenoid component in the limited available bone stock of the lateral scapula is exceptionally difficult. At the present time the arthroplastic technique described by Neer, which, admittedly requires virtually an intact rotator cuff, is the optimal

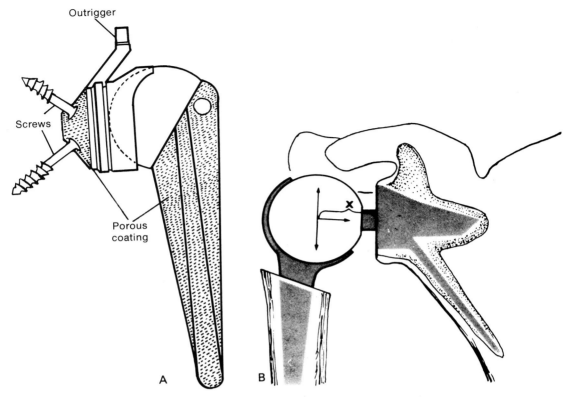

Figure 14-13. *A.* The total shoulder joint replacement devised by Macnab and English for resurfacing the glenohumeral joint in the presence of a deficient rotator cuff is shown. *B.* The total shoulder joint replacement devised by Fenlin for reconstruction of the glenohumeral joint with a compromised rotator cuff is shown. (*B*, reproduced with permission of J. M. Fenlin.[175])

form of reconstruction and therefore is described in detail.

Indications for its use as a hemi- or total joint arthroplasty include a painful, stiff shoulder secondary to trauma, or rheumatoid arthritis, osteoarthritis, and avascular necrosis of the humeral head. Specific contraindications include a neuropathic or infected shoulder joint.

The Neer[171] Technique for Total Shoulder Joint Replacement

The patient is placed in a semireclining position under general anesthesia with a small pad placed under the ipsilateral shoulder. A gentle curved incision is made which extends from the lateral acromion across the tip of the coracoid process and obliquely across the deltopectoral groove (Fig. 14-14*A*). The deltopectoral groove is developed and the cephalic vein is identified. The vein is retracted in a medial direction along with the pectoralis major. The interval between

pectoralis major and deltoid is opened from the clavicle distal for about 5 to 7 inches. With finger dissection, the deep surface of deltoid is separated from underlying tissues, after which the pectoralis major is treated in a similar fashion. For excision of the medial insertion of the deltoid muscle, the clavicle is osteotomized with a narrow osteotome in a longitudinal fashion along the origin of the deltoid muscle. Flakes of clavicle remain attached to the muscle for rapid reattachment to the principal portion of bone during the closure. Similarly, the acromion is osteotomized with flakes of bone attached to muscle to the posterolateral extent of the cutaneous wound (Fig. 14-14*B*). The deltoid is reflected in a superolateral direction to reveal the rotator cuff and the coracoid process. The tendinous portion of the subscapularis is incised about 1 inch medial to its insertion of the humerus (Fig. 14-14*C*). Stay sutures are secured to the main portion of the subscapularis *prior* to its division for rapid repair of the muscle. After incision of the capsule the glenohumeral articular surfaces are examined for the extent of degenerative change. With an osteotome, the humeral head is divided through the anatomical neck of the humerus (Fig. 14-14D). A humeral rasp may be inserted to prepare the intramedullary canal. A tight fit of the stem within the medullary canal is essential. Four stem sizes of different dimensions are currently available. Where the glenoid surface is badly eroded, a central drill hole is prepared for anchorage of the glenoid component as shown in Figure 14-14E. The wound is irrigated and carefully dried for optimal insertion of cement. A batch of cement is mixed and impacted into the glenoid surface. The glenoid component is inserted and impacted into position. Subsequently, a humeral component of appropriate size is inserted so that the articular surface faces in 30° of anatomical retroversion to provide stability against dislocation (Fig. 14-14F). A trial range of motion is undertaken to ensure optimal positioning of the implant and adequate motion. If excessive limitation of motion is observed adhesions around the shoulder joint are lysed, primarily with finger dissection, between the rotator cuff and superficial structures in the posterior, superior, lateral, anterior and medial aspects of the shoulder joint. Marked increase in the range of shoulder motion may follow such dissection, although the procedure must be undertaken with care in view of the numerous neurovascular structures around the shoulder joint. Figure 14-14G reveals the prostheses *in situ* after total shoulder joint arthroplasty.

In Figure 14-14H, proximal humeral arthroplasty for a 4-part fracture dislocation of the shoulder is revealed. The operative technique of Neer[170] approximates that previously described with two principal exceptions. The initial entry into the shoulder joint is made through the fracture sites in the lesser and greater tuberosities rather than through a separate incision in the subscapularis. Secondly, for the reconstruction of the tuberosities two 20 s.w.g. (standard wire gauge) wires are used for their reattachment to appropriate drill holes in the humeral prosthesis.

The rotator cuff and subscapularis are repaired with interrupted 2-0 Tevdek sutures. Drill holes are prepared in the distal acromion and clavicle, 0 Tevdek sutures are inserted through the drill holes by the use of a straight needle. A free end of each suture is passed around the flakes of bone attached to the detached portion

of the deltoid muscle. The deltoid muscle is sutured in place, after which subcutaneous tissues and skin are closed in a conventional manner. Closed suction irrigation may be used for the first 24 hours. The shoulder is immobilized with a Velpeau-type sling.

Postoperative Management. Two or 3 days after surgery, when the patient is comfortable, we initiate the elaborate therapeutic regime described by Neer which he withholds for a few more days. On the first day of therapy the patient is instructed in gentle passive external rotation. On the following day he continues that exercise and initiates gentle passive internal rotation. On the next day, gentle passive assisted flexion is undertaken by the use of the patient's contralateral extremity. All of the exercises are performed with the patient in a supine position so that minimal tension is applied to the anterior repair and the rotator cuff. The exercises are continued for the first postoperative week. At the end of this period, extremely gentle passive assisted abduction is initiated, again with the patient in the supine position; motion is restricted to 40°. The therapy should be undertaken on at least four occasions during the day for periods of not less than 20 minutes. At this time the patient is discharged home with continued outpatient supervision over the daily therapeutic regime. Upon discharge the patient should possess 90° of passive assisted flexion and 40° of passive assisted abduction with about 30° of internal and external rotation. Three weeks after surgery, pendulum exercises are begun. Six weeks after surgery, strengthening exercises of the upper extremity are first encouraged. Also at that time, greater amounts of forward flexion and abduction are undertaken.

As Neer has emphasized, the therapeutic regime required for a successful result from shoulder joint replacement requires diligent effort by the patient for many months after surgery. It is perhaps ironical that the shoulder continues to provoke modest pain until a substantial recovery of shoulder motion is regained.

Complications of Total Shoulder Joint Replacement

Surgical errors provide the greatest source of complications, followed by errors in the rehabilitation program. The common surgical errors include disruption of the deltoid muscle with residual weakness of its anterior or lateral portion. The subscapularis and rotator cuff may have unsatisfactory repairs with residual rotator cuff weakness and instability of the humeral

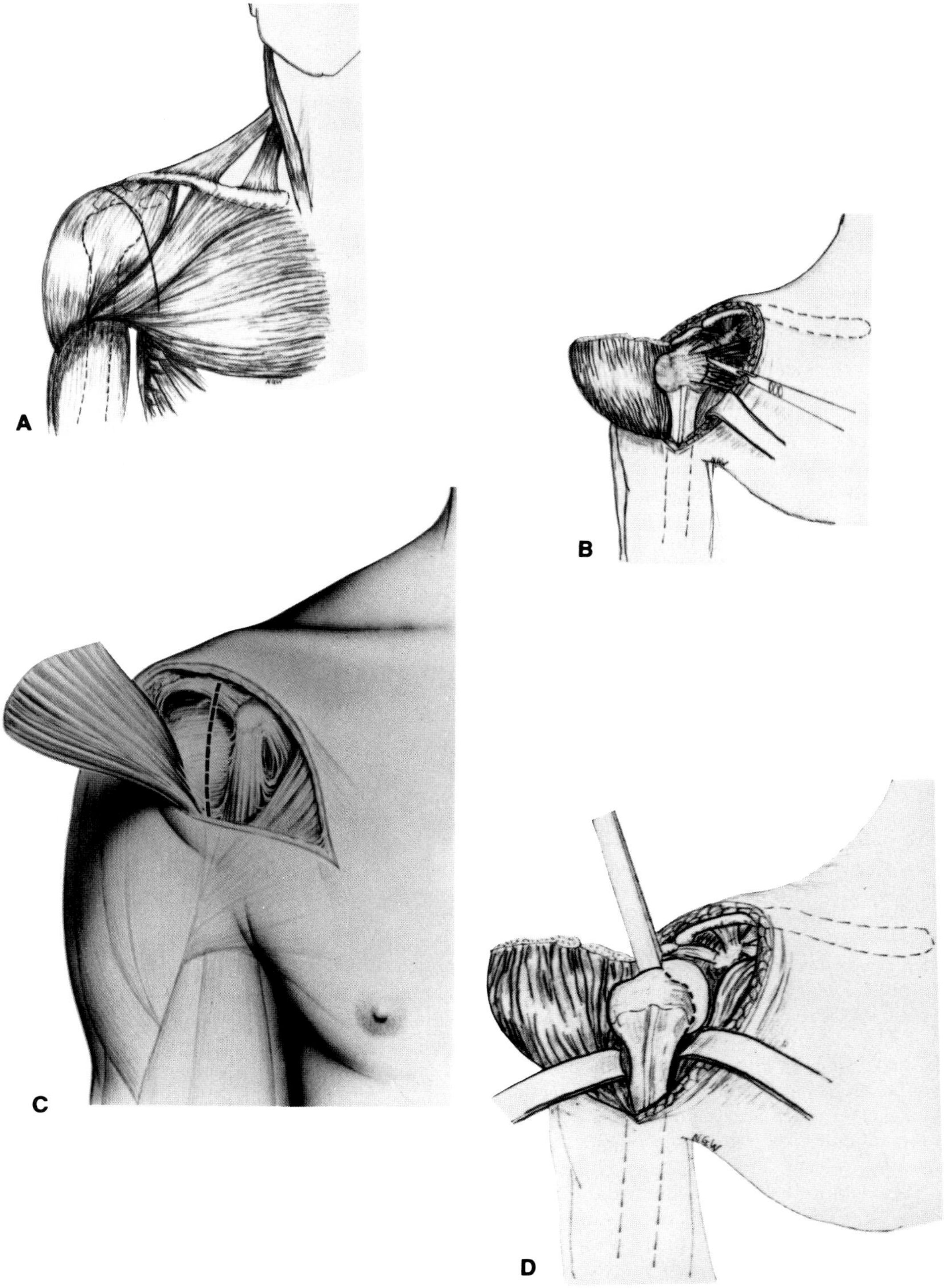

Figure 14-14. *A* to *H*. Technique for insertion of the Neer total shoulder joint replacement. (Figures 14-14*C*, *G* and *H*, reproduced with permission of C. S. Neer.)

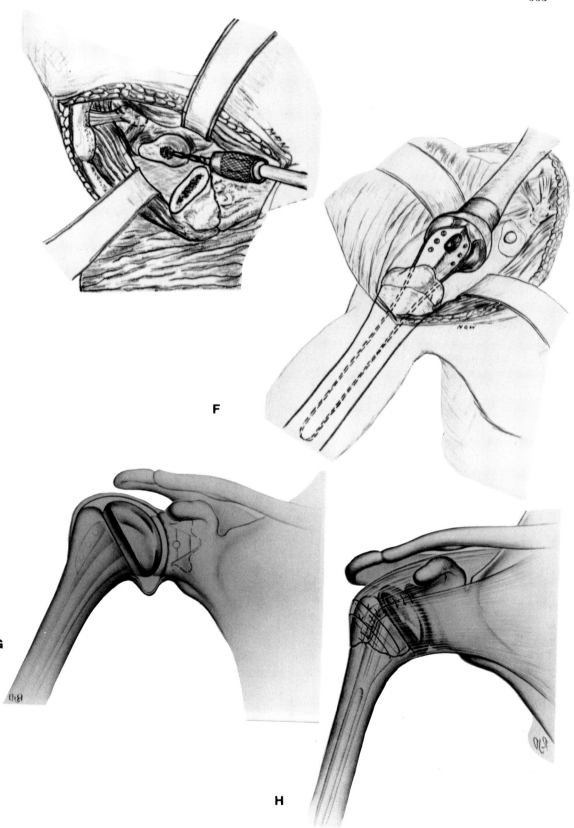

F

H

head. Neurovascular injury to the brachial plexus, the circumflex-humeral vessels and adjacent nerves may accompany the exposure. Fractures of the glenoid or of the proximal humerus are not unknown. Unless the glenoid component is carefully anchored subsequent loosening is likely to occur. Malrotation of the humeral component with postoperative subluxation readily occurs unless the surgeon achieves 30° of retroversion of the articular surface. Where the anatomy of the proximal humerus is distorted by previous fractures or other pathological conditions, particular care is required in the insertion of the stem of the prosthesis. The surgeon should consider preliminary insertion of a Kirschner wire and radiological documentation of the intramedullary cavity. The postoperative therapeutic regime requires careful collaboration between the patient and the therapist. Premature excessive passive range of motion may compromise the soft tissue repair while delayed resumption of shoulder motion is likely to yield a painful, stiff shoulder. If a patient presents to a surgeon many months after arthroplastic surgery with a painful, stiff shoulder a closed manipulation under general anesthesia can be attempted. Where closed manipulation is unsuccessful surgical lysis of adhesions between the capsule of the shoulder and superficial structures may be extremely helpful to regain passive motion of the glenohumeral joint. Afterward the therapeutic regime of Neer must be closely followed until active shoulder motion is restored. Other complications of total shoulder joint replacement such as infection are uncommon.

TOTAL ELBOW JOINT REPLACEMENT

Attempts to develop total elbow joint replacements have been thwarted by the imposing anatomical constraints which are described in Chapter 13. The elbow is a polycentric hinge with a complex arc of rotation somewhat similar to that of the knee joint. Until recently, the available arthroplastic devices have been unicentric hinges which inevitably fail to replicate the anatomical motion.[178] With the soft tissues that constrain and motor the joint all designed for a complex polycentric motion, it is not surprising that considerable fatigue forces are imposed upon a unicentric prosthesis. Loosening, and migration or mechanical failure of the implant could be predicted. In view of the limited soft tissue covering around the implant the relatively high incidence of infection secondary to total elbow joint replacement, also, is not surprising. Nevertheless, for certain patients with a

painful, stiff elbow who possess appropriate muscle strength to power the elbow the available hinge-like devices may be the best available treatment and superior to the alternatives of hemiarthroplasty,[179] interpositional arthroplasty or arthrodesis. More recently, Ewald* has designed an unconstrained device in which the opposing surfaces of the distal humerus and proximal ulna are resurfaced with polyethylene and metal components. His preliminary clinical observations have been encouraging and help to direct future work. The following operative procedure describes the insertion of a currently available hinge-like device, the GSB (Gschwend, Scheier, Bähler prosthesis, DePuy Co., Warsaw, Ind.) elbow endoprosthesis.[180] A similar technique is used for the insertion of most of the other implants.

Technique

At least three surgical approaches to the elbow joint have been described for replacement arthroplasty. Dee[181, 182] prefers a posterolateral approach while Schlein[183] uses a posteromedial approach and Gschwend[180] prefers to use a true posterior approach. In the following description the posteromedial approach and the true posterior approach are described for the treatment of a moderately and a severely disrupted elbow respectively.

For the posteromedial approach the patient is placed in a supine position with the arm draped freely. A tourniquet is applied to the upper arm and the limb is exsanguinated. A long curved medial incision is made (Fig. 14-15A) which permits visualization and careful retraction of the ulnar nerve (Fig. 14-15B). The medial epicondyle is osteotomized (Fig. 14-15B) and the flexor muscle mass is retracted in a distal direction. The triceps tendon is sharply reflected from the medial aspect of its insertion on the olecranon. The capsule of the elbow joint is reflected from the anteromedial incision (Fig. 14-15C) around both the anterior and posterior aspects of the proximal ulna. With an air drill the olecranon and coronoid process are fashioned into the appropriate shapes (Fig. 14-15D). At this stage dislocation of the elbow joint in a medial direction is readily achieved without excessive distraction on the ulnar nerve (Fig. 14-15E). The center of the trochlear notch and the capitellum are trimmed with the air drill until the medullary cavity is broached. At this time the radial head is sharply excised. The medullary cavity in

---

* F. C. Ewald, personal communication.

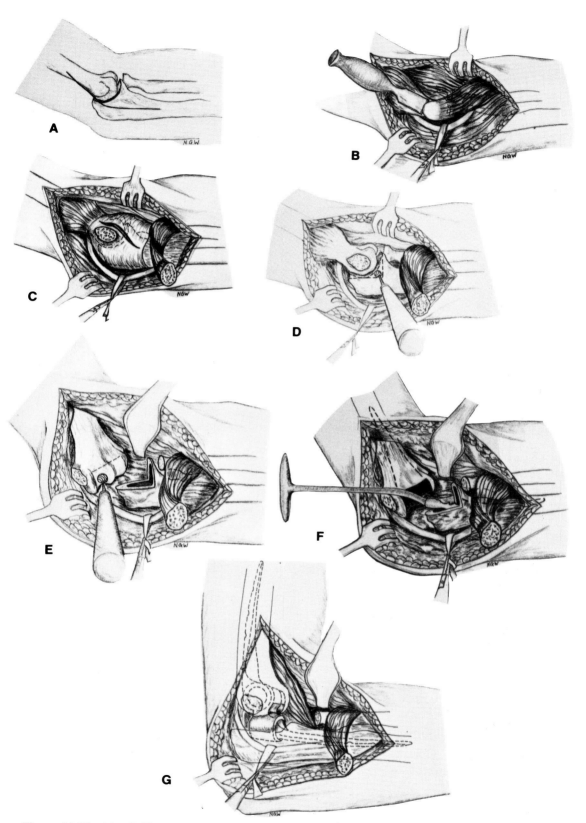

Figure 14-15. *A* to *G*. The technique for total elbow joint replacement with a GSB prosthesis through a posteromedial approach.

the proximal ulna is reamed in slow, progressive stages. Reaming, as viewed in Figure 14-15F, is performed slowly and carefully so that adjacent soft tissues are not damaged and the cortex of the ulna is not breached. Special rasps are available for this process which can be supplemented by the use of an air drill. The implants are inserted for a trial fit and a range of motion is performed. Appropriate adjustments in the bone are made until satisfactory positioning is achieved. For the GSB prosthesis the humeral components should not project beyond the medial or lateral humeral epicondyles. The ulnar and subsequently the humeral components are cemented in separate stages (Fig. 14-15G). Molten cement in adequate quantity should be injected or impacted into the medullary cavities of the humerus and ulna. The ulnar portion of the prosthesis should be carefully inserted to achieve proper rotational alignment and depth. The humeral component should be wholly surrounded by bone apart from its exposed articular surface which should not extend distally beyond the humeral condyles. The implants are connected by the retaining screw and the wound is irrigated with antibiotic solution. The triceps aponeurosis is carefully repaired and the medial epicondyle is reattached with a malleolar or cancellous screw. The cutaneous wound is closed with minimal tension.

Alternatively, for elbows with marked flexion or angular deformities or with bony ankylosis, the posterior approach of Gschwend is preferred. The patient is placed in a prone position under general anesthesia with intubation. The arm is supported with a pillow under the elbow with 60 to 90° of elbow flexion. The tourniquet is inflated after the limb is exsanguinated. A curvilinear dorsal longitudinal incision (Fig. 14-16A) is made which extends about 10 cm proximal to the tip of the olecranon and 8 cm distal to the olecranon. The central portion of the incision is displaced somewhat toward the ulnar aspect to facilitate visualization of the radial head. The ulnar nerve is identified, isolated and gently retracted as in Figure 14-16 B and C. The triceps aponeurosis is incised in the shape of a V with the base at the tip of the olecranon (Fig. 14-16 B and C). The length of the V depends upon the magnitude of the flexion deformity. Each limb of the V should exceed 8 cm so that good visualization of the olecranon fossa is achieved.

Alternatively, the triceps can be retracted proximally by osteotomy of the olecranon as in Figure 14-16D. The olecranon is drilled for reattachment prior to its excision. The drill hole is placed somewhat closer to the dorsal surface of the ulna than is described in Chapter 10. The osteotomized portion of olecranon should possess the minimal area of articular surface. For the repair procedure the drill hole is extended through the osteotomized portion into the cement dorsal of the ulnar prosthetic stem. The cement hole is tapped and a 4.5 mm screw is inserted with a lag technique.

The subsequent stages are comparable to those described in Figure 14-15 D to G. Rheumatoid patients with proliferative synovitis may require a synovectomy.

The radial head is excised with an oscillating blade. Hohmann retractors are placed around the ventral surface of the distal humerus to protect the vital soft tissues and neurovascular structures. The articular surface of the proximal ulna is removed with an oscillating blade and the medullary cavity is opened with a curet. A special intramedullary reamer is inserted into the ulna. Serial trial fits with the ulnar component are undertaken until optimal alignment is achieved. With the elbow dislocated the middle third of the humeral articular surface is removed with the oscillating blade. The saw cut extends immediately proximal to the level of the coronoid fossa. The medial and lateral epicondyles of the humerus are carefully preserved. The medullary canal of the humerus is breached with a curet and enlarged with an intramedullary reamer. Serial trial fits with the humeral component are undertaken until the metallic portion of the humeral component ceases to project beyond the medial or lateral humeral epicondyles. The humeral and ulnar components are inserted and articulated and a trial range of motion of the elbow is performed. When optimal alignment of the components is realized, they are cemented in place as previously described. Either the olecranon is replaced with a cancellous lag screw or the triceps aponeurosis is carefully repaired. When the preoperative elbow shows a marked flexion deformity the repair in the triceps aponeurosis must be adjusted to permit full extension of the elbow. Again the cutaneous closure is undertaken with minimal tension.

After total elbow joint replacement a bulky compression with a posterior splint is applied with the elbow at 45° of flexion. A closed suction drainage may be used. A course of prophylactic systemic antibiotics as previously described is advised.

Postoperative Treatment. Forty-eight hours after surgery, the suction drainage system is

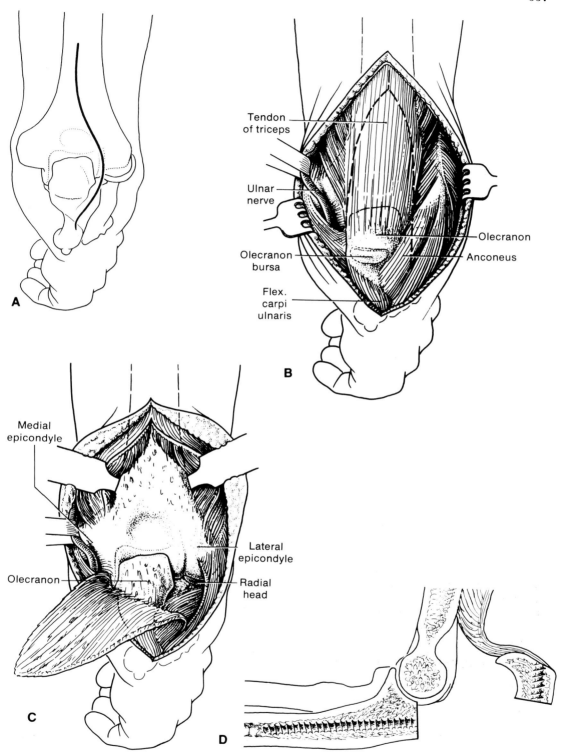

Figure 14-16. *A* to *D*. The posterior approach of Gschwend for total elbow joint replacement. (*A* to *D*, reproduced with permission of U. Heim and K. M. Pfeiffer.[184])

removed and active range of motion of the fingers and shoulder are encouraged. One week after surgery the dressing and splint are removed. If the wound shows satisfactory healing, active flexion and extension of the elbow as well as pronation and supination are initiated. No passive exercises, however, are performed. Three weeks after surgery strengthening exercises of adjacent muscle groups are carefully initiated. Heavy lifting is discouraged until full motion of the elbow and moderate strength of adjacent muscle groups have returned.

Complications of Elbow Joint Replacement

The most frequently encountered problems after total elbow arthroplasty have been loosening and migration of the implants. If the surgeon fails to align the implant in the anatomical axis of motion or if he applies inadequate amounts of cement, loosening and migration are particularly likely to occur. The patient presents with mechanical elbow pain, a decrease in the range of elbow motion or obvious crepitus with elbow motion. Clinical examination may readily confirm the presence of a loose and unstable implant. Surgical reconstruction is advisable prior to further destruction of bone adjacent to a loose implant. In rheumatoid patients with severe osteoporosis, loosening and migration of the implant are particularly likely to occur. Ultimately, removal of the implant and arthrodesis may be necessary. Another important complication, infection, usually culminates in the removal of the implant, debridement of the joint and arthrodesis. The fusion may be technically difficult in view of the substantial loss of available bone stock. External fixation as described in Chapter 11 may be helpful. Dee[181] has described avascular necrosis of the olecranon secondary to excessive stripping of soft tissues and failure of the triceps repair. In one case he undertook a full thickness rotational flap graft to cover the site where metal protruded from the wound.

TOTAL WRIST JOINT REPLACEMENT

Attempts to develop total wrist joint replacements have lagged substantially behind the efforts devoted to other joints. While fusion of the wrist is admittedly disabling it does not provide nearly the incapacity that fusion of a variety of other joints instills. In the present state of knowledge, where the clinical experience with total wrist joint replacement is small, the indications for such surgery must be limited. In view of the fragile nature of available implants, manual laborers with heavy physical demands upon their upper extremity should not be considered for arthroplastic surgery. Perhaps the optimal indication is a rheumatoid patient with bilateral disease and involvement of his elbows as well as his hands and fingers. Even a few degrees of wrist motion may greatly improve the functional potential of the fingers. Arthroplastic surgery provides an opportunity to realign the wrist which may further improve function of the hand. Indeed, the realignment of the wrist is essential to enable a hand surgeon to undertake subsequently reconstruction in the hand and to lessen the substantial bending moments that otherwise would be imposed upon the implant with a great likelihood for it to fracture, loosen or migrate. As reviewed in Chapter 13 two concepts of arthroplastic device have been developed. Swanson[185] has designed an intramedullary, stemmed flexible hinge of silicone rubber. The core of the implant possesses a Dacron reinforcement to augment axial and rotational stability. The implants are available in five sizes. Meuli[186] has devised a metal and polymeric device in which a trunnion bearing concept is employed. Two metallic components composed of Protasul-10 and a polyester ball are available in two sizes. A metallic trunnion is implanted into the distal radius with the polyester ball inserted onto the trunnion. A metallic socket possesses two intramedullary stems which are embedded into the medullary cavity of the second and third metacarpals. The socket articulates with the ball to restore wrist motion. The techniques for insertion of the Meuli and Swanson devices are now described. Another prosthesis developed by Volz at the Arizona Medical Center, the AMC total wrist (AMC Total Wrist Prosthesis, Howmedica Inc., Rutherford, N.J.), is similar to the design by Meuli.

Technique of Meuli

Total wrist joint replacement after the technique of Meuli requires exacting attention to detail if a satisfactory result is to be achieved.[186] The principle indications have been wrist pain, stiffness and deformity secondary to traumatic or rheumatoid arthritis. Prior to surgery, X-rays of the wrist are carefully examined so that the surgeon determines the necessary realignment to restore the physiological axis of motion of the wrist joint. The accurate radiological realignment technique of Hamas, described in Chapter 13, is strongly recommended. The normal axis resides approximately at the center of the capitate bone. Failure to restore this axis greatly increases the likelihood of loosening, migration or mechanical failure of the implant. Meuli has prepared two plastic templates of the implant in its two sizes. The templates can be superimposed upon the X-rays to select the appropriate size of the implant. The surgeon determines whether the intramedullary stems of the cup portion of the implant will be inserted into the second and third or second and fourth or third and fourth metacarpals.

With the patient in a supine position, under general or regional anesthesia, a tourniquet is inflated after exsanguination of the limb. A curved dorsal incision across the wrist is made as shown in Figure 14-17A. The incision extends in a proximal direction for about 5 inches from the middle of the second metacarpal. The extensor retinaculum (Fig. 14-17B) is incised to prepare a narrow proximal and a broad distal, radially based flap. Where necessary, synovectomy of the extensor compartments is performed but the capsule of the ligamentous structures are carefully preserved for subsequent reconstruction. Part of the proximal carpal row is usually destroyed and resorbed with the residual remnants displaced in a volar direction on the radius. Resection of the residual lunate and scaphoid bones (Fig. 14-17C) is performed with an air drill or a rongeur. The proximal tip of the capitate is resected. The radial styloid is removed to prepare a transverse distal end of the radius. The distal 2 cm of ulna is resected. At this stage the radiocarpal subluxation should be completely reduced. The intramedullary canal of the radius is prepared with an air drill, a curet or a broach (Fig. 14-17D). A hole is prepared in the appropriate bones of the distal carpal row that penetrates the opposing metacarpals. Usually the second and third metacarpals are employed although, as previously described, other combinations may be necessary to restore the physiological axis of the wrist. Radiological control may be applied to ensure intramedullary alignment of the implant. The special broach is used to enlarge the hole in the distal carpal row and the two metacarpals. Alternatively, in an osteoporotic rheumatoid patient a straight hemostat suffices for preparation of the holes. The intramedullary stems of the cup prosthesis are inserted into a hollow metallic rod to bend them into appropriate alignment (Fig. 14-17E). The two metallic components are inserted into the metacarpals and the radius respectively. The polyester ball is placed on the trunnion and the implant is reduced. The wrist joint is inspected for axial alignment and appropriate length. A trial range of motion is undertaken and minor adjustments are performed as necessary. Cement is inserted into the distal radius and into the two metacarpals with appropriate care to achieve adequate penetration of the cement. The implants are inserted (Fig. 14-17F) and immobilized until the cement has solidified. Excessive cement is removed and the joint is reduced after the addition of the polyester ball.

The capsule and ligamentous structures are firmly sutured over the implant. Capsular repair may be augmented by the passage of sutures through small drill holes in the dorsal radial cortex. The repair should be examined with the wrist joint in 45° of extension and flexion and 10° of ulnar and radial deviation. The distal extensor retinacular flap is interposed between the wrist joint and the extensor tendons to supplement the capsular repair. The extensor tendons are examined for tension or balance and appropriate adjustments are made by shortening or by tendon transfers. Extension of the wrist without lateral deviation should be achieved. Where necessary supplementary tendon transfers or repairs may be performed to reconstruct ruptured tendons. The proximal retinacular flap is sutured superficially to the extensor tendons to prevent bow stringing. The wound is closed in layers and a suction drain is inserted. A bulky hand dressing with a dorsal plaster splint is applied with the wrist in a neutral position. The extremity is elevated for 3 to 5 days after which time a short arm cast is applied with the wrist in a neutral position. Where extensor tendons have been repaired dynamic outriggers are employed to anchor rubber band slings on the fingers. Immobilization persists for 4 to 6 weeks to provide adequate stabilization of the wrist. Upon removal of the cast, active flexion and extension exercises are initiated. Where extensor tendons have been repaired a dynamic brace[187] may be necessary to support extension of the fingers.

Complications of Meuli Total Wrist Joint Replacement

Most of the complications that occur after other arthroplastic procedures may occur after total wrist joint replacement. The two notable examples are fracture and late progressive subluxation and malalignment of the Meuli device.[188] Both complications may be avoided or greatly reduced in incidence if great care is taken during surgery to accurately align the implant along the anatomical axis of motion of the intact wrist joint. The complications are corrected by

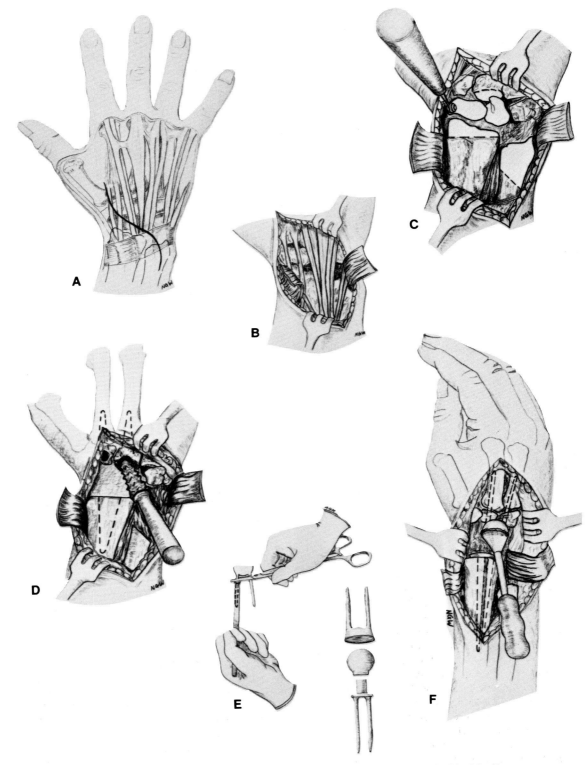

Figure 14-17. *A* to *F*. Technique for total wrist joint replacement devised by Meuli.

replacement of the arthroplasties with realignment of the wrist or by arthrodesis. To fuse the wrist, Meuli[188] recommends the application of autogenous cancellous or corticocancellous bone graft and a dynamic compression plate that is attached to the dorsal surface of the distal radius and the second metacarpal.

Flexible Implant Arthroplasty of the Radiocarpal Joint—Surgical Technique and Long Term Results*

Rheumatoid arthritis is a frequent cause of severe wrist impairment. It may affect the soft tissues and the joints of the wrist, including the radiocarpal, intercarpal and radioulnar, singly or in combination. The destructive rheumatoid synovitis causes loosening of ligaments and erosive changes of bones, disturbing the multiple link system of the wrist joint. In some cases spontaneous fusion of the wrist may occur before subluxation. In severe cases complete dislocation of the wrist may result. Loosening of the ligaments on the radial aspect of the joint is common and allows ulnar displacement of the proximal carpal row; radial deviation of the hand on the forearm may follow. The associated subluxation of the distal radioulnar joint provokes a loss of stability on the ulnar aspect of the wrist. Loosening of the palmar radiocarpal ligament allows collapse of the long axis and buckling of the radiocarpal link system. However, palmar subluxation of the proximal row on the radius is more common.

Arthrodesis of the wrist has been the accepted procedure for treatment of the severely involved rheumatoid arthritic wrist under the concept that a stable wrist is needed for transmission of forces to the digits to provide a strong grip and thereby a functional hand. A mobile wrist, however, is necessary for the performance of activities of daily living particularly in the placement of the hand on the diverse surfaces of the body. The ideal solution with the provision of both stability and mobility clearly entailed the development of a reliable and simple arthroplasty for the radiocarpal joint.

Functional adaptations of the hand are greatly facilitated by wrist motion, especially flexion, even of a small arc of motion. A few degrees of wrist movement will increase the reach of the fingers by 5 to 6 cm in space and thereby improve considerably their functional potential. The need for some degree of wrist motion, especially flexion, is particularly important if disabilities of the finger or of other proximal joints

of the upper extremity are present such as those often seen in the rheumatoid arthritic patient. Personal hygiene can be a problem for patients with fused wrists, especially if the wrists are fixed in extension. The most functional postures of the hand are associated with forearm supination and wrist flexion.

In the past Swanson has fused only markedly unstable wrists when adequate rotation of the forearm and flexion and extension of the fingers were present to compensate for the loss of wrist motion. The wrist was usually fused in a neutral position or in slight flexion. When a small degree of pain-free wrist movement is present but in a nonfunctional arc of motion, an osteotomy of the radius is indicated to provide a more useful arc of motion.

Moderately satisfactory results are observed after the use of a pseudarthrosis procedure for wrist stabilization. In this method the surgical technique for a wrist arthrodesis is performed, but the postoperative immobilization period is deliberately foreshortened to achieve a fibrous and somewhat mobile union instead of an immobile bony union; this method, however, has been unreliable because it is difficult to determine the optimal duration of immobilization to achieve a satisfactory pseudarthrosis. Other procedures, such as palmar shelf arthroplasty, also, have been performed in an attempt to retain some wrist movement. In this technique the carpus is transposed dorsally over a shelf prepared from the anterior cortex of the radius. While the method is designed to prevent palmar dislocation of the carpus, it has not provided highly reproducible results. Resection of the proximal carpal row is another method of treatment for certain severely impaired osteoarthritic wrists with destruction of the proximal carpal row or subluxation of the radiocarpal joint although the results, too, are of variable quality.

Concept and Method

Stability of the wrist is a prerequisite for normal function of the extrinsic muscles of the fingers. In a disabled wrist the reconstructive procedure must provide moderate stability and strength with enough mobility to assist in hand adaptations. In light of the experience gained with finger joint implants, the concept of a flexible intramedullary stemmed hinged implant was applied to the wrist joint. A double stemmed flexible hinge of silicone rubber for the radiocarpal joint was developed in 1967 to be used as an adjunct to resection arthroplasty of the wrist. The proximal stem of the implant is inserted in

* This section was provided by A. B. Swanson.

the intramedullary canal of the distal radius and the distal stem is inserted through the capitate into the intramedullary canal of the third metacarpal. Four different types of implants were designed and tested in order to determine the best possible configuration of the midsection. The best model has a barrel-shaped midsection, slightly flattened on the dorsal and volar surfaces. The core of the implant contains a Dacron reinforcement to provide axial stability and resistance to rotatory torque. Since 1974, this implant model has been made of high performance silicone elastomer available in five anatomical sizes. It has been mechanically tested to more than 200 million flexion repetitions to 90° without evidence of material fatigue or fracture. The implant contains barium sulfate to improve its radiopacity. The implant functions as a flexible hinge to allow vertical and lateral movements through its flexible midsection and stems. At the time of implantation, a proximal carpal row resection including a resection of the base of the capitate is performed. The distal stem of the implant is directed through the capitate into the third metacarpal and the proximal stem is positioned in the intramedullary cavity of the radius. With this alignment the implant is well situated in respect to the anatomical site for wrist flexion. It has been shown that the axis of motion of the wrist occurs at the level of the head of the capitate bone. Most of the diseased wrists, however, show marked alterations in radiocarpal and intercarpal movements. The flexible hinge possesses an advantage over rigid implants because its inherent flexibility permits it to adjust to the pathological axis of rotation with minimal resistance; the mobility of the arthroplastic stems confirmed by cinefluoroscopy permits further adjustments in the position and alignment of the implant. Swanson's observation of cases over a period of more than 7 years has confirmed excellent tolerance by the host tissues to the implant which is an excellent indication of its biomechanical acceptability. At surgery reinforcement of the joint capsule, and balancing the musculotendinous system are essential provisions to realize a stable and durable arthroplasty.

The implant has been used as an adjunct to resectional arthroplasty of the wrist in patients who have demonstrated marked instability of the wrist joint with absorptive changes of the proximal carpal row and subluxation of the radiocarpal joint. The implant serves as a temporary scaffold to maintain an adequate joint space with appropriate alignment during the regeneration of a new capsuloligamentous system. So far the degree of stability and mobility, durability and biological tolerance obtained with this technique has been most encouraging.

Indications. The wrist implant arthroplasty is indicated in cases of instability of the wrist due to subluxation or dislocation of the radiocarpal joint, severe deviation of the wrist causing musculotendinous imbalance of the digits, stiffness or fusion of the wrist in a nonfunctional position, and stiffness of a wrist when motion is a requirement for hand function.[185]

Reconstruction of the wrist should be performed prior to any reconstructive surgery on the finger joints. The procedure is contraindicated in young patients with open epiphyses, in those with inadequate skin, bone or neurovascular system and those who show irreparable tendon damage. The technique is not recommended for patients who are heavy manual workers.

Procedure. A straight longitudinal or a gentle curved incision seen in Figure 14-17A is made over the dorsum of the wrist, with careful preservation of the superficial sensory nerves. The extensor retinaculum is incised to provide a radially based flap between the first and second dorsal compartments (Fig. 14-18A). Another retinacular ligament flap can be prepared to relocate the extensor carpi ulnaris tendon in associated implant reconstructions of the ulnar head. Synovectomy of the extensor compartments is performed with minimal disruption or removal of adjacent soft tissues. The dorsal capsuloligamentous structures are reflected carefully from the radius as a distally based flap for the subsequent capsular repair.

A part of the proximal carpal row is usually resorbed and the remnants are displaced palmarward on the radius. Resection of the residual lunate and scaphoid bones is carefully done with a rongeur or air drill (Fig. 14-17B). In certain cases the distal pole of the scaphoid can be left *in situ*. Injury to the underlying tendons and neurovascular structures should be avoided. The end of the radius is squared off to abut against the distal carpal row (Fig. 14-18B). A portion of the base of the capitate and the triquetrum is removed. The distal row of carpal bones should be left intact because of their vital stabilization of the metacarpal bases. The radiocarpal subluxation should be completely reduced.

The intramedullary canal of the radius is prepared with a broach, curet or air drill to receive the proximal stem of the implant. If there has been a marked radiocarpal dislocation with subsequent soft tissue contracture, it is preferable

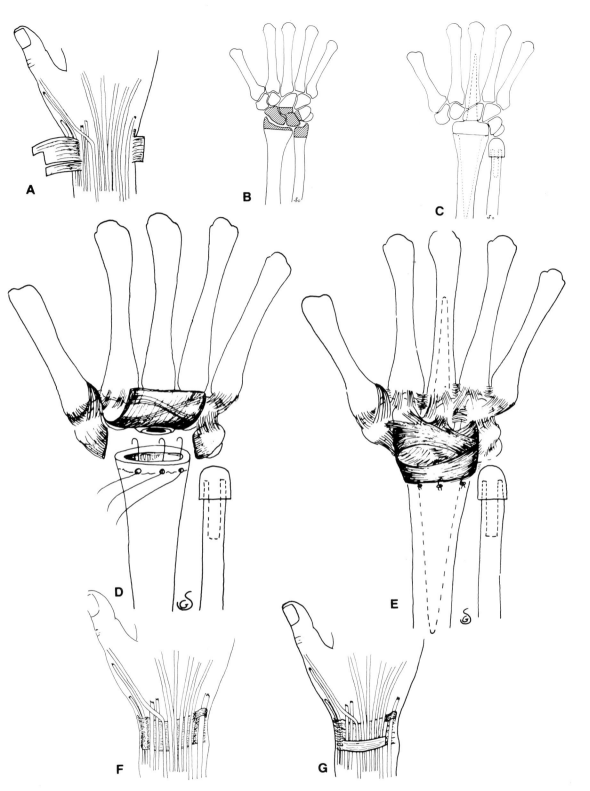

Figure 14-18. *A* to *G*. Technique for total wrist joint replacement devised by Swanson. Figure 14-18*D* A distally based radiocarpal flap is made by careful elevation of the dorsal capsuloligamentous structures from the underlying radius and carpal bones. For the subsequent repair procedure small drill holes are prepared in the dorsal cortex of the radius. Figure 14-18*E* The radiocarpal capsuloligamentous flap is firmly sutured over the wrist implant by the use of 3-0 Dacron sutures with an inverted knot technique. (*A* to *G*, reproduced with permission of A. B. Swanson.[185])

to shorten the distal radius rather than remove more of the carpal bones. The distal stem of the implant fits through the capitate bone into the intramedullary canal of the third metacarpal (Fig. 14-18C). The intramedullary canal of the third metacarpal is prepared by carefully passing a wire or thin broach through the capitate bone, the base of the metacarpal and into its canal. A Kirschner wire can be passed into the metacarpal and out through its head to verify the intramedullary orientation. The bones are usually thin and this preparation is performed quite easily. An air drill may be used for the final reaming procedure.

The distal ulna is trimmed about 1 cm shorter than the distal end of the radius and capped with a silicone rubber ulnar head implant (Fig. 14-18C). The hand is then centralized over the radius. The proximal stem of the wrist joint implant is inserted first into the intramedullary canal of the radius and the distal stem is then introduced through the capitate and into the intramedullary canal of the third metacarpal. Enough bone should have been removed so that extension of the wrist is possible on passive manipulation. Usually 1.0 to 1.5 cm of separation between the bone ends is adequate. The capsuloligamentous structures are firmly sutured over the implant. Sutures are passed through small drill holes in the dorsal cortex of the radius (Fig. 14-18 D and E) to assure a good capsular fixation. On passive manipulation the repair should permit approximately 45° of extension and flexion and 10° of ulnar and radial deviation.

The previously prepared extensor retinacular flap is replaced over the wrist joint and under the extensor tendons where it is sutured to augment capsular support (Fig. 14-18F). The tension in the extensor tendons across the wrist joint is evaluated. The tendons are shortened or transferred as necessary to obtain wrist extension without lateral deviation. The extensor carpi radialis longus tendon may be transferred under the extensor carpi radialis brevis tendon and attached to the third metacarpal by a suture through the bone or interwoven into the brevis tendon's distal attachment. The extensor tendons of the digits are repaired if necessary. A tendon transfer of a flexor superficialis muscle readily permits the reconstruction of a ruptured extensor digitorum communis tendon. If isolated extensor tendons are ruptured, side-to-side anastomosis can be performed. A ruptured extensor pollicis longus tendon can be repaired by transferring the extensor indicis proprius tendon. The reconstruction of the distal radioulnar joint is completed by using a retinacular flap from the sixth dorsal compartment to relocate dorsally the extensor carpi ulnaris tendon (Fig. 14-18G). Figure 14-19 A and B show radiological views of a rheumatoid wrist prior to and after a wrist arthroplasty.

The wound is closed in layers and a drain or a suction drainage system is inserted subcutaneously. The usual voluminous conforming hand dressing including a plaster splint is applied with the wrist in neutral position. The extremity is maintained in an elevated position for 3 to 5 days with an arm sling, while the patient remains at bed rest. A short arm cast, with the wrist in a neutral position, is then applied. If tendons have been repaired the cast is fitted with outriggers and rubber band slings to maintain the fingers in extension. About 2 to 4 weeks of immobilization provides a satisfactory compromise of stability and mobility with an optimum of about 50% of normal flexion and extension.

Postoperative Care. Following removal of his cast the patient starts an exercise problem to encourage active flexion and extension of the wrist. If the wrist is excessively tight gentle active and passive stretching exercises are undertaken. If extensor tendons have been repaired, extension of the fingers is maintained by the outrigger devices attached to the cast or a dynamic brace.

Materials and Method

A series of 76 wrists reconstructed with the flexible hinge radiocarpal implant arthroplasty method is presented in this study. The procedures were performed in 59 patients, 17 with bilateral wrist reconstructions. There were 45 female and 14 male patients whose ages ranged from 20 to 74 years with an average age of 53. There were 63 cases of rheumatoid arthritis, 3 of psoriatic arthritis, 2 of scleroderma, 6 of osteoarthritis, and the sequelae of poliomyelitis in one wrist and of arthrogryposis in another. The duration of the pathological processes ranged from 4 to 52 years for an average duration of 19 years. Follow-up was less than 6 months in 8 cases, from 6 months to 1 year in 12 wrists, 1 to 2 years in 21 wrists, 2 to 3 years in 17 wrists and greater than 3 years in 18 wrists. For this group of 56 cases in whom the follow-up ranged from 12 to 91 months, the average follow-up was 34 months. Before and after surgery the patients were thoroughly assessed on specially prepared forms. The anatomical evaluation included measurements of grasp strength and range of motion.

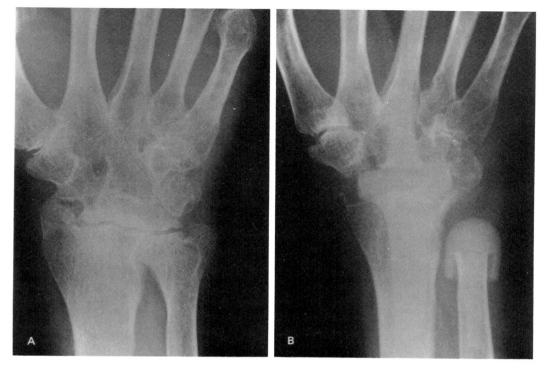

Figure 14-19. *A.* The preoperative X-ray of a painful rheumatoid arthritic wrist joint in a 40-year-old male is seen. *B.* The postoperative X-ray was taken 1 year after the patient underwent proximal row resection and flexible implant arthroplasty of the radiocarpal and distal radioulnar joints. At that time the patient has returned to a useful occupation with a pain-free wrist that shows a functional range of motion. (*A* and *B*, reproduced with permission of A. B. Swanson[185].)

The functional evaluation included rating and questioning the patients on their performance of activities of daily living, as well as on pain and cosmetic improvement. Radiograms and cinefluoroscopy taken before surgery and serially after surgery also were available for analysis.

A total of 30 wrists were operated with implants made of silicone elastomer No. 372 and 46 with implants made of high performance silicone elastomer. The ulnar head implant was not used in 23 of the 76 reconstructed wrists, including five osteoarthritic wrists and one wrist deformed by poliomyelitis but with preservation of the distal radioulnar joint. Three rheumatoid wrists presented with severe resorption of the distal ulna equivalent to a Darrach procedure while four rheumatoid wrists showed no significant disability of this joint. Ten rheumatoid wrists had had a previous resectional arthroplastic procedure of the distal radioulnar joint with relatively good results of which two later presented with pain and instability. At present it appears that arthroplasty should be undertaken concurrent with the ulnar head implant radiocarpal joint reconstruction in the rheumatoid wrist.

Associated Tendon Surgery. Associated tendon reconstruction was required in 24 of the 76 wrists with the following procedures: repair of the extensor carpi radialis brevis and longus tendons in two cases; transfer of the brachioradialis tendon to the wrist extensors in one case; transfer of the extensor carpi radialis longus to the base of the third metacarpal in one case; transfer of the extensor carpi radialis longus to the extensor carpi radialis brevis by interweaving the tendons in three cases; repair of a ruptured extensor pollicis longus by transfer of the indicis proprius tendon in three wrists; transfer of the extensor carpi ulnaris to the extensor digitorum in three wrists; transfer of the flexor superficialis tendon of the ring finger to the extensor digitorum in four cases; side-to-side transfer of the tendons of the extensor digitorum in three cases; rerouting of the extensor carpi ulnaris as a routine in all cases; repair of the ruptured extensor carpi ulnaris in two cases; lengthening of a contracted flexor carpi ulnaris in two wrists.

Results

Pain. The pain was classified according to the degree which it interferes with the individual's performance of his activities as follows: (1) Minimal, an annoyance; (2) mild, interferes with activity; (3) moderate, prevents activity; (4) severe, prevents activity and also causes distress.

Preoperatively there was no pain in 16% of the wrists, mild pain in 20%, moderate pain in 49% and severe pain in 15% of the wrists. After surgery a remarkable improvement was noted: 89% of the operated wrists were pain free, while 8% had mild pain and 3% moderate pain on prolonged activity while none had severe pain.

Cosmetic. The cosmetic improvement was rated numerically at rest and with activity by both the patient and the examiner. A minimum improvement was given 1 point, moderate improvement 2 points, and marked improvement 3 points. The maximum of 12 points corresponds to a marked improvement (3 points) both at rest and with activity from the patient's and examiner's observations. In the 76 operated wrists, the postoperative cosmetic improvement ranged from 6 to 12 points for an average of 9.8 points.

Range of Motion. The preoperative and postoperative ranges of motion for the 76 reconstructed wrists have been documented in detail elsewhere.[189] Extension showed the greatest improvement with a gain of 15°. The average degree of pronation, radial deviation and flexion were also improved postoperatively. The average supination of 57° and ulnar deviation of 18° show little or no change as compared to the preoperative values and are highly functional values.

Strength of Grasp. The grasp strength, measured before and after surgery with a Jamar hydraulic dynamometer, averaged 7 lb preoperatively and 12 lb postoperatively. This group of rheumatoid arthritics possessed a variable degree of digital and tendinous involvement which can compromise substantially the power of grasp. The moderate increase of recorded strength is related to the improved position, stability and freedom of pain of the wrist.

Radiological Survey. Postoperative radiograms of the wrist were routinely reviewed and compared at 3 months, 6 months and yearly intervals. The films were evaluated for evidence of recurrent deformity, loss of the joint space, bone resorption around the stems or at the junc-

tion of the implant midsection. Bone production around the stems or at the midsection level was evaluated.

The development of a thin bone plate around the intramedullary stems of the implant and a smooth remodeling of bone next to the midsection was seen routinely. There was one case with bone growth across the midsection of the implant to form a fusion of the wrist in a scleroderma patient. An adequate joint space was maintained in all the other wrists. There were no cases of increasing bone absorption around a stem or midsection of an implant. In two cases the distal stem of the implant was not properly fitted in the third metacarpal and protruded through its side wall. There were no significant clinical or radiological consequences from this technical error.

Complications and Revision Procedures. There were no postoperative infections. A delay in wound healing requiring no secondary procedure was noted in three wrists, two with rheumatoid arthritis and one with psoriatic arthritis.

Postoperative problems requiring a revision procedure were necessary in eight wrists among seven patients. There were three fractured implants made of the original elastomer, one case of tendon imbalance with recurrent ulnar deviation and four cases of tendon imbalance and recurrent synovitis.

Discussion

The flexible intramedullary stemmed wrist joint implant is a worthwhile adjunct to resectional arthroplasty procedures in cases of severely involved and unstable rheumatoid arthritic wrists. Clinically, it maintains the relationship of the carpus and radius and allows motion of the wrist joint in all planes. The formation of a surrounding capsuloligamentous system provides adequate stability of the rheumatoid wrist. The functional adaptation of the rheumatoid hand is facilitated by the movement and good stability of the arthroplastic wrist.

A stable essentially pain-free wrist was obtained in all of the cases. The average motion recorded was 21° of extension and 41° of flexion. One patient had 50° of dorsiflexion and 60° of palmar flexion. Ideally, a range of motion of 45° of dorsiflexion and 45° of palmar flexion, with 10° of radial and ulnar deviation should be achieved. Where finger joint reconstruction is indicated arthroplasty of the wrist should precede them. While some of the patients have returned to manual occupations in factory and office jobs not requiring heavy lifting, arthroplasty of the wrist in heavy laborers has been discouraged. One patient with bilateral wrist arthroplasties for degenerative arthritis has returned to his job as a welder.

Between 1972 and 1978 more than 600 cases have been performed elsewhere which are documented in a variable degree. They indicate mostly satisfactory results as reported by both patients and physicians. These patients have had a pain-free wrist with functional mobility and stability. An important and unique asset of silicone implant arthroplasty is the absence of methylmethacrylate cement or of significant bone resection so that infected or failed arthroplasties may be treated by removal or replacement of the implant, as indicated, or they may be fused with the addition of bone graft.

Flexible implant resection arthroplasty of the wrist appears to have an established place in the reconstruction of the upper extremity with decided advantages over arthrodesis, pseudarthrodesis, or other arthroplasty procedures.

METACARPOPHALANGEAL JOINT REPLACEMENTS

Metacarpophalangeal joint arthroplasty using the flexible silicone rubber prosthesis or certain hinge-type prostheses is a reliable and effective method for the treatment of various painful and deforming conditions affecting the metacarpophalangeal joint. Initially the technique was developed for the treatment of rheumatoid arthritis although more recently the operation has been extended to various other arthritides. For over a decade the use of the inert flexible silastic rubber implant has proven to be both effective and long lasting. While the optimal results of surgery do not recreate the extraordinary capabilities of normal metacarpophalangeal joints, nevertheless the results of surgery are impressive when the formidable problems of soft tissue reconstruction around the damaged joints are considered.[190] Unlike the reconstruction of an arthritic hip, comparable procedures on finger joints rest heavily on the surgeon's capacity to restore alignment of the joint and to correct a variety of deforming forces. The history of metacarpophalangeal joint arthroplasty is outlined in Chapter 13. Several general considerations arise before planning implant arthroplasty for the hand especially in patients with rheumatoid arthritis. Prior to surgical reconstruction the rheumatoid patient should receive appropriate medical management with careful supervision. As a general rule major reconstruction of the

lower extremities should be complete prior to reconstruction of the hand.[187] If the patient requires crutches for walking platform crutches should be used in preference to axillary crutches to limit the otherwise severe deforming forces that act across the wrist joints. Reconstruction of the upper extremity and the hand should be started proximally with distal progression. The shoulder and elbow should be painfree and mobile so that the hand can be effectively placed by the patient. Where necessary these joints should be reconstructed with synovectomy, debridement or arthroplasty. The wrist must be stable, anatomically aligned and functional. Where necessary, fusion or arthroplasty should be performed. A prominent painful ulnar head should be realigned or excised in view of its deleterious effects on forearm rotation and participation in extensor tendon rupture. Significant flexor or extensor tenosynovitis with or without tendon rupture should be treated with appropriate surgery prior to implant arthroplasty in the hand. Functional musculotendinous units are essential if postoperative exercises after implant arthroplasty are to be performed satisfactorily.

The surgeon must be realistic both with himself and with the patient in the goals that are to be realized. Many rheumatoid patients with multiple deformities in their upper extremities achieve remarkable "trick" movements whereby their functional status is surprisingly good despite severe destruction of their musculoskeletal elements. Previously many surgeons have undertaken numerous reconstructive procedures in such extremities which provided superior cosmesis but with markedly impaired functional capacity of the limb. Even in the presence of grotesque deformities of a rheumatoid hand, the surgeon should strongly consider the likelihood for *functional* improvement before embarking upon extensive reconstructive surgical procedures.

Millender and Nalebuff[191] have devised a useful preoperative classification of metacarpophalangeal joint deformities which is shown in Table 14-4. The classification provides both a useful preoperative evaluation and a realistic prediction for the postoperative result. Type A represents the simple type which gives the best postoperative results. While ulnar deviation may be present the remainder of the hand is minimally involved. After surgery 60 to 80° of metacarpophalangeal joint flexion may be achieved with nearly full extension and excellent alignment and stability. Type B represents the complicated

Table 14-4
Classification of Metacarpophalangeal Joint Deformities

Type A
  Simple (metacarpophalangeal joint dislocation without complicating factors)
Type B
  Complicated
    B-1 Metacarpophalangeal joint dislocation with stiff proximal interphalangeal joints
    B-2 Metacarpophalangeal joint dislocation with proximal interphalangeal joint destruction
    B-3 Metacarpophalangeal joint dislocation with fixed flexion contractures and proximal migration of the proximal phalanx
    B-4 Metacarpophalangeal joint dislocation with extensor tendon ruptures
    B-5 Metacarpophalangeal joint arthroplasty after previous metacarpophalangeal joint surgery
    B-6 Metacarpophalangeal joint arthroplasty with postoperative infection

problems associated with metacarpophalangeal joint dislocation. The associated problems can range from minor to exceedingly complicated with markedly deformed hands. Occasionally only salvage surgery is practical as a realistic goal. Millender and Nalebuff have delineated the appropriate ancillary procedures that should be undertaken for each of the types of complicating factors. Surgeons are strongly advised to familarize themselves with such a format before they undertake metacarpophalangeal joint reconstruction. A more critical analysis of the anatomy and kinesiology of the hand is fully documented elsewhere.[192-195]

Indications and Contraindications for Metacarpophalangeal Joint Replacement[196]

For patients with rheumatoid arthritis the indications are: (1) Pain; (2) destruction of the articular surfaces; (3) volar subluxation and ulnar deviation that is not passively correctable; and (4) loss of functional motion.

In patients with degenerative arthritis of the hand the interphalangeal joints are much more frequently involved than the metacarpophalangeal joints. Occasionally prosthetic replacement of the metacarpophalangeal joints is indicated after traumatic arthritis. The particular indications include pain, complete articular destruction, severe loss of functional motion and gross instability. Resectional arthroplasty is contrain-

dicated after the presence of infection in the joint. Other prerequisites for implant arthroplasty include healthy skin, a co-operative patient, intact neurovascular structures of the digit, functional extensor and flexor tendons or alternative methods for their reconstruction, and a surgeon knowledgeable in reconstructive hand surgery.

The contraindications for implant arthroplasty include unhealthy dorsal or volar skin, inadequate bone stock such as is seen in patients with Still's disease, rapidly progressive or ankylosing types of rheumatoid arthritis, stiff finger joints associated with various types of mucopolysaccharidoses and severely deformed hands that are painless and functional.

Surgical Technique. Metacarpophalangeal joint arthroplasty requires a complete set of instruments with a full complement of prostheses and testers, medullary canal reamers and small plastic surgical instruments.[196] The surgery may be performed under general or regional anesthesia but a pneumatic tourniquet should be employed. A transverse incision is made over the metacarpophalangeal joints as seen in (Fig. 14-20*A*). In nonrheumatoid patients where a single joint is involved, a longitudinal incision is used. The dorsal neurovascular structures are preserved and the extensor mechanism is carefully cleared of areolar tissue. Where the extensor tendon is dislocated into the intermetacarpal valley it is elevated with a sharp skin hook and the ulnar saggital fibers are cut. Subsequently the extensor tendon usually can be released easily from its dislocated position. The ulnar border of the extensor tendon (Fig. 14-20*B*) is incised proximally to free the tendon from any inner tendinous connections to the next ulnar tendon. A small curved hemostat is placed under the ulnar wing intrinsic tendon which is divided (Fig. 14-20*C*). After adequate release of the ulnar intrinsic tendons each extensor tendon can be dissected easily from the underlying capsule to which it may have become adherent. The extensor mechanisms are retracted radially into the adjacent intermetacarpal spaces. As seen in Figure 14-20*D*, proliferative synovium is sharply excised.

In some instances bony erosion and destruction of the phalanx by synovial proliferation provokes erosion of the dorsal cortex of the phalanx and the formation of an exostosis along the lateral border of the phalanx. In these cases, the phalangeal base must be flattened to receive the prosthetic stem and to lessen the likelihood of its subsequent dislocation.

After the ulnar intrinsic muscles have been sectioned and the metacarpal head and the proximal end of the adjacent phalanx have been excised (Fig. 14-20E) the proximal interphalangeal joint stiffness can be evaluated (type B-1 complications after Millender and Nalebuff[191]). Usually gentle manipulation of the proximal interphalangeal joint liberates the adhesions of the lateral band and permits the joint to be flexed to 90°. Subsequently the proximal interphalangeal joints are placed in flexion and held with a percutaneous Kirschner wire. In more difficult cases, formal lateral band releases seen in Figure 14-20F, are required to mobilize the proximal interphalangeal joints.

After soft tissue release has been completed the medullary cavity of the metacarpal is reamed and the cartilaginous end plate of the phalanx is perforated with an awl and the medullary cavity is reamed. Alternatively a small straight hemostat may be inserted forcefully into the intramedullary cavity to shape it appropriately (Fig. 14-20F). The ends of the medullary canal should be squared with a rectangular instrument or osteotome to inhibit rotation of the implant within the canal. The prosthesis is tested and the largest prosthesis that fits loosely into the intramedullary cavity is chosen. The stem of the implant should fit loosely into the canal with its base abutting the bony end plate. Adjustments in the seating can be undertaken by further reaming or selection of the next smaller size of implant. The alignment of the finger should be scrutinized and the digit should be manipulated through a complete range of motion. After the correct size of implant is selected the space is irrigated with antibiotic solution and a silastic prosthesis is inserted with a no-touch technique (Fig. 14-20G). The no-touch technique prevents contamination with lint or talc which might provoke a late foreign body reaction. The prosthesis is handled with smooth forceps to prevent superficial scratching that could initiate subsequent fatigue fracture.[198]

After insertion of all of the prostheses the digits should be correctly aligned. If a deformity is observed the implant is removed and appropriate adjustments are made. With the prosthesis properly seated and the digit aligned closure is undertaken. If adequate capsule is available it is closed to supplement the stability of the digit. The radial portion of the capsule including the radial collateral ligament is repaired to the dorsal aspect of the periosteum. The repair maintains the digit in neutral alignment with extension of the joint. The extensor tendon is aligned over the center of the joint and the attenuated radial sagittal fibers are reefed (Fig. 14-20H).

The tourniquet is released and hemostasis is obtained by electrocautery, irrigation and pressure. The skin is closed with minimal tension by the use of interrupted 5-0 nylon sutures. A bulky soft dressing is applied with a volar plaster splint across the wrist. The wrist is positioned in slight extension and the digits are aligned with the metacarpal joints in increasing flexion from the index to the small finger.

Postoperative Care. A meticulous postoperative program is essential for metacarpophalangeal joint arthroplasty. Initially the hand is elevated for 24 to 48 hours although proximal interphalangeal joint motion may be encouraged. By the fifth postoperative day swelling has subsided and a molded plaster resting splint and a dynamic splint are fabricated.[199] The resting splint secures the metacarpophalangeal joints with an increasing amount of flexion from the index to the fourth fingers. The dynamic splint is adjusted to maintain proper alignment of the digits and enables the patient to exercise against a dorsal outrigger. The resting splint is worn by night while the dynamic splint is worn most of the day. Exercises are recommended several minutes every hour and are prolonged as the postoperative period continues. The splinting regimen is maintained for 3 to 4 weeks. Subsequently, if the fingers are well aligned and show no tendency toward an extension lag or axial deviation, splinting is gradually decreased over the next 2 to 3 weeks. The resting splint should be used for at least 8 weeks after surgery while the dynamic splint is recommended for three to four applications per day for 10 to 12 weeks after surgery.

The most unpredictable result of surgery is the range of flexion that may be achieved. A result of 40 to 80° of flexion may be anticipated. Variable factors include the patient's propensity to form scar tissue and the surgeon's adherence to operative details and the extent of rheumatoid or traumatic damage to extra-articular soft tissues.

By the use of a somewhat similar technique, silicone-Dacron (Niebauer-Cutter) finger joint prostheses have been developed in which anchorage of the prosthesis is achieved by ingrowth of tissue into the porous Dacron sleeve. As Urbaniak[197] relates the general principles of reconstruction are similar to the use of silicone spacers and the same attention to soft tissue reconstruction is essential. The surgical exposure of the joints is comparable to that previously de-

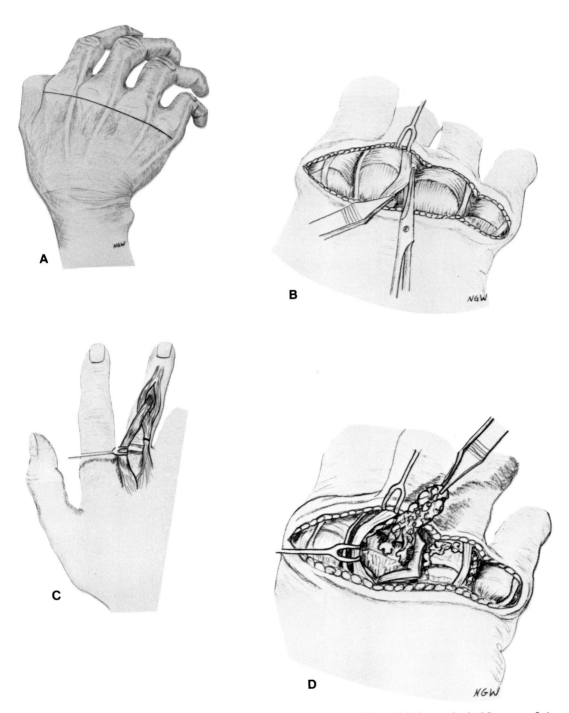

Figure 14-20A to H. Technique for metacarpophalangeal joint arthroplasty with the method of Swanson. I. A method for anchorage of the extensor tendon after metacarpophalangeal joint arthroplasty. A is the metacarpal head, B is the proximal end of the proximal phalanx, C is the extensor tendon, and D is a tongue of dorsal capsule. (I, reproduced with permission of J. R. Urbaniak.[197])

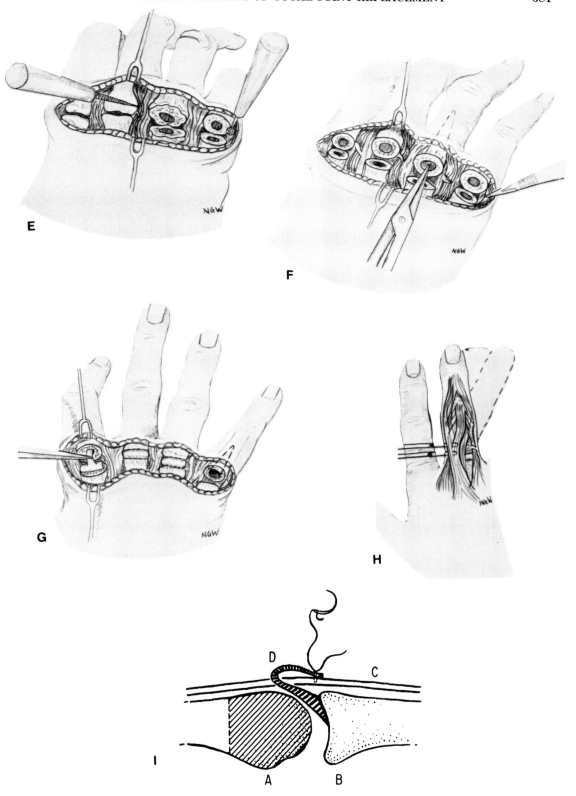

scribed. The implants may be anchored by the insertion of a nonabsorbable suture through the Dacron portion of the stem and into the periosteum or through small drill holes of the metacarpal or phalanx just proximal to the shoulder of the implant. This step prevents subsequent subluxation or dislocation of the implant which may follow closure of the wound or application of the postoperative dressing. Urbaniak,[197] also describes a method for anchorage of the extensor tendon in the midaxis of the joint. A portion of the dorsal capsule (Fig. 14-20I) is tapered until it fits through a slit in the extensor tendon to which it is sutured. This procedure, originally described by McCollum et al.,[200] provides an upward stabilizing force on the proximal phalanx and helps to centralize the extensor tendon while permitting functional excursion of the extensor mechanism.

Insertion of the Steffie Prosthesis in Metacarpophalangeal Joints*

The relative merits of fully stabilized articulations, such as a cemented hinge, and a mobile, flexible spacer, such as a Swanson prosthesis, are fully reviewed in Chapter 13. The former provides superior stability for the digit. It is essential, however, that the rigorously stabilized arthroplasty shows an axis of rotation concentric with that of the supporting soft tissues. Otherwise excessive bending moments are imposed upon the functional digit and mechanical failure or migration of the prosthesis is likely to occur. The Steffie prosthesis is a cemented hinge-like articulation for reconstruction of the metacarpophalangeal joint. In light of its polycentric concept, it replicates abduction and adduction of the extended anatomical joint. While its period of application has been insufficient to provide a well documented clinical series, nevertheless, the early clinical impressions suggest highly satisfactory results. The indications and contraindications for its application are comparable to those for the use of silicone spacers.

Procedure. A dorsal transverse skin incision is made superficial to the metacarpal necks. The incision is extended through the subcutaneous tissue to the extensor tendons. During the dissection, care is taken to preserve the dorsal veins. The extensor hood mechanism is exposed over each of the metacarpal heads and necks. The distal skin flap is elevated to the base of the proximal phalanges. Each extensor tendon is

retracted in a radial direction. A longitudinal incision is made in the extensor hood on its ulnar aspect, parallel to the tendon. The tendon is elevated sharply from the underlying joint capsule and retracted to the radial aspect of the joint. The ulnar lateral band is dissected from adjacent soft tissues and sharply released. While the extensor tendon is retracted to the radial side of the joint, a longitudinal incision is made in the capsule and synovium of the metacarpophalangeal joint. The capsule is dissected sharply to the radial and ulnar aspects respectively. Each metacarpal neck is dissected free of soft tissues and transected with either an osteotome or an air drill. After a metacarpal head has been removed, any tight soft tissues on the palmar or ulnar aspects of the base of the proximal phalanx are released. The abductor digiti minimi and flexor digiti minimi tendons inserting on the ulnar aspect of the proximal phalanx of the small finger are incised sharply and released. At the completion of the soft tissue release the fingers should not deviate spontaneously into ulnar drift. When the soft tissue release is completed the proximal phalanges can be exposed by flexion of the digits and retraction of the extensor mechanisms. With an osteotome or air drill, the canal of each proximal phalanx is penetrated. The canal is reamed using a burr on the air drill. Once the bone has been prepared, the Steffie implant can be tested both in the metacarpal and in the proximal phalanx. After the proper size has been selected, methylmethacrylate cement is mixed and placed down the metacarpal shaft and the shaft of the proximal phalanx simultaneously. As the cement hardens, the implant is positioned in the metacarpal shaft and then in the proximal phalanx. At this stage, prior to solidification of the methylmethacrylate, it is crucial to ensure correct rotational alignment of the finger.

When arthroplasties are performed on multiple digits, the cement may be inserted simultaneously into two of the digital bones with adequate time to seat the prostheses. Once the cement has hardened and the prostheses are stabilized, each extensor hood is reefed on its radial side with two or three overlapping mattress sutures of 4-0 nylon. Subsequently, the tourniquet is deflated, bleeding is controlled, and the skin is closed with interrupted 5-0 nylon sutures. The patient is placed in a bulky soft dressing with a plaster splint surrounded by bias cut stockinet or an ace bandage. At 5 days the dressings are changed and active motion exercises of the digits are started. The vigorous ex-

---

* This section was provided by Joseph E. Imbriglia.

ercise program is supervised by a trained therapist.

Figure 14-21A to D shows preoperative and intraoperative photographs and an X-ray of a rheumatoid hand with ulnar drift and destruction of the metacarpophalangeal joints. In Figure 14-21D, a postoperative X-ray reveals the presence of the Steffie prostheses in the realigned fingers.

Proximal Interphalangeal Joint Implant Arthroplasty

Generally proximal interphalangeal implant arthroplasty is employed for patients with degenerative or traumatic arthritis. In patients with rheumatoid arthritis who show severe involvement of the metacarpophalangeal and proximal phalangeal joints replacement arthroplasty of the metacarpal joints and soft tissue reconstruction or fusions of the proximal interphalangeal joints is usually preferred.[199] If the metacarpophalangeal joints are functional and painless the severely affected proximal interphalangeal joints may be reconstructed by implant arthroplasty. Rarely is there an indication for implant arthroplasty of both the metacarpophalangeal and proximal interphalangeal joints in the same digit. In fact, patients with metacarpophalangeal joint implant arthroplasty with limited proximal interphalangeal joint motion commonly obtain greater motion at the metacarpophalangeal joints.

For patients with degenerative arthritis of the hands which involves proximal interphalangeal joints implant arthroplasty is indicated if there is instability, articular destruction, lateral deviation, subluxation or pain. If the patient is young and requires a strong grip for his occupation, interphalangeal joint arthrodesis is usually preferable. In the young patient with post-traumatic arthritis of the proximal interphalangeal joint, a volar capsule interposition arthroplasty may restore motion and function. If severe destruction of the tendon complex and neurovascular structures exists, deletion of the digit provides a more useful hand. Other prerequisites and contraindications for proximal interphalangeal joint arthroplasty are similar to those listed for metacarpophalangeal joints.

Surgical Technique Devised by Swanson. A curved longitudinal incision (Fig. 14-22A) is made over the dorsum of the joint with care taken to protect the dorsal veins. A midlateral incision is employed when associated surgery of the flexor tendon mechanism is also indicated.

The extensor mechanism is exposed by blunt atraumatic dissection. The extensor tendon is identified and incised longitudinally (Fig. 14-22B) from its insertion on the base of the middle phalanx proximally along the distal two-thirds of the proximal phalanx. When there is a flexion deformity of the joint, each half of the extensor mechanism can be gently dislocated volarward as the joint is flexed. The collateral ligaments are released from their attachments to the proximal phalanx but the insertion of each half of the central tendon into the middle phalanx is not disturbed. If there is a contracture of the joint so that the extensor mechanism cannot be readily dislocated, the head of the proximal phalanx may be excised first by making a transverse osteotomy through the neck with an air drill and then moving the fragmented phalangeal head. Adequate release of the joint is essential. A moderate flexion contracture is released by incision of the volar plate and collateral ligaments at their insertions proximally. If there is a severe contracture of the collateral ligament, the accessory collateral ligaments and palmar plate are carefully and completely excised.

After resection of the head of the proximal phalanx (Fig. 14-22C) and soft tissue release the intramedullary canal of the proximal phalanx is carefully reamed with an air drill of special configuration to avoid perforation through the cortex. The canal is shaped to accept the rectangular stem of the implant. The intramedullary cavity of the middle phalanx is prepared in a similar way. The base of the middle phalanx is not resected but osteophytes are trimmed if present.

The proximal stem of the Swanson prosthesis is inserted after which the joint is flexed and the distal stem is inserted into the middle phalanx (Fig. 14-22D). The implant sizes 0, 1, 2, 3 are used most frequently for the proximal interphalangeal joint arthroplasty. The largest implant size that will fit properly is employed. The bone ends are trimmed smoothly to remove sharp edges that might damage the implant. The midsection of the implant should seat well against the adjacent surfaces of the phalanges. With the joint in extension the bone ends should not impinge on the midsection of the implant. Impingement is corrected by further soft tissue release or additional bony resection. Once an implant is well fitted throughout a passive range of motion of the joint, the incised extensor tendon mechanism is reapproximated and sutured with 4-0 Dacron or other nonabsorbable suture (Fig. 14-22E). The tourniquet is released and

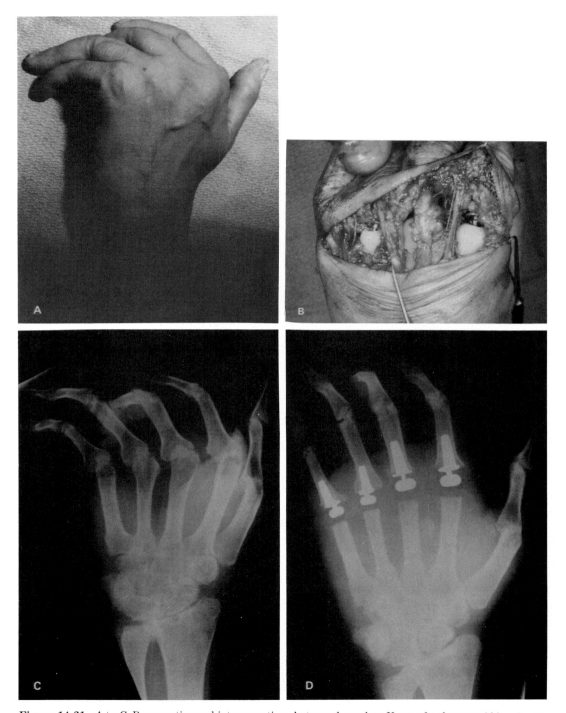

Figure 14-21. *A* to *C.* Preoperative and intraoperative photographs and an X-ray of a rheumatoid hand with ulnar drift and destruction of the metacarpophalangeal joints. *D.* The postoperative X-ray reveals the hand after arthroplastic reconstruction of the metacarpophalangeal joints with Steffie prostheses. (Reproduced with permission of J. E. Imbriglia.)

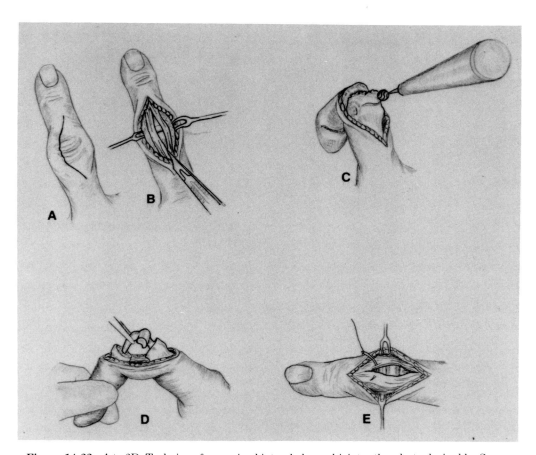

Figure 14-22. *A* to 2D. Technique for proximal interphalangeal joint arthroplasty devised by Swanson.

hemostasis is obtained prior to skin closure. The digit is splintered and a bulky compression dressing with the proximal interphalangeal joint in full extension and the metacarpophalangeal joint in flexion.

Postoperative Management. The bulky dressing can be removed on the third day and active movements of flexion and extension are started within 3 to 5 days after surgery. The objective of arthroplastic surgery is an active range of motion from 0° of extension to 70° of flexion. For the exercises the proximal phalanx is supported with a modified lumbrical bar attached to a dynamic brace or cast. The exercise device hinders motion at the metacarpophalangeal joint and augments the flexion power of the proximal interphalangeal joint. A padded aluminum resting splint is used to hold the digit in extension when the dynamic splint is removed. The resting splint is used at night for 3 to 6 weeks after surgery. Active flexion exercises and isometric exercises are continued for at least 3 months after surgery.

Complications after Arthroplasty of the Metacarpophalangeal or the Proximal Interphalangeal Joints

Most of the complications after implant resection arthroplasty arise as a result of errors in preoperative assessment or from technical limitations in the soft tissue reconstruction. Residual deformities around the arthroplastic joint are likely to progress, particularly if more proximal joints such as the wrist have not previously been adequately realigned. Excessive soft tissue trauma or damage to the critical dorsal veins may culminate in a slough of skin superficial to the implant; adjacent soft tissue structures also can be damaged at surgery. Infection of the arthroplastic joint is uncommon unless the dorsal skin flaps are compromised. Late fracture of the silicone implants occurs primarily when inadequate realignment of the digit is realized.[197] Fractured implants are readily replaced although appropriate realignment should be undertaken to correct preoperative deformity.

REFERENCES

1. Charnley, J., and Cupic, Z. *Clin. Orthop., 95:*9, 1973.
2. Muller, M. E. Late complications of total hip replacement. In *The Hip* p. 319, edited by W. H. Harris, C. V. Mosby Co. St. Louis, 1974.
3. Eftekhar, N. S. *Clin. Orthop., 121:*120, 1976.
4. DeHaven, K. E., Evarts, C. M., Wilde, A. H., Collins, H. R., Nelson, C., and Razzano, C. D. *Orthop. Clin. N. Am., 4:*465, 1973.
5. Gschwend, N., and Debrunner, H. U. (editors). *Total Hip Prosthesis,* p. 95, H. Haber Verlag, Berne, 1977.
6. Charnley, J. *J. Bone Jt. Surg., 54B:*61, 1972.
7. Halley, D. K., and Charnley, J. *Clin. Orthop., 112:*180, 1975.
8. McKee, G. K. *Clin. Orthop., 72:*85, 1970.
9. Watson-Farrar, J. Total hip replacement in rheumatoid arthritis and Marie-Strümpell arthritis of the hip. In *Surgery of Rheumatoid Arthritis,* p. 69, edited by R. L. Cruess and N. S. Mitchell, J. B. Lippincott, Philadelphia, 1971.
10. Amstutz, H. C. The biomechanics of total hip replacement. In *Surgical Management of Degenerative Arthritis of the Lower Limb* p. 82, edited by R. L. Cruess and N. S. Mitchell, Lea & Febiger, Philadelphia, 1975.
11. Amstutz, H. C. Total hip replacement. In *Surgery of the Hip Joint,* p. 656, edited by R. G. Tronzo, Lea & Febiger, Philadelphia, 1973.
12. Harris, W. H. Indications for major elective reconstructive surgery of the hip in the adult. In *Instructional Course Lectures, A.A.O.S., 23:* 143, 1974.
13. Chandler, H. P. and Dickson, D. B. Total hip replacement in the young patient. In *Instructional Course Lectures, A.A.O.S., 23:*184, 1974.
14. Müller, M. E. Intertrochanteric osteotomies in adults. In *Surgical Management of Degenerative Arthritis of the Lower Limb,* edited by R. L. Cruess and N. S. Mitchell, p. 53, Lea & Febiger, Philadelphia, 1975.
15. Tronzo, R. G., and Okin, E. M. *Clin. Orthop., 106:*94, 1975.
16. Harris, W. The role of cup arthroplasty in contemporary reconstructive surgery of the hip. In *Surgical Management of Degenerative Arthritis of the Lower Limb,* p. 79, edited by R. L. Cruess and N. S. Mitchell, Lea & Febiger, Philadelphia, 1975.
17. Tronzo, R. G., and Lowell, J. D. Cup arthroplasty. In *Surgery of the Hip Joint,* p. 726, edited by R. G. Tronzo, Lea & Febiger, Philadelphia, 1973.
18. Leach, R. E., and Deweese, J. Arthrodesis in the treatment of degenerative arthritis of the hip. In *Surgical Management of Degenerative Arthritis of the Lower Limb,* p. 114, edited by R. L. Cruess and N. S. Mitchell, Lea & Febiger, Philadelphia, 1975.
19. Weber, B. G. Hip arthrodesis. In *Surgery of the Hip Joint,* p. 759, edited by R. G. Tronzo, Lea & Febiger, Philadelphia, 1973.
20. d'Aubigne, R. M., and Postel, M. *J. Bone Jt. Surg., 36A:*451, 1954.
21. Harris, W. H. *J. Bone Jt. Surg., 51A:*737, 1969.
22. Wilson, P. D., Jr., Amstutz, H. C., Czerniecki, A., Salvati, E. A., and Mendes, D. G. *J. Bone Jt. Surg., 54A:*206, 1972.
23. Charnley, J. *J. Bone Jt. Surg., 54B:*61, 1972.
24. Amstutz, H. C. Total hip replacement. In *Surgery of the Hip Joint* p. 656, edited by R. G. Tronzo, Lea & Febiger, Philadelphia, 1973.
25. Janecki, C. J., DeHaven, K. E., and Benton, J. W. *Orthop. Clin. N. Am., 4:*523, 1973.
26. Amstutz, H. C. Treatment of sepsis in total hip replacement. In *Instructional Course Lectures, A.A.O.S., 23:*248, 1974.
27. Eftekhar, N. S. Sepsis in total hip replacement. In *Instructional Course Lectures, A.A.O.S., 23:*253, 1974.
28. Kolczun, M. C., and Nelson, C. L. Antibiotic

concentration in human bone. In *The Hip,* p. 207, edited by W. H. Harris, C. V. Mosby Co., St. Louis, 1974.

29. Eftekhar, N. S. Controversy of clean air and total hip replacement. In *The Hip,* p. 266, edited by W. H. Harris, C. V. Mosby Co., St. Louis, 1974.

30. Eftekhar, N. S., Bush, D. C., Freeman, M. A. R., and Stinchfield, F. E. *Ortho. Rev., 3:*17, 1974.

31. Acton, R. K. Surgical approaches to the hip joint. In *Surgery of the Hip Joint,* p. 79, edited by R. G. Tronzo, Lea & Febiger, Philadelphia, 1973.

32. Tronzo, R. G., and Whittaker, R. Endoprosthetic arthroplasties. In *Surgery of the Hip Joint,* p. 722, edited by R. G. Tronzo, Lea & Febiger, Philadelphia, 1973.

33. Harris, W. H. *J. Bone Jt. Surg., 49A:*891, 1967.

34. Coventry, M. B. *Orthop. Clin. N. Am., 4:*473, 1973.

35. Müller, M. E. Technique of total hip replacement. In *Surgery of the Hip Joint,* p. 688, edited by R. G. Tronzo, Lea & Febiger, Philadelphia, 1973.

36. Evarts, C. M., Nelson, C. L., Collins, H. R., and Wilde, A. H. *Orthop. Clin. N. Am., 4:*449, 1973.

37. Harris, W. H. Total hip replacement for congenital dysplasia of hip. In *The Hip* p. 251, edited by W. H. Harris, C. V. Mosby Co., St. Louis, 1974.

38. Lazansky, M. G. Low-friction arthroplasty for the sequelae of congenital and developmental hip disease. In *Instructional Course Lectures, A.A.O.S., 23:*194, 1974.

39. Ferguson, A. B., Jr. *J. Bone Jt. Surg., 55A:*671, 1973.

40. Harris, W. H. *Clin. Orthop., 128:*176, 1977.

41. Harris, W. H., and Jones, W. N. *Clin. Orthop., 106:*117, 1975.

42. Dunn, H. K. and Hess, W. E. *J. Bone Jt. Surg., 58A:*838, 1976.

43. Dupont, J. A., and Charnley, J. *54B:*77, 1972.

44. Jackson, C. T., and Charnley, J. The results of low friction arthroplasty of the hip performed in Paget's disease. In *Charnley Low Friction Arthroplasty,* Internal Publ. Wrightington Hospital, no. 47, Leeds (Thackray), 1974.

45. Ferrari, A., and Charnley, J. *Clin. Orthop., 121:*12, 1976.

46. Harris, J., and Curry, H. L. F. Sexual problems due to disease of the hip joint: Its relevance to hip surgery. In *Total Hip Replacement,* p. 144, edited by M. Jayson, J. B. Lippincott Co., Philadelphia, 1971.

47. Williams, R. E. O., Blowers, R., Garrod, G., and Shooter, R. A. *Hospital Infection,* p. 7, Lloyd Luke, London, 1966.

48. Amstutz, H. C. *Cleveland Clin. Quar., 40:*125, 1973.

49. Morris, L. V., French, M. L. V., Ritter, M. A., Hart, J. B., and Eitzer, H. E. *Cleveland Clin. Quar., 40:*221, 1973.

50. Charnley, J., and Eftekhar, N. *Br. J. Surg., 56:* 641, 1969.

51. Harris, W. H., Salzman, E. W., Athanasoulis, C., Wattmur, A. C., Baum, S., and DeSanctis, R. W. *J. Bone Jt. Surg., 56A:*1552, 1974.

52. Convery, F. R., Barnes, R. W., Krogmire, R. B. Jr., and Strandness, D. E. Jr. Case against drug prophylaxis of thromboembolism in total hip replacement. In *The Hip,* p. 173, edited by W. H. Harris, C. V. Mosby Co., St. Louis, 1974.

53. Evarts, C. M. Prevention of thromboembolism by use of low molecular weight dextran. In *The Hip* p. 182, edited by W. H. Harris, C. V. Mosby Co., St. Louis, 1974.

54. Beckenbaugh, R. D., Coventry, M. B., and Nolan, D. R. Prophylactic anticoagulation with sodium warfarin in total hip arthroplasty. In *The Hip,* p. 190, edited by W. H. Harris, C. V. Mosby Co., St. Louis, 1974.

55. Goldner, J. L., Hopkins, J. E., and Weiker, G. G. Therapeutic low-dose heparin for prevention of thromboembolism. In *The Hip,* p. 195, edited by W. H. Harris, C. V. Mosby Co., St. Louis, 1974.

56. Sakai, D. N., and Amstutz, H. C. *Clin. Orthop., 121:*108, 1976.

57. Amstutz, H. C. Total hip replacement. In *Surgery of the Hip Joint,* p. 669, edited by R. G. Tronzo, Lea & Febiger, Philadelphia, 1973.

58. Patterson, F. P., and Brown, C. S. *Orthop. Clin. N. Am., 4:*503, 1973.

59. Lowell, J. D. Complications of total hip replacements. In *Instructional Course Lectures, A.A.O.S., 23:*209, 1974.

60. Amstutz, H. C. *Clin. Orthop., 72:*123, 1970.

61. Johnson, B. L. *Instructional Course Lectures, A.A.O.S., 23:*246, 1974.

62. Salvati, E. A. Infection complicating total hip replacement. In *The Hip,* p. 200, C. V. Mosby Co., St. Louis, 1976.

63. Amstutz, H. C. *Instructional Course Lectures, A.A.O.S., 23:*248, 1974.

64. Müller, M. E. Preservation of septic total hip replacement *versus* Girdlestone operation. In *The Hip,* p. 308, C. V. Mosby Co., St. Louis, 1974.

65. Girdlestone, G. R. *J. Bone Jt. Surg., 6:*519, 1924.

66. Duthie, R. B., and Ferguson, A. B., Jr. *Mercer's Orthopaedic Surgery,* p. 723, Edward Arnold, London, 1973.

67. Hamblin, D., Haw, C. S., and Gray, D. H. *J. Bone Jt. Surg., 58B:*44, 1976.

68. Amstutz, H. C. Skeletal fixation and loosening of total hip replacements. In *Instructional Course Lectures, A.A.O.S., 23:*201, 1974.

69. Marmor, L. *Clin. Orthop., 121:*116, 1976.

70. Markolf, K. L., and Amstutz, H. C. *Clin. Orthop., 121:*99, 1976.

71. Eftekhar, N. S. *Clin. Orthop., 121:*120, 1976.

72. Harris, W. H. *J. Bone Jt. Surg., 51A:*737, 1969.

73. Wilson, P. D., Amstutz, H. C., Czerniecki, A., Salvati, E., and Mendes, D. G. *J. Bone Jt. Surg., 54A:*207, 1972.

74. Brooker, A. F., Bowerman, J. W., Robinson, R. A., and Riley, L. H., Jr. *J. Bone Jt. Surg., 55A:*1629, 1973.

75. DeLee, J., Ferrari, A., and Charnley, J. *Clin. Orthop., 121:*53, 1976.

76. Lazansky, M. G. *Clin. Orthop., 95:*96, 1973.

77. Russell, R. G. G., and Fleisch, H. *Clin. Orthop., 108:*241, 1975.

78. Bijvoet, O. L. M., Nollen, A. J. G., Slooff, J. J., and Feith, R. *Acta Orthop. Scand., 45:*926, 1974.

79. Lazansky, M. G. Trochanteric osteotomy in total hip replacement. In *The Hip,* p. 237, edited by W. H. Harris, C. V. Mosby Co., St. Louis, 1974.

80. Nicholson, O. R. *Clin. Orthop., 95:*217, 1973.

81. Charnley, J. *Clin. Orthop., 95:*9, 1973.

82. Bronson, J. L. *Clin. Orthop., 121:*50, 1976.

83. Sledge, C. B. Osteotomy of the greater trochanter. In *The Hip*, p. 247, edited by W. H. Harris, C. V. Mosby Co., St. Louis, 1974.

84. Coventry, M. B., Beckenbaugh, R. D., Nolan, D. R., and Ilstrup, D. M. *J. Bone Jt. Surg., 56A:* 273, 1974.

85. Shires, G. T., and Canizaro, P. C. Fluid, electrolyte and nutritional management of the surgical patient. In *Principles of Surgery*, p. 65, edited by S. I. Schwartz, R. C. Lillehei, G. T. Shires, F. C. Spencer, and E. H. Storer, McGraw-Hill Book Co., New York, 1974.

86. Hollander, A., Barny, F., Monteny, E., and Donkerwolcke, M. *Acta Orthop. Scand., 47:*86, 1976.

87. Feith, R. *Acta Orthop. Scand., Suppl. 161:*17, 1975.

88. Lowell, J. D., Davies, J. A. K., and Bennett, A. H. *Clin. Orthop., 111:*131, 1975.

89. Hirsch, S. A., Robertson, H., Gorniowky, M. *Arch. Surg., 111:*204, 1976.

90. Salama, R., Stavorsky, M. M., Pellin, A., and Weissman, S. L. *Clin. Orthop., 89:*143, 1972.

91. Mallory, T. H. *J. Bone Jt. Surg., 54A:*276, 1972.

92. Tkaczuk, A. *Acta Orthop. Scand., 47:*317, 1976.

93. Kroese, A., and Møllerud, A. *Acta Orthop. Scand., 46:*119, 1976.

94. Scullin, J. P., Nelson, C. L., and Beven, E. G. *Clin. Orthop., 113:*145, 1975.

95. Clarke, I. C., Black, K., Rennie, C., and Amstutz, H. C. *Clin. Orthop., 121:*126, 1976.

96. Evans, E. M., Freeman, M. A. R., Miller, A. J. and Vernon-Roberts, B. *J. Bone Jt. Surg., 56B:*626, 1974.

97. Jones, D. A., Lucas, H. K., O'Driscoll, M., Price, C. H. G., and Wibberley, B. *J. Bone Jt. Surg., 57B:*289, 1975.

98. Weber, F. A., and Charnley, J. *J. Bone Jt. Surg., 57B:*297, 1975.

99. Salvati, E. A., Freiberger, R. H., and Wilson, P. D. *J. Bone Jt. Surg., 53A:*701, 1971.

100. Salvati, E. A., Ghelman, B., McLaren, R. T., and Wilson, P. D. *Clin. Orthop., 101:*105, 1974.

101. Bergstrom, B., Lidgrew, L., and Lindberg, L. *Clin. Orthop., 99:*95, 1974.

102. DeLee, J. G., and Charnley, J. *Clin. Orthop., 121:*20, 1976.

103. Patterson, F. P., and Brown, C. S. *Orthop. Clin. N. Am., 4:*503, 1973.

104. Schwartz, S. I., and Troup, S. B. Hemostasis, surgical bleeding and transfusion. In *Principles of Surgery*, p. 97, edited by S. I. Schwartz, R. C. Lillehei, G. T. Shires, F. C. Spencer, and E. H. Storer. McGraw-Hill Book Co., New York, 1974.

105. Hardy, J. D. Surgical complications. In *Davis-Christopher Textbook of Surgery*, p. 398, edited by D. C. Sabiston Jr., W. B. Saunders Co., Philadelphia, 1972.

106. Mallory, T. H. *Orthop. Rev., 4:*21, 1975.

107. Davis, N. J., Jennings, J. J., and Harris, W. H. *Clin. Orthop., 101:*93, 1974.

108. Johnson, R., Green, J. R., and Charnley, J. *Clin. Orthop., 127:*123, 1977.

109. Sabiston, D. C., Jr., and Wolfe, W. G. Pulmonary embolism. In *Gibbon's Surgery of the Chest*, p. 591, edited by D. C. Sabiston, Jr., and F. C. Spencer, W. B. Saunders Co., Philadelphia, 1976.

110. Moser, K. M. Pulmonary thromboembolism. In *Harrison's Principles of Internal Medicine"*,

8th ed., p. 1401, edited by G. W. Thorn, R. D. Adams, E. Braunwald, K. J. Isselbacher, and L. G. Petersdorf. McGraw-Hill Book Co., New York, 1977.

111. Webb, W. R. Post-operative pulmonary complications. In *Management of Surgical Complications*, p. 93, (edited by C. P. Artz and J. D. Hardy, W. B. Saunders Co., Philadelphia, 1975.

112. Daniel, W. W., Coventry, M., and Miller, W. *J. Bone Jt. Surg., 54A:*282, 1972.

113. Herndon, J., Bechtol, C. O., and Crickenberger, O. *J. Bone Jt. Surg., 56A:*1350, 1974.

114. Kallos, T., Evis, J., Gollan, F., and Davis, J. *J. Bone Jt. Surg., 56A:*1363, 1974.

115. Dandy, D. J. *Injury, 3:*85, 1971.

116. McLaughlin, R. E., DiFazio, C. A., Hakala, M., Abbott, B., MacPhail, J. A., Mack, W. P., and Sweet, D. E. *J. Bone Jt. Surg., 55A:*1621, 1973.

117. Spengler, D. M., Costenbader, M., and Bailey, R. *Clin. Orthop., 121:*105, 1976.

118. Feith, R. *Acta Orthop. Scand., Suppl. 161,* 15, 1975.

119. Radin, E. L. *Ortho. Clin. N. Am., 4:*539, 1975.

120. Kummer, B. Biomechanics of the hip and knee joint. In *Advances in Artificial Hip and Knee Joint Technology*, p. 24, edited by M. Schaldach and D. Hohmann, Springer-Verlag, Berlin, 1976.

121. Kettelkamp, D. B., and Nasca, R. *Clin. Orthop., 94:*8, 1973.

122. Gariepy, R., DeRome, A., and Laurin, C. A. Tibial osteotomy in the treatment of degenerative arthritis in the knee. In *Surgical Management of Degenerative Arthritis of the Lower Limb*, p. 155, edited by R. L. Cruess and N. S. Mitchell, Lea & Febiger, Philadelphia, 1975.

123. Kettlekamp, D. B. *Clin. Orthop., 101:*74, 1974.

124. MacIntosh, D. L. Arthroplasty of the knee in rheumatoid arthritis using the hemiarthroplasty prosthesis. In *Surgery of Rheumatoid Arthritis*, p. 29, edited by R. L. Cruess and N. Mitchell, J. B. Lippincott Co., Philadelphia, 1971.

125. Siller, T. N. Arthrodesis in the treatment of degenerative arthritis of the knee. In *Surgical Management of Degenerative Arthritis of the Lower Limb*, p. 203, edited by R. L. Cruess and N. S. Mitchell, Lea & Febiger, Philadelphia, 1975.

126. Duthie, R. B., and Ferguson, A. B. Jr., *Mercer's Orthopaedic Surgery*, p. 661, Edward Arnold, London, 1973.

127. Crenshaw, A. H. (editor). *Campbell's Operative Orthopaedics*, p. 1056, C. V. Mosby Co., St. Louis, 1971.

128. Insall, J., and Walker, P. *Clin. Orthop., 120:*83, 1976.

129. Marmor, L. *Clin. Orthop., 122:*181, 1977.

130. Engelbrecht, E., Siegel, A., Rotter, R., and Buchholz, H. W. *Clin. Orthop., 120:*54, 1976.

131. Marmor, L. *Clin. Orthop., 94:*242, 1973.

132. Kettlekamp, D. B., and Thompson, M. S. *Clin. Orthop., 107:*93, 1975.

133. Ranawat, C. S., and Shine, J. J. *Clin. Orthop., 94:* 185, 1973.

134. Waugh, T. R., Smith, R. C., Orofino, C. F., and Anzel, S. M. *Clin. Orthop., 94:*196, 1973.

135. Evanski, P. M., Waugh, T. R., Orfino, C. F., and Anzel, S. H. *Clin. Orthop., 120:*33, 1976.

136. Insall, J., Ranowat, C. S., Scott, W. N., and Walker, P. *Clin. Orthop., 120:*149, 1976.

137. Coventry, M. B., Upshaw, J. E., Riley, L. H., Finerman, G. A. M., and Turner, R. H. *Clin. Orthop., 94:*171, 1973.
138. Turner, R. H. *Instructional Course Lectures, A.A.O.S., 23:*20, 1974.
139. Peterson, L. F. A., Bryan, R. S., and Combs, J. J., Jr., *Instructional Course Lectures, A.A.O.S., 23:*6, 1974.
140. Cracchiolo, A. *Clin. Orthop., 94:*140, 1973.
141. Bargren, J. H., Freeman, M. A. R., and Swanson, S. A. V. *Clin. Orthop., 120:*65, 1976.
142. Freeman, M. A. R., Sculco, T., and Todd, R. C., *J. Bone Jt. Surg., 59B:*64, 1977.
143. Habermann, E. T., Deutsch, S. D., and Rovere, G. D. *Clin. Orthop., 94:*72, 1973.
144. Merryweather, R., and Blundell Jones, G. *Orthop. Clin. N. Am., 4:*585, 1973.
145. Phillips, R. S. *Clin. Orthop., 94:*122, 1973.
146. Mazas, F. B., and the Guepar, *Clin. Orthop., 94:*211, 1973.
147. Matthews, L. S., Sonstegard, D. A., and Kaufer, H. *Clin. Orthop., 94:*234, 1973.
148. Sonstegard, D. A., Kaufer, H., and Matthews, L. S. *J. Bone Jt. Surg., 59A:*602, 1977.
149. McKeever, D. C. *J. Bone Jt. Surg., 43B:*752, 1961.
150. Levitt, R. L. *Clin. Orthop., 97:*153, 1973.
151. Murray, J. W. G. *Orthop. Rev., 4:*33, 1975.
152. Ewald, F., and Sledge, C. In *Symposium—The Surgical Aspects of Rheumatoid Arthritis,* Robt. B. Brigham Hospital, Boston, Mass., May 18, 1973,
153. Chrisman, O. D., and Snook, G. A. *Clin. Orthop., 101:*40, 1974.
154. Kaushal, S. P., Galante, J. O., McKenna, R., and Bachmann, F. *Clin. Orthop., 121:*181, 1976.
155. Walker, P. S., and Shoji, H. *Clin. Orthop., 94:*222, 1973.
156. Arden, G. P. *Clin. Orthop., 94:*92, 1973.
157. Gunston, F. H., and MacKenzie, R. I. *Clin. Orthop., 120:*11, 1976.
158. Blauth, W., Skripitz, W., and Bontemps, G. Problematics of current hinge-type artificial knee joints. In *Advances in Artificial Hip and Knee Joint Technology* p. 374, edited by M. Schaldach and D. Hohmann, Springer-Verlag, Berlin, 1976.
159. Wilde, A. H., Collins, H. R., Evarts, C. M., and Nelson, C. L. *Orthop. Clin. N. Am., 4:*547, 1973.
160. Walker, P. S., and Hsieh, H. H. *J. Bone Jt. Surg., 59B:*222, 1977.
161. Jackson, J. P., and Elson, R. A. *Clin. Orthop., 94:*104, 1973.
162. Laurin, C. A. The surgical management of degenerative lesions of the foot and ankle. In *Surgical Management of Degenerative Arthritis of the Lower Limb,* p. 215, edited by R. L. Cruess and N. S. Mitchell, Lea & Febiger, Philadelphia, 1975.
163. Johnson, E. W., and Boseker, E. H. *Arch. Surg., 97:*766, 1968.
164. Lance, E. M., Pavel, A., Patterson, R. L., Jr.,
165. Evanski, P. M., and Waugh, T. R. *Clin. Orthop., 122:*110, 1977.
166. Manes, H. R., Alvarez, E., and Levine, L. S. *Clin. Orthop., 127:*200, 1977.
167. Sammarco, G. J., Burstein, A. H., and Frankel, V. H. *Ortho. Clin. N. Am., 4:*75, 1973.
168. Morris, J. M. *Clin. Orthop., 122:*10, 1977.
169. Haliburton, R. A., Sullivan, C. R., Kelly, P. J., and Peterson, L. F. A. *J. Bone Jt. Surg., 40A:*1115, 1958.
170. Neer, C. S. *J. Bone Jt. Surg., 37A:*215, 1955.
171. Neer, C. S. *J. Bone Jt. Surg., 56A:*1, 1974.
172. Neer, C. S. *J. Bone Jt. Surg., 46A:*1607, 1964.
173. Marmor, L. *Clin. Orthop., 122:*201, 1977.
174. Macnab, I., and English, T. *Gleno-humeral Prosthesis,* p. E 1 Medishield, Paramus, N. J., 1976.
175. Fenlin, J. M. *Orthop. Clin. N. Am., 6:*565, 1975.
176. Letten, A. W. F., and Scales, J. T. *Proc. R. Soc. Med., 65:*373, 1972.
177. Letten, A. W. F., and Scales, J. T. *J. Bone Jt. Surg., 55B:*217, 1973.
178. Ewald, F. C. *Orthop. Clin. N. Am., 6:*685, 1975.
179. Street, D. M., and Stevens, P. S. *J. Bone Jt. Surg., 56A:*1147, 1974.
180. Gschwend, N., Scheier, H., and Bähler, A. *Arch. Orthop. Unfall-Chir., 73:*316, 1972.
181. Dee, R. *Orthop. Clin. N. Am., 4:*395, 1973.
182. Dee, R. *J. Bone Jt. Surg., 54B:*88, 1972.
183. Schlein, A. P. *Clin. Orthop., 121:*222, 1976.
184. Heim, U., and Pfeiffer, K. M. *Small Fragment Set Manual,* Springer-Verlag, Berlin, 1974.
185. Swanson, A. B. *Orthop. Clin. N. Am., 4:*383, 1973.
186. Meuli, H. C. *Ann. Chir., 27:*527, 1973.
187. Barton, R. I. *Orthop. Clin. N. Am., 4:*313, 1973.
188. Meuli, H. C. *Z. Orthop., 113:*476, 1975.
189. Swanson, A. B. *Orthop. Clin. N. Am., 4:*373, 1973.
190. Flatt, A. E. *The Care of the Rheumatoid Hand,* p. 78, C. V. Mosby Co., St. Louis, 1974.
191. Millender, L. H., and Nalebuff, E. A. *Ortho. Clin. N. Am., 4:*349, 1973.
192. Motamed, H. A. *Color Anatomy and Kinesiology of the Hand,* p. 115, H. A. Motamed, Chicago, 1973.
193. Pieron, A. P. *Acta Orthop. Scand., Suppl. 148,* 7, 1973.
194. Flatt, A. E. *The Care of the Rheumatoid Hand,* p. 12, C. V. Mosby Co., St. Louis, 1974.
195. Swanson, A. B., and Swanson, G. de G. *Orthop. Clin. N. Am., 4:*1039, 1973.
196. Swanson, A. B. *Flexible Implant Resection Arthroplasty in the Hand and Extremities,* p. 147, C. V. Mosby Co., St. Louis, 1973.
197. Urbaniak, J. R. *Clin. Orthop., 104:*9, 1974.
198. Swanson, A. B., Meester, W. D., Swanson, G. de G., Rangaswamy, L., and Schut, G. E. D. *Orthop. Clin. N. Am., 4:*1097, 1973.
199. Swanson, A. B. A dynamic brace for finger joint reconstruction in arthritis. In *Surgery of Rheumatoid Arthritis,* p. 205, edited by R. L. Cruess and N. Mitchell, J. B. Lippincott Co., Philadelphia, 1971.
200. McCollum, D. E., Goldner, J. L., Rhangus, W. C., and Aidem, H. P. Surgery of the Hand in Rheumatoid Arthritis, presented to the American Academy of Orthopaedic Surgeons, New York, N. Y., Jan. 10, 1965.
Fries, L., and Larsen, I. J. *J. Bone Jt. Surg., 53A:*1030, 1971.

15

Supplementary Implants in Musculoskeletal Surgery

As demonstrated in Chapters 13 and 14, the vast majority of implants employed in reconstruction of the musculoskeletal system function in articular joints. Their proliferation over the past decade is attributable to the ubiquitous nature of the arthritides and of the relative success encountered in the resurfacing of articular joints with man-made materials.

A variety of other implants, however, have been devised to reconstruct other musculoskeletal organs such as tendons, ligaments and muscles. While their application has not enjoyed such striking success as the use of total hip joint replacements, nevertheless, they represent a serious attempt by surgeons and bioengineers to solve what technically may entail even more complex problems than innovations in total joint replacements. One formidable example is the development of a prosthetic weight-bearing ligament, such as the medial collateral ligament of the knee. In contrast, the attempts to develop artificial tendons have been rewarded by notable success in the elucidation of most of the technical hurdles. In the present chapter this diverse array of reconstructive problems is reviewed. The reader should recognize that future developments in this area may enjoy even greater clinical success and recognition than total joint replacements have witnessed.

SILASTIC IMPLANT ARTHROPLASTY

During the past 15 years, Swanson[1] and his colleagues have undertaken research on a variety of flexible implants for reconstructive surgery of the extremities. In fact, the attempt to utilize resilient implants of silicone rubber followed the previous decade of labor when they had attempted unsuccessfully to employ metallic hemiarthroplastic devices such as a hemispherical cap to replace the proximal side of the first metatarsophalangeal joint. The adjacent bone frequently showed resorption with loss of stability of the arthroplastic joint. The failures were attributed to the dynamic shear stresses imposed by weight-bearing forces on the rigid implant-bone interface. The flexible "silastic" devices did not share this liability, at least for most applications. Silicone rubber implants have evolved as flexible, self-centering hinges for the reconstruction of joints and as spacers for use in hemiarthroplasties or as a replacement for the entirety of the small carpal bones. A variety of the silastic joints are described in Chapters 13 and 14, while a discussion of several silastic spacers follows here.

IMPLANT ARTHROPLASTY FOR THE GREAT TOE

Initially Swanson[2] attempted to replace the proximal, weight-bearing end of the metatarsophalangeal joint. For the many adults who develop a painful, stiff or deformed proximal, metatarsophalangeal joint in the great toe, the most widely employed surgical procedure is the Keller resectional arthroplasty. The proximal end of the proximal phalanx is removed, along with the medial exostosis in the distal end of the metatarsal and the joint capsule is reefed to realign a valgus deformity of the great toe. Occasionally, certain technical considerations compromise the results of what, otherwise, is usually a highly successful operation. Excessive foreshortening of the proximal phalanx may result in a cosmetic deformity, and instability of the toe with diminished power in the take-off phase of gait. Inadequate removal of bone may predispose the patient to a painful, stiff pseudoarthrosis. Swanson wondered whether the application of a resilient spacer might augment the predictability of the operation. When an intramedullary stemmed implant was employed for replacement of the weight-bearing articular surface on the metatarsal bone, tolerance of the flexible device was superior to that observed when a metal implant was employed but was still inadequate. Subsequently the spacer was used to resurface the bone of the proximal phalanx. The implant served as an articular surface and as a spacer to support the regeneration of a stabilizing capsuloligamentous system. With its smooth articular surface, the implant facilitated the return of good mobility of the joint. With the weight-bearing portion of the distal metatarsal *in situ,* the transfer of flexion power to the great toe in take-off was increased and a normal walking pattern was restored. Improved cosmesis was realized with the preservation of length of the great toe.

Swanson and his colleagues have undertaken various mechanical tests on the implants, in which the mechanical environment of the first metatarsophalangeal joint is simulated with dynamic stress, comparable to the forces imposed upon the joint in an adult human. The implants have withstood more than 250 million stress cycles through an excursion of 90° without evidence of fatigue failure or other deterioration.

The indications for silicone rubber implant has included hallux valgus, hallux rigidus, rheumatoid arthritic deformities, and unstable or painful, stiff metatarsophalangeal joints following a Keller[3, 4] or Mayo-type[4, 5] bunionectomy.

Procedure. The joint is exposed through a slightly curved longitudinal incision made over the dorsomedial aspect of the first metatarsophalangeal joint (Fig. 15-1*A*). A Hoffmann[6] or Clayton[7] procedure may be conducted at the same time as the great toe arthroplasty. The lateral metatarsals may be exposed through a dorsal transverse (Fig. 15-1*B*), longitudinal, or a plantar transverse incision with resection of a wedge of skin. The dorsal sensory nerves and veins are carefully preserved. The fascia and medial capsule of the joints are dissected and incised with the preparation of a distally based flap on the proximal phalanx. Alternatively, if the distal capsuloligamentous attachments are compromised, the flap is based proximally on the metatarsal head. If a bursa is present it is resected and the metatarsophalangeal joint is incised.

The proximal third of the proximal phalanx is resected with an osteotome or air drill (Fig. 15-1*C*). Irregularities or excessive length of the metatarsal may be resected along with medial or plantar exostoses. With an air drill or broach, the canal of the proximal phalanx is shaped to accept the stem of the implant. A precise fit is essential with the stem fitting snugly in the intramedullary canal and the collar abutting the cut surface of the proximal phalanx. Implants are available in five sizes and the correct size is essential.

Using the sizing set as a guide, the largest implant that the bone can accommodate is selected. Prior to insertion, the implant is thoroughly rinsed with saline solution and it is handled with a blunt instrument to avoid damaging it or contaminating it with foreign bodies. While the stem may be shortened to enable it to fit in the phalanx the residual portion of the implant should not be reshaped because the modification of the implant might weaken it.

If the implant is contaminated prior to insertion it is washed thoroughly in a hot soapy solution to remove superficial contaminants. Synthetic detergents or oil-based soaps are discouraged because they may be absorbed and subsequently released in tissues to provoke an undesirable biological reaction. Next the implant is rinsed in hot water followed by distilled water after which it is autoclaved in a conventional way.

Complete correction of a hallux valgus deformity may require release of the lateral capsule, incision of the attachments of the adductor muscles, lengthening or rerouting the long extensor tendon or shortening the metatarsal head (Fig. 15-1*D*). Prior to closure an unrestricted anatomical range of passive motion of the joint must be realized and rotational or angular deformities must be eliminated.

With the toe held in a neutral position, the medial fasciocapsular flap is sutured to the metatarsal head with 3-0 Dacron inserted through a drill hole (Fig. 15-1*E*). If a proximally based flap is present it is sutured to the proximal phalanx in a similar way. The aponeurosis of the long extensor tendon is sutured to the medial capsule with 4-0 Dacron also with a buried knot technique. The cutaneous incision is closed and a bulky conforming dressing is applied to the foot. A longitudinal splint, such as a tongue-blade, is incorporated into the dressing to support the great toe. Radiological views before and after insertion of a great toe prosthesis are seen in Figure 15-2.

From 3 to 5 days after surgery the dressing is removed and a dynamic splint is applied to maintain the alignment of the toe while early active flexion and extension exercises are begun. Swanson recommends the use of the splint by day and night for 3 to 4 weeks followed by its application at night for an additional 3 weeks. Initially, the patient walks with a heel gait and about 3 weeks after surgery he gradually proceeds to full weight bearing. Conventional nonrestrictive shoes are recommended.

Results. Swanson[2] has published the results of 55 cases in which 73 arthroplastic procedures

Figure 15-1. *A*. When surgery is restricted to arthroplasty of the great toe, a longitudinal curvilinear approach is used through the dorsomedial aspect of the toe. (Reproduced with the permission of Dow Corning Corp. Midland, Mich.) *B*. Alternatively when resection of the other metatarsal heads is indicated a transverse dorsal extension of the incision across the metatarsophalangeal heads is recommended. *C*. For great toe arthroplasty the proximal third of the proximal phalanx is resected. Exostoses on the medial and plantar surfaces are excised. With a curet, broach or drill the intramedullary cavity of the proximal phalanx is shaped to receive the stem of the implant. *D*. For the correction of marked hallux valgus deformity or with marked irregularity of the distal first metatarsal, the metatarsal head may be shortened and reshaped. Where indicated the four lateral metatarsal heads, also, may be resected. *E*. The stem of the implant should fit tightly into the intramedullary cavity with the collar of the implant abuting the osteotomized surface of the phalanx. With the great toe anatomically realigned, the medial flap of the fascia and capsule is sutured firmly to the metatarsal through small drill holes.

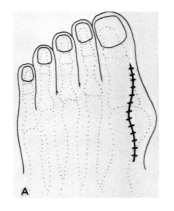

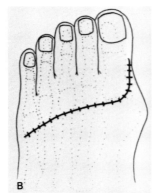

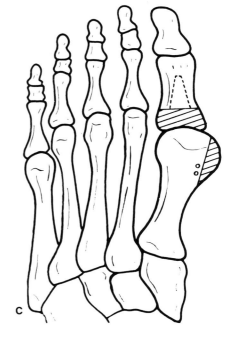

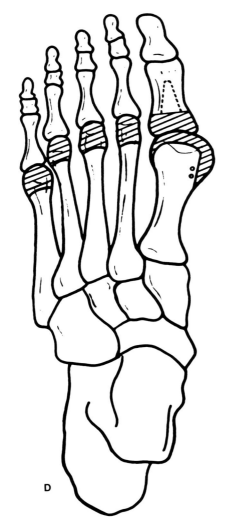

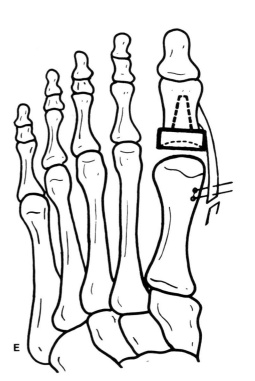

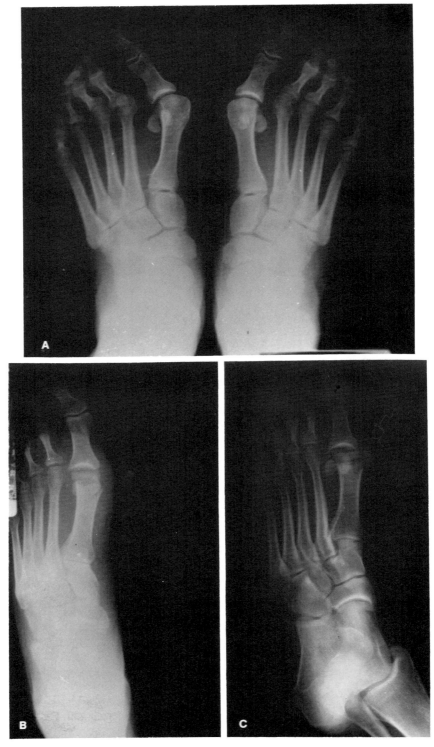

Figure 15-2. *A* and *B*. Radiological views present a patient with a painful hallux rigidus deformity before and after arthroplasty of the proximal joint with a Swanson prosthesis. (Reproduced with permission of Dow Corning Corp., Midland, Mich.)

were performed. Forty-one patients were rheumatoid arthritics and 32 patients were osteoarthritics. In 39 patients arthroplasty of the great toe was performed while the others had additional procedures. After surgery the average range of motion of the great toe was 60° of extension, and 5° of flexion. All of the patients had minimal discomfort and were pleased with the functional and cosmetic results. No implants underwent fracture or dislocation or showed evidence of infection. In view of these preliminary encouraging results, a report on more prolonged follow-up is eagerly awaited.

THE USE OF SILASTIC IMPLANTS IN THE UPPER EXTREMITY

Silastic Radial Head Implant

With the provisional success observed by the use of silastic spacers in the great toe, Swanson[2, 8, 9] was encouraged to undertake similar types of procedures in the upper extremity. One of the conspicuous sites for application was the radial head after it had been resected for rheumatoid, degenerative or traumatic arthritis, or as a primary replacement following radial head resection for fractures. A pliable spacer with an intramedullary stem was developed to restore the radiohumeral articulation. The implant was available in three diameters of radial head and a special model with an exceptionally long head for use where extensive resection of the proximal radius previously has been undertaken. Where the above mentioned pathologies provoked persistent mechanical pain or subluxation of the residual head, or after comminuted fractures of the radial head or after established traumatic arthritis, the implant was applied by Swanson in 120 cases.[10] As with other silastic spacers the primary contraindications include inadequate skin, bone or neurovascular status or irreparable damage to muscles and tendons.

Procedure. The radial head is approached through a dorsolateral incision and the joint is entered between the anconeus and extensor carpi ulnaris muscles. The motor branch of the radial nerve must be protected where it courses across the radial neck. The radial head is resected with a preservation of the bulk of the annular ligament (Fig. 15-3A). Where necessary a synovectomy of the elbow joint may be performed. With a curet, broach or air drill the intramedullary canal of the radius is shaped to accommodate the prosthetic stem. The flange on the implant should overlap the cut surface of the radius and the stem should fit snugly into

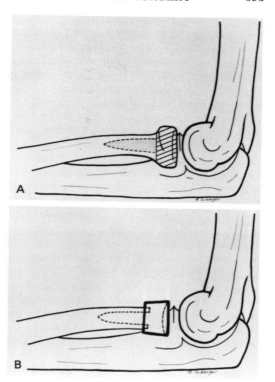

Figure 15-3. *A.* Excision of the radial head with preparation of the intramedullary cavity of the radial neck in preparation for the insertion of a silicone prosthesis is shown. *B.* The schematic diagram indicates the appropriate fit of a silicone prosthesis to replace the radial head. (*A* and *B*, reproduced with permission of Dow Corning Corp., Midland, Mich.)

the canal (Fig. 15-3*B*). One of the three available sizes of implant is selected and inserted by the use of a no-touch technique as with other silicone implants. Subsequently, pronation and supination of the forearm is performed while the implant is examined for evidence of smooth rotation and articulation with the distal humerus.

The capsule, anconeus and extensor carpi radialis are sutured with nonabsorbable sutures after which the fascial layers and the skin are closed. A compression dressing with a long-arm plaster splint is applied.

On the third postoperative day the dressing is reduced and the splint is removed. Active motion of the elbow is cautiously encouraged while full activities are resumed after 6 weeks.

Silicone Ulnar Head Implant Arthroplasty

For proper function of the hand, the wrist joint serves both as a stabilizing element and as a mobile unit. Smooth rotational movements of the wrist joint require integrity of the distal radioulnar joint. Disabilities of the distal radioulnar joint, therefore, can impair normal adaptations of the wrist and function of the hand. The function of the distal radioulnar joint may be compromised by traumatic insults such as a Colles' fracture or a dislocation of the wrist joint, or impairment may be secondary to proximal displacement of the radial shaft that may follow resectional arthroplasty of the radial head, particularly in children. Dysfunction of the radioulnar joint, however, occurs most frequently as a sequel to destructive proliferative synovitis with rheumatoid arthritis. Frequently rheumatoid patients undergo progressive subluxation of the hand on the forearm which is characterized by a dorsal prominence and instability of the ulnar head with weakness of the wrist joint, painful crepitant motion, limited in both rotation and dorsiflexion.[11] The fourth and the fifth metacarpals may show exaggerated flexion in view of the abnormal function of the flexor carpi ulnaris with its volar displacement. Concomitantly, the extensor tendons of the little, ring and middle fingers may undergo rupture over the irregular ulnar head to produce drop of the involved fingers. A variety of other musculoskeletal structures in the hand and forearm may be compromised as fully characterized by Swanson.[12]

As the proliferative synovitis provokes further destruction, the ligamentous support of the distal ulna especially the triangular fibrocartilage, the ulnar collateral ligament and the adjacent capsule undergo attritional changes. The ulnar head becomes prominent on the dorsum of the wrist as the hand subluxes in a volar direction. X-rays may reveal the apparent dorsal subluxation of the ulnar head with erosive changes and, subsequently, progressive irregularity and destruction of the ulnar head. The ulnar styloid may diminish in size and disappear secondary to destructive change.

Resection of the ulnar head with various disabilities of the distal radioulnar joint was popularized by Darrach[13] in 1912. It has been widely performed often with good results provided that less than 2 to 3 cm of the distal ulna is excised.[14] If a greater amount of bone is removed, the pronator quadratus and interosseous membrane cease to provide adequate stabilization of the residual distal ulna. In rheumatoid arthritis instability of the distal ulna is more common because of the destruction of the ligamentous support by the proliferative synovitis. After resectional arthroplasty of the distal ulna, progressive ulnar carpal shift may occur. Some workers have

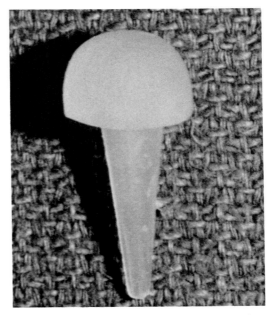

Figure 15-4. A photograph reveals a silicone ulnar head replacement.

attempted to perform soft tissue repairs although successful stabilization of the subluxed rheumatoid carpus is uncommon. Alternatively, in 1966, Swanson[8] developed an ulnar head replacement of silicone rubber which is seen in Figure 15-4. The implant was designed to supplement the Darrach type of resectional arthroplasty to preserve the anatomical relationship of the distal radioulnar articulation. By the application of the implant, a minimal amount of distal ulna can be excised to provide maximal stability of the wrist. A smooth articular surface opposes the radius and carpus to encourage greater motion of the distal radioulnar and carpoulnar articulations as well as the overlying extensor tendons. Not least, the cosmetic appearance of the wrist is improved. The implant is available in seven sizes with a pretied polyester retention cord.

Procedure. The specific indications for the application of an ulnar head implant replacement arthroplasty include pain and weakness of the wrist joint not improved by conservative treatment and instability of the ulnar head with X-ray evidence of apparent dorsal subluxation and erosive change in the distal ulna.

A 6 to 8 cm longitudinal incision is centered over the ulnar head (Fig. 15-5A). The dorsal cutaneous branch of the ulnar nerve is carefully preserved. The extensor retinaculum of the sixth dorsal compartment is incised with preparation

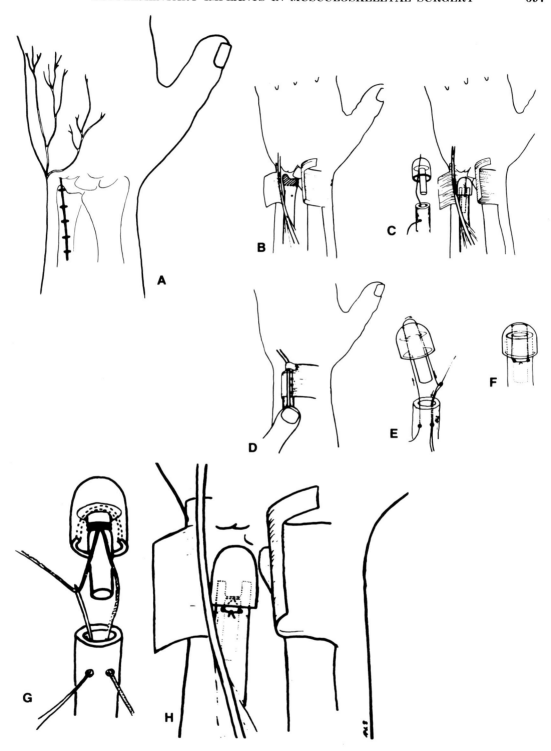

Figure 15-5. *A.* The dorsal longitudinal incision recommended for ulnar head replacement is shown. The dorsal cutaneous branches of the ulnar nerve, seen here, are carefully protected. *B* to *F.* The schematic views reveal the stages in ulnar head replacement. (*B* to *F*, Reproduced with permission of A. B. Swanson.[15]) *G* and *H.* Insertion of the newer model of implant with its pretied polyester cord can be observed.

of a narrow radial-based distal flap and a broad ulnar-based proximal flap (Fig. 15-5B). Where indicated a synovectomy of the dorsal compartment is performed. The extensor carpi ulnaris which is usually subluxed volarward off the ulnar head is retracted. By subperiosteal dissection the distal ulna is exposed and retractors are positioned to protect the overlying neurovascular structures. With an air drill or bone cutting forceps, the bone is sectioned at the neck. Muscular attachments on the anterior surface of the ulna are released for the distal 2 cm although periosteum on the distal ulna is carefully preserved. The ulnar head and attached synovium are excised and complete synovectomy of the joint is undertaken. With the rongeur the cut end of the distal ulna is trimmed to provide a highly regular smooth surface.

The ulnar intramedullary canal is prepared with a curet or broach to receive the stem of the implant. The stem of the trial prosthesis of appropriate size should fit snugly into the intramedullary canal and the cuff should fit loosely over the bone.

Two centimeters proximal to the resected end of the ulna a small drill hole is made (Fig. 15-5C). Previously a 2-0 Dacron or nylon suture was passed through the cap of the implant and the bone to stabilize the position of the prosthesis (Fig. 15-5 C and E). The stem of the implant was introduced into the medullary cavity and the longitudinal suture was tied securely. While the insertion of the sutures through the silicone rubber implant was a potential source of a mechanical defect that might propagate in service with the formation of a crevice or tear, no frank mechanical failures were encountered. Nevertheless, the implant has been modified by the addition of a pretied polyester retention cord so that the need for puncturing the implant is circumvented. Insertion of the newer type of implant is seen in Figure 15-5 G and H.

The hand is located on the distal ulna and the retinacular flaps are sutured as shown in Figure 15-5D. The broad proximal retinacular flap is placed under the extensor carpi ulnaris tendon and sutured over the ulna into the residual ligaments of the distal radioulnar joint and the retinaculum of its dorsal compartment with five or six 3-0 Dacron sutures. Where necessary the sutures may be secured through drill holes in the radius. The narrow distal retinacular flap is looped under and around the extensor carpi ulnaris tendon and sutured to itself. It serves as a pulley to maintain the tendon dorsal to the ulnar head. The wound is closed with interrupted sutures and a large conforming dressing with a volar plaster splint is applied. On the third postoperative day the wound is inspected, and if satisfactory, a short-arm cast or splint is applied for 3 to 4 weeks.

Results. Swanson[8] has provided a detailed report on the results of 73 operated wrists on 54 patients of which 68 operations were performed as treatment for rheumatoid arthritis. Frequently, other reconstructive procedures were performed concurrently on the same extremity. These procedures were notable for relief of pain and crepitation and additional functional and cosmetic improvements. In a relatively short period of follow-up progressive postoperative subluxation of the ulnar head replacements has not been observed. Obviously further observations will be necessary.

Two complications have been reported with the use of ulnar head prostheses. In 5 cases distal migration of the implant has been noted in which the cup of the implant ceased to cover the resected end of the ulna. Apparently, this problem did not effect the clinical result. Subsequently, the implants were sutured into bone as described in the present operative report. Since then migration of the implant has not been noted. In 2 other cases X-rays revealed resorption of bone in the distal centimeter of the ulna around the implant. After these observations the design of the implant was modified somewhat in anticipation of alleviation of this complication. More recently Swanson has undertaken a long term follow-up on 225 wrist procedures performed in his clinic. The study showed marked improvement in wrist function in terms of stability, mobility and relief of pain.

Silicone Rubber Implant Arthroplasty for the Trapezium (Greater Multangular)

One of the most common sites of degenerative arthritis is the carpometacarpal joint[16] at the base of the thumb. Previously fusions have been undertaken although motion of the joint is necessarily eradicated. While a variety of arthroplastic procedures have been devised frequently residual subluxation of the joint has occurred. The replacement of the trapezium with a silicone rubber implant, seen in Figure 15-6, has served to restore and maintain motion at the base of the thumb, to function as a space filler and to prevent relative instability and subluxation which otherwise tend to follow simple resectional arthroplasty.[17] Nevertheless, subluxation of the implant on the residual carpus has remained a problem to the present time. Various

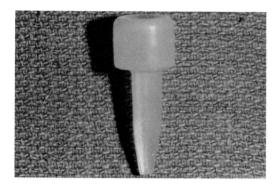

Figure 15-6. A photograph reveals a silicone rubber trapezium replacement.

supplementary soft tissue reconstructive procedures have been attempted with limited success in an effort to maintain the implant in a located position. At present the silicone trapezium implant appears to have a role for the treatment of patients with degenerative, rheumatoid or post-traumatic arthritis involving the carpometacarpal joint of the thumb. The indications include localized pain and crepitation of the joint, loss of motion with diminished strength of pinch and grip and X-ray evidence of arthritic change of the trapeziometacarpal or trapezioscaphoid joint with or without subluxation.

Procedure. A straight radial longitudinal incision of 2 to 3 inches is made parallel to the extensor pollicus brevis tendon centered over the trapezium (Fig. 15-7A). The branches of the superficial radial nerve are identified, mobilized and carefully retracted (Fig. 15-7B). The bases of the metacarpal and the trapeziometacarpal joint are identified and a longitudinal capsular incision is made at the metacarpal base. By sharp dissection the capsule is reflected from the base of the metacarpal in a proximal direction until the scaphoid is observed. The capsule is carefully preserved for subsequent closure. An elevator is placed into the trapezioscaphoid joint which protects a superficial branch of the radial artery. The dissection proceeds in a volar direction to detach the transverse carpal ligament from the trapezium.

The entire trapezium is removed usually in fragments by the use of an osteotome or a rongeur. In this procedure branches of the radial artery and the flexor carpi radialis longus tendon are carefully preserved. The scaphoid is examined for osteophytes or other irregularity which are trimmed.

The proximal end of the metacarpal is flattened with the rongeur. A central hole is pre-

pared in the flat surface which violates the intramedullary canal. An appropriate size of implant is selected so that the stem of the implant fits easily into the intramedullary cavity of the first metacarpal. The residual portion of the implant should comfortably fill the site of the resected trapezium and it should permit unrestricted abduction of the thumb.

With a no-touch technique the stem of the implant is inserted into the intramedullary canal of the first metacarpal. The collar of the implant rests firmly on the base of the metacarpal (Fig. 15-7C). With the thumb held in abduction the capsule is sutured with 3-0 Dacron. If possible a capsular imbrication is performed. The capsule may be strengthened with a slip of the abductor pollicus longus tendon (Fig. 15-7 D to G). The tendinous slip is incised 2 inches proximal from its attachment to the base of the metacarpal and is dissected distally to its metacarpal attachment. It is placed deep to the capsule and sutured back over the capsule during the closure. The soft tissue repair may be further strengthened by the reconstruction of an ulnar oblique ligament between the first and second metacarpals with a slip of the flexor carpi radialis tendon (Fig. 15-7H). This procedure is advisable in heavy laborers and in patients with chronic subluxation of the trapeziometacarpal articulation. The skin is closed in layers in conventional fashion although the sensory branches of the radial nerve must not be violated by the sutures. A bulky conforming dressing with a plaster splint is applied. A roll of cotton is placed between the first and second metacarpals to maintain 40 to 60° of palmar adduction. After 3 to 4 days a scaphoid-type forearm cast is applied. At 4 to 6 weeks after surgery the cast is removed when the capsular repair is usually stable. At that time abduction and opposition movements at the base of the thumb are encouraged. Unprotective movements of the arthroplastic joint should be possible in 6 to 10 weeks after surgery. Special surgical problems include marked abduction or adduction contractures of the thumb with or without swan-neck or boutonniere deformities. Unless such secondary deformities are corrected resection implant arthroplasty is unlikely to provide a satisfactory result. Abduction contractures of the thumb must be released after which a Kirschner wire should be placed between the first and second metacarpals to provide maintenance of wide palmar abduction during the healing phase. The wire is removed 6 weeks after surgery. Severe swan-neck deformities are treated by fusion of the metacarpophal-

Figure 15-7. *A.* Typical incisions for trapeziometacarpal arthroplasty are shown, of which the longitudinal incision parallel to the extensor pollicis brevis tendon is preferred. (Reproduced with permission of A. B. Swanson.) *B.* The principal anatomical structures to be carefully identified and retracted in the approach to the trapeziometacarpal joint are shown. (Reproduced with permission of A. B. Swanson.[18]) *C.* A schematic view of the trapezial stemmed implant *in situ* is seen. (Reproduced with permission of Dow Corning Corp., Midland, Mich.) *D.* The stages in reinforcement of the capsule around the trapezial implant with a slip of abductor pollicus longus are reviewed. A tendinous slip, 5 cm in length, is left attached at its distal end, *D*, and placed directly over the implant, *E.* The weakened capsule is plicated or overlapped and sutured over the tendon slip, *F.* The remainder of the slip is folded back over the capsule, *G*, and sutured with 3-0 Dacron. (*D* to *G*, reproduced with permission of A. B. Swanson.[19]) *H.* An ulnar restraint ligament can be reconstructed from a slip of the flexor carpi radialis. The procedure is particularly useful for patients with chronic dislocation of the trapeziometacarpal joint and for patients who may undertake heavy labor. (Reproduced with permission A. B. Swanson.[20])

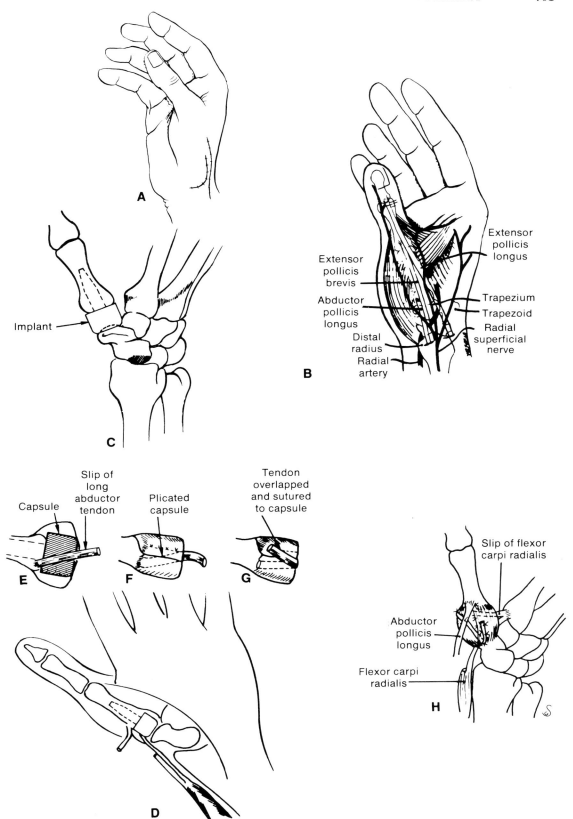

A

C

Implant

B

Extensor
pollicis
brevis

Abductor
pollicis
longus

Distal
radius

Radial
artery

Extensor
pollicis
longus

Trapezium

Trapezoid

Radial
superficial
nerve

Capsule

Slip of
long
abductor
tendon

Plicated
capsule

Tendon
overlapped
and sutured
to capsule

E

F

G

D

Slip of flexor
carpi radialis

Abductor
pollicis
longus

Flexor carpi
radialis

H

angeal joint in a position of 0 to 10° of flexion with the use of small cancellous bone grafts from the resected bone and Kirschner wire fixation. If the swan-neck deformity is moderate the metacarpophalangeal joint is temporarily pinned in 20° of flexion. If the swan-neck deformity is mild, surgical treatment may be unnecessary. Moderate or severe boutonniere deformity is treated by fusion of the metacarpophalangeal joint with release of the extensor tendon and capsule at the interphalangeal joint. Kirschner wires are used to transfix both joints for a period of immobilization of about 6 weeks. Severe adduction deformities also must be corrected. If 45° of abduction between the first and second metacarpals cannot be realized the adductor muscle of the thumb should be released from its origin on the third metacarpal through a separate palmar incision.

The Application of Silicone Rubber Implants to Replace Carpal Bones

The treatment of fractures of the scaphoid bone has remained a problem to the present time. Most fractures of the bone are readily treated by closed reduction and a long-arm cast. In view of the somewhat unique vascular supply of the proximal end of the bone, however, a substantial number of fractures, particularly where anatomical reduction is not realized, culminate in a painful pseudarthrosis.[21] If the fracture is comminuted or if the fragments are grossly displaced or if an avascular necrotic fragment is present incongruity of the radioscaphoid or intercarpal joints may ensue. In all of these cases patients may present with a complaint of a painful wrist and hand which greatly compromises their function. When conservative treatment with limitation of activity or the use of a splint is unsuccessful one of several surgical procedures may be undertaken, all of which have considerable limitations. A variety of resectional arthroplasties of the scaphoid and partial excision of the radial styloid have been attempted to eliminate carporadial impingement and fusion. None of the procedures provides a predictable satisfactory result. Replacement arthroplasty, therefore, has been attempted by several workers[22] of whom Swanson[23] is the best recognized. A silicone rubber spacer with a stabilizing trapezial peg has been devised which replaces the entire scaphoid.

The procedure is an attractive method to improve stability, to preserve or restore the alignment of several adjacent joints and to improve the range of motion of the wrist and carpus. The principal liability of the procedure has been the limited means available to stabilize the position of the implant. Subluxation of the spacer is not uncommon and is almost inevitable if the patient previously has had partial excision of the radial styloid. At present the role of the silicone rubber scaphoid arthroplasty remains unclear. Perhaps the best indications are in elderly patients with traumatic arthritis involving the scaphoid and others who will not undertake heavy laboring activities after surgery.

Procedure. A dorsolateral approach over the scaphoid, along the anatomical snuff box of the wrist is preferred (Fig. 15-7A). A longitudinal incision courses between the tendons of extensor pollicis longus and extensor carpi radialis longus. Sensory branches of the radial nerve and the radial artery shown in Figure 15-7B, are carefully protected. The capsule of the trapezioscaphoid joint is incised in a longitudinal plane and carefully preserved. The entire scaphoid bone is excised after X-ray confirmation of its identity. By the use of an air drill or a curet a hole is prepared in the trapezium to receive the stem of the implant. The hole is directed so that the implant will be anatomically oriented. The stabilizing peg fits into the trapezium. Of the several carpal articulations involving the scaphoid, this one shows the least motion. The correct size of the implant is determined by a trial fit with sizing units. The implant should fit comfortably into the space (Fig. 15-8A). With a no-touch technique the appropriate size of right or left handed implant is inserted into the space with its retaining peg embedded into the trapezium. The capsule is carefully repaired with 3-0 Dacron and the skin is closed in a conventional manner. A bulky pressure dressing is applied with a posterior molded plaster splint.

About 3 days after surgery a short-arm thumb spica cast is applied with the wrist in a neutral position. From 4 to 6 weeks after surgery the cast is removed and limited activity of the wrist and hand is encouraged. Twelve weeks after surgery full activity of the arm is permitted.

Silicone Rubber Lunate Arthroplasty

Traumatic arthritis of the lunate is considerably less common than that involving the scaphoid bone. Unfortunately, traumatic dislocation of the lunate is often unrecognized in the first post-traumatic evaluation. Frequently it presents several weeks after the accident when a painful stiff wrist is evident. Subsequently traumatic arthritis of the lunate may ensue irrespective of the method of treatment. Alternatively,

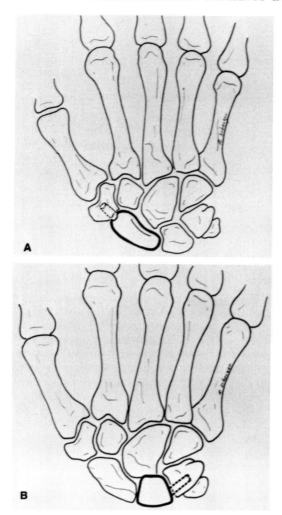

Figure 15-8. *A.* A schematic view of a scaphoid silicone implant after insertion is shown. *B.* A lunate prosthesis *in situ* is revealed.

Procedure. For a located lunate a dorsal approach is made through a curvilinear or an S-shaped cutaneous incision. Alternatively, when the lunate bone is dislocated a volar approach is recommended. The capsule of the wrist joint is incised transversely between the third and the fourth dorsal compartments. It is carefully preserved for the closure. Exposure is made between the tendons of the extensor pollicus longus and extensor digitorium communus. The lunate bone should be positively identified by X-rays. Usually it is removed by fragmentation. One of the three available sizes of implants is selected. The proper size should fill the cavity left by the excised lunate (Fig. 15-8*B*). With an air drill or small curet a small hole is prepared in the triquetrum to receive the stem of the implant. The triquetrum is used for stabilization because the triquetrial-lunate interface undergoes less motion than any other articulation of the lunate. The placement of the stem should permit accurate reduction of the prosthesis. The implant of correct size is inserted with a no-touch technique and the capsule is repaired with nonabsorbable sutures. The skin is closed in conventional fashion and a bulky pressure dressing with a posterior molded splint is applied.

About 3 days after surgery when postoperative swelling has decreased the dressing is replaced with a short-arm cast in which the wrist is positioned in neutral. About 4 to 6 weeks after surgery the cast is removed and limited motion of the forearm is permitted. Twelve weeks after surgery full activity is resumed.

SILICONE INTERPOSITIONAL ARTHROPLASTY FOR THE RECONSTRUCTION OF INTEROSSEOUS MEMBRANES

In both the forearm and the lower leg two parallel osseous structures move on one another with constraint provided by an interosseous membrane. The extraordinary range of motion in the forearm is recognized as 180° of combined pronation and supination. Perhaps less well recognized is the considerable longitudinal migration of the fibula on the tibia during gait. As Scranton *et al.*[25] have emphasized, motion of the fibula is essential to permit a change in the size and shape of the ankle mortise and thereby permit motion of the talus. If during plantar flexion and dorsiflexion of the ankle joint the distal fibula ceases to migrate proximally and distally, arthritis of the ankle joint rapidly ensues. Scranton *et al.*[25] have documented a number of patients in whom traumatic mineraliza-

avascular necrosis of the lunate of unclear origin is a well recognized entity that may culminate in arthritis of the carpus. Treatment of these problems has included fusion and proximal row carpectomy, although neither type of procedure is entirely satisfactory. The development of a silicone rubber replacement of the lunate was an obvious sequel of the evolution of the scaphoid prosthesis. The indications for its application include a painful or stiff wrist secondary to traumatic arthritis or avascular necrosis of the lunate. Swanson[23] and Aggerholm and Goodfellow[24] have reported satisfactory results of replacement arthroplasty of the lunate with different polymeric materials.

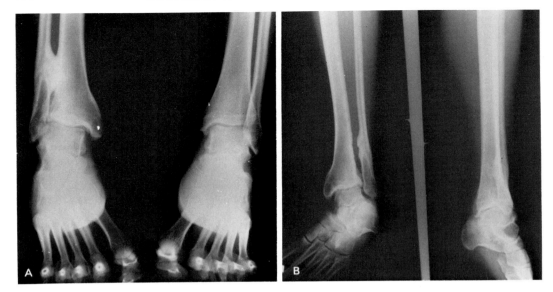

Figure 15-9. *A* and *B*. Pre- and postoperative radiological views taken prior to and after the excision of a bony bar between the distal tibia and fibula are revealed. The patient, a female of 21 years, previously had sustained a fracture dislocation of her ankle joint that was treated by plaster immobilization. Her symptoms of a painful effusion of her ankle were greatly alleviated by excision of the bar. The postoperative X-ray was taken 1 year after the surgical procedure. The bar is replaced by a somewhat mobile sheet of silicone rubber which attaches to the anterior surface of one bone and the posterior surface of the other.

tion of the interosseous membrane proximal to the ankle joint was followed by arthritis of the ankle joint. The author, also, has observed a group of 10 similar patients. The patients have been treated by resection of the bony union between the tibia and fibula and insertion of a silicone rubber interpositional barrier. After surgery, motion of the ankle joint is dramatically improved and the symptoms of pain with swelling and stiffness of the ankle joint are alleviated. Initially a silicone rubber barrier of minimal dimensions was inserted between the tibia and fibula. After the use of small barriers bone was observed to grow around either side of the implant to reform the bony union between the tibia and fibula. Subsequently a lengthy sheet of silicone rubber was used for the surgical reconstructions. One end of the sheet was attached to the anterior surface of the tibia. The sheet possessed a loose fold of rubber anterior to the interosseous membrane. A second loose fold was positioned posterior to the site of the interosseous membrane and the free end of the sheet was attached to the posterior fibula. During gait the sheet shows a substantial degree of motion and thereby seems to discourage formation of a continuous barrier between the two bones (Fig. 15-9). The patients have been followed for more than 2 years without recurrence of their bony

bridge. Clearly further follow-up will be necessary to document the long term results of this type of surgery.

In the upper extremity, similar silicone rubber interpositional barriers have been implanted between the radius and ulna after excision of bony bars of traumatic origin or those associated with congenital anomalies of the forearm. The results of surgery have not been notably successful possibly in view of the extraordinary range of motion of the intact radioulnar articulation. Also the osseous syndesmoses between the radius and ulna, especially in patients with congenital abnormalities, frequently are much longer than those encountered in the lower extremity and they may be accompanied by other deformities of bone and soft tissues.

THE USE OF SILICONE RUBBER SHEETS IN BONE

It will be recalled from Chapter 5 that the long bones grow primarily at highly discrete sites, the physes or growth plates. As a result of trauma, infection or other insult, the growth plate may be partly or wholly damaged. When the growth plate is entirely destroyed further growth is terminated. When a substantial limblength discrepancy necessitates surgical correction, a shortening procedure of the contralateral extremity may be undertaken with epiphysiodesis or, after skeletal maturity, a shortening osteotomy. Alternatively, the damaged bone may be lengthened by the more hazardous limb lengthening procedures as described in Chapter 11. Where part of the growth plate is injured the residual undamaged portion of growth plate continues to grow while the damaged portion shows partial or complete cessation of growth. The injured bone, therefore, shows a disturbance of subsequent growth with the presentation of an angular deformity. Several workers have questioned how the angular displacement could be prevented so that subsequent corrective osteotomy would not be necessary. For over 20 years Langenskiold[26, *] has excised the damaged osseous part of the growth plate and replaced it with subcutaneous fat. Where the osseous defect thereby created is less than approximately 25% of the cross-sectional area of the bone, subsequent growth of the growth plate is unrestricted so that the bone elongates without deformity. Where the defect in the physis is substantially greater than 25% of the cross-sectional area, subsequent growth of the bone is likely to be abnormal to a variable degree depending upon the area and the configuration of the defect.

The clinical documentation by Langenskiold *et al.* rests on an elegant laboratory investigation performed on juvenile rabbits femora.[27] A series of epiphyseal defects were made in the distal growth plate. When a peripheral defect is made, a bony bridge appears at the site of the defect, which is well seen by the 20th day after surgery (Fig. 15-10). With subsequent growth the bone shows progressive deformity as seen in Figure 15-11. The outcome is markedly different if the bony defect is filled with an autogenous graft of fat tissue (Fig. 15-12). The defect does not ossify and subsequent growth of the bone shows a normal configuration.

Other workers have utilized a silicone rubber sheet to fill the defect in the physis instead of the subcutaneous fat. For small defects in the physis substantially less than 25% of the cross-sectional area, the results of silicone rubber interposition rival those where fat is used. For larger defects, however, the use of fat shows superior results to the use of the man-made material. In view of the superior success of fatty interposition and of the ability of the fat to undergo biological remodeling and to resist infection, the author prefers to employ subcutaneous fatty interposition.

---

* A. Langenskiold, personal communication, 1976.

ATTEMPTS TO DEVELOP ARTIFICIAL TENDONS AND TENDON SHEATHS

Lacerations or attrition of tendons secondary to tenosynovitis[31] such as is encountered in rheumatoid arthritis are one of the more common types of injuries to the musculoskeletal system. The highly variable healing capacity of tendons has been of great interest to many workers. Some tendons such as the extensor tendons of the digits or the peroneal tendons show considerable propensity for spontaneous healing of traumatic lacerations with restitution of apparently normal function. Other tendons particularly the long flexor tendons in the hand show minimal tendency toward spontaneous restitution. When the superficial and profundus tendons in the hand are lacerated at one site in the extremity even after surgical repair, the two tendons are apt to unite to form one common unit with the loss of their independent motion. After more extensive hand injuries with destruction of a tendon and its sheath, the innate healing mechanisms are unlikely to restore a mobile musculotendinous unit. Many workers, therefore, have attempted to develop superior methods of treatment for tendinous injuries.[32, 33]

One direction of the newer work has been a study of the results that are achieved after different types of suture and suture technique are employed to repair lacerated tendons. The healing property of the tendons including biomechanical assessment of the tensile strength and the mobility of the tendons has been carefully studied by Hirsch and others. During the healing phase certain types of suture technique such as the criss-cross method of Bunnell, provide greater strength of the anastomosis although after the tendon has united the method used to provide provisional stability with sutures is immaterial. As Kleinert *et al.*[32] have emphasized, a suturing technique which provides a tendon repair of constant diameter rather than an acute "bulge" at the repair site provides a lower incidence of cross-union between a deep and superficial flexor tendon. Despite these and other experimental observations many clinical situations require a tendon graft to fully replace a tendon or to alter the site of a suture line, usually to the distal bone and to the proximal musculotendinous junction. Liabilities of tendon grafts include the need for a donor tendon and failures of the anastomoses. For these and other reasons, Hunter and Salsbury,[34] Hunter and Jaeger,[35] with others[36] have attempted to develop artificial tendons which are described below.

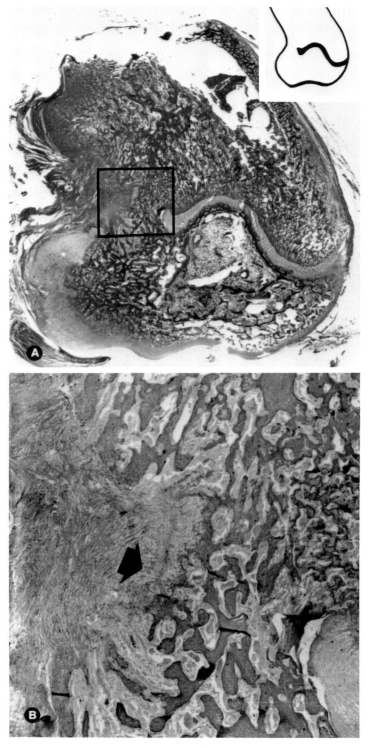

Figure 15-10. *A* and *B*. A histological section of a distal femoral physis in a juvenile rabbit taken 20 days after a peripheral defect has been made. The epiphyseal plate shows growth activity but a bony bridge has appeared at the site of the defect (*A*, ×7; *B*, ×40). (Reproduced with permission of K. Osterman.[28])

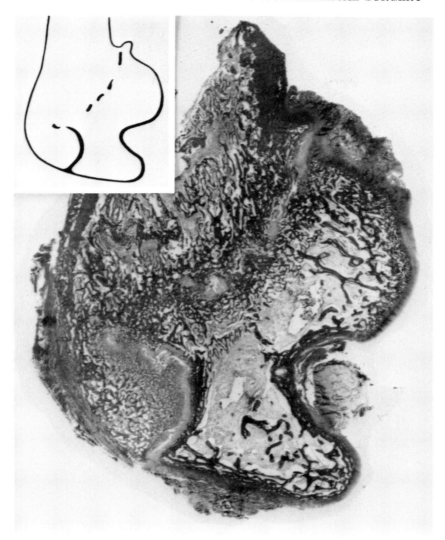

Figure 15-11. A histological section from an experiment similar to that shown in Figure 15-10 shows a comparable distal femur prepared 66 days after the provocative procedure. Gross deformity, cartilaginous islets and fibrous tissue replace the defective region of the epiphyseal plate and provoke progressive deformity (×7). (Reproduced with permission of K. Osterman.[29])

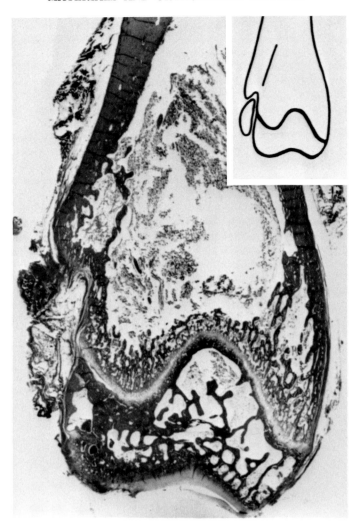

Figure 15-12. The histological section of a rabbit femur similar to those shown in Figures 15-10 and 15-11 with an epiphyseal injury treated by resection of the bony bridge and implantation of fat tissue is seen 84 days after the corrective operation. The transplant has remained at the level of the epiphyseal plate adjacent to the growing region. The epiphyseal plate is active and shows a normal configuration. The fat tissue is living but possesses some fibrotic changes (×7). (Reproduced with permission of K. Osterman.[30])

Prior to the insertion of a tendon graft or an artificial tendon a suitable receptive tissue bed is necessary in which to place the tendon or failure is assured. Hunter was one of the first workers to investigate the criteria of a suitable tendinous bed. He and his colleagues inserted flexible semirigid polymeric rods into spinal musculature and other sites of experimental animals. Histological evaluation of the regenerative tissues around the static nongliding implants revealed an orderly development of a new sheath remarkably similar to that surrounding an intact flexor tendon. These observations initiated the development of a silicone rubber rod which is widely employed to promote the formation of a tendon sheath after a long flexor tendon and its sheath has been severely traumatized. The damaged flexor tendon is excised and a rod is inserted into the hand from the palm distal to the distal phalanx. After surgery passive motion of the relevant finger is encouraged to assist in the formation of a highly organized tendon sheath. Within about 6 weeks a suitable bed has regenerated to receive a tendon graft replacement. Hunter *et al.*[35] next studied tendon sheath formation in response to limited active gliding around artificial tendons implanted in experimental animals. In the forepaw of a dog the extensor carpi radialis tendon was replaced with an active gliding flexor tendon. The artificial tendon was attached to bone and to the appropriate musculotendinous junction to restore active motion. Within 20 days histological observations revealed the conversion of a nonspecific bed of connective tissue or scar tissue into a well differentiated living envelope comparable to a tendon sheath system. The envelope was capable of lubricating and supporting a gliding implant to implement normal tendon function. At a later time the artificial tendon was replaced by a long free tendon graft. The latter structure is nourished in part by fluid and filmy adhesions between the tendon and the regenerative bed that resided between the proximal and distal anastomoses.

For these experiments the tendon and tendon sheath were primarily excised. A polymeric or metal loop was inserted through the tendinous stump at the musculotendinous junction to provide a loop-to-loop anastomosis and the distal end was anchored in bone. The cast was used to immobilize the extremity for the first 4 weeks after surgery. The sheaths and prosthesis were removed at periods of 4 to 12 months after insertion.

By gross observation the tendon sheath had remarkably normal appearance. Photomicroscopy revealed a smooth cell superficial layer on the surface of the gliding implants of about five cells in thickness. Superficial to this cellular layer was a secondary mobile plane, surrounded by a dense outer layer of connective tissue. The outer layer showed a linear arrangement of collagen comparable to a normal tendon. In summary, the mobile artificial tendinous unit appears to provoke the formation of a biological envelope similar to the surface of a living tendon. In turn, the biological layer is coated with connective tissue; eventually the two cylindrical structures undergo spontaneous separation to form a mobile interface between the tendon and the new tendon sheath. Hunter and Salsbury[34] and their colleagues have undertaken further morphological studies on the neosheath development around artificial tendons. As a model, Hunter et al.[34] used the flexor tendons and sheaths in chickens. A flexor tendon sheath in a toe was excised and replaced with a U. S. Army artificial tendon. The tendon consisted of a knitted Dacron tape coated with silicon rubber. The anastomosis of the tendon was secured with 6-0 Ethaflex (Ethicon, Inc., Somerville, N. J.) sutures. Four weeks later the animal was sacrificed and the tendon with its accompanying sheath was subjected to light microscopy and transmission electron microscopy. Evaluation of the sheath reveals a folded and pleated surface comparable to that of an intact synovial layer around a joint. An inner areolar and an outer fibrous synovial layer were observed similar to that visualized around an intact tendon sheath. The intimal layer of alveolar synovium consisted of cuboidal cells, two to four cells in thickness, with dark staining ovoid nuclei by hematoxylin and eosin preparations. The deep layer consisted of a loose filmy collagenous membrane with small capillaries resting above a thick layer of tightly packed collagen. The outer fibrous synovial layer consisted of a unicellular layer of fibroblasts superficial to dense collagen tissue. Transmission electron microscopy revealed the presence of type A and type B cells that are seen in intact synovial sheath or synovium around an articular joint. The A cells consist of phagocytes while the B cells show abundant ergastoplasm which indicates the synthesis and secretion of protein.

All of these elegant studies confirm the formation of a mobile flexor tendon sheath around an artificial tendon which is comparable to the intact human organ. A porous artificial tendon which is secured to the site of an intact flexor tendon after removal of a living flexor tendon and its sheath can provoke the formation of a surrounding flexor tendon sheath after the infiltration of living cells into the porous surface of the implant. These observations give great encouragement for the subsequent development of clinically useful artificial tendons. In fact the question arises why such striking provisional success has not culminated in widespread application of artificial tendons. To date the clinical problem has been the inability of surgeons and research workers to devise satisfactory union between an artificial tendon and a musculotendinous junction. When an artificial tendon, even one with a porous coated surface, is sutured to a musculotendinous junction, the sutures provide temporary stabilization. Fibroblasts infiltrate the implant to provide a collagenous medium for biological attachment. Ultimately the sutures undergo fatigue failure and the strength of the bond rests upon the mechanical properties of the collagenous scar tissue.[37] Subsequently mechanical failure of the scar is observed. To date no one has discovered a satisfactory method to regenerate a tendinous-like material to impregnate the artificial tendon. The distal site of attachment of an artificial tendon to bones such as the phalanx, has proved to be a lesser problem. The growth of bone into a porous matrix provides firm anchorage of the prosthetic unit. Perhaps the optimal form of union is the application of a porous titanium plug on the distal end of the artificial tendon. Semple and Murray* have tested such porous titanium plugs for anchorage of prosthetic replacements of the Achilles' tendon in dogs. With the preparation of titanium plugs that lock in the bone with a mortise fit, a distal anastomosis is provided which can withstand full activity of the tendon unit immediately after surgery. The porous material is described fully in Chapter 16.

Another attempt to develop artificial tendons has been reported by Amstutz et al.[38] These workers have employed Dacron mesh and silicone prostheses for the reconstruction of canine Achilles' and patellar tendons. Dacron No. 6-0 and 5-0 mesh (U. S. Catheter Instrument Co.), is rolled into a tube of 6 to 10 mm in diameter. The tube is secured with 5.0 Dacron sutures. A silicone rubber sheet of 0.10 or 0.02 inch in thickness (Dow-Corning) is secured around the Dacron mesh. Such artificial tendons were implanted in 15 mature beagle dogs. Ultimately the animals were sacrificed and both histological and biomechanical evaluations of the prosthetic tendinous units were performed. The principal practical problem was that observed by other workers namely mechanical failure of the prosthetic tendinous interface.

In every example, tendon formation outside the Dacron tube was observed. For implants that remained in situ for more prolonged periods of time a progressive diminution in the cellular content of the matrix was observed while concomitant maturation of the matrix was evident. Focal areas of accumulation of acid mucopolysaccharide were noted.

While there was rapid re-establishment of functional continuity in the patellar tendons, mechanical failure at the musculotendinous junctions of the Achilles' tendons presented a much greater problem. Walter et al.[38] undertook a biomechanical evaluation of the regenerative canine tendons. Mechanical tests with an Instron were performed within 24 hours after sacrifice of the animals. During the tests the tendons were immersed in physiological solution. The regenerative tendons appear to remodel rapidly in dimensions and structure so that their

mechanical properties were remarkably similar to those of normal intact tendons, as ascertained by a load-extension parameter. Normal tendons were somewhat stiffer than regenerative units. The modulus of elasticity of the normal patellar tendon was measured at 1000 to 2000 kg./cm.[2]

The observations of Amstutz and Walker reaffirm those of Hunter and Salsbury[34] and further confirm that the body's propensity to form new gliding units around flexible polymeric materials provides the mechanism for prosthetic and biological reconstitution of tendons. To date, however, this exciting observation cannot be realized as a clinical solution until a novel technique for attachment of the prosthetic tendon to the musculotendinous junction is developed.

ATTEMPTS TO DEVELOP NEW ARTIFICIAL LIGAMENTOUS PROSTHESES

One of the greatest limitations in presently available orthopaedic needs is the limited success in attempts to repair or reconstruct human ligaments. In weight-bearing joints such as the knee, surgical approximation of torn ligaments with the use of sutures is notoriously unsuccessful.[39] The reconstructed ligaments are rarely comparable to intact ligaments. Where a part of an intact ligament such as the medial collateral ligament in the knee is fully disrupted, attempts to provide a biological substitute such as a graft of fascia lata, usually, are unsatisfactory. No other biological tissue possesses the same mechanical properties as intact ligament. At the site of union between surfaces of a disrupted ligament or at the site of repair between a portion of the ligament and a graft of fascia or other biological material, a collagenous scar develops which fails to provide sufficient mechanical stability for the restitution of normal joint function. For a full discussion on the mechanical properties of intact ligaments such as the anterior cruciate ligament the reader is referred to several useful reviews elsewhere.[40-45]

One of the first clinically tested ligamentous prostheses has been developed by the Richards Manufacturing Company for replacement of the anterior cruciate ligament. Previous biological reconstructions of the anterior cruciate ligament with tendons such as the gracilis or the semitendinosis have failed to show satisfactory results. Thus the impetus for the development of an artificial tendon was readily provided. The ligamentous prostheses are fabricated from Hercules 1900 medical-grade ultra high molecular

---

* C. Semple, and G. A. W. Murray, personal communication, 1977.

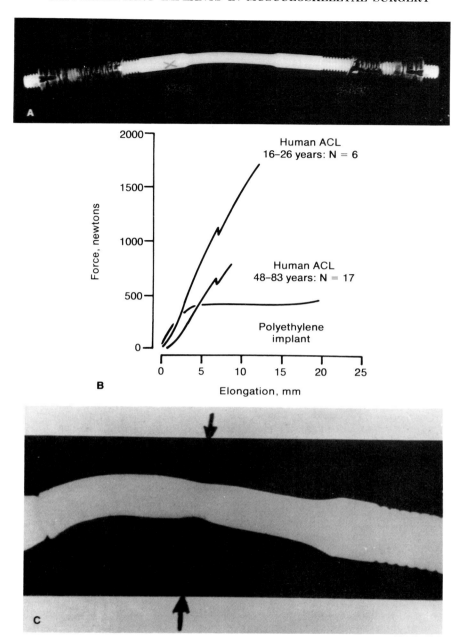

Figure 15-13. *A.* The photograph shows the Richards anterior cruciate ligament replacement, about two-thirds of its actual size. *B.* A comparison of the load-elongation behavior of the anterior cruciate implant and the comparable human ligament is presented. Summary curves are presented for preparations from both younger and older human patients. The dips in the curve represent the onset of observable macroscopic failure. The largest force values at the end of the curve represent the average maximum loads supported by the preparations prior to complete failure. The polyethylene implant yields and deforms plastically at a force which is only one-half and one-fourth the maximum strength of the specimens from older and younger human patients, respectively. (Reproduced with permission of E. S. Grood and F. R. Noyes.[46]) *C.* A cruciate ligament implant removed after 10 months *in vivo* for fixation failure is shown. The implant exhibits a neck, indicated by *arrows*, showing that it was subjected to forces above its elastic limit to provoke permanent elongation. The defect seen near the left end of the implant was made at the time of removal. (Reproduced with permission of E. S. Grood and F. R. Noyes.[47])

weight polyethylene. They are 6.35 mm in diameter and 178 mm in length. They have a reduced central cross-section 4.76 mm in diameter and 35 or 40 mm in length. Each end of the implant is formed into an 0.25 by 20 thread for a distance of 50 mm to be fitted into a threaded knot which is used for fixation of the implant in the bone with supplementary polymethylmethacrylate cement (Fig. 15-13A). Recently Noyes and Grood[40] undertook a detailed mechanical analysis of the cruciate ligament prosthesis. The tests were performed under a variety of *in vitro* experimental conditions and the results were compared with the behavior of human anterior cruciate ligaments. The mechanical attributes of tensile strength, residual elongation, creep and bending fatigue were measured. Also the effect of strain rate and temperature on the load-elongation properties of the implant were investigated.

When tested at an elongation rate of 100% per sec, the polyethylene prosthesis yields under the imposition of a force of 420 newtons (94 lb) and plastically deforms at about 10% elongation. The implant shows considerable viscoelastic behavior so that the amount of elongation depends upon the force applied and the duration of both loading and recovery. It is possible that a change in implant length induced by cyclic loading *in vivo* might alter the joint mechanics considerably. A comparison of load-elongation behavior of the implant and the human tibia anterior cruciate ligament-femoral preparation are shown in Figure 15-13B. The polyethylene implant yields and deforms plastically at a force which is about one-half and one-fourth the maximum strength of the intact ligament in older and younger human patients, respectively. Noyes and Grood[40] estimate that under normal conditions biological tissues are subjected to forces of about one-tenth to not more than one-fifth of their breaking loads. They estimate that forces applied to the anterior cruciate ligament *in vivo* in young adults typically range from 200 to 400 newtons (50 to 100 lb) and from 80 to 160 newtons (20 to 40 lb) in older people. In comparison the polyethylene implant shows a yield point with permanent deformation at loads of 420 newtons (94 lb).

Morrison[45] used a combined experimental and analytical approach to calculate the forces acting on the anterior cruciate ligament during level walking (169 newtons), ascent of stairs (67 newtons) and descent of stairs (445 newtons). During the descent of stairs a force in excess of the yield point of the implant (420 newtons) was achieved.

From these studies it should be apparent that the margin of safety of the polyethylene component of the Richards implant is low in terms of its ability to resist anticipated *in vivo* forces without sustaining permanent deformation. The data suggests that the implant may function adequately in older patients with restricted activities but not in younger individuals exposed to high *in vivo* loads.

The manufacturer of the prosthesis (Richards Manufacturing Co., Memphis, Tenn.) has reported the failure of four implants *in vivo* through mechanical failure of the polyethylene component. The four failures are believed to represent 4.6% of the total number of implants inserted. One of the failed implants was subjected to mechanical tests after its removal. Gross observation revealed a region of necking where the implant was subjected to stress above its yield limit. An example is seen in Figure 15-13C. Tensile tests conducted on the prosthesis indicate the material in the neck region has a higher strength and a lower ductility than is found with undeformed polyethylene. Such local changes in the polymer affect its fatigue life in a deleterious way.

At the present time the clinical application for the prosthetic cruciate ligaments would appear to be very limited. In common with other prosthetic devices the insertion of the cruciate implant compromises the ability of the joint to resist infection. Infection after such a procedure could severely compromise the functional capacity of the knee when, with the absence of an anterior cruciate ligament, without other abnormality, the knee may show surprisingly normal function. Since the prosthetic device is most unlikely to withstand the vigorous mechanical environment imposed upon the knees of competitive athletes, the implant is specifically contraindicated in such individuals.

Procedure. The optimal incision depends upon the need for supplementary ligamentous repair procedures in addition to replacement of the anterior cruciate ligament. If ligamentous replacement is the sole procedure, a medial parapatellar incision from the superior pole of the patella distal to the anterior tibial tubercle will suffice. Alternatively, if the surgeon elects to undertake a posteromedial capsular reefing or a pes anserinus transfer, as well as the prosthetic replacement, an oblique medial incision from above the medial femoral condyle to the anterior tibial tubercle is preferred. Alternatively, if a lateral ligamentous repair is necessary, a lateral parapatellar incision is recommended. Irrespective of the incision, the wound is extended in layers through the capsule and synovium. For the tibial attachment of the prosthesis a ³/₃₂-inch guide wire is inserted into the tibial metaphysis (Fig. 15-14A). If a medial incision has been used, the guide wire is inserted medial to the tibial tubercle and at least 4 cm (1⁹/₁₆″) distal to the joint line. The pin is aimed in a somewhat lateral direction so that its tip exits from the bone in the intercondylar region 2 cm (²⁵/₃₂″) from the anterior rim. Alternatively, if a lateral incision has been made the tibial hole can be introduced lateral to the tibial tubercle and at least 4 cm distal to the joint line (Fig. 15-14B). Again it is angled toward the intercondylar region, 2 cm from the anterior rim. The ⁷/₁₆-inch diameter cannulated reamer is inserted over the guide wire and a hole is prepared (Fig. 15-14C). A curet should be placed over the protruding guide wire within the knee to prevent the reamer from damaging other structures within the knee. A trial sleeve, seen in Figure 15-14D, is inserted into the exit hole in the intercondylar region to determine the optimal length and angle of the final sleeve implant.

Through a separate cutaneous incision along the lateral parapatellar region, preparation is made for the lateral femoral condylar hole. The incision is extended through the capsule and synovium with exposure of the lateral compartment. Alternatively if the initial cutaneous incision is made through the lateral parapatellar region it can be used to prepare the lateral femoral condylar hole. A ³/₃₂-inch guide wire is inserted with a power drill into the lateral aspect of the lateral femoral condyle (Fig. 15-14E). It should be introduced at least 2 cm proximal to the articular cartilaginous rim. The guide wire is aimed toward the intercondylar notch and about 1.5 cm (⁵/₈″) posterior to the articular cartilaginous rim. A ⁷/₁₆-inch diameter cannulated reamer is placed over the guide wire and the hole is prepared. A curet is placed over the tip of the guide wire to protect the articular cartilage. A trial sleeve is placed in the intercondylar hole to measure the optimal length and angle of the final sleeve implant. Subsequently, the countersink reamer (Fig. 15-14F) is used to prepare a countersink in the femoral entrance hole, on the lateral femoral condyle and the tibial entrance hole. Fixation nuts are placed in the entrance holes (Fig. 15-14G). At this time a length of the sleeve should be examined to ensure that it is not excessively long, thereby to prevent adequate insertion of the fixation nut, for the fixation nut should fit in the countersunk hole with-

out any protrusion above the surface of bone.

A trial Polyflex ligament (Fig. 15-14H) is inserted from the tibial hole to the femoral hole to determine the length of the prosthetic ligament. The measurement refers to the length from one tapered end to the other tapered end on the trial prosthesis. The trials are color coded with lengths of 3.0, 3.5 and 4.0 cm (1¼″, 1⅜″ and 1⁹/₁₆″). The prosthetic ligament should be somewhat too long rather than too short.

Methylmethacrylate cement is prepared and the coating of cement is applied to the tibial sleeve. The sleeve is inserted into the interarticular portion of the tibial hole (Fig. 15-14I). A sleeve pusher is applied to the sleeve to ensure adequate impaction of the implant. A Teflon probe is inserted through the sleeve to remove excessive cement. A second sleeve is coated with cement and inserted into the interarticular end of the femoral hole. The sleeve is impacted and excessive cement is removed by insertion of the Teflon probe. After the cement has solidified, the Teflon probes are removed. As shown in Figure 15-14J, the prosthetic ligament is inserted through the extra-articular end of the tibial hole. Alternatively a 2-0 nylon suture can be inserted through a hole in the end of the prosthetic ligament. The suture can be inserted through the hole with a tendon passer to facilitate introduction of the prosthetic ligament. The trial fixation nuts (Fig. 15-14K) are advanced onto each end of the ligament until the nuts abut against cortical bone. The knee is tested for stability and range of motion.

Another unit of methylmethacrylate cement is mixed and the tibial and femoral exit holes are filled. The metallic fixation nuts are threaded onto the exposed ends of the prosthetic ligaments with the use of wrenches (Fig. 15-14L). The fixation nuts are advanced simultaneously until they are flush with the cortical surface. This procedure is performed while the knee is flexed between 60 and 80°. Again the knee joint is tested for range of motion and stability. At this time the surgeon may elect to augment stability by a supplementary extra-articular soft tissue repair procedure.

The knee joint is irrigated with triple antibiotic solution and a suction drain is inserted. The knee joint is closed in layers in conventional fashion as described under total knee joint replacement. A bulky dressing is applied with anterior and posterior plaster splints.

Postoperative Course. The postoperative regime for physical therapy varies considerably depending upon the supplementary soft tissue

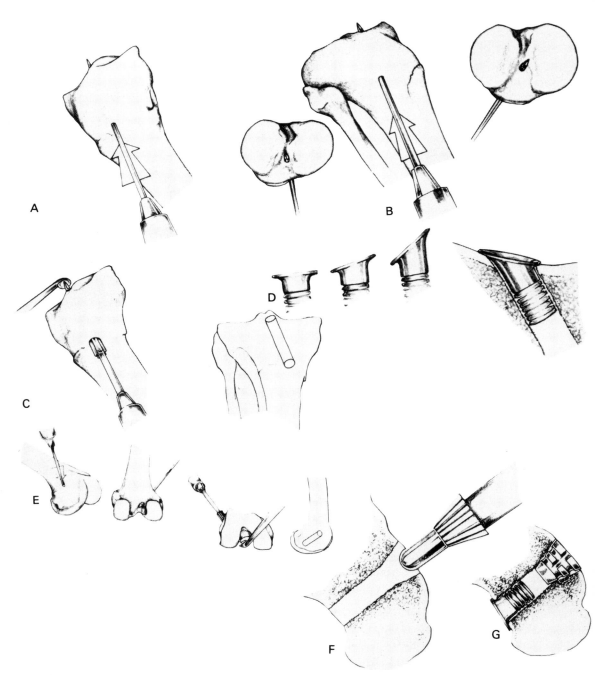

Figure 15-14. A series of schematic diagrams reveals the stages of insertion of an anterior cruciate ligament prosthesis. *A,* A ³⁄₃₂-inch guide wire is inserted with a power drill medial to the anterior tibial tubercle and at least 4 cm below the joint line. The guide wire is directed toward the intercondylar region about 2 cm (²⁵⁄₃₂″) from the anterior rim. Alternatively, as shown in *B,* a similar tibial hole can be prepared through a lateral parapatellar incision. *C.* A ⁷⁄₁₆-inch diameter cannulated reamer is inserted over the guide wire and a protective cover such as a curet or periosteal elevator is placed over the protruding end of the wire in the knee joint. *D.* A trial sleeve is placed in the intercondylar end of the drill hole to determine the appropriate length and angle of the final sleeve implant. *E.* Using the same technique a femoral hole is prepared in the lateral femoral condyle. The hole starts along the lateral aspect of the lateral femoral condyle at least 2 cm superior to the articular cartilaginous rim. The guide wire should exit in the intercondylar notch about 1.5 cm (⅝″) posterior to the articular cartilaginous rim. *F.* With a countersink reamer, the femoral entrance hole in the lateral femoral condyle and the tibial entrance hole are countersunk. *G.* A fixation nut is placed in the entrance holes to ensure proper seating and length of the sleeve. *H.* A trial ligament is inserted to select the appropriate length for the prosthetic ligament. The prosthetic ligament should be a little too long rather than too short. *I.* A sleeve is

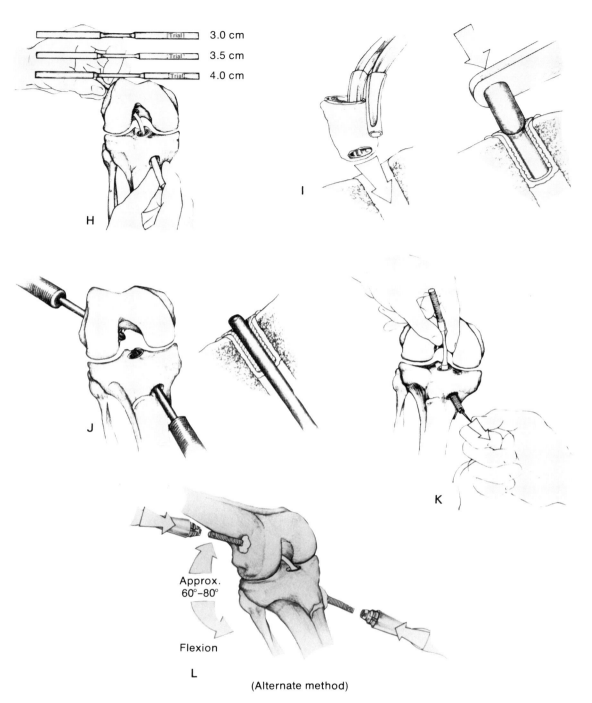

H

3.0 cm
3.5 cm
4.0 cm

I

J

K

Approx.
60°–80°

Flexion

L

(Alternate method)

coated with methylmethacrylate and inserted into the interarticular tibial hole. A sleeve pusher instrument is used which prevents cement from plugging the sleeve or tibial hole. Another sleeve is inserted in a similar fashion into the interarticular aspect of the femoral hole. *J.* The prosthetic ligament is inserted into the interarticular aspect of the tibial hole. A heavy suture and a tendon passer can be used to facilitate this step. A similar maneuver is undertaken to pass the ligament through the femoral hole. *K.* Black Delrin trial fixation nuts are advanced on each end of the ligament and secured against the cortical bone by hand pressure. Then the knee is tested for stability and range of motion. *L.* The tibial and femoral exit holes are filled with another bolus of methylmethacrylate cement. Metallic fixation nuts are advanced onto the ends of the prosthetic ligament by the use of two nut wrenches. Both fixation nuts are advanced synchronously with the knee flexed at 60 to 80° until the nuts are flush or below the cortical limit level of the outer holes. Alternatively, the metallic fixation nuts can be advanced individually and cemented in turn. (*A* to *L*, reproduced with permission of R. Heros and C. Lawler, Richards Manufacturing Co., Memphis, Tenn.)

repairs undertaken at the time of anterior cruciate ligament replacement. Where no supplementary procedures are undertaken, within a few days after surgery the patient may be instructed in quadriceps and hamstring exercises and active range of motion. Where supplementary repairs are performed a variety of alterations in the therapeutic program may be indicated depending upon the nature of the repair. The reader is referred elsewhere[48] for a more detailed account.

ATTEMPTS TO DEVELOP ARTIFICIAL MUSCLES

The attempts to develop internal replacements of muscles remain at an exceptionally primitive stage. In 1934 Voelcker[49] described the insertion of steel springs for replacement of muscles. These and comparable attempts to use elastic bands were unsuccessful. The steel springs underwent corrosion and fracture. Subsequently the same author attempted to employ stainless steel springs in five patients with peroneal paralysis secondary to anterior poliomyelitis. The springs were inserted between the tibia and the foot or as a substitute for the gastrocnemius muscle. Apparently modest success was achieved for at least a limited period of time. More recently Strach has employed springs to supplement paralyzed muscles in children with myelodysplasia. Success has been compromised by limitations of currently available materials and tissue infiltration. In a somewhat similar way Gruca[50] and White et al.[51] have inserted springs into the paravertebral region to supplement weakened trunk muscles and attempt to correct spinal deformity. Mooney* has replicated this procedure by the use of Wyss springs in patients with kyphosis of certain etiologies with similar good results.

As a biological alternative solution to replace one or more impaired muscles, recent workers[52, 53] have concentrated on autogenous muscle transfers by the use of muscles on a neurovascular pedicle. The crucial surgical problem is the microsurgical anastomosis of the small nutritional artery and the accompanying nerve which innervates the muscle transplant. With the early successes recorded in these attempts it seems not unlikely that free muscle transplants on a neurovascular pedicle will provide a markedly superior concept to attempts to develop prosthetic muscles. The biological solution permits continuous biological repair and the body's innate defenses against infection. Furthermore

it provides a simple method to control contractility of the transplanted muscle.

IMPLANTS IN SURGICAL RECONSTRUCTION OF AMPUTATION STUMPS

Several workers have attempted to use implantable materials for improvement in the function of amputation stumps. The implantable materials have been used to augment the end-bearing capabilities of stumps both for cushioning impulsive loads and for providing the optimal configuration of the end-bearing endoskeletal structure. The implants, also, have been used to limit the relative overgrowth of diaphyseal bone that is frequently observed in transdiaphyseal amputations in children. Also, implants have been employed as a means by which artificial limbs might be attached to the endoskeleton of an amputation stump. These efforts are described briefly in turn.

Swanson's first clinical studies on the use of silicon implants was an assessment of intramedullary stemmed silicone rubber implants for insertion in the distal end of the bone at an amputation site.[54] It was hoped that the implant would serve to provide a pain-free smooth stump with optimal shape for uniform distribution of impulsive loads over the adjacent soft tissues. In a similar way it was hoped that after surgery, the artificial limb would possess a simpler and superior fit to facilitate walking. The silicone implants were used in the distal end of the femur and tibia although otherwise the surgical preparation of the stump was according to conventional format. The reader is referred to the detailed description by Swanson. The study suggested that the patients who underwent the insertion of this flexible implant showed improved tolerance to end bearing. Swanson reported a detailed follow-up on 49 patients of which 19 adults had bilateral procedures. The principal complication was breakdown of the wound which required removal of the implant in five amputated limbs. Extrusion of the implant did not seem to be a problem when careful surgical technique was followed. Despite Swanson's encouraging results other workers do not appear to accept the use of the silicone rubber implants.

The Control of Bone Overgrowth in Juvenile Amputees with Silicone Rubber Implants

A well recognized problem in transdiaphyseal amputation in children is subsequent bone ov-

---

* V. Mooney, personal communication, 1977.

ergrowth which exceeds the rate of growth of skin and soft tissue at the stump site.[54] The precise explanation for the relative overgrowth of bone has remained obscure. The problem is obviated if juvenile amputations are performed as a disarticulation rather than as a transection through a long bone. Also special care must be taken to ensure adequate soft tissue coverage of the stump. Nevertheless in certain instances a transdiaphyseal amputation becomes the optimal form of management in certain children. Swanson inserted the silicone rubber intramedullary stemmed implant into the stump sites of a group of juvenile amputees. The implants appear to have been remarkably successful in the control of relative bone overgrowth. Despite the successful results reported by Swanson the technique has not gained widespread popularity.

The Use of Transcutaneous Porous Graphite Implants for the Attachment of Artificial Limbs

Most presently available limbs attach to the amputation stump by means of a close-fitting socket.[55, 56] The socket may be of the end-bearing type and have supplementary straps or cups to stabilize the limb on the stump. For at least a decade the more popular method of attachment has been the use of a closely fitting total contact socket whereupon the forces of weight bearing are distributed uniformly around the area of contact between the socket and the stump. Optimal contact between the skin and the socket is realized by the use of a system of valves that permits elimination of air between the two surfaces. Even with the optimal system, however, substantial weight-bearing forces are imposed upon the skin at the stump site which may provoke stump pain, ulceration or other clinical problems. Mooney* and others have attempted to employ porous coated implantable materials such as graphite which could be inserted into the distal end of the diaphysis of the transected bone to protrude through the skin at the stump site and provide a means for rigid attachment of the prosthesis. In theory the method would eliminate weight-bearing forces on the skin at the stump site. Also it would provide a much simpler method for attachment of any artificial limb or for a variety of limbs to one stump site each with a peculiar functional or cosmetic attribute. As will be discussed in Chapter 16, the ingrowth of bone into a porous substrate is now recognized as an excellent method for attachment of a va-

riety of implants to bone. The principal limitation with the protruding implants is the grave liability for infection at the margin between the protruding portion of the implant and skin. To the present time this problem has remained unsolved so that the technique is not available for clinical application.

ATTEMPTS TO REPLACE LUMBAR INTERVERTEBRAL DISCS

For thousands of years low back pain has hampered the productivity of man. In 1934, Mixter and Barr[57] published their classic explanation for the source of low back and leg pain previously recognized as lumbago and sciatica. As the annulus fibrosus, the peripheral resilient portion of the intervertebral disc, undergoes characteristic biochemical changes with advancing age, it weakens. Ultimately, upon minor provocation the central, gelatinous nucleus pulposus herniates through a defect in the annular protrusion. Posterior displacement of the nucleus pulposus may occur in several directions to culminate in a variety of clinical pictures. If a large volume of disc material exudes into the spinal canal, a profound neurological catastrophe may ensue. More commonly the extrusion is a gradual and intermittent process, usually in a posterolateral direction. The process is fully described elsewhere.[58] The extruded material may impinge upon a nerve root to provoke the characteristic radicular pain, weakness and diminution in sensation of the appropriate cutaneous distribution, or dermatome. Concomitant degenerative changes in the facetal joints, also may contribute to nerve impingement with further symptomatic upset.[59]

Treatment of acute or chronic lumbar disc disease is perhaps the single most common problem to which the typical orthopaedic surgeon must address himself. Irrespective of the available therapeutic methods the convalescent period tends to be prolonged.[58] Most heavy laborers require at least 3 months of unemployment and many never return to arduous endeavor. The hallmark of management is a variable period of bedrest followed by restricted activity. Pelvic traction, heat, exercises and other forms of physical therapy are widely employed; medications such as analgesics and muscle relaxants also are used. Patients who present with acute neurological catastrophe, severe pain refractory to conservative treatment and those with chronic lumbar disc disease that fails to respond to conservative methods may be treated by laminectomy and discectomy. Even after surgery,

---

* V. Mooney, personal communication, 1976.

their convalescence prior to return to work usually persists for a few months or longer.

As a sequel of lumbar disc disease treated by conservative or operative means, many patients develop mechanical low back pain. The origin of the pain is believed to originate in the facetal joints at the degenerative site.[59] Routine lumbar or lumbosacral fusion at the time of discectomy has been employed with limited success as a method to prevent the subsequent mechanical low back pain.

For these and other reasons several workers have attempted to develop artificial lumbar discs to replace symptomatic degenerative ones. While the previous attempts have not yet provided a useful clinical method, nevertheless they serve as a stimulant for future work.

Urbaniak et al.[60] replaced lumbar discs in chimpanzees with a silicone-Dacron composite. The artificial discs consisted of a central core of Dacron mesh with silicone elastomer. The peripheral surfaces to oppose the vertebral bodies possessed vulcanized layers of Dacron mesh for ingrowth of bone. Through a left permedian incision a retroperitoneal approach to the lumbosacral spine was made. The anterior longitudinal ligament was elevated as a flap. A lumbar disc was excised, and in some animals, the adjacent end plates of bone were removed to expose cancellous bone. A countersink of several millimeters was made on the anterior portion of the vertebral body. An artificial disc of precisely anatomical dimensions was selected and carefully keyed into place. The anterior longitudinal ligament was repaired to assist in anchorage of the disc.

The animals were sacrificed after variable periods of time up to a year after surgery. Two disc space infections occurred of which one artificial disc was removed at 4 months and another at 6 months. One implant of excessive size was found to be tilted 1 month after surgery. Five months later it was recovered surgically at which time it was firmly stabilized to the adjacent bone. The residual implants appeared to be rigidly incorporated into the adjacent spinal elements. There was no evidence of bony resorption nor of instability of the spine when X-rays of the spine were taken in flexion and extension. In a few cases biomechanical tests were performed after the animals were sacrificed and the discs were removed. For these studies, the vertebral bodies adjacent to the artificial disc were divided in their midportion so that a segment of bone, disc and bone was removed as an intact specimen. The specimen was embedded in methylmeth-

acrylate and surrounded by a steel case. Subsequently the bending, torsional and compressive properties of the artificial disc were measured and compared with normal anatomical intervertebral discs. The results show remarkable similarity provided that the replacement disc was of the correct size. Histological observations on the discs also indicate satisfactory tolerance of the implant by the host.

More recently Schneider and Oyen[61] have published a preliminary report on the replacement of lumbar discs with silicone rubber in human patients. After discectomy and currettage of the disc a fluid-activated polysiloxan is injected into the space formerly occupied by the nucleus pulposus. The silicone polymerizes in situ to form an elastic silicone rubber which wholly fills the cavity. The silicone rubber becomes firmly embedded and immobilized in the annulus fibrosus. After surgery the reconstructed disc appears to restore the normal motility and stability of the relevant portion of the lumbar spine. A more detailed clinical account is eagerly awaited.

REFERENCES

1. Swanson, A. B. *Flexible Implant Resection Arthroplasty in the Hand and Extremities*, p. 1, C. V. Mosby Co., St. Louis, 1973.
2. Swanson, A. B. *Flexible Implant Resection Arthroplasty in the Hand and Extremities*, p. 296, C. V. Mosby Co., St. Louis, 1973.
3. Keller, W. L. *N.Y. Med. J., 80:*701, 1904.
4. Crenshaw, A. H. (editor), *Campbell's Operative Orthopaedics*, p. 18, 115, C. V. Mosby Co., St. Louis, 1971.
5. Mayo, C. H. *Ann. Surg., 48:*300, 1908.
6. Hoffman, P. *Am. J. Orthop. Surg., 9:*441, 1911.
7. Clayton, M. L. *J. Bone Jt. Surg., 42a:*523, 1970.
8. Swanson, A. B. *Orthop. Clin. Am., 4:*383, 1973.
9. Swanson, A. B. *Orthop. Clin. Am., 4:*373, 1973.
10. Swanson, A. B. *Flexible Implant Resection Arthroplasty in the Hand and Extremities*, p. 265, C. V. Mosby Co., St. Louis, 1973.
11. Flatt, A. E. *The Care of the Rheumatoid Hand*, p. 52, C. V. Mosby Co., St. Louis, 1974.
12. Swanson, A. B. *Flexible Implant Resection Arthroplasty in the Hand and Extremities*, p. 71, C. V. Mosby Co., St. Louis, 1973.
13. Darrach, W. *Ann. Surg., 56:*802, 1912.
14. Goldstein, L. A., and Dickerson, R. C. *Atlas of Orthopaedic Surgery*, p. 188, C. V. Mosby Co., St. Louis, 1974.
15. Swanson, A. B. *Orthop. Clin. N. Am., 4:*373, 1973.
16. Pieron, A. P. *Acta Orthop. Scand., Suppl. 148,* 8, 1973.
17. Swanson, A. B. *Flexible Implant Resection Arthroplasty in the Hand and Extremities*, p. 218, C. V. Mosby Co., St. Louis, 1973.
18. Swanson, A. B. *Flexible Implant Resection Arthroplasty in the Hand and Extremities*, p. 220 C. V. Mosby Co., St. Louis, 1973.

19. Swanson, A. B. *J. Bone Jt. Surg., 54A:*456, 1972.
20. Swanson, A. B. *Flexible Implant Resection Arthroplasty in the Hand and Extremities,* p. 231, C. V. Mosby Co., St. Louis, 1973.
21. Dobyns, J. H., and Linscheid, R. L. Fractures and dislocations of the wrist. In *Fractures,* p. 385, edited by C. A. Rockwood and D. P. Green, J. B. Lippincott Co., Philadelphia, 1975.
22. Agerholm, J. C., and Lee, M. L. *Acta Orthop. Scand., 37:*67, 1966.
23. Swanson, A. B. *Flexible Implant Resection Arthroplasty in the Hand and Extremities,* p. 240, C. V. Mosby Co., St. Louis, 1973.
24. Aggerholm, J. C., and Goodfellow, J. W. *J. Bone Jt. Surg., 45B:*110, 1963.
25. Scranton, P. E., McMaster, J. H., and Kelly, E. *Clin. Orthop., 118:*76, 1976.
26. Langenskiold, A. *Acta Ortho.Scand., 38:*267, 1967.
27. Osterman, K. *Acta Orthop. Scand., Suppl. 147,* 24, 1973.
28. Osterman, K. *Acta Orthop. Scand., Suppl. 147,* 33, 1973.
29. Osterman, K. *Acta Orthop. Scand., Suppl. 147,* 1973.
30. Osterman, K. *Acta Orthop. Scand., Suppl. 147,* 41, 1973.
31. Flatt, A. E. *The Care of the Rheumatoid Hand,* p. 96, C. V. Mosby Co., St. Louis, 1974.
32. Kleinert, H. E., Kutz, J. E., Atasoy, E., and Stormo, A. *Orthop. Clin. N. Am.,* 4:865, 1973.
33. Tubiana, R. *Orthop. Clin. N. Am.,* 4:877, 1973.
34. Hunter, J. M., and Salsbury, R. E. *Plast. Reconstruct. Surg.,* 45:564, 1970.
35. Hunter, J. M., and Jaeger, S. H. *Orthop. Clin. N. Am.,* 8:473, 1977.
36. Carroll, R. E., and Bassett, C. A. L. *J. Bone Jt. Surg., 45A:*884, 1963.
37. Hirsch, G., *Acta Orthop. Scand., Suppl. 153,* 12, 1974.
38. Amstutz, H., Coulson, W. F., Walker, P., and Rubinfeld, M., *J. Biomed. Mater. Res., 10:*47 and 61, 1976.
39. Larson, R. L. Dislocations and ligamentous injuries of the knee. In *Fractures,* p. 1227, edited by C. A. Rockwood and D. P. Green, J. B. Lippincott Co., Philadelphia, 1975.
40. Noyes, F. R., and Grood, E. S. *J. Bone Jt. Surg., 58A:*1074 and 1083, 1976.
41. Alm, A., Ekstrom, H., and Stromberg, B. *Acta Chir. Scand., Suppl. 445,* 15, 1974.
42. Benedict, J. v., Walker, L. B., and Harris, E. H., *J. Biomech., 1:*53, 1968.
43. Galante, J. O. *Acta Ortho. Scand., Suppl. 100,* 5, 1967.
44. Kennedy, J. C., Hawkins, J. R., Willis, R. B., and Daynlchuk, K. D. *J. Bone Jt. Surg., 58A:*350, 1976.
45. Morrison, J.B. *J. Biomech., 3:*51, 1970.
46. Grood, E. S., and Noyes, F. R. *J. Bone Jt. Surg., 58A:*1087, 1976.
47. Grood, E. S., and Noyes, F. R. *J. Bone Jt. Surg., 58A:*1088, 1976.
48. Goldstein, Z. A., and Dickerson, R. C. *Atlas of Orthopaedic Surgery,* pp. 736–742, C. V. Mosby Co., St. Louis, 1974.
49. Voelcker, H. *Arch. Clin. Chir., 180:*347, 1934.
50. Gruca, A. *J. Bone Jt. Surg., 39A:*699, 1957.
51. White, A. A., Panjaband, M. M., and Thomas, C. L. *Clin. Orthop., 128:*8, 1977.
52. O'Brien, B. M. *Microvascular Reconstructive Surgery,* p. 290, Churchill-Livingstone, Edinburgh, 1977.
53. Ikuta, Y. Free muscle transfer. In *Reconstructive Microsurgery,* p. 270, edited by R. K. Daniel and J. K. Terzis, Little, Brown & Co., Boston, 1977.
54. Swanson, A. B., *Flexible Implant Resection Arthroplasty in the Hand and Extremities,* p. 306, C. V. Mosby Co., St. Louis, 1973.
55. Duthie, R. B., and Ferguson, A. B., Jr., *Mercer's Orthpaedic Surgery,* p. 1159, Edward Arnold, London, 1973.,
56. Stavos, A., and Le Blanc, M., Orthotic components and systems. In *Atlas of Orthotics, A.A.O.S.,* p. 184, C. V. Mosby Co., St. Louis, 1975.
57. Mixter, W. S., and Barr, J. S., *N. Eng. J. Med., 211:*210, 1934.
58. Rothman, R. H., and Simeone, F. A., Lumbar disc disease in the spine. In *The Spine,* p. 443, edited by R. H. Rothman and F. A. Simeone, W. B. Saunders Co., Philadelphia, 1975.
59. Macnab, I. *J. Bone Jt. Surg., 53A:*891, 1971.
60. Urbaniak, J. R., Bright, D. S., and Hopkins, J. E. *J. Biomed. Mater. Res., 4:*165, 1973.
61. Schneider, P. G., and Oyen R., *Z. Orthop., 112:*1078, 1974.

16
Future Developments

As the previous 15 chapters have attested, orthopaedic surgery has undergone numerous striking advances during the past 20 years. Many of these innovations pertain to the use of implantable materials in the body. If the previous rate of progress is to be maintained in the future, a number of urgent problems will require considerable attention. Solutions to these problems, such as elucidation of the causes of degenerative and rheumatoid arthritis, will require the close scrutiny of cell pathophysiology and biochemistry. Solving many other problems, however, will necessitate additional studies on the use and application of implantable materials. In the following pages the author explores the principal objectives for orthopaedic research as they appear to him. The solution to one problem, however, may necessitate or encourage a redirection of future work in other areas. For example, elucidation of the etiologies and the prevention of rheumatoid and osteoarthritis could greatly diminish the need for surgical reconstruction of joints. Despite these limitations in the ability to predict future needs, the author believes that a brief description of the principal problems in orthopaedic surgery that involve the use of surgical implants, may serve as a challenge and, simultaneously, as a source of direction for research workers and surgeons. These principal problems are presented in the order in which the related topics were discussed in the previous chapters.

FUTURE DEVELOPMENTS IN IMPLANTABLE MATERIALS

Mechanical Considerations

Previously, surgical materials employed for fixation of fractures were selected primarily for their attributes of high strength and inertness. Without a detailed knowledge of the mechanical forces imposed upon various parts of the musculoskeletal system, early workers attempted to prevent mechanical failure of implants by providing great mechanical strength. As discussed in Chapters 2 and 3, strong, useful metals possess a high modulus of elasticity quite unlike that of biological tissues. In the past decade the unde-

sirable biological side-effects associated with the use of extremely rigid materials adjacent to bone has become evident.[1] The relief of stress from the plated bone induces osteoporosis secondary to the so called "stress-protection". The undesirable aspects of cyclic load transmission, through an interface between living hard tissues and an inanimate material that possesses widely differing moduli of elasticity, also was discussed in Chapters 5 and 13. The bone or cartilage was liable to resorption and fibrosis. The recent search for superior implantable materials has been redirected toward the discovery of inert substances that possess moduli of elasticity comparable to the tissues that they augment or replace. For segmental replacement of bone, the β-titanium alloys with niobium, tantalum or molybdenum provide a source of inert materials with an elastic modulus similar to that of intact bone. Polymeric materials may be encountered that permit reconstruction of ligaments and tendons with appropriate mechanical counterparts that possess immense resistance to fatigue.

An ideal substitute for the hard tissues may be the new composite materials wherein two dissimilar materials can be combined to provide a material of mechanical properties that differ greatly from the isolated constituents. Such a composite material may possess both high strength and a relatively low modulus of elasticity. At present, several laboratories are exploring this possibility. The recent introduction of carbon fiber reinforced high density polyethylene by the Zimmer Company (Warsaw, Ind.) for the manufacture of a portion of a total ankle joint replacement is one example.

For a variety of endoskeletal reconstructive procedures, surgeons could employ advantageously a material that may change its size, shape or surface area after the time of implantation. The Nitinol alloys, mentioned in Chapter 3, provide such a possibility.[2] By adjustment of the temperature of the metal, a specimen may undergo a change in its shape which also alters its size and surface area. At present, Nitinol is receiving intense scrutiny as a means to provide progressive correction of spinal deformity.[3] If fixation devices comparable to Harrington rods or Dwyer instrumentation were available in Nitinol, a slow, superior correction of spinal deformity might be undertaken with less likelihood of damage to the spinal cord, its nerve roots and blood supply. Fixation of fractures in osteoporotic bone remains one of the great problems in fracture surgery. Fractures of the femoral neck present a particular problem in a weight-bearing bone of many geriatric patients. A fixation device composed of Nitinol might possess numerous small projections which underwent deformation after implantation so that the principal osteoporotic fragment was stabilized by an implant of very large surface area and correspondingly low force transmission per unit area of interface.

Wear Resistance. With the introduction of total hip joint replacement, the wear resistance of implantable materials initially was assumed to be the primary limitation in the longevity of the functional arthroplasty. After about 12 years of clinical experience, the favorable wear resistance of high density polyethylene in the hip joint has exceeded all expectations. It is unclear, of course, whether this surprisingly good state of erosion resistance will be maintained indefinitely. In other joint replacements such as the knee joint, where the mechanical environment is more harsh, the wear resistance of polyethylene has not been as good. The minute polymeric wear particles have proven to be elusive in the attempts to follow them around the body. While no evidence of systemic toxicity of polyethylene wear particles has been accumulated, nevertheless, the possibility remains that ultimately it may be documented. For these and other reasons, numerous attempts are underway to discover superior wear resistance in inert materials of low coefficients of friction. The recently introduced carbon fiber reinforced high density polyethylene provides a modest improvement in wear resistance over the pure polymeric material. Future studies should focus primary attention on organic polymers or graphite of superior wear resistance and hardness to oppose a metallic or graphite surface. The provision for living tissues as bearing surfaces for joint arthroplasties is discussed below.

Corrosion Resistance. In the past decade few total failures of implants have been encountered which can be attributed solely or primarily to corrosion. Crevice and fretting corrosion can be observed on many implants although the magnitude of the problem, at least from mechanical considerations, renders it under the category of an academic curiosity. Nevertheless, the biological significance of minute accumulations of metallic dissolution products should not be wholly discounted until further information is available. As will be described shortly, the possibility remains that dissolution of wear products may encourage bacterial ingrowth by the inhibition of host resistance. Various laboratory tests, such as the use of galvanic protection of implants in experimental animals might reveal whether the complete absence of dissolution products alters the behavior of tissues around metallic implants.

Nondestructive Tests for Implants *in Vivo*

With the innovation of total joint replacements, the projected duration of service of foreign implant devices has altered from a short period, usually less than 1 or 2 years, to an indefinite period of many decades. Until recently, however, the only methods available to determine the state of the implant *in vivo,* were clinical evaluation and X-rays. These methods permit an assessment that the implant is functioning satisfactorily or that it has undergone mechanical failure. What obviously has been needed is a test which permits an accurate record of subtle changes in an implant indicative of incipient mechanical failure. In Chapters 3 and 8, ferrographic analyses of synovial fluid from artificial joints was described. With this technique, 1 or 2 ml of joint fluid may be aspirated and subjected to an analysis of its wear particles. From the morphology and numbers of particles, an estimation of the current rate of wear of the articulating surfaces can be made. From a concomitant study of the biological cells in the joint fluid and from cells in the adjacent synovium, the effect of the wear particles on the joint can be determined. Ferrographic and synovial fluid analyses permit sequential assessments in individual patients which will enable material scientists to ascertain the function of new designs for total joint replacements or for implants constructed of previously untried materials. Also, it will enable surgeons to determine when implants undergo changes from previously slow and acceptable rates of wear to states of rapid deterioration. Replacement of the implant should be performed prior to the accumulation of large amounts of potentially toxic wear particles that serve to accelerate the subsequent rate of wear of the joint. Further nondestructive methods to assess the mechanical integrity of implants *in situ,* however, are needed. Perhaps ultrasonic techniques could provide one supplementary technique.

Accelerated Laboratory Tests. For the study of previously untried implantable materials, the optimal method of study is a simulated human environment that accurately replicates the magnitude of forces and the duration of useful life. An accelerated laboratory test becomes essential in view of the many decades of service which man-made replacement parts may need to function satisfactorily. Accelerated laboratory tests that accurately reflect conditions of service for a great range of mechanical contrivances have proved to be extraordinarily difficult to devise. Their elucidation would greatly facilitate the study of new surgical implants.

PROPERTIES OF MUSCULOSKELETAL TISSUES

Biomechanical Attributes

The application of implantable materials in the human body rests heavily upon a sound knowledge of the biomechanical properties of musculoskeletal tissues and the kinematics of articular joints. Unless a bioengineer possesses a precise tabulation of the mechanical properties of a tissue which he is requested to replace, he is hard pressed to provide a suitable man-made alternative. Similarly, for the development of total joint replacements an engineer requires a rigorous description of the planes of motion of an articular joint, the magnitude, direction and frequency of application of weight-bearing forces, and the mechanisms of lubrication. The mechanical failures currently seen in presently available total joint replacements can be explained in large part by faulty or limited knowledge of complex human joints such as the knee or the elbow.

Previously, workers assumed that the hard tissues showed homogenous mechanical properties which could be replicated in prosthetic counterparts. Brown[4] and others[5] have reassessed the intimate local variations in the mechanical properties of bone and articular cartilage of the hip and knee. These workers have employed finite element analysis and allied techniques which permit the detection of local variations in mechanical properties at sites that are 1 or 2 mm apart. Figure 16-1A illustrates local variations in the mechanical properties of one cross-section of the human femoral head. In Figure 16-1B, a method to determine similar variations in the contact forces and the modulus of elasticity of the articular cartilage on the femoral head is shown. This method is currently in use in the author's laboratory. It employs novel pressure sensitive materials such as pressure sensitive paint and pressure sensitive con-

ductive silicone whose electrical resistance changes with applied pressure. The pressure sensitive units, seen in Figure 16-1B, are 0.020 inch in thickness and permit an accurate record of loads applied at a frequency up to 5 per second. These studies indicate that the mechanical properties of the bone and possibly of the articular cartilage in the femoral head may vary by 5-fold from one site to another within the same structure. As will be described shortly future attempts to design superior total joint replacements must rely heavily on such information.

Healing and Regeneration

After the implantation of any type of surgical implant, the future function of the device is largely determined by the healing processes that occur in juxtaposition to it. In the past there have been very limited capabilities for alteration of healing mechanisms. Most of the known methods for influencing regeneration and tissue repair, such as the effect of corticosteroids on the healing of bone or fibrous tissue have been an academic curiosity or an undesirable side-effect of the pharmacological agent. A few recent observations, however, have provided insight into how regeneration of musculoskeletal tissues may be influenced in ways that have a therapeutic effect.

Earlier workers[6] recognized the limited capacity of articular cartilage to undergo healing or regeneration. The rate at which articular cartilage undergoes formation of matrix is inherently low. When isolated segments of articular cartilage are transplanted, the boundary between the graft and the host shows a limited remodeling capacity to provide solid incorporation of the graft. The observations of Mankin[6] and others confirm that the rate of metabolism of chondrocytes in vivo is slow compared to many other cell types. Over the past decade, Green[7, 8] has questioned the influence of articular cartilaginous matrix on the metabolism of the chondrocytes. This worker isolated chondrocytes from articular cartilage and cultivated the isolated cells both in vivo and in vitro. Initially, the cells were grown in vitro on glass surfaces. Subsequently, they were implanted into porous Gelfoam and decalcified bony fragments. After infusion of cells into the matrices, the specimens were implanted into articular defects in the knees of rabbits. Histological observations were performed on the specimens after implantation for a period of up to 16 months. The studies indicated that isolated chondrocytes cultured in vitro undergo rapid cell division and the forma-

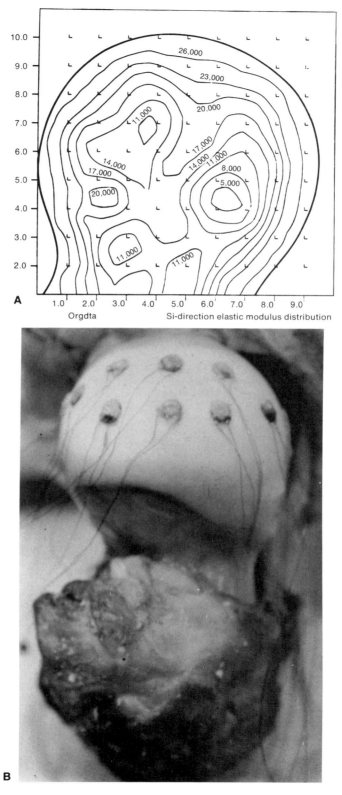

Figure 16-1. *A*. A schematic diagram of the femoral head with isoelastic lines shows the wide variations in the elastic moduli in different regions of bone. *B*. For the measurement of the distribution of joint contact forces, thin piezoelectric transducers are attached to the articular surface of a fresh cadaveric femoral head, as shown in the photograph. Considerable local variations in the stresses at the surface are observed. (*A* and *B*, reproduced with permission of Dr. T. D. Brown.)

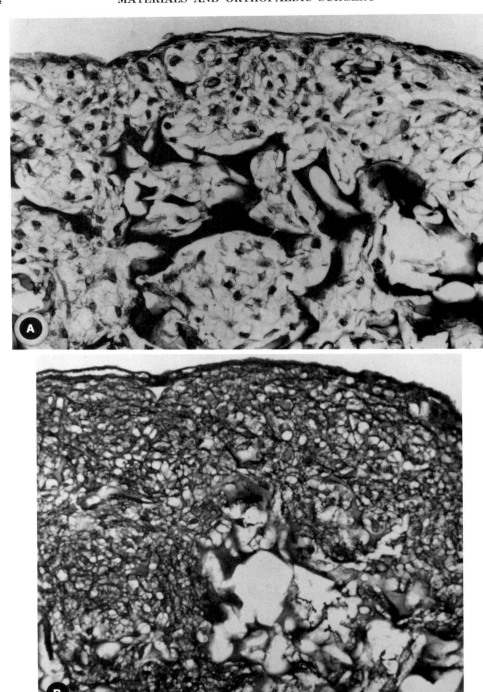

Figure 16-2. *A.* A histological section of a gelatin sponge culture of articular chondrocytes is shown in this photomicrograph 7 days after the initial culture. The cells are dispersed deeply within the sponge and are widely separated by a pale chondromyxoid material (H & E, ×220). *B.* Another histological section of a gelatin sponge culture at 7 days shows the cells widely separated by metachromatic chondromyxoid matrix. The cells have grown down into the substance of the sponge (toluidine blue, ×220). (*A* and *B*, reproduced with permission of W. T. Green, Jr.[8])

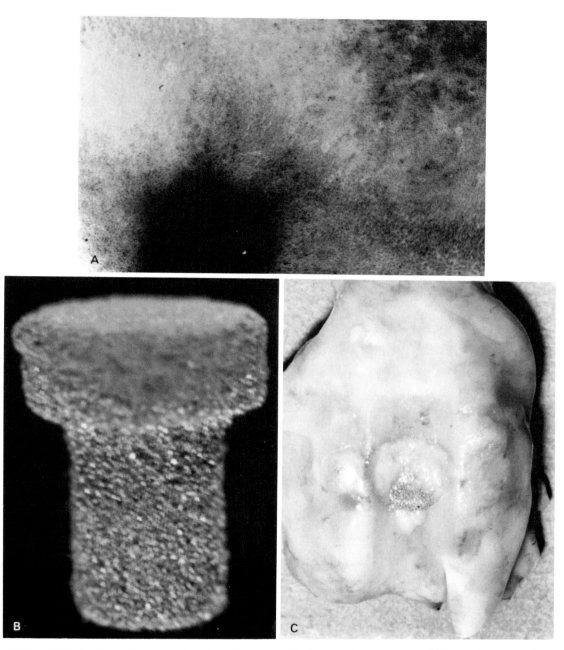

Figure 16-3. In the author's experiments, autogenous articular chondrocytes from rabbits are isolated and cultured *in vitro*. *A.* A photomicrograph of a clonal culture is shown (H & E, ×6.5). *B.* The porous sintered coated implants of cobalt-chromium alloy are implanted into the intercondylar region of the distal femur to articulate with the patella. The smaller diameter portion for attachment to bone possesses a surface with larger interstices while the flat surface of large diameter possesses smaller interstices for ingrowth of cartilage (×1.25). *C.* After insertion with the exposed metallic surface level of the articular surface, a suspension of the chondrocytes is applied to the implant. One to two months later, the animal is sacrificed when the implant is covered with an intact layer of articular cartilage (×½).

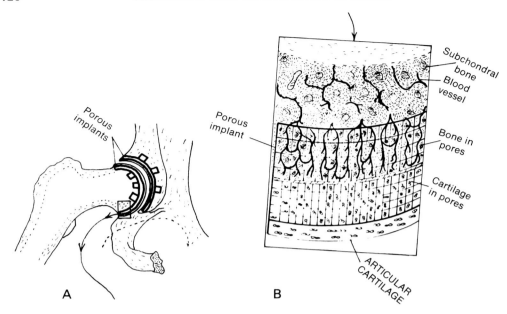

Figure 16-4. Schematic diagrams reveal the concept of total joint replacement which the author foresees for use in the future. *A.* The implant is attached to bone by ingrowth into an open pore network. *B.* The enlarged view shows the vascularized bone within large interstices while autologous articular cartilage is seen within small interstices and on the exposed porous surface of the implant. The small interstices occlude small blood vessels, including capillaries and thereby prevent the ingrowth of bone that would otherwise occur. (Reproduced with permission of D. C. Mears.[11])

tion of matrix which seems to be articular cartilage. As seen in Figures 16-2*A* and *B,* after infusion into a porous matrix, the cells continue to divide and to produce matrix until the entire porous network is filled with the biological material. The exposed articular surface of the porous matrix is covered with a layer of articular cartilage that is remarkably similar to intact cartilage. The boundary between the specimen and the host shows a tightly interlocking interface. Other workers have undertaken somewhat similar studies which support these observations.[9, 10]

More recently the author has repeated these studies with the application of porous specimens made of pure titanium or of cobalt-chromium alloy. After the infusion of autogenous articular chondrocytes, cultured *in vitro,* into the porous specimen, the specimen was inserted into a defect in the knees of rabbits (Fig. 16-3). Within 4 to 6 weeks after implantation, the specimen showed coverage of the articular surface of the implant with articular cartilage.

From these and other observations the author foresees future total joint replacements of a type shown schematically in Figure 16-4. The im-

plantable material represents a thin porous surface whose geometry corresponds to that desired in the reconstructed joint. On the surface opposing bone the pores are of appropriate size and geometry to provide optimal encouragement for ingrowth of bone and attachment of the implant to the osseous system. The interstices on the opposing articular surface of the implant provide optimal geometry for ingrowth of autogenous chondrocytes. To prevent the conversion of the articular cartilage into bone the interstices must be of sufficiently small size to prohibit the ingrowth of capillaries. The regenerative cartilaginous surfaces would provide the optimal bearing surfaces for reconstructed joints. They would show a low coefficient of friction and the optimal modulus of elasticity to dampen impulsive loads. If the surfaces underwent the erosion of cartilaginous wear particles such as normal anatomical joints undergo, the wear debris would be of a biological nature and unlikely to provoke any toxic side-effects. Upon such wear the living cartilaginous surface would have the potential for regeneration quite unlike any man-made material. Also in the event of transient bacterial invasion into the joint, the living cartilage would

Table 16-1

The Characteristics and Parameters of Prosthesis Attachment by Tissue Ingrowth

Attachment characteristic	Structural parameter
1. Rate of bone ingrowth	Pore size
2. Strength of porous material	Volume fraction pores
3. Depth of tissue viability	Interconnection pore size
4. Attachment strength	Volume fraction pores at surface
5. Bone/porous material interface deformation	Pore size, pore morphology and pore volume

Table 16-2

Engineering Properties of Porous Materials

Material	Porosity (%)	Y.T.S.*[a] U.T.S.[b] (psi)	U.C.S. (psi)	Flexural strength (psi)	Elastic modulus (psi)
Co-Cr-Mo	0	75,000*	—	—	30×10^6
Co-Cr-Mo	44	10,500	—	43,500	4×10^6
Ti	0	80,000*	—	—	16×10^6
Ti	40	7,000	—	—	6×10^5
Al$_2$O$_3$	0	30,000	400,000	50,000	50×10^6
Al$_2$O$_3$	50	—	15,000	56,000	9×10^6
PMMA[c]	0	10,000	15,000	16,000	3.5×10^5
PMMA	32	1,200	2,750	1,800	5.5×10^4

[a] Y.T.S.,
[b] U.T.S.,
[c] PMMA, polymethylmethacrylate.

possess a greater degree of host resistance than man-made materials. Currently, this concept is under scrutiny in the author's laboratory, with the use of implants in rabbits and sheep.

Previous workers[12] have characterized the optimal shapes and sizes of interstices for the ingrowth of bone. A brief outline of their results is tabulated in Table 16-1. The engineering properties of a variety of porous materials currently under scrutiny is given in Table 16-2.

The implants attached by porous ingrowth do not require intramedullary stems, as seen in the Meuli total wrist joint prosthesis in Figure 16-5. Such intramedullary stems provide susceptible sites for fatigue failures. They limit the surgeon's ability to make minor alterations of alignment at surgery and they compromise his capacity to direct the implant so that it is concentric with the forces imposed by ligaments and musculotendinous units.[13] Salzer et al.[14] have studied a ceramic femoral cap endoprosthesis which is intended for use in osteoarthritic hips. The implant, seen in Figure 16-6, is attached by bony ingrowth. It possesses a supporting plate to augment the distribution of weight-bearing forces. More recently, two types of total hip joint replacements have been used which eliminate the femoral stem. One design by Wagner[15] and an-

other by Amstutz et al.,[16] as shown in Figure 16-7, employ concentric shells which are attached to bone at the acetabulum and femoral head, respectively, with polymethylmethacrylate cement. For 6 months the author has used a porous sintered coated cobalt-chromium total hip joint replacement (Medishield, Inc., Paramus, N. J.) which possesses a femoral stem. In most of the patients, methylmethacrylate is not used to insert the femoral component. To date, no implants have shown clinical or radiological evidence of loosening. The results after prolonged implantation are eagerly awaited. Nevertheless, the results of studies in experimental animals, especially dogs, reveal excellent coadaptation of bone to the porous implant.[17,]* Figures 16-8 to 16-10 show similar porous coated specimens removed from a canine femur 3 months after implantation. In Figure 16-3, a light micrograph reveals the cross-section of the stem of the cobalt-chromium alloy implant embedded within the bone. Regenerative bone has surrounded the stem to provide rigid stabilization. Figures 16-8 to 16-10 present transmission and reflection optical micrographs and a scanning electron micrograph at various magnifications, all of which

---

* R. M. Pilliar, personal communication, 1977.

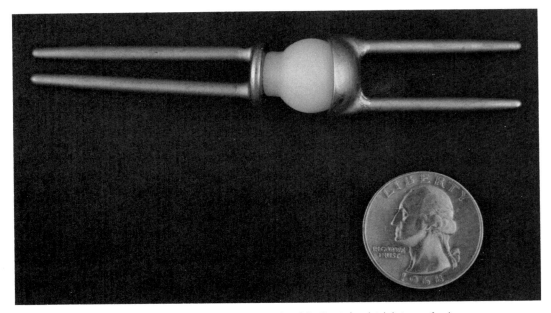

Figure 16-5. The photograph reveals a Meuli total wrist joint prosthesis.

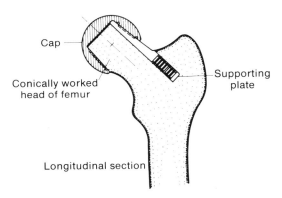

Cap

Conically worked head of femur

Supporting plate

Longitudinal section

Figure 16-6. The schematic diagram reveals a ceramic femoral cup endoprosthesis designed for use in osteoarthritic hips. (Reproduced with permission of M. Salzer *et al.*[14])

confirm the ingrowth of bone into minute interstices without a fibrous tissue barrier between metal and bone.

In Chapter 15 the use of silicone rubber rods to stimulate the formation of new tendon sheaths and of an apparently normal biological coating on tendons is described. From those observations and from the studies on regenerative articular cartilage, it seems likely that the healing process of numerous musculoskeletal tissues can be manipulated in a highly productive way to facilitate the reconstruction of numerous organs and tissues. A concentrated effort should

be made to explore the regenerative capabilities of isolated cells from tendons and ligaments to discern whether a satisfactory musculotendinous junction and an intact ligament can be made. Combinations of isolated cells with porous materials of peculiar mechanical properties also may facilitate reconstruction of the musculoskeletal system. The recent observations by Hunter and Jaeger[18] and by Eskeland *et al.*[19] on the formation of artificial tendons with biological surfaces lend preliminary support to this concept. Semple and Murray* have devised an artificial tendon which anchors to bone with a porous titanium plug, as seen in Figure 16-11A. The tapered plug is keyed into place to provide immediate fixation. The artificial tendon itself is porous Dacron velour and Dacron cord. An X-ray showing its application in a dog to replace the Achilles' tendon, is revealed in Figure 16-11B. These workers have observed favorable results in their animal experiments. In Figure 16-11C, a photomicrograph of one of their histological preparations shows a titanium plug after the ingrowth of bone reveals excellent coadaptation of bone to the surface of the implant. Nevertheless, if their device were used in human subjects, late failure of the junction between the implant and the musculotendinous junction would be anticipated.

---

* C. Semple and G. A. W. Murray, personal communication, 1977.

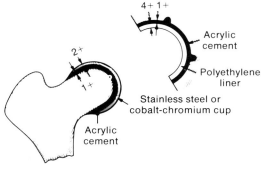

ITEM	MINIMUM THICKNESS (mm)
Acetab. cement	2
PE liner	8
Metal cup	4
Femoral cement	2
TOTAL	16

Figure 16-7. A schematic drawing shows total hip replacement by "interval eccentric shells". With minimal dimensions for the cemented interface and the replacement components at least 16 mm of joint space is required for adequate fitting with bone coverage of the polyethylene (PE) liner. (Reproduced with permission of H. C. Amstutz, I. C. Clarke, J. Christie and A. Graff-Radford.[16]

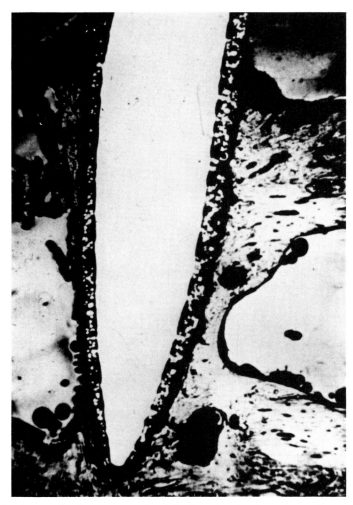

Figure 16-8. A photomicrograph of porous coated cobalt-chromium implants shows the specimens 3 months after insertion into a canine femur. A cross-section of the implant stem with its sintered coating and ingrowth of bone is revealed. (× 10) (Reproduced with permission of R. M. Pilliar.)

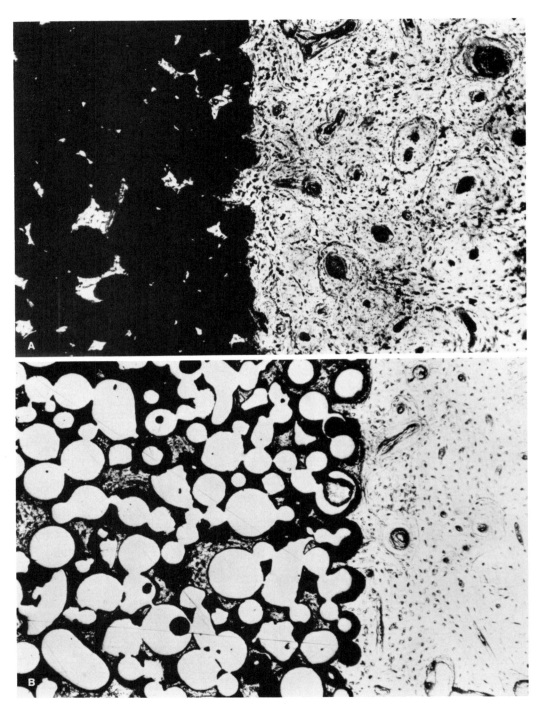

Figure 16-9. *A* and *B*. Transmission and reflection optical micrographs show the implant-bone interface with extensive ingrowth of bone 3 months after insertion of porous coated cobalt-chromium implants into canine femora. (× 83) (Reproduced with permission of R. M. Pilliar.)

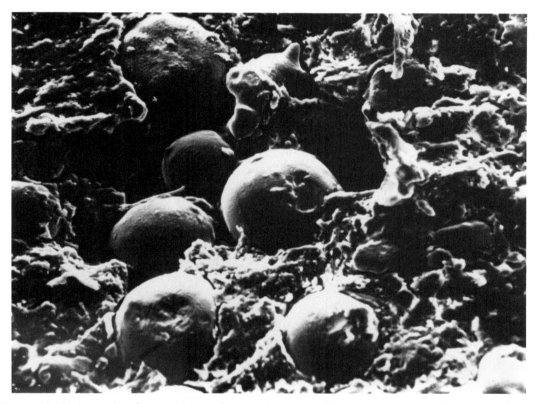

Figure 16-10. A scanning electron micrograph shows the surface of the porous coating and bone ingrowth of cobalt-chromium implants 3 months after insertion into canine femora. The spherical particles of metallic powder are readily distinguished and possess a diameter of about 150 μm. (Reproduced with permission of R. M. Pilliar.)

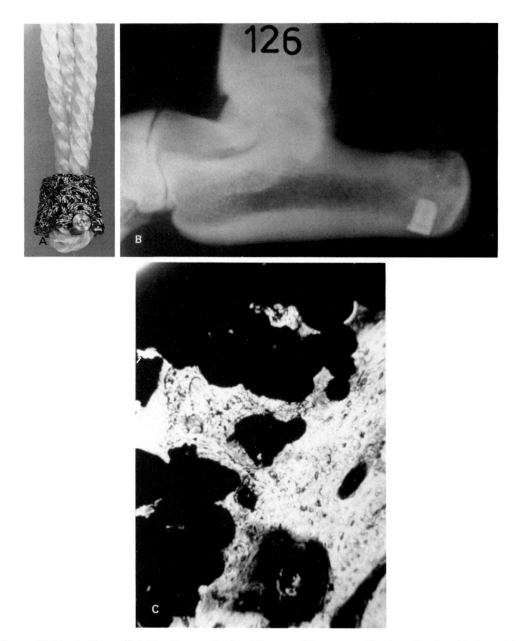

Figure 16-11. *A.* The artificial tendon prosthesis of Dacron with a porous titanium plug for attachment to bone is inserted into dogs to replace the Achilles' tendon. *B.* An X-ray shows the metal implant in a greyhound at 126 days after surgery. The implant is well anchored in the os calcis although resorption of bone is evident where the Dacron cord passes through the bone. *C.* Shown is a histological preparation of the porous interface of a similar implant removed after 203 days *in vivo*. The sintered titanium wire is black and shows bony ingrowth with a lamellar structure. The bone has grown to the metallic interface without intervening tissue (polarized light, ×6). (Reproduced with permission of G. A. W. Murray and C. Semple.)

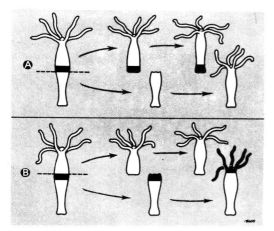

Figure 16-12. The schematic diagrams reveal the Hydra observations of Abraham Trembley (1710–1784) on a green Hydra (*Chlorohydra viridissima*) when the animal is transected. Depending upon the level of division the animal can regenerate a basal disc, as in *A*, or tentacles and hypostome, as in *B*, from the same tissue. (Reproduced with permission of G. B. Moment.[21])

The goal of surgeons who attempt to reconstruct the musculoskeletal system should be guided by the observations of Trembley[20, 21] in his classic study of the hydra, which he undertook over 100 years ago. If the primitive animal was transected it could regenerate two new terminal portions (Fig. 16-12) of appropriate size and shape. It has been recognized that human bone, skin and liver display a somewhat similar regenerative capacity, but now it should be evident that many other tissues possess extraordinary regenerative capacity if the appropriate stimulus can be applied.

Several recent studies represent attempts to stimulate the growth of immature tissues which might be employed at sites of traumatic, or other insults. Epiphyseal stimulation of bone has received special scrutiny. Langenskiold[22] and Osterman,[23] on fatty interposition, and Brighton,[24] Bassett[25] and Becker *et al.,*[26] with electrical stimulation, have demonstrated that epiphyseal growth can be influenced toward a therapeutic end. Comparable studies on the growth of other musculoskeletal tissues merit comparable study. The ability of surgeons to influence growth in predictable ways would alter immeasurably the opportunities to undertake ancillary reconstructive methods such as arthroplastic procedures.

In recent years the reconstruction of musculoskeletal tissues has been extended by autogenous grafts of bone, skin and muscle on neurovascular pedicles by the advent of microvascular anastomoses.[27] One example of this technique, the transfer of vascular pedicle grafts of fibula and anterior iliac crest is discussed in Chapter 11. This field is clearly in its infancy and further developments can be anticipated. It lends itself to complementary reconstruction with surgical implants. For example, after an extensive resection of bone, an articular joint and surrounding soft tissues, a prosthetic joint might be applied in juxtaposition to bone and muscle grafts on neurovascular pedicles.

Resistance to Infection

Another biological attribute of unclear nature is the resistance of tissues to infection in the presence of implantable materials. As described in Chapters 13 and 14, the tissues adjacent to large foreign implants such as total joint replacements show a propensity for infection which is much greater than that possessed by intact tissues. The infections may result from intraoperative contamination or from organisms which disseminate through the body *via* the blood stream after surgery. Infections at the site of a total joint replacement represent a major catastrophy for which usually the treatment ultimately requires removal of the implant. The precise role of the implant in the provocation of this diminished bacteriological resistance of the host is unclear. In Chapter 8, the current knowledge in this field is described. Future study might take several directions. If a metallic implant is rendered wholly immune from dissolution, the possible toxicity of dissolution products on adjacent tissues with compromise of resistance to infection might be eliminated. At least as an experimental observation, the bacterial resistance of tissues adjacent to galvanically protected metals which display absolutely no dissolution should be studied. While the clinical implementation of galvanic protection would be cumbersome, nevertheless it could be employed for the clinical application of implants with a notably high risk of infection and its associated morbidity. Incidentally, it should not be forgotten that Von Baeyer[28, 29] suggested such a therapeutic application for galvanic effects in 1908.

As an alternative concept for elimination of bacterial infection associated with the use of large implants, scrutiny of the bacterial resistance of the hard tissues might be rewarding. In intact bone or articular cartilage, the inanimate matrix seemingly provides no resistance to infection. The living cells, including elements of the blood in bone, must possess the principal site of defense mechanisms. If this concept is correct, it implies that an inert porous implant provided by a continuous network of living cells should possess a resistance to infection that rivals that of intact bone or cartilage. Admittedly, this resistance to infection would not prevail until the implant had been permeated by the cells with or without blood vessels. If the concept is valid, however, it provides a fairly simple way for improvement of total joint replacements and other large implants.

Another concept in the provision of resistance to bacterial infection has been the addition of antibiotics to implantable materials such as methylmethacrylate cement.[30, 31] At least for a period of months after implantation, the antibiotic is slowly released from the cement to augment local resistance to infection. While the effectiveness of this technique remains unclear, nevertheless, it provides insight into a way that future work might be directed.

Toxicity

A most disturbing gap in present knowledge concerning the use of surgical implants is the limited understanding of the mechanisms by which small amounts of dissolution or wear products influence local and distant tissues. The intracellular mechanisms of toxicity of the musculoskeletal tissues remain largely obscure.[32] Future studies would require elaborate experimental methods and a solid foundation in cell biology. The possible significance of immune mechanisms in the response of the body to wear particles has been questioned but not satisfactorily answered. The recent interest expressed by governmental regulatory agencies in the use of present and future surgical implants is an additional impetus for further studies in this field.

SURGICAL TOOLS AND IMPLANTS

Surgical Tools

For the orthopaedic surgeon who employs hand and power tools in the operating room on a daily basis, a number of glaring deficiencies are evident. Perhaps the single greatest source of frustration is the noisy cast cutter, inevitably with a dull, loose oscillating blade that terrifies countless children in fracture clinics. In many instances, assessment of the noise emitted by the device in clinics exceeds local safety regulations and puts Concorde to shame. Future studies should consider ultrasonic and oscillating

tools that act with an impulsive force on the cast, either of which might propagate a crack in the cast to provoke brittle fracture without damaging the skin.

The most widely employed power tools for use on bone utilize compressed air for their power source. Admittedly, the devices are superior to previous models, although they have several shortcomings. In comparison with electrical drills or other tools of comparable size, they provide considerably less power. In attempts to cut the hard cortical bone of young adults, presently available air tools are observed to possess barely adequate cutting capability. Also, the tools require a bulky air hose, large connectors and a suitable source of gas under pressure. The battery powered electrical tools circumvent the need for a supply of bottled gas and a suitable pressure line, but these assets are offset by the need for large batteries because compact batteries possess inadequate power and duration of charge. Admittedly, recent research in rechargable batteries has made immense strides so that future tools powered in this way may be highly satisfactory. Further scrutiny of electrical tools powered by 110 volts AC, however, seem to be warranted. Explosive anesthetics which circulate in the operating room were a hazard of the previous generation. Routine monitoring of patients by most anesthesiologists includes the application of a variety of electrical devices to continuously document heart and ventilation rates, an electrocardiographic record, body temperature and other biological indices. Volatile anesthetic gases have been suggested as the provocative agent of a greatly elevated incidence of birth defects in the offspring of female anesthetic personnel. For all of these reasons, volatile and potentially explosive anesthetic gases currently are rigorously excluded from the circulating air in the operating room. By consideration of these and other factors, including the potentially low cost of electrically powered tools, further study on their widespread introduction appears to be indicated. One interchangeable electric tool could be developed to serve as an electrocautery, a reciprocating saw, drill, tap and screwdriver, and probably in other capacities.

The tools utilized to cut bone are liable to become dull after brief periods of use. If the cutting edge encounters a metal obstacle such as a screw or other implant hidden within the substance of bone, a single application may terminate its functional life. The introduction of prepackaged and sterilized disposable utensils is mentioned as a possible solution, provided that widespread application could facilitate an acceptably low cost per unit item.

Surgical Implants

Previous discussions have described the likely future developments in reconstructive devices and implants for internal fixation of appendicular fractures. Recently, external fixation has begun to be widely used. Further improvements in these techniques appear to be inevitable. Simpler devices that retain the capacity for 3-plane correction of fractures and osteotomies are needed. The devices should be provided with polycentric hinges so that highly unstable and open fractures in or near joints may be treated with the early postoperative resumption of active range of motion of the joints. The methods are likely to see further application on the axial skeleton. The author is exploring the use of a haloexternal fixation system for use on the cervical and upper thoracic spine that obviates the need for body jackets and vests. At St. Gallen, Switzerland, Magerl and his colleagues* have introduced a technique of external fixation for the management of unstable fracture dislocations of the lower thoracic and lumbosacral spine that restores adequate stability for substantial early mobilization of the patient. The preliminary results have been highly encouraging. For all of the external fixation devices, superior types of transfixing pins are needed which resist loosening and the predilection for pin tract infections. One solution would appear to be the application of porous coated pins that encourage the ingrowth of bone, skin and other tissues.

ORTHOPAEDIC EDUCATION FOR THE USE OF IMPLANTABLE DEVICES

Orthopaedic surgery has led the surgical disciplines in its attempts to standardize the system of testing residents in training on their comprehension of the field. While the elaborate system developed by the American Board of Orthopaedic Surgery and its sister organizations deserves credit, it has overlooked the attempts to teach residents or postgraduate surgeons the manipulative skills that are used in fracture or reconstructive surgery of the appendicular and axial skeleton. It has been widely believed that those individuals who have demonstrated adequate intellectual capacity and clinical acumen in their early medical training, can master the

use of orthopaedic operative techniques by the time-honored method of observing senior surgeons. In certain instances this method promotes the perpetuation of ineffective surgical techniques.

During the past decade the AO group[33] in Switzerland has developed a comprehensive educational system to acquaint surgeons in all parts of the world with their sophisticated operative techniques for internal and external fixation of fractures. The instructional courses include lectures, audio tapes, live demonstrations and the application of tools and implants on cadaveric and artificial bones. In the future such courses should be made available for virtually all residents as well as postgraduate surgeons.[34] As with any other manual skills, such as tennis or golf, the time to learn the correct manipulative techniques is at the introductory stage, before faulty habits are established. Comparable courses are needed for spinal instrumentation, microsurgical techniques and total joint replacements. With the universal adoption of such teaching methods, the general standard of application of surgical implants should improve substantially.

In summary, for the optimal use of surgical implants, both the bioengineers who develop them and the surgeons who employ them must fully understand the mechanical and biological attributes of the musculoskeletal system. Continued close cooperation and understanding between surgeons and bioengineers will be necessary if the use of materials in orthopaedic surgery is to continue to provide superior methods of treatment for mankind.

REFERENCES

1. Morscher, E., Mathys, A., and Henche, H. R. Isoelastic endoprosthesis—A new concept in artificial joint replacement. In *Advances in Artificial Hip and Knee Joint Technology*, p. 403, edited by M. Schaldach and D. Hohmann, Springer-Verlag, Berlin, 1976.
2. Castleman, L. S., Motzkin, S. M., Aliandri, F. P., Bonawit, V. L., and Johnson, A. A. *J. Biomed. Mater. Res.,* 10:695, 1976.
3. Schmerling, M. A., Wilkov, M. A., Sanders, A. E., and Woosley, J. E. *J. Biomed. Mater. Res.,* 10:879, 1976.
4. Brown, T. D., and Ferguson, A. B. Jr. *J. Bone Jt. Surg.,* 60A: 619, 1978.
5. Harris, L. S., Chao, R., Bloch, R., and Weingarten, V. A three-dimensional finite element analysis of the proximal third of the femur. In press, 1978.
6. Mankin, H. J. *N. Eng. J. Med.,* 291:1285, 1974.
7. Green, W. T., Jr. *Clin Orthop.,* 124:237, 1977.
8. Green, W. T., Jr. *Clin Orthop.,* 75:248, 1971.

---

* F. Magerl, personal communication, 1978.

9. Karagianes, M. T., Wheeler, K. R., and Nilles, J. L. *Arch. Pathol., 99:*398, 1975.
10. Chvapil, M. *J. Biomed. Mater. Res., 11:*721, 1977.
11. Mears, D. C. *Orthop. Surv., 1:*64, 1977.
12. Klawitter, J. J., Weinstein, A. M., Hulbert, S. F., and Sauer, B. W. Tissue ingrowth and mechanical locking for anchorage of prosthesis in the locomotor system. In *Advances in Artificial Hip and Knee Joint Technology*, p. 422, edited by M. Schaldach and D. Hahmann, Springer-Verlag, Berlin, 1976.
13. Gschwend, N. Design criteria, present indication and implantation techniques for artificial knee joints. In *Advances in Artificial Hip and Knee Joint Technology*, p. 90, edited by M. Schaldach and D. Hohmann, Springer-Verlag, Berlin, 1976.
14. Salzer, M., Locke, H., Plenk, H., Jr., Punzet, G., Stark, N., and Zweymuller, K. Experience with bioceramic endoprostheses of the hip joint. In *Advances in Artificial Hip and Knee Joint Technology*, p. 459, edited by M. Schaldach and D. Hohmann, Springer-Verlag, Berlin, 1976.
15. Wagner, H. *Arch. Orthop. Unfallchir., 82:*101, 1975.
16. Amstutz, H. C., Clarke, I. C., Christie, J., and Graff-Radford, A. *Clin. Orthop., 128:*261, 1977.
17. Pilliar, R. M., Cameron, H. U., and Macnab, I. *Biomed. Eng., 126:*10, 1975.
18. Hunter, J. M., and Jaeger, S. H. *Orthop. Clin. N. Am., 8:*473, 1977.
19. Eskeland, G., Eskeland, T., Hovig, T., and Teigland, J. *J. Bone Jt. Surg., 59B:*206, 1977.
20. Moment, G. B. *General Zoology*, p. 91, Riverside Press, Cambridge, Mass., 1958.
21. Moment, G. B. *General Zoology*, p. 102, Riverside Press, Cambridge, Mass., 1958.
22. Langenskiold, A. *Acta Orthop. Scand., 38:*267, 1967.
23. Osterman, K. *Acta Orthop. Scand., Suppl. 147:*24, 1973.
24. Brighton, C. T. *J. Bone Jt. Surg., 57A:*368, 1975.
25. Bassett, C. A. L. *Sci., 184:*575, 1974.
26. Becker, R. O., Spadero, J. A., and Marino, A. A. *Clin. Orthop., 124:*75, 1977.
27. O'Brien, B. M. *Microvascular Reconstructive Surgery*, p. 50, Churchill-Livingstone, Edinburgh, 1977.
28. Von Baeyer, H. *Muchen. Med. Wchnschr., 56:*2416, 1909.
29. Von Baeyer, H. *Beitr. Klin. Chir. 58:*1, 1908.
30. Hill, J., Klenerman, L., Trustey, S., and Blowers, R. *J. Bone Jt. Surg., 59B:*197, 1977.
31. Elson, R. A., Jephcott, A. E., McGechie, D. B., and Verettas, D. *J. Bone Jt. Surg., 59B:*200, 1977.
32. Luckey, T. D., and Venugopal, B. *Metals Toxicity in Mammals*, p. 103, New Plenum Press, New York, 1977.
33. Müller, M. E., Allgöwer, M., and Willenegger, H. *Manual of Internal Fixation*, p. 14. Springer-Verlag, Berlin, 1970.
34. Kapta, J. A. *Clin. Orthop., 75:*80, 1971.

Index

Manufacturers' List

PROSTHESIS	COMPANY
Proximal Femoral Endoprostheses	
Judet hip prosthesis	(No longer available)
Moore prosthesis	Zimmer
Thompson prothesis	Zimmer
Bateman UPF (University Proximal Femur)	Wright Dow Corning
Gilberty Bipolar Endoprosthesis	Zimmer
Total Hip Replacement	
Charnley	Thackray, Ltd.
Bechtol	Richards
Harris	Howmedica
TR-28 (Trapezoidal-28)	Zimmer
Anfranc-Turner	Howmedica
Muller	Protek
McKee-Farrar	Howmedica
CAD (Computer Aided Design)	Howmedica
Weber Trunnion (and with ceramic socket)	AlloPro Ag
Sivash	US Surgical Corp.
Tharies	Zimmer
Molded Polyethylene Acetabular Cups	Zimmer
Buchholz total hip joint replacement	Richards
Smith-Petersen Cup	Zimmer
I.C.L.H. Double Cup Arthroplasty	Depuy
Wagner Resurface Prosthesis	Synthes
Total Knee Replacements	
Femoral mold arthroplasty (MGM knee)	(No longer available)
UCI	Deloro Surgical Co.
Geometric	Howmedica
Freeman-Swanson	Deloro Surgical Co.
Guepar	BGC (Benoist Girard & Cie)
Sheehan	Deloro Surgical Co.
Polycentric	Howmedica
Stabilocondylar	Codman Co.
Total condylar	Codman Co., Howmedica
Unicondylar, Duocondylar	Codman Co., Howmedica
Charnley	Thackray, Ltd.
Goodfellow	Downs Surgical

PROSTHESIS	COMPANY
Attenborough	Medishield
Bechtol	Richards
Kenna	Medishield
McKeever prosthesis	(No longer available)
Patello-femoral Replacement Systems	Richards, Link America, Inc.
Deane Prosthesis	
Spherocentric	Howmedica
Marmor modular	Richards
Waldieus	(No longer available)
Guepar	BGC (Benoist Girard & Cie)
Herbert	(No longer available)
Richards Anterior Cruciate Ligament Prosthesis	Richards

Total Ankle Joint Replacement

Oregon ankle	Zimmer
St. Georg	Richards
Newton	Howmedica
TPR (Thompson-Parkridge-Richards)	Richards
Smith	Wright

Toe Joint Replacements

Great toe	Dow-Corning, Cutter
Swanson Prosthesis	Dow-Corning

Total Shoulder Joint

Neer	Howmedica-Zimmer
Stanmore	Zimmer G.B.
Fenlin	
MacNab	Medishield

Total Elbow Joint Replacement

Gschwend (GSC)	Depuy
Dee	Howmedica, Zimmer Great Britain, OEC
Shiers	Down's Surgical Ltd.
Ewald	Codman-Cintor
Schlein	Howmedica
Swanson	Dow-Corning

Total Wrist Replacement

Meuli	JRI, Protek
Volz A. M. C. (Arizona Medical Center)	Howmedica
Swanson	Dow-Corning

PROSTHESIS	COMPANY

Finger Joint Replacement

Swanson	Dow-Corning
Steffee	Depuy
Calnan-Nicolle	Zimmer G.B.

Flexor Tendon Replacement

Hausner Passive Tendon Implant	Holter-Hauser International
Hunter Artificial Tendons	Dow-Corning

Tools

Oscillating power saw, reamer and drill	3M, Zimmer, Stryker, Howmedica, Codman-Cintor Synthes

Implants for Internal Fixation of Fractures and Osteotomies

Müeller-Harris nail plate	Zimmer, Howmedica, Synthes
Kuntscher	Zimmer/AO, OEC
Hansen-Street IM Rod	Zimmer, Howmedica
Schneider IM Rod	Zimmer, Howmedica
Sampson IM Rod	3M
Rush Rod	Zimmer, Howmedica
Enders Nail	B.G. Orthopedic Corp.
Phillips Cross-Slotted screws	Pauwell's (JRI)
Woodruff Cross-Slotted screws	Pauwell's (JRI)
AO-hexagonal recessed screw	Synthes
AO-4.5 mm cortical screw	Synthes
Kirschner wire	Richards, Zimmer, Howmedica
AO 6.5 mm. cancellous screw	Synthes
Drill Guides (neutral, load)	Synthes
AO 4.0 mm. self-tapping screw	Synthes
AO/ASIF Compression plate	Synthes
AO Semi-tubular plate	Synthes
Dynamic Compression plate (DCP)	Synthes
AO 6.5 self-tapping malleolar screw	Synthes
AO Sunken hexagonal screw head	Synthes
Phillips screw head	Zimmer
Müller compression device	Synthes
T or buttress plate	Synthes
Jewett nail	Howmedica, Zimmer, Richards
Richards hip screw	Richards
Zickel nail	Howmedica
Sampson-subtrochanteric nail	3M
Steinmann pins	Richards, Zimmer, Howmedica

PROSTHESIS	COMPANY
H beam nail, and McLaughlin side plate	Zimmer
AO screw set	Synthes
Schanz screws	Synthes
AO leg lengthening plate (Wagner)	Synthes
MacIntosh plates	Zimmer
Wainwright spline	Zimmer
Müller-Harris osteotomy blade plate	Synthes, Zimmer Orthopaedic Ltd.
Kuntscher (clover-leaf) intramedullary nail	Synthes, Zimmer, Howmedica
AO broad plate	Synthes
Schneider	Howmedica, Zimmer
Hansen-Street (diamond shaped nail)	Howmedica, Zimmer
Lottes tibial intramedullary nail	Zimmer, Richards
Rush rod	Howmedica, Zimmer
Hackenthal rod	Synthes
Ender's condylocephalic nail (for trochanteric femoral fractures)	Ortomed, B.G. Orthopaedic Corp., American Orthomed Co.
Venables plate	(No longer available)
Bending press	Synthes
Templates for onlay plates	Synthes
T-plate	Synthes
Tri-flanged (Smith-Petersen) stainless steel nail	Zimmer
Deyerle device (hip fixation)	OEC
Holt hip nail	Howmedica
Sampson fluted hip nail	3M
Massie slide hip nail	Howmedica, Zimmer
Pugh sliding hip nail	Zimmer
AO distraction device	Synthes
Cerclage wire	Synthes
Condylar blade plate	Synthes
Richards compression screw (90°)	Richards
Rush rods	Howmedica, Zimmer
Sampson fluted humeral nail/rod	3M
Malleolar screws	Synthes
Small fragment set	Synthes
Cobra	Synthes
AO IM Nail	Synthes
AO Flexible reamer set	Synthes
Steinmann pins	Howmedica, Zimmer, Richards
Neufeld pins	Richards
Compression hip screw	Richards, Zimmer
Sampson fluted pediatric hip nail	3M
AO pediatric hip nail	Synthes
Leinbach screw	Zimmer
Ti or Co-Cr mesh	3M

PROSTHESIS	COMPANY
X-ray image intensification	Picker, Siemens, Philips, Saab

Implants for External Fixation of Fractures

Charnley external fixation device	Zimmer, Richards
AO external fixation	Synthes
Ilisarov external fixation device	Medexport
Hoffmann external fixation device	Ets Jaquet Freres
Wagner external fixation device	Synthes

Spinal Instrumentation

Harrington instrumentation	Zimmer
Halo and Pins	Zimmer
Halo-pelvic distraction	Medishield
Dwyer apparatus	Zimmer, Downs Surgical

Cast Material

Plaster of Paris	Zimmer
Plastic sockets for cast brace	

Clean-Air Systems

Charnley Howarth Enclosure	Howarth Surgicair
Clean-air systems	AlloPro AG
GEL-OT laminar air flow unit	Gelman Hawksley Ltd.

Cement

Methylmethacrylate	Simplex P—Howmedica Zimmer
Polyethylene (RCH-1000)	Hoechst, West Germany

Miscellaneous

Gortex woven dacron vascular graft	USCI

Addresses for Manufacturers' List

1. Thackray, Ltd.
   P.O. Box 171 Park Street
   Leeds LS1 IRQ England

2. Richards Manufacturing Company, Inc.
   1450 Brooks Road
   Memphis, Tennessee 38116

3. Howmedica, Inc.
   Orthopaedics Division
   359 Veterans Boulevard
   Rutherford, N. J. 07070

4. Zimmer USA
   Warsaw, Indiana 46580

5. Protek, Ltd.
   P.O. Box 2016
   3001 Berne, Switzerland

6. AlloPro Ag
   Baar/Zug
   Switzerland

7. U.S. Surgical Corporation
   New York, New York

8. Deloro Surgical Co.
   Lancaster, N.Y.

9. Codman Shirtiff Company
   Randolph, Mass.

10. Medishield Inc.
    Surgical Division
    600 Industrial Avenue
    Paramus, New Jersey 07652

11. Wright Manufacturing Company
    Memphis, Tennessee

12. Dow-Corning
    Midland, Michigan

13. 3M
    P.O. Box 33211
    Eagan, Minn. 55121

14. Synthes LTD (U.S.A.)
    P.O. Box 529
    Wayne, Pa. 19087

15. Ets Jaquet Freres,
    5 Routes des Jeunes
    1211 Genevea 26
    Switzerland

16. Stryker Corporation
    420 Alcott Street
    Kalamazoo, Mich 49001

17. Downs Surgical
    Church Path
    Mitchum Surrey, England

18. Benoist Girard & Cie
    1 Rue Pascal
    Cachan 95, France

19. Howarth Surgicair
    Lorne Street
    Farnworth Bolton BL47LZ
    England

20. Joint Replacement Instruments Ltd. (JR1)
    51 Brixton Water Lane
    London SW2 INX

21. Zimmer Orthopaedic Ltd.
    Bridgend, Glam. U.K.

22. B. G. Orthopedic Corp.
    P.O. Box 518
    Cheshire, Conn. 16410

23. Ortomed
    P.O. Box 306
    Schiedam, Netherlands

24. American Ortomed Corp.
    P.O. Box 3184 4 Nobile Lane
    Poughkeepsie, N.Y. 12603

25. London Splint Co. Ltd.
    50–52 New Cavendish Street
    London England

26. Holter-Hausner International
    3rd & Mill Streets
    P.O. Box 1,
    Bridgeport, Pa. 19405

27. Link America, Inc.
    10 Gt. Meadow Lane
    E. Hanover, N.J. 07936

28. Medexport
    Moscow, G-200
    USSR

29. Zimmer Great Britain
    180 Brompton Road
    Lond SW3 1 HN

30. (OEC) Orthopaedic Equipment Co.
    Bourbon, Ind. 46504

31. Zimco Industries, Inc.
    3724 Park Place, P.O. Box 567
    Montrose, Cal., 91020

32. Saab-Scania AB
    Aerospace Division
    Medical Products
    S-581 88 Linköping
    Sweden

33. Gelman Hawksley Ltd.
    10 Harrowden Road, Brackmills,
    Northampton
    England

The manufacturer's list provides an abbreviated tabulation of the sources of most of the surgical tools and implants described in the previous chapters. It is not meant to be a complete list of all the available implants nor a list of all of the suppliers.

/